Pediatric and Adolescent Gynecology

Fourth Edition

Pediatric and Adolescent Gynecology

Fourth Edition

Sarah Jean Herriot Emans, M.D.
Associate Professor of Pediatrics
Harvard Medical School
Chief of Division of Adolescent/Young Adult Medicine
Children's Hospital
Boston, Massachusetts

Marc Reed Laufer, M.D.
Assistant Professor of
Obstetrics, Gynecology, and Reproductive Biology
Harvard Medical School
Chief of Gynecology
Children's Hospital
Department of Obstetrics and Gynecology
Brigham and Women's Hospital
Boston, Massachusetts

Donald Peter Goldstein, M.D.
Clinical Professor of
Obstetrics, Gynecology, and Reproductive Biology
Harvard Medical School
Emeritus Chief of Gynecology
Children's Hospital
Department of Obstetrics and Gynecology
Brigham and Women's Hospital
Boston, Massachusetts

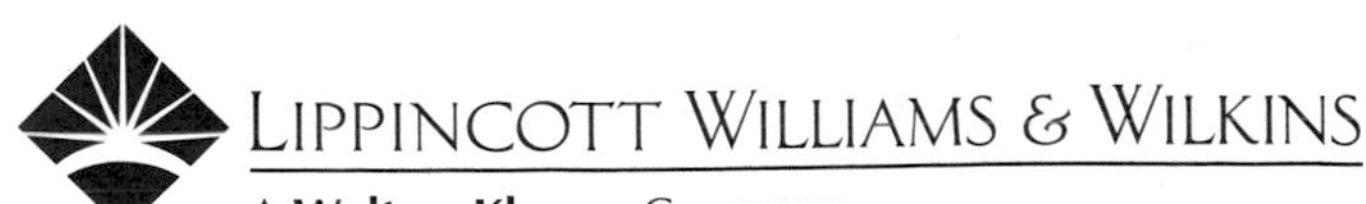
LIPPINCOTT WILLIAMS & WILKINS
A **Wolters Kluwer** Company
Philadelphia • Baltimore • New York • London
Buenos Aires • Hong Kong • Sydney • Tokyo

Acquisitions Editor: Paula Callaghan
Developmental Editor: Michelle LaPlante
Manufacturing Manager: Dennis Teston
Production Manager: Larry Bernstein
Production Editor: Liane Carita
Cover Designer: Wanda Lubezska
Indexer: Lisa Mullenneaux
Compositor: Lippincott Williams & Wilkins Electronic Production
Printer: RR Donnelley Crawfordsville

Printed in the United States of America

9 8 7 6 5 4 3

Library of Congress Cataloging-in-Publication Data

Pediatric and adolescent gynecology / edited by S. Jean Herriot Emans, Marc R. Laufer, Donald P. Goldstein. — 4th ed.

p. cm.

Rev. ed. of: Pediatric and adolescent gynecology / S. Jean Herriot Emans, Donald Peter Goldstein.

Includes bibliographical reference and index.

ISBN 0-316-23395-1

1. Pediatric gynecology. 2. Adolescent gynecology. I. Emans, S. Jean Herriot. II. Laufer, Marc R. III. Goldstein, Donald Peter.

[DNLM: 1. Genital Diseases, Female—in adolescence. 2. Genital Diseases, Female—in infancy & childhood. WS 360 P37076 1997]

RJ478.E46 1997
618.92′098—DC21
DNLM/DLC
for Library of Congress 97-21996
CIP

Care has been taken to confirm the accuracy of the information presented and to describe generally accepted practices. However, the authors, editors, and publisher are not responsible for errors or omissions or for any consequences from application of the information in this book and make no warranty, express or implied, with respect to the contents of the publication.

The authors, editors, and publisher have exerted every effort to ensure that drug selection and dosage set forth in this text are in accordance with current recommendations and practice at the time of publication. However, in view of ongoing research, changes in government regulations, and the constant flow of information relating to drug therapy and drug reactions, the reader is urged to check the package insert for each drug for any change in indications and dosage and for added warnings and precautions. This is particularly important when the recommended agent is a new or infrequently employed drug.

Some drugs and medical devices presented in this publication have Food and Drug Administration (FDA) clearance for limited use in restricted research settings. It is the responsibility of the health care provider to ascertain the FDA status of each drug or device planned for use in their clinical practice.

To our spouses (John, Sue, and Connie), families, friends, and colleagues who have lived through the stacks of references and manuscripts and provided us with love and support.

Contents

Contributing Authors

Richard Bourne, J.D., Ph.D. *Office of the General Counsel, Children's Hospital, 300 Longwood Avenue, Boston, Massachusetts 02115*

Lauren R. Brown, M.D. *Instructor in Obstetrics and Gynecology, Harvard Medical School; Assistant in Gynecological Surgery, Assistant in Medicine, Children's Hospital, 300 Longwood Avenue, Boston, Massachusetts 02115; Associate Obstetrician and Gynecologist, Brigham and Women's Hospital, 75 Francis Street, Boston, Massachusetts 02115*

Janet S. Donovan, R.N., B.S.N. *Clinic Coordinator, Division of Gynecology, Children's Hospital, 300 Longwood Avenue, Boston, Massachusetts 02115*

S. Jean Emans, M.D. *Associate Professor of Pediatrics, Harvard Medical School; Chief of Division of Adolescent/Young Adult Medicine, Children's Hospital, 300 Longwood Avenue, Boston, Massachusetts 02115*

Donald P. Goldstein, M.D. *Clinical Professor of Obstetrics, Gynecology, and Reproductive Biology, Harvard Medical School; Emeritus Chief of Gynecology, Children's Hospital, 300 Longwood Avenue, Boston, Massachusetts 02115; Department of Obstetrics and Gynecology, Brigham and Women's Hospital, 75 Francis Street, Boston, Massachusetts 02115*

Ingrid A. Holm, M.D. *Instructor of Pediatrics, Harvard Medical School; Assistant in Medicine, Division of Endocrinology, Division of Genetics, Children's Hospital, 300 Longwood Avenue, Boston, Massachusetts 02115*

Marc R. Laufer, M.D. *Assistant Professor of Obstetrics, Gynecology, and Reproductive Biology, Harvard Medical School; Department of Obstetrics and Gynecology, Brigham and Women's Hospital, 75 Francis Street, Boston, Massachusetts 02115; Chief of Gynecology, Children's Hospital, 300 Longwood Avenue, Boston, Massachusetts 02115*

Joan F. Mansfield, M.D. *Assistant Professor of Pediatrics, Harvard Medical School, Boston, Massachusetts; Divisions of Endocrinology and Adolescent/Young Adult Medicine, Children's Hospital, 300 Longwood Avenue, Boston, Massachusetts 02115*

Maurice W. Melchiono, R.N., M.S., F.N.P. *Clinical Instructor of Pediatrics, Harvard Medical School, Boston, Massachusetts; Nursing and Patient Services Director, Division of Adolescent/Young Adult Medicine, Children's Hospital, 300 Longwood Avenue, Boston, Massachusetts 02115*

Anne Jenks Micheli, R.N., M.S. *Director, Perioperative Program and Allied Services, Children's Hospital, 300 Longwood Avenue, Boston, Massachusetts 02115*

Amy B. Middleman, M.D., M.P.H., M.S.Ed. *Assistant Professor of Pediatrics, Department of Pediatrics, Baylor College of Medicine, 6621 Fannin Street, MC3-3340, Houston, Texas 77030*

Sally E. Perlman, M.D. *Instructor of Obstetrics, Gynecology, and Reproductive Biology, Harvard Medical School, Boston, Massachusetts; Department of Obstetrics and Gynecology, Brigham and Women's Hospital, 75 Francis Street, Boston, Massachusetts 02115; Division of Gynecology, Children's Hospital, 300 Longwood Avenue, Boston, Massachusetts 02115*

Cathryn L. Samples, M.D., M.P.H. *Instructor of Pediatrics, Harvard Medical School, Boston, Massachusetts; Department of Medicine, Children's Hospital, Martha Eliot Health Center, Jamaica Plain, Massachusetts 02130*

Victoria A.M. Smith, M.D. *Resident, Department of Family Medicine, Louisiana State University Medical Center, 1542 Tulane Avenue, New Orleans, Louisiana 70112-2822*

Preface

With the publication of the fourth edition of *Pediatric and Adolescent Gynecology*, we hope to provide for pediatricians, obstetrician–gynecologists, family practitioners, internists, nurse practitioners, and residents/fellows a practical text to address the common gynecologic problems of children and adolescents. Drawing from the experience of the three editors and the many contributing authors, we present medical and surgical approaches to the pediatric and adolescent gynecologic patient.

Many gynecologic problems can be diagnosed on the basis of the history and physical examination. Step-by-step descriptions of the techniques for examining the child and the adolescent are included in Chapter 1. A positive, nontraumatic examination will help girls seek future care. In Chapter 4, the physiology of puberty is reviewed as a background to the assessment of the child with signs of sexual precocity (Chapter 5) and to the evaluation of menstrual problems in the adolescent (Chapters 6 and 7). The importance of growth charts is underscored throughout these sections, as they often provide the clue to the differential diagnosis. Case studies are presented to help health care providers formulate appropriate evaluations. The special gynecologic and reproductive endocrine issues related to girls and young women with diseases such as diabetes, cystic fibrosis, and cancer are addressed in a new chapter that also discusses long-term followup of these patients relating to fertility and pregnancy outcomes. An updated chapter on sexuality education reviews the controversy and advances in this important field. The diagnosis and management of vulvovaginal complaints, sexually transmitted diseases, human papillomavirus, and human immunodeficiency virus have been expanded to include new management choices and strategies. Surgical issues related to the treatment of gynecologic congenital anomalies, ovarian masses, and breast diseases are important for the obstetrician–gynecologist, the pediatric surgeon, and primary care providers. We have added a new chapter on preoperative and postoperative care.

The evaluation and management of the child with a disclosure or suspicion of sexual abuse remains an area of controversy and ongoing research. The latest classification systems and data are included to provide the essential elements of examination and potential involvement with the legal system. Legal issues have assumed increasing importance and are discussed in a practical format. Finally, the appendices provide additional references and resources for contraception, pamphlets and books on sexuality for patients and families, sexual abuse terminology, estimations of percentage body fat, calcium intake, and the use of bone age determinations to estimate final height.

We have markedly expanded this edition to include more diagnostic dilemmas and solutions, enhanced by the expertise of new chapter authors, who helped provide an in-depth approach to many clinical problems. As editors and authors, our goal is to stimulate readers to become more knowledgeable and proficient in the gynecologic care of the child and adolescent. We are grateful to the pediatricians, family practice physicians, obstetrician–gynecologists, nurse practitioners, and others with whom we have worked. We are also indebted to Dr. Alvin Goldfarb, founder of the North American Society of Pediatric and Adolescent Gynecology. The dialogue between medical and surgical specialties at Children's Hospital, fostered by our Chiefs, Drs. David Nathan, Phillip Pizzo, Hardy Hendren, and Robert Barbieri, has been an essential factor in providing excellent gynecologic care to children and adolescents, and we are grateful to be able to work with these world leaders.

S.J.H.E.
M.R.L.
D.P.G.

Acknowledgments

We want to acknowledge and thank the many people who have helped with this and previous editions: Sally Perlman, M.D., Joan Mansfield, M.D., Ingrid Holm M.D., Anne Jenks Micheli, R.N., M.S., Janet S. Donovan, R.N., B.S.N., Lauren R. Brown, M.D., Cathryn Samples, M.D., M.P.H., Victoria Smith (HMS '98), Richard Bourne, J.D., Ph.D., Amy Middleman, M.D., M.Ed., M.P.H., Maurice Melchiono, R.N., F.N.P., Marian Craighill, M.D., M.P.H., John Crigler, M.D., Samir Najjar, M.D., Stuart Bauer, M.D., Jane Share, M.D., Carol Barnewolt, M.D., Elizabeth Woods, M.D., M.P.H., Trina Anglin, M.D., Susan Pokorny, M.D., Mary Aruda, R.N., P.N.P., Phaedra P. Thomas, R.N., B.S.N., Vicki J. Burke, R.N., B.S.N., Beverly Hector-Smith, R.N.C., M.S., Sara Forman, M.D., Ann J. Davis, M.D., Joyce Adams, M.D., David Muram, M.D., Arnold Cologny, M.D., Astrid Heger, M.D., Robert L. Barbieri, M.D., and W. Hardy Hendren, III, M.D.

Our special thanks to Ann Barrett, R.N., M.S.N., Patricia Bartels, R.N., P.N.P., and Lola Moore, R.N., B.S.N., for their encouragement of the role of nurses in our programs; to Laurette Langlois, Beth Ingraham, and most especially Paul Andriesse for his artistic contribution; to Jim Koefler for his much appreciated and always timely help with photography and preparation of figures; to Children's Hospital Media Services; to Alison Clapp, Hospital Librarian (for this edition), and Miriam Geller, Radiology Librarian (for past editions), for tireless searching of the medical literature; to Annette Luongo, Ruth Connors, Robin Guilfoy, Michael Richards, and Cathy DeLucca for invaluable assistance in preparing the manuscript; and to Michelle LaPlante, Paula Callaghan, and Liane Carita for sticking with us through multiple revisions. We are also indebted to our Maternal and Health Bureau Interdisciplinary Adolescent Health Training Grant MCJ259195 (S.J. Emans), and to the HRSA Grant (970155-04-0) (E.R. Woods, Cathryn Samples, Maurice Melchiono), which have allowed us the time to write and publish in the fields of adolescent health and human immunodeficiency virus disease.

Pediatric and Adolescent Gynecology

Fourth Edition

1

Office Evaluation of the Child and Adolescent

OFFICE EVALUATION OF THE INFANT AND CHILD

Gynecologic assessment and inspection of the external genitalia of the infant and child provide an opportunity to give the child preventive health care and to diagnose important clinical conditions. Although gynecologic problems are uncommon in young girls, inspection of the external genitalia and palpation of the breasts should be part of the routine physical examination. The clinician may note smegma or feces in the labial folds, indicating inadequate perineal hygiene. During or after the examination, instructing the parents and child about hygiene may prevent the later occurrence of nonspecific vulvovaginitis. The presence of a cyst, clitoromegaly, early signs of puberty, *Candida* vulvitis, vulvar dermatoses, or an abnormality of or change in the configuration of the hymen may be a clue to other problems. Errors in diagnosis often stem from a lack of simple inspection.

A healthy dialogue between parents and children on issues of sexuality should begin during the prepubertal years. Parents should be encouraged to answer the questions of their young children with simple facts and correct anatomic terminology (see Chapter 22). Appendix 1 contains a list of pamphlets that may help parents become more comfortable in talking with their children about sex. The clinician's knowledge of the educational materials available at the local library and of how to select appropriate pamphlets and videos for the clinical setting is helpful to parents and children.

Obtaining the History

Vaginal discharge or bleeding, pruritus, signs of sexual development, or an allegation of sexual abuse should prompt a more thorough evaluation. The nature of the history depends on the presenting complaint. If the problem is vaginitis, questions should focus on the timing of the onset of symptoms; the type of discharge; perineal hygiene; antibiotic therapy; recent infections in the patient or other members of the family, including streptococcal infection and pinworm infestation; masturbation; and the possibility of sexual abuse (see Chapter 20). Behavioral changes and somatic symptoms such as abdominal pain, headaches, and enuresis may suggest the possibility of abuse. Information on the caretaker(s) should always be elicited. If the problem is vaginal bleeding, the history should include information about recent growth and development, signs of puberty, the use of hormone creams or tablets, trauma, vaginal discharge, and any previous finding of foreign bodies in the vagina or other orifices. Although the history is usually obtained chiefly from a parent, the child should first be asked questions about toys or school to put her at ease. Then, questions may be asked about genital complaints, genital contact, and, depending on the complaint, whether she has ever placed something in her vagina. Eye contact with the child should be maintained, and she should be told that she is an important part of the team. Questions focusing on what has bothered the child, such as itching or discharge, can help her understand why the examination is important. She should be given the opportunity to ask her own questions. A questionnaire can be used to speed the intake process so that the young child does not become fidgety while the history is being taken. However, this history-taking time can be used advantageously to put the child at ease and to promote the understanding that the clinician is acting in her best interests.

Gynecologic Examination

The gynecologic examination should be carefully explained in advance to the parent and the child. It is extremely important to tell the parent that the size of the vaginal opening is quite variable and that the examination will in no way alter the hymen. A diagram showing the vulva is often helpful, as many parents still believe that the virginal introitus is totally covered by the hymen (Fig. 1). For the most part, gynecologic assessment of the child involves inspection of the genitalia and not instrumentation.

Both parent and child should be told that the instruments to be used are specially designed for little girls. The otoscope or hand lens to be used for external examination should be shown to the child with an assurance that the clinician will use these instruments "to look." The child may look through the lens of the otoscope. If a colposcope will be used for an evaluation of sexual abuse, the child should have a chance to look at the instrument, turn the light on and off, and view fingers or jewelry through the binocular eyepieces so that she will feel more comfortable with the examination.

The child can then be offered her choice of gown color and asked whether she wishes to have her parent lift her onto the table or climb "up the big stairs." In our clinic, the parent typically stays in the room to talk with the young child

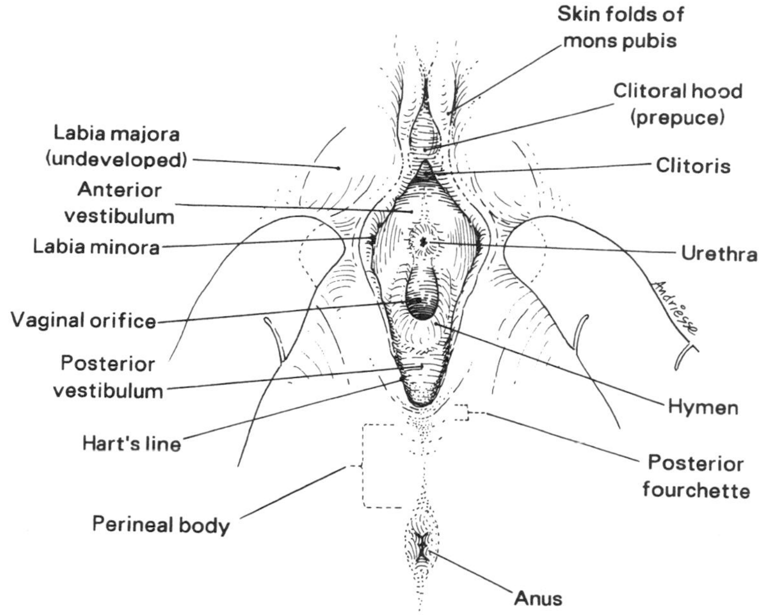

FIG. 1. External genitalia of the prepubertal child. (From Goldstein DP, Laufer MR, Davis AJ. *Gynecologic surgery in children and adolescents: a text atlas.* New York: Springer-Verlag (in preparation); with permission.)

and assist in the examination. Although the father, mother, both parents, or a relative may accompany the child for the assessment, most commonly the mother plays an active role during the examination. The older child should be asked whom she prefers to have in or out of the room during the examination. Most children and many young adolescents prefer their mothers in the room; almost all middle adolescents and late adolescents prefer their mothers out of the examining room.

The majority of children are comfortable on the examining tables with the mother (or father or other caretaker) sitting close by or holding a hand. Some girls are quite fearful, especially if they have previously been sexually abused or had a painful genital examination. In this case, the mother or other caretaker can sit on the table in a semireclined position with her feet in stirrups and have the child's legs straddle her thighs. A hand mirror can help the child relax and allows her to become an active participant in the examination. The mirror can be used for both education and distraction. If the clinician is confident and relaxed, the patient usually responds with cooperation. An abrupt or hurried approach will precipitate anxiety and resistance in the child. Sometimes it is necessary to leave the room and return when the patient feels ready. Occasionally, a child needs to return several days later to have the examination completed. The tempo of the examination depends on the urgency of evaluating a problem and the degree of cooperation that can be elicited. For example, if a child has had a discharge for months, the examination can occur over several visits if necessary so that the clinician can gain the confidence of the child. If a child has significant vaginal bleeding and cooperation cannot be elicited, then an examination under anesthesia may be necessary.

The examination of any child with gynecologic complaints should include a general pediatric assessment of the child's weight and height, head and neck, chest wall, heart, lungs, and abdomen. The breasts should be carefully inspected and palpated. The increasing diameter of the areola or a unilateral tender breast bud is often the first sign of puberty. The abdominal examination is often easier if the child places her hands on the examiner's hand; she is then less likely to tense her muscles or complain of being "tickled." The inguinal areas should be carefully palpated for a hernia or gonad; occasionally, an inguinal gonad is the testis of an undiagnosed male pseudohermaphrodite.

The complete gynecologic examination of the child includes inspection of the external genitalia, visualization of the vagina and cervix, and rectoabdominal palpation. This examination is usually possible without anesthesia if the child has not been traumatized by previous examinations and if the clinician proceeds slowly. The child should be explicitly told that the exam will not hurt. The young child should be in a supine position with her knees apart and feet touching in the

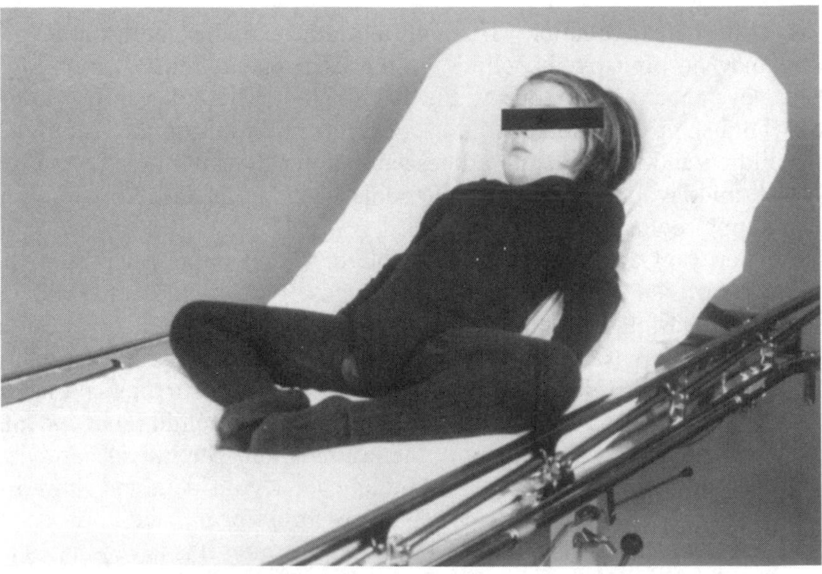

FIG. 2. Positioning the prepubertal child in the frog-leg position. She can lie horizontally or with the head of the examining table raised. [Courtesy of Dr. Trina Anglin, Office of Adolescent Health, Health Resources and Services Administration (HRSA), Washington, DC]

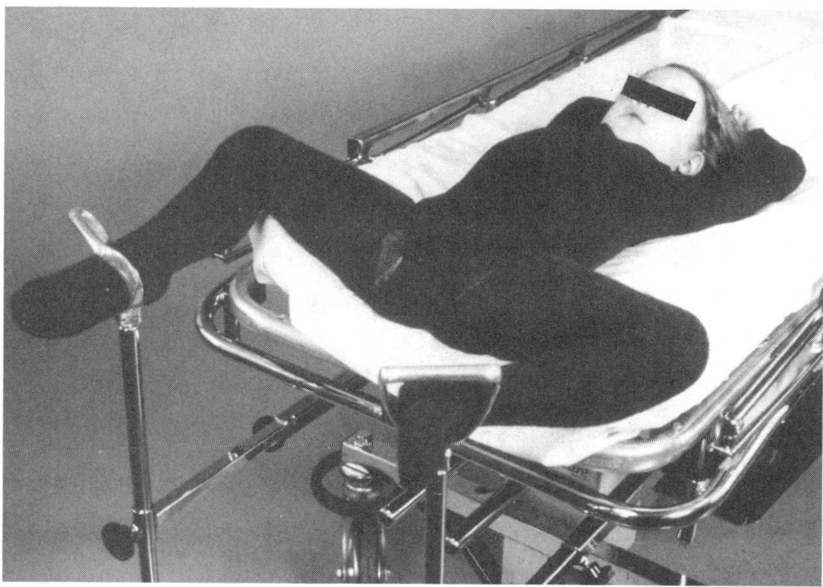

FIG. 3. Positioning the child in the lithotomy position with the use of stirrups. (Courtesy of Dr. Trina Anglin, Office of Adolescent Health, HRSA, Washington, DC)

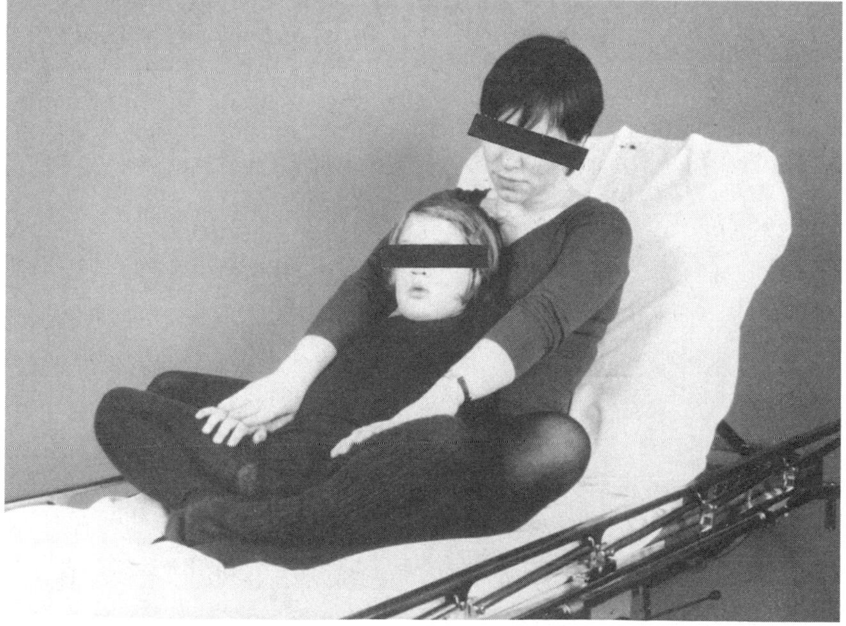

FIG. 4. Positioning the child in the frog-leg position with the aid of her mother. (Courtesy of Dr. Trina Anglin, Office of Adolescent Health, HRSA, Washington, DC)

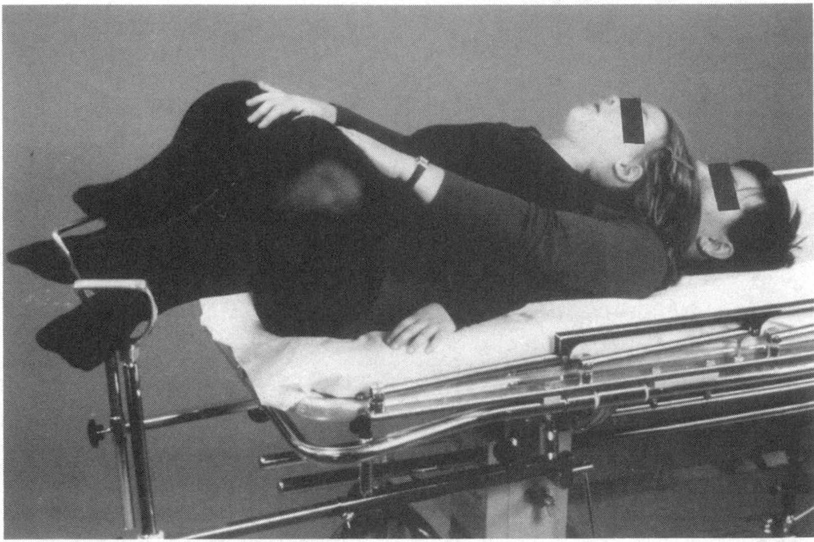

FIG. 5. Positioning the child in the lithotomy position with the aid of her mother. (Courtesy of Dr. Trina Anglin, Office of Adolescent Health, HRSA, Washington, DC)

frog-leg position, or in the lithotomy position with the use of adjustable stirrups (Figs. 2 to 5). Asking a child whether she has ever seen a frog and whether she can say "ribbit" will often put her at ease so she can assume the correct position "like a frog." During inspection of the external genitalia, the young child may be less anxious if she assists the physician by holding the labia apart. The physician should note the presence of pubic hair, the size of the clitoris, the configuration of the hymen, signs of estrogenization of the vagina and hymen, and perineal hygiene. Friability of the posterior fourchette as the labia are separated can occur in children with vulvitis or a history of sexual abuse, or if the labia are separated too widely (1). If the hymenal orifice and edges of the hymen are still not visible, the labia can be gently gripped and pulled forward in a traction maneuver to enable viewing of the anterior vagina (Fig. 6). The normal clitoral glans in the premenarcheal child is on average 3 mm in length and 3 mm in transverse diameter (2). The vaginal mucosa of the prepubertal girl appears thin and red in contrast with the moist, dull pink, estrogenized mucosa of the pubertal girl. Frequently, the perihymenal tissue is erythematous. The hymen will often gape open if the child is asked to cough or take a deep breath; if not, the labia should be gently pulled downward and laterally so that the hymenal edges and the anterior vagina can be viewed.

The configuration of the hymen should be noted (Figs. 7 and 8; see also Color Plate 1). A hand lens or the light and magnification of an otoscope, without a speculum, can be used (Fig. 9). Hymens can be classified as posterior rim (or

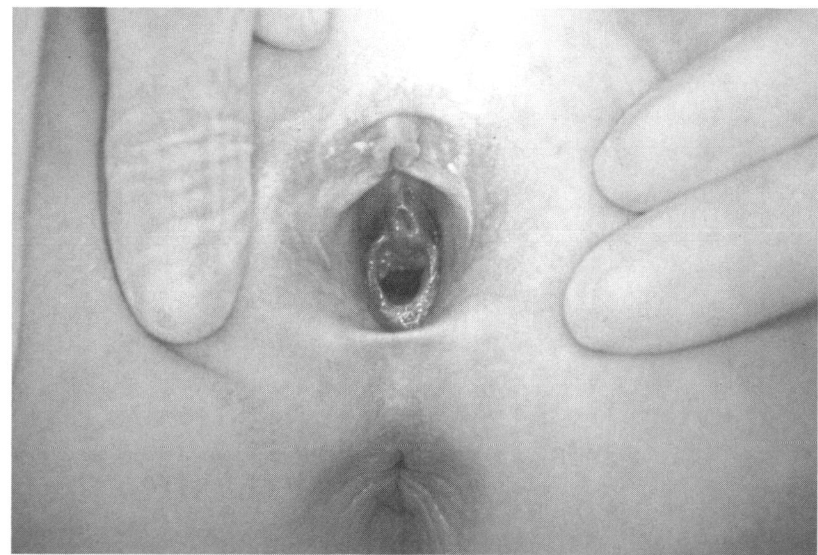

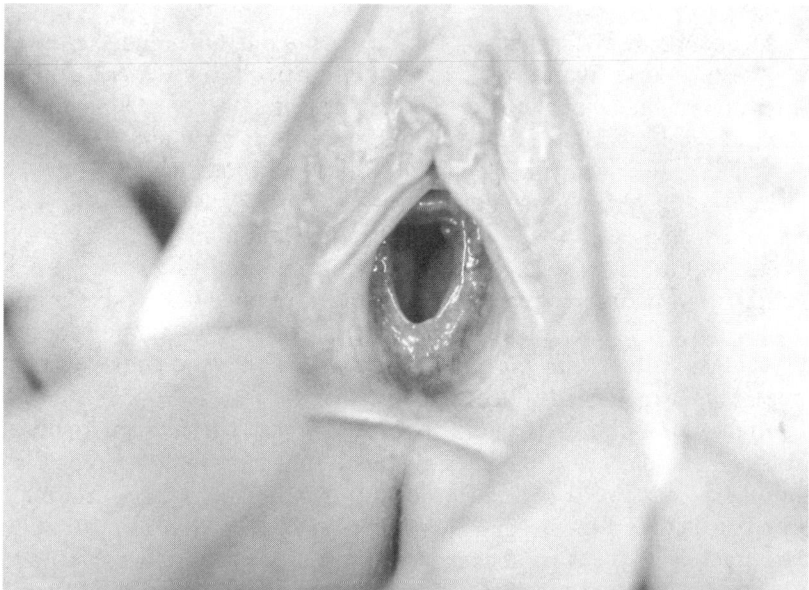

FIG. 6. Examination of the vulva, hymen, and anterior vagina by gentle lateral retraction **(A)** and gentle gripping of the labia and pulling anteriorly **(B)**

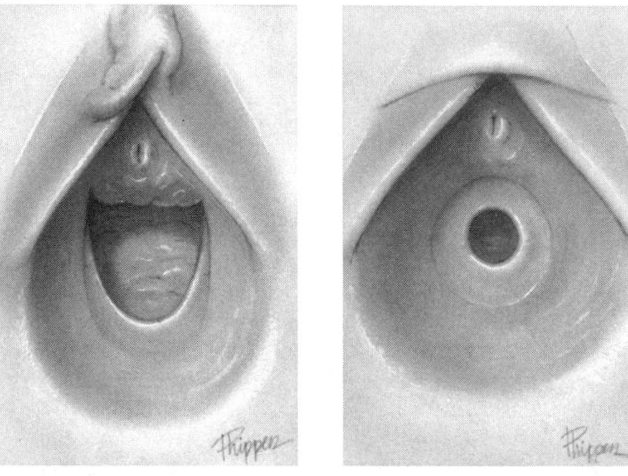

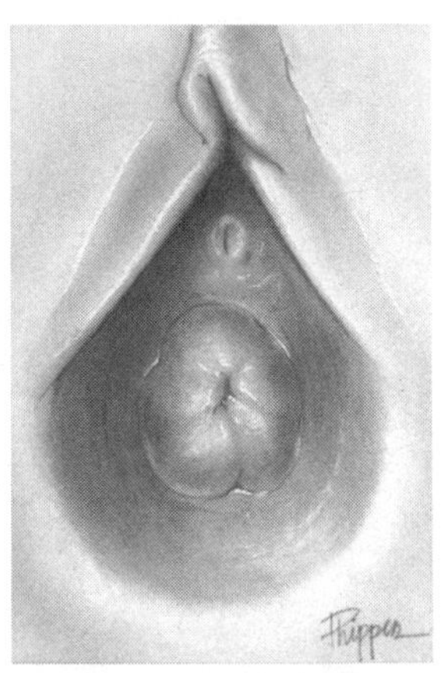

A,B C

FIG. 7. Configurations of hymens in prepubertal girls. **(A)** Posterior rim or crescentic hymen. **(B)** Circumferential or annular hymen. **(C)** Fimbriated or redundant hymen. (From Pokorny SF. Configuration of the prepubertal hymen. *Am J Obstet Gynecol* 1987;157:950; with permission.)

crescent), annular, or redundant (3). In girls with a redundant hymen, the edges of the hymen and the anterior vagina are often difficult to visualize. Congenital abnormalities of the hymen, especially microperforate and septate hymens, are not uncommon (Figs. 10 to 17; see also Chapter 8). It may initially be difficult to establish the presence of an opening in a microperforate hymen. Several techniques are useful: a small amount of warm water or saline can be squirted with a syringe or an angiocath, or the young girl can be placed in the knee-chest position (Fig. 18). Probing can also be done with a small urethral catheter or feeding tube (Fig. 16), or a nasopharyngeal Calgiswab moistened with saline. Applying a small amount of lidocaine jelly may reduce discomfort if probing is necessary and if vaginal cultures are not needed as part of the evaluation. Congenital absence of the hymen has not been documented (4,5).

Acquired abnormalities of the hymen usually result from sexual abuse and rarely from accidental trauma (see Chapters 3 and 20; see also Color Plates 9 through 18). Chapter 20 reviews the most current literature on normal and abnormal anogenital findings and the signs associated with sexual abuse. Signs of acute trauma from sexual abuse include hematomas, abrasions, lacerations, hymenal transections, and vulvar erythema and irritation. Physical healing from trauma is often complete by 10 to 14 days. Signs of previous sexual abuse may include acute and healed trauma, erythema, hymenal remnants, scars, and hymenal transections, which may heal in a V-shape or a U-shape. It should be remembered that in most girls with a history of substantiated sexual abuse, the findings on genital examination are normal. Clinicians seeing girls for annual physical examinations should be encouraged to inspect the genitalia and the

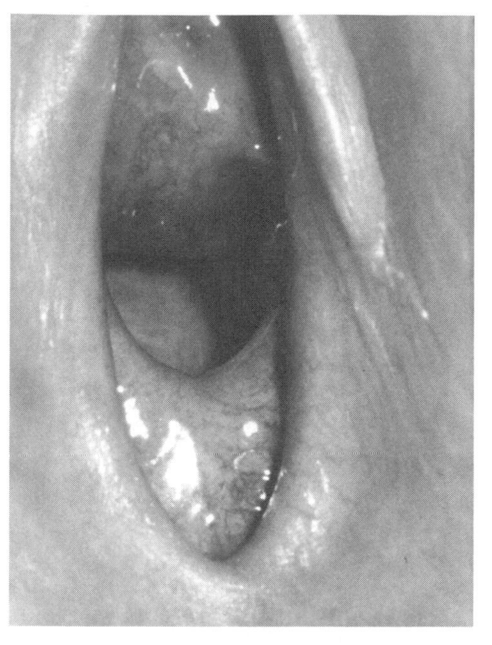

A

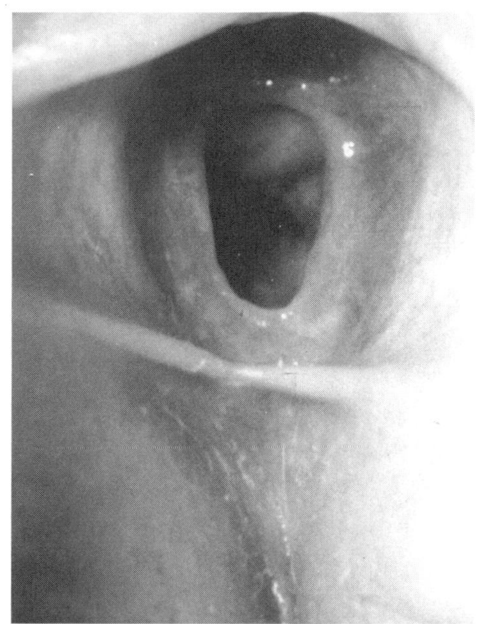

B

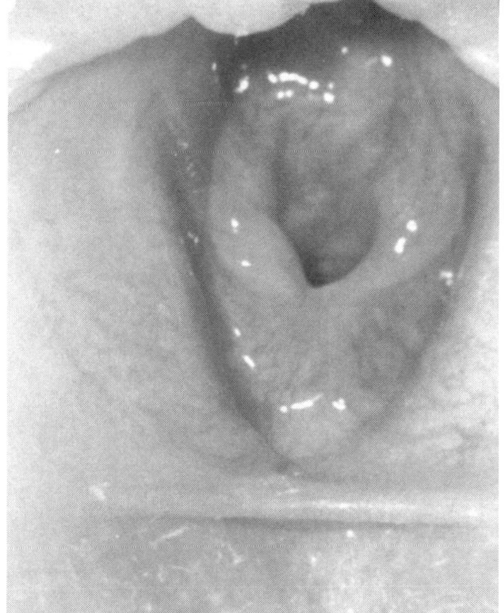

C

FIG. 8. Types of hymens, photographed through a colposcope. **(A)** Crescentic hymen. **(B)** Annular hymen. **(C)** Redundant hymen with crescent appearance after retraction.

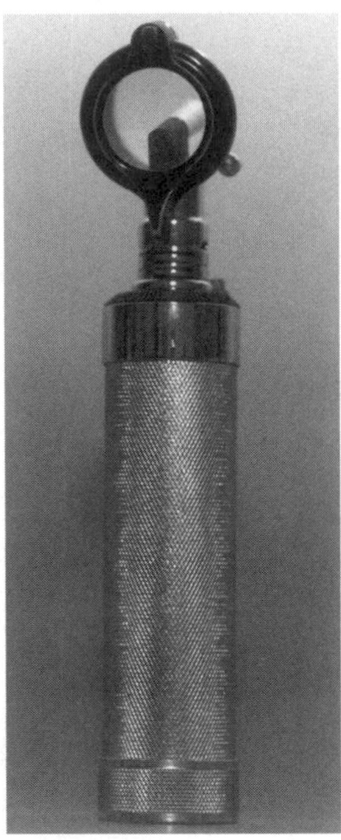

FIG. 9. Otoscope (without a speculum) for visualizing hymen and vagina.

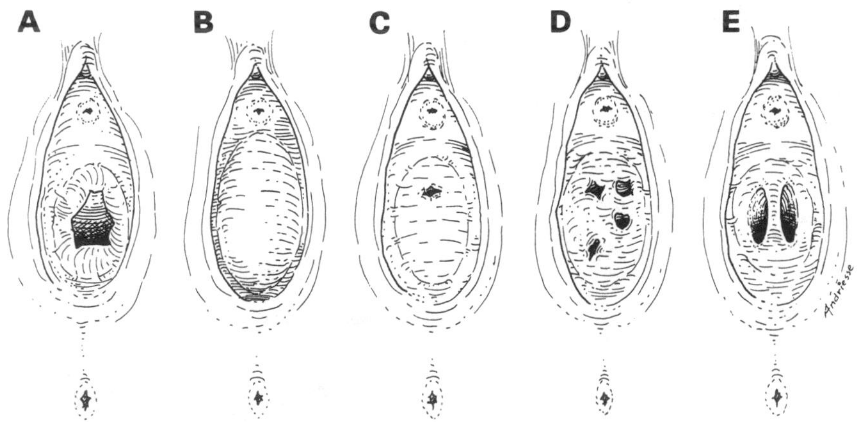

FIG. 10. Types of hymens. **(A)** Normal. **(B)** Imperforate. **(C)** Microperforate. **(D)** Cribriform. **(E)** Septate. (From Goldstein DP, Laufer MR, Davis AJ. *Gynecologic surgery in children and adolescents: a text atlas.* New York: Springer-Verlag (in preparation); with permission.)

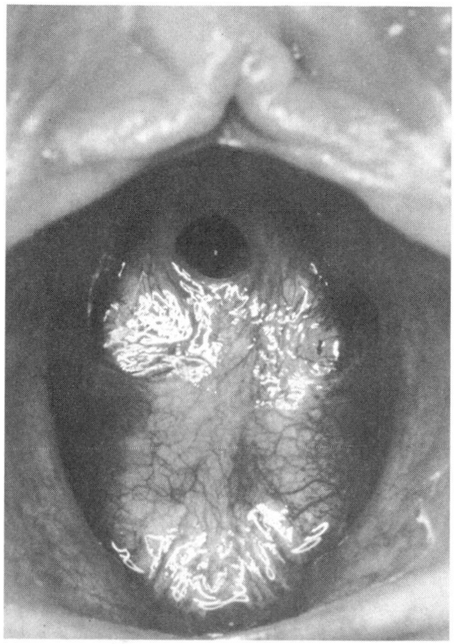

FIG. 11. Microperforate hymen.

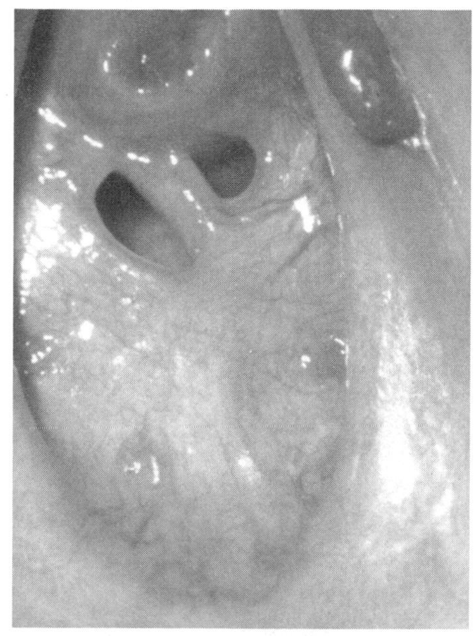

FIG. 12. Microperforate septate hymen.

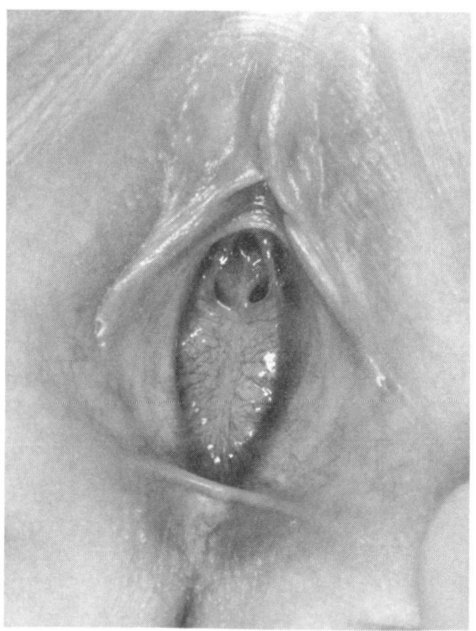

FIG. 13. Microperforate septate hymen.

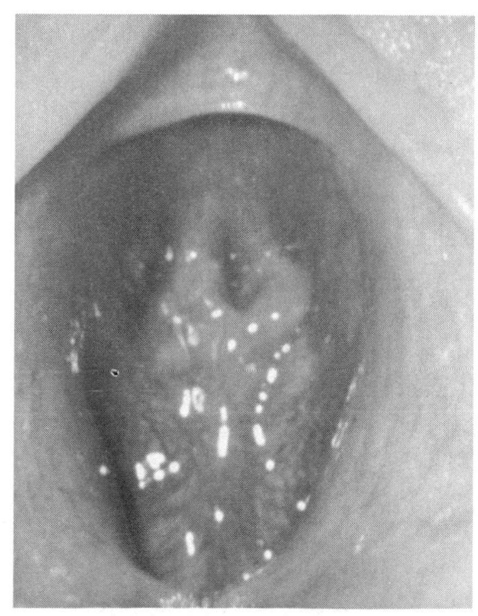

FIG. 14. Imperforate hymen.

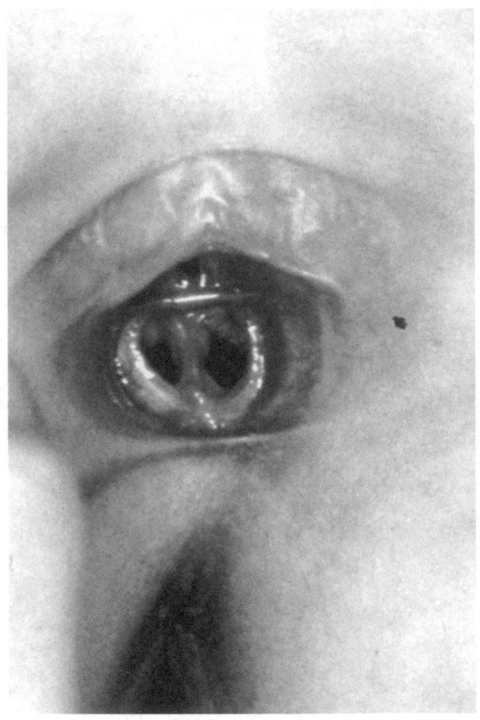

FIG. 15. Septate vagina.

hymen and to make drawings in the office notes of their configuration. A change from previously noted anatomy could provide an important clue to sexual abuse.

The significance of measuring the diameter of the hymenal orifice is controversial and is discussed below and in Chapter 20. The transverse and anterior–posterior measurements are influenced by age, relaxation of the child, method of examination and measurement, and type of hymen. The older the child and the more relaxed she is, the larger the opening. The opening is larger with retraction on the labia and when the child is in the knee-chest position than with gentle separation alone when the supine position is used. The orifice of a posterior rim hymen appears larger than the opening of a redundant hymen. Measurements can be obtained with a tine test 5-cm ruler, a small clear plastic centimeter ruler, or a colposcope. Our study of 3- to 6-year-old girls found a mean transverse measurement of 2.9 ± 1.3 mm (range 1 to 6 mm) and mean anterior-posterior measurement of 3.3 ± 1.5 mm (range 1 to 7 mm) (1) (see Chapter 20 for additional measurements). A large hymenal orifice may be consistent with a history of sexual abuse, but it is not the absolute criterion and should only be considered as part of the evaluation.

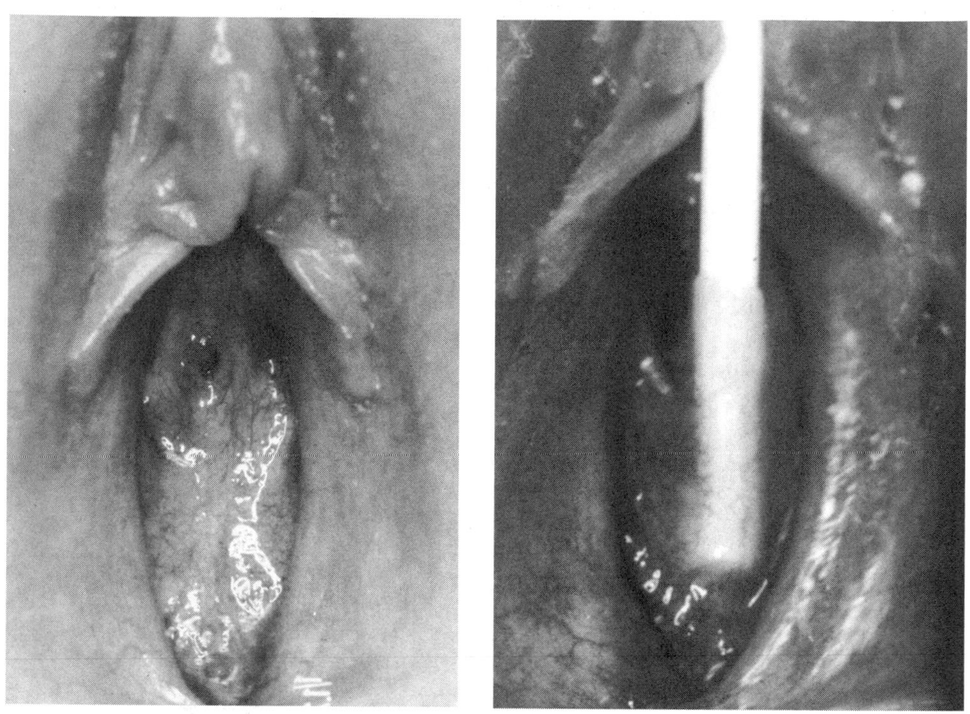

FIG. 16. Microperforate hymen. **(A)** Opening difficult to visualize. **(B)** Opening gently probed.

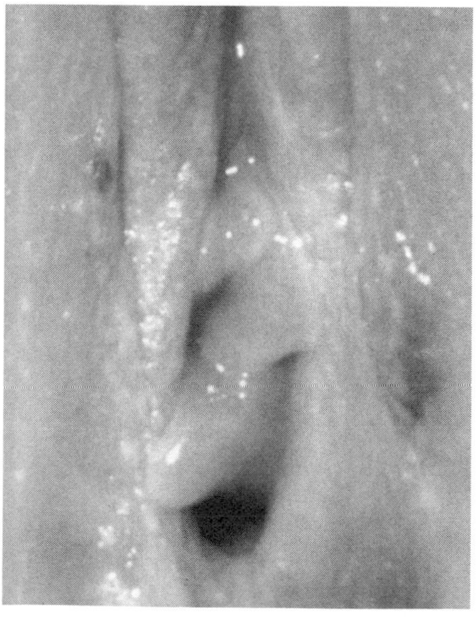

FIG. 17. Hymenal tags.

The anus and labia should always be examined for cleanliness, excoriations, and erythema. Perianal excoriation is often a clue to pinworm infestation. Normal findings, as well as those associated with sexual abuse, are noted in Chapter 20.

Once the external genitalia have been carefully examined, the clinician should proceed with visualization of the vagina if there is discharge, bleeding, or any other complaint that may be of vaginal origin. For example, the child who presents with vulvar itching and is found to have lichen sclerosus (see Color Plates 3 and 4) on external examination does not need a vaginal assessment. In contrast, visualization of the vagina in a girl with bleeding is essential.

In girls over 2 years old, the knee-chest position provides a particularly good view of the vagina and cervix without instrumentation (6). The patient is told that she should lie with her chest on the table and her "bottom in the air." She is reassured that the examiner plans to "take a look at her bottom" but will not put anything inside her. In the knee-chest position, the child rests her head to one side on her folded arms and supports her weight on bent knees (6–8 inches apart). With her buttocks held up in the air, she is encouraged to let her spine and stomach "sag downward." Some girls like to hear that they may have slept in this position when they were "little." Also they may think of themselves as "hopping like a bunny." A pillow can be placed under the girl's abdomen if she desires. A sheet can also be used so that she feels covered. An assistant or the mother helps hold the buttocks apart, pressing laterally and slightly upward. As the child takes deep breaths, the vaginal orifice falls open for examination (Fig. 18). In 80% to 90% of prepubertal girls, an ordinary otoscope head, used without a speculum (Fig. 9), provides the magnification and light necessary to enable visualization of the lower vagina and usually the upper vagina and cervix. The child's anxiety will be allayed if she is again shown the otoscope light and efforts are made to gain her full confidence before this part of the examination. A running conversation of small talk about school, toys, and siblings often diverts the child's attention and helps her maintain this position for several minutes without moving or objecting. Since the vagina of the prepubertal child is quite short, a foreign body or a lesion is often easily detected.

A supine position with the child's legs flexed on her abdomen also enhances visualization of the hymen, vagina, and anus. The use of a small vaginoscope, cystoscope, hysteroscope, or flexible fiberoptic scope with water insufflation of the vagina can be considered for other methods of visualization. The child is examined in a supine position with her knees held apart. A step-by-step method of inserting the vaginoscope in the young child was originally described by Capraro (7). The child is first allowed to touch the instrument and is told that it feels "slippery, funny, and cool." The instrument is then placed against her inner thigh and the same words are repeated. Next, the instrument is placed against her labia, again with the words "This feels slippery, funny, and cool." As the vaginoscope is inserted through the hymen, the examiner repeats the words and presses the child's buttocks firmly with the other hand to divert her attention. The application of lidocaine jelly or some other anesthetic cream to the introitus

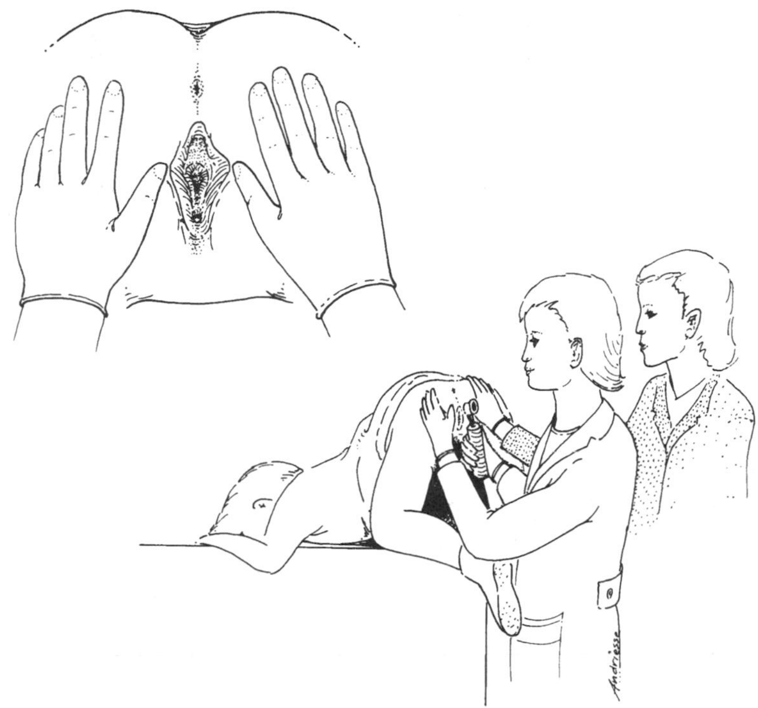

FIG. 18. Examination of the prepubertal child in the knee-chest position. (From Goldstein DP, Laufer MR, Davis AJ, *Gynecologic surgery in children and adolescents: a text atlas.* New York: Springer-Verlag (in preparation); with permission.)

makes insertion easier. Good visualization of the cervix and vagina is thus possible without general anesthesia. Others have used a narrow veterinary otoscope speculum with the child in the supine (lithotomy) position (8). Rarely, a narrow vaginal speculum can be useful in examining the older child if insertion does not cause pain or trauma.

If a vaginal discharge is present, samples should be obtained for culture and for saline and potassium hydroxide (KOH) preparations (see section on wet preparation). Gram stain can also be done if samples are easy to obtain and the discharge is purulent. Usually, the child prefers to lie on her back with her knees apart and with her feet together or in the stirrups so that she can watch the procedure without becoming excessively anxious. The child should be allowed to feel a cotton-tipped applicator, Calgiswab, eyedropper, feeding tube attached to a syringe, or catheter on her skin before a similar sterile device is inserted into her vagina. For example, a cotton-tipped applicator can be gently stroked over the back of her hand to allow her to feel it as "soft" or "ticklish." For the prepubertal child, we usually use a nasopharyngeal Calgiswab moistened with nonbacteriostatic saline (Fig. 19A); individual ampules of nebulizer saline are convenient for office use.

The swab can be inserted into the vagina painlessly if the clinician avoids touching the hymenal edges. The child can be asked to cough as the examiner inserts the swab. This action distracts the child and makes the hymen gape open. Several Calgiswabs can be used in rapid succession without discomfort. If indicated, the specimen for *Chlamydia* culture can be obtained by using a Dacron male urethral swab, gently inserting it through the hymenal opening, and scraping the lateral vaginal wall gently. If multiple samples are needed, as in an evaluation for rape, a small feeding tube attached to a syringe (a small amount of saline being used for vaginal wash and aspiration), a soft plastic eyedropper (such as a Clinitest or Medi sterile clinic dropper), or a glass eyedropper with 4 to 5 cm of intravenous plastic tubing attached (9) can be gently inserted through the hymen to aspirate secretions. Occasionally a small amount of lidocaine solution applied to the hymenal edges can be used to facilitate insertion. Another method of obtaining samples has been used by Pokorny and Stormer (10) and consists of a modified syringe and urethral catheter (Fig. 19B). The proximal 4-inch end of an intravenous butterfly catheter is inserted into the 4-inch endpiece of a No. 12 bladder catheter, and a syringe is attached. The catheter is slid into the vagina, similarly to catheterizing the bladder. Sterile saline (0.5 to 1 ml) is injected into the vagina and aspirated. This device is commercially available as the Pediatric Vaginal

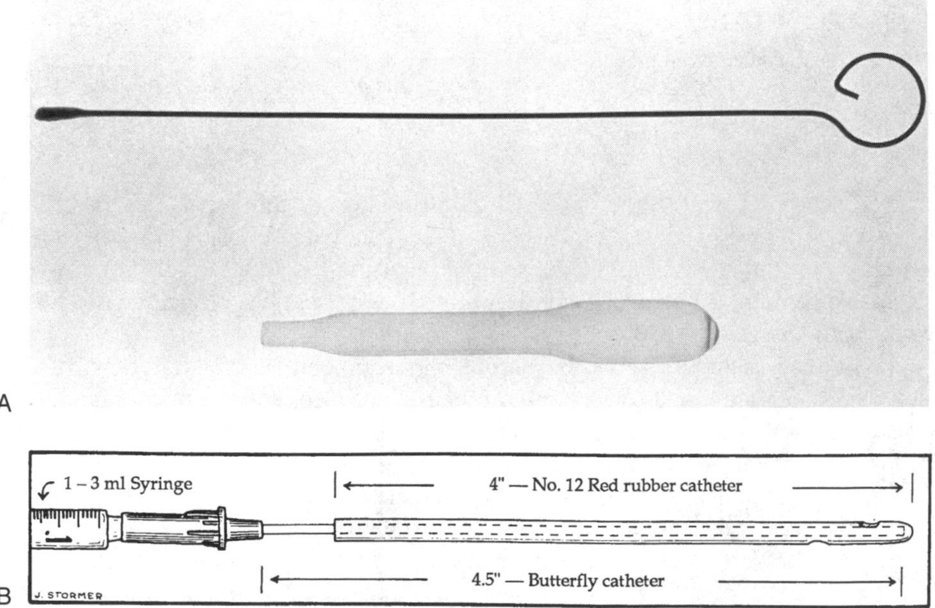

FIG. 19. **(A)** Soft plastic eyedropper and Calgiswab for obtaining vaginal specimens in the prepubertal girl. **(B)** Assembled catheter-within-a-catheter, for obtaining specimens from a prepubertal child. (From Pokorny SF, Stormer LVN. Atraumatic removal of secretions from the prepubertal vagina. *Am J Obstet Gynecol* 1987;156:581; with permission.)

Aspirator from Cook ObGyn (Spencer, IN). For the child who will not allow an intravaginal sampling, Muram has used a technique of squirting saline to fill the vagina followed by holding three swabs perpendicular just outside the vagina with the labia held closed over the swabs by the examiner. The child is asked to cough and the wet swabs are used for the needed tests.

A culture for *Neisseria gonorrhoeae* should be done on modified Thayer-Martin-Jembec medium at the time of the examination. Cultures for other organisms are done by placing the moistened Calgiswab into a transport Culturette II with medium. The bacteriology laboratory should plate the swab on the standard genitourinary media, which usually include blood agar, MacConkey, and chocolate media. The laboratory should be notified that the Thayer-Martin-Jembec medium being processed is from the vagina of a *prepubertal* child so that if a *Neisseria* species grows, it is properly and unequivocally identified as *N. gonorrhoeae* for medicolegal purposes. The Centers for Disease Control reported that 14 of 40 bacterial isolates identified as *N. gonorrhoeae* from children under 15 years of age during 1983 to 1984 proved to be other *Neisseria* species; they included *N. lactamica*, *N. meningitidis*, and *N. cinerea* as well as *Branhamella catarrhalis* (11,12). Cultures for *Chlamydia trachomatis* are recommended rather than indirect tests and slide immunofluorescent tests in the prepubertal child because of the possibility of false-positive test results and the association of this organism with sexual abuse (see Chapters 3, 12, and 20). Nonculture tests are not currently approved for vaginal or rectal samples in prepubertal children. The newest ligase chain reaction (LCR) and polymerase chain reaction (PCR) *Chlamydia* tests need further evaluation in vaginal or urine samples in sexually abused and nonabused prepubertal girls. For patients who complain of itching or have suspected yeast infection, a Biggy agar culture can be incubated and read in the office.

After the samples have been obtained, a gentle rectoabdominal examination is performed with the patient in stirrups or supine with her legs apart. For bimanual palpation, the examiner places the index or little finger of one hand into the rectum and the other hand on the abdomen. The child can be reassured that this examination will feel somewhat like having her temperature taken rectally or having a bowel movement. She should be reassured that a finger has a smaller diameter than a bowel movement.

Except in the newborn infant, in whom the uterus is enlarged secondary to maternal estrogen, the rectal examination in the prepubertal child reveals only the small "button" or thickening of the cervix and uterus. Since the ovaries are not palpable in the child and are located higher in the pelvis than in the adult, masses should alert the physician to the possibility of a cyst or tumor. At the end of the rectal examination, as the finger is removed from the rectum, the vagina should be gently "milked" to promote the passage of any discharge or extremely rare polypoid tumors.

After assessing a patient's chief complaint and the results of the examination, the clinician should spend time with the parents and child to discuss the diagnosis, the proposed therapy, and the necessity of followup. Praising the young child

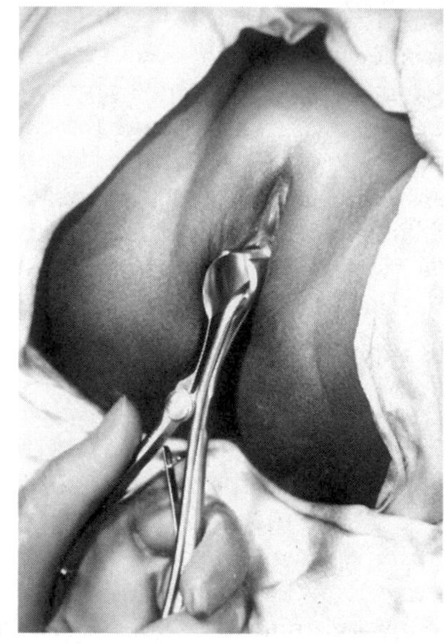
A

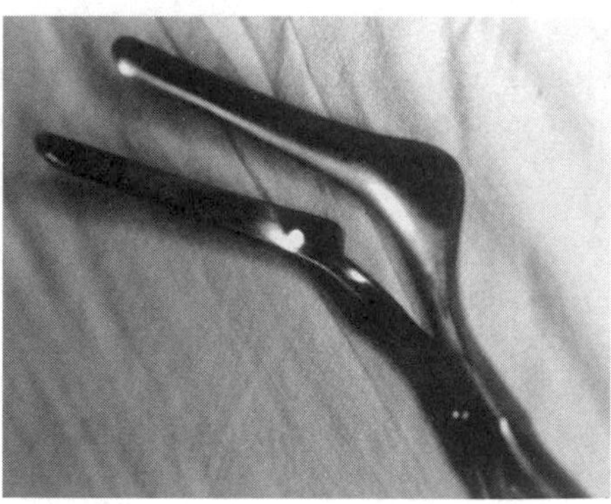
B

FIG. 20. (A) Examination of patient under anesthesia, **(B)** using a Killian nasal speculum with fiberoptic light (obtained from Codman and Shurtleff, Inc., Pacella Drive, Randolph, MA).

for her cooperation and bravery helps establish the clinician–patient relationship so important during future examinations.

If a child is unable to cooperate with the evaluation, she may need to be examined under anesthesia to facilitate adequate assessment of the chief complaint. If vulvar dystrophies are suspected, a biopsy specimen can be obtained, and if vaginitis or vaginal bleeding is present, a thorough evaluation can be undertaken as outlined above. The use of a hysteroscope, cystoscope, or flexible narrow-diameter fiberoptic scope can be helpful for magnification and identification of vaginal or cervical lesions. In addition, a nasal speculum with a light source can be helpful for direct visualization of the vagina and cervix (Fig. 20).

OFFICE EVALUATION OF THE ADOLESCENT

Evaluation of the adolescent requires different technical skills, including speculum examination of the vagina, rectal–vaginal–abdominal palpation, and an office environment that is welcoming to the adolescent patient. It is most important that the clinician have the interpersonal skills, sensitivity, and time to establish a primary relationship with the adolescent herself. The clinician must be willing to see the teenager alone and listen to her concerns. For example, the patient with oligomenorrhea may ask at each return visit, “Why am I not normal?” Listening to her describe her feelings is just as important as drawing diagrams of the hypothalamic–pituitary–ovarian axis. The statement “Your pelvic exam is normal” answers few of the adolescent’s questions.

The office setting should have a welcoming group of secretaries and clinical aides. A seating area for teens is optimal, since they may not feel comfortable sitting with babies in the pediatrician's office, or with pregnant women older than themselves in the gynecologist's office. Special times can sometimes be reserved in the evening or late afternoon to respond to the needs of teens. In addition, a mechanism to receive phone calls from teens needs to be arranged by the office staff. In a pediatric, internal medicine, family medicine, or gynecologic practice, examination rooms should be neutral. In a practice limited to adolescents, the office can have posters and pamphlets (see Appendix 1) that are pertinent to their concerns and, for example, give information on birth control, sexually transmitted diseases (STDs), human immunodeficiency virus (HIV), nutrition, and how to say "no" to premature sexual activity.

When a girl reaches the age of 11 or 12 years, the clinician can discuss with her and her family the need for adolescent preventive health care, the opportunities for confidentiality, and the importance of communication among the health care provider, the patient, and her family. The parents should be educated about giving their adolescents the special time they need to discuss concerns with the health care provider about peer relations, school, family, drugs, alcohol, and sexuality. The well teenager should have at least an annual visit; a patient with medical or psychosocial concerns should be seen more frequently. The American Medical Association (AMA) has published a set of 24 recommendations for annual preventive health care for adolescents (13) (Table 1). A project under the sponsorship of the Maternal Child Health Bureau with representatives from the American Academy of Pediatrics, Medicaid, Health Care Financing Administration, and other groups has resulted in similar guidelines for children from birth to 21 years of age, with the title *Bright Futures—Guidelines for Health Supervision of Infants, Children, and Adolescents* (14).

Parents should be included as much as possible in important medical decisions, but the adolescent's need for medical privacy and confidentiality should be respected. Parents should be encouraged to call in advance of an appointment if they have special concerns, since an adolescent may sometimes be strikingly nonverbal about troubling issues at home or in school. At the same time, parents may need help communicating more effectively with their adolescent. Clinicians should be explicit with both parents and adolescents about the extent of confidentiality. An excellent monograph and potential letters and policies have been developed by the AMA (15). In a survey of high school students, Cheng and colleagues (16) reported that 25% of teens would forgo health care in some situations if their parents found out, and only 57% of teens would go to their regular physician for questions about pregnancy. Although explicit confidentiality is important, it is essential that teens know the limits of confidentiality and that the clinician needs to involve others in conditions that are life threatening or carry a significant health risk. Letting teens know that the clinician will work with them if there are issues that need to be shared can alleviate many of their concerns.

TABLE 1. *Summary of recommendations of the American Medical Association Guidelines for Adolescent Preventive Services (GAPS)*

General
1. Annual preventive services visit
2. Age and developmentally appropriate preventive services
3. Office policies regarding confidentiality

Health guidance
4. For parents or other adult caregivers at least twice during child's adolescence
5. Physical growth, psychosocial and psychosexual development
6. Reduction of injuries
7. Dietary habits and safe weight management
8. Exercise
9. Responsible sexual behaviors (including abstinence), prevention of sexually transmitted diseases, and contraception
10. Avoidance of tobacco, alcohol, other abusable substances, and anabolic steroids.

Screening
11. Hypertension
12. Hyperlipidemia
13. Eating disorders and obesity
14. Use of tobacco products
15. Use of alcohol and other abusable substances
16. Sexual behaviors
17. Screening for sexually transmitted diseases
18. Access to confidential human immunodeficiency virus testing
19. Pap test
20. Depression and risk of suicide
21. Emotional, physical, or sexual abuse
22. Learning or school problems
23. Tuberculin testing

Immunizations
24. Appropriate immunizations

The transition from girlhood to adolescence involves biologic, cognitive, and psychological changes. The prepubertal latency-age girl of 10 years undergoes tremendous body changes as she develops into the sexually mature young woman of 20. The appearance of pubic hair and breast development, over which the girl has no control, can be exciting but also distressing. She may view asymmetry of breasts, acne, or normal weight gain as problems. The fact that her pubertal changes occur at the same rate as in her peer group may offer some reassurance; to be early or late can provoke considerable anxiety. A 12-year-old girl who looks 16 may be confronted with sexual demands; a 16-year-old girl who looks 10 may be embarrassed to undress for physical education class or to interact with her peer group. Girls with lesbian attractions may feel uncomfortable in schools and office settings that speak only to the needs and questions of heterosexual girls (17). Since the young adolescent has many fantasies about her body and its changes, she may ask the same questions at each visit. The older teenager is usually more capable of coping intellectually with the physical examination, the diagnosis, and the treatment plan. Young adolescents are concrete thinkers; thus, explanations and directions for medications must take this into account. Even when an older teen, who is more capable of abstraction and orientation to the future, is prescribed oral contraceptives, it is helpful to have the actual pill package in front of her so she can see how the pills look and learn the calendar system of the individual package.

The clinician must be sensitive to the different needs of each patient and respond to her issues during assessment, physical examination, and treatment plan.

Obtaining the History

The source of the medical history depends on the medical setting and the age of the patient. The older adolescent tends to seek gynecologic care on her own initiative. In a clinic setting, the clinician may first see the mother (and/or the father or other caretaker) to ascertain the nature of the chief complaint and to ask about the girl's medical history, school problems, and psychosocial adjustment. Most of the visit should be devoted to seeing the teenager alone, since her presenting complaint is quite often different from her parent's concerns. In other settings, the parent may make the appointment by telephone, and then the teenager may appear alone for the examination.

The history should relate not only to gynecologic issues but to general health concerns, risk behaviors, and a review of systems. The information can be gathered by the clinician, a computer-aided questionnaire, or a health history form. Private space is important if honest answers are expected. A girl should be told that the clinician asks these questions of *all* patients so that she does not feel singled out. Family history and psychosocial history are just as important as the usual medical history. With adolescents, it is best to first ask them why they are in the office for an evaluation that day. Otherwise, the presenting complaint can be lost in the review of systems, attention to birth control needs, and other issues. The clinician should proceed from neutral areas such as review of systems, allergies, gastrointestinal problems, diet, and weight changes to menstrual history and then finally to risky behaviors, sexual preference, and sexual activity. It is often helpful to ask the patient first about risky behaviors in the peer group: "Do your friends smoke? Do your friends use drugs? Are your friends having sex? Have any of your friends been pregnant?" An adolescent's sexual and drug-taking behavior frequently is similar to that of her friends. Even if she is not currently involved in such behaviors, she may be influenced by her peers to experiment in the near future. She may also need assistance with ways to resist the pressure and later reassurance that she is making a sound decision: "From what you are telling me, you have made a healthy choice to avoid . . . ."

In questioning the patient, the clinician can start with more neutral risk behaviors: "Do you smoke? Do you use a seat belt? Have you ever been in a car with someone drinking? Do you have a sexual partner? Tell me about your partner. Have you ever had sex? Have you ever been forced or pressured into having sex? What would you do if you were feeling pressured to have sex? Have you ever had a sexually transmitted infection? Do you need birth control?" It is important that questions be carefully worded so they are not overly heterosexually biased or convey the assumption that all patients are sexually active. The clinician should be discouraged from writing down answers during the interview when asking about risky behaviors such as drugs and alcohol, because the teen may then feel reluctant to give honest answers and the dialogue may be interrupted. Other good questions might be "If you make a decision to have sexual relations, would you know how to protect yourself from pregnancy? If you had a girl friend who didn't want to get pregnant, could you help her?" If she says, "Yes," ask, "How?" Such discussions require skillful handling, because adolescents who are not sexually active often benefit from support in maintaining their choice. Since many adolescents assume that "everyone" is sexually active, they are often reassured when they learn that many teens choose to postpone having sex until they are older or in a permanent relationship. The messages conveyed are important: the clinician usually wants to encourage young women to postpone sexual intercourse but also wants to be there to help the patient with sexual decision making and contraceptive choices. The question "Tell me the things you are doing to stay healthy" also assures the teen that she can make healthy decisions for herself.

Risky behaviors often occur in clusters, and adolescents who begin smoking and using alcohol early are also frequently involved in early sexual activity. For example, a 13- or 14-year-old girl who has problems in school, is in conflict with her mother, and has a history of running away is likely to engage in unprotected intercourse. She also may have been previously sexually molested. The young adolescent often does not consider the consequences of her actions and may become pregnant or acquire an STD. The older teenager of 16 or 17 is more likely to consider the future outcomes of her actions, but nevertheless, she too may fail to obtain birth control. Defining the issues and identifying alternatives may direct the adolescent to an acceptable solution. Concerned medical care that is sensitive to the patient's needs will hopefully assist her in the development of a healthy body image and responsible sexuality.

As clinicians ask these questions, many feel frustrated by the time constraints of the office setting and the slowness of behaviorial change. It is useful to know what curricula are being taught in the local school system so that messages can be built into community-wide norms. Office interventions can then use the framework of the school, church, or other community groups. Many clinicians find the GAPS algorithms (Table 2) and an understanding of the "stages of

TABLE 2. *GAPS algorithm for office interventions for high-risk behaviors*

G = Gather information
A = Assess further
P = Problem identification
S = Solutions

change" useful in planning strategies for interventions with adolescents. The GAPS algorithms have been formulated for many of the 24 recommendations of the AMA guidelines for preventive services (Table 1) (18). The clinician gathers initial information by means of the office interview and/or questionnaires (19), makes a further assessment to determine the level of risk, and then identifies problems. The adolescent's goals and perception of risk are sought. It is important to find out whether the teen is interested in change and what she is willing to do. Finally, the clinician works with the adolescent to seek solutions. The "S" in Table 2, which represents Solutions, can also be thought of standing for Self-efficacy (can the patient make a change?) and Solving barriers.

For example, to address the problem of smoking, which is common in teen women, the clinician gathers information (does the patient smoke?), assesses the level of risk (age started, packs per day, efforts to quit), problem-solves (presents choices, discusses with the teen such problems as impaired athletic performance, stains on fingers and teeth, bad breath, respiratory disease, and cost), and finds solutions (sets a quit date; supports the teen in avoiding activities associated with smoking; recommends chewing gum, exercise, or possibly nicotine patches or other pharmacologic therapy; and arranges followup).

Many clinicians have also found an understanding of the stages of change, originally described as a transtheoretical model of how substance abusers change addictive behaviors, with or without formal treatment (Fig. 21), to be valuable in conceptualizing interventions for teens (20). In order to move an adolescent toward a particular behavior change, the clinician determines that stage of change for that adolescent and then assists the adolescent to move from one stage to the next over several visits. The clinician helps to personalize the risk for the individual adolescent. *Precontemplators* do not consider the behavior in question to be a problem; it is neither relevant nor a risk to their health. To move

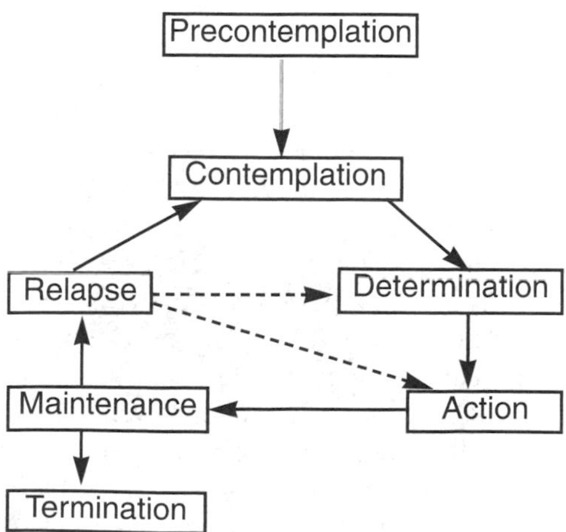

FIG. 21. Stages of change. (Adapted from Prochaska JO, DiClemente CC. Transtheoretical therapy: toward a more integrative model of change. *Psychother Theory Res Pract* 1982;19:276; with permission.)

an adolescent to the next stage, the provider should give information about the health consequences and promote the benefits of change. *Contemplators* consider that they may indeed have a problem, realize that there are pros and cons to the behavior, and begin to weigh the feasibility of change. The provider needs to address the teen's barriers and concerns about behavior change and to assist with achieving change in steps. "What would happen if you quit smoking? What would happen if you used a condom? How do you imagine your life could improve if you gave up using drugs?"

At the *Determination* or *Preparation* stage, the adolescent recognizes the need to change (within a month), although the behavior itself remains unchanged. The health care provider assists by emphasizing the importance of the pros and deemphasizing the value of the cons. In the *Action* stage, the adolescent is actively changing behavior. The action should be reinforced through visits and telephone calls. In *Maintenance*, the adolescent refrains from the risky behavior and is confident in having made a change, which may lead to either a permanent exit (*termination* or *recovery*) from the cycle, or a *relapse* and entry into another cycle. Relapse should be treated as a learning experience, not a failure. This framework provides the clinician with the opportunity to think about a variety of interventions for the risky or unhealthy behaviors noted during the interview.

The clinician providing gynecologic health care to adolescents needs to consider not only the chief complaint for a visit but the more general psychological and health needs of the teen. Often, the interventions and recommendations for therapy must be focused on life issues beyond those yielding to simple hormonal or antibiotic therapy.

Gynecologic Examination

Once the history has been obtained and the problems have been identified, the patient should be given a thorough explanation of a pelvic examination. The use of diagrams or a plastic model of the pelvis is helpful. If she has ever used tampons or is sexually active, she will find her first examination easier. However, a previous examination that was uncomfortable or a history of sexual assault may make the examination much more difficult. In explaining the first examination, the clinician should acknowledge the feelings of the adolescent. Good communication can be established by a statement such as this: "Some girls I see are worried about pain or embarrassment." It helps to acknowledge that adolescents can be nervous: "A lot of patients I see because of irregular periods are pretty nervous about these exams. It takes only 2 or 3 minutes, and I will explain everything to you now, and then again as I do the exam. I can't do a good exam unless you are really relaxed, so it's my job to help you feel comfortable. You are welcome to have someone in the room with you during the exam." Millstein and colleagues (21) noted that messages from friends about pelvic examinations were usually negative and referred to pain, self-consciousness, fear, anxiety, and physical or psychological discomfort. In contrast, messages from mothers and health care providers were primarily descriptions of procedures and their importance. The study underscored the necessity for clinicians to discuss the physical sensations associated with the procedure and to suggest methods of cognitive control. Such a discussion may include the use of imagery, a complete explanation before and during the examination, a mirror, or distraction. Each patient needs individualized attention, and adequate drapes and gowns are important. Allowing the adolescent to control the tempo of the examination is important to alleviate her concerns.

After the explanation, the patient should be asked if she needs to empty her bladder. She should then be given a gown and asked to remove all her clothes, including brassiere and underpants. If she is covered appropriately and approached in a relaxed manner, she will feel more able to cooperate with the examination. The young adolescent may request that her mother stay with her during a pelvic examination. Most older patients prefer their mothers to stay in the waiting room. The patient's wishes should be respected. Male clinicians should be accompanied by a female chaperone, who can aid in reassuring the patient and helping with samples. A chaperone should always be present if the patient desires one or needs support during the examination, or if medical or legal issues are a factor.

The general physical examination of a teenage girl should always include inspection of the skin, palpation of the thyroid gland, examination of the breasts, and a careful notation of the Tanner stages of breast and pubic hair development (see Chapter 4).

Demonstrating self-examination of the breast to the patient during the actual breast examination (see Chapter 16) often puts the young woman at ease. Since breast cancer is not a disease of teenagers, breast self-examination can be taught as part of self-awareness and health promotion to the older teen, but it should not be thought of as an effort to detect cancer and should not increase the anxiety of the young teen. It is essential not to overload the adolescent with guilt when she does not follow instructions for breast self-examination.

Inspection of the genitalia in the adolescent is an important part of the physical examination. Several medical conditions may be detected: *Candida* vulvitis, which can be the first sign of diabetes; vulvar dermatoses; obstructive congenital anomalies such as an imperforate hymen; a labial, periurethral, or hymenal cyst; or clitoromegaly. The actual examination frequently elicits questions that the teenager was embarrassed to ask, such as queries about a vaginal discharge, a lump, or irregular periods.

When is a pelvic examination indicated? A bimanual rectoabdominal examination, with the patient in the lithotomy position, should be performed on any teenager with gynecologic complaints or unexplained abdominal or pelvic pain. A vaginal examination enables assessment of irregular bleeding, severe dysmenorrhea, vaginal discharge, STDs, and amenorrhea. For the teen with a vaginal discharge who has never been sexually active, samples of the discharge can be obtained with a cotton-tipped applicator and the diagnosis made without a full speculum examination. For a patient with primary amenorrhea, a determination of vaginal length using a cotton-tipped applicator, followed by a one–finger vaginal–abdominal examination or rectoabdominal examination can assist in the identification of a normally patent vagina and confirm the presence of a cervix and uterus. The least invasive examination that will answer the question should be performed. On the other hand, examinations should not be omitted solely because of the age of the patient. It is important to recognize cultural issues surrounding vaginal examinations. Some families and adolescents are reluctant to permit examination with a speculum because of the misconception that it will alter the hymenal anatomy and impair virginity. After careful explanation that pelvic examinations have not been shown to be associated with changes in hymens (22), the patient may allow the examination. With some patients, the examination may have to be a rectoabdominal examination, or sometimes a visualization of the external genitalia and ultrasonography of the pelvis. Flexibility is the key to good rapport.

Sexually active patients should have a routine vaginal examination and a Papanicolaou (Pap) smear annually. Tests for *N. gonorrhoeae* and *C. trachomatis* are usually done at least annually, and more frequently when the patient has changed sexual partners, experiences vaginal symptoms, has been exposed to or

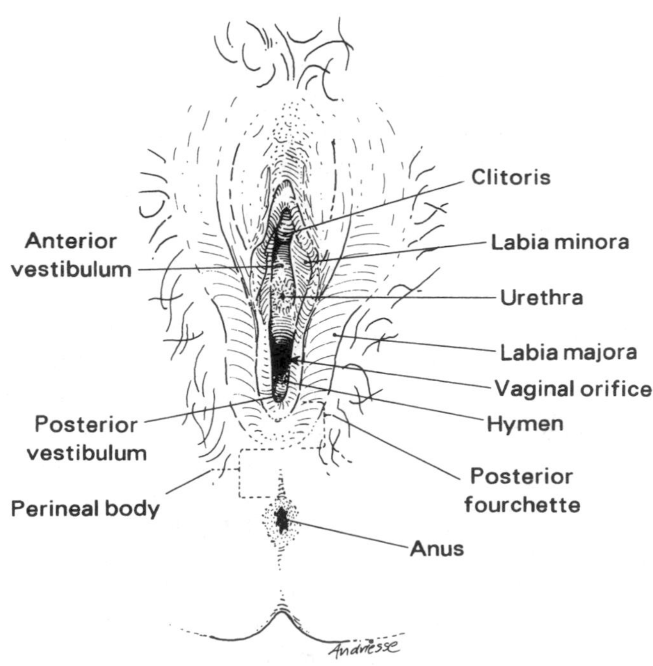

FIG. 22. External genitalia of the pubertal female. (From Goldstein DP, Laufer MR, Davis AJ. *Gynecologic surgery in children and adolescents: a text atlas.* New York: Springer-Verlag (in preparation); with permission.)

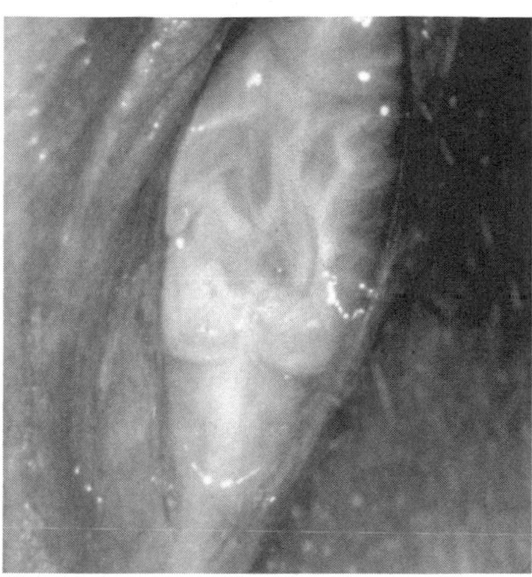

FIG. 23. Normal estrogenized hymen. (From Heger A, Emans SJ. *Evaluation of the sexually abused child.* New York: Oxford University Press, 1992; with permission.)

has a history of STDs, or engages in high-risk behaviors (see Chapter 12 for a discussion of cervical and urine screening tests for STDs).

An adolescent who is not sexually active can begin to have routine annual examinations whenever she feels comfortable about the procedure, with the hope that around the age of 18 years, she will have initiated routine gynecologic care. Contrary to popular belief, rarely is a patient unable to be fully cooperative during a pelvic examination if she has received a careful explanation about the procedure and its importance in evaluating her individual problem. Using tampons before a first examination is helpful for the virginal patient and increases the ease of the examination for the patient (22).

The pelvic examination is done with the patient in the lithotomy position and her feet in stirrups. A mirror can be offered to her. The external genitalia are inspected first; the type of hymenal opening, estrogenization of the vaginal mucosa, the distribution of pubic hair, and the size of the clitoris are assessed. The pubic hair should be inspected for pediculosis pubis if itching is present. The inguinal areas should be palpated for evidence of lymphadenopathy. The estrogenized vagina has a moist or thickened dull pink mucosa in contrast to the thin red mucosa of the prepubertal child. The normal clitoral glans is 2 to 4 mm wide; a width of 10 mm is considered to indicate significant virilization. In a study of 200 consecutive normal women, Verkauf and colleagues (23) reported a mean transverse diameter of the clitoral glans of 3.4 ± 1.0 mm, a longitudinal diameter of 5.1 ± 1.4 mm, and a total clitoral length, including glans and body, of 16.0 ± 4.3 mm. The mean clitoral index (the product of the glans width times glans length) was 18.5 mm^2.

The normal anatomy of the postpubertal external genitalia is illustrated in Figs. 22 and 23. The hymen in the adolescent girl is estrogenized and thickened. Minor changes due to sexual abuse or minor trauma that might have been easily

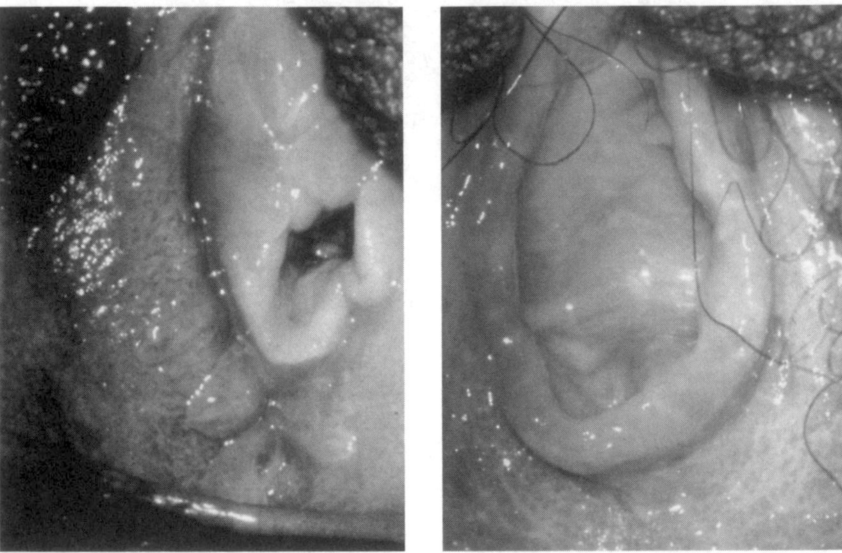

FIG. 24. Adolescent hymens. **(A)** Complete cleft at 4 o'clock from prior sexual abuse. **(B)** Dilated hymenal opening from consensual sexual activity (no clefts on hymen). (From Heger A, Emans SJ. *Evaluation of the sexually abused child.* New York: Oxford University Press, 1992; with permission.)

seen in the thin unestrogenized hymen of the prepubertal child may be difficult to visualize or may have disappeared in the estrogenized vulva and hymen of the adolescent. As the normal hymen is elastic, tampons can be inserted by most adolescents. Tampon use does not cause lacerations of the hymen (22). In the virginal adolescent, the hymenal opening is usually large enough to allow the insertion of a small Huffman speculum or a finger for palpation of the cervix, uterus, and ovaries. An adolescent who has been sexually active may have a hymen without any obvious changes or may have transections ("complete clefts" down to the base of the hymen), a narrow rim of hymen, or myrtiform caruncles (small bumps of residual hymen along the lower edge) (Fig. 24).

The examination of the sexually abused adolescent should involve a careful assessment of the vulva and hymen. The hymenal edges can be carefully examined by running a saline-moistened cotton swab around the edges (Fig. 25). Another method used by some clinicians to facilitate examination of the hymen is the use of a 12- or 14-gauge Foley bladder catheter with a 5- to 10-ml balloon and a 10-ml syringe. The catheter is inserted into the vagina, the balloon filled to capacity, usually to 10 ml, with water and the catheter pulled back gently (avoiding extreme traction) just to the hymenal edge to enhance observation of hymenal disruptions, one side at a time (24). After the examination is completed, the catheter is deflated and removed.

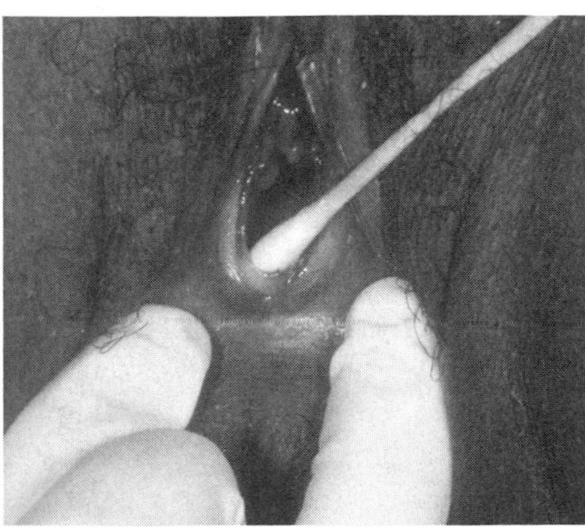

FIG. 25. Cotton swab used to examine the edge of the hymen.

As with the prepubertal child, different configurations of hymens may be seen in adolescents (Fig. 10). A simple hymenotomy is required for the imperforate hymen (type B) at the time of diagnosis and for microperforate, cribriform, and septate hymens (types C, D, and E) prior to tampon use or sexual intercourse. The septal band may be excised in the office or in an outpatient operating room with the patient being given intravenous sedation or general anesthesia; it may also break when a tampon is removed or during coitus. It is important for the adolescent with any of the latter three types to be aware of her anatomy so she is not traumatized by difficulty in the use of tampons or in having intercourse. The timing of intervention should be decided by the patient after discussion with her physician.

To avoid surprising the patient during the bimanual or speculum examination, the clinician should precede the examination by a statement such as "I'm now going to touch your bottom," or "I'm now going to place this cool metal speculum first against your thigh and then in your vagina." In the virginal teenager, a slow, one-finger examination will demonstrate the size of the hymenal opening and the location of the cervix, and will allow subsequent easy insertion of the speculum. It is helpful to warm the speculum and then touch it to the patient's thigh to allow her to feel its "cool metal" quality. The speculum should be inserted posteriorly with a downward direction to avoid the urethra. Applying pressure to the inner thigh at the same time the speculum or finger is inserted into the vagina is helpful. Experts have varying opinions about the value of showing the adolescent the speculum before the examination. In our experience, the adolescent is often much more fearful if she is shown the speculum in advance and does better if she merely feels it initially against her thigh. The patient's wishes should always be respected if she wishes to view or handle a speculum.

If the hymenal opening is small, a Huffman speculum (1/2 × 4 1/4 inches) is used to visualize the cervix. Occasionally, a latex glove with the tip cut off and placed over the narrow speculum or a condom over a longer speculum is needed to keep the vaginal walls from obstructing the view of the cervix. In the sexually active teenager, a Pederson speculum (7/8 × 4 1/2 inches) or occasionally (in the postpartum adolescent) a Graves speculum (1 3/8 × 3 3/4 inches) is appropriate. A child's speculum (5/8 × 3 inches or 7/8 × 3 inches) is rarely useful because of its inadequate length and excessive width (Figs. 26 and 27). A plastic speculum with an attached light source (Welch Allen) is also useful for facilitating the examination.

The stratified squamous epithelium of the cervix is usually a homogeneous dull pink color; however, in many adolescents an erythematous area surrounding the os is noted. The so-called ectropion is caused by endocervical columnar epithelium on the cervix. The squamocolumnar junction, instead of being inside the endocervical canal, is visible on the portio of the cervix; it does not represent a disease process and may persist throughout the adolescent years, especially if the patient is taking oral contraceptives. The ectropion gradually disappears through the process of squamous metaplasia. Mucopurulent discharge from the endocervix and ectropion characterizes cervicitis and is typical of infections with gonorrhea, *C. trachomatis*, herpes virus, or cytomegalovirus. Small pinpoint hemorrhagic spots on the cervix ("strawberry cervix") can be seen with *Trichomonas* infection. The character of any discharge present should be noted (see Chapter 11). Samples for the Pap smear, cultures, pH determination, and saline and KOH preparations are taken with the speculum in place; the techniques are described in the section on diagnostic tests, below. The optimal sequence for

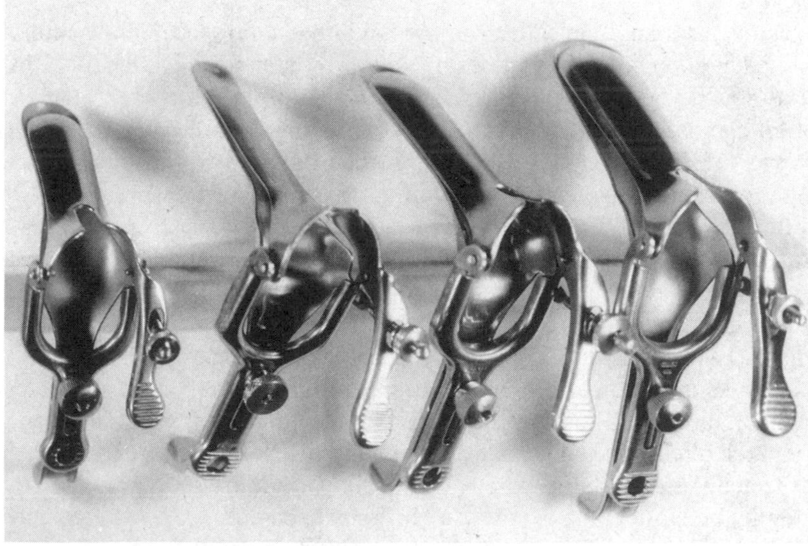

FIG. 26. Types of specula *(from left to right)*: infant, Huffman, Pederson, and Graves.

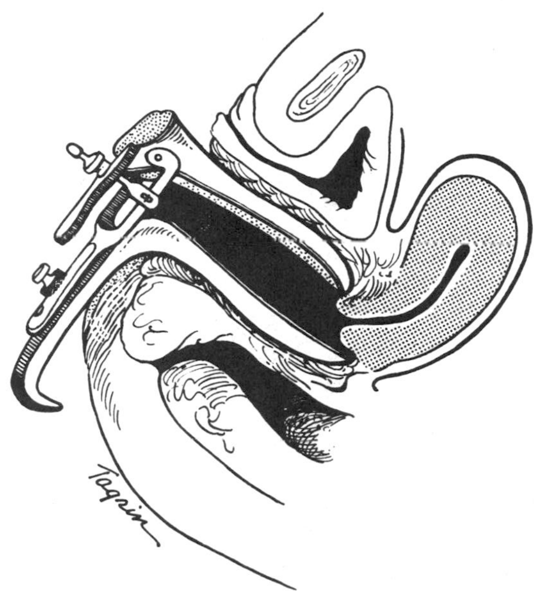

FIG. 27. Speculum examination of the cervix. (From Clarke-Pearson D, Dawood M. *Green's gynecology: essentials of clinical practice*, 4th ed. Boston: Little, Brown, 1990; with permission.)

endocervical tests is Pap smear, followed by a test for *N. gonorrhoeae* and then a test for *C. trachomatis*. After the vagina and cervix have been visualized, the speculum is removed, and the uterus and adnexa are carefully palpated with one or two fingers in the vagina and the other hand on the abdomen (Fig. 28) (25). Normal ovaries are usually <3 cm long and are rubbery. The adolescent may complain of discomfort with palpation.

A rectovaginal abdominal examination performed with the index finger in the vagina, the middle finger in the rectum, and the other hand on the abdomen permits palpation of a retroverted uterus and assessment of the mobility of the adnexa and uterus (Fig. 29). The uterosacral ligaments and cul-de-sac should be palpated carefully in patients with pain or dysmenorrhea, since tenderness may be experienced by patients with endometriosis (see Chapter 9). The patient is usually less anxious if she is told in advance that the rectal examination may cause the somewhat uncomfortable sensation that she is "moving her bowels" or "going to the bathroom." Allaying this fear usually elicits better relaxation and cooperation. In patients with a narrow hymenal opening, a simple bimanual rectoabdominal examination with the index finger pushing the cervix upward allows palpation of the uterus and adnexa. In a relaxed patient, an examination revealing no abnormalities rules out the possibility of large ovarian masses or uterine enlargement.

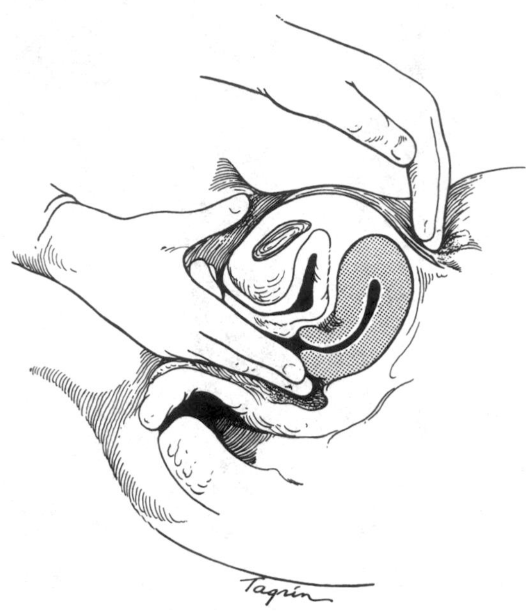

FIG. 28. Bimanual abdominal vaginal palpation of the uterus. (From Clarke-Pearson D, Dawood M. *Green's gynecology: essentials of clinical practice, 4th ed.* Boston: Little, Brown, 1990; with permission.)

If the adolescent has orthopedic or other disabilities, special attention may be needed for proper positioning during a pelvic examination. The patient's legs may need to be held by one or two assistants rather than supported by her feet in the stirrups. Other positions that may be helpful include the frog-leg position, the knee-chest position for patients with extreme spasticity, a V position (with the legs abducted and straight or slightly bent), or a side-lying position with an assistant helping to elevate the uppermost leg and the speculum inserted with the handle toward the front or back of the body (see Appendix 1 for Ortho Videotapes and monographs). An electric examination table that is accessible for adolescents with disabilities is particularly helpful in providing gynecologic care, although with skillful lifting, regular tables can be successfully used. If the adolescent is mentally challenged, the clinician needs to proceed slowly and accomplish as much of the examination as possible to answer the concerns of the patient, family, or caregivers. This may include a bimanual examination, cotton-swab samples of the vaginal secretions, or a Pap smear, depending on the age of the patient and her chief complaint. Often an office examination can be accomplished by gaining the confidence of the adolescent with an unhurried, calm approach. Preparation at home before the examination is helpful, and during the examination the adolescent can be encouraged to help with holding the labia or a mirror. It is usually possible to insert a small Huffman speculum. If the young woman will not tolerate a speculum examination, a sample for Pap smear can be obtained by inserting a gloved finger moistened with water into the vagina, palpating the cervix, and guiding a cotton-tipped applicator over the finger to the cervical os. However, the percentage of samples with endocervical cells present is much lower than when the standard Pap technique is used. In our experience, the aid of a friendly caretaker who can assist by giving reassurance is preferred to sedation, although other centers have successfully used ketamine and midazolam. Ultrasound examination can help with the differential diagnosis of some conditions. If vaginal examination is imperative and cooperation cannot be elicited, then examination with the patient under anesthesia is necessary (26–28). Most centers use an ambulatory operating room; some have developed specific services within the gynecology clinic (26).

After the examination has been concluded and the patient has dressed, the clinician should sit down and discuss in detail her complaint and the findings

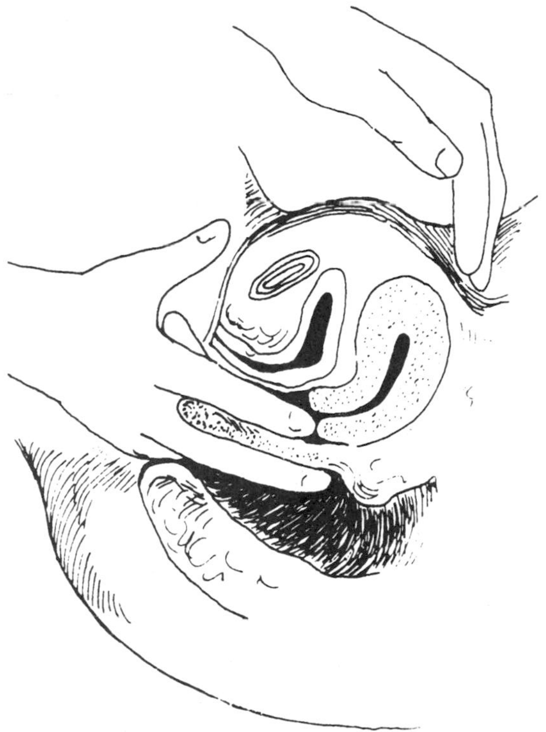

FIG. 29. Bidigital rectovaginal examination. (Adapted from Clarke-Pearson D, Dawood M: *Green's gynecology: essentials of clinical practice, 4th ed.* Boston: Little, Brown, 1990; with permission.)

from the examination. It is essential that the adolescent be treated as an adult capable of understanding the explanation. If her parent or other caregiver has accompanied her, the patient should be asked whether she would like to tell that person the findings herself or whether she would prefer to have the clinician discuss the diagnosis in her presence. It is extremely important for the patient to know that the clinician and her parent will not have a "secret" about her and that confidential information will not be divulged to her parent.

DIAGNOSTIC TESTS

Papanicolaou Smear

A Papanicolaou (Pap) smear is obtained during the speculum examination. Any adolescent who has ever been sexually active, is 18 years old or older, or has ever been exposed to human papillomavirus (HPV) should have an initial Pap smear screening that is repeated annually (see Chapter 13). Cervical dysplasia and, rarely, carcinoma *in situ* can occur during adolescence, especially in adolescents who become sexually active with multiple partners shortly after menarche or who have been exposed to HPV. The results of Pap smears may be falsely negative, and an abnormal growth on the cervix (regardless of Pap smear results) should therefore be assessed with colposcopy and biopsy as indicated.

For cytologic diagnosis to be accurate, the sample must be collected in such a way as to be representative of normal and abnormal cell populations and must include the squamocolumnar junction and the endocervix. The sample for Pap smear should be collected before samples for STD tests, and lubricant should not be used. Ideally, the entire portio of the cervix should be visible. The sample should not be taken during the menses. If vaginal discharge is present in a large amount, it should be carefully removed without disturbing the epithelium before the sample is obtained. With the speculum in place, an Ayer spatula is rotated with pressure around the cervix in a circular motion, and the collected material is spread thinly on a slide, both sides of the spatula being applied. In addition, an endocervical specimen should be obtained by using a cytobrush, which is inserted into the os and gently rotated (a cotton-tipped applicator is used by some clinicians for pregnant patients) (29). The sample is rolled onto a second glass slide, or a slide with a line down the middle can be used for both the endocervical and exocervical samples. The slides from the exocervix and endocervix must be fixed immediately with a spray fixative held 10 inches from the slide to prevent dispersal of the cells, or by placing the slides in a bottle of Pap fixative (95% ethyl alcohol). Slides with a frosted end are preferred for easy labeling. The laboratory should be given the patient's essential history, such as the date of the last menstrual period, the use of oral or other hormonal contraceptive methods, the presence of an intrauterine device, and a prior abnormal Pap smear or treatment.

Clinicians are encouraged to use the collection and fixation methods that are standard in their communities and to communicate with their cytologists regarding the classification systems used (see Chapter 13 for new Pap techniques).

Vaginal Smear to Determine Estrogenization

In the absence of inflammation, a vaginal smear is useful for evaluating the patient's estrogen status. The sample for the smear is best obtained by inserting a speculum and then scraping the side wall of the upper vagina with a wooden tongue depressor or cotton-tipped applicator moistened with saline. A sample can also be obtained without using a speculum by inserting a moistened cotton-tipped applicator or, in a small child, a moistened Calgiswab through the hymenal opening and scraping the upper lateral side wall of the vagina. The cells obtained are rolled onto a glass slide, and the slide is sprayed with Pap fixative. The cytologist reads the smear by the number of parabasal, intermediate, and superficial cells, and a percentage of each cell type is determined. The greater the estrogen effect, the more superficial cells there are. The patient with little or no estrogen, such as the prepubertal child or the adolescent with amenorrhea due to anorexia nervosa, will have predominantly parabasal cells. The relationship between the percent of superficial cells and the level of estrogenization can be characterized as follows:

<5%	Poor estrogen effect
5–10%	Slight estrogen effect
10–30%	Moderate estrogen effect
>30%	Marked estrogen effect

The smear can be correlated with the clinical situation (Table 3).

The maturation index reports the number of cells as a ratio of parabasal/intermediate/superficial. In the interpretation, the clinician should remember that the vaginal epithelium is influenced by estrogens, androgens, progestins, and

TABLE 3. *Percentage of parabasal, intermediate, and superficial cells in the vaginal smear*

State	Parabasal	Intermediate	Superficial
Childhood	60–90	10–20	0–3
Early puberty	30	50	20
Stage 5 puberty			
Proliferative phase	0	70	30
Secretory phase	0	80–95	5–20
Pregnancy	0	95	5
Anorexia nervosa (depends on clinical status)	75	25	0
Isosexual precocity	20	50	30
Premature thelarche	60	30	5–10
Premature adrenarche	60–90	10–20	0–3

adrenal hormones and that different patients respond differently to the same level. A preponderance of intermediate cells does not make a diagnosis in the absence of clinical information; thus, similar maturation indices in different patients could be associated with pregnancy, the luteal phase of the cycle, secondary amenorrhea, or long-term administration of a low-dose estrogenic preparation.

A scoring system has also proved useful if it is combined with clinical information, especially in the followup of girls evaluated and treated for precocious puberty. The original system proposed by Meisels (30) gave a score of 1.0 for superficial cyanophilic cells, 0.6 for large intermediate cells, 0.5 for small intermediate cells, and 0 for parabasal cells. The points are multiplied by the percentage of that type of cell. A score of 90 to 100 is seen in hyperestrogenic patients, 31 to 55 in hypoestrogenic patients, 60 to 70 in newborns, 50 to 60 in pubertal girls, and 0 to 30 in prepubertal girls. Meisels has subsequently modified the system to give 1 point to superficial cells, 0.5 to intermediate cells, and 0 to parabasal cells.

Some clinicians find it extremely useful to perform the assessment of the vaginal smear at the time of the examination. A stain can be formulated by combining 83 ml of light green (5% aqueous solution) with 17 ml of eosin Y (1% aqueous solution). A saline-moistened cotton-tipped applicator is used to obtain the vaginal sample and is then placed in a test tube with 2 ml of saline and 3 drops of the stain. The tube is gently shaken, and a large drop is applied to a slide and covered with a coverslip for examination under a microscope (31).

Since the epithelial cells in urine show the same hormonal changes, the urine of a prepubertal child can be collected for a urocytogram. The first morning urine specimen is centrifuged, and the sediment is spread on a slide. The cytologist records the percentage of superficial, intermediate, and parabasal cells. Two methods of collection and staining have been described (32,33).

Cervical Mucus

An examination of the cervical mucus is another method of evaluating a patient's estrogen status. The cervix is gently swabbed with a large cotton-tipped applicator, and a small sample of cervical mucus is obtained with a saline-moistened cotton-tipped applicator. Profuse, clear, elastic mucus is seen in the preovulatory period and at ovulation. The elastic quality decreases rapidly following ovulation. Thick, sticky mucus is characteristic of the secretory phase of the cycle (see Chapter 4).

The mucus is spread on a glass slide and allowed to air dry for 5 minutes. Under the microscope, beautiful ferning patterns will be seen in the smear taken from the late proliferative phase of the cycle (Fig. 30). Ferning does not occur in the presence of progesterone.

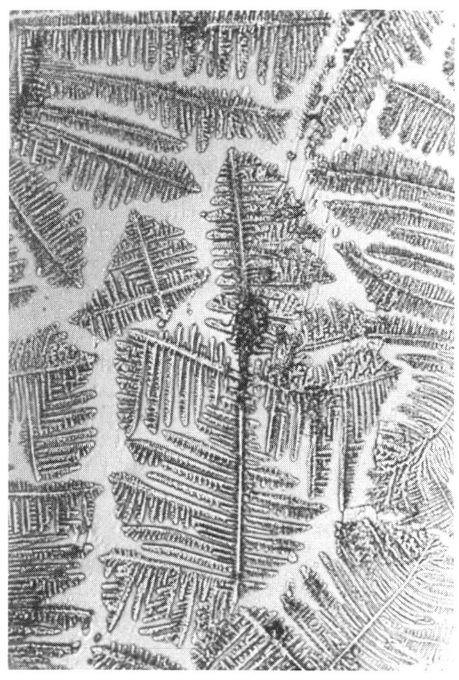

FIG. 30. Microscopic evaluation of cervical mucus; ferning during late proliferative phase of the normal menstrual cycle.

Wet Preparations

The so-called wet preparations are useful in defining the etiology of a vaginal discharge. In the prepubertal child, the discharge is collected with a saline-moistened Calgiswab, an eyedropper, or a catheter. In adolescents, a cotton-tipped applicator is inserted into the vaginal pool with the speculum in place or, for the virginal adolescent, directly into the vagina. The applicator is mixed first with one drop of saline on a glass slide and then with one drop of 10% KOH on another slide. A coverslip is then applied, and the slides are examined under the microscope (low and high dry power) (Fig. 31; see also Figs. 2 and 3 in Chapter 11). On the saline slide, trichomonads appear as lively, flagellated organisms, slightly larger than white blood cells. In bacterial vaginosis, a saline preparation typically shows many refractile bacteria within large epithelial cells (so-called clue cells) and rare leukocytes; mixing this discharge with 10% KOH may liberate an amine-like fishy odor (a positive "whiff" test result). In contrast, physiologic leukorrhea is characterized by numerous epithelial cells without evidence of inflammation. On the KOH slide, the presence of budding pseudohyphae and yeast forms is evidence of *Candida* vaginitis.

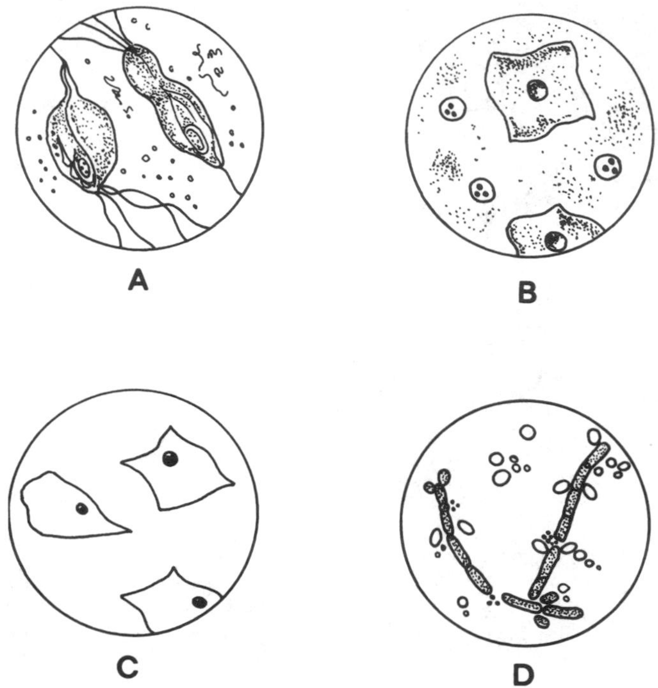

FIG. 31. Fresh vaginal smears. **(A)** *Trichomonas.* **(B)** Clue cells of bacterial vaginosis. **(C)** Leukorrhea. **(D)** *Candida.* **A**, **B**, and **C** are saline preparations; **D** is a KOH preparation.

pH

The pH of the prepubertal vagina is neutral. In contrast, the pH of the vagina of the pubertal adolescent is acid (<4.5). A higher than normal pH (>4.5) occurs with bacterial vaginosis and *Trichomonas* vaginitis. Testing postpubertal vaginal secretions with pH paper can be very helpful in diagnosing the cause of the vaginal discharge (see Chapter 11).

Gram Stain

In symptomatic gonorrhea, a Gram stain of a vaginal or cervical discharge may reveal polymorphonuclear leukocytes and gram-negative intracellular diplococci. Although a positive Gram stain is highly suggestive of gonorrhea, only a positive culture is conclusive evidence of this diagnosis in females. The Gram stain may also show an increased number of polymorphonuclear leukocytes in chlamydial infections (see Chapter 12) as well as *Trichomonas* vaginitis and herpetic cervical infections.

Cultures and Tests for *N. gonorrhoeae* and *C. trachomatis*

Sexually active teenage girls should have screening tests for sexually transmitted infections, including *N. gonorrhoeae* and *C. trachomatis*, at least annually. Such tests should be obtained more frequently if they change sexual partners, engage in high-risk behaviors, have had an STD or a history of exposure, or have symptoms of cervicitis, breakthrough bleeding on the oral contraceptive pill, or lower abdominal pain. In some low-risk suburban populations, less frequent screening for *N. gonorrhoeae* may be indicated. *C. trachomatis* is epidemic in all adolescent populations, and thus screening is essential.

In screening for gonorrhea, either a culture method or a DNA probe is recommended. For culture, a cotton-tipped applicator is inserted into the cervical os and then streaked directly onto modified Thayer-Martin-Jembec or Thayer-Martin medium. The use of plain Thayer-Martin plates requires immediate transportation of the culture to a bacteriology laboratory and incubation under increased carbon dioxide tension. The Jembec medium, with a small carbon dioxide–generating tablet inserted into a well of the plastic case, is easy to use and reliable; the medium can be transported after an incubation of 24 to 48 hours or processed in the office. For DNA probes (GenProbe), the test is sent directly to the laboratory (see Chapter 12).

For *C. trachomatis,* endocervical samples can be screened using cultures, direct immunofluorescent smears (MicroTrak), enzyme immunoassays (Chlamydiazyme, Abbott; IDEIA, Dako), DNA probes (Pace 2, Gen-Probe), ligase chain reaction (LCR, Abbott), polymerase chain reaction (PCR) (Amplicor, Roche), and transcription mediated amplification (TMA) (Gen-Probe Amplified) (see Table 2 in Chapter 12 for sensitivities and specificities of each test). LCR and PCR techniques provide marked amplification of specific DNA sequences, and TMA is an amplified RNA assay; all three have yielded a new standard for chlamydial detection. Several of these tests are also approved for screening of urine in adolescents, and thus noninvasive screening for *Chlamydia* is possible. In addition, some methods allow for detection of *Chlamydia* and gonorrhea simultaneously. Culture techniques remain important for confirmation of *Chlamydia* in sexually abused girls although they are less sensitive than the newer methods.

Other Cultures

Nickerson Biggy agar medium (PML Microbiologicals, Portland, OR) helps confirm a *Candida* vaginitis if the result of KOH preparation is negative. A sample of the discharge is streaked on the medium, and the tube is incubated at 35°C. The appearance of brown colonies 3 to 7 days later is a positive result for yeast; however, a positive culture suggests but does not prove infection, since *Candida* may be part of the normal flora.

Cultures for *Trichomonas* are significantly more sensitive than the "wet prep" but are not widely available (see Chapter 11).

Aerobic cultures of the vagina are useful in the diagnosis and treatment of vaginitis in prepubertal girls when respiratory pathogens such as *Streptococcus pyogenes* play a major role, but such cultures are rarely indicated in the diagnosis of vaginal discharge in the adolescent. Normal flora are discussed in Chapters 3 and 11.

Progesterone Test

The patient is given medroxyprogesterone (Provera, Cycrin), 10 mg orally once a day for 5 or 10 days, or progesterone-in-oil, 50 to 100 mg intramuscularly once. If the patient has an estrogen-primed endometrium and is not pregnant, she will have a period 3 to 10 days after the last medroxyprogesterone tablet. Progesterone withdrawal is used as a diagnostic test for the evaluation of primary and secondary amenorrhea (see Chapter 6).

Pregnancy Tests

Several highly sensitive, rapid pregnancy tests are available. Qualitative kits used on urine samples are the most practical for office use (34–36). The newer kits use specific monoclonal antibodies to human chorionic gonadotropin (hCG) and enzyme-linked immunoassay techniques. For example, the positivity of ICON II HCG (Hybritech) kits is associated with hCG levels of 20 mIU/ml or more; the tests are not affected by blood or protein and have a built-in control (Fig. 32). In studies of ectopic pregnancies, 26 of 27 and 95 of 95 ectopic pregnancies were detected by ICON (34,35). Very low levels of hCG (10 to 20 mIU/ml), especially in urine with low specific gravity (<1.015), may be missed.

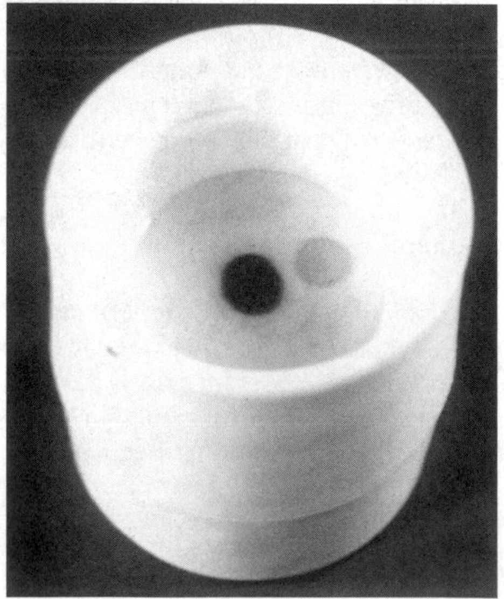

FIG. 32. ICON office pregnancy test. The center dot indicates a positive result; the dot on the outer circle is the positive control.

TABLE 4. *Mean serum human chorionic gonadotropin levels throughout normal gestation*

Weeks after last menstrual period	Mean (mIU/ml)	SEM (mIU/ml)[a]
3–3.5	22	6
4–4.5	353	9
5–5.5	2270	390
6–6.5	6640	1160
7–7.5	13,610	2740
8–8.5	46,830	4710
9–9.5	44,710	3690
10–10.5	37,750	5420
11–11.5	38,360	8100

[a]SEM, standard error of the mean.

(Adapted from Braunstein GD, Rasor J, Adler D, et al. Serum human chorionic gonadotropin levels throughout normal pregnancy. *Am J Obstet Gynecol* 1976;126:678–681.)

Testpack (Abbott) offers similar advantages. Because of the sensitivity of such tests, the detection of early pregnancies and ectopic pregnancies is significantly enhanced. Pregnancy tests should always be correlated with clinical information and examination (Table 4) (see Chapter 18).

Blood tests for measuring hCG can be qualitative or quantitative. For example, Tandem ICON can be used on serum to determine a positive or negative pregnancy test. Quantitative hCG levels are important in the diagnosis of ectopic pregnancy and some spontaneous abortions and threatened abortions and for the followup of molar pregnancies and choriocarcinomas. Because not all laboratories use the same units or methods in reporting hCG levels, sequential measures in a patient should use the same laboratories. Two international systems for hCG can be reported: the newer International Reference Preparation (IRP) or the older Second International Standard, which is roughly half the IRP levels. Although urine hCG can also be quantitated, blood measurements are preferred for serial measures (see Chapter 18 for evaluation of disorders of early pregnancy).

Over-the-counter pregnancy tests have improved significantly, and most use monoclonal antibody technology, which yields sensitive and specific results at the time of a missed period or shortly thereafter. However, adolescents may misread the instructions and the results and should therefore be encouraged to use primarily office and laboratory tests and to confirm the results of at-home tests with a medical assessment and a repeat office test.

Bone Age

The bone age is determined by comparing radiographs of the patient's wrist and hand (carpal and phalangeal ossification centers) with the standards in Greulich and Pyle (37) or by applying the Tanner-Whitehouse method (38). A radiograph of the iliac crest can be used in a similar way. At puberty, the epiphysis along the iliac crest undergoes ossification. During adolescence, the ossification progresses from the lateral to the medial part, and fusion occurs at 21 to 23 years of age.

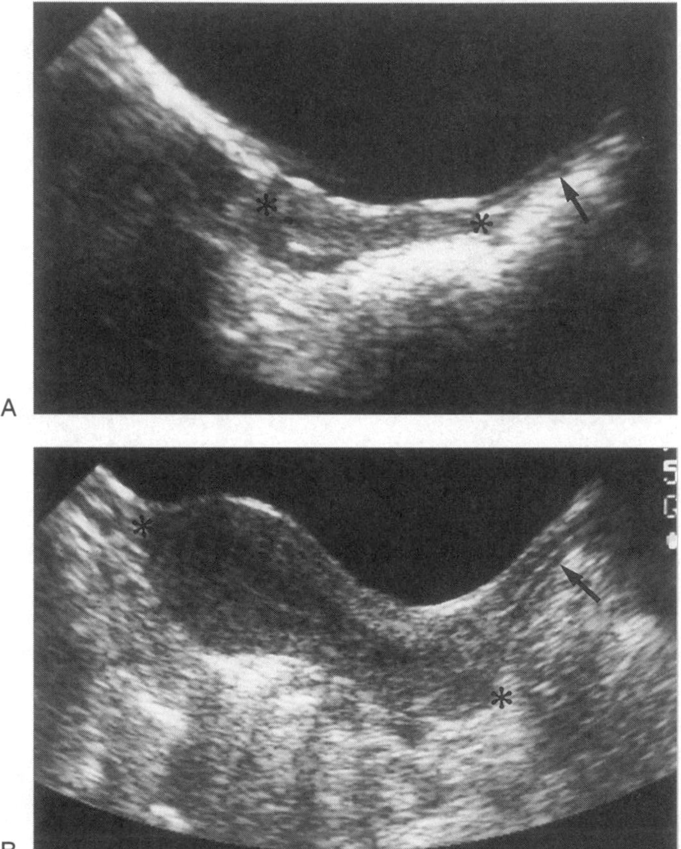

FIG. 33. Ultrasound images of prepubertal and pubertal girls. **(A)** Longitudinal view of a normal prepubertal uterus, between the asterisks (patient's head to the right). The fundus and cervix are approximately the same size. The *arrow* points to the vagina. **(B)** With puberty, the fundus enlarges. This is the longitudinal scan of a normal teenage girl with the fundus shown between the asterisks. The *arrow* points to the vagina.

Growth hormone and thyroid deficiencies, glucocorticoid excess, delayed puberty, and malnutrition result in delayed maturation; androgens produce an advanced bone age. In the absence of sex steroids (for example, in sexual infantilism associated with Turner's syndrome), the bone age will not advance beyond 13 years.

Imaging Techniques

Ultrasonography of the pelvis is useful for evaluating suspected and known gynecologic problems such as ovarian masses, pregnancy, and pelvic anomalies (39–49). Because an ill-defined adnexal mass in an adolescent may represent a

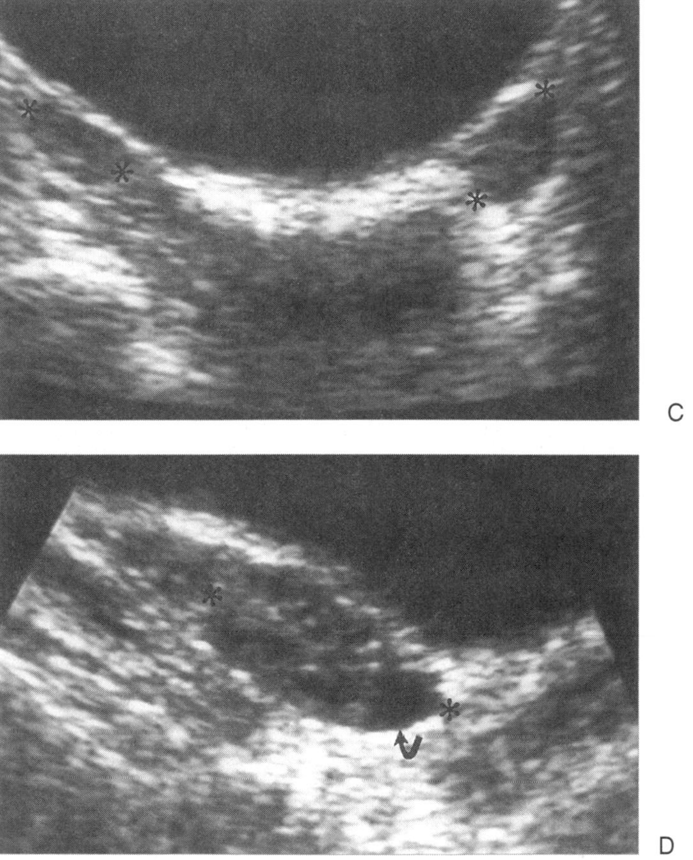

FIG. 33. *Continued* **(C)** Both normal ovaries (between the *asterisks*) are seen on the transverse scan of this prepubertal girl. It is not uncommon to see tiny areas of low density in the ovary, presumably representing follicles. **(D)** Longitudinal view of a normal ovary (between the *asterisks*) in a postpubertal girl. The *curved arrow* indicates a normal follicle. (Courtesy of Dr. Jane Share, Children's Hospital, Boston.)

congenital abnormality of the müllerian system, ultrasonography should also include views of the kidneys, as there is a high correlation of müllerian with renal anomalies. Although ultrasonography is an extremely helpful technique, false–positive findings do occur, as when bowel gas is read as an ovarian cyst.

The uterus should be identified in the prepubertal child, with measurements of 2.0 to 3.3 cm in length and 0.5 to 1.0 cm in width. The fundus and cervix are the same size. With puberty, the fundus increases in size; the postpubertal uterus is 5 to 8 cm in length, and the fundus is 1.6 to 3.0 cm in width. In the prepubertal girl, the ovaries are usually <1 cm^3 in volume (0.13 to 0.9 cm^3) (Fig. 33). In the pubertal girl, the ovaries are 1.8 to 5.7 cm^3, with a mean of 4 cm^3

(42). The average reproductive ovary varies from 2.5 to 5 cm in length, 1.5 to 3.0 cm in width, and 0.7 to 1.5 cm in thickness. Prepubertal girls can have follicles up to 7 mm in diameter. A progressive increase in the proportion of normal girls with more than six follicles in each ovary ("multicystic ovaries") occurs after the age of 8 1/2 years (43). Follicles of 1 to 3 cm occur normally in adolescent girls, and girls in early and midpuberty may have enlarged ovaries with multiple small "cysts" throughout the ovarian stroma. Small amounts of fluid in the cul-de-sac may be seen in normal girls and with ovulation. Cul-de-sac fluid may also occur with bleeding, retrograde menstruation, a ruptured ovarian cyst, or infection.

Ultrasonography is useful when bimanual examination is difficult, when a mass is palpated, and to define the anatomy in patients with probable congenital anomalies. A patient with gonadal dysgenesis should have her renal status assessed by ultrasonography. A patient thought to have uterine agenesis can also be assessed by this technique; the absence of the uterus can be confirmed, the presence of normal ovaries established (in Mayer-Rokitansky-Küster-Hauser syndrome), and the kidneys examined (see Chapter 8). In patients with androgen insensitivity, the testes may sometimes be visualized as soft tissue densities behind the bladder or in the inguinal areas.

Ultrasonography is also helpful in establishing the presence of uterine, cervical, and vaginal anomalies with or without obstruction. Magnetic resonance imaging (MRI), however, is usually the definitive test in assessing the complexities of the anatomic abnormalities and planning potential operative approaches.

In the assessment of müllerian abnormalities, the kidneys should be scanned for unilateral agenesis, horseshoe kidney, and crossed fused ectopia. Skeletal anomalies are also common in patients with müllerian anomalies; they include abnormalities of segmentation and rudimentary and wedge vertebrae. Conversely, patients with cervical spine anomalies or congenital scoliosis, or both, should undergo ultrasonography to screen for renal and pelvic anomalies in midpuberty before the menarche. A renal screen can be done much earlier, but pelvic screening is easier in the pubertal child. The girl with unilateral renal agenesis should undergo ultrasonography and gynecologic assessment before menarche.

Uterine hypoplasia, as well as ovarian failure, often occurs in patients treated with pelvic radiation therapy for childhood malignancies. Uterine leiomyomas are rare in adolescents; ultrasonography may show uterine enlargement and alterations in the texture and contour.

Ultrasound imaging may also be indicated in establishing the gestational age of an intrauterine pregnancy or to sort out abnormalities such as ectopic pregnancy, threatened abortion, and trophoblastic disease (see Chapter 18).

Ovarian enlargement and pelvic pain are often evaluated with ultrasonography. The ovaries of patients with polycystic ovaries may be of normal size or enlarged, with multiple cysts and a thickened capsule. Unlike the girl in early adolescence, who may have "multicystic" ovaries, the adolescent with polycystic ovary syndrome may have the small cysts in a "string of pearls" configuration just underneath the cortex (see Chapter 7). Simple ovarian cysts are very common in adolescents. They are usually 3 to 6 cm in diameter, unilocular, and without internal debris, and they often resolve spontaneously. Complex ovarian cysts may be a corpus luteum cyst, a cystadenofibroma, a cystadenoma, a teratoma, a hemorrhagic ovarian cyst, ovarian torsion (see Chapters 9 and 15 for discussion of Doppler ultrasound), ectopic pregnancy, tuboovarian abscess, ovarian tumor, or periappendicular abscess. Hemorrhagic ovarian cysts have quite variable findings depending on when they are scanned; most are heterogenous with mixed solid and cystic areas, which may become more cystic as the clot resorbs. The ultrasound findings in ovarian torsion are also variable; classically, there is a large solid mass with peripheral follicular cysts. Pelvic inflammatory disease (PID) with tuboovarian abscess may produce edema and loss of anatomic planes, giving a disorganized pattern and adnexal enlargement, but PID alone cannot be distinguished by ultrasound (39,50). An ovarian tumor with a cystic component may be easier to visualize than a solid teratoma, which can be obscured by bowel gas. A radiograph of the abdomen may help identify fat, calcifications, or teeth in these tumors (see Chapter 15).

Transvaginal ultrasonography is used frequently in the evaluation of intrauterine and ectopic pregnancy, spontaneous and incomplete abortion (see Chapter 18), pelvic masses, PID, and uterine abnormalities. Signs of abnormal early gestation include irregular decidua, pathologic double ring, subchorionic bleeding, degenerative changes of fetal pole and yolk sac, and absence of fetal heartbeat. Tuboovarian disease can also be assessed and the actual tube examined in greater detail in cases of both PID and ectopic pregnancy. The vaginal probe can be easily inserted into the vagina of the sexually active adolescent. It can also be used for selected girls who have never been sexually active but who have used tampons and do not experience pain with insertion of the probe.

Computed tomography (CT) and MRI are important additional tests in pathologic conditions of the pelvis when ultrasonography has not yielded sufficient diagnostic information. CT is useful in staging malignancies and in defining abscesses. MRI has become the prime modality for assessing congenital pelvic anomalies. It has advantages over CT because of its greater tissue definition, as well as the the lack of radiation and risk of the allergic reactions caused by contrast media. However, the disadvantages of MRI are the high cost and long imaging times.

Detection of Ovulation

Several methods have been used to detect ovulation. Most are used primarily in the evaluation and treatment of infertility. Occasionally, in older adolescents with conditions such as oligomenorrhea or Turner's syndrome with normal gonadotropin levels, or after exposure to chemotherapy or radiation therapy, the clinician may wish to establish whether ovulatory cycles are occurring. The methods include measurement of basal body temperature charts, determination of serum progesterone levels during the luteal phase, testing for luteinizing hormone (LH), ultrasonography, and endometrial sampling.

In using basal body temperature charts, the patient is instructed to take her temperature every morning as soon as she awakens. For accurate recording, a basal thermometer is kept at the bedside, and the patient is told not to go to the bathroom, drink fluids, or have sexual activity before taking her temperature. The temperature is recorded on a special chart. The typical ovulatory and anovulatory cycles are shown in Fig. 34. Basal body temperature charts are useful if the patient shows a classic pattern, but some ovulatory patients may not have a biphasic chart, may be ill during the recording, or may fail to use the proper method. The use of basal body temperatures during the placebo week of oral contraceptives can also be helpful in managing a lack of withdrawal flow; for example, a low temperature of 97°F is consistent with pill amenorrhea, not pregnancy (see Chapter 17).

Home kits are available for testing the urine to detect the midcycle rise of LH (49). These kits, which use monoclonal antibody technology, are helpful in infertility evaluations, since the time from the detected surge to ovulation is typically about 12 to 24 hours. However, as will be noted in Chapter 4, an LH surge in an

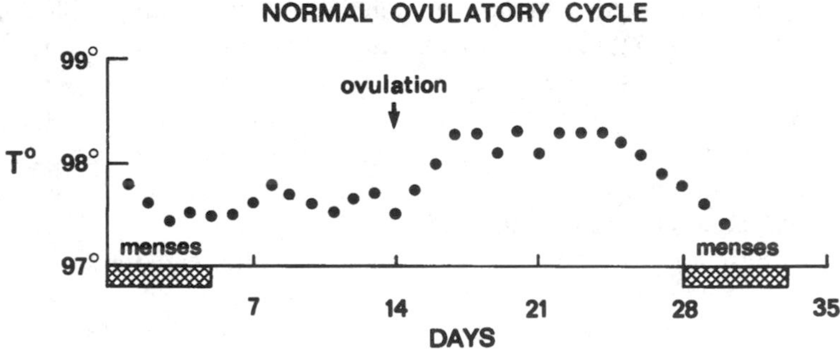

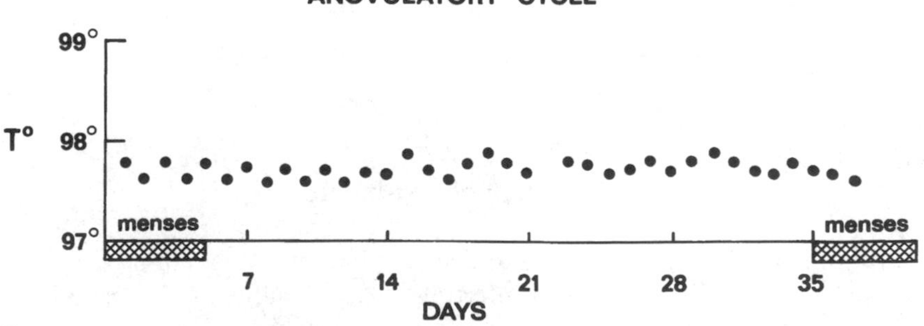

FIG. 34. Basal body temperature charts.

adolescent may not be evidence of normal ovulation and a normal luteal phase. Similarly, a random serum progesterone level may be suggestive but not definitive evidence of a normal luteal phase. A luteal progesterone level >10 ng/ml establishes ovulation with normal corpus luteum function. Endometrial sampling, with a small catheter (e.g., Pipelle endometrial suction curette), can be difficult for the physician to perform in the virginal patient. It is uncomfortable for the adolescent and is rarely indicated.

Clearly, the use of any of these tests necessitates discussion with the patient of the problems and likely benefits from the results.

REFERENCES

1. Emans SJ, Wood ER, Flagg NT, et al. Genital findings in sexually abused symptomatic and asymptomatic girls. *Pediatrics* 1087;79:778.
2. Huffman JW, Dewhurst CJ, Capraro VJ. *The gynecology of childhood and adolescence.* Philadelphia: WB Saunders, 1981.
3. Pokorny SF. Configuration of the prepubertal hymen. *Am J Obstet Gynecol* 1987;157:950.
4. Jenny C, Kuhns MLD, Arakawa F. Hymens in newborn female infants. *Pediatrics* 1987;80:399.
5. Mor N, Merlob P. Congenital absence of the hymen only a rumor? *Pediatrics* 1988;82:679.
6. Emans SJ, Goldstein DP. The gynecologic examination of the prepubertal child with vulvovaginitis: use of the knee-chest position. *Pediatrics* 1980;65:758.
7. Capraro V. Gynecologic examination in children and adolescents. *Pediatr Clin North Am* 1972; 19:511.
8. Billmire ME, Farrell MK, Dine MS. A simplified procedure for pediatric vaginal examination: use of veterinary otoscope specula. *Pediatrics* 1980;65:823.
9. Capraro V, Capraro E. Vaginal aspirate studies in children. *Obstet Gynecol* 1971;37:462.
10. Pokorny SF, Stormer J. Atraumatic removal of secretions from the prepubertal vagina. *Am J Obstet Gynecol* 1987;156:581.
11. Alexander ER. Misidentification of sexually transmitted organisms in children: medicolegal implications. *Pediatr Infect Dis* 1988;7:1.
12. Whittington WL, Rice RJ, Biddle JW, et al. Incorrect identification of *Neisseria gonorrhoeae* from infants and children. *Pediatr Infect Dis* 1988;7:3.
13. American Medical Association. *Guidelines for Adolescent Preventive Services (GAPS).* Chicago: Department of Adolescent Health, American Medical Association, 1993.
14. Green M, ed. *Bright futures—guidelines for health supervision of infants, children, and adolescents.* Arlington, VA: National Center for Education in Maternal and Child Health, 1994.
15. American Medical Association. *Confidential health services for adolescents.* Chicago: Department of Adolescent Health, American Medical Association, 1994.
16. Cheng TL, Savageau JA, Sattler AL, et al. Confidentiality in health care: a survey of knowledge, perceptions, and attitudes among high school students. *JAMA* 1993;269:1404.
17. Roberts SJ, Sorenson L. Lesbian health care: a review and recommendations for health promotion in primary care settings. *Nurse Pract* 1995;20:42–47.
18. American Medical Association. *Clinical evaluation and management handbook.* Chicago: Department of Adolescent Health, American Medical Association, 1995.
19. American Medical Association. *Implementation forms.* Chicago: Department of Adolescent Health, American Medical Association, 1995.
20. Prochaska JO, DiClemente CC. Transtheoretical therapy: toward a more integrative model of change. *Psychother Theory Res Pract* 1982;19:276.
21. Millstein SG, Adler NE, Irwin CE. Sources of anxiety about pelvic examinations among adolescent females. *J Adolesc Health Care* 1984:5:105.
22. Emans SJ, Woods ER, Allred EN, Grace E. Hymenal findings in adolescent women: impact of tampon use and consensual sexual activity. *J Pediatr* 1994;125:153.
23. Verkauf BS, Von Thron J, O'Brien WF. Clitoral size in normal women. *Obstet Gynecol* 1992;80:41.
24. Starling S, Jenny C. Forensic examination of adolescent female genitalia: the Foley catheter technique. *Arch Pediatr Adolesc Med* 1997;151:102.

25. Green T. *Gynecology: essentials of clinical practice*, 3rd ed. Boston: Little, Brown, 1977.
26. Rosen DA, Rosen KR, Elkins TE, et al. Outpatient sedation: an essential addition to gynecologic care for persons with mental retardation. *Am J Obstet Gynecol* 1991;164:825.
27. Elkins TE, McNeeley SG, Rosen D, et al. A clinical observation of a program to accomplish pelvic exams in difficult-to-manage patients with mental retardation. *Adolesc Pediatr Gynecol* 1988; 1:195.
28. Muram D, Elkins TE. Reproductive health care needs of the developmentally disabled. In: Sanfilippo JS, ed. *Pediatric and adolescent gynecology*. Philadelphia: WB Saunders, 1994.
29. Germain M, Heaton R, Erickson D, et al. A comparison of the three most common Papanicolaou smear collection techniques. *Obstet Gynecol* 1994;84:168.
30. Meisels A. Computed cytohormonal findings in 3,307 healthy women. *Acta Cytol* 1965;9:328.
31. Rakoff AE. Hormonal cytology in gynecology. *Clin Obstet Gynecol* 1961;4:1045.
32. Lencioni LJ, Staffieri J. Urocytogram diagnosis of sexual precocity. *Acta Cytol* (*Baltimore*) 1969; 13:302.
33. Preeyasombat C, Kenny F. Urocytogram in normal children and various abnormal conditions. *Pediatrics* 1966;38:436.
34. Cartwright PS, Victory DG, Moore RA, et al. Performance of a new enzyme-linked immunoassay urine pregnancy test for the detection of ectopic gestation. *Ann Emerg Med* 1986;15:1198.
35. Norman RJ, Buck RH, Rom L, et al. Blood or urine measurement of human chorionic gonadotropin for detection of ectopic pregnancy? A comparative study of quantitative and qualitative methods in both fluids. *Obstet Gynecol* 1988;71:315.
36. Klee G. Human chorionic gonadotropin. *Mayo Clin Proc* 1994;69:391.
37. Greulich WW, Pyle S. *Radiographic atlas of skeletal development of the hand and wrist.* Stanford, CA: Stanford University Press, 1959.
38. Tanner JM, Whitehouse RH, Cameron N, et al. *Assessment of skeletal maturity and prediction of adult height (TW2 method)*. New York: Academic Press, 1983.
39. Share J, Teele R. Ultrasonography in adolescent gynecology. *Clin Pract Gynecol* 1989;1:72.
40. Sanfilippo JS, Lavery JP. The spectrum of ultrasound: antenatal to adolescent years. *Semin Reprod Endocrinol* 1988;6:45.
41. Salardi S, Orsini IF, Cacciari E, et al. Pelvic ultrasonography in premenarcheal girls: relation to puberty and sex hormone concentration. *Arch Dis Child* 1985;60:120.
42. Lippe BM, Sample WF. Pelvic ultrasonography in pediatric and adolescent endocrine disorders. *J Pediatr* 1978;92:897.
43. Stanhope R, Adams J, Jacobs HS, et al. Ovarian ultrasound assessment in normal children, idiopathic precocious puberty, and during low dose pulsatile gonadotropin releasing hormone treatment of hypogonadotrophic hypogonadism. *Arch Dis Child* 1985;60:116.
44. Wu A, Siegel MJ. Sonography of pelvic masses in children: diagnostic predictability. *AJR* 1987; 148:1199.
45. Baltarowich OH, Kurtz AB, Pasto ME, et al. The spectrum of sonographic findings in hemorrhagic ovarian cysts. *AJR* 1987;148:901.
46. Bass IS, Haller JO, Friedman AP, et al. The ultrasonographic appearance of the hemorrhagic ovarian cyst in adolescents. *J Ultrasound Med* 1984;3:509.
47. Warner MA, Fleischer AC, Edell SL, et al. Uterine adnexal torsion: sonographic findings. *Radiology* 1985;154:773.
48. Graif M, Shalev J, Strauss S, et al. Torsion of the ovary: sonographic features. *AJR* 1984;143:1331.
49. Swayne LC, Love MB, Karasick SR. Pelvic inflammatory disease: sonographic-pathologic correlation. *Radiology* 1984;151:751.
50. Rebar RW. Practical appreciations of home diagnostic products: a symposium. *J Reprod Med* 1987; 32(9S):705.

Suggested Videotapes for Examination

See Appendix 1.

2

Ambiguous Genitalia in the Newborn

Although most clinicians rarely see an infant with ambiguous genitalia at birth, the need to assess the situation as quickly as possible makes this subject essential. Any deviation from the normal appearance of male or female genitalia should prompt investigation, since apparent but incomplete male or female external genitals may be associated with the gonads and genotype of the opposite sex. Even a slight doubt that arises during the initial examination of the newborn should be pursued systematically to prevent the possibility of later confusion. Bilateral cryptorchidism, unilateral cryptorchidism with incomplete scrotal fusion or hypospadias, labial fusion, or clitoromegaly require evaluation.

DETERMINING SEX ASSIGNMENT

Abnormal sexual differentiation is a medical and psychological emergency. Two major issues need to be immediately addressed: the relationship of the sexual ambiguity to a possible life-threatening disease, and the sex of rearing. In the delivery room, it is critical *not* to make a gender assignment but to postpone that determination until the necessary data have been collected. Clearly, most parents will react with dismay and anxiety. It is important to reassure the parents that they have a healthy baby, but that the development of the external genitals is incomplete, and tests are necessary to determine the sex. They should be reassured that tests will show the cause of the problem and identify the baby as a girl or a boy, and that a definite answer should be possible within a few days, or at most in 1 or 2 weeks. The possibility of an intersex disorder (hermaphroditism) should not be raised at this time. Speculation about the possible assignment of sex could be psychologically damaging to the parents. The child should be referred to by all caretakers as *the baby* rather than as a boy or girl. The physician should examine the baby in the presence of the parents, explain the common genital anlage for boys and girls, and educate the family about normal sexual development. Once the sex of rearing has been determined, the physician should help the family put aside issues of sexual ambiguity (1). Parents should be encouraged to use the names previously selected for a boy or girl. Names that are definitely male or female help the family see the child unequivocally as belonging to that sex. As long as parental attitudes toward the child's sex remain unequivocal, the child usually assumes his or her gender role without difficulty, regardless of the genotype. Finally, parents should be encouraged to tell other family members and friends, when they ask about the sex of the baby, that the baby is sick, and to delay sending out birth announcements until the gender has been decided upon.

Although a diagnosis of the patient's condition requires knowledge of the genotype (karyotype), sex assignment is based on other criteria as well. The main issues are the potential for an unambiguous appearance, the potential for normal sexual functioning, and fertility. The female pseudohermaphrodite has normal ovaries and uterus, is potentially capable of bearing children, and thus should always be given a female gender identity. The male pseudohermaphrodite, on the other hand, may not be adequately virilized to allow for reconstruction of male external genitalia. In addition, the defect in the male pseudohermaphrodite may limit the potential for adequate virilization at puberty. In gonadal disorders in which fertility is not possible, the decision regarding sex assignment is based on the potential for reconstructive surgery. In general, surgical techniques are more suited to reduction of the size of the phallus and, later, the creation of a vagina than to the construction of a normal male phallus.

REVIEW OF EMBRYOGENESIS

Prior to the seventh week of gestation, the fetal gonads are bipotential. Maleness is imposed on the innate tendency of the fetal gonads to develop along female lines. There are three major components to sex determination: chromosomal sex, gonadal sex, and hormonal sex. Chromosomal sex refers to the karyotype, 46,XY or 46,XX, which under normal circumstances determines whether the individual is male or female. More specifically, the chromosomal sex refers to genes important in sex determination. The first critical gene in the cascade of genes involved in sexual differentiation is the sex-determining region of the Y chromosome (SRY), which is located on the short arm of the Y chromosome (Yp) just centromeric to the pseudoautosomal region (the region where the X and Y chromosomes pair during meiosis) (Fig. 1). The SRY is required for differentiation of the gonad into a testis (2,3). If it is absent or abnormal, the gonad differentiates into an ovary. The importance of SRY in sex determination is demonstrated by the 46,XX males who have SRY present (3) and 46,XY females with mutations or deletions in SRY (2,5). The SRY protein activates transcription of genes on the sex chromosomes and autosomes that are important in sex determination (2,6,7). Defects in genes activated by SRY are

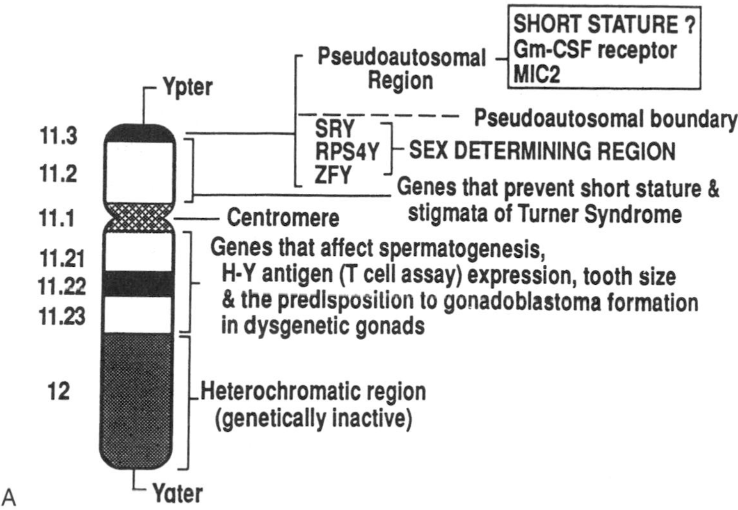

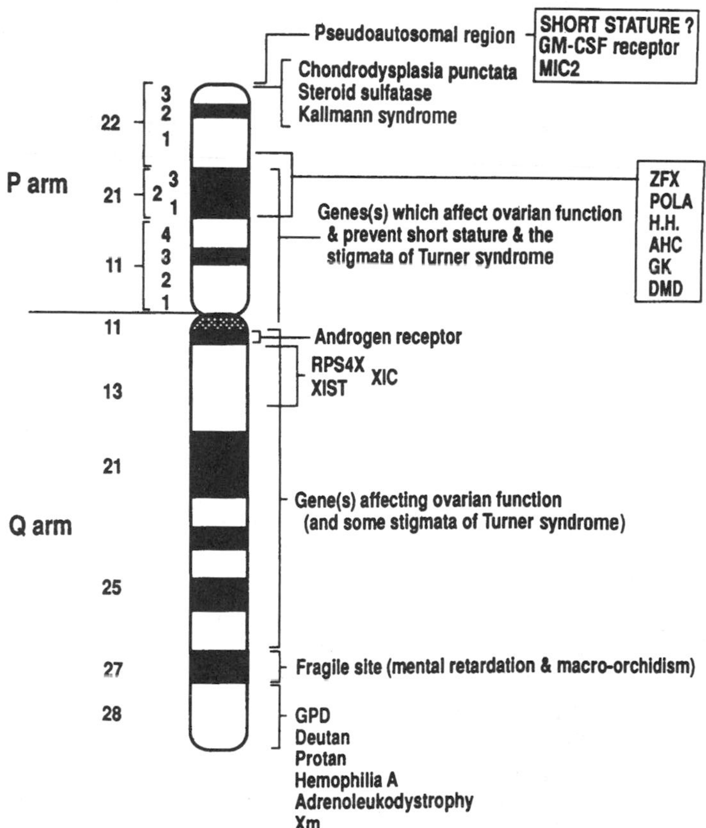

FIG. 1. Diagrammatic representation of the G-banded Y and X chromosomes. Functional regions and loci involved in sex determination and differentiation are shown. **(A)** The Y chromosome. SRY, sex determining region; RPS4Y, ribosomal protein S4; ZFY, zinc finger protein. **(B)** The X chromosome. RPS4X, ribosomal protein S4 on X; XIST, Xi-specific transcript; XIC, X-inactivation center. (From Grumbach MM, Conte FA. Disorders of sex differentiation. In: Wilson JD, Foster DW, eds, *Williams textbook of endocrinology*, 8th ed. Philadelphia: WB Saunders, 1992; with permission.)

postulated to be responsible for sex reversal in 46,XX males who have no Y sequences detectable (4,8,9), including no SRY (10), and in 46,XY females with normal SRY. Sex reversal occurs in patients with abnormalities in chromosomes other than the Y, and in patients with mutations in genes other than SRY (11–16).

The presence of two X chromosomes appears to be important for development of the ovary. 46,XX and 45,X fetuses initially have oocytes. However, in the 45,X fetus, oocyte atresia is accelerated in the second half of intrauterine life and in the prepubertal years. This suggests that two copies of genes on the X chromosome are necessary for oocyte maintenance. Mapping of the X chromosome has identified regions of the X chromosome responsible for short stature, ovarian function, and some of the stigmata of Turner's syndrome (see Chapter 6 and Fig. 1). Mapping of the Y chromosome has identified regions involved in spermatogenesis (17). Autosomes also play a role in normal ovarian differentiation.

At 5 to 6 weeks of gestation, the undifferentiated gonad is bipotential and is capable of differentiating into either a testis or an ovary. At this time, under the influence of the chromosomal sex, the gonadal sex is established. The first sign of gonadal differentiation occurs in the male with the appearance of Sertoli cells at 6 to 7 weeks (18); Leydig cells appear at about 8 weeks. In the female at this stage, the only sign of ovarian differentiation is the absence of Sertoli and Leydig cells. The ovarian cortex does not begin to develop until 12 weeks, and primordial follicles appear at $13^1/_2$ weeks (18). In contrast to the male, in whom testicular cords form in the absence of germ cells, the ovary does not develop if germ cells are not present.

The gonadal sex determines the third component of sex determination: the phenotypic sex. Testosterone and antimüllerian hormone (AMH), secreted from the Leydig cells and the Sertoli cells of the testes, respectively, induce differentiation of the genital primordia into the male phenotype (Fig. 2). In the absence of a functioning testis, whether or not an ovary is present, the genital primordia will differentiate into the female phenotype. However, although the presence of a functioning testis is necessary, it is not sufficient for the development of a male phenotype. Normal androgen metabolism is also required, including normal androgen receptors and 5α-reductase activity.

The internal genitalia are derived from the müllerian ducts in the female and the wolffian ducts in the male. The first phenotypic sign of differentiation of the male internal genitalia is the regression of müllerian ducts at 8 weeks of gestation, mediated by AMH (19). This hormone, a high-molecular-weight glycoprotein secreted from the Sertoli cells, prevents the differentiation of the müllerian duct structures (the fallopian tubes, uterus, and upper vagina); the müllerian duct structures are almost completely absent by 10 weeks. Testosterone secreted from the Leydig cells is responsible for the differentiation of the wolffian ducts (the vas deferens, seminal vesicles, and epididymis). High concentrations of antimüllerian hormone and testosterone are required locally around the müllerian and wolffian ducts, respectively, and androgen receptors must be functional for dif-

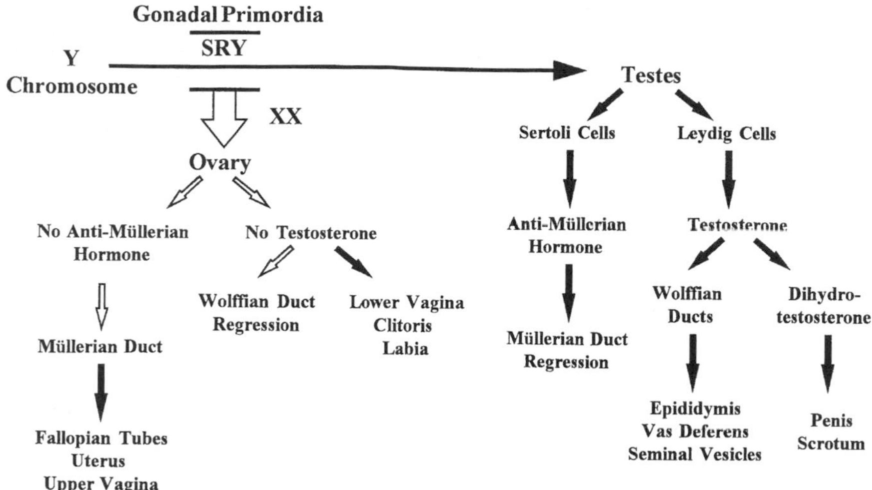

FIG. 2. Male and female gonadal differentiation. Gonadal primordia, under the influence of the sex-determining region (SRY), become a testis; the presence of antimüllerian hormone (AMH) and testosterone causes the regression of müllerian ducts and the formation of male internal and external genitalia. In the absence of SRY, an ovary differentiates, and in the absence of AMH and testosterone, female internal and external genitalia are formed.

ferentiation of the male internal genitalia to occur. In the female, or in the absence of testicular tissue secreting AMH and testosterone locally, müllerian duct differentiation and wolffian duct regression occur. This explains why female pseudohermaphrodites, who do not have testes, develop female internal genital structures.

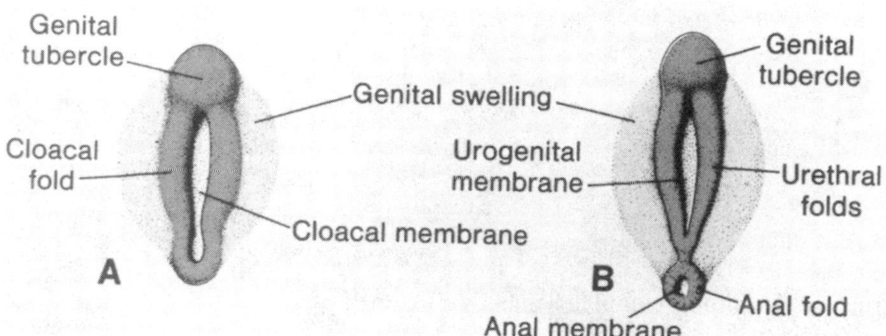

FIG. 3. The indifferent stage of the external genitalia. **(A)** At approximately 4 weeks. **(B)** At approximately 6 weeks. (From Sadler TW. *Langman's medical embryology*, 6th ed. Baltimore: Williams & Wilkins, 1990; with permission.)

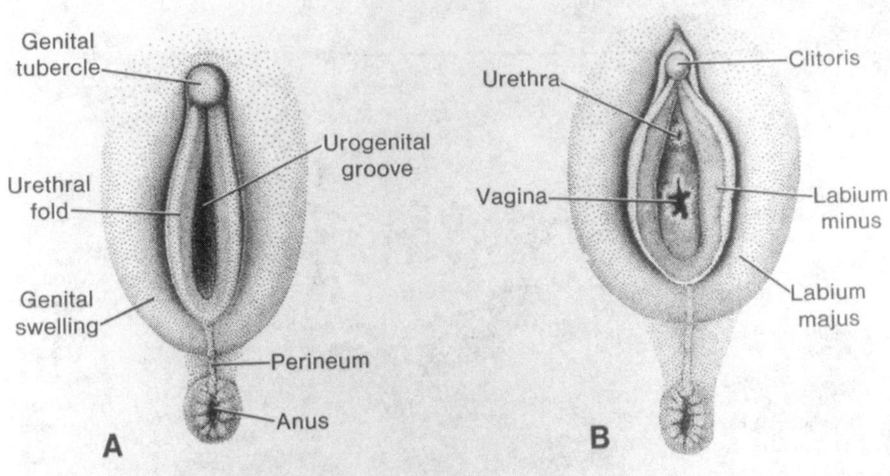

FIG. 4. Development of the external genitalia in the female **(A)** at 5 months and **(B)** in the newborn. (From Sadler TW. *Langman's medical embryology*, 6th ed. Baltimore: Williams & Wilkins, 1990; with permission.)

External genital development occurs between the 8th and 12th weeks of gestation, and in the male does not require high local concentrations of testosterone. Normal differentiation of the male external genitalia requires the conversion of testosterone to dihydrotestosterone (DHT) by 5α-reductase in the target organs, and requires functional androgen receptors. In the male, under the influence of DHT, the urogenital sinus gives rise to the prostate, the genital tubercle forms the glans penis, the labiourethral folds form the urethra and ventral shaft of the penis, and the labioscrotal folds fuse to form the scrotum. In the female, or in the absence of testicular tissue secreting bioactive testosterone, functioning androgen receptors, or 5α-reductase, the genital tubercle forms the clitoris, the labiourethral folds form the labia minora, and the labioscrotal folds form the labia majora. An outline of normal development is shown in Figs. 3 and 4 and in Chapter 8.

Thus, from this brief review of embryogenesis, it is clear that defects in any one of many steps along the pathway of sexual differentiation can result in ambiguous genitalia.

ASSESSMENT OF THE NEONATE

The initial evaluation of the newborn with ambiguous genitalia includes a careful history, physical examination, karyotype determination, serum hormone analyses, and radiographic studies (Fig. 5). The direction of further studies, including the performance of a human chorionic gonadotropin (hCG) stimula-

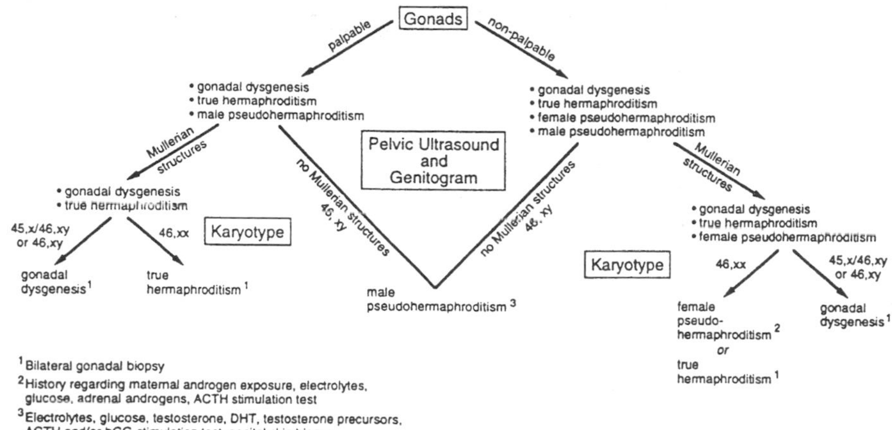

FIG. 5. An approach to the evaluation of ambiguous genitalia in the newborn. ACTH, adrenocorticotropic hormone; DHT, dihydrotestosterone; hCG, human chorionic gonadotropin. (From Meyers-Seifer CH, Charest NJ. Diagnosis and management of patients with ambiguous genitalia. *Semin Perinatol* 1992;16:322–339; with permission.)

tion test, more extensive hormone analyses, DNA studies in a search for SRY, laparoscopy, or gonadal biopsy, depends on the results of the initial evaluation. Tables 1, 2, and 4 provide summaries of clinical information regarding gonadal abnormalities and androgen abnormality/insensitivity syndromes.

History

A careful history should be obtained from the parents, particular attention being given to the following points:

TABLE 1. *The androgen abnormality/insensitivity syndromes*

Syndrome	5α-reductase	Complete	Incomplete	Reifenstein	Infertile
Inheritance	Autosomal recessive	X-linked recessive	X-linked recessive	X-linked recessive	X-linked recessive
Spermatogenesis	Decreased	Absent	Absent	Absent	Decreased
Müllerian	Absent	Absent	Absent	Absent	Absent
Wolffian	Male	Absent	Male	Male	Male
External	Female	Female	Female clitoromegaly	Male hypospadias	Male
Breasts	Male	Female	Female	Gynecomastia	Gynecomastia

(Adapted from Griffin JE. Androgen resistance—the clinical and molecular spectrum. *N Engl J Med* 1992;326:611–618; and Kim HH, Laufer MR. Developmental abnormalities of the female reproductive tract. *Curr Opin Obstet Gynecol* 1994;6:518–525; with permission.)

TABLE 2. *A clarification of the terminology for gonadal abnormalities*

Event	Time of event (days after fertilization)	Nomenclature	Müllerian duct	Wolffian duct	External genitalia
Early embryonic testicular regression	<43	Pure gonadal dysgenesis	Present	Absent	Female
Late embryonic testicular regression	43–59	Swyer's syndrome	Present	Absent	Female
Early fetal testicular regression	60–69	Agonadism	Present	Absent	Ambiguous
	70–75	Testicular dysgenesis	Present	Present	Ambiguous
	75–84	Testicular regression	Absent	Present	Ambiguous
Midfetal testicular regression	90–120	Rudimentary testis	Absent	Present	Male infantile
Late fetal testicular regression	>140	Vanishing testis, anorchia	Absent	Present	Male infantile

(Adapted from Speroff L, Glass RH, Kase NG. Normal and abnormal sexual development. In: Mitchell C, ed. *Clinical gynecologic endocrinology and infertility*, 5th ed. Baltimore: Williams & Wilkins, 1994; and Kim HH, Laufer MR. Developmental abnormalities of the female reproductive tract. *Curr Opin Obstet Gynecol* 1994;6:518–525; with permission.)

1. Family history (see Tables 1 and 3 for a summary of the inheritance of disorders leading to ambiguous genitalia) (21,23–25).
   a. Other family members, especially siblings, with congenital adrenal hyperplasia (CAH).
   b. A history of early neonatal death. The diagnosis of CAH may be missed in males, since there are often no physical signs at birth except, occasionally, increased scrotal rugae, pigmentation, or a large phallus. Thus, a brother may have died in early infancy of vomiting and dehydration, not recognized as secondary to adrenal insufficiency.

TABLE 3. *Patterns of inheritance: ambiguous genitalia*

Disorder	Heredity
Female pseudohermaphroditism	
Congenital adrenal hyperplasia	Autosomal recessive
Male pseudohermaphroditism	
Testosterone biosynthetic defects	Autosomal recessive
Leydig cell hypoplasia	Autosomal recessive
5α-reductase deficiency	Autosomal recessive
Androgen insensitivity syndrome	X-linked recessive
Gonadal disorders	
Gonadal dysgenesis	Sporadic and familial
True hermaphroditism	Sporadic and rarely familial

TABLE 4. *Differential diagnosis of ambiguous genitalia in the newborn*

Female pseudohermaphroditism
Congenital adrenal hyperplasia
21-hydroxylase deficiency
11β-hydroxylase deficiency
3β-hydroxysteroid dehydrogenase deficiency
Exogenous androgens
Drugs
Maternal congonital adrenal hyperplasia or a virilizing tumor
Idiopathic
Male pseudohermaphroditism
Leydig cell hypoplasis or agenesis
Defects in testosterone biosynthesis
20,22-desmolase (congenital lipoid adrenal hyperplasia)
3β-hydroxysteroid dehydrogenase
17α-hydroxylase
17,20-lyase (17,20-desmolase)
17β-hydroxysteroid dehydrogenase (17-ketosteroid reductase)
End-organ resistance to androgens (androgen insensitivity syndrome)
Defects in the intracellular metabolism of testosterone (5α-reductase deficiency)
Persistent müllerian duct syndrome
Maternal ingestion of progestogens or estrogens
Disorders of gonadal differentiation
True hermaphroditism
Pure gonadal dysgenesis
Mixed gonadal dysgenesis

   c. Consanguinity, which makes an autosomal recessive disorder, such as CAH or 5α-reductase deficiency, more likely.
   d. Aunts or other relatives with amenorrhea and infertility, which suggest male pseudohermaphroditism.
2. Maternal history.
   a. Maternal ingestion of drugs during pregnancy (particularly androgens or progestational agents).
   b. Maternal history of virilization or CAH.

Physical Examination

The physical examination of the infant starts with a general examination and a search for the stigmata of a malformation syndrome (e.g., intrauterine growth retardation, dysmorphic features, abnormal body proportions). If a malformation syndrome is identified, further hormonal evaluation may not be necessary, for example, if the suspected diagnosis is trisomy 13. Other signs to look for on the general examination include hypertension, areolar hyperpigmentation, and signs of dehydration, all suggestive of CAH.

The genitalia should be carefully examined. The number of gonads and the size, symmetry, and position are crucial. A palpable gonad below the inguinal canal is almost always a testis, and if present, generally rules out the diagnosis of female pseudohermaphroditism. An undescended gonad could be a testis, ovary, or ovotestis. Asymmetric labioscrotal folds with a unilateral gonad make mixed gonadal dysgenesis or true hermaphroditism more likely. The infant should be examined for the presence of a hernia, as it may contain a uterus, ovary, or testis. Precise measurements of the phallus should be made, including the stretch penile length (along the dorsum of the stretched phallus from the pubic ramus to the tip of the glans) and the midshaft diameter. The mean stretched penile lengths in normal males are as follows (± 1 standard deviation):

2.5 (± 0. 4) cm for a 30-week newborn
3.0 (± 0. 4) cm for a 34-week newborn
3.5 (± 0. 4) cm for a full-term newborn
3.9 (± 0. 8) cm for a 0- to 5-month-old
4.3 (± 0. 8) cm for a 6- to 12-month-old

A good rule of thumb in evaluating the full-term newborn is that the normal male penis should be >2.5 cm (2.5 standard deviations below the mean).

The thickness and degree of development of the corpora should be assessed. If a clitoris is present, the length and breath should be measured. The location of the urethral opening should be noted. In first-degree hypospadias, the urethra opens on the glans of the phallus, in second degree on the shaft, and in third degree on the perineum. Hypospadias is usually accompanied by chordee, a tethering of the phallus due to incomplete closure of the tissue layers that constitute the covering over the urethra. Any child with hypospadias or a small phallus, bilateral cryptorchism, and a neonatal hernia should be evaluated for the possibility of an intersex disorder. It should be determined whether or not a vaginal opening or urogenital sinus is present. The labioscrotal folds should be examined for hyperpigmentation, the presence of gonads, and the degree of labial fusion. Labioscrotal folds range in phenotype (from the least to most virilized) from normal labia majora, to labia majora with posterior fusion, to a bifid scrotum, to a fully fused scrotum. Fusion of the labioscrotal folds is an androgen effect and can be assessed by measuring the anogenital ratio: the distance from the anus to the fourchette (AF) divided by the distance from the anus to the base of the clitoris (AC) (i.e., AF/AC). An anogenital ratio greater than 0.5 falls outside the 95% confidence limits (25) and represents fusion of the labioscrotal folds. A rectal examination should always be performed, since if a uterus is present, it is often easily palpable at birth because of uterine stimulation in utero by placental and maternal estrogens.

Laboratory and Radiographic Tests

The most important tests in the initial evaluation include the determination of the blood karyotype, 17-hydroxyprogesterone (17-OHP), dehydroepiandrosterone (DHEA), luteinizing hormone (LH), follicle-stimulating hormone (FSH), testosterone, and dihydrotestosterone (DHT), and performing radiographic studies. The results of the blood karyotype determination are usually available in 2 to 3 days if the laboratory is alerted and processes the blood expediently. Buccal smears should not be performed, as they are inaccurate. In primary gonadal defects, and possibly in androgen-resistant states, LH and FSH are elevated. To define the internal structures, an ultrasound examination and either a retrograde genitogram (retrograde injection of contrast material via the urogenital orifice) or a voiding cystourethrogram are performed. A contrast study will delineate the anatomy of the urethra and vagina (if present), the urogenital sinus, and at times, the cervix. The location of the gonads and the presence of a uterus and endometrial stripe can be determined by ultrasound examination. Once it has been determined whether the infant is a male or female hermaphrodite, or has a disorder of gonadal differentiation, other studies are usually indicated.

The most common cause of ambiguous genitalia is female pseudohermaphroditism with CAH, and the majority of patients with this condition have 21-hydroxylase deficiency resulting in a markedly elevated 17-OHP level. If gonads are not palpable, 17-OHP and DHEA determinations should be obtained after 24 hours of life. In the normal infant, 17-OHP is elevated in cord blood but decreases to 100 to 200 ng/dl after 24 hours of life; this decrease may take longer in premature infants. The early-morning 17-OHP is generally greater than 1000 ng/dl in infants with 21-hydroxylase deficiency. If the 17-OHP is not diagnostic, and CAH is suspected, a repeat level should be obtained a few days later, and fluid and electrolyte balance monitored daily. In infants with 21-hydroxylase deficiency, androstenedione and DHEA are elevated, serum cortisol may be very low or at the lower end of the normal range, and adrenocorticotropic hormone (ACTH) is elevated. Given the frequency of the CAH gene in the population (varying from 1:300 in Alaskan Eskimos to an average of 1:14,500 worldwide), screening of newborns for 21-hydroxylase deficiency has been implemented in some states by measurement of 17-OHP in the neonatal blood filter specimens (26). If the patient is a female pseudohermaphrodite but the etiology is unclear, other steroid precursor levels are measured after ACTH (Cortrosyn) stimulation and may delineate a specific adrenal enzyme defect.

In the male pseudohermaphrodite, testosterone is low in any defect in testosterone production. The testosterone/DHT ratio is elevated in 5α-reductase deficiency. AMH correlates with the degree of müllerian duct development and is a reliable marker for the presence of functional testicular tissue (27–29,30). AMH is nondetectable in normal females, detectable in normal males, and detectable but low in true hermaphrodites and patients with other disorders of testicular dysgenesis (31). In patients with androgen insensitivity syndrome (AIS) and those with defects in testosterone production (32), AMH is elevated. In the persistent müllerian duct syndrome, AMH is nondetectable in patients with defects in AMH and detectable in patients with end-organ resistance to AMH.

An hCG stimulation test is useful for determining the defect in the male pseudohermaphrodite. Several protocols for intramuscular hCG administration are available, including 3000 U/m^2/dose once a day for 3 to 5 days (33), 2000 U/m^2 a day for 3 days (34), and 5000 U/m^2 for 1 day (35,36). Testosterone and DHT are measured 24 hours after hCG; they increase in the normal male, and a sample of serum should be saved for further hormone analyses. In patients with 5α-reductase deficiency, the basal testosterone/DHT ratio may be normal, but elevated after hCG stimulation. Failure of testosterone and DHT to rise after hCG stimulation suggests either a defect in testosterone biosynthesis or Leydig cell hypoplasia, and steroid hormone precursors should be measured in the serum saved from the test. Fibroblasts from a scrotal skin biopsy can be assayed for 5α-reductase activity if 5α-reductase deficiency is suspected, or for androgen receptor binding capacity if AIS is suspected. If the patient has a primary gonadal abnormality, a skin biopsy or scrotal skin biopsy may be indicated to rule out mosaicism on a karyotype analysis. A gonadal biopsy may be indicated to determine whether ovarian or testicular tissue is present, or to confirm Leydig cell hypoplasia.

Several genetic studies are now available that may aid in the evaluation of ambiguous genitalia in the infant. A DNA probe for SRY will demonstrate whether SRY is present in the 46,XX male, and it is useful in determining whether Y material is present in a 45,X individual, placing the patient at risk for gonadoblastoma (see section on gonadal abnormalities below, and Chapter 6). Mutations have been identified in the 21-hydroxylase gene in CAH, the 5α-reductase 2 gene in patients with 5α-reductase deficiency, the androgen receptor gene in AIS when prenatal diagnosis has been performed, and the AMH gene in persistent müllerian duct syndrome.

DIFFERENTIAL DIAGNOSIS OF AMBIGUOUS GENITALIA IN THE NEWBORN

The differential diagnosis of the newborn with ambiguous genitalia can be divided into four broad categories:

1. Female pseudohermaphroditism
2. Male pseudohermaphroditism
3. Disorders of gonadal differentiation
4. Malformation syndromes

The female pseudohermaphrodite has a 46,XX karyotype, ovaries, no wolffian duct structures, well-developed müllerian duct structures, and virilized external genitalia. The male pseudohermaphrodite has a 46,XY karyotype; wolffian duct structures that are normal, hypoplastic, or absent; no müllerian duct structures; and undervirilized external genitalia. Patients with disorders of gonadal differentiation have either both ovarian and testicular tissue (true hermaphrodite) or one dysgenetic testis, one streak gonad, and no ovarian tissue (mixed gonadal dysgenesis [MGD]) (see Table 4 for the differential diagnosis of the infant with ambiguous genitalia).

FEMALE PSEUDOHERMAPHRODITISM

Congenital Adrenal Hyperplasia

Congenital adrenal hyperplasia is the most common cause of ambiguous genitalia in the 46,XX newborn. It is caused by a deficiency in one of the adrenal cortical enzymes involved in the synthesis of cortisol (Fig. 6) and is inherited in an autosomal recessive manner. The results are inadequate cortisol synthesis, inadequate negative feedback to the hypothalamus and pituitary, and increased ACTH secretion. High levels of ACTH stimulate adrenal gland hyperplasia, and the block in adrenal cortisol production results in shunting of the adrenal steroid precursors toward adrenal androgen production. The enzyme blocked and the degree of block vary, and ambiguity may range from labial fusion, with or without slight clitoromegaly, to a male-type phallus with labial fusion and rugae on the labioscrotal folds (Fig. 7).

More than 95% of CAH is due to 21-hydroxylase deficiency in the adrenal cortex (37). Classic 21-hydroxylase deficiency occurs in the newborn period, and salt losing is seen in about three-quarters of patients. In salt-losing CAH, the enzyme deficiency is more severe, and aldosterone secretion from the adrenal glomerulosa is decreased as well. Decreased aldosterone secrction decreases renal electrolyte exchange, resulting in hyponatremia, hyperkalemia, and metabolic acidosis. The extent of virilization is not a reliable indicator of the degree of adrenal insufficiency. Thus, the electrolyte status of all infants with 21-hydroxylase deficiency should be monitored.

Congenital adrenal hyperplasia can also be due to 11β-hydroxylase deficiency. Levels of 11-deoxycortisol and 11-deoxycorticosterone levels are high, and these moderately salt-retaining compounds result in salt retention, volume expansion, and hypertension. A rare form of CAH, 3β-hydroxysteroid dehydrogenase deficiency, results in severe adrenal insufficiency and increased ACTH. Pregnenolone, 17-hydroxypregnenolone, and DHEA are increased. Virilization is quite mild, since the block occurs in the initial steps of hormone synthesis so that only the weak androgen DHEA can be produced in excess. Aldosterone deficiency can lead to salt wasting. Testosterone biosynthesis is decreased; therefore, 3β-hydroxysteroid dehydrogenase deficiency is also a cause of male pseudohermaphroditism.

Glucocorticoid treatment should be instituted as soon as possible in the female pseudohermaphrodite once the laboratory studies have been obtained. Hydrocortisone, 2.5 mg two or three times daily (10 to 20 $mg/m^2/day$), is the usual initial treatment. Since salt losing does not occur until day 6 to day 14 of

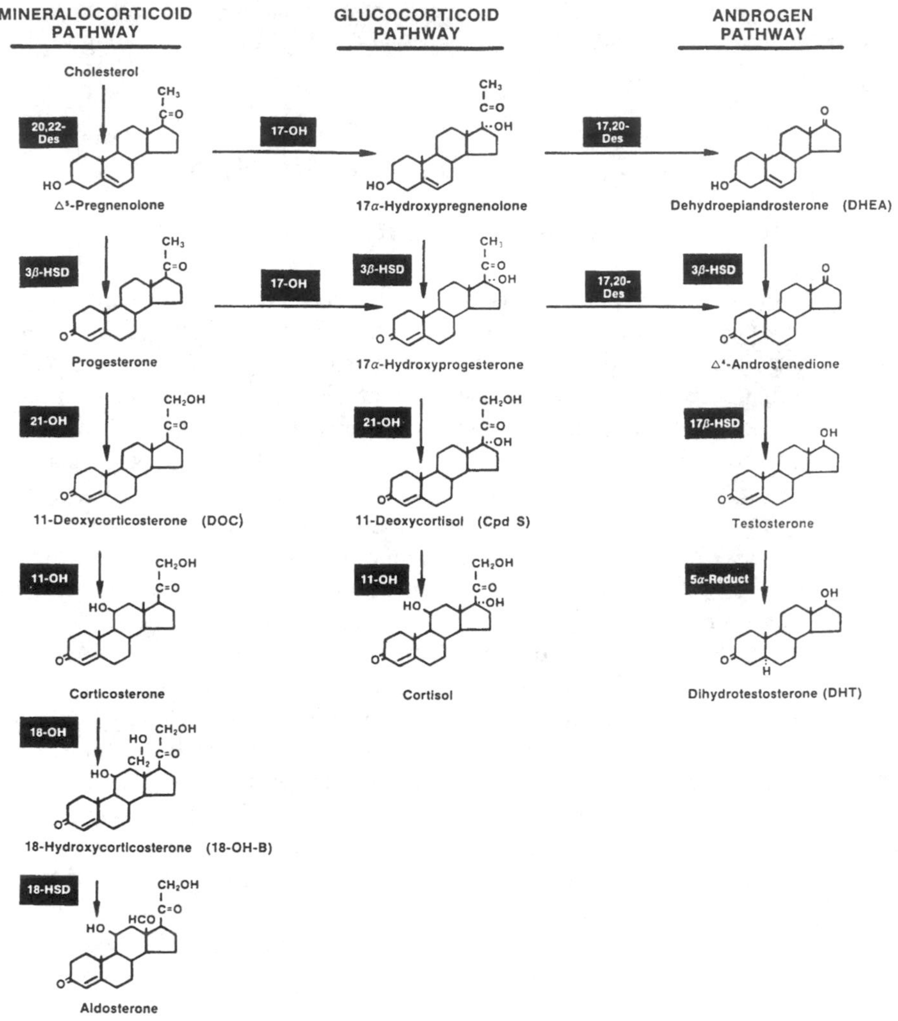

FIG. 6. Pathways of steroid biosynthesis. (Courtesy of Endocrine Sciences, 18418 Oxnard Street, Tarzana, CA 91356; with permission.)

life, the baby's weight, electrolytes, fluid status, and plasma renin activity (PRA) should be closely monitored. Salt losing is demonstrated by decreased serum sodium, increased serum potassium, decreased aldosterone, and elevated PRA; the elevated PRA is the most sensitive indicator of aldosterone deficiency. If salt losing is documented, salt (2 to 4 g/day) should be added to the formula, and a mineralocorticoid, fludrocortisone acetate (Florinef) 0.05 to 0.1 mg daily should be given. In some children, the PRA is elevated in the absence of low aldosterone levels and salt wasting. In these children, the addition of flu-

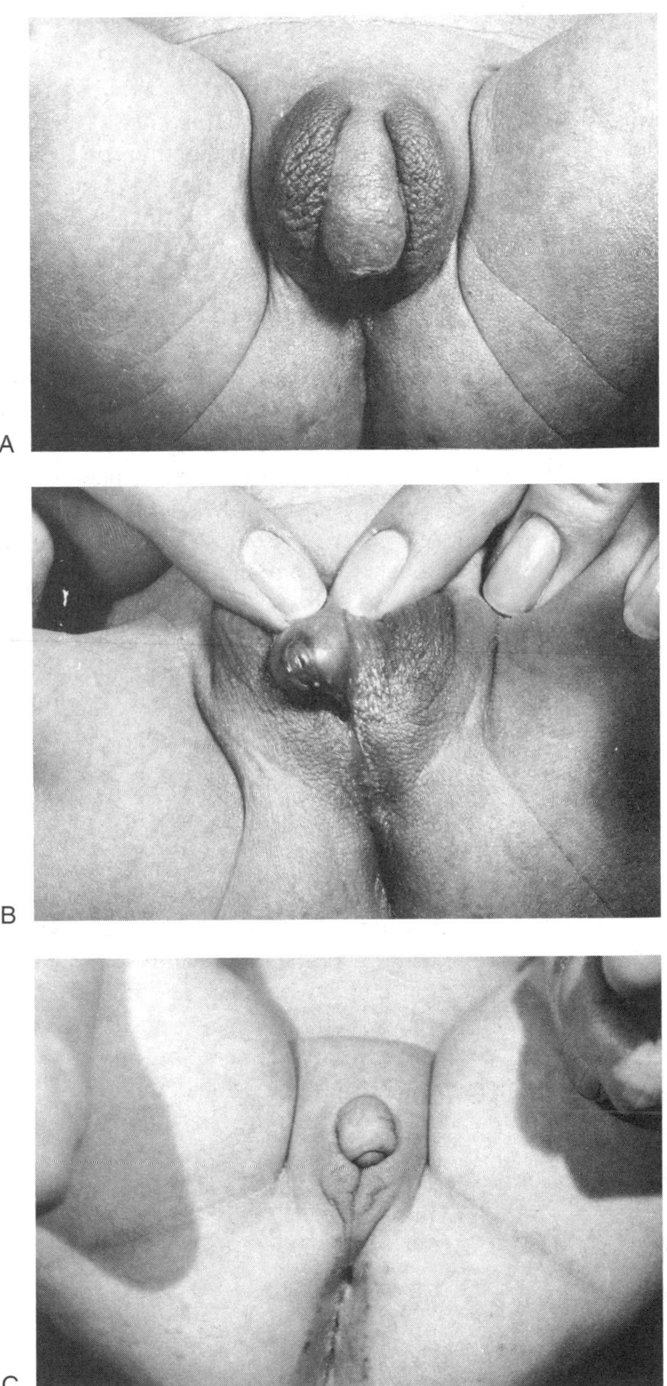

FIG. 7. Two newborn girls with virilization and salt-losing congenital adrenocortical hyperplasia. **(A)** and **(B)** patient S.C.; **(C)** patient M.T.

drocortisone acetate normalizes the PRA and thus improves hormonal control and growth.

Hydrocortisone dosage is adjusted on the basis of growth parameters (length, weight, skeletal maturation) and adrenal steroid precursor levels, including serum 17-OHP, Δ^4-androstenedione, DHEA, DHEA sulfate (S), and (except in infants and adolescent boys) testosterone. Therapy should be aimed at keeping the 17-hydroxyprogesterone well below 1000 ng/dl; levels <200 ng/dl in the morning usually indicate oversuppression. In patients in good control, Δ^4-androstenedione is normal, and DHEAS is below the normal range. However, DHEAS is not sensitive for detecting overtreatment. Twenty-four-hour urinary 17-ketosteroid determinations can be used to monitor therapy in older children, and should be in the low normal range (for bone age). Overtreatment with glucocorticoids results in growth retardation and delayed skeletal maturation. Undertreatment leads to accelerated skeletal maturation and virilization. The glucocorticoid dosage must be increased at times of stress, such as during illness and in the event of surgery (see Chapter 7 for further discussions of CAH). The adequacy of mineralocorticoid replacement is most accurately determined by measuring the PRA. New approaches using antiandrogens are being investigated (38).

It should be emphasized that female pseudohermaphrodites with CAH are females with ovaries and are potentially fertile. Thus, regardless of the appearance of the external genitalia, the sex assignment should be female. Surgery, which may include clitoroplasty, labioplasty, and vaginoplasty, is discussed in Chapter 8 (23).

Exogenous Androgens

The 46,XX infant with no evidence of CAH may have been exposed to exogenous androgens from maternal ingestion or production. Androgens, danazol, and synthetic progestins (in doses much higher than in oral contraceptive pills) given before the 14th week of gestation can cause labial fusion and clitoromegaly; such therapy after the 14th week causes clitoromegaly only. If the maternal drug history is noncontributory, the mother should undergo a careful physical examination and laboratory testing for hyperandrogenism. In the absence of a maternal history of virilization or hormone ingestion, the internal genital anatomy should be evaluated to determine whether there is a primary gonadal abnormality (see below).

MALE PSEUDOHERMAPHRODITISM

Understanding the steps involved in the development of normal male genitalia facilitates the diagnosis of the specific defect in the male pseudohermaphrodite (Figs. 2 to 5 and Tables 1 and 3). If the testis is unresponsive to hCG and LH because of absence of LH receptors or abnormal Leydig cell development (Leydig cell hypoplasia or agenesis) (39), wolffian duct structures do not differentiate owing to lack of testosterone. Müllerian duct structures regress under the stimulus of AMH, which comes from the Sertoli cells, and testes are present in the abdomen. Testosterone is low, LH is elevated, and testosterone does not rise in response to exogenous hCG. The external genital phenotype is usually female, with a urogenital sinus and a short vaginal pouch. Biopsy of the testicles reveals no distinct Leydig cells, normal Sertoli cells, and spermatogenic arrest in the seminiferous tubules.

Defects in testosterone biosynthesis can be due to deficiencies in one of five enzymes in the pathway toward testosterone synthesis, and all are inherited in an autosomal recessive manner. Also involved in adrenal steroid synthesis are the enzymes 20,22-desmolase (congenital lipoid adrenal hyperplasia), 3β-hydroxysteroid dehydrogenase, and 17α-hydroxylase, and defects in any of these enzymes are associated with CAH (Table 5). The enyzymes 17,20-lyase (17,20-desmolase) and 17β-hydroxysteroid dehydrogenase (17-ketosteroid reductase) (40) are involved only in testosterone biosynthesis. Defects in testosterone production result in absence of wolffian duct structures, regression of müllerian duct structures (AMH is normal), and external genitalia that are either female or ambiguous. Testosterone and DHT are low and do not increase in response to hCG. The specific defect can be determined by measuring steroid hormone precursors after hCG stimulation. Enzyme deficiencies that also lead to CAH can be confirmed by an ACTH (Cortrosyn) stimulation test.

Defects in androgen-dependent target tissues include AIS and 5α-reductase deficiency. In AIS, binding of testosterone and DHT to the androgen receptor is impaired because of a receptor defect (20,39) (see Table 1 for a summary of findings). Complete AIS gives the classic picture of testicular feminization and is not manifested by ambiguous genitalia at birth, although occasionally testes may be noted in a hernia sac early in life. The phenotypic female infant with a hernia should undergo an evaluation to determine what is in the hernia; 7% of females with a hernia have no cervix by palpation or vaginoscopy; they are either male pseudohermaphrodites (usually AIS) or have mixed gonadal dysgenesis. In AIS, the testes function normally, producing AMH (müllerian ducts regress) and testosterone, which is converted into DHT. However, since androgen-dependent target tissues are unresponsive to testosterone and DHT, wolffian duct structures do not develop, and the external genitalia develop along female lines (Table 1). Partial AIS, on the other hand, results in a spectrum of ambiguous genitalia syndromes (41); they include the Gilbert-Dreyfus, Reifenstein, Rosewater, and Lubs syndromes. Patients with partial AIS have some degree of wolffian development and labioscrotal fusion. The androgen receptor has been well characterized, and molecular defects in AIS have been described. The androgen receptor gene is located on the short arm of the X chromosome, and AIS is inherited in an X-linked recessive manner.

5α-Reductase deficiency is an autosomal recessive disorder in which the enzyme that converts testosterone to DHT in androgen-dependent tissues is

TABLE 5. *Defects of adrenal steroidogenesis*[a]

Deficiency	Syndrome	Ambiguous genitalia	Postnatal virilization	Salt metabolism	Steroids increased	Steroids decreased	Enzyme	Chromosome	Frequency[b]
Cholesterol desmolase	Lipoid hyperplasia	Males	No	Salt wasting	None	All	p450scc	15	Rare
3β-OH-steroid dehydrogenase	Classic	Males and ? females	Yes	±Salt wasting	DHEA, 17-OH-pregnenolone	Aldo, cortisol, T	3β-OH-steroid dehydrogenase	?	Rare
	Nonclassic	No	Yes	Normal	DHEA, 17-OH-pregnenolone	—	3β-OH-steroid dehydrogenase	?	? Frequent
17-Hydroxylase	—	Males	No	Hypertension	DOC, corticosterone	Cortisol, T	p450c17	10	Rare
17,20-Lyase	—	Males	No	Normal	—	DHEA, T, androstenedione	p450c17	10	Rare
21-Hydroxylase	Salt wasting	Females	Yes	Salt wasting	17-OHP, androstenedione	Aldo, cortisol	p450c21	6p (HLA)	1/10,000
	Simple virilizing	Females	Yes	Normal	17-OHP, androstenedione	Cortisol	p450c21	6p (HLA)	1/20,000
	Nonclassic	No	Yes	Normal	17-OHP, androstenedione	—	p450c21	6p (HLA)	0.1–1% (3% in European Jews)
11-Hydroxylase	Classic	Females	Yes	Hypertension	DOC, 11-deoxycortisol	Cortisol, ±aldo	p450c11	8q	1/100,000
	Nonclassic	No	Yes	Normal	11-deoxycortisol, ±DOC	—	p450c11	8q	? Frequent
Corticosterone methyl oxidase II	—	No	No	Salt wasting	18-OH-corticosterone	Aldo	p450c11	8q	Rare (except in Iranian Jews)

[a]Deficiency of 17,20-lyase is expressed in the gonads but is included here because it apparently involves the same gene as 17-hydroxylase deficiency. DHEA, dehydroeprandrosterone; DOC, deoxycorticosterone; 17-OHP, 17-hydroxyprogesterone; aldo, aldosterone; T, testosterone.

[b]"Rare" denotes a syndrome accounting for <1% of reported cases of congenital adrenal hyperplasia, which has an overall frequency of about 1 of 5000 births. "? Frequent" syndromes may occur at frequencies similar to that of nonclassic 21-hydroxylase deficiency, but prevalence data are not available.

(From White PC, New MI, Dupont B. Congenital adrenal hyperplasia. *N Engl J Med* 1987;316:1580; with permission.)

defective (42). Since DHT is responsible for the masculinization of the external genitalia, patients with 5α-reductase deficiency have undervirilized external genitalia but develop normal male internal genitalia (wolffian duct structures differentiate, and müllerian duct structures regress). The phenotype is characterized by a bifid scrotum, a clitoris-like phallus, hypospadias, a urogenital sinus that opens onto the perineum, and a blind vaginal pouch. In some families, children with this condition have been initially raised as females but due to masculinition at puberty (the testes descend, the scrotum enlarges, and the phallus lengthens) take on a male gender identity (43).

The persistent müllerian duct syndrome occurs in a 46,XY individual with testes and either defective AMH or end-organ resistance to AMH (44). Such a patient does not often have ambiguous genitalia but may have cryptorchidism or hernia uteri inguinale (presumably due to the mobilization of müllerian derivatives during testicular descent into the inguinal canal or scrotum). Wolffian duct development varies among individuals. Few males are fertile, and there is a high incidence of postnatal testicular degeneration.

As discussed in the section on laboratory and radiographic testing, the evaluation of the 46,XY male with ambiguous genitalia should include an hCG stimulation test. An increased testosterone/DHT ratio is characteristic of 5α-reductase deficiency and can be confirmed by measurement of 5α-reductase activity in cultured genital skin fibroblasts. If the testosterone and DHT are both low, steroid precursors in the testosterone biosynthetic pathway should be measured. If a testosterone biosynthesis defect that also leads to CAH is suspected, an ACTH stimulation test can confirm the diagnosis. If all hormone levels are low, and there is no adrenal insufficiency, Leydig cell hypoplasia is likely and can be verified by testicular biopsy. If hormone levels are normal, the diagnosis of AIS is suggested and can be confirmed by identification of a mutation in the androgen receptor gene or by measurement of androgen receptor binding in scrotal skin.

Sex assignment is based on the patient's potential to achieve unambiguous appearance of the external genitalia and normal sexual function after reconstructive surgery and hormonal therapy. Some patients with a micropenis and testes respond to a 3- to 5-day hCG stimulation test with adequate penile growth, achieving a length of >2.0 cm (45); they should be assigned a male gender. However, sex assignment may need to be delayed until the patient is given a longer course of hCG (3000 U/m^2/dose biweekly for about 5 weeks) (33), or a course of intramuscular testosterone enanthate, propionate, or cypionate 25 to 75 mg/m^2/dose every 3 to 4 weeks for 2 to 3 months (33). If testosterone does not rise after hCG stimulation, testosterone should be used. Three monthly intramuscular injections of testosterone enanthate, 25 to 50 mg, should produce lengthening of the penis by 2.0 ± 0.6 cm (46), and in this case, the patient is assigned a male gender. In patients with 5α-reductase deficiency, topical DHT cream applied to the external genitalia causes phallic growth (47). If the male phallus is so small that the patient cannot possibly function in the male sexual role, or if the response to testosterone is poor, a female identity should be chosen regardless of the genotype. The phallus will not grow at puberty in patients with androgen insensitivity who do not respond to testosterone in the newborn period. If the sex assignment is female, the gonads should be electively removed early once the diagnosis has been made.

DISORDERS OF GONADAL DIFFERENTIATION

The true hermaphrodite has both testicular and ovarian tissue (with follicles) and represents the rarest intersex disorder. The gonads consist of either one ovary and one testis, two ovotestes, or one ovotestis and one ovary or testis. About half of patients have a 46,XX karyotype (48), one-third are chimeric 46,XX/46,XY (two distinct populations of cells with different genetic origins) or mosaic (46,XY/47,XXY or 45,X/46XY), and only a few have a 46,XY karyotype (48). Although a few 46,XX true hermaphrodites have detectable SRY, the etiology in the majority who lack SRY is unclear (49,50). Differentiation of the internal ducts depends on the amount and location of functional testicular tissue; wolffian duct structures differentiate on the side with testicular tissue, and müllerian duct structures on the side with no testicular tissue. A uterus (frequently hypoplastic or abnormal) is present in 90% of patients. Although a few patients have normal female external genitalia or have a penile urethra, the majority have ambiguous genitalia. In the past, most have been reared as males. At puberty, three-quarters of patients develop gynecomastia, and one-half menstruate. Decisions about sex assignment should be based on the internal and external genitalia, and the organs of the opposite sex should be removed. If the patient is to be reared as a male, the phallus must be adequate in size and the testis or testes brought down into the scrotum.

Patients with pure gonadal dysgenesis are phenotypical females, lack the stigmata of Turner's syndrome (see Chapter 6), and do not have ambiguous genitalia at birth (Tables 1 and 2). The karyotype is either 46,XX or 46,XY; individuals with a 46,XY karyotype are sometimes referred to as having complete gonadal dysgenesis (49). Individuals with pure gonadal dysgenesis have dysgenetic (streak) gonads consisting of ovarian stroma, fibrous tissue, and no primordial follicles. Pure gonadal dysgenesis is usually diagnosed during adolescence when a girl presents with primary amenorrhea and is found to have elevated gonadotropins. In the past, pure gonadal dysgenesis has been referred to as Swyer's syndrome. Although a few 46,XY females have a mutation in the SRY, in most patients the SRY is intact (51) and the etiology is unknown.

MGD is characterized by one normal or dysgenetic testis and one streak ovary. All patients have a Y chromosome, and the karyotype is usually 45,X/46,XY mosaic but can be 46,XY (sometimes referred to as partial gonadal dysgenesis) (49). The phenotype reflects the level of functioning of the fetal dysgenetic testis. The internal genitalia are usually asymmetric, with müllerian duct differentiation on the side with the streak ovary and variable wolffian duct differentiation on the side with the testis. Approximately one-half of patients with MGD are born with ambiguous external genitalia, which may be asymmetric with an enlarged labioscrotal fold on the side with the testis. The dysgenetic testis is not capable of completely virilizing the external genitalia, but it is capable of producing androgen levels sufficient to virilize an apparent female at puberty (52). Most patients have been raised as females.

The choice of gender in gonadal disorders depends on the external genitalia and the possibility for future coital adequacy. Once the sex assignment has been made, the gonads that conflict with the assignment are electively removed. Any patient with a dysgenetic gonad and a Y-bearing cell line is at high risk for developing a gonadal tumor (48). Even if a Y chromosome is not visible cytogenetically, DNA probes for SRY may detect Y material. Gonadoblastomas occur in 20% to 30% of 46,XY patients with pure gonadal dysgenesis and one-third of patients with MGD, and they may develop into malignant tumors (dysgerminomas or seminomas) in about one-third of patients (47) (see Chapter 15 for a further discussion of ovarian masses). True hermaphrodites are also at risk for developing gonadoblastomas, although the risk is lower. All patients with a dysgenetic gonad and a Y-bearing cell line should have the intraabdominal dysgenetic gonads removed in infancy. Dysgenetic testes may be left in place *only* in the child with bilateral descended dysgenetic testes given a male sex assignment; in this case, the risk of malignancy is less, and the testes should be routinely examined (48).

MALFORMATION SYNDROMES

Chromosomal abnormalities that can be associated with ambiguous genitalia include trisomy 13 and 18, triploidy, and 4p- syndrome (53). Monogenic disorders can be associated with ambiguous genitalia, including Smith-Lemli-Opitz and Camptomelic dysplasia (53,54). Associations of defects, such as the CHARGE association (**C**oloboma, **H**eart defect, **A**tresia choanae, **R**etarded growth and development with or without central nervous system anomalies, **G**enital anomalies with or without hypogonadism, and **E**ar anomalies with or without deafness) can include ambiguous genitalia (52) (see Table 6 for a summary of malformation syndromes associated with genital ambiguity). Finally, genital abnormalities can be associated with other anomalies, especially those of the urinary tract (see Chapter 8).

HYPOSPADIAS AND CRYPTORCHIDISM

The incidence of hypospadias in newborn males ranges from 1 in 300 to 1 in 800. Familial clustering has been reported, and hypospadias is present in a sec-

TABLE 6. *Conditions associated with genital ambiguity*

Chromosomal
Trisomy 13
Trisomy 18
Triploidy
4p-, 13q-
Aniridia-Wilms
Single gene
Ellis van Creveld
Smith-Lemli-Opitz
Opitz
Opitz-Frias
Rieger
Robinow
Carpenter
Meckel-Gruber
Camptomelic dysplasia
Androgen insensitivity
Congenital adrenal hyperplasia
Associations
CHARGE
Vater

ond individual in 21% of families (55). Variable modes of inheritance suggest that familial hypospadias represents a heterogeneous group of disorders. Some patients with hypospadias have defects in the androgen receptor gene (39); usually, these patients have perineoscrotal hypospadias, with or without cryptorchidism, although penoscrotal hypospadias associated with decreased androgen receptor binding has been described (56). The majority of patients with hypospadias have normal androgen receptors. Severe forms of hypospadias, especially if accompanied by unilateral or bilateral cryptorchidism, defects in scrotal fusion, or a cervix palpable by rectal examination, necessitate a complete evaluation.

Cryptorchidism occurs in 2.7% of full-term newborn males and in 21% of premature infants. The incidence decreases to 0.8% by 1 year of age, and descent is unlikely after that time. Malignancy is 12 to 40 times more common in undescended testes than in scrotal testes (31,41). These two facts have led to the recommendation that evaluation for cryptorchidism occur by 9 to 12 months of age (58,59). It should be noted that both the cryptorchid testis and the contralateral testis have an increased risk of cancer even with surgery. Cryptorchidism can occur in Kallmann's syndrome, hormonal deficiencies, dysgenetic or "vanishing" testes, persistent müllerian duct syndrome (43), and >40 congenital syndromes (57). Thus, disorders of sexual differentiation need to be considered in the infant with cryptorchidism.

If one testis is absent but the genitalia are otherwise completely normal, a rectal examination should be performed to rule out the remote possibility that there is a cervix or large utricle. If a midline structure is not palpated, ultrasonography of the pelvis will rule out the presence of müllerian duct structures. If this is normal, no further evaluation is indicated. If both testes are missing, but the genitalia appear to be that of a normal male, karyotype determination and hormone analysis should be performed to rule out female pseudohermaphroditism. If the karyotype is 46,XY and the genitals adequate for male function, the infant should be raised as a male. An hCG stimulation test should be performed to determine whether or not functional testes are present; a lack of rise in testosterone indicates primary testicular failure or an agonadal state. Some of these patients may have congenital anorchia, in which the testes presumably functioned at least until the 16th week of gestation and then disappeared. In these patients, serum LH and FSH are elevated, and testosterone and AMH are low (29). Testosterone therapy at puberty is necessary for the development of secondary sexual characteristics. Testicular implants may be helpful as well. Other patients may have bilateral undescended testes that are capable of function. A 4- to 6-week course of hCG or gonadotropin-releasing hormone can be given to induce descent of the testes. However, this therapy remains controversial; success rates are low with truly cryptorchid testes in contrast to retractile testes, which usually descend with hormonal stimulation (59). Laparoscopy is useful in locating intraabdominal testes or cord structures entering the inguinal canal, which suggests a descended but probably atrophic organ (60). If the testes do not descend by 9 to 12 months of age, the testes should undergo orchidopexy, either open or using laparoscopic techniques. There seems to be an inverse correlation between the age of surgery and the degree of fertility; the younger the patient is at surgery, the higher the rate of fertility (33).

REFERENCES

1. Rock JA, Katz E. Ambiguous genitalia. *Semin Reprod Endocrinol* 1987;5:327.
2. Sinclair AH, Berta P, Palmer MS, et al. A gene from the human sex-determining region encodes a protein with homology to a conserved DNA-binding motif. *Nature* 1990;346:240.
3. Berta P, Hawkins JR, Sinclair AH, et al. Genetic evidence equating SRY and the testis-determining factor. *Nature* 1990;348:448.
4. Fechner PY, Marcantonio SM, Jaswaney V, et al. The role of the sex-determining region Y gene in the etiology of 46,XX maleness. *J Clin Endocrinol Metab* 1993;76:690.
5. Poulat F, Soullier S, Goze C, et al. Description and functional implications of a novel mutation in the sex-determining gene SRY. *Hum Mutat* 1994;3:200.
6. Harley VR, Jackson DI, Hextall PJ, et al. DNA binding activity of recombinant SRY from normal males and XY females. *Science* 1992;255:453.
7. Dubin RA, Ostrer H. Sry is a transcriptional activator. *Mol Endocrinol* 1994;8:1182.
8. Kuhnle U, Schwarz HP, Lohrs U, et al. Familial true hermaphroditism: paternal and maternal transmission of true hermaphroditism (46,XX) and XX maleness in the absence of Y-chromosomal sequences. *Hum Genet* 1993;92:571.
9. McElreavey K, Vilain E, Abbas N, et al. A regulatory cascade hypothesis for mammalian sex determination: SRY represses a negative regulator of male development. *Proc Natl Acad Sci USA* 1993; 90:3368.
10. Tsutsumi O, Iida T, Taketani Y, et al. Intact sex determining region Y (SRY) in a patient with XY pure gonadal dysgenesis and a twin brother. *Endocr J* 1994;41:281.

11. Bennett CP, Docherty Z, Robb SA, et al. Deletion 9p and sex reversal. *J Med Genet* 1993;30:518.
12. Arn P, Chen H, Tuck-Muller CM, et al. SRVX, a sex reversing locus in Xp21. 2-p22. 11. *Hum Genet* 1994;93:389.
13. Wagner T, Wirth J, Meyer J, et al. Autosomal sex reversal and campomelic dysplasia are caused by mutations in and around the SRY-related gene SOX9. *Cell* 1994;79:1111.
14. Foster JW, Dominguez-Steglich MA, Guioli S, et al. Campomelic dysplasia and autosomal sex reversal caused by mutations in an SRY-related gene. *Nature* 1994;372:525.
15. Haber DA, Buckler AJ. WT1: a novel tumor suppressor gene inactivated in Wilms tumor. *New Biol* 1991;4:97.
16. Van Heyningen V, Hastie ND. Wilms' tumor: reconciling genetics and biology. *Trends Genet* 1992; 8:16.
17. Moore CCD, Grumbach MM. Sex determination and gonadogenesis: a transcription cascade of sex chromosome and autosome genes. *Semin Perinatol* 1992;16:266.
18. Voutilaninen R. Differentiation of the fetal gonad. *Horm Res* 1992;38(suppl 2):66.
19. Josso N. Hormonal regulation of sexual differentiation. *Semin Perinatol* 1992;16:279.
20. Brown TR. Male pseudohermaphroditism: defect in androgen-dependent target tissues. *Semin Reprod Endocrinol* 1987;5:243.
21. Griffin JE. Androgen resistance—the clinical and molecular spectrum. *N Engl J Med* 1992;326:611.
22. Speroff L, Glass RH, Kase NG. Normal and abnormal sexual development. In: Mitchell C, ed. *Clinical gynecologic endocrinology and infertility*, 5th ed. Baltimore: Williams & Wilkins, 1994.
23. Kim HH, Laufer MR. Developmental abnormalities of the female reproductive tract. *Curr Opin Obstet Gynecol* 1994;6:518.
24. Meyers-Seifer CH, Charest NJ. Diagnosis and management of patients with ambiguous genitalia. *Semin Perinatol* 1992;16:322.
25. Callegari C, Everett S, Ross M, et al. Anogenital ratio: measure of fetal virilization in premature and full-term newborn infants. *J Pediatr* 1987;111:240.
26. Thompson R, Seargeant L, Winter JS. Screening for congenital adrenal hyperplasia: distribution of 17 α-hydroxyprogesterone concentrations in neonatal blood spot specimens. *J Pediatr* 1989;114:400.
27. Gustafson ML, Lee MM, Asmundson L, et al. Müllerian inhibiting substance in the diagnosis and management of intersex and gonadal abnormalities. *J Pediatr Surg* 1993;28:439.
28. Josso N, Lamarre I, Picard JY, et al. Anti-müllerian hormone in early human development. *Early Hum Dev* 1993;33:91.
29. Josso N. Anti-müllerian hormone and Sertoli cell function. *Horm Res* 1992;38(suppl 2):72.
30. Lee MM, Donahoe PK, Silverman BL, et al. Measurement of serum müllerian inhibiting substance in the evaluation of children with nonpalpable gonads. *N Engl J Med* 1997;336:1480.
31. Carrol WA. Malignancy in cryptorchidism. *J Urol* 1949;61:396.
32. Rey R, Mebarki F, Forest MG, et al. Anti-müllerian hormone in children with androgen insensitivity. *J Clin Endocrinol Metab* 1994;79:960.
33. Lanes RL. Ambiguous genitalia, micropenis, and cryptorchidism. In: Lifshitz F, ed. *Pediatric Endocrinology,* 3rd ed. New York: Marcel Dekker, 1995:353.
34. Almaguer MC, Saenger P, Linder BL. Phallic growth after hCG. A clinical index of androgen responsiveness. *Clin Pediatr* 1993;32:329.
35. Hughes IA, Williams DM, Batch JA, Patterson MN. Male pseudohermaphroditism: clinical management, diagnosis and treatment. *Horm Res* 1992;38(suppl 2):77.
36. Dunkel L, Huhtaniemi I. Testicular responsiveness to hCG during infancy measured by salivary testosterone. *Acta Endocrinol* 1990;123:633.
37. New MI. Female pseudohermaphroditism. *Semin Perinatol* 1992;16:299.
38. Merke DP, Cutler GB. New approaches to the treatment of congenital adrenal hyperplasia. *JAMA* 1997;277:1073.
39. Kupfer SR, Quigley CA, French FS. Male pseudohermaphroditism. *Semin Perinatol* 1992;16:319.
40. Givens JR, Wiser WL, Summitt RL, et al. Pseudohermaphroditism and deficient testicular 17-ketosteroid reductase. *N Engl J Med* 1974;291:938.
41. Imperato-McGinley J, Gautier T, Pichardo M, et al. The diagnosis of a 5α-reductase deficiency in infancy. *J Clin Endocrinol Metab* 1986;63:1313.
42. Imperato-McGinley J, Peterson RE, Gautier T, et al. Androgen and the evolution of male-gender identity among male pseudohermaphrodites with 5α-reductase deficiency. *N Engl J Med* 1979;300:1233.
43. Josso N, Picard JY, Imbeaud S, et al. The persistent müllerian duct syndrome: a rare cause of cryptorchidism. *Eur J Pediatr* 1993;152(suppl 2):S76.

44. Donahoe PK, Ito Y, Morikawa Y, et al. Müllerian inhibiting substance in human testes after birth. *J Pediatr Surg* 1977;12:323.
45. Almaguer MC, Saenger P, Linder BL. Phallic growth after HCG. A clinical index of androgen responsiveness. *Clin Pediatr* 1993;32:329.
46. Villee D, Najjar S. Endocrinology. In: Avery ME, First L, eds. *Pediatric medicine*, 2nd ed. Baltimore: Williams & Wilkins, 1994;978.
47. Odame I, Donaldson MD, Wallace AM, et al. Early diagnosis and management of 5 alpha-reductase deficiency. *Arch Dis Child* 1992;67:720.
48. Savage MO, Lowe DG. Gonadal neoplasia and abnormal sexual differentiation. *Clin Endocrinol* 1990;32:519.
49. Berkovitz GD. Abnormalities of gonadal determination and differentiation. *Semin Perinatol* 1992; 16:289.
50. Berkovitz GD, Fechner PY, Marcantonio SM, et al. The role of the sex-determining regin of the Y chromosome (SRY) in the etiology of 46,XX true hermaphroditism. *Hum Genet* 1992;88:411.
51. Mittoch U. Sex determination and sex reversal: genotype, phenotype, dogma and semantics. *Hum Genet* 1992;89:467.
52. Gantt PA, Byrd JR, Greenblatt RB. A clinical and cytogenetic study of fifteen patients with 45X/46XY gonadal dysgenesis. *Fertil Steril* 1980;34:216.
53. McGillivray BC. The newborn with ambiguous genitalia. *Semin Perinatol* 1992;16:365.
54. Aarskog D. Syndromes and genital dysmorphology. *Horm Res* 1992;38(suppl 2):82.
55. Bauer SB, Retik AB, Colodny AH. Genetic aspects of hypospadias. *Urol Clin North Am* 1991;8:565.
56. Evans BA, Williams DM, Hughes IA. Normal postnatal androgen production and action in isolated micropenis and isolated hypospadias. *Arch Dis Child* 1991;66:1033.
57. Murphy AA, Zacur HA. Unclassified forms of abnormal sexual development. *Semin Reprod Endocrinol* 1987;5:295.
58. Colodny AH. Undescended testes: is surgery necessary? [editorial] *N Engl J Med* 1986;314:510.
59. Rajfer J, Handelsman DJ, Swerdloff RS, et al. Hormonal therapy of cryptorchidism: a randomized, double-blind study comparing human chorionic gonadotropin and gonadotropin-releasing hormone. *N Engl J Med* 1986;314:466.
60. Moore RG, Peters CA, Bauer SB, et al. Laparoscopic evaluation of the nonpalpable testis: a prospective assessment of accuracy. *J Urol* 1994;151:728.

3

Vulvovaginal Problems in the Prepubertal Child

VULVOVAGINITIS

Vulvovaginitis is a common gynecologic problem in prepubertal girls. Vulvar inflammation—vulvitis—may occur alone or may be accompanied by a vaginal inflammation—vaginitis. A child may acquire a primary vaginal infection, and the discharge may cause maceration of the vulva and secondary vulvitis. The prepubertal child is particularly susceptible to vulvar and vaginal infections because of the physiology of the genital tract. In the newborn period, the vagina is well estrogenized from maternal hormones. For several months to several years beyond the newborn period, the infant has fluctuating gonadotropin levels, which can result in stimulation of the ovaries to produce low levels of estrogen. The estrogen influences the hymenal configuration and the vaginal flora. As the hormone levels wane, the hymen becomes thin and the vagina atrophic. The vaginal pH is 6.5 to 7.5.

In order to interpret the results of vaginal cultures taken from girls with vaginitis, the clinician needs to be knowledgeable about the data published on normal flora of the prepubertal vagina (1–5). The early study of Hammerschlag and colleagues (1) included a wide range of ages of pubertal and prepubertal girls from an urban hospital clinic. Paradise et al (2,5) cultured specimens from 52 premenarcheal girls without genitourinary signs or symptoms (Table 1); 11 of 40 had *Bacteroides* species (*B. bivius, B. fragilis, B. melaninogenicus*) (2). *Bacteroides* species were as commonly found in control subjects as in those with vulvovaginitis. Gardner (3) studied a group of 77 girls, 3 to 10 years of age, having general anesthesia for minor surgical procedures. She defined normal flora as lactobacilli, *Staphylococcus epidermidis*, enteric organisms (*Streptococcus faecalis*, *Klebsiella* species, *Proteus* species, *Pseudomonas* species), and viridans species of streptococci other than *Streptococcus milleri*. Additional isolates from the control group included *Escherichia coli* (2), *Streptococcus pneumoniae* (3), *Staphylococcus aureus* (2), *S. milleri* (1), and

TABLE 1. *Aerobic bacteria and yeasts recovered from vaginal cultures of 52 girls without genitourinary symptoms or signs*

Microorganisms isolated	No. (%)
Normal flora[a]	52 (100)
β-Hemolytic streptococci (not group A or B)	2 (4)
Escherichia coli	4 (8)
Group B streptococcus	1 (2)
Coagulase-positive staphylococcus	1 (2)
Candida tropicalis or "yeast"[b]	2 (4)

[a]Includes diphtheroids, α-hemolytic streptococci, and lactobacilli.
[b]If fewer than one-third of the colonies in a culture are yeasts, the laboratory did not identify their species.
(Source: J. Paradise. Unpublished data; with permission.)

Gardnerella vaginalis (1); no isolates of *Haemophilus influenzae*, *Streptococcus pyogenes*, or mycoplasmas were identified. However, since 43% of girls among the 108 controls in all age groups were undergoing ear, nose, and throat procedures and 14% had received antibiotics during the previous month, it is unclear whether the underlying diagnosis or antibiotic therapy given to some girls more than a month previously (percent not specified) may have influenced the flora of the vagina. Another study of vaginal flora in prepubertal girls (mean age 9 years, range 3 months to 16 years) found that the most common aerobic organisms were *S. epidermidis*, enterococcci, *E. coli*, lactobacilli, and *Streptococcus viridans*. The anaerobes included *Peptococcus* species, *Peptostreptococcus* species, *Veillonella parvula*, *Eubacterium* species, *Propionibacterium* species, and *Bacteroides* species (4). Other organisms found in asymptomatic girls included *Proteus mirabilis* (3.2%), *Pseudomonas* species (6.5%), and *Candida albicans* (3.2%).

Etiology

The prepubertal child is susceptible to both nonspecific and specific vaginal infections and a variety of vulvar skin abnormalities (dermatoses) (Table 2). Contributing factors are poor hygiene, the proximity of the vagina to the anus, the lack of protective hair and labial fat pads, and the lack of estrogenization. The vulvar skin is susceptible to irritation and is easily traumatized by chemicals, soaps, medications, and clothing.

Nonspecific vulvovaginitis accounts for 25% to 75% of diagnoses of vulvovaginitis of prepubertal girls seen in referral centers (2,6–10). The pathogenesis and associated alteration in vaginal flora have not been well defined, but the absolute number of colonies of fecal aerobes or an overpopulation with anaerobes may contribute to the symptoms of odor and discharge. Gertner (4) found *Candida*, *Peptococcus*, *Peptostreptococcus*, and *Bacteroides* species more commonly in girls with vaginal discharge and/or vulvovaginitis than in asymptomatic girls. The vaginal culture from girls with vaginitis typically grows normal

TABLE 2. *Etiology of vulvovaginal symptoms in the prepubertal child*

"Nonspecific" vulvovaginitis
Specific vulvovaginitis
  Respiratory pathogens
    Streptococcus pyogenes (Group A β-streptococcus)
    Staphylococcus aureus
    Haemophilus influenzae
    Streptococcus pneumoniae
    Branhamella catarrhalis
    Neisseria meningitidis
  Enteric
    Shigella
    Yersinia
    Other flora
  Candida
  Sexually transmitted diseases
    Neisseria gonorrhoeae
    Chlamydia trachomatis
    Herpes simplex
    Trichomonas
    Condyloma accuminata (human papillomavirus)
Pinworms, other helminths
Foreign body
Polyps, tumors
Systemic illness: measles, chickenpox, scarlet fever, Stevens-Johnson syndrome, mononucleosis, Kawasaki's disease, histiocytosis, Crohn's disease
Vulvar skin disease: lichen sclerosus, seborrhea, psoriasis, atopic dermatitis, scabies, contact dermatitis (nickel allergy), zinc deficiency, bullous pemphigoid
Trauma
Psychosomatic vaginal complaints
Miscellaneous: draining pelvic abscess, prolapsed urethra, ectopic ureter, disposable diapers

flora (lactobacilli, diphtheroids, *S. epidermidis,* or α-streptococci) or gram-negative enteric organisms (usually *E. coli*). The significance of *E. coli* and other enteric organisms is unclear. Gertner and colleagues (4) found that 23% of asymptomatic girls had *E. coli* in the vagina, compared with 36% of girls with vaginitis. Hammerschlag and coworkers (1) reported that 90% of girls under 3 years of age had vaginal colonization with *E. coli* but that in 3- to 10-year-old asymptomatic girls, the *E. coli* colonization rate was only 15%. In our clinic, we found that 47% of 3- to 10-year-old girls with nonspecific vaginitis had *E. coli* on culture (6), which suggests that poor hygiene and contamination with bowel flora may play an important role in the persistence of symptoms.

Nonabsorbent nylon underpants, nylon tights, nylon bathing suits, close-fitting blue jeans, and ballet leotards may result in maceration and infection, particularly in hot weather. Little girls who are overweight are more likely to experience these symptoms. The vulvar irritation of the child with vaginitis may appear similar to the diaper dermatitis seen in infants who wear infrequently changed cloth diapers or plastic-covered paper diapers. Bubble baths and harsh soaps may cause vulvitis and a secondary vaginitis. It is possible (although to our knowledge, studies have not been done) that either a high hymenal opening that does not allow normal vaginal drainage or a gaping hymenal opening that allows easy contamination of the vagina can predispose a girl to nonspecific vaginitis. In addition, girls typically urinate on the toilet with their knees together, increasing the possibility that urine will reflux into the vagina. Pinworms appear to be a major contributor to nonspecific infections in some populations. In a British study, 32% of girls with vulvovaginitis who were tested for pinworms had these helminths detected (10). Children susceptible to recurrent vulvovaginitis may also have other factors that promote adherence of bacteria to epithelial cells.

The specific infections that occur in the prepubertal child are often respiratory, enteric, or sexually transmitted pathogens. The respiratory pathogens include *S. pyogenes* (group A β-hemolytic streptococci), *H. influenzae*, *S. aureus*, *Branhamella catarrhalis*, *S. pneumoniae,* and rarely *Neisseria meningitidis* (2,6,10–18). Vaginal *S. pyogenes* infections may occur as a result of direct inoculation from nasopharygeal infections, fecal carriage, or skin infections. Although throat cultures from approximately 75% of girls with *S. pyogenes* vaginitis are positive, only 25% have respiratory symptoms (15). Scarlet fever can also be associated with streptococcal vaginitis. In England, a winter peak of *S. pyogenes* isolates from both the throat and the vagina has been reported. Overall, *S. pyogenes* is isolated from 7% to 20% of girls with vulvovaginitis (10,16). The vulva and perianal areas often have a distinctive bright red appearance.

In most series, *H. influenzae* has not been found to be part of normal flora (18). In the Pierce and Hart study (10), this organism was the most commonly isolated organism among girls with vulvovaginitis and was found in three high vaginal swabs obtained from patients under anesthesia. *S. aureus* can also cause a vaginal infection and can be associated with impetiginous lesions on the vulva and the buttocks.

Shigella infection can result in a mucopurulent, sometimes bloody discharge; in up to one-fourth of cases, the discharge occurs in association with an episode of diarrhea (19). Between 70% and 90% of *Shigella* vaginitis is caused by *S. flexneri*, and prolonged treatment is sometimes necessary (20,21). *Yersinia entercolitica* has also been reported to be associated with vaginitis (22); whether *Campylobacter* species and other enteric pathogens play a role is not known.

Although *Candida* vulvovaginitis is common in pubertal girls, it is uncommon in prepubertal children unless the girl has recently finished a course of antibiotics, has diabetes mellitus, is immunosuppressed, is still in diapers, or has other risk factors. *Candida* appears to be present in the normal flora of 3% to 4% of girls.

Sexually acquired vulvovaginal infections occurring in the prepubertal child include *Neisseria gonorrhoeae*, *Chlamydia trachomatis*, *Trichomonas,* herpes simplex, and human papillomavirus (condyloma acuminata) (these infections are also discussed in Chapters 12, 13, and 20) (23–36). Gonococcal infection in the prepubertal child usually causes a green purulent vaginal discharge; occasionally the discharge is mucoid. Confirmatory tests are crucial in prepubertal girls whose vaginal culture appears to be positive for *N. gonorrhoeae* (see Chapter 12). Most cases of gonococcal vaginal infections in prepubertal girls are identified by culturing samples from girls with vaginal discharge, not from asymptomatic victims of sexual abuse (32). Overall, 2.8% of 1538 children evaluated for sexual abuse were found to have gonococcal infections (35) (see Chapter 20). Siblings of individuals with known gonococcal infections are also at risk of infection and should be cultured. The perpetrator is often a family member who is identified only by culturing samples taken from the entire family. Clusters of several children with gonorrhea have been identified (34). All children with *N. gonorrhoeae* vaginitis should be reported to local authorities that deal with child abuse so that adequate evaluation can be carried out (23–28,35).

The presence of *C. trachomatis* in the vagina of prepubertal girls is associated with a history of sexual abuse, but the finding in infants can occur because of perinatal maternal–infant transmission (26,29,30,37–42). Schachter and associates (37) found that 14% of infants born to *Chlamydia*-positive mothers had vaginal/rectal colonization; none of these infants still had positive cultures at 12 months of age. Bell and colleagues (38) reported that among 120 infants born vaginally to infected women, 22% had positive cultures from the conjunctiva and 25% from the pharynx in the first month of life. Initial positive rectal and vaginal cultures were seen only during the third and fourth month of life. All initial vaginal cultures were associated with positive rectal cultures. In a study of 22 infants in Seattle, positive rectal and vaginal cultures were not seen beyond 383 and 372 days, respectively, but positive cultures from the nasopharynx, oropharynx, and conjunctiva persisted up to 866 days (40). Persistence of ocular infection has also been reported for 3 to 6 years (33); persistence of genital infections for more than 12 to 24 months (rarely 36 months) is unlikely. Because the majority of girls will have been treated with antibiotics to which *Chlamydia* is sensitive by the age of 2 or 3 years (e.g., erythromycin, trimethoprim/sulfamethazole), the issue of persistence often becomes much less likely and the need to identify the source of the sexual transmission greater. Bell (41) has suggested that serologic testing, if available, could provide additional information, since the presence of IgM antibody against the serovar of either the suspect's serovar or the child's own or a fourfold rise in IgG titer could provide presumptive evidence of recent contact.

Despite all the data collected on maternal–infant transmission, it is important to remember that most cases of *Chlamydia* infections in prepubertal girls beyond the age of 2 years are sexually acquired. Ingram and associates (29) reported that 10 of 124 sexually abused girls and 0 of 90 control subjects had a positive introital culture for *C. trachomatis*. A subsequent study of a larger population reported that 1.2% of 1538 children evaluated for possible sexual abuse had *Chlamydia* infections (35). *C. trachomatis* can occur as a coexisting infection in girls with *N. gonorrhoeae* (43).

How frequently *C. trachomatis* is responsible for signs of vaginitis is a subject of controversy. In a study of 622 girls under 12 years of age who were evaluated for sexual abuse or who had a sexually transmitted disease, six girls had *Chlamydia* without gonorrhea and only one had a discharge on examination (although four gave a history of discharge) (31). Ingram et al (35) found that only 6 of 17 girls with positive *Chlamydia* cultures had a vaginal discharge at presentation or a history of vaginal discharge in the previous 6 months. Culture tests should be used in the diagnosis of prepubertal infections, since false-positive results can occur with some nonculture tests, especially if the nonculture kits are used for rectal samples. Common bowel organisms such as *E. coli*, *Proteus* species, *G. vaginalis*, and even *S. pyogenes* have resulted in positive reactions with enzyme immunoassay tests (26,44). Using a vaginal wash technique in 138 prepubertal girls being evaluated for sexual abuse, Embree and colleagues (45) tested samples both by culture and by polymerase chain reaction (PCR) for *Chlamydia.* Two children had positive tests on both PCR and culture and two by PCR alone. Further studies with these techniques are needed.

Herpes simplex type 1 (oral-labial herpes) can cause lesions in the mouth and vulva of young girls with the vulvar infection occurring through self-inoculation. Both types 1 and 2 can be acquired by sexual abuse, although type 2 is more likely to be secondary to abuse. In a study of six cases of genital herpes (five type 1 and one type 2), Kaplan and colleagues (46) reported that infection resulted from sexual abuse in four of six patients. Recurrent lesions may occur with either type of herpes but are more likely with type 2. Varicella-zoster infections in the genital area have been confused with herpes simplex (47). Condyloma acuminata (venereal warts) are caused by human papillomavirus, usually type 6 or type 11 (see Chapter 13).

Trichomonas vaginalis can be transmitted from the mother to the child at birth and rarely can cause urethritis and vaginitis, which usually resolves spontaneously with the waning of estrogen levels. Occasionally, persistent symptoms require treatment (36). This pathogen is rarely seen in the prepubertal child because the unestrogenized vagina is relatively resistant to infection. It occurs primarily in the pubescent sexually active teenager (see Chapter 11). Although *Trichomonas* can theoretically be spread by wet towels and washcloths, it is primarily a sexually transmitted infection.

The role of *G. vaginalis* in causing vaginitis in the child has been controversial (3,48–50). Bartley and coworkers (48) found that the isolation of *G. vaginalis* from the vaginas of prepubertal girls appeared to be more likely in sexually abused girls (14.6%) than in control subjects (4.2%) or in patients with genitourinary complaints (4.2%). However, they did not find any association of this organism with vaginal erythema or discharge. In a study of 238 girls 1.5 to 16.1 years old (including pubertal patients), Steele and de San Lazaro (49) isolated *G. vaginalis* from 19% of girls who had disclosed sexual abuse, 3% of those in whom sexual abuse was suspected, and 3% of girls with vulvovaginitis. By contrast, Ingram and associates (50) found *G. vaginalis* in the vaginal cultures of 5.3% of 191 sexually abused girls, 4.9% of 144 girls evaluated for possible sexual abuse and found to have no such history or infection with gonorrhea or *Chlamydia*, and 6.4% of girls (daughters of friends of the authors) without such a history or infection with gonorrhea or *Chlamydia*. The diagnosis of bacterial vaginosis should not be confused with the isolated finding of *G. vaginalis* on vaginal culture. Bacterial vaginosis is characterized by an alteration of the bacterial flora with the presence of increased concentrations of *G. vaginalis* and anaerobes, and in adolescents is characterized by a high vaginal pH and clue cells (see Chapter 11). Bacterial vaginosis has been reported to occur in girls who presented with vaginal odor after an episode of rape; the diagnosis was made by the observation of clue cells on microscopic examination of the discharge and the presence of a characteristic amine (fishy) odor on the "whiff" test (1 drop of discharge is mixed with 1 drop of 10% potassium hydroxide [KOH] on a slide).

Other causes of vulvovaginal complaints include vaginal foreign bodies; vaginal and cervical polyps and tumors; cavernous lymphangioma; urethral prolapse; systemic illnesses such as measles, chickenpox (47,51), scarlet fever, mononucleosis, Crohn's disease, Kawasaki's disease (52), or histiocytosis; anomalies such as double vagina with a fistula, pelvic abscess or fistula, or ectopic ureter; and vulvar skin diseases such as seborrhea, psoriasis, atopic dermatitis, lichen sclerosus, scabies, contact dermatitis, or autoimmune bullous diseases (7,53). Zinc deficiency from insufficient intake (54), urinary loss, or malabsorption (acrodermatitis enteropathica) can result in vulvar dermatitis. Seborrheic dermatitis is associated with seborrhea in other parts of the body; fissures within the folds of the labia can lead to bleeding. Both psoriasis and seborrheic dermatitis can become secondarily infected. Atopic dermatitis usually occurs in other parts of the body as well as the vulva; vulvar lesions are pruritic, dry, papular, scaly patches (53). Bullous pemphigoid occasionally occurs in young children; two girls with symmetric ulcers responded to fluocinonide 0.05% cream (55). Vesicular lesions in the perineum secondary to nickel allergy from an enuresis alarm has also been reported (56). Histiocytosis can present with firm, yellow, and often purpuric papules in the vulvar area and also has been associated with a persistent 2 × 2-cm labial ulcer (57). Epstein-Barr virus infection has been associated with labial ulcers in children (58); we have identified a small number of early pubescent girls with vulvar ulcers who were found on further evaluation to have mononucleosis. Lymphedema of the clitoral hood and labia may occur from hypoproteinemia resulting from renal failure or gastrointestinal disease. Crohn's disease may present with painful asymmetric swelling of the labia, perineal induration (59), and ulcers. Gelatin-like beads from superabsorbent disposable diapers can simulate vaginal discharge (60,61).

An ectopic ureter may cause daytime wetness, sometimes in quite minimal amounts (Fig. 1); occasionally ectopic ureters can present in late childhood or adolescence with purulent discharge and without enuresis (62). If the kidney is infected, purulent perineal discharge will result, and the initial diagnosis may be vaginal discharge. The ectopic ureter usually empties on the perineum adjacent to the normal urethra, but it may also open into the vagina, cervix, uterus, or ure-

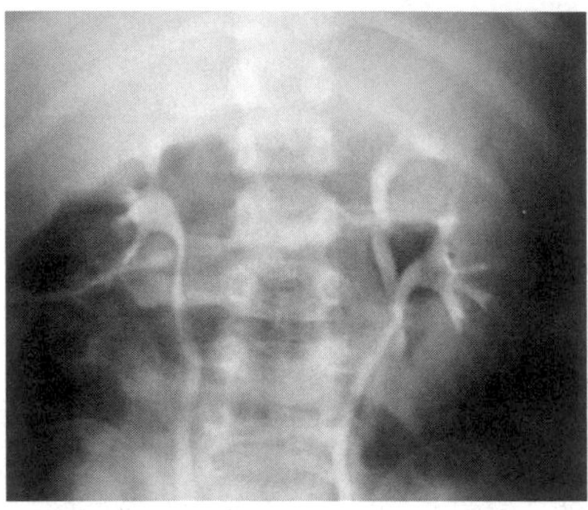

FIG. 1. Double collecting system of the left kidney in a 4-year-old girl with an ectopic ureter and a history of persistent vulvovaginitis.

thra. The clinician should look for a small drop of urine (or pus) adjacent to the urethra after the child drinks a large amount of a beverage, especially one containing caffeine. Ultrasonography of the kidneys will suggest the anomaly in most cases with obstruction and a purulent discharge. An intravenous pyelogram (IVP) is particularly helpful as an initial test if daytime "dampness" or dribbling (not purulent discharge) is the presenting complaint. Even if the double collecting system cannot be visualized because of poor function in the upper pole, the contour of the kidney is likely to provide the key to diagnosis.

Occasionally, children have vaginal or vulvar complaints of itching, tingling, or tickling, sometimes associated with posturing, scissoring, and masturbation. The behavioral changes can precipitate great concern in parents. Psychosomatic complaints may also occur in the absence of any definable signs of vulvovaginal change.

True vulvovaginitis should not be confused with physiologic leukorrhea. Newborns and pubescent girls often have copious secretions from the effect of estrogen on the vaginal mucosa. In newborns, since maternal estrogen is primarily responsible for the discharge, the leukorrhea typically disappears within a few weeks after birth.

Obtaining the History

In most cases of vulvovaginitis, the parent brings the child to the clinician with a complaint of discharge, dysuria, pruritus, or redness. A complete history is obtained before the examination; a questionnaire may speed the process so that the child does not become fidgety or nervous before the examination. The clinician should elicit information on the quantity, duration, odor, and type of discharge; perineal hygiene; recent use of medications or bubble baths; symptoms of anal pruritus (associated with pinworm infection); enuresis; history of atopic dermatitis or allergies; and recent infections in the patient or family. A history of recent infections is important because, for example, group A β-hemolytic streptococcal (*S. pyogenes*) vaginitis, perianal cellulitis, or, rarely, proctocolitis may follow a streptococcal upper respiratory or skin infection in the child or other family members. Overvigorous cleansing of the vulva in a girl with mild vaginal symptoms or odor can lead to significant vulvitis. Questions about caretakers that may give a clue to ongoing sexual abuse should be asked. The parent should be asked about behavioral changes, nightmares, fears, abdominal pain, headaches, and enuresis, all of which may suggest the possibility of abuse or other stressors. The vaginal discharge may be copious and purulent, or it may be thin and mucoid.

The child should be included in the history taking by being asked what she has noticed and about bathing, use of soaps, tights, and perineal hygiene. She can be asked to demonstrate her motion of wiping and whether she has ever placed anything within her vagina. A child's scratching because of vulvar pruritus may cause conflict between parent and child. Compulsive masturbation may also cause vulvar irritation and erythema and guilty feelings for the child and parents. A cycle of itching and scratching may have started with a vaginal infection and then persisted with resultant chronic vulvitis. The child should be asked about the possibility that someone has touched her in the vaginal area.

The history may give a clue to the diagnosis. For example, a foul-smelling discharge may result from a foreign body (usually toilet paper), a necrotic tumor (rare), or vaginitis. Both *Shigella* and group A β-streptococcal infections can cause bleeding. An odorless, bloody discharge may result from vulvar irritation (from scratching or masturbation), trauma (from playground equipment, bicycle, or sexual abuse), precocious puberty, a foreign body, vaginitis, condyloma acuminata, or, rarely, a tumor (adenocarcinoma, sarcoma botryoides) (20,63). A greenish discharge is usually associated with a specific cause of the vaginitis, such as *N. gonorrhoeae,* group A β-streptococci, *H. influenzae*, *S. aureus*, *Shigella*, or a foreign body. Itching and redness are usually nonspecific signs of irritation. In our experience (6), a short duration of symptoms (<1 month) is associated more often with specific diagnoses, perhaps because the parent notices an abrupt change in the vulvovaginal area. Girls with nonspecific vaginitis often have symptoms that have lasted for months or, in some cases, for years before clinical presentation. Nonetheless, even a long history of symptoms calls for a careful examination.

Physical Examination

For children with symptoms of vulvitis, a brief history and external genital examination in the office and instructions to the parent on improved hygiene, avoidance of irritants, and/or treatment of pinworms is all that is needed. A similar approach is appropriate for many little girls with vulvitis and minimal vaginal discharge. The only findings on external examination are usually a scanty mucoid discharge and an erythematous introitus. The cause is usually poor perineal hygiene, which results in infection with mixed bacterial flora. Cultures are unnecessary if the condition responds promptly to improved hygiene.

Any child with persistent, purulent, or recurrent vaginal discharge deserves a thorough gynecologic assessment. The physical examination of the prepubertal child is described in Chapter 1. To diagnose the vaginal complaints, the physician should undertake a stepwise approach: (a) do a general physical examination; (b) inspect the perineum, vulva, and vaginal introitus with the patient supine; (c) visualize the vagina and cervix with the patient in the knee-chest position; (d) obtain specimens for wet preparations, Gram stain (optional), and cultures; and (e) if indicated, do a rectoabdominal examination with the patient supine, knees apart, and feet together or in stirrups. Providing a mirror for the child, asking her to assist in the examination, or encouraging the parent to engage in conversation with the child can help her relax. A colorful poster on the ceiling or wall is a good distraction. A visible discharge at the time of the examination increases the likelihood that the vaginal culture will be positive for a specific pathogen (2). If the knee-chest position does not allow adequate visualization *and* the symptoms are significant or persistent, visualization can be accomplished in the cooperative child by use of a veterinary otoscope, hysteroscope, cystoscope, or flexible endoscope with the patient supine. Anesthetic ointment can be applied to the vulva prior to insertion, after cultures have been obtained. An examination with the child under general anesthesia, using a Killian nasal speculum or flexible endoscope, is often necessary for complete assessment of the young child with persistent discharge and inadequate office evaluation. It should be remembered that although visualization of the vagina and cervix is optimal and usually easily performed, this part of the examination can be deferred if mild symptoms of vulvovaginitis improve in 2 to 3 weeks of good perineal hygiene. The rectal examination is important for girls with persistent discharge, bleeding, or pelvic/abdominal pain. The rectal examination can help to express a discharge from the vagina not previously seen, can allow palpation of hard foreign bodies, and can detect abnormal masses.

Laboratory Tests

If the discharge is persistent or purulent at the initial office visit, cultures and, if possible, wet preparations should be done. A nasopharyngeal Calgiswab moistened with nonbacteriostatic saline, a soft plastic eyedropper, a glass eyedropper with plastic tubing attached, a small feeding tube, or a small urethral catheter attached to a syringe can be gently inserted through the hymenal opening to aspirate secretions or a vaginal wash sample (see Chapter 1). If a small saline-moistened Calgiswab is used, care should be taken to place it into the vagina without touching the edges of the hymen. The child will be amazed that no discomfort is felt, and the three samples (one with a Dacron male urethral swab if a sample for vaginal *Chlamydia* culture is desired) can be quickly obtained and directly plated or sent for culture. If no discharge is apparent, one or two drops of saline can be squeezed into the vagina with an eyedropper and then aspirated.

The sample of vaginal secretions is mixed first with one drop of saline on a glass slide and then with one drop of 10% KOH on another slide. A coverslip is applied, and the slides are examined under the microscope for *Candida* and trichomonads. A culture for *N. gonorrhoeae* is done on modified Thayer-Martin-Jembec medium at the time of the examination. Cultures for other organisms are done by sending the small Calgiswab, a moistened cotton-tipped applicator (used only if easily inserted without discomfort), or a small amount of aspirated secretions to the bacteriology laboratory for plating on genitourinary media (blood, MacConkey, and chocolate media). The swab can be kept moist in a Culturette II transport tube during transport to the laboratory. Samples for *Chlamydia* culture are generally obtained from girls with persistent symptoms and those with a history of sexual abuse. Samples for Biggy agar culture can be obtained from girls with itching or suspected yeast infections; this culture is incubated in the office and observed for the growth of brown colonies 3 to 7 days later. Patients with vulvar or anal pruritus can be screened for pinworm infestation. Material is obtained in the morning by pressing the sticky side of a piece of cellophane tape against the perineal area. The tape is affixed to a slide and examined under the microscope for the characteristic eggs (Fig. 2). The parent should also check the child's anus late at night (with

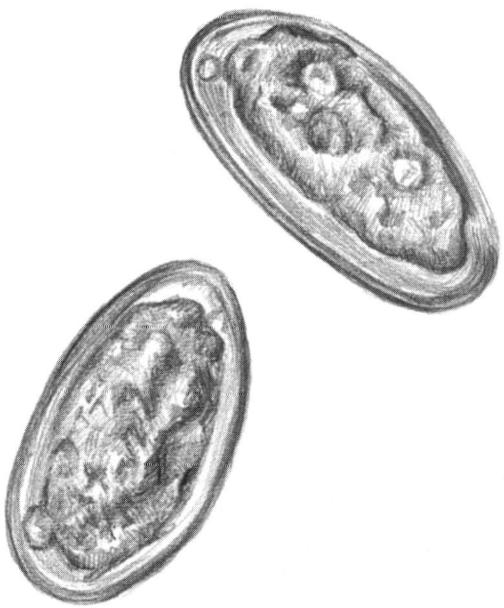

FIG. 2. Pinworm eggs (*Enterobius vermicularis*).

a flashlight) for adult pinworms. Radiography of the pelvis in a search for foreign bodies should be avoided, since most foreign bodies are not radioopaque.

Treatment

As noted in the section on etiology, no specific cause is found in a substantial portion of prepubertal girls with vulvovaginal symptoms, so-called "nonspecific vulvovaginitis." The culture may grow gram-negative enteric organisms such as *E. coli* or normal flora. Treatment of nonspecific vulvovaginitis should focus on improved hygiene (white cotton underpants or cotton crotch, front-to-back wiping, loose-fitting skirts, no nylon tights or tight blue jeans, avoidance of prolonged sitting in nylon bathing suits), handwashing, and sitz baths. The child should be asked to urinate with her knees spread apart so the labia are separated and urinary reflux into the vagina is minimized. The vulvar skin of the prepubertal child is extremely sensitive to drying, chapping, and irritants, including heat, medications, and soaps.

The child should be instructed to sit in a tub of clear, warm (not hot) water for 10 to 15 minutes once or twice daily. At the end of that time, she should be washed with a bland soap (such as Basis, unscented Dove, Lowila, Oilatum, Aveeno, or Neutrogena), with little or preferably no soap being applied to the vulva. The vulva should not be scrubbed. Hair should be shampooed over a sink or in the shower, rather than in the bathtub while the child is bathing. If neither is possible, the shampooing should occur at the end of the bath and the child rinsed in clear water. A hand-held sprayer is helpful. If the child is not afraid of showers, the optimal course is for her to soak for 10 to 15 minutes in several inches of clean water in the tub, and then stand up to wash her body in the shower. Some clinicians prefer cleaning the perineum gently with cotton pledgets and Cetophil. Bubble bath crystals and solutions should not be used, since the irritant soap may exacerbate the symptoms. After a bath, the child should pat the vulva dry or air-dry it with the legs spread apart; a hair dryer on cool setting for 10 to 15 seconds can aid drying. Sleeper pajamas should not be used if possible, since the associated heat and poor air circulation frequently cause maceration of the vulva. Underwear should be washed in a mild detergent and double-rinsed in clear water, and no rinse or dryer additives should be used.

A small amount of A and D ointment, Vaseline, or Desitin can be used to protect the vulvar skin. Topical medications such as triple sulfa cream, clindamycin cream, metronidazole gel, and mupirocin ointment or cream (Bactroban) have been used empirically but have not been subjected to controlled clinical trials. Different children appear to tolerate preparations differently, and it may be necessary to try several creams. Loose-fitting clothes such as skirts and knee socks or loose pants or shorts should be worn during the daytime. During the summer, the girl should not spend long periods of time in a wet swimsuit; a change to a pair of shorts or a dry suit should be suggested. Some girls without vaginal discharge have recurrent episodes of vulvar irritation and dysuria (transient vulvitis). Symptoms usually last for 12 to 24 hours and respond to tepid sitz baths and one or two applications of hydrocortisone cream 1%. These episodes are often triggered by irritants or a long period of time in tights, leotards, or sleeper pajamas.

Some girls have persistent vaginal discharge despite enhanced hygienic and other measures. Generally, if a discharge persists more than 2 or 3 weeks after such measures have been undertaken, the possibility of pinworms should be excluded or, in the girl with perianal or vulvar itching, empirically treated with mebendazole. A trial of oral antibiotics, such as amoxicillin, amoxicillin/clavulanate, or a cephalosporin, may be given for 10 days. Other clinicians have used oral or topical metronidazole or clindamycin.

Some children have persistent or frequently recurring symptoms even though a specific cause has been excluded. A variety of measures have been advocated, but none have been studied in clinical trials. We often prescribe a 1-month course of a small dose of an antibiotic at bedtime or even 3 nights a week, similar to suppression of urinary tract infections. Occcasionally, estrogen-containing creams (Premarin cream) can be used to thicken the epithelium, making it more resistant to infection; the cream is applied to the vulva but should be used only briefly (2 to 3 weeks at a time). This cream can also be applied for a brief course to the periclitoral area if erythema and adhesions from a previous inflammation appear to cause sensations of pulling and tingling. The parent should not be given a refillable prescription, since systemic absorption of estrogen does occur. Hygiene needs to be emphasized to all these girls, since the prescription of medication sometimes suggests to parents and child that the other measures can be discontinued.

Intravaginal medications are rarely indicated and may be difficult for the parent and child to administer. In some unusually persistent cases, irrigation of the vagina with a 1% povidone-iodine solution, using a syringe and a small infant feeding tube or urethral catheter, may be helpful.

Nonspecific vaginitis often recurs when the child develops an upper respiratory infection or has poor hygiene. Obese girls with inadequate hygiene are particularly prone to recurrences. Other causes of recurrent discharge, though rare, need to be considered, including pelvic abscess and ectopic ureter. Thus, the child with recurrent vaginitis often needs a careful reexamination and a search for a foreign body or an ectopic ureter. Other tests, such as pelvic ultrasonography, IVP, vaginoscopy, or cystoscopy, may be necessary to establish the more unusual diagnosis.

Recurrence of vaginitis may become a source of considerable anxiety for the parent, who may express fear that the child's future reproductive capacity will be harmed. In particular, the mother may have concerns about whether her own gynecologic problems of recurrent vaginitis, pelvic infection, or abnormal bleeding are hereditary or are related to the child's symptoms. The clinician can offer important reassurance by performing an adequate physical examination, obtaining vaginal cultures, and outlining a treatment plan.

Specific causes of vulvovaginitis are listed in Table 2, and treatment is outlined in Table 3 (6,64).

TABLE 3. *Treatment of vulvovaginal infections in the prepubertal child*

Etiology	Treatment
Streptococcus pyogenes	Penicillin V 250 mg t.i.d. p.o. for 10 days
Haemophilus influenzae	Amoxicillin 20–40 mg/kg/day p.o. for 7 days For resistant strains: amoxicillin/clavulanate, cefixime, cefuroxime axetil, trimethoprim/sulfamethoxazole, erythromycin-sulfamethaxazole
Staphylococcus aureus	Cephalexin 25–50 mg/kg/day p.o. for 7–10 days Dicloxacillin 25 mg/kg/day p.o. for 7–10 days Amoxicillin-clavulanate 20–40 mg/kg/day (of the amoxicillin) p.o. for 7–10 days Cefuroxime axetil oral suspension 30 mg/kg/day p.o. divided b.i.d. (max 1 g) for 10 days (tablets: 250 mg b.i.d.)
Streptococcus pneumoniae	Penicillin[a], erythromycin, trimethoprim/sulfamethoxazole, clarithromycin
Shigella	Trimethoprim/sulfamethoxazole 8 mg/40 mg/kg/day p.o. for 5 days For resistant organisms: cefixime, ceftriaxone
Chlamydia trachomatis	Erythromycin 50 mg/kg/day p.o. for 10–14 days; or azithromycin 20 mg/kg (max 1 g) single dose Children ≥8 years of age, doxycycline 100 mg b.i.d. p.o. for 7 days or azithromycin 1g p.o. single dose
Neisseria gonorrhoeae	Ceftriaxone 125 mg IM[b] (alternative: spectinomycin 40 mg/kg (max 2 g) IM once, *plus* treatment for *Chlamydia* as above Children ≥45 kg can be treated with adult regimens
Candida	Topical nystatin, miconazole, clotrimazole or terconazole cream; ?fluconazole p.o. in immunosuppressed children
Trichomonas	Metronidazole 15 mg/kg/day given t.i.d. (max 250 mg t.i.d.) for 7–10 days or 40 mg/kg (max 2 g) single dose
Pinworms (*Enterobius vermicularis*)	Mebendazole (Vermox), 1 chewable 100 mg tablet, repeated in 2 weeks

[a]With increased resistance, high-dose penicillin or alternative therapy may be needed.
[b]Given the effectiveness of oral therapies in adults, it is likely that the same regimens can be used in children.

The treatment of group A β-streptococci (*S. pyogenes*) is oral penicillin. Perianal streptococcal infection may occur with a vaginal infection or alone and may require a longer treatment course of 14 to 21 days if symptoms recur. *H. influenzae* and *S. aureus* can be treated effectively with any of several antibiotics, although symptoms do not always clear up even when the organism has been eradicated. *S. pneumoniae* is increasingly resistant to penicillin, and alternative therapy may be necessary if the symptoms do not resolve and the organism is resistant. The finding of *N. gonorrhoeae* should prompt careful evaluation for sexual abuse and mandated reporting. The girl should be examined for *C. trachomatis* as a coinfection and given appropriate treatment to cover both infections (see Chapter 12). Since sexual abuse often involves genital fondling, oral sex, or vulvar coitus rather than vaginal penetration in young girls, normal findings on examination of the girl with *N. gonorrhoeae* or *C. trachomatis* should not be taken as evidence against sexual abuse (see Chapter 20). A history of prior antibiotic therapy that would have been expected to eradicate *Chlamydia* transmitted at birth can help establish the likely timing of acquisition.

In contrast to the frequent occurrence of *Candida* vaginitis in the estrogenized pubescent (pre- or postmenarcheal) girl, the presence of this infection in the toilet-trained prepubertal girl who has not recently taken systemic antibiotics should prompt laboratory tests to exclude diabetes mellitus. Topical antifungal creams for the external genitalia should be tried first and are usually successful. If not, the diagnosis should be reassessed and intravaginal or oral antifungal therapy suggested. An intravaginal application can usually be accomplished by using a small urethral catheter attached to a syringe filled with an antifungal cream. Alternatively, 1 ml of nystatin (100,000 units/ml) can be instilled with a small eyedropper three times daily. To our knowledge, oral fluconazole has not been studied in prepubertal girls with *Candida* vulvovaginitis, but it has been used in immunocompromised children with oropharyngeal infections (65). Generally, it is used primarily in children who are immunocompromised or in whom topical medications are contraindicated or have failed.

Pinworms (*Enterobius vermicularis*) always need to be kept in mind as a specific cause of recurrent nonspecific vaginitis and are easily treated with oral medication. Mebendazole is not recommended for children under the age of 2 years. Family members may also need to be treated. Occasionally, other helminthic infections require treatment.

A purulent and/or bloody discharge is often the presenting complaint in a girl with a vaginal foreign body, most commonly toilet paper. The child should be questioned alone to determine whether another child or an adult placed the object in her vagina, since sexual abuse may be involved. If the child herself repeatedly places objects in her vagina, a psychosocial assessment is important. Toilet paper in the bathroom can be replaced with witch hazel pads (Tucks) to prevent accidental or purposeful shredding of toilet paper.

Summary of Therapy for Nonspecific Vulvovaginitis

General Measures

1. Good perineal hygiene (including wiping from front to back after bowel movements).
2. Frequent changes of white cotton underpants to absorb discharge.
3. Avoidance of bubble baths, harsh soaps, and shampooing hair in the bathtub.
4. Loose-fitting skirts; no nylon tights or tight blue jeans.
5. Sitz baths one to three times daily with plain warm water. The vulva should be gently washed (no soap) using soaking alone if possible. If soap is needed, only a mild, nonscented soap (Basis, unscented Dove, Lowila, Oilatum, Aveeno, or Neutrogena) should be applied. The bath should be followed by

careful drying (patting, not rubbing). The child should then lie with her legs spread apart for approximately 10 minutes to complete the drying, or a hair dryer used on the cool or low setting for 10 to 15 seconds. Even after the discharge clears up, daily sitz baths should be continued.

6. Urination with legs spread apart and labia separated.

Therapy for Acute Severe Edematous Vulvitis

1. Sitz baths every 4 hours (with plain water or with a small amount of Aveeno colloidal oatmeal or baking soda added). Soap should not be used, and the vulva should be air-dried. Powders should be avoided.
2. Witch hazel pads (Tucks) give soothing relief to most girls (although some complain of discomfort with their use) and may be used in place of toilet paper for wiping. After the acute phase of 1 to 2 days has passed, if there is no oozing, the sitz baths can be alternated every 4 hours with painting on a bland solution such as calamine lotion. In this phase, infection may need to be treated with oral antibiotics; topical antibacterials should be avoided.
3. In the subacute phase, topical creams such as hydrocortisone cream 1%, an antibacterial cream (triple sulfa cream, mupirocin), or A and D ointment can be applied.

Occasionally, an oral medication to lessen pruritus is indicated, such as hydroxyzine hydrochloride (Atarax), 2 mg/kg/day divided in four doses, or diphenhydramine hydrochloride, 5 mg/kg/day divided in four doses.

Therapy for Persistent Nonspecific Vulvovaginitis

1. Oral antibiotics, such as amoxicillin, amoxicillin/clavulanate, or a cephalosporin for 10 to 14 days; a 1- to 2-month low dose of bedtime cephalexin, cefuroxime axetil, amoxicillin/clavulanate, or trimethoprim/sulfamethoxazole may be helpful in the child with many recurrences; or
2. Antibacterial cream or ointment applied locally (mupirocin, metronidazole, clindamycin, triple sulfa cream); or
3. Estrogen-containing cream (Premarin cream), applied nightly to the vulva for 2 weeks and then every other night for 2 weeks; a repeat course may be necessary.
4. Hygiene must be emphasized.

LICHEN SCLEROSUS

Lichen sclerosus is uncommon in prepubertal children but should be recognized by the clinician (66–78). Patients usually complain of itching, irritation, soreness, bleeding, and dysuria. Less commonly, they may have bowel symptoms and a vaginal discharge. Some girls have painful defecation, constipation, encopresis, or anal stenosis (72). The vulva characteristically has white, atrophic, parchment-like skin and evidence of chronic ulceration, inflammation, and subepithelial hemorrhages. As the disease progresses there is loss of normal vulvar architecture: loss of the demarcation of the labia, scarring of the clitoral hood, and thickening of the posterior fourchette. Bleeding without a history of trauma has often caused suspicions of sexual abuse. The friction involved with bike riding can produce bleeding. Often, the involvement of the perianal area along with the labia may give the affected area an hourglass (or so-called figure-of-eight) configuration. Secondary infection may occur. The condition should be distinguished from vitiligo, which causes loss of pigmentation but not inflammation or atrophy. The occurrence of vulvar lichen sclerosus in monozygotic twin girls suggests a genetic factor (8).

The diagnosis of lichen sclerosus is made clinically and, if necessary, by examining a biopsy specimen (Fig. 3; see also Color Plates 3 and 4). Since the etiology is unknown, the best form of therapy is controversial. A graded approach based on the symptoms and clinical appearance seems best. For mild to moderate cases, treatment is aimed at elimination of local irritants and improved hygiene. Soaps should be minimally used in the vulvar area; the child should be encouraged to wear cotton underpants and loose-fitting pants or skirts to minimize local maceration and irritation. A protective ointment such as A and D ointment is helpful, and oral hydroxyzine hydrochloride is given 1 hour before

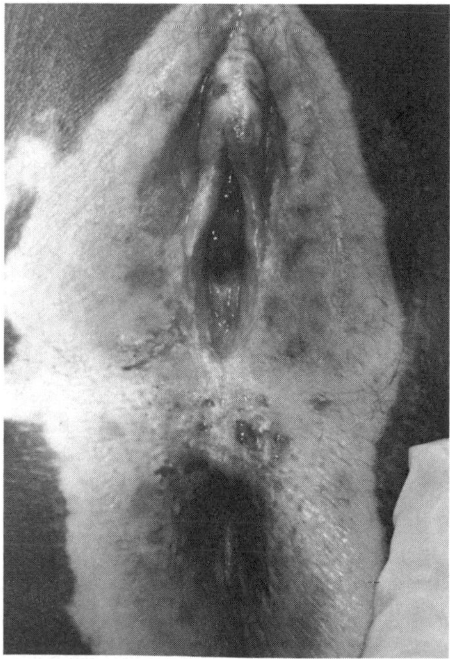

FIG. 3. Vulva of girl with lichen sclerosus.

bedtime to lessen the child's nocturnal scratching. The child is encouraged to become an active participant by applying the ointment and avoiding scratching. If this therapy is not adequate, a 1- to 3-month course of a low-potency topical steroid cream or ointment such as hydrocortisone 1% or 2.5% can be used with close followup. If the response is good, the hydrocortisone 1% can be continued for several additional months and then discontinued in favor of scrupulous hygiene and emollients. If flareups occur or symptoms continue, hydrocortisone cream can be reapplied. Oral antibiotics are prescribed for significant superinfections.

For more severe symptoms, a short course (2 to 4 weeks) of a moderate-potency ointment such as fluocinolone acetonide 0.025% can be used, followed by hydrocortisone 1%. Berth-Jones and colleagues (4) have used fluocinonide 0.05% as long as 2 weeks and then changed to hydrocortisone. Mometasone furoate (Elocon) has also been used successfully for short courses. The most recent treatment is clobetasol cream (Temovate), which has been used for 12 weeks in studies of adult women and then replaced by a lower potency steroid with clobetasol used as needed (2,76–78). Ridley (73) has suggested that a course of the potent steroid clobetasone propionate 0.05% is justifiable for severe symptoms in children and adolescents and for girls in whom there is a tendency to gross destruction of the vulval architecture; close supervision is mandatory to prevent adverse effects from the topical steroids. We have also used clobetasol gel twice a day for 2 weeks, and then, after a followup visit, generally tapered the application to once a day for another 2 weeks, and then once every other day for 2 weeks.

Topical progesterone has been used at some centers with variable reports of success. Micronized progesterone powder as a 2% application in a hydrophilic petrolatum base has been used twice daily for 3 months (72). Approximately 5 mg of progesterone is delivered as a pea-sized amount on a fingertip. Progesterone solution in Aquaphor has also been used by some. Testosterone cream (2% in petrolatum) applied nightly for several months has been used in postmenopausal women, but most clinicians do not currently favor its use in the prepubertal child because of the occurence of side effects, including induction of pubic hair. Controlled studies are lacking. A few children with severe intractable disease have been treated at our institution and in other centers with laser brushing of the vulva with the child under general anesthesia (79); long-term data are needed, and the use of clobetasol has essentially obviated the need for this surgical approach.

In some girls, lichen sclerosus improves with puberty; in many, the symptoms and signs persist (67–73). Among 15 girls (aged 18 months to 9 years) followed up for more than 43 months, 7 improved, 7 showed no change, and 1 was worse; there was a trend toward improvement with increasing age (75). Ridley (73) has questioned whether the absence of active lesions really represents disappearance of the condition. The long-term risks of vulvar malignancy in girls with lichen sclerosus have not been studied, and only a few anecdotal cases have been reported (73,75).

VAGINAL BLEEDING

Vaginal bleeding in the prepubertal child should always be carefully assessed. In the neonate, vaginal bleeding sometimes occurs in the first week of life secondary to withdrawal from maternal estrogen. After that, the causes to be considered include vaginitis, lichen sclerosus (Color Plates 3, 4, and 19), condyloma (Fig. 4 and Color Plate 8); trauma (80) (Color Plates 9–18), foreign body (Fig. 7), tumor (Color Plate 7), precocious puberty, hypothyroidism, blood dyscrasia, hemangioma (Fig. 5) (81), polyp, and urethral prolapse (Fig. 8) (Table 4). A good history and physical examination are important to the differential diagnosis. Acceleration of height and weight or signs of pubertal development before the age of 8 years suggest precocious puberty (see Chapter 5). A history of foreign bodies in the ears or vagina may implicate another foreign body, which may have been placed by the child or by an abuser. Patients with blood dyscrasias typically have other signs of bleeding, such as epistaxis, petechiae, or hematomas.

The physical examination should include a general assessment and a careful gynecologic examination. Trauma, vulvovaginitis, and hemangiomas (Fig. 5) are usually evident on inspection. A straddle injury typically causes ecchymoses in the vulva and periclitoral folds. A laceration of the labia minora and periurethral tissue may be seen (Color Plate 17). It is extremely uncommon for a child to have a tear in the hymen without having suffered a penetrating injury (e.g., from

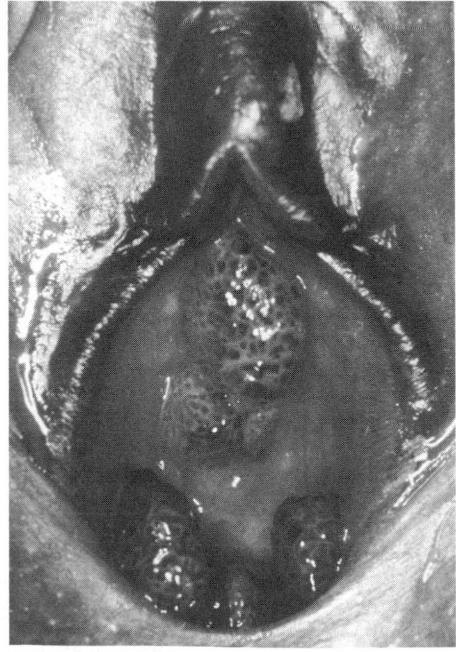

FIG. 4. Condyloma accuminata, presenting as vaginal bleeding.

TABLE 4. *Differential diagnosis of vaginal bleeding in the prepubertal girl*

Trauma
Accidental
Sexual abuse
Vulvovaginitis
Irritation, pinworms
Nonspecific vulvovaginitis
Streptococcus pyogenes, Shigella
Endocrine abnormalities
Newborn bleeding due to maternal estrogen withdrawal
Isosexual precocious puberty
Pseudoprecocious puberty
Precocious menarche
Exogenous hormone preparations
Hypothyroidism
Dermatoses
Lichen sclerosus
Condyloma accuminata (human papillomavirus)
Foreign body
Urethral prolapse
Blood dyscrasia
Hemangioma
Tumor
Benign
Malignant

a nail, a broom handle, a bedpost). Therefore, in the absence of an appropriate history, sexual abuse should be strongly considered when a hymenal tear is noted (Color Plate 16 and Chapter 20) (80,82). Significant vaginal tears, however, can occur with water-skiing injuries (83).

Some suggestions for examining the child who has active bleeding from the vulva are to wipe 2% lidocaine jelly over the cut, place warm water in a syringe to irrigate the tissue gently, and/or irrigate using IV tubing and solution. The child can also assist by holding cool compresses with strong pressure. As noted

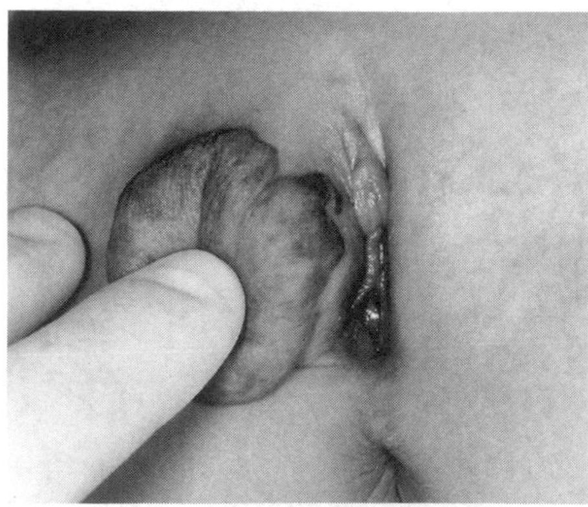

FIG. 5. Hemangioma of the vulva.

in Fig. 6, the irrigation allows blood that may have collected in the vagina from a labial laceration to be washed out and the source of bleeding to be identified. If an abrasion is oozing, it can often be treated with ice and compression. If the oozing continues, then Gelfoam or Surgicel can be applied. If only a few stitches are necessary for repairing a vulvar laceration, some emergency wards have a protocol for anesthesia (conscious sedation). Lidocaine 1% to 2% with epinephrine can then be injected locally with a 25-gauge needle and the repair done with No. 4 chromic or vicryl interrupted sutures. If cooperation is not possible and a hymenal or intravaginal tear or a periurethral laceration is noted, an examination and repair should be done while the child is under general anesthesia. Straddle injuries may cause deep lacerations in the periurethral tissue; repair requires the placement of a Foley catheter and meticulous suturing. Significant penetrating injuries may have occurred to the upper vagina without obvious symptoms or signs other than a hymenal tear at presentation. Many vulvar injuries heal after repair with little or no residual scarring or other sequelae.

Most bleeding in the prepubertal girl occurs not because of major trauma but because of vulvovaginitis, scratching due to pinworm infection, or a vaginal foreign body. Vaginitis caused by group A β-streptococci or *Shigella* is especially likely to be accompanied by bleeding. If drops of blood have only recently been seen on the underwear, it is important to visualize the vagina (e.g. with the patient in the knee-chest position) and to obtain specimens for vaginal culture before anesthesia examination is recommended. If excoriations are noted around

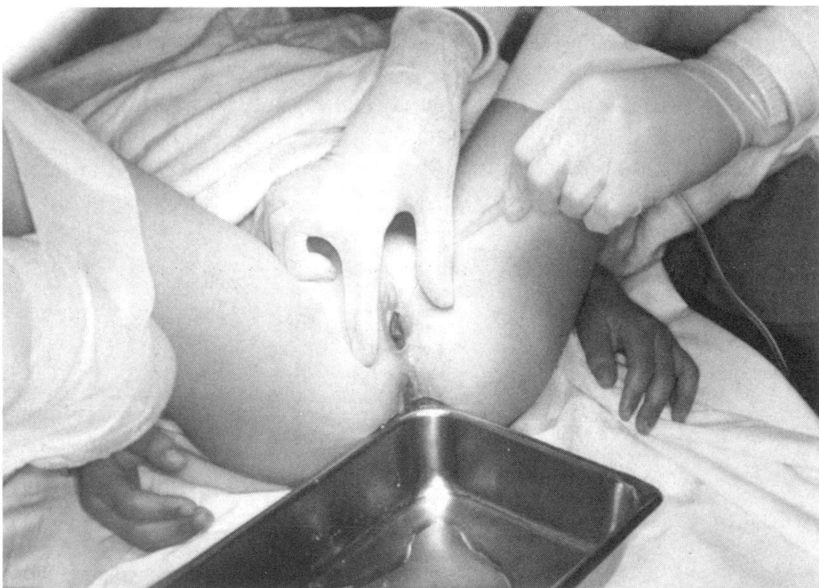

FIG. 6. Irrigation of the vulva and vagina with saline to identify the source of bleeding.

the anus and vulva, a cellophane tape test should be done to search for pinworms, or the patient should be treated empirically if pinworms are strongly suspected. Intravaginal foreign bodies are usually wads of toilet paper (Fig. 7) but may be pins, paper clips, tampon cartons, beads, marker tips, crayons, or batteries. An irritative vulvitis with sharp demarcation of redness on the vulva may occur secondary to the chronic discharge associated with a foreign body. The upper vaginal mucosa may show a papillary response with small projections of 1–2 mm (53). A study by Paradise and Willis (63) found that 18% of girls under 13 years with vaginal bleeding with or without discharge, and 50% of those with vaginal bleeding and *no* discharge, had a foreign body. Most girls with a foreign body do not have a foul-smelling discharge with the bleeding. A tumor is a rare cause of bleeding, but the possibility of this diagnosis makes adequate assessment of the vagina important in the child with unexplained bleeding.

Urethral prolapse usually presents with bleeding, often thought by the parent to be vaginal bleeding, but the examination reveals the characteristic friable red-blue (doughnut-like) annular mass (Fig. 8). Cyclic vaginal bleeding without signs of pubertal development is rare; Heller and associates (84,85) have termed this entity precocious menarche (see Chapter 5). Although we have seen several girls with this problem, one of whom has a mother who had the same pattern of bleeding, full examination, with the girl under anesthesia if necessary, is essential before vaginal bleeding can be considered an idiopathic or benign disorder.

Bleeding secondary to vulvitis should respond promptly to local measures. Vaginitis due to organisms such as group A β-hemolytic streptococci or *Shigella* requires oral antibiotics.

A foreign body may be removed in the outpatient setting if the patient is cooperative. Soft foreign bodies can often be easily removed by twirling a dry cotton-tipped applicator within the vagina with the patient in the lithotomy or knee-chest position. Gentle irrigation of the vagina with saline or water can usually be accomplished with the child supine, using a small urethral catheter or infant feeding tube attached to a 25-ml syringe or an angiocath attached to

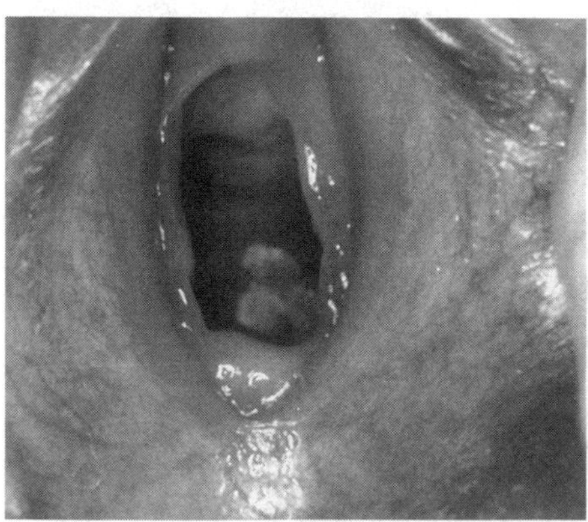

FIG. 7. Wad of toilet paper within the vagina, visualized through an irregular hymenal orifice of a prepubertal girl.

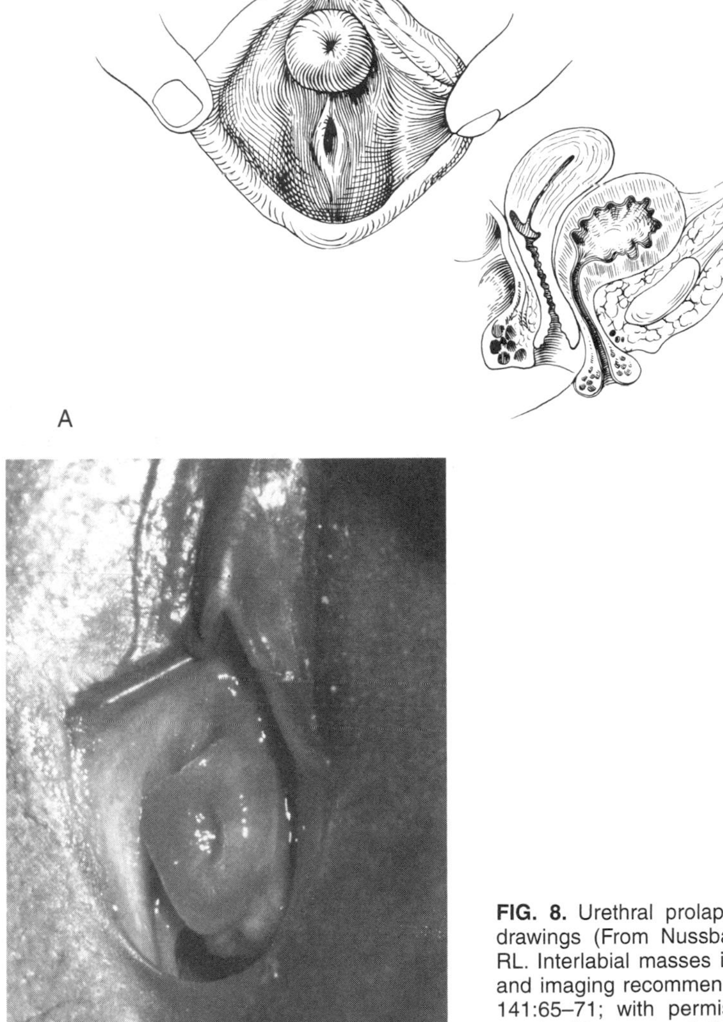

FIG. 8. Urethral prolapse. **(A)** Schematic drawings (From Nussbaum AR, Lebowitz RL. Interlabial masses in little girls: review and imaging recommendations. *AJR* 1983; 141:65–71; with permission.) **(B)** Photograph. (Courtesy of Dr. Arnold Colodny, Children's Hospital, Boston.)

a syringe. Lubricant or lidocaine jelly (or liquid) can be applied to the introitus to aid in insertion of the small catheter. It may be possible to remove metallic items such as safety pins or hymenal edges with bayonet forceps. If the child is frightened or the foreign body cannot be easily removed, general anesthesia is necessary. Some clinicians apply estrogen cream following the removal of a foreign body, but sitz baths alone are generally adequate to clear the residual symptoms.

Therapy for a tumor depends on the extent of the lesion and requires referral to a tertiary care medical center.

INTERLABIAL MASSES

The causes of interlabial masses include urethral prolapse, paraurethral cyst (Fig. 9), hydro(metro)colpos, rhabdomyosarcoma of the vagina (botryoid sarcoma) (Color Plate 7), prolapsed ectopic ureterocele (Fig. 10), condyloma acuminata (see Fig. 4 and Chapter 13), urethral polyp, and vaginal or cervical prolapse (86–97).

Urethral prolapse (Fig. 8) usually presents with bleeding, and the characteristic friable red-blue (doughnut-like) annular mass is visible in the perineum. The vaginal orifice is sometimes obscured and may be visualized only when the girl is in the knee-chest position. The patient may complain of dysuria, bleeding, and pain that has occurred after coughing or straining or following trauma. The peak age of prolapse is 5 to 8 years; for unclear reasons the condition appears to occur more commonly in black girls. The youngest case reported was in a 5-day-old infant (95). Prolapse usually resolves with nonsurgical treatment. Methods used in (uncontrolled) series of patients include sitz baths, plain or with the addition of antiseptic soap (povidone-iodine or hexachlorophene); topical estrogen cream or topical antibiotics; and systemic oral antibiotics. Topical estrogen cream is used at most centers. Resolution takes 1 to 4 weeks. Prolapse with tissue necrosis requires surgical resection of the necrotic distal urethra.

Paraurethral cysts (Fig. 9) may occur in children, especially during the newborn period, and arise from obstruction or cystic degeneration of embryonic remnants

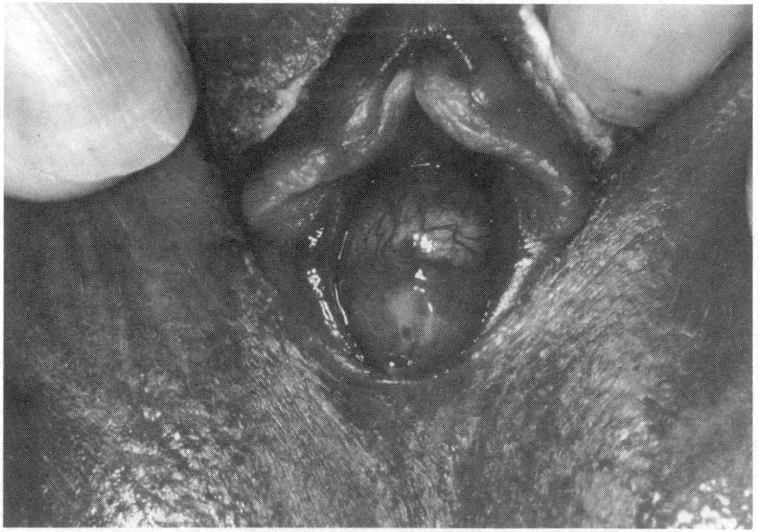

FIG. 9. Paraurethral cyst in a neonate.

of the urogenital sinus: paraurethral glands, Skene's duct, mesonephric duct (Gartner's duct), or müllerian duct (95). In the newborn, the cysts usually disappear or spontaneously rupture without requiring any treatment. Before surgery is undertaken, the possibility of a urologic or gynecologic problem such as urethral diverticulum, ectopic ureterocele, hymenal or vaginal cyst, or obstructed hemivagina should be excluded by preoperative examination and ultrasonography of the kidneys and bladder. Intraoperatively, radioopaque dye such as Renografin should be injected into the cyst and imaged to enable detection of an anomaly.

A *prolapsed ectopic ureterocele* (Fig. 10) is a congenital anomaly that includes cystic dilatation of the terminal (intramural) part of a ureter; 90% are associated with a duplex collecting system (95).

Hydro(metro)colpos (Fig. 11) may present in the nursery with a bulging imperforate hymen or obstruction from a low vaginal septum (a mid or high vaginal septum will not usually present with an interlabial mass). An imperforate hymen is not usually associated with other anomalies, but a transverse septum is often associated with genitourinary and gastrointestinal anomalies (95).

Neonatal vaginal prolapse has been reported in a healthy neonate. The mass was restored to normal position with the examiner's small finger, and the mother

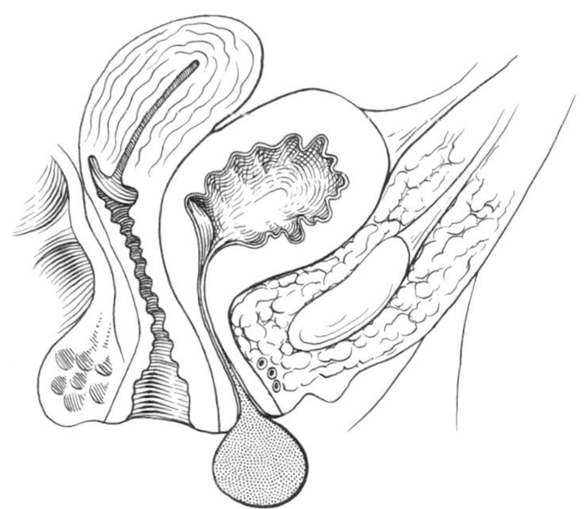
A

FIG. 10. Prolapsed ectopic ureterocele. Schematic drawings. **(A)** Cross section of pelvis. **(B)** View from vulva. (From Nussbaum AR, Lebowitz RL. Interlabial masses in little girls: review and imaging recommendations. *AJR* 1983;141:65–71; with permission.) **(C)** Photograph of prolapse.

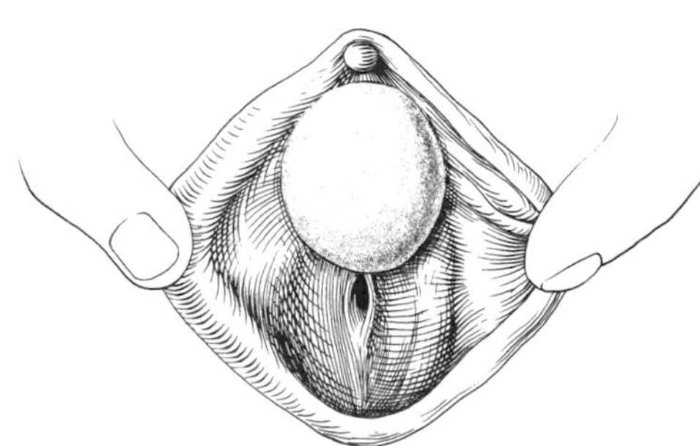
B

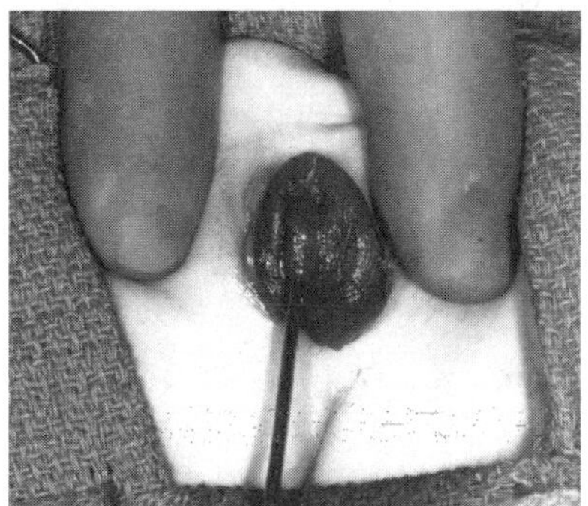
C

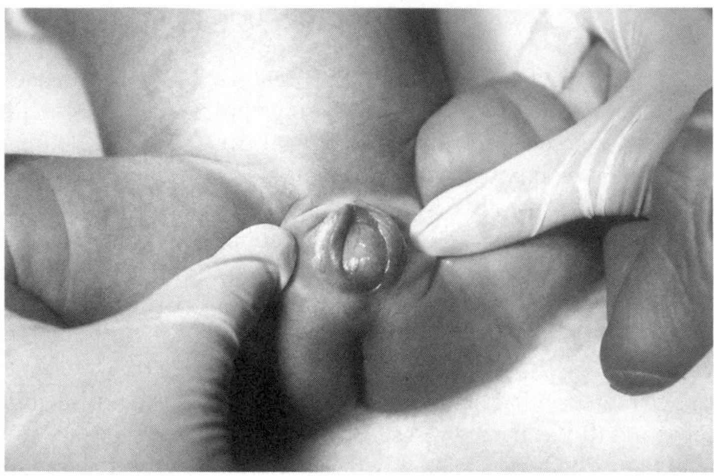

FIG. 11. Hydrocolpos in a newborn.

was trained to reinsert the vagina subsequently; after 6 months there was no further prolapse (96,97).

Sarcoma botryoides (Color Plate 7) is a malignant tumor that involves the vagina, uterus, bladder, and urethra of very young girls and is also known as embryonal rhabdomyosarcoma. The symptoms include vaginal discharge, bleeding, abdominal pain or mass, or the passage of grape-like lesions. The peak incidence is in the first 2 years of life, and 90% of cases occur before the child is 5 years old. The tumor usually originates in the lower vagina or urethra in younger girls. In those diagnosed when they are older, the growth usually starts on the anterior vaginal wall near the cervix, and as the tumor grows larger it fills the vagina.

On examination, the tumor appears as a prolapse of grape-like masses through the urethra or vagina. If a vaginal tag is seen on vaginal examination, it should never be assumed to be benign. Growth of the tumor is rapid, and the prognosis is poor unless the diagnosis is made early. A combination of chemotherapy and aggressive surgery, along with radiation therapy for some patients, can result in a survival rate of 80% to 90% in girls with localized pelvic rhabdomyosarcoma (90–93). Copeland and associates (90) reported the survival of 11 of 14 patients with sarcoma botryoides of the female genital tract. The 3-year survival rate for localized botryoid tumors in the Intergroup Rhabdomysarcoma Study-II was 86% (93). In early-stage vulvovaginal rhabdomyosarcoma, systemic vincristine, dactinomycin, and cyclophosphamide have resulted in high cure rates and retention of fertility (92). The prognosis is poorer in patients with regional or distant spread or recurrences.

CLITORAL LESIONS

The clitoral hood may occasionally develop an infection with intense edema and erythema. An antibiotic such as dicloxacillin or a cephalosporin with antistaphylococcal efficacy should be given orally, and warm soaks should be applied. Surgical incision and drainage are necessary if the abscess becomes fluctuant.

Hemorrhages may occur around the clitoris in girls with lichen sclerosus, and synechiae in the vulvar area may be apparent even after the condition has improved. An ecchymotic clitoris may also be caused by trauma.

Edema of the clitoris may occur with hypoproteinemia in conditions such as the nephrotic syndrome. Hypertrophy of the clitoral hood and clitoris can be due to neurofibromatosis (98,99), congenital hemangiopericytoma (a rare vascular tumor) (100), or rhabdomyosarcoma (101). A "clitoral tourniquet syndrome" has been described in which a hair had become wrapped around the clitoris, resulting in edema and severe pain (102). After removal of the hair, the clitoris returned to normal size. The syndrome is similar to strangulation by hair of other parts of the body, such as fingers, toes, or the penis. Clitorism, a persistent painful erection of the clitoris, has been reported in one 11-year-old with acute nonlymphocytic leukemia and extremely elevated leukocyte count (196,000/mm^3) (103).

LABIAL ADHESIONS

Agglutination of the labia minora, termed labial adhesions or, in the lower half, vulvar adhesions, occurs primarily in young girls aged 3 months to 6 years (Fig. 12 and Color Plate 2). Occasionally, adhesions occur for the first time after

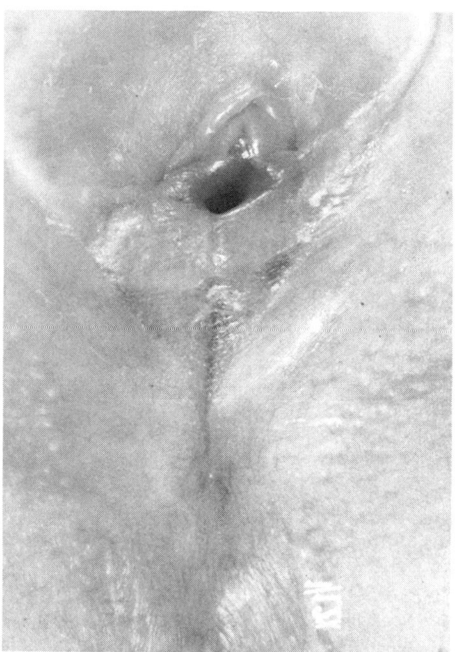

FIG. 12. Labial/vulvar adhesions with small opening below the clitoris.

age 6, and adhesions presenting at any age may persist to the time of puberty. It is possible that poor hygiene and vulvar irritation can cause an initially small posterior adhesion to progress to a near-total fusion. The vaginal orifice may be completely covered, causing poor drainage of vaginal secretions. Parents often become alarmed because the vagina appears "absent." It has been suggested (although not proved) that fondling and the irritation from sexual abuse may predispose the older girl to labial agglutination (104,105).

The diagnosis of labial adhesions is made by visual inspection of the vulva. The treatment of labial adhesions remains controversial. Spontaneous separation may occur, particularly with small vulvar adhesions at the posterior fourchette and with estrogenization at puberty. If the opening in the agglutination is large enough for good vaginal and urinary drainage, lubrication of the labia with a bland ointment such as A and D ointment, and gentle separation applied by the mother over several weeks, may be helpful. For adhesions that impair vaginal or urinary drainage, the most effective treatment is the application of an estrogen-containing cream (106). We prescribe estrogen (Premarin) cream twice daily for 3 weeks and then at bedtime for another 2 to 3 weeks. The adhesion may lyse in 2 to 3 weeks, and therapy can then be changed to A and D ointment. The parent must be shown exactly where the labial adhesion is ("a line") and shown how to rub in the cream with gentle separation. The use of a long cotton-tipped applicator may facilitate correct application of the cream and gentle separation (the child may appreciate that the cream is "painted on"). Most failures result when the par-

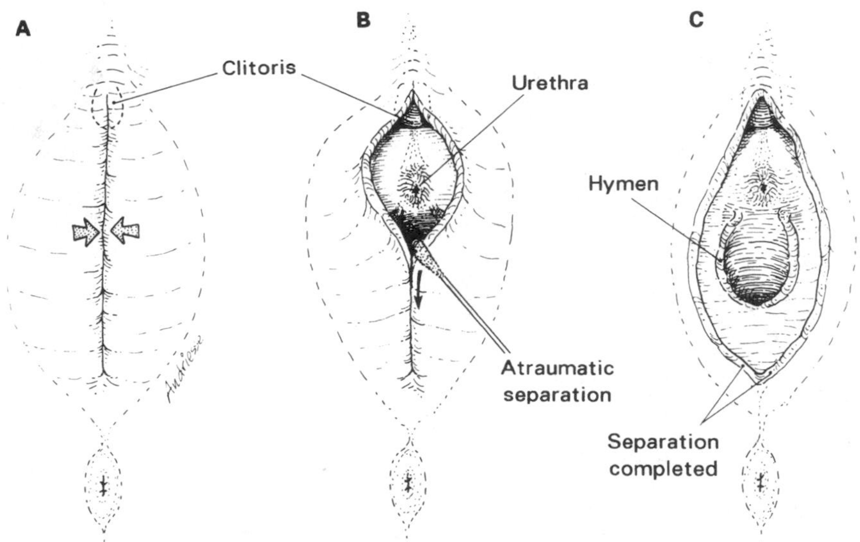

FIG. 13. Atraumatic separation of a labial adhesion that failed to separate. (From Goldstein DP, Laufer MR, Davis AJ. *Gynecologic surgery in children and adolescents: a text atlas.* New York: Springer-Verlag (in preparation); with permission.)

ent applies the cream over the entire vulva without specific attention to the adhesion. After separation has occurred, the labia should be maintained apart by daily baths, good hygiene, and the application of a bland ointment (such as A and D ointment) at bedtime for 6 to 12 months. Forceful separation is generally contraindicated because it is traumatic for the child and may cause the adhesions to form again.

In occasional patients, the extensive, dense labial adhesions fail to respond to estrogen cream, even when proper technique is used. Separation can be accomplished in the cooperative patient in the office at the end of the 6-week course of estrogen cream. Approximately 5 minutes after the application of 5% lidocaine ointment, or 30 minutes after EMLA (a eutectic mixture of local anesthetics, lidocaine, and prilocaine) application, the physician can slide a Calgiswab gently along the adhesions thinned by the estrogen cream, teasing them apart in an anterior-to-posterior direction (Fig. 13). If this is not easily accomplished or if the girl has acute urinary retention, separation in an ambulatory surgical setting is recommended. Rarely, early adolescents who have had labial adhesions since early childhood do not have the usual spontaneous separation, either with their endogenous estrogen or with topically applied estrogen, seemingly because of the thick bands that have formed over time. Our oldest patient with persistent adhesions was 16 years old and required general anesthesia for separation.

MISCELLANEOUS ENTITIES

Three other entities that should be recognized by the physician are labial abscesses, lipomas, and congenital failure of midline fusion.

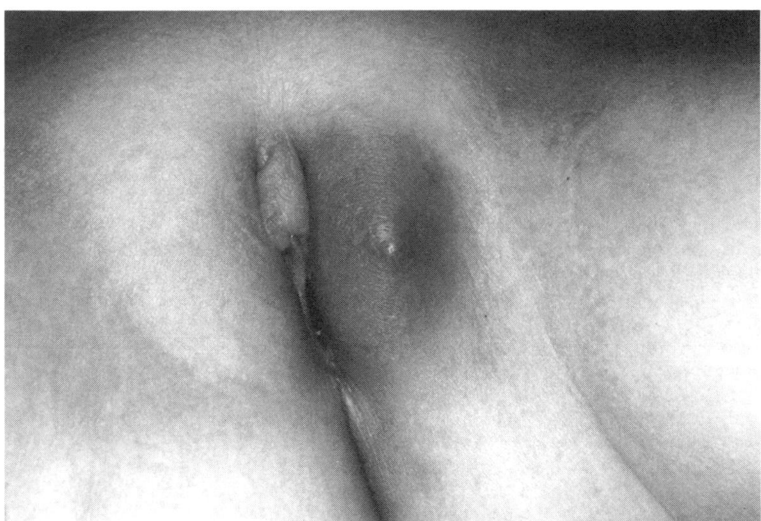

FIG. 14. Labial abscess.

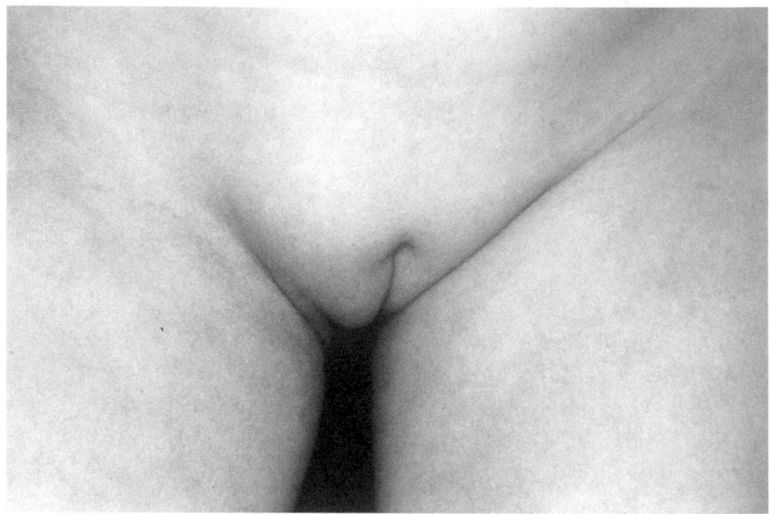

FIG.15. Lipoma of labia in an 8-year-old girl who had had a labial mass for 1 year.

Labial abscesses (Fig. 14) in immunocompetent girls are usually caused by infections with *S. aureus* or *S. pyogenes*. The abscesses are treated with antibiotics, sitz baths, and, as indicated, incision and drainage.

A lipoma (Fig. 15) may occur in the labia majora and present with a mass that may initially be mistaken for a hernia. Treatment is observation or excision.

Failure of midline fusion is congenital and may be confused with trauma or sexual abuse; the child in Color Plate 6 underwent excision of the base of the separation, and suturing of the edges to give a normal vulvar appearance, at the age of 4 years.

REFERENCES

1. Hammerschlag MR, Albert S, Rosner I, et al. Microbiology of the vagina in children: normal and potentially pathogenic organisms. *Pediatrics* 1978;68:57.
2. Paradise JE, Compos JM, Friedman HM, et al. Vulvovaginitis in premenarchal girls: clinical features and diagnostic evaluation. *Pediatrics* 1982;70:193.
3. Gardner JJ. Comparison of the vaginal flora in sexually abused and nonabused girls. *J Pediatr* 1992; 120:872.
4. Gertner GJ, Grunberger W, Boschitsch E, et al. Vaginal organisms in prepubertal children with and without vulvovaginitis. *Arch Gynecol* 1982:231:247.
5. Paradise J. Unpublished data.
6. Emans SJ, Goldstein DP. The gynecologic examination of the prepubertal child with vulvovaginitis: use of the knee-chest position. *Pediatrics* 1980;65:758.
7. Altchek A. Pediatric vulvovaginitis. *J Reprod Med* 1984;29:359.
8. Capraro VJ. Vulvovaginitis and other local lesions of the vulva. *Clin Obstet Gynecol* 1974;1:533.
9. Heller RH, Joseph JH, David HJ. Vulvovaginitis in the premenarchal child. *J Pediatr* 1969;74:370.
10. Pierce AM, Hart CA. Vulvovaginitis: causes and management. *Arch Dis Child* 1992;67:509.
11. Ginsburg CM. Group A streptococcal vaginitis in children. *Pediatr Infect Dis* 1982;1:36.

12. Figeroa-Colon R, Grunow JE, Torres-Pinedo R, et al. Group A streptococcal proctitis and vulvovaginitis in a prepubertal girl. *Pediatr Infect Dis* 1984;3:439.
13. Spear RM, Rithbaum RJ, Keating JP, et al. Perianal streptococcal cellulitis. *J Pediatr* 1985;107:557.
14. Kokx NP, Comstock JA, Facklam RR. Streptococcal perianal disease in children. *Pediatrics* 1987; 80:659.
15. Straumanis JP, Bocchini JA. Group A beta-hemolytic streptococcal vulvovaginitis in prepubertal girls: a case report and review of the past twenty years. *Pediatr Infect Dis* 1990:9:845.
16. Donald FE, Slack RCB, Colman G. *Streptococcus pyogenes* vulvovaginitis in children in Nottingham. *Epidemiol Infect* 1991;106:459.
17. Zeiguer NJ, Galvano A, Comparato MR, et al. Vulvar abscesses caused by streptococcus pneumoniae. *Pediatr Infect Dis J* 1992;11:335.
18. Macfarlane DE, Sharma DP. *Haemophilus influenzae* and genital tract infections in children. *Acta Paediatr Scand* 1987;76:363.
19. Murphy TV, Nelson JD. Shigella vaginitis: report of 38 patients and review of the literature. *Pediatrics* 1979;63:511.
20. Yanovski JA, Nelson LM, Willis ED, Cutler GB. Repeated childhood vaginal bleeding is not always precocious puberty. *Pediatrics* 1992;89:149.
21. Gryngarten MG, Turco ML, Ewcobar ME, et al. Shigella vulvaginitis in prepubertal girls. *Adolesc Pediatr Gynecol* 1994;7:86.
22. Watkins S, Quan L. Vulvovaginitis caused by *Yersinia* enterocolitica. *Pediatr Infect Dis* 1984;3:444.
23. Heger AH, Emans SJ, et al, eds. *Evaluation of the sexually abused child: a medical textbook and photographic atlas.* New York: Oxford University Press, 1992.
24. Jenny C. Sexually transmitted diseases and child abuse. *Pediatr Ann* 1992;21:497.
25. Ingram DL. Neisseria gonorrhoeae in children. *Pediatr Ann* 1994;23:341.
26. Hammerschlag MR. Chlamydia trachomatis in children. *Pediatr Ann* 1994;23:349.
27. Farrell MK, Billmire ME, Shamroy JA, et al. Prepubertal gonorrhea: a multidisciplinary approach. *Pediatrics* 1981;67:151.
28. Folland DS, Burke RE, Hinman AR, et al. Gonorrhea in preadolescent children: an inquiry into source of infection and mode of transmission. *Pediatrics* 1977;60:153.
29. Ingram DL, White ST, Occhiuti AC, et al. Childhood vaginal infections: association of *Chlamydia trachomatis* with sexual contact. *Pediatr Infect Dis* 1986;5:226.
30. Fuster CD, Neinstein LS. Vaginal *Chlamydia trachomatis* prevalence in sexually abused prepubertal girls. *Pediatrics* 1987;79:235.
31. Shapiro RA, Schubert CJ, Myers PA. Vaginal discharge as an indicator of gonorrhea and chlamydia infection in girls under 12 years old. *Pediatr Emerg Med* 1993;9:341.
32. Sicoli RA, Losek JD, Hudlett JM, et al. Indications for *Neisseria gonorrhoeae* cultures in children with suspected sexual abuse. *Arch Pediatr Adolesc Med* 1995;149:86.
33. Goh BT, Forster GE. Sexually transmitted diseases in children: chlamydial oculo-genital infection. *Genitourin Med* 1993;69:213.
34. Desenclos JA, Garrity D, Wroten J. Pediatric gonococcal infection, Florida 1984 to 1988. *Am J Public Health* 1992;82:426.
35. Ingram DL, Everett VD, Lyna PR. Epidemiology of adult sexually transmitted disease agents in children being evaluated for sexual abuse. *Pediatr Infect Dis J* 1992;11:945.
36. Danesh IS, Stephen JM, Gorbach J. Neonatal trichomonas vaginalis infection. *J Emerg Med* 1995; 13:51.
37. Schachter J, Grossman M, Sweet RL, et al. Prospective study of perinatal transmission of *Chlamydia trachomatis. JAMA* 1986;255:3374.
38. Bell TA, Stamm WE, Kuo CC, et al. Delayed appearance of *Chlamydia trachomatis* infection acquired at birth. *Pediatr Infect Dis* 1987;6:928.
39. Hammerschlag MR. *Chlamydia* and suspected sexual abuse. *Pediatrics* 1988;81:600.
40. Hammerschlag M. Chlamydial infections. *J Pediatr* 1989;114:727.
41. Bell TA. *Chlamydia trachomatis* infections in infants: perinatal or sexual transmission? *Infect Med* 1993;10:32
42. Bell AC, Bell TA, Stamm WE, et al. Chronic *Chlamydia trachomatis* infections in infants. *JAMA* 1992;267:400.
43. Patamasucon P, Rettig PJ, Nelson JD. Cefuroxime therapy of gonorrhea and coinfection with *Chlamydia trachomatis* in children. *Pediatrics* 1981;68:534.
44. Hammerschlag MR, Rettig PJ, Shields ME. False positive result with the use of *Chlamydia* antigen detection tests in the evaluation of suspected sexual abuse in children. *Pediatr Infect Dis* 1988;7:11.

45. Embree JE, Lindsay D, Williams T, et al. Acceptability and usefulness of vaginal washes in premenarcheal girls as a diagnostic procedure for sexually transmitted diseases. *Pediatr Infect Dis J* 1996;15:662–7.
46. Kaplan KM, Fleisher GR, Paradise JE, et al. Social relevance of genital herpes simplex in children. *J Pediatr* 1984;104:243.
47. Simon HK, Steele DW. Varicella: pediatric genital/rectal vesicular lesions of unclear origin. *Ann Emerg Med* 1995;25:111.
48. Bartley DL, Morgan L, Rimsza ME. *Gardnerella vaginalis* in prepubertal girls. *Am J Dis Child* 1987;141:1014.
49. Steele AM, de San Lazaro C. Transhymenal cultures for sexually transmissible organism. *Arch Dis Child* 1994;71:423.
50. Ingram DL, White ST, Lyna PR, et al. *Gardnerella vaginalis* infection and sexual contact in female children. *Child Abuse Neglect* 1992;16:847.
51. Simon HK, Steele DW. Varicella: pediatric genital/rectal vesicular lesions of unclear origin. *Ann Emerg Med* 1995;25:111.
52. Fink CW. A perineal rash in Kawasaki disease. *Pediatr Infect Dis* 1983;2;140.
53. Pokorny SF. Prepubertal vulvovaginopathies. *Obstet Gynecol Clin North Am* 1992;19:39.
54. Khoshoo V. Zinc deficiency in a full-term breast-fed infant: unusual presentation. *Pediatrics* 1992; 89:1094.
55. Guenther LC, Shum D. Localized childhood vulvar pemphigoid. *J Am Acad Dermatol* 1990;22:762.
56. Hanks JW, Venters WJ. Nickel allergy from a bed-wetting alarm confused with herpes genitalis and child abuse. *Pediatrics* 1992;90:458.
57. Otis CN, Fischer RA, Johnson N, et al. Histiocytosis X of the vulva: a case report and review of the literature. *Obstet Gynecol* 1990;75:555.
58. Wilson RW. Genital ulcers and mononucleosis. *Pediatr Infect Dis J* 1993;12:418.
59. Tuffnell D, Buchan PC. Crohn's disease of the vulva in childhood. *Br J Clin Prac* 1991;45:159.
60. Rimsza ME, Chun JJ. Vaginal discharge of "beads" and the new diapers. *Pediatrics* 1988;81:332.
61. Tudor RB. Disposable diaper damper. *Pediatrics* 1988;81:471.
62. See WA, Mayo M. Ectopic ureter: a rare cause of purulent vaginal discharge. *Obstet Gynecol* 1991; 78:552.
63. Paradise JE, Willis ED. Probability of vaginal foreign body in girls with genital complaints. *Am J Dis Child* 1985;139:472.
64. Vandeven A, Emans SJ. Vulvovaginitis. *Pediatr Rev* 1993;14:141.
65. Flynn PM, Cunningham CK, Kerkering T. Oropharyngeal candidiasis in immunocompromised children: a randomized, multicenter study of orally administered fluconazole suspension versus nystatin. *J Pediatr* 1995;127:322.
66. Muramatsu T, Kitamura W, Sakamoto K. Lichen sclerosus et atrophicus in children. *J Dermatol* 1985;12:377.
67. Kaufman RH, Gardner HL. Vulvar dystrophies. *Clin Obstet Gynecol* 1978;21:1081.
68. Clark JA, Muller SA. Lichen sclerosus et atrophicus in children. *Arch Dermatol* 1967;95:476.
69. Meyrick Thomas RH, Kennedy CT. The development of lichen sclerosus et atrophicus in monozygotic twin girls. *Br J Dermatol* 1986;114:337.
70. Redmond CA, Corvell CA, Krafchik B. Genital lichen sclerosus in prepubertal girls. *Adolesc Pediatr Gynecol* 1988;1:177.
71. Loening-Bauecke V. Lichen sclerosus et atrophicus in children. *Am J Dis Child* 1991;145:1058.
72. Parks G, Growdon WA, Mason GD, et al. Childhood anogenital lichen sclerosus. *J Reprod Med* 1990;191.
73. Ridley CM. Genital lichen sclerosus in childhood and adolescence. *J R Soc Med* 1993;69.
74. Ridley CM. Vulvar disorders. In: Sanfilippo JS. *Pediatric and adolescent gynecology*. Philadelphia: WB Saunders, 1994.
75. Berth-Jones J, Graham-Brown RA, Burns DA. Lichen sclerosus et atrophicus—a review of 15 cases in young girls. *Clin Exp Dermatol* 1991;16:14.
76. Wilkinson EJ, Stone IK. *Atlas of vulvar disease*. Baltimore: Williams & Wilkins, 1995.
77. Dalziel KL, Millard PR, Wojnarowska F. The treatment of vulval lichen sclerosus with a very potent topical steroid (clobetasol propionate 0.05%) cream. *Br J Dermatol* 1991;124:461.
78. Dalziel KL, Wojnarowska F. Long-term control of vulval lichen sclerosus after treatment with a potent topical steroid cream. *J Reprod Med* 1993;38:25.
79. Davis A, Goldstein DP. Treatment of pediatric lichen sclerosus with the CO_2 laser. *Adolesc Pediatr Gynecol* 1989;2:71.

80. Pokorny S, Pokorny W, Kramer W. Acute genital injury in the prepubertal girl. *Am J Obstet Gynecol* 1992;166:1461.
81. Hostetler BR, Muram D, Jones CE. Capillary hemangiomas of the vulva mistaken for sexual abuse. *J Pediatr Adolesc Gynecol* 1994;7:44.
82. Hostetler BR, Muram D, Jones CE. Sharp penetrating injury to the hymen. *J Adolesc Pediatr Gynecol* 1994;7:94.
83. Perlman SE, Hertweck SP, Wolfe WM. Water-ski douche injury in a premenarcheal female. *Pediatrics* 1995;96;782.
84. Heller ME, Dewhurst J, Grant DB. Premature menarche without other evidence of precocious puberty. *Arch Dis Child* 1979;54:472.
85. Heller ME, Savage MO, Dewhurst J. Vaginal bleeding in childhood: a review of 51 patients. *Br J Obstet Gynaecol* 1970;85:721.
86. Mercer LJ, Mueller CM, Hajj SN. Medical treatment of urethral prolapse in the premenarchal female. *Adolesc Pediatr Gynecol* 1988;1:181.
87. Capraro VJ, Bayonet MP, Magoss I. Vulvar tumors in children due to prolapse of urethral mucosa. *Am J Obstet Gynecol* 1970;108:572.
88. Owens SB, Morse WH. Prolapse of the female urethra in children. *J Urol* 1968;100:171.
89. Fernandes ET, Dekermacher S, Sabadin MA, Vaz F. Urethral prolapse in children. *Urology* 1993;41: 240–242.
90. Copeland LJ, Gershenson DM, Saul PB, et al. Sarcoma botryoides of the female genital tract. *Obstet Gynecol* 1985;66:262.
91. Hendren WH, Lillehei CS. Pediatric surgery. *N Engl J Med* 1988;319:86.
92. Hicks ML, Piver MS. Conservative surgery plus adjuvant therapy for vulvovaginal rhabdomyosarcoma, diethylstilbestrol clear cell adenocarcinoma of the vagina, and unilateral germ cell tumors of the ovary. *Obstet Gynecol* 1992;19:219.
93. Raney RB, Gehan EA, Hays DM, et al. Primary chemotherapy with or without radiation therapy and/or surgery for children with localized sarcoma of the bladder, prostate, vagina, uterus, and cervix. *Cancer* 1990;2072.
94. Klee LW, Rink RC, Gleason PE, et al. Urethral polyp presenting as interlabial mass in young girls. *Urology* 1993;41:132.
95. Nussbaum AR, Lebowitz RL. Interlabial masses in little girls: review and imaging recommendations. *AJR* 1983;141:65.
96. Bayatpour M, McCann J, Harris T, Phelps H. Neonatal genital prolapse. *Pediatrics* 1992;90:465.
97. Bayatpour M, McCann J, Harris T, Phelps H. Neonatal genital prolapse [Letter]. *Pediatrics* 1993;91: 854.
98. Griebel ML, Redman JF, Kemp SF, Elders MJ. Hypertrophy of clitoral hood: presenting sign of neurofibromatosis in female child. *Urology* 1991;37:337.
99. Nonomura K, Kanno T, Tanaka M, et al. A case of neurofibromatosis associated with clitoral enlargement and hypertension. *J Pediatr Surg* 1992;27:110.
100. Brock JW 3rd, Morgan W, Anderson TL. Congenital hemangiopericytoma of the clitoris. *J Urol* 1995;153:468.
101. Bond SJ, Seibel N, Kapur S, Newman KD. Rhabdomyosarcoma of the clitoris. *Cancer* 1994;73: 1984.
102. Press S, Schachner L, Paul P. Clitoris tourniquet syndrome. *Pediatrics* 1980;66:781.
103. Williams DL, Bell BA, Ragab AH. Clitorism at presentation of acute nonlymphocytic leukemia. *J Pediatr* 1985;107:754.
104. Berkowitz CD, Elvik SL, Logan MK. Labial fusion in prepubescent girls: a marker for sexual abuse? *Am J Obstet Gynecol* 1987;156:16.
105. McCann J, Voris J, Simon M. Labial adhesions and posterior fourchette injuries in childhood sexual abuse. Am J Dis Child 1988;142:659.
106. Ariberg A. Topical oestrogen therapy for labial adhesions in children. *Br J Obstet Gynaecol* 1975; 82:424.

Further Reading

AAP Committee on Infections Diseases. Peter G, ed. *1997 red book*. 24th ed., Elk Grove IL: AAP, 1997.

4

The Physiology of Puberty

Puberty is the natural life transition from childhood to adulthood. Change can be stressful, and puberty is no exception. As a young woman proceeds through this time of change she, her parents, guardians, or teachers may have questions about what is normal and what is abnormal. In order to gain the needed information, she may approach the family pediatrician, gynecologist, or other health care provider. An understanding of the physiology of puberty and menarche is essential for all health care providers so that they can dispense accurate information and help dispel myths. Once normal development is understood, the foundation is set for the diagnosis and management of precocious puberty (see Chapter 5), menstrual abnormalities (see Chapter 6), and other growth problems (see Chapter 19) of the adolescent.

HORMONAL CHANGES AT PUBERTY

Normal female pubertal development requires an elaborate orchestration of the hypothalamic–pituitary–gonadal axis. The physical signs of puberty in girls are an acceleration of growth and the appearance of secondary sex characteristics. Before the visible signs of puberty appear, hormonal changes result from the activation of the hypothalamic pituitary unit and the secretion of sex steroids from the ovary. The hypothalamus is responsible for the synthesis and release of gonadotropin-releasing hormone (GnRH), historically referred to as luteinizing hormone–releasing hormone (LHRH) (Fig. 1). GnRH is a decapeptide with a serum half-life of 2 to 4 minutes and is released in a pulsatile fashion into the pituitary portal plexus. Higher cortical centers and the limbic system influence the synthesis and secretion of GnRH. In addition, neurotransmitters, sex steroids, and gonadal peptides also affect the synthesis and secretion of GnRH. This hormone binds to surface receptors on anterior pituitary gonadotrophs, which synthesize and store the glycoprotein gonadotropins: follicle-stimulating hormone (FSH) and luteinizing hormone (LH). Pulses of electric activity have been recorded from the hypothalamus coincident with LH pulses (1). The pulsatile GnRH stimulation results in a pulsatile secretion of

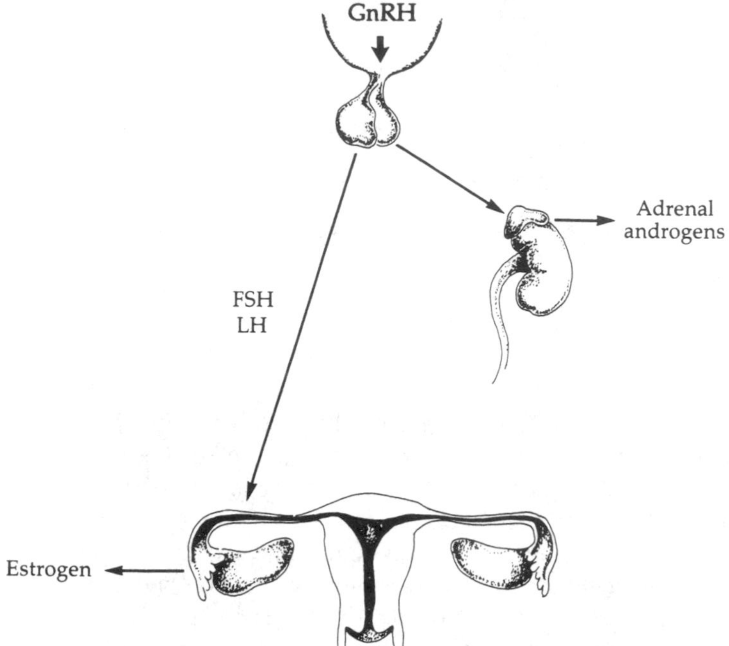

FIG. 1. Hormones responsible for the onset of puberty. GnRH, gonadotropin releasing hormone; FSH, follicle-stimulating hormone; LH, luteinizing hormone. The stimulus for the rise in adrenal adrogens is unclear.

gonadotropins, as has been demonstrated by pulsatile versus continuous administration of GnRH to oophorectomized rhesus monkeys (Fig. 2) (2). The pulsatile release of gonadotropins is thus responsible for the stimulation of the ovary and the resultant maturation of the germinal epithelium and synthesis of gonadal steroid hormones.

Sex steroids are produced in the ovarian follicles and the thecal component of the ovary. In addition, the ovary produces insulin-like growth factor (IGF), inhibin, activin, and cytokines. These ovarian products exert a feedback effect upon gonadotropin secretion (Fig. 3). The feedback occurs both at the level of the hypothalamus, modulating the frequency and amplitude of GnRH release, and at the level of the pituitary, affecting the amount of LH and FSH released in response to the GnRH pulses. Estrogen from the ovary suppresses gonadotropin secretion by negative feedback. Although both FSH and LH are released in pulses, the pulses of LH are recognizable by minute-to-minute serum measurements, as the half-life of LH is approximately 30 minutes compared with the 300-minute half-life of FSH.

The hypothalamic–pituitary–ovarian system is remarkably well developed at the time of birth. In fact, the hypothalamic portal system is intact by 14 weeks

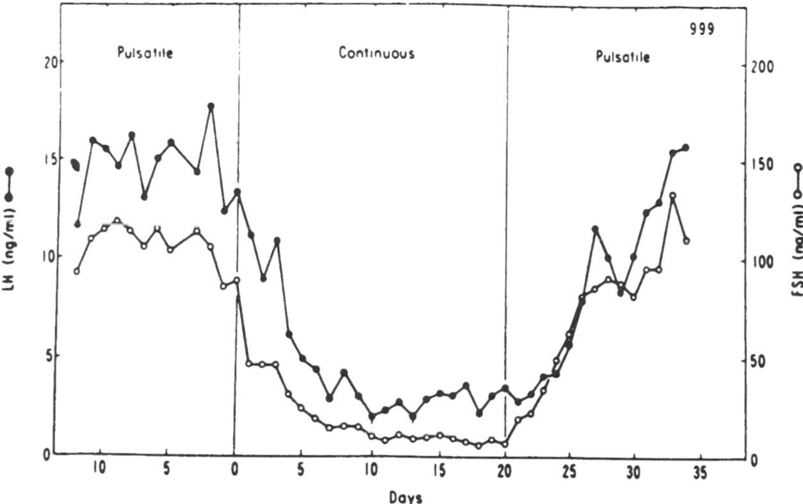

FIG. 2. Effect of pulsatile administration of luteinizing hormone releasing hormone (LHRH) in contrast to continuous infusion of LHRH in adult oophorectomized rhesus monkeys in which gonadotropin secretion has been abolished by lesions that ablated the medial basal hypothalamic LHRH pulse generator. Note the high concentrations of plasma luteinizing hormone (LH) and follicle-stimulating hormone (FSH) in monkeys given one LHRH pulse per hour, the suppression of gonadotropin secretion by continuous infusion of LHRH even though the total dose of LHRH was the same, and the restoration of FSH and LH secretion when the pulsatile mode of LHRH administration was reinitiated. (From Belcheltz PE, Plant TM, Nakai Y, et al. Hypophysial responses to continuous and intermittent delivery of hypothalamic gonadotropin releasing hormone. *Science* 1978;202:631–633; with permission.)

of gestation. The negative feedback effect of gonadal steroids on the hypothalamus and pituitary is apparent by midgestation. The production of gonadotropins and ovarian sex steroids is important in stimulating germ cell division and follicular development. By 5 to 6 months of gestation, 6 to 7 million oocytes are present, and through the process of atresia, the neonate has approximately 1 to 2 million at birth; by puberty only 0.3 to 0.5 million oocytes remain (Fig. 4) (3). By 5 days after birth, gonadotropin levels rise sharply to levels considerably higher than those found in the prepubertal child, probably in response to the fall in placental estrogen (Fig. 4). A transient rise in plasma estradiol is apparent in female infants, especially during the first 3 months of life. Preantral and antral follicles are seen in the ovary. Thereafter, gonadotropin levels gradually fall to prepubertal levels, although FSH levels may not be maximally suppressed for 1 to 4 years. Girls have an elevated FSH/LH ratio compared with boys (4).

During the prepubertal childhood years, there is a downregulation of the hypothalamic–pituitary system, with reduction of the amplitude and frequency of GnRH pulses (Fig. 5) and a decreased pituitary responsiveness to a GnRH stimulation test (single 2.5–mg/kg IV dose of native GnRH) (5). Table 1 (6) shows the method and Fig. 6 the normal adult response to GnRH stimulation testing. Figure

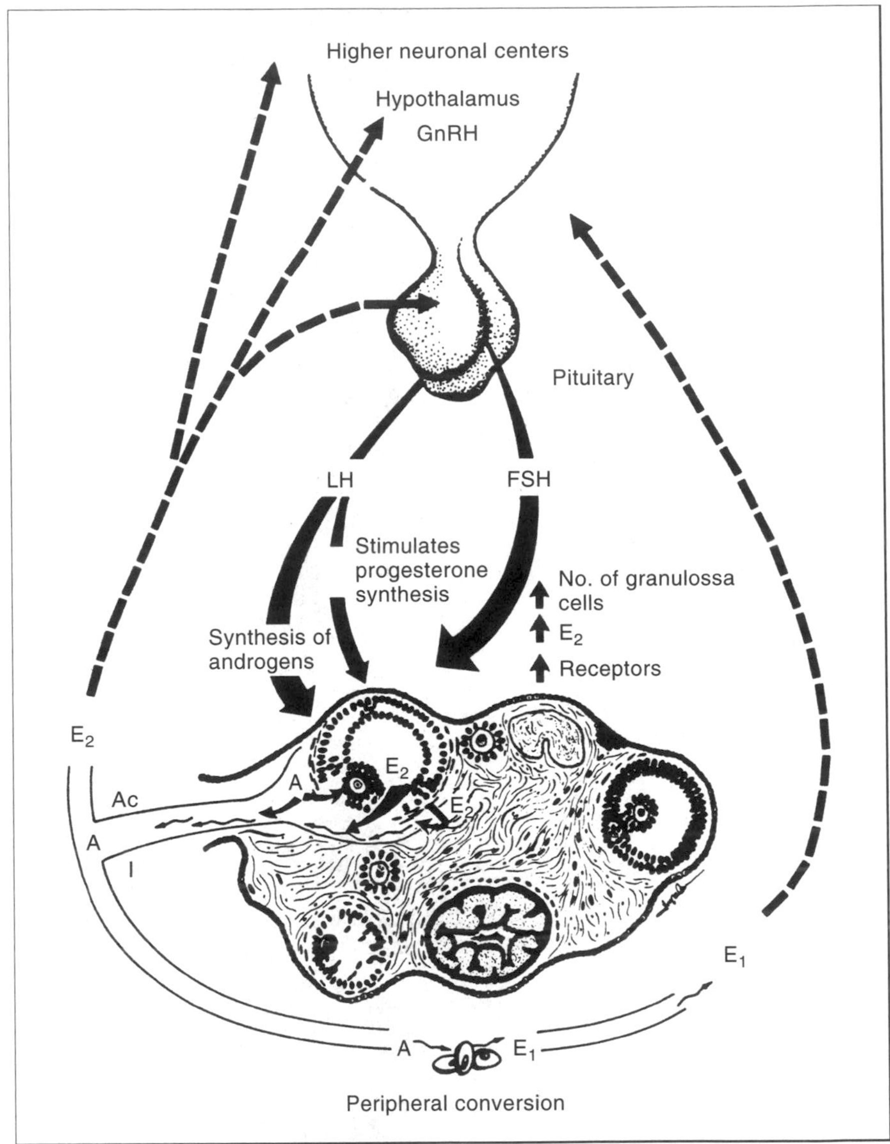

FIG. 3. Hypothalamic-pituitary-ovarian axis interaction in the regulation of follicular maturation and steroid biosynthesis. GnRH, gonadotropin releasing hormone; LH, luteinizing hormone; FSH, follicle-stimulating hormone; E2, estradiol; A, androstenedione; E1, estrone; I, inhibin; Ac, activin. The ovary shows the various stages of growth of the follicle and the formation and regression of the corpus luteum.

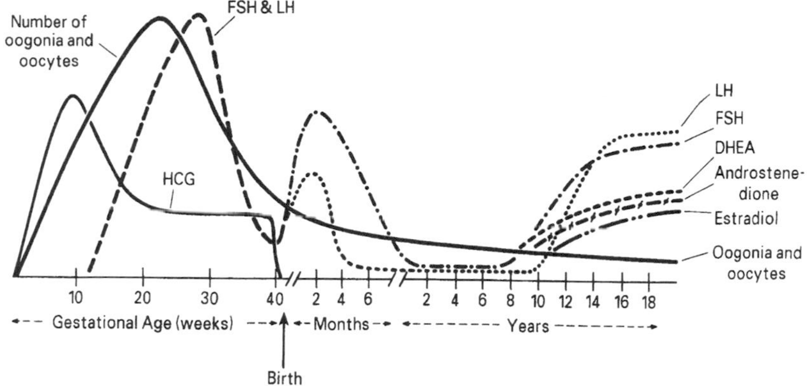

FIG. 4. Variations in number of oogonia and oocytes, and fluctuations in levels of hormones throughout gestational, neonatal, childhood, pubertal, adolescent, and adult life. DHEA, dehydroepiandrosterone; FSH, follicle-stimulating hormone; HCG, human chorionic gonadotropin; LH, luteinizing hormone. (Adapted from Speroff L, Glass RH, Kase NG. *Clinical gynecologic endocrinology and infertility*, 5th ed. Baltimore: Williams & Wilkins, 1994.)

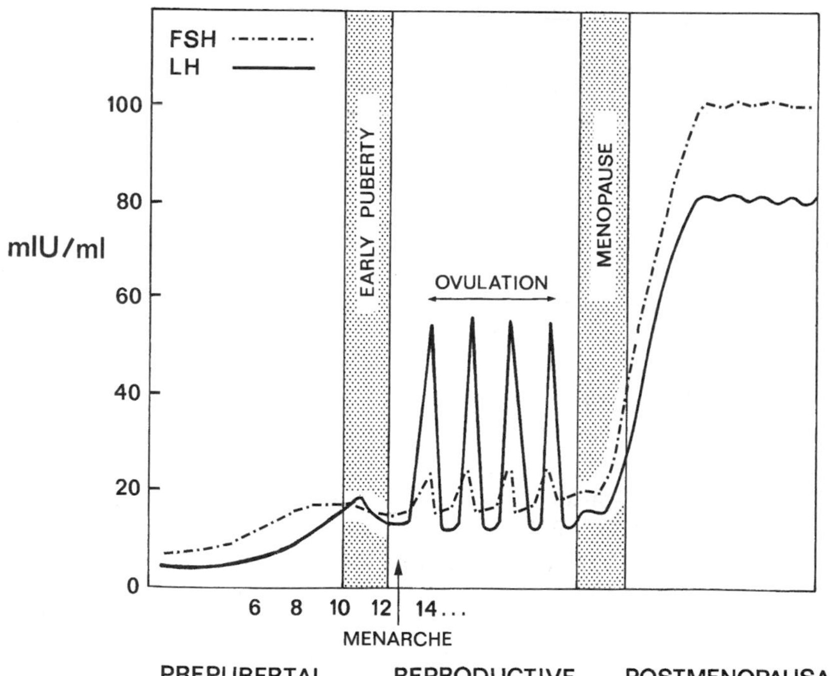

FIG. 5. Gonadotropin levels from the age of 6 years to menopause. FSH, follicle-stimulating hormone; LH, luteinizing hormone.

TABLE 1. *Normal responses to luteinizing hormone (LH) in adult women following Factrel administration in the early follicular phase (days 1–7) of the menstrual cycle*

Subcutaneous administration
- LH peak: mean 67.9 ± 27.5 mIU/ml
  - 100% ≥ 12.5 mIU/ml
  - 90% ≥ 39.0 mIU/ml
- Maximum LH increase: mean 52.8 ± 26.4 mIU/ml
  - 100% ≥ 7.5 mIU/ml
  - 90% ≥ 23.8 mIU/ml
- LH % response: mean 374 ± 221%, range 108–981%
  - 90% ≥ 185%
- Time to peak: mean 71.5 ± 49.6 min

Intravenous administration[a]
- LH peak: mean 57.6 ± 36.7 mIU/ml
  - 100% ≥ 20.0 mIU/ml
  - 90% ≥ 24.6 mIU/ml
- Maximum LH increase: mean 44.5 ± 31.8 mIU/ml
  - 100% ≥ 7.5 mIU/ml
  - 90% ≥ 16.2 mIU/ml
- LH % response: mean 356 ± 282%; range 60–1300%
  - 90% ≥ 142%
- Time to peak: mean 36 ± 24 min

[a]The results are based on 31 tests in women between the ages of 20 and 35 years, inclusive.
LH peak (mIU/mL) = highest LH value after Factrel administration.
Maximum increase (mIU/mL) = peak LH value − LH baseline value.

$$\text{LH \% response} = \left(\frac{\text{peak LH} - \text{baseline LH}}{\text{baseline LH}}\right) \times 100\%$$

Time to peak (minutes) = time required to reach LH peak value.
(Adapted from Ayerst Laboratories, Inc., Factrel (gonadorelin hydrochloride) package insert. New York, 1990.)

7 shows a prepubertal versus a pubertal response to GnRH stimulation testing. This inactivity appears to be in response to a central nervous system signal, since it occurs even in agonadal patients (7). For example, levels of FSH and LH in Turner's syndrome, which are markedly elevated in the neonatal period, are suppressed between the ages of 4 and 10 years, although the mean levels are higher than in normal children of similar ages. In some agonadal children between the ages of 5 and 11 years, basal levels of LH and FSH and responses to GnRH are comparable to those in normal prepubertal children; this similarity precludes a definitive diagnosis of gonadal failure by hormonal tests alone at this age (8).

In prepubertal girls, GnRH pulses continue to persist at low levels with enhancement during sleep, and the FSH/LH ratio is higher than in earlier or later stages. Prepubertal girls often show very little LH response to a single dose of GnRH but a considerable rise in FSH; however, if GnRH is administered in a physiologic manner over the course of time, the pituitary is then "primed" and capable of a pubertal response.

The ovary increases in size during the prepubertal years and demonstrates evidence of active follicular growth and atresia. The vagina, which is approximately 4 cm long at birth, grows only 0.5 to 1.0 cm during early childhood but increases in length to 7.0 to 8.5 cm in late childhood. The uterus is about 2.5 cm long in infancy. The corpus/cervix ratio is slightly <1:1; it reaches 1:1 at menarche and the adult ratio of 3:1 postmenarcheally.

An early change associated with pubertal maturation is the secretion of adrenal androgens—dehydroepiandrosterone (DHEA), its sulfate (DHEAS), and androstenedione—between the ages of 6 and 8 years. Termed *adrenarche*, this process involves the regrowth of the zona reticularis (the zone that was large in the fetal adrenal cortex and regressed after birth) of the adrenal cortex with increases in activity of the microsomal enzyme p450c17. Adrenal androgens continue to rise through ages 13 to 15 years and are primarily responsible for the appearance of pubic and axillary hair in girls (*pubarche*) (9,10). Acne vulgaris may be an early sign of puberty, resulting from rising levels of DHEAS (11,12). The ovarian androgens, androstenedione and testosterone, also stimulate growth of pubic and axillary hair.

At approximately 8 years of age or thereafter, although no physical changes are present, GnRH secretion is enhanced, at first during sleep (13). There is a resultant increase in pituitary responsiveness and increased secretion of LH and FSH (see Fig. 5) (14). Luteinizing hormone and responsiveness to exogenous GnRH testing also increase at this time and allow differentiation between a pubertal and prepubertal pattern (Fig. 7). It also appears that the increase in LH bioactivity at puberty exceeds the changes seen in studies that examine the more commonly used

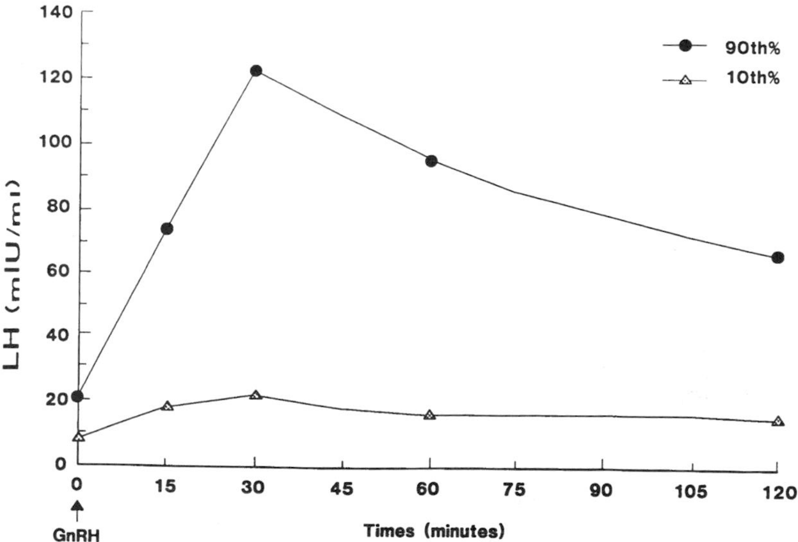

FIG. 6. Normal response of luteinizing hormone (LH) to exogenous gonadotropin-releasing hormone (GnRH). (Adapted from Ayerst Laboratories Inc., Factrel (gonadorelin hydrochloride) package insert. New York: 1990.)

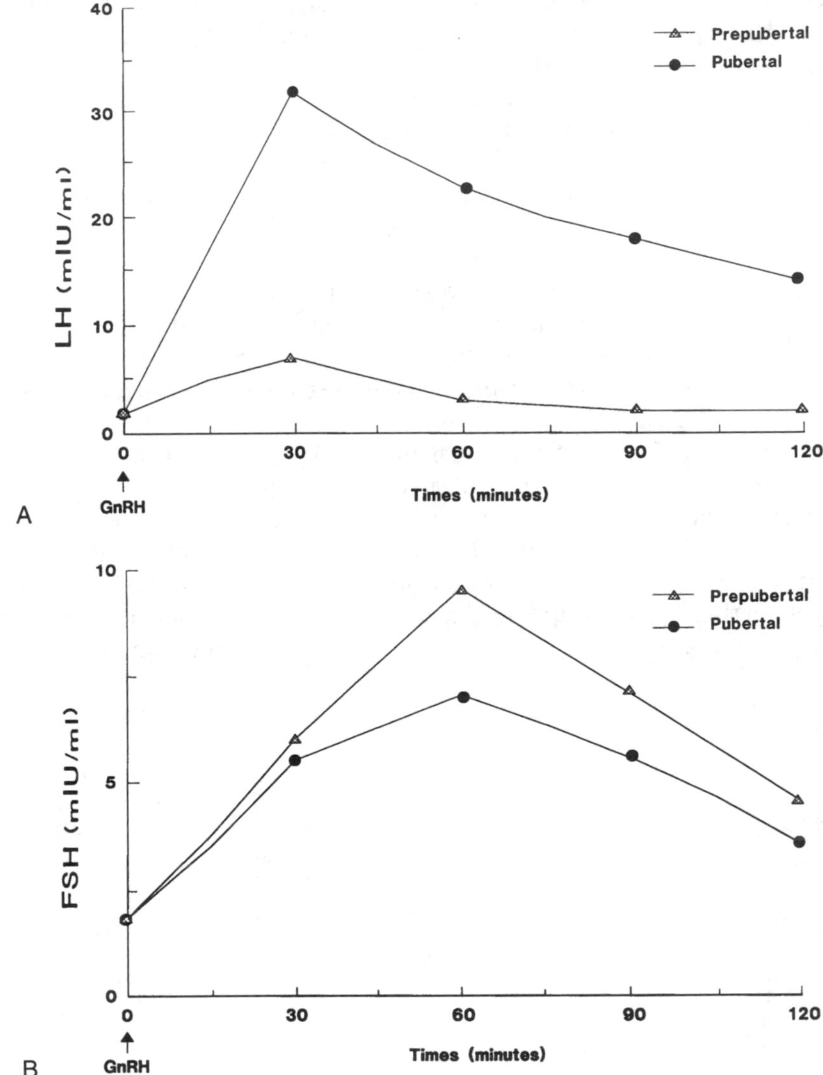

FIG. 7. Serum luteinizing hormone (LH) **(A)** and follicle-stimulating hormone (FSH) **(B)** responses as measured following an intravenous bolus of gonatropin-releasing hormone in prepubertal and pubertal girls.

radioimmunoassay. Lucky and associates (15) found that bioactive LH increased 23.1-fold, while immunoreactive LH increased only 4-fold during puberty, which suggests a role of the pituitary in controlling the maturational process of puberty.

The age-related rise in gonadotropins with an initial sleep enhancement also occurs in patients with Turner's syndrome, and menopausal levels of LH and FSH pulses occur at this time (7). It does not appear that ovarian sex steroids play a critical role in the onset of puberty, since patients with Turner's syndrome experience adrenarche (the rise of adrenal androgens) and an age-related rise in gonadotropins. Prepubertal patients with Addison's disease can experience normal *gonadarche* (the activation of the hypothalamic–pituitary–ovarian axis) but not adrenarche. Patients in whom precocious puberty begins before age 6 typically exhibit gonadarche but not adrenarche. Patients with constitutional delay of puberty frequently have delays of both adrenarche and gonadarche (16). Sex steroids are important for the development of functional feedback mechanisms (4).

During late prepuberty and early puberty, there is a gradual augmentation of episodic peaks of LH and FSH during sleep. The onset of puberty is associated with a greater increase in LH pulse amplitude than frequency (17). There is a gradual increase in daytime pulsatility. LH pulsatility is GnRH dependent at all ages, while there is a decrease in GnRH regulation of FSH pulsatility as there is an increase in ovarian activity (18). Luteinizing hormone stimulates the theca interna cells of the ovary to synthesize precursors, and FSH increases the enzyme aromatase, which is responsible for the conversion of androgen precursors to estrogen. Estrogen peaks 10 to 12 hours after the gonadotropin secretion

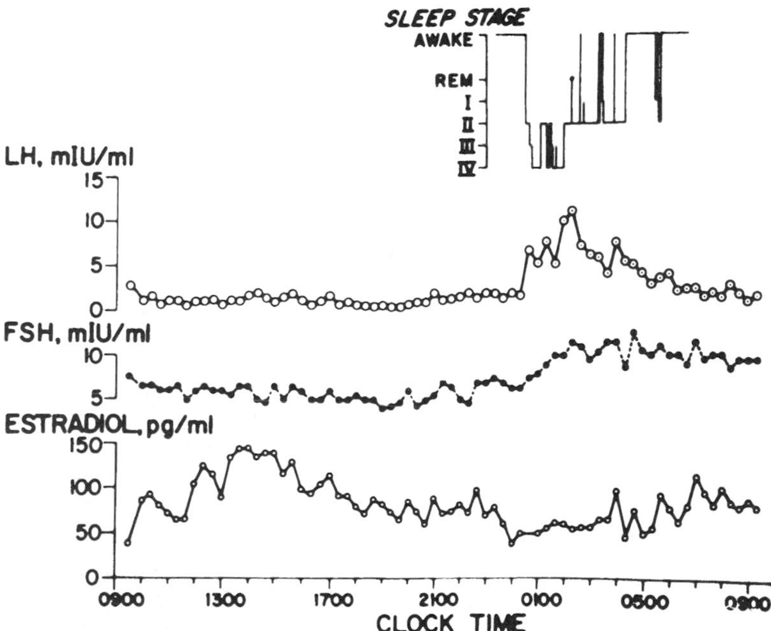

FIG. 8. LH, FSH, and estradiol levels in a premenarcheal girl, 13 7/12 years old (Tanner stage 3), showing a rise in LH and FSH during sleep and a rise in plasma estradiol during the afternoon. LH, luteinizing hormone; FSH, follicle-stimulating hormone. (From Boyar RM, Wu RH, Roffwarg H, et al. Human puberty: 24-hour estradiol patterns in pubertal girls. *J Clin Endocrinol Metab* 1976;43:1418.)

(Fig. 8) (14). In addition, inhibin, activin, and follistatin interact in this complex regulatory system. These peptides are secreted in the highest levels by the gonads and act to increase (activin) or decrease (inhibin and follistatin) FSH biosynthesis and secretion at the level of the pituitary. They also act locally in the gonad, affecting steroid biosynthesis and gametogenesis (19–22). During puberty, inhibin levels increase in a manner corresponding to the pubertal stage and sex steroid production (19). Circulating levels of follistatin are not found to change during puberty, but they increase with the establishment of regular menstrual cycles (21). The ovaries are marked by increased follicular growth and on ultrasonography may appear as "enlarged and multicystic" ovaries. As puberty progresses, the ovaries amplify the gonadotropin message and release greater amounts of sex steroids for a given amount of gonadotropins.

Breast budding, estrogenization of the vaginal mucosa, and lengthening and enlargement of the uterus occur with estrogen exposure. The physiologic vaginal discharge of puberty, leukorrhea, is the desquamation of epithelial cells and mucus from the estrogenized mucosa. The pubertal process is accompanied by a growth spurt; both growth hormone and sex steroids appear to contribute to the growth spurt. The levels of growth hormone and IGF-1 (previously termed somatomedin-C) increase during puberty as estrogen levels rise (23–26). The effect of estrogen on growth hormone and growth is dose related; low doses of estrogen stimulate growth, growth hormone, and IGF-1, while high doses of estrogen decrease them. This observation has led to the use of large pharmacologic doses of estrogen in an attempt to diminish final adult height in girls who are predicted to have excessively tall stature. In contrast, low doses of estrogen replacement in hypogonadal patients result in increased IGF-1 levels and growth. Since bone age, as determined by the Greulich and Pyle standards (27), correlates best with pubertal age, when an individual with delayed or advanced puberty is evaluated, it is important to obtain a radiograph of the wrist and hand for bone age interpretation. An increase in weight accompanies the growth spurt in normal girls, and body composition changes through late childhood and adolescence with a particularly apparent increase in percentage of body fat.

As puberty progresses, the levels of FSH and LH reached at night are gradually carried over into the waking hours until the sleep augmentation disappears. Even before menarche, circulating estrogen concentrations in pubertal girls have some cyclicity; eventually, these periodic fluctuations are sufficient to result in uterine bleeding. The first 1 to 2 years following menarche are often characterized by anovulatory menses (28–33). This time period coincides with the rapid growth of the uterus, vagina, fallopian tubes, and ovaries. With maturation, a mechanism known as the biphasic positive feedback system develops; in this system, a rise in plasma estrogen during the latter part of the follicular phase of the menstrual cycle triggers the surge of LH and FSH, which is responsible for ovulation. Historically, the change in the sensitivity of the feedback system was demonstrated by the use of clomiphene citrate, a nonsteroidal, agonist–antagonist estrogen, which when administered to prepubertal and early pubertal girls caused further suppression of gonadotropin levels (34–36). However, in late pubertal adolescents and adults, clomiphene causes a rise in gonadotropin levels and ovulation, a property that makes it useful as a fertility drug. It is noteworthy that this test is no longer used to determine the normal pubertal status, but the clomiphene challenge test is now used as a predictor of ovarian reserve for women desiring to conceive (37).

STAGES OF BREAST AND PUBIC HAIR DEVELOPMENT

In 1969, Marshall and Tanner (38) recorded the rates of progress of pubertal development of 192 English schoolgirls. These stages can be important guidelines in assessing whether an adolescent is developing normally. The Tanner stages—also termed Sexual Maturity Rating (SMR)—for breast development are as follows (Fig. 9) (38,39):

Stage B1 (preadolescent): elevation of the papilla only.
Stage B2 (breast bud stage): elevation of the breast and papilla as a small mound, enlargement of the areolar diameter.
Stage B3: further enlargement of the breast and areola with no separation of their contours.
Stage B4: further enlargement with projection of the areola and papilla to form a secondary mound above the level of the breast.
Stage B5 (mature stage): projection of the papilla only, resulting from recession of the areola to the general contour of the breast.

The pubic hair stages are as follows (Fig. 10) (38,39):

Stage PH1 (preadolescent): the vellus over the pubes is not further developed than that over the anterior abdominal wall; no pubic hair.

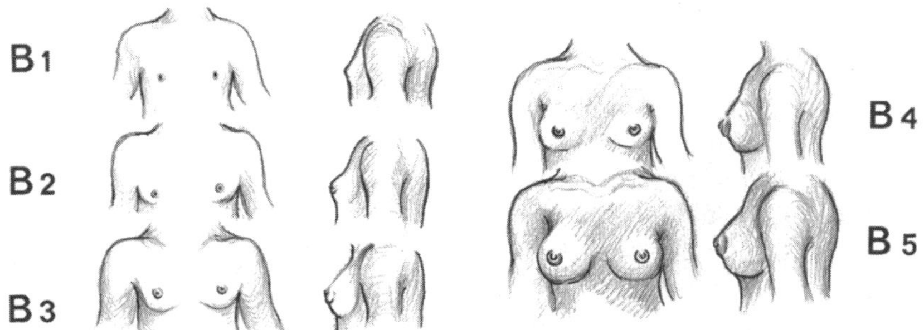

FIG. 9. The Tanner stages of human breast development. (Adapted from Grumbach MM, Styne DM. Puberty: ontogeny, neuroendocrinology, physiology, and disorders. In: Wilson JD, Foster DW, eds. *Williams textbook of endocrinology*, 8th ed. Philadelphia: WB Saunders, 1992; and from Marshall WA, Tanner JM. Variations in pattern of pubertal changes in girls. *Arch Dis Child* 1969;44:291.)

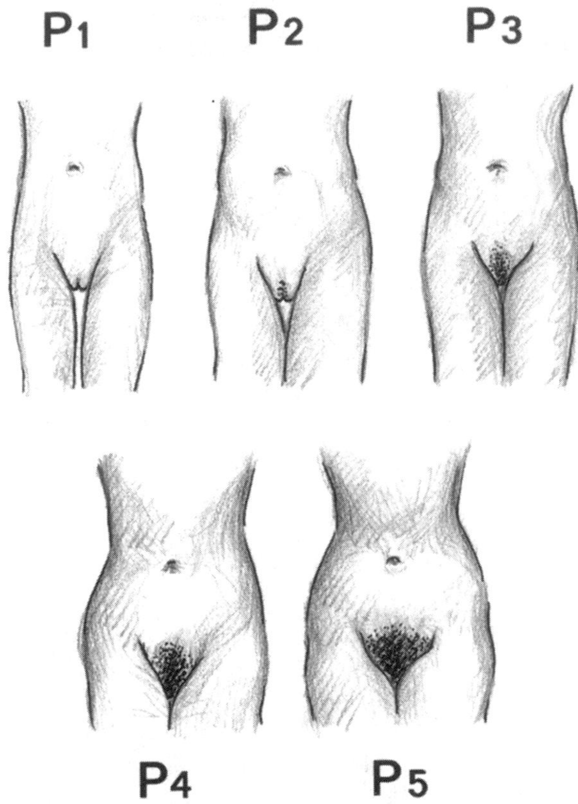

FIG. 10. The Tanner stages for the development of female pubic hair. (Adapted from Grumbach MM, Styne DM. Puberty: ontogeny, neuroendocrinology, physiology, and disorders. In: Wilson JD, Foster DW, eds. *Williams textbook of endocrinology*, 8th ed. Philadelphia: WB Saunders, 1992; and from Marshall WA, Tanner JM. Variations in pattern of pubertal changes in girls. *Arch Dis Child* 1969;44:291.)

Stage PH2: sparse growth of long, slightly pigmented, downy hair, straight or only slightly curled, appearing chiefly along the labia.

Stage PH3: hair darker, coarser, and curlier; spreads to extend sparsely over the junction of the pubes.

Stage PH4: hair adult in type; spreads over the mons pubis but not to the medial surface of the thighs.

Stage PH5 (mature stage): hair adult in quantity and type; spreads to the medial surfaces of the thighs; distribution in an inverse triangle forms the classic feminine pattern.

The mean age of each stage of puberty for British girls is shown in Figs. 11 and 12 (38). The ages of normal sexual development from American data are shown in Table 2 (40).

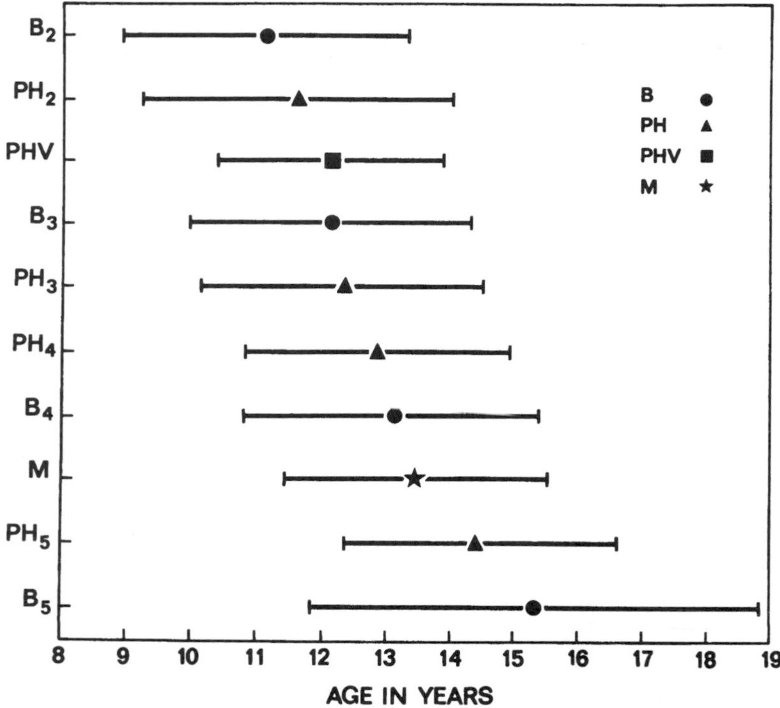

FIG. 11. Mean age at each stage of puberty in English girls. B, breast; PH, pubic hair; M, menarche; PHV, peak height velocity. The center of each symbol represents the mean; the length of the symbol is equivalent to 2 standard deviations on either side of the mean. (Adapted from Marshall WA, Tanner JM. Variations in pattern of pubertal changes in girls. *Arch Dis Child* 1969;44:291.)

The first sign of puberty in 85% to 92% of white girls is breast budding, which may initially be unilateral. Some girls pass from stage B3 directly to stage B5, and some remain in stage B4. Developmental stages are assessed most accurately by observation of sequential changes in an individual girl. In the series of Marshall and Tanner (38), the mean interval from stage B2 to stage B5 was 4.2 years. Pubic hair development usually lags by about 6 months and appears at an average age of 11 to 12 years. Pubic hair as the first sign of development may be a normal variant (especially in those of African-American descent), but in some girls, it may reflect an excess of androgens that later may cause hirsutism and menstrual irregularity (see Chapters 6 and 7). The mean interval from stages PH2 to stage PH5 is 2.7 years. Generally, pubic hair will not advance beyond stage PH2 or PH3 in the absence of gonadal sex steroids. The beginning of breast development usually corresponds to the onset of the growth spurt. The timing of these events is variable, but 98.8% of girls have the first signs of sexual development between the ages of 8 and 13 years. Harlan and associates (41) have

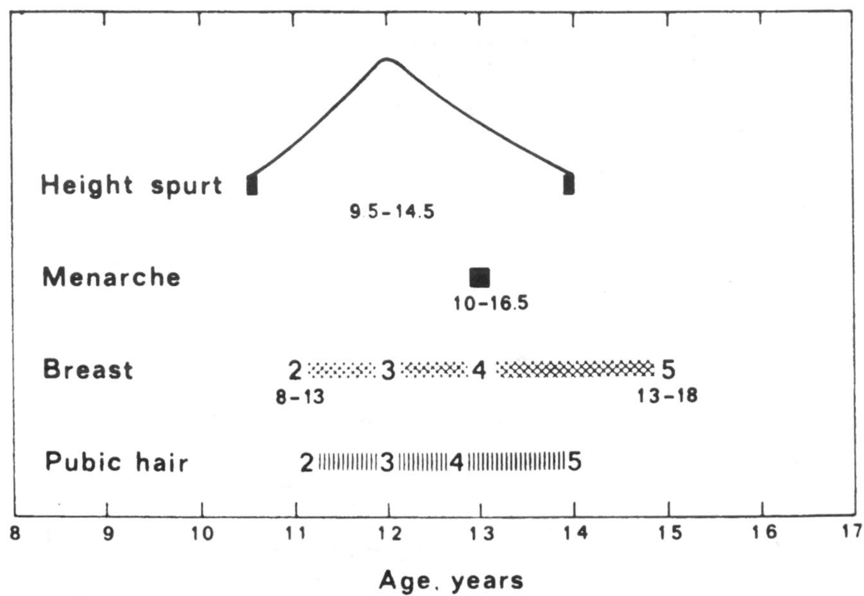

FIG. 12. The sequence of events at puberty in females. (Adapted from Marshall WA, Tanner JM. Variations in pattern of pubertal changes in girls. *Arch Dis Child* 1969;44:291.)

reported a high concordance between breast and pubic hair stage (within one ordinal rank) for both black and white girls, with black girls being consistently more advanced in Tanner stages than white girls for each chronologic age.

Recent data from a large cross-sectional observational study of more than 17,000 girls by community pediatricians noted an even earlier age of pubertal development (42). They noted that among 8- to 9-year-old girls, 7.7% of white girls and 34.3% of African-American girls had Tanner stage 2 or greater pubic hair, and that 5% of white girls and 15.4% of African-American girls had Tan-

TABLE 2. *The mean (±SD) ages of various pubertal events in American adolescents*

Pubertal event (Tanner stage)	Age (yr)
B2	11.2 ± 1.6
PH2	11.9 ± 1.5
B3	12.4 ± 1.2
PH3	12.7 ± 0.5
B4	13.1 ± 0.7
PH4	13.4 ± 1.2
B5	14.5 ± 1.6
PH5	14.6 ± 1.1

(Adapted from Lee PA. Normal ages of pubertal events among American males and females. *J Adolesc Health Care* 1980;1:26-29.)

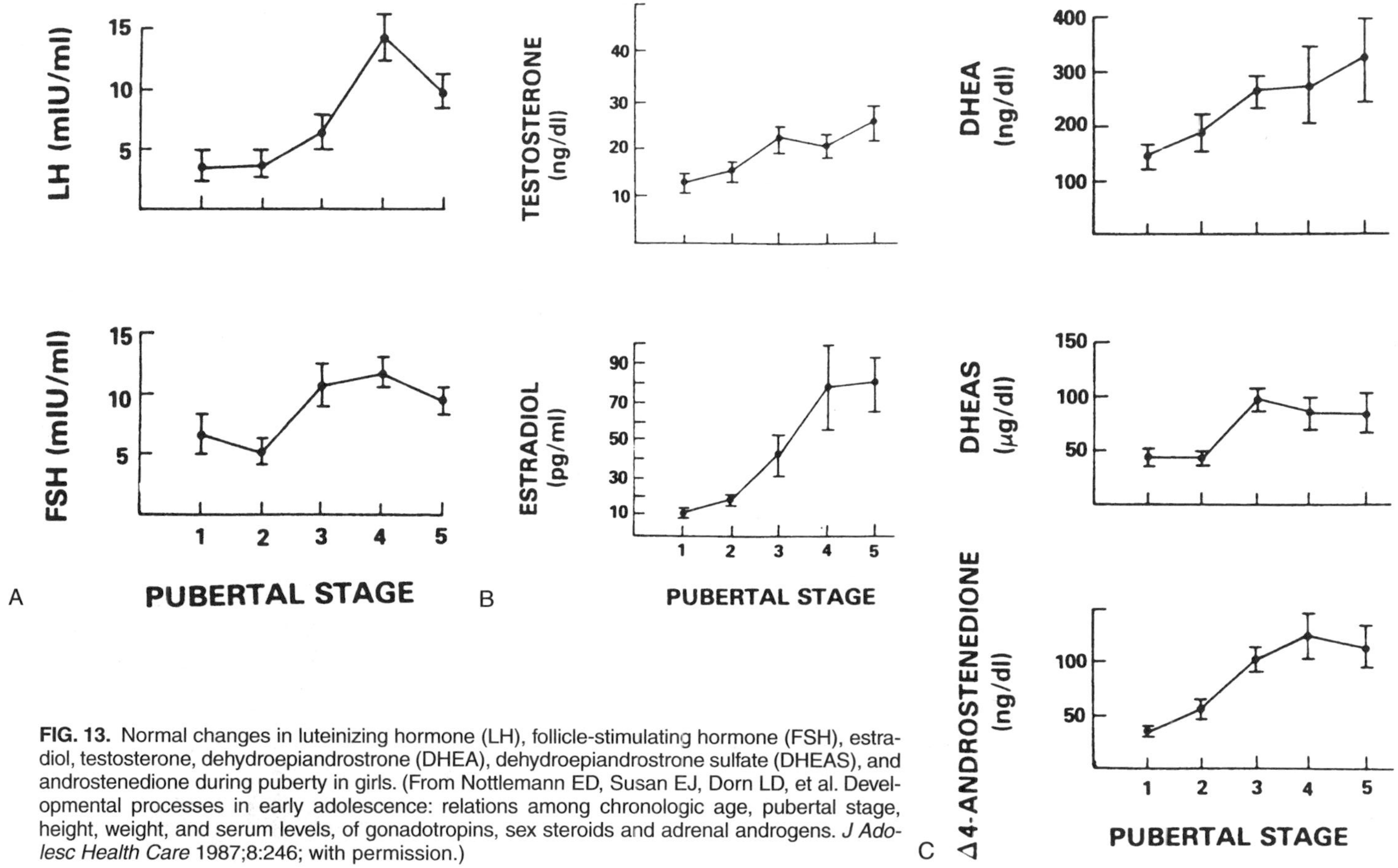

FIG. 13. Normal changes in luteinizing hormone (LH), follicle-stimulating hormone (FSH), estradiol, testosterone, dehydroepiandrostrone (DHEA), dehydroepiandrostrone sulfate (DHEAS), and androstenedione during puberty in girls. (From Nottlemann ED, Susan EJ, Dorn LD, et al. Developmental processes in early adolescence: relations among chronologic age, pubertal stage, height, weight, and serum levels, of gonadotropins, sex steroids and adrenal androgens. *J Adolesc Health Care* 1987;8:246; with permission.)

ner stage 2 or greater breast development. Among girls 12 to 13 years of age, 96% of white girls and 99% of African-American girls had breast development, and 92% of white girls and 99% of African-American girls had pubic hair development. However, it should be noted that Tanner stage 2 breast development may be difficult to identify in obese prepubertal girls, and Biro and colleagues (43) have suggested the utility of the Garn-Falkner system for staging areola. With this system, four areolar stages are identified on the basis of areolar diameter, pigmentation, and contour, with areolar stage 1 being prepubertal. Areolar stage 2 displays palpable subareolar tissue, an increase in size and pigmentation of the areola, and little development of the papilla. Areolar stage 3 has a further increase in size and pigment of the areola, with separation of the areola and papilla from the contour of the breast. Areolar stage 4 has an elevation of the papilla and regression of the areola, with a mature size and color of the areola (not all women develop stage 4). Comparison is made to staging plates. Biro (43) reported that 9 of 15 girls in breast Tanner stage 2 were in areolar stage 1. Thus longitudinal data from the National Heart, Lung, and Blood Institute Growth and Health Study will yield additional information on normal ages of pubertal development in U.S. girls.

Breast development before 8 years of age is generally considered precocious and will require further evaluation (see Chapter 5). A girl who has experienced no breast development by the age of 13 is 2 standard deviations from the norm, has delayed development, and should be evaluated to determine the specific cause of the delay (see Chapter 6). It is also extremely unlikely for a young woman to achieve full stage B5 breast development without pubic hair development; this occurrence raises the question of an androgen insensitivity (testicular feminization) syndrome or adrenal insufficiency (see Chapters 2, 6, and 8). The development of pubic hair without any evidence of breast development suggests the presence of androgens alone and raises the possibility of either estrogen deficiency such as Kallmann's syndrome or a virilized state such as an intersex disorder. The normal changes in LH, FSH, estradiol, testosterone, DHEA, DHEAS, and androstenedione are shown in Fig. 13 (44).

GROWTH PATTERNS

The growth spurt is dependent on the onset of puberty. Growth charts, such as those illustrated in Figs. 14 (45) and 15 (46) are helpful in evaluating normal development. Special growth charts for Turner's syndrome patients (see Chapter 6) can be obtained from Genentech or its representatives.* The inserts (the increment curves) on the charts in Fig. 14 (45) represent velocities, that is, the peak is at the maximum rate of linear growth and weight gain. The peak height velocity is

*Genentech, Inc., 460 Pt Bruno Blvd, San Francisco, CA 94080.

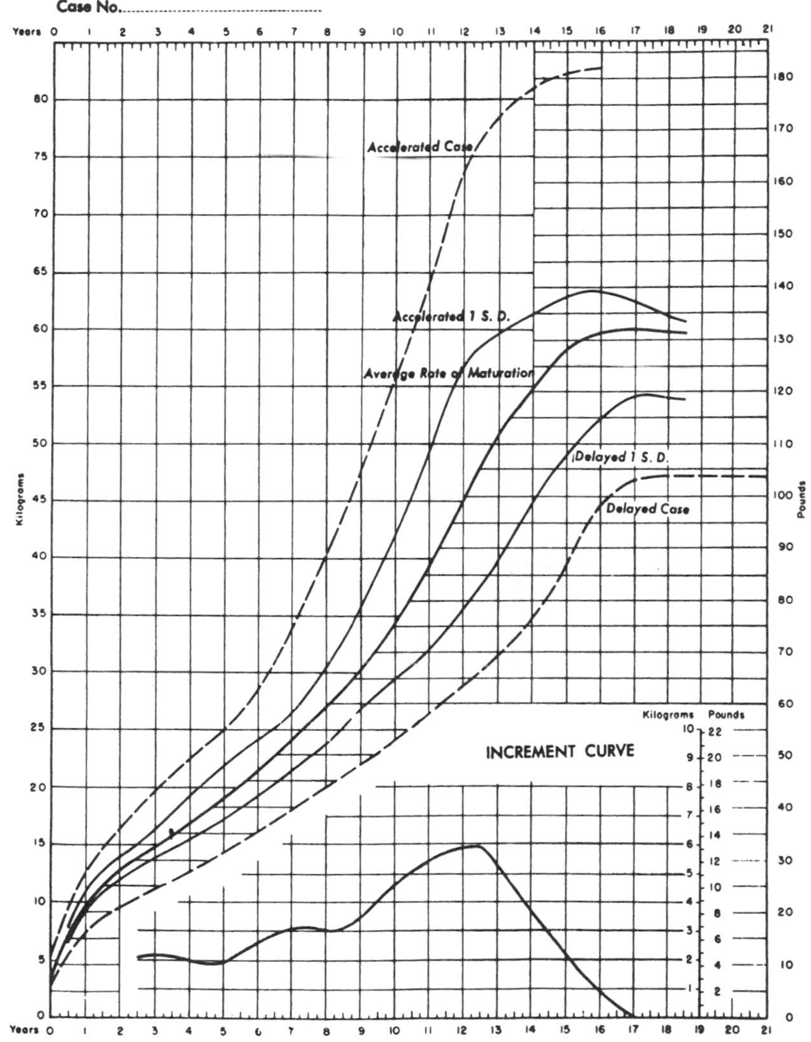

FIG. 14. Growth charts. **(A)** Weight.

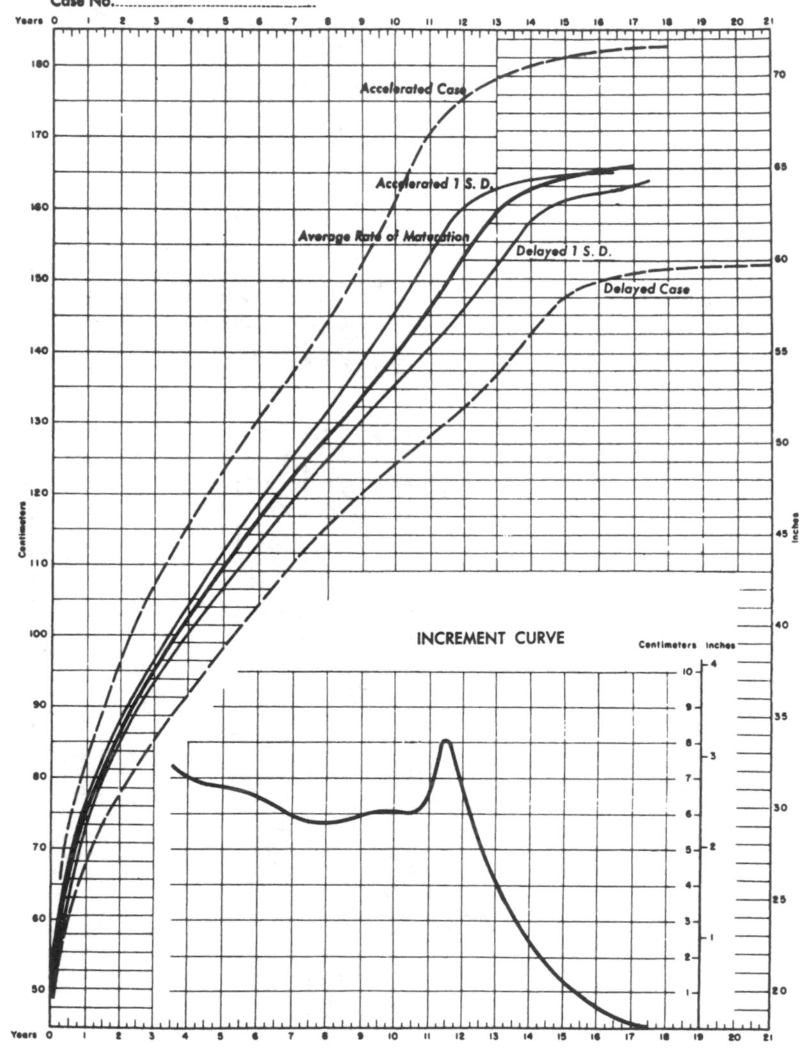

FIG. 14. *Continued.* **(B)** Height. (From Bayley N. Growth curves of height and weight by age for boys and girls, scaled according to physical maturity. *J Pediatr* 1956;48:187.)

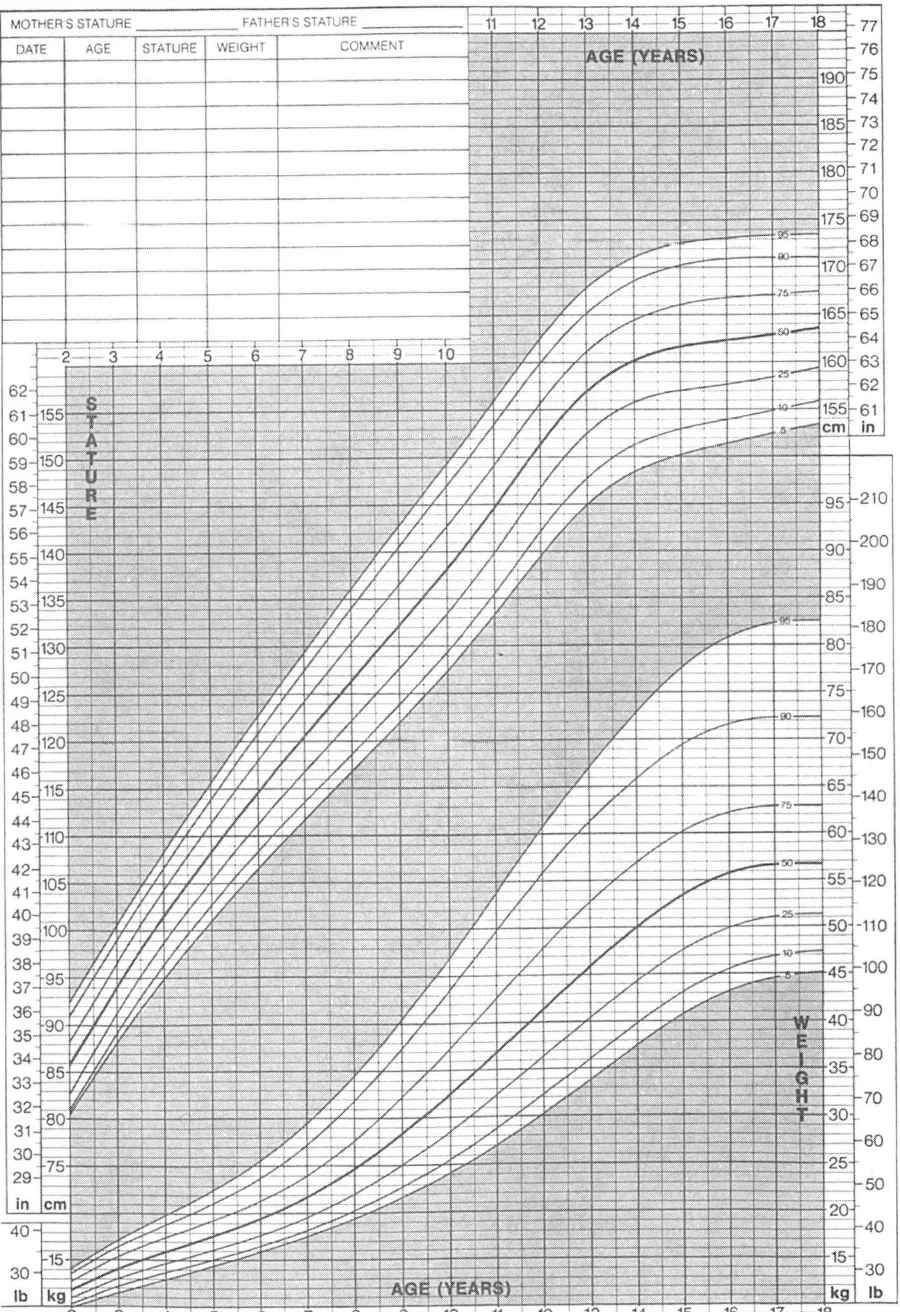

FIG. 15. Growth Chart. Height and weight percentiles. (Adapted from Hamill PVV, et al. Physical growth: National Center for Health Statistics percentiles. *Am J Clin Nutr* 1979;32:607. Data from the National Center for Health Statistics (NCHS), Hyattsville, MD.)

attained in the majority of girls before they reach Tanner stages B3 and PH2. The growth chart in Fig. 15 (46) represents data from the National Center for Health Statistics. Because the data in Fig. 15 (46) are cross-sectional rather than longitudinal, as in Fig. 14 (45), the pubertal growth spurt is not seen clearly on Fig. 15. The average girl grows 2 to 3 inches during the 2 years following menarche.

Skeletal proportions are determined by the rate of pubertal development. The upper/lower (U/L) body ratio is approximately 1.0 by the age of 10 years, L being the distance from the patient's symphysis pubis to the floor, with the patient standing, and U the height minus L. At puberty, the extremities rapidly increase in length, while the vertebral column lengthens more gradually. Initially, the U/L ratio may dip to 0.9. As the epiphyses of the legs close, the vertebrae continue to add height, and thus the final adult U/L ratio approximates 1.0. In patients with hypogonadism, the lower segment becomes relatively longer because of delayed fusion; thus, the U/L ratio may be approximately 0.8. Span (the distance between the fingertips of outstretched arms) usually reflects the same clinical situation; if the span is more than 2 inches greater than the height, the patient has eunuchoid proportions. Athletes who have undergone intensive training during the prepubertal years may have delayed development and menarche, along with delayed epiphyseal closure, and therefore may have arm spans longer than normal.

MENARCHE

The mean age at menarche in Tanner's series in England was 13.46 ± 0.46 years with a range of 9 to 16 years. In a study by Zacharias and Wurtman (28), the mean age of menarche among student nurses in the United States was 12.65 ± 1.2 years. The National Health Examination Survey (29) estimated the median age at menarche to be 12.77 years (12.8 years for white girls and 12.56 for black girls). In a large study, Herman-Giddens reported that by age 12 to 13, 35% of white girls and 62% of African-American girls had initiated menses (42). Table 3 (38) shows that most patients had attained stage 4 breast

TABLE 3. *Percentage of patients in stages 1 through 5 at time of menarche*

Stage	Breast (% of patients)	Pubic hair (% of patients)
1	0	1
2	1	4
3	26	19
4	62	63
5	11	14

(Adapted from WA Marshall and Tanner JM. Variations in pattern of pubertal changes in girls. *Arch Dis Child* 1969;44:291.)

and pubic hair development at the time of menarche. In Tanner's series, the mean interval from breast development to menarche was 2.3 ± 0.1 years, but the range was 0.5 to 5.75 years. A late onset of pubertal development did not appear to change the intervals between the stages of pubic hair and breast development. Frisch (47) established a nomogram predicting the age of menarche based on height and weight at the ages of 9 to 13 years, using her observation that menarche was associated with the attainment of a critical body weight (an average of 46 to 47 kg for American and most European girls), the percentage of body fat being the important determinant. According to this theory, a minimum fatness level of about 17% of body weight is necessary for the onset of menstrual cycles, and a minimum of 22% fat is necessary to maintain regular ovulatory cycles (48). Early- and late-maturing girls begin their adolescent growth spurt with a weight of about 30 kg. The apparent decline in the age of menarche from the late 1800s to the mid-1900s has been attributed to improved nutrition and in the past two decades, the lack of a further age decline is attributed to the attainment of optimal nutrition (49). Gymnasts, ballet dancers, and long-distance runners with reduced weights and (calculated) percentages of body fat often experience significant delays in development and menarche, especially if their training began in the prepubertal years. Since estrogens are also produced by aromatization of androgen precursors in fat, a low percentage of body fat may contribute less estrogen, which is necessary for hypothalamic pituitary regulation and the onset of vaginal bleeding. The theory remains controversial, however, because the secretion of GnRH and gonadotropins begins many years before menarche, percentages of body fat are often only calculated figures, and weight at the time of menarche can show tremendous variation in individual girls. Gonzales and Villena (50) reported that the association of body weight, body mass index, or height with menarche is coincidental instead of critical for menarche.

In a retrospective series, Zacharias and Wurtman (28,51) found that the interval between menarche and regular periods was approximately 14 months, and the interval between menarche and painful (presumably) ovulatory cycles was approximately 24 months. However, ovulatory cycles can begin during the first year following menarche and may be associated with shortened luteal phases. Data from Finland (18) demonstrated that in the first 2 years after menarche, 55% to 82% of cycles were anovulatory (the figure depends on whether only samples drawn <10 days until the next menstrual bleeding or all samples drawn on days 20 to 23 of the menstrual cycle were considered). By 3 years after menarche, the percentage of anovulatory cycles decreased to 50%, and by 5 years to 10% to 20% (9,18). It appears that the later the age of menarche the longer the interval before 50% of cycles are ovulatory. Apter and Vihko (52) found that this interval was 1 year if menarche occurred before the age of 12 years, 3 years when menarche occurred at 12.0 to 12.9 years, and 4.5 years when menarche was after 13 years of age.

HORMONE LEVELS IN NORMAL OVULATORY CYCLES

The establishment of ovulatory cycles depends on the maturation of a positive feedback mechanism in which rising estrogen levels trigger an LH surge at midcycle. Understanding the hormone changes responsible for ovulation allows the health care provider to understand the pathophysiology of polycystic ovary syndrome (see Chapter 7), amenorrhea, and dysfunctional uterine bleeding (see Chapter 6). Figure 3 demonstrates the complex interactions between the changes in the ovary during ovulation and gonadotropins.

The menstrual cycle is divided into a follicular phase, an ovulatory phase, and a luteal phase. In the early follicular phase of the menstrual cycle (Fig. 16), pulsatile GnRH released from the hypothalamus stimulates the secretion of FSH and LH from the pituitary. In turn, FSH increases the number of granulosa cells in the ovarian follicle, increases the number of receptors for FSH on the granulosa cells, and induces the granulosa cells to acquire an aromatizing enzyme that provides the essential step for the conversion of androgen precursors to estradiol. Estradiol also increases the number of granulosa cells and the number of FSH receptors, which thus leads to further amplification of the effect of FSH. The theca cells, under LH stimulation, secrete androstenedione, testosterone, and estradiol into the bloodstream and also into the follicle as substrate. Usually, a single dominant follicle emerges by day 5 to day 7 of the cycle. The rising estradiol level increases the number of glandular cells and stroma in the endometrium of the uterus. By the midfollicular phase, FSH is beginning to decline, in part because of estrogen-mediated negative feedback. Inhibin, which is secreted by granulosa cells and blocks FSH synthesis and release, rises in the late follicular phase of the cycle, paralleling the rise of estradiol. The highest levels are found during the luteal phase and, together with estradiol and progesterone, appear to play a role in the regulation of FSH in that phase of the cycle as well. Serum FSH and inhibin levels are inversely related in the middle to late follicular phase and in the luteal phase (53). Activins, also secreted by the granulosa cells, stimulate FSH secretion. The dominant follicle has the richest blood supply and the most estrogen production and granulosal aromatase. The increased number of FSH receptors on the dominant follicle allows it to continue to respond even as rising estrogen levels lower the FSH. Locally, in the dominant follicle, estradiol levels are greater than androstenedione levels, whereas androstenedione levels are greater than estradiol levels in the atretic follicles.

Crowley's group at the Massachusetts General Hospital (54) has characterized the sleep latency changes in LH that occur during the normal ovulatory menstrual cycle. The LH interpulse interval decreased from a mean of 94 minutes in the early follicular phase to 71 minutes in the late follicular phase, with a change in the mean pulse amplitude from 6.5 mIU/ml in the early follicular phase, to 5.1 mIU/ml in the midfollicular phase, to 7.2 mIU/ml in the late follicular phase. In the luteal phase, the LH pulse interval progressively increased from a mean of 103 minutes in the early luteal phase to 216 minutes in the late luteal phase. The

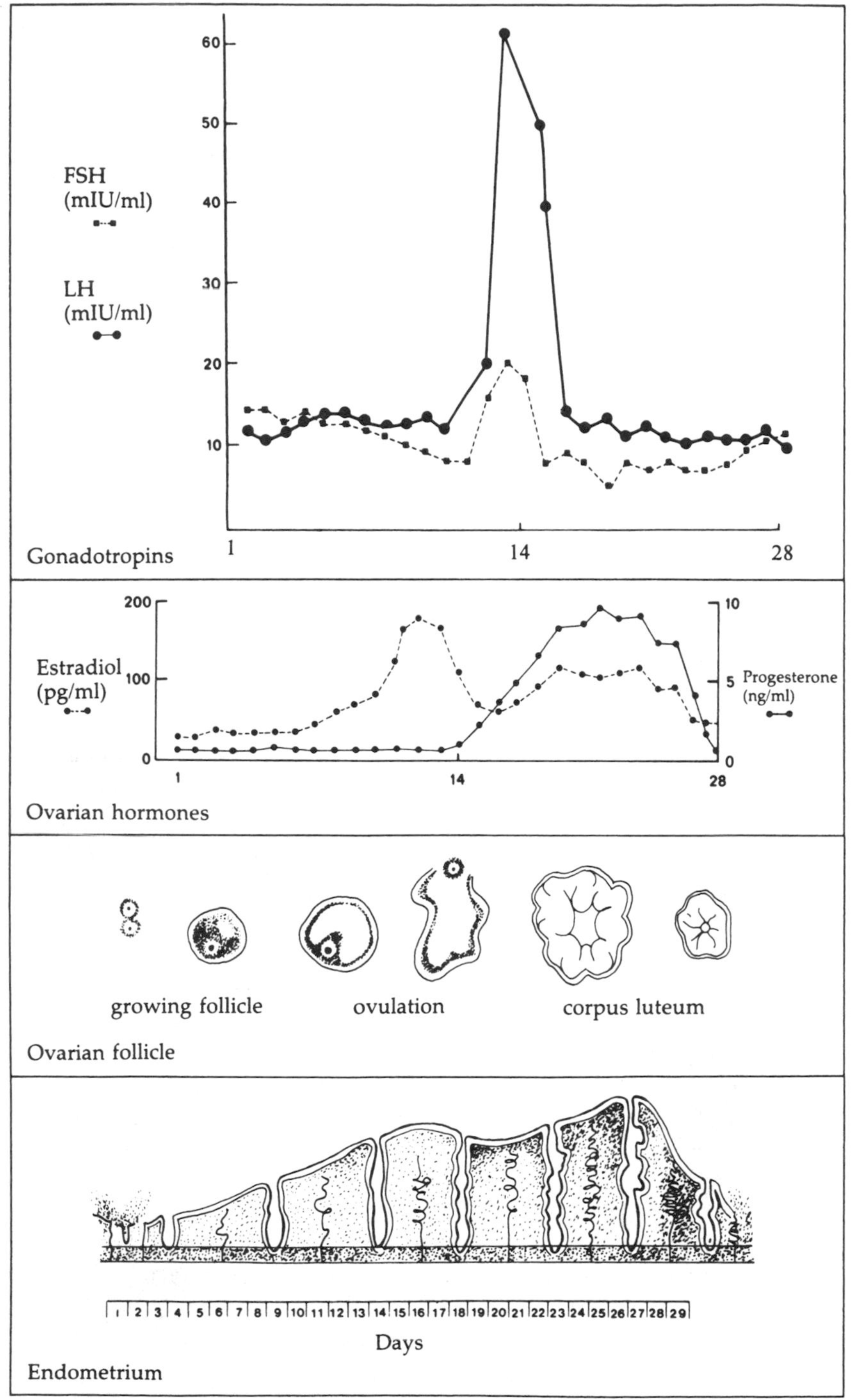

FIG. 16. Physiology of the normal ovulatory menstrual cycle: gonadotropin secretion, ovarian hormone production, follicular maturation, and endometrial changes during one cycle. FSH, follicle-stimulating hormone; LH, luteinizing hormone.

mean pulse amplitude was highest in the early luteal phase (14.9 mIU/ml) and decreased to 12.2 mIU/ml in the midluteal phase and to 7.6 mIU/ml by the late luteal phase. FSH was closely correlated to LH secretion.

In the periovulatory phase of the cycle, the dominant follicle is clearly evident; it has increased receptors for LH and secretes increasing levels of estradiol. The rising estrogen levels produce a further proliferation of the endometrium, with increasing length of the glands. The rising LH levels appear to induce a block in steroid pathways, which initiates secretion of 17-hydroxyprogesterone and progesterone and the gradual luteinization of the granulosa cells. The exact mechanism for the positive feedback effect of rising estrogen and progesterone levels on the midcycle release of multiple pulses of LH is unknown. By midpuberty, the hypothalamic–pituitary unit is capable of this positive feedback response. Following the surge of LH, follicular rupture and expulsion of the oocyte occur (ovulation).

The development of the corpus luteum is affected by levels of LH and the rupture of the follicle. As noted, GnRH and thus LH are released in slower pulses. The corpus luteum secretes progesterone and 17-hydroxyprogesterone. Plasma progesterone concentrations are stable over 24-hour studies in the early luteal phase and show no relationship to LH pulses; however, in the middle and late luteal phases, progesterone levels rapidly fluctuate during 24-hour studies from levels as low as 2.3 ng/ml to peaks of 40.1 ng/ml, and they correlate with LH pulses (55). Thus, a single progesterone level in the middle to late luteal phase of the cycle may not always predict the adequacy of the corpus luteum.

Under the influence of rising progesterone and estrogen levels, the endometrium enters the secretory phase, which is characterized by coiling of the endometrial glands, increased vascularity of the stroma, and increased glycogen content of the epithelial cells. Maturation of the endometrium is reached within 8 or 9 days after ovulation, and if fertilization does not occur, regression begins. Exact dating of the endometrium is possible because of the date-specific changes in the structure of the endometrial cells. Evidence for ovulation and the occurrence of a luteal phase may be obtained by endometrial biopsy, basal body temperature charts, and measurement of serum progesterone levels (>10 ng/ml).

Without pregnancy and the concomitant rise in placental human chorionic gonadotropin (hCG) levels, luteolysis begins, and progesterone and estrogen levels begin to decline. Unlike hCG, the luteotropic support of LH cannot extend the life of the corpus luteum beyond 14 days. In contrast to the variable length of the follicular phase, the luteal phase is usually constant at 14 days. Thus, the life span of the corpus luteum is determined by a preset "clock" with time to allow implantation and retention until trophoblastic hCG intervenes. With the waning of progesterone and estrogen levels, the endometrium undergoes necrotic changes that result in menstrual bleeding. The stage for the new cycle is in fact set in the late luteal phase when plasma FSH begins to rise to initiate follicular development.

Several researchers have studied adolescent cycles as they pass from anovulatory to ovulatory cycles (30,31,56). Apter and coworkers (56) reported that in adolescents, follicular development was slower and eventual ovulation took place from a smaller follicle than in older women (age 25 to 35 years). In adults, the concentration of FSH decreased from day 4 to day 10 of the cycle, whereas in adolescents the FSH level increased. The selection of the dominant follicle seemed disturbed, with seven of eight adolescent patients studied still having several follicles of 8 to 14 mm on days 12 to 15 of the cycle. In the last 3 days before ovulation, the mean increase in the diameter of the dominant follicle was 2.9 mm in the adolescent group and 5.6 mm in the adult group. Ovulation occurred later in the cycle in adolescents than in adults (mean of 5 days longer). Apter and coworkers (31) had previously shown a negative correlation between the FSH concentration on days 3 to 4 of the cycle and the length of the follicular phase. In comparison with adolescents, the adults had slightly but significantly higher mean maximal progesterone levels during the luteal phase.

Apter and coworkers (56) found several patterns in adolescents with anovulatory cycles. One pattern was characterized by low estradiol levels without LH at midcycle and minor or no follicular growth. A second pattern was characterized by developing follicles, slightly higher estradiol, and minor increases in LH at midcycle. A third pattern was identical to an ovulatory pattern, with an increase in follicular development, increased estradiol levels, and an LH surge but no evidence of ovulation (no rise in progesterone, no cul-de-sac fluid by ultrasound, menses 3 to 4 days after the LH surge). Others have found similar patterns in adolescents and adult women involved in strenuous athletic competition. Bonen and associates (57) found that competitive swimmers may have an LH surge at midcycle but no rise in serum progesterone; abnormal FSH secretion during the first half of the cycle may inadequately prepare the follicle for ovulation. The time from the LH surge to menstruation was 4 or 5 days, resembling the third pattern described by Apter and coworkers. Shangold and associates (58) determined that the luteal phase in a healthy adult runner shortened as she increased her weekly mileage.

In adolescents, the gonadotropin response to a dose of exogenous GnRH appears to change during the follicular phase in the first 2 postmenarcheal years toward that observed in adult women and in the luteal phase from the third to the fifth postmenarcheal year (Fig. 17) (58,59). Another pattern that appears to occur early in the adolescent years in association with menstrual irregularity is the overproduction of adrenal and ovarian androgens. Venturoli and associates (60,61) found that adolescents with persistent anovulatory menses maintained marked hyperandrogenism, increasingly high LH levels, and enlarged multicystic ovaries. Mean testosterone and androstenedione were higher than in ovulatory cycles and in adult controls. The persistence of this pattern sets the stage for classic polycystic ovary syndrome (see Chapter 7) with rapid pulses of GnRH and LH. In contrast, adolescents with anovulatory cycles and normal LH levels were more similar to ovulatory adolescents. Venturoli and associates (60) have suggested that the pulsatile pattern of GnRH and gonadotropin secretion accounts for the endocrine differences in these groups of postmenarcheal adolescents. In addition, they have

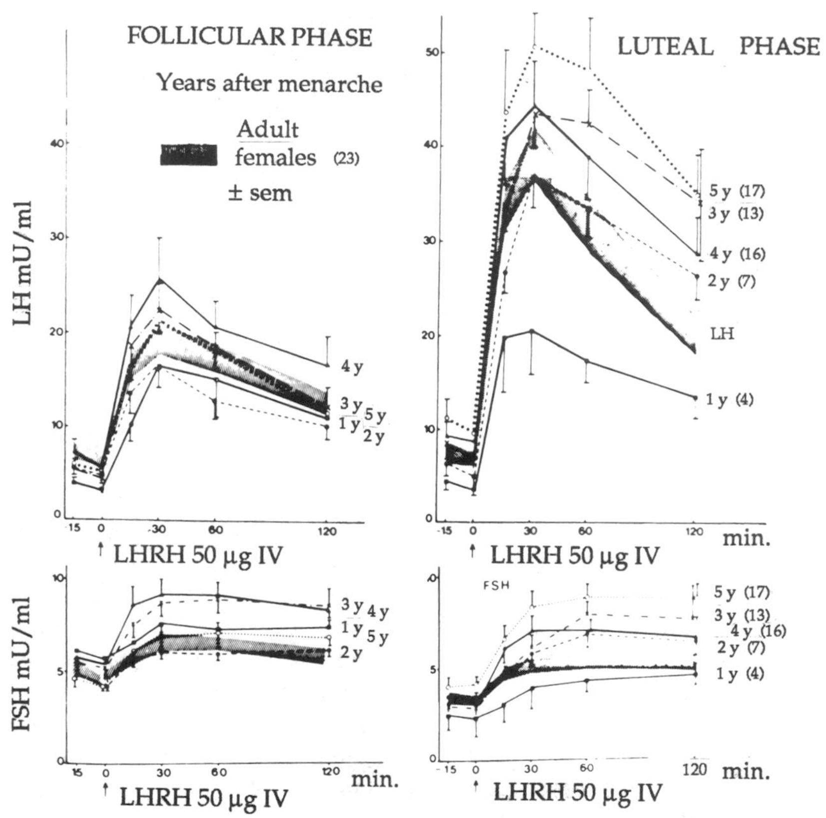

FIG. 17. Gonadotropin responses to luteinizing hormone-releasing hormone (LHRH) in adolescent girls distributed according to gynecologic age (years after menarche). Upper panels: Luteinizing hormone (LH) responses during the follicular and luteal phases. Lower panels: Follicle-stimulating hormone (FSH) responses in the same girls. ■–■, first postmenarcheal year; ●–●, second postmenarcheal year; X__.__X, third year; ▲–▲, fourth year; 0. . .0, fifth year. The hatched area represents the mean ± SEM gonadotropin responses in 23 normally cycling adult women. LH and FSH are expressed as milliunits per milliliter MRC international standards 68/40 and 68/39, respectively. The number of subjects is in parentheses. (From Lemarchand-Beraud T, Zufferey M, Reymond M, et al. Maturation of the hypothalamic-pituitary-ovarian axis in adolescent girls. *J Clin Endocrinol Metab* 1982;54:241.)

suggested that in the postmenarcheal period, progesterone, by modulating LH and FSH pulsatility and thus reducing androgen levels and their action on producing atresia of follicles, may be a regulatory factor in enhancing normal cyclicity.

The term *hypothalamic amenorrhea* has been used to apply to the common problem in which, despite a normal pituitary and ovaries, normal cyclic changes do not occur. Recent studies have suggested that abnormalities in pulsatile GnRH are involved and may include a spectrum of changes. The frequency of LH pulses is reduced in most women with hypothalamic amenorrhea (62), which suggests that GnRH pulses are too infrequent to stimulate normal follicular maturation. Santaro and associates (63) have offered a classification of hypogonadotropic hypogonadism based on a comparison of the LH pulse pattern (90-minute intervals) found in the early follicular phase. One pattern was an apulsatile pattern associated with the most profound clinical abnormalities (often primary amenorrhea). A second pattern showed pulses of abnormally low amplitude but a normal number of pulses. A third pattern showed pulses of normal or greater than normal amplitude but low frequency, resembling the normal luteal phase. A fourth group showed no discernible differences in LH in spite of amenorrhea. This last group may have a difference in night–day secretion or lower levels of circulating bioactive gonadotropins. Since patients in the last group have a significant incidence of spontaneous resumption of normal menses, this pattern may represent a transition.

Central nervous system opioids appear to play an inhibitory role, and catecholamines a stimulatory role, on GnRH secretion. Clomiphene citrate appears to be active in promoting fertility by increasing the frequency of LH pulses; the better response to this drug by women with higher estradiol levels can be explained by its ability to increase GnRH pulse frequency in patients with less impairment of GnRH secretion (62). The ability to deliver pulses of GnRH at physiologic doses of amplitude and frequency has enhanced the ability to induce ovulation and normal female and male sexual maturation in hypogonadal patients (64,65).

Clinical Applications

An understanding of the normal cycle is useful in the clinical management of patients with menstrual problems. In patients with anovulatory cycles, the ovary produces continuous levels of estrogen, and thus the endometrium remains in the proliferative phase; menstrual periods may be heavy and irregular. Regulation can often be obtained with medroxyprogesterone (Provera) given 14 days each month to produce a secretory endometrium; 1 to 7 days after taking medroxyprogesterone, the patient then has a menstrual period. In the evaluation of the patient with amenorrhea, a withdrawal flow after intramuscular progesterone or oral medroxyprogesterone has been given implies that the endometrium has been adequately primed with estrogen (see Chapter 6).

Quantification of serum FSH and LH by radioimmunoassay is readily available; laboratories vary both in normal values and in units per milliliter (mIU/ml or ng/ml). Because gonadotropins are released in a pulsatile fashion, a single random serum value of LH and FSH may not be helpful in distinguishing between low and normal levels of these hormones. In Fig. 13 (44), the variability of values in normal cycles is evident. In this assay, levels of 5 to 25 mIU/ml are in the normal range; consistently low values of 2 to 4 mIU/ml may imply hypothalamic or pituitary hypofunction (see Chapter 5 for discussions of other assays of FSH and LH). An FSH level >50 to 60 mIU/ml and an LH level >40 mIU/ml in a prepubertal or poorly estrogenized female imply ovarian failure; such high levels are also found in the postmenopausal woman. Newer assays have reference levels of >30 mIU/ml for the postmenopausal or ovarian failure range. In addition, an elevated serum LH with normal FSH in an amenorrheic or oligomenorrheic adolescent may suggest an androgen excess/polycystic ovary syndrome (see Chapter 7). Gonadotropin levels and serum androgen levels should be measured in the oligomenorrheic patient who has hirsutism, acne, or signs of virilization. It is always important to know when the blood samples for FSH and LH levels were drawn in relation to the menstrual cycle, if any. The last menstrual period should be recorded at the time of the office visit, and the patient should be instructed to keep a calendar and call with the date of the next menses. If no menses have occurred by 4 weeks after the visit, the clinician should record this fact to aid in interpreting the levels.

Frequent sampling of the serum for LH and FSH levels over a 24-hour period or over a menstrual cycle has been useful in research settings for investigating normal and abnormal physiology. Clinically, pituitary function can also be studied by the administration of a GnRH stimulation test. A single dose of GnRH is given intravenously or subcutaneously, and serum LH and FSH levels are measured at frequent intervals over a 4-hour period. The LH values should increase 150% *above* baseline in normal pubertal patients (6) (see Table 1 for normal responses and Fig. 17 for variations with menarcheal age). Girls with isosexual central precocious puberty will respond with a pubertal LH and FSH response, whereas those with premature thelarche or puberty secondary to an ovarian tumor respond with a prepubertal response. Patients with anorexia nervosa and craniopharyngiomas usually have little response to GnRH, whereas those with prolactin-secreting pituitary microadenomas have a normal pubertal response. Patients with Kallmann's syndrome (hypogonadotropic hypogonadism) have heterogeneous responses to GnRH; some may have minimal response to the single dose of GnRH and require longer administration of pulsatile GnRH to cause normal release of LH and FSH. Even patients with anorexia nervosa and amenorrhea can be stimulated to secrete LH and FSH and to ovulate with long-term pulsatile GnRH (66). As previously mentioned, the administration of physiologic pulses of GnRH can be used clinically to induce ovulation in infertile women with normal ovarian function and to stimulate normal pubertal maturation in men.

The observation (2,67,68) that pulsatile GnRH results in secretion of LH and FSH but that the continuous infusion of GnRH results in the suppression of LH and FSH has led to new treatment modalities for precocious puberty in children (see Chapter 5). The use of long-acting GnRH analogs offers the possibility of reversing the pubertal activation of gonadotropins and sex steroids. GnRH analogs are also potentially useful for ovarian suppression in the treatment of endometriosis, polycystic ovary syndrome, severe premenstrual syndrome, and, possibly, hormonally dependent malignancies. In addition, the ovarian suppression also results in amenorrhea, which may be helpful in the treatment of some medical diseases (see Chapter 19).

The measurement of serum estrogen, progesterone, and androgen levels is now possible in many laboratories, although variation in quality control and normal levels makes interpretation, especially of androgen levels, problematic at times. In addition, the fact that most of these levels vary during the day and during the menstrual cycle must be kept in mind when one is drawing conclusions from these levels. For example, girls in the early stages of puberty may have low daytime FSH and LH levels and undetectable or very low estradiol levels in spite of normal maturation. As noted, progesterone is secreted in pulses, and thus a single level cannot assess the adequacy of the luteal phase in infertile patients. The importance of the physical examination should not be underestimated, despite the ability to measure many hormone levels. The response of the target organs to these hormones is essential to a correct diagnosis. Pubertal breast development, a pink moist vaginal mucosa, and watery cervical mucus are all signs that suggest functional ovaries and the secretion of estrogen. From the presence of normal axillary and pubic hair, the physician can infer functioning adrenal glands and circulating androgens. Hirsutism and clitoromegaly are signs of androgen excess; a patient with these signs will require an evaluation of her hormone status (see Chapter 7). The assessment of many gynecologic problems depends on a careful physical examination (see Chapter 1) combined with a thorough understanding of normal pubertal development. Primary and secondary amenorrhea, menorrhagia, and virilization can then be evaluated in terms of the hypothalamic-pituitary-ovarian-adrenal axis.

REFERENCES

1. O'Bryne KT, Thalabard J-C, Grosser PM, et al. Radiotelemetry monitoring of hypothalamic gonadotropin releasing hormone pulse generator activity throughout the menstrual cycle of the Rhesus monkey. *Endocrinology* 1991;129:1207.
2. Belchetz PE, Plant TM, Nakai Y, et al. Hypophyseal responses to continuous and intermittent delivery of hypothalamic gonadotropin-releasing hormone. *Science* 1978;202:631.
3. Speroff L, Glass RH, Kase NG. *Clinical gynecologic endocrinology and infertility*, 5th ed. Baltimore: Williams & Wilkins, 1994.
4. Lee PA. Neuroendocrinology of puberty. *Semin Reprod Endocrinol* 1988;6:13.
5. Besser GM, McNeilly AS, Anderson DC, et al. Hormonal responses to synthetic luteinizing hormone and follicle stimulating hormone in man. *Br Med J* 1972;3:267.
6. Ayerst Laboratories Inc. Factrel (gonadorelin hydrochloride) package insert. New York: Ayerst, 1990.
7. Conte FA, Kaplan SL, Grumbach MM. A diphasic pattern of gonadotropin secretion in patients with the syndromea of gonadal dysgenesis. *J Clin Endocrinol Metab* 1975;40:670.
8. Conte FA, Grumbach MM, Kaplan SL, et al. Correlation of luteinizing hormone-releasing factor-induced luteinizing hormone and follicle stimulating hormone release from infancy to 19 years with the changing pattern of gonadotropin secretion in agonadal patients: relation to the restraint of puberty. *J Clin Endocrinol Metab* 1980;50:163.
9. Apter D, Pakarinen A, Hammond GL, et al. Adrenocortical function in puberty. *Acta Paediatr Scand* 1979;68:599.
10. Styne DM, Grumbach MM. Puberty in the male and female: its physiology and disorders. In: Yen SSC, Jaffe RB, eds. *Reproductive endocrinology*. Philadelphia: WB Saunders, 1986.
11. Lucky AW, Biro FM, Huster GA, et al. Acne vulgaris in premenarchal girls. An early sign of puberty associated with rising levels of dehydroepiandrosterone. *Arch Dermatol* 1994;130:308.
12. Leyden JJ. Therapy for acne vulgaris. *N Engl J Med* 1997;336:1156.

13. Landy H, Boepple PA, Mansfield MJ, et al. Sleep modulation of neuroendocrine function: developmental changes in gonadotropin-releasing hormone during sexual maturation. *Pediatr Res* 1990;28:213.
14. Boyar RM, Wu RH, Roffwarg H, et al. Human puberty: 24-hour estradiol patterns in pubertal girls. *J Clin Endocrinol Metab* 1976;43:1418.
15. Lucky AW, Rich BH, Rosenfield RL, et al. LH bioactivity increases more than immunoreactivity during puberty. *J Pediatr* 1980;97:205.
16. Sklar CA, Kaplan SL, Grumbach MM. Evidence for dissociation between adrenarche and gonadarche: studies in patients with idiopathic precocious puberty, gonadal dysgenesis, isolated gonadotropin deficiency, and constitutionally delayed growth and adolescence. *J Clin Endocrinol Metab* 1980;51:548.
17. Yen SSC, Apter D, Bhtzow T, Laughlin GA. Gonadotropin releasing hormone pulse generator activity before and during sexual maturation in girls: new insights. *Hum Reprod* 1993;8:66.
18. Apter D, Bhtzow TL, Laughlin GA, Yen SCC. Gonadotropin releasing hormone pulse generator activity during pubertal transition in girls: pulsatile and diurnal patterns of circulating gonadotropins. *J Clin Endocrinol Metab* 1993;76:940.
19. Burger HG, McLachlan RI, Bangah M, et al. Serum inhibin concentrations rise throughout normal male and female puberty. *J Clin Endocrinol Metab* 1988;67:689.
20. Burger HG, Yamada Y, Bangah ML, et al. Serum gonadotropin, sex steroid, and immunoreactive inhibin levels in the first two years of life. *J Clin Endocrinol Metab* 1991;72:682.
21. Kettel LM, Apter D, DePaolo LV, et al. Circulating levels of follistatin from puberty to menopause. *Fertil Steril* 1996;65:472.
22. Halvorson LM, DeCherney AH. Inhibin, activin, and follistatin in reproductive medicine. *Fertil Steril* 1996;65:459.
23. Rosenfield RL, Frulanetto R. Physiologic testosterone in estradiol induction of puberty increases plasma somatomedin-C. *J Pediatr* 1985;107:415.
24. Moll GW, Rosenfield RL, Fang VS. Administration of low-dose estrogen rapidly and directly stimulates growth hormone production. *Am J Dis Child* 1986;140:124.
25. Zachmann M, Prader A, Sobel EH, et al. Pubertal growth in patients with androgen insensitivity: indirect evidence for the importance of estrogens in pubertal growth of girls. *J Pediatr* 1986; 108:694.
26. Rose SR, Municchi G, Barnes KM, et al. Spontaneous growth hormone secretion increases during puberty in normal girls and boys. *J Clin Endocrinol Metab* 1991;73:428.
27. Greulich WW, Pyle S. *Radiographic atlas of skeletal development of the hand and wrist.* Stanford, CA: Stanford University Press, 1959.
28. Zacharias L, Wurtman R. Age at menarche: genetic and environmental influences. *N Engl J Med* 1969;280:868.
29. MacMahon B. *National health examination survey: age at menarche.* DHEW Publication 74-1615, Series 11, No. 133, November 1973.
30. Apter D. Serum steroids and pituitary hormones in female puberty: a partly longitudinal study. *Clin Endocrinol* 1980;12:107.
31. Apter D, Viinikka L, Vihko R. Hormonal pattern of adolescent menstrual cycles. *J Clin Endocrinol Metab* 1978;47:944.
32. World Health Organization Task Force on Adolescent Reproductive Health. World Health Organization multicenter study on menstrual and ovulatory patterns in adolescent girls: I. A multicenter cross-sectional study of menarche. *J Adolesc Health Care* 1986;7:229.
33. World Health Organization Task Force on Adolescent Reproductive Health. World Health Organization multicenter study on menstrual and ovulatory patterns in adolescent girls: II. Longitudinal study of menstrual patterns in the early postmenarcheal period, duration of bleeding episodes and menstrual cycles. *J Adolesc Health Care* 1986;7:236.
34. Wentz AC, Jones GS, Sapp KC. Effect of clomiphene citrate on gonadotropin responses to LRH administration in secondary amenorrhea and oligomenorrhea. *Obstet Gynecol* 1976;47:677.
35. Wentz AC, Schoemaker J, Jones GS, Sapp KC. Studies of pathophysiology in primary amenorrhea. *Obstet Gynecol* 1977;50:129.
36. Wentz AC, Jones GS. Prognosis in primary amenorrhea. *Fertil Steril* 1978;29:614.
37. Scott RT, Hofmann GE. Prognostic assessment of ovarian reserve. *Fertil Steril* 1995;63:1.
38. Marshall WA, Tanner JM. Variations in pattern of pubertal changes in girls. *Arch Dis Child* 1969;44: 291.

39. Grumbach MM, Styne DM. Puberty: ontogeny, neuroendocrinology, physiology, and disorders. In: Wilson JD, Foster DW, eds. *Williams textbook of endocrinology*, 8th ed. Philadelphia: WB Saunders, 1992.
40. Lee PA. Normal ages of pubertal events among American males and females. *J Adolesc Health Care* 1980;1:26.
41. Harlan WR, Harlan EA, Grillo GP. Secondary sex characteristics of girls 12 to 17 years of age: the U.S. Health Examination Survey. *J Pediatr* 1980;96:1074.
42. Herman-Giddens ME, Slora EJ, Wasserman RC, et al. Secondary sexual characteristics and menses in young girls seen in office practice: a study from the Pediatric Research in Office Settings Network. *Pediatrics* 1997;99:505.
43. Biro FM. Areolar and breast staging in adolescent girls. *Adolesc Pediatr Gynecol* 1992,5:271.
44. Nottelmann ED, Susan EJ, Dorn LD, et al. Developmental processes in early adolescence: relations among chronologic age, pubertal stage, height, weight, and serum levels of gonadotropins, sex steroids, and adrenal androgens. *J Adolesc Health Care* 1987;8:246.
45. Bayley N. Growth curves of height and weight by age for boys and girls, scaled according to physical maturity. *J Pediatr* 1956;48:187.
46. Hamill PVV, et al. Physical growth: National Center for Health Statistics percentiles. *Am J Clin Nutr* 1979;32:607.
47. Frisch RE. A method of prediction of age and menarche from height and weight at ages nine through thirteen years. *Pediatrics* 1974;53:384.
48. Frisch RE, McArthur JW. Menstrual cycles: fatness as a determinant of minimum weight necessary for their maintenance or onset. *Science* 1974;185:949.
49. Wyshak G, Frisch RE. Evidence for a secular trend in age of menarche. *N Engl J Med* 1982;306:1033.
50. Gonzales GF, Villena A. Critical anthropometry for menarche. *J Pediatr Adolesc Gynecol* 1996;9:139.
51. Zacharias L, Wurtman RJ, Schatzoff M. Sexual maturation in contemporary American girls. *Am J Obstet Gynecol* 1970;108:833.
52. Apter D, Vihko R. Serum pregnenolone, progesterone, 17-hydroxyprogesterone, testosterone, and 5 α-dihydrotestosterone during female puberty. *J Clin Endocrinol Metab* 1977;45:1039.
53. Tsonis CG, Messinis IE, Templeton AA, et al. Gonadotropic stimulation of inhibin secretion by the human ovary during the follicular and early luteal phase of the cycle. *J Clin Endocrinol Metab* 1988;66:915.
54. Filicori M, Santoro N, Merriam GR, et al. Characterization of the physiological pattern of episodic gonadotropin secretion throughout the human menstrual cycle. *J Clin Endocrinol Metab* 1986;62:1136.
55. Filicori M, Butler JP, Crowley WF. Neuroendocrine regulation of the corpus luteum in the human: evidence for pulsatile progesterone secretion. *J Clin Invest* 1984;73:1638.
56. Apter D, Raisanen I, Ylostalo P, et al. Follicular growth in relation to serum hormonal patterns in adolescent compared with adult menstrual cycles. *Fertil Steril* 1987;47:82.
57. Bonen A, Belcastro AN, Ling WY, et al. Profiles of selected hormones during menstrual cycles of teenage athletes. *J Appl Physiol* 1981;50:545.
58. Shangold M, Freeman R, Thysen B, et al. The relationship between long distance running, plasma progesterone and luteal phase length. *Fertil Steril* 1979;31:130.
59. LeMarchand-Berand T, Zafferey M-M, Reymond M, et al. Maturation of the hypothalamic-pituitary-ovarian axis in adolescent girls. *J Clin Endocrinol Metab* 1982;54:241.
60. Venturoli S, Porcu E, Fabbri R, et al. Postmenarchal evolution of endocrine pattern and ovarian aspects of adolescents with menstrual irregularities. *Fertil Steril* 1987;48:78.
61. Venturoli S, Porcu E, Gammi L, et al. Different gonadotropin pulsatile fashions in anovulatory cycles of young girls indicate different maturational pathways in adolescence. *J Clin Endocrinol Metab* 1987;65:785.
62. Marshall JC, Kelch RP. Gonadotropin-releasing hormone: role of pulsatile secretion in the regulation of reproduction. *N Engl J Med* 1986;315:1459.
63. Santaro N, Filicori M, Crowley W Jr. Hypogonadotropin disorders in men and women: diagnosis and therapy with pulsatile gonadotropin releasing hormone. *Endocrinol Rev* 1986;7:11.
64. Hurley DM, Brian R, Outch K, et al. Induction of ovulation and fertility in amenorrheic women by pulsatile low-dose gonadotropin-releasing hormone. *N Engl J Med* 1984;310:1069.
65. Hoffman AR, Crowley WF Jr. Induction of puberty in men by long-term pulsatile administration of low-dose gonadotropin-releasing hormone. *N Engl J Med* 1982;307:1237.

66. Nillius SJ, Wide L. Gonadotropin-releasing hormone treatment for induction of follicular maturation and ovulation in amenorrheic women with anorexia nervosa. *Br Med J* 1975;3:405.
67. Knobil E, Plant TM, Wildt L, et al. Control of the rhesus monkey menstrual cycle: permissive role of hypothalamic gonadotropin-releasing hormone. *Science* 1980;207:1371.
68. Crowley WF Jr, Comite F, Vale W, et al. Therapeutic use of pituitary desensitization with a long-acting LHRH agonist: a potential new treatment for idiopathic precocious puberty. *J Clin Endocrinol Metab* 1981;52:370.

FURTHER READING

Herman-Giddens ME, Bourdony CJ. *Assessment of sexual maturity in girls. Pediatric Research in Office Settings,* Elk Grove IL: American Academy of Pediatrics, 1995.

5

Precocious Puberty

A thorough understanding of the normal progression of puberty (see Chapter 4) is essential in the evaluation of precocious puberty, premature thelarche, and premature adrenarche. In normal adolescence, estrogen is responsible for breast development; for maturation of the external genitalia, vagina, and uterus; and for the initiation of menses. An increase in adrenal androgens is associated with the appearance of pubic and axillary hair. Excess androgens of either ovarian or adrenal origin may cause acne, hirsutism, voice change, increased muscle mass, and clitoromegaly. Thus, precocious puberty in girls can be divided into two categories: isosexual precocity, in which the patient has normal pubertal development; and contrasexual precocity, in which the patient has evidence of androgenization or true virilization with or without the changes characteristic of normal puberty.

Premature thelarche is defined as the appearance of breast development in the absence of other signs of puberty, growth spurt, or acceleration of skeletal maturation. Premature pubarche is the appearance of pubic or axillary hair without signs of estrogenization and is usually associated with increased secretion of adrenal androgens (adrenarche). Although generally self-limited, isolated breast budding or pubic hair development may be the first sign of a true precocious puberty. Isolated premature menarche without breast development may represent precocious puberty or a benign ovarian cyst, but local vaginal lesions as a source of bleeding (trauma, infection, tumor) should be ruled out (see Chapter 3).

The workup of precocious puberty requires fairly sophisticated endocrine studies and management. Thus, referral to an endocrinologist is advisable. However, the primary care clinician can initiate the investigation and diagnosis.

ISOSEXUAL PRECOCIOUS PUBERTY

Over the past century, the age of onset of pubertal development and menarche has declined in the United States and western Europe, perhaps in part because of improved nutrition (1). Currently, breast or pubic hair development in girls under

8 years of age is defined as precocious. However, in a recent study of 17,000 girls aged 3 to 12 years in the United States, Herman-Giddens and colleagues reported that a group of pediatric practitioners found breast or pubic hair development to be present at age 7 to 8 years in 6.7% of white and 27.2% of African-American girls seen in office practices (2). Isosexual precocious puberty can be divided into two categories: true isosexual precocity and isosexual pseudoprecocity.

In true isosexual precocity (central precocious puberty), the stimulus for development is gonadotropin-releasing hormone (GnRH) secreted in pulses by the hypothalamus. The pituitary gland responds to the GnRH pulsations with the production and release of pituitary gonadotropin (follicle-stimulating hormone [FSH], and luteinizing hormone, LH) pulses, which in turn stimulate the ovarian follicles to produce estrogen. In response to estrogen, the young girl has a growth spurt, develops breasts, and may begin menstruation. With the establishment of positive estrogen feedback resulting in the cyclic midcycle LH peak, the child may ovulate and thus becomes potentially fertile. Thus, in central precocious puberty, the hormonal process is that of an entirely normal puberty occurring at an early age (3–6).

Precocious puberty is much more common in girls than boys, with a ratio of about 23:1 (7). Although the large majority of cases of central precocious puberty in girls are idiopathic, computed tomography (CT) and magnetic resonance imaging (MRI) of the central nervous system (CNS) have identified small CNS abnormalities, such as hypothalamic hamartomas in some children with the onset of sexual precocity before the age of 3 years (8–11). In isosexual pseudoprecocity (peripheral precocious puberty), an ovarian tumor or cyst or rarely an adrenal adenoma produces estrogen autonomously.

Although the etiology of most cases of precocious puberty in girls is idiopathic, the differential diagnosis includes many organic disorders that need to be considered in the evaluation of the girl with early isosexual development (12–21).

True Isosexual Development

Idiopathic. This is a diagnosis of exclusion.

Cerebral disorders. These disorders include space-occupying lesions such as congenital malformations (hypothalamic hamartomas), brain tumors (e.g., glioma, astrocytoma, ependymoma, neuroblastoma), neurofibromatosis (optic nerve glioma or hypothalamic glioma), brain abscess, hydrocephalus (sometimes secondary to myelomeningocele), tuberous sclerosis, suprasellar cysts, infiltrative lesions such as sarcoid or other granulomatous disease, sequelae of cellular damage from prior infections (meningitis, encephalitis), head trauma, cerebral edema, or cranial radiation.

Secondary central precocious puberty. Prolonged exposure to sex steroids from any source, resulting in the advancement of skeletal maturation to a bone age of 11 to 13 years, can trigger central precocity. Patients with undertreated or late treated congenital adrenocortical hyperplasia (CAH) or androgen-secreting tumors may develop early central puberty (20).

Pseudoprecocious Puberty

Ovarian tumors. Approximately 60% of ovarian tumors that cause sexual precocity are granulosa cell tumors; the remainder are cystadenomas, gonadoblastomas, carcinomas, arrhenoblastomas, lipoid cell tumors, thecomas, and benign ovarian cysts. Ovarian tumors can secrete estrogens and androgens, thus resulting in both breast and pubic hair development.

Adrenal disorders. Adrenal adenomas may secrete estrogen alone and cause sexual precocity. Adrenal carcinomas that secrete estrogen also produce other hormones that cause contrasexual precocity and sometimes Cushing's syndrome. Patients with untreated CAH may have virilization as well as some breast development.

Gonadotropin-independent sexual precocity (autonomous follicular ovarian cysts). Recurrent ovarian follicular cysts may occur independently but are often associated with McCune-Albright syndrome. Girls with McCune-Albright syndrome have recurrent follicular cysts, polyostotic fibrous dysplasia, and large irregular café au lait spots (21–26). In these girls, ovarian volumes by ultrasonography are often asymmetric and fluctuate in size over time (24). The mechanism of gonadotropin-independent follicular cyst development in McCune-Albright syndrome is now believed to be due to a dominant somatic mutation in certain cell lines, which results in an overactivity of the cyclic adenosine monophosphate pathway owing to a mutation of the Gs alpha gene (25,26). The fluctuating estrogen levels produced by cysts result in sexual development and anovulatory menses.

Gonadotropin-producing tumors. Tumors that secrete both LH-like substances, such as human chorionic gonadotropin (hCG) and estrogen (primary ovarian choriocarcinoma), can cause precocious development. The production of LH or hCG alone will cause isosexual precocity in boys but not in girls.

Iatrogenic disorders. The prolonged use of estrogen-containing creams for labial adhesions may cause transient breast development. Oral estrogen intake (oral contraceptive ingestion) is a rare cause of breast development. It has been speculated that the ingestion of estrogen-like compounds in certain meat or plant foods may play a role in clusters of cases of premature breast development, but this has not been well defined (27).

Primary hypothyroidism. Ovarian cysts may develop in the presence of severe primary hypothyroidism, perhaps because of cross-reaction of high levels of thyroid-stimulating hormone (TSH) with ovarian FSH receptors (15–17). Premature breast development or vaginal bleeding usually regresses following thyroid hormone replacement. Absence of a statural growth spurt and delayed skeletal maturation accompanying breast development may be a clue to hypothyroidism as a cause of premature development.

Patient Assessment

The initial assessment of the patient with precocious development should include a careful history and physical examination. There is often a history of mildly early development in relatives of children with idiopathic central puberty between the ages of 6 and 8 years. Adopted children with a previous history of poor nutrition may have an increased chance of developing precocious puberty (28). A complete family history must include inherited conditions such as neurofibromatosis or CAH.

On reviewing the child's own history, the clinician should look for a history suggestive of CNS damage such as birth trauma, encephalitis, meningitis, CNS irradiation, seizures, headaches, visual symptoms, or other neurologic symptoms. Increased appetite, growth spurt, and emotional lability suggest a significant estrogen effect. The time course of precocious puberty is similar to that of normal puberty, whereas an abrupt and rapid course of development suggests an estrogen-secreting lesion. Abdominal pain, urinary symptoms, or bowel symptoms may be present in patients with abdominal masses.

Vaginal bleeding may be the first sign of precocity in patients with both true precocity and pseudoprecocity. Some children have no signs of puberty but have recurrent menses. This may be a benign, self-limited condition, although this is a diagnosis of exclusion (29,30).

Growth charts should be accurate and up to date, since the growth spurt often correlates with the onset of development in precocious puberty. The finding of accelerated growth and advanced skeletal maturation is important in distinguishing between true precocious puberty and premature thelarche. The photograph and growth charts of an untreated patient with idiopathic precocious puberty are shown in Fig. 1.

The physical examination should include height and weight measurements. A neurologic assessment, including visualization of the optic discs for evidence of papilledema, and evaluation of visual fields by confrontation, should be done. The skin should be assessed for acne, apocrine odor, café au lait spots, and pubic or axillary hair. In patients with neurofibromatosis, café au lait spots are multiple brown macules with smooth edges, whereas in those with McCune-Albright syndrome, one or more large macules with irregular borders may be found. The thyroid should be palpated and clinical signs suggestive of severe hypothyroidism (hair and skin changes, low pulse) noted. The breast dimensions and staging of breast development should be recorded. The external genitalia should be examined for evidence of estrogen effect (enlargement of the labia minora, thickening of the vaginal mucosa, and leukorrhea). Signs of virilization such as clitoromegaly, deepening of the voice, increased muscularity, or hirsutism should alert the examiner to the possibility of contrasexual precocity due to androgen excess. The normal prepubertal clitoral glans is 3 mm in diameter. A clitoral glans width >5 mm, or an index (clitoral length × width) >35 suggests significant androgen exposure (31). If the young child is approached in a relaxed

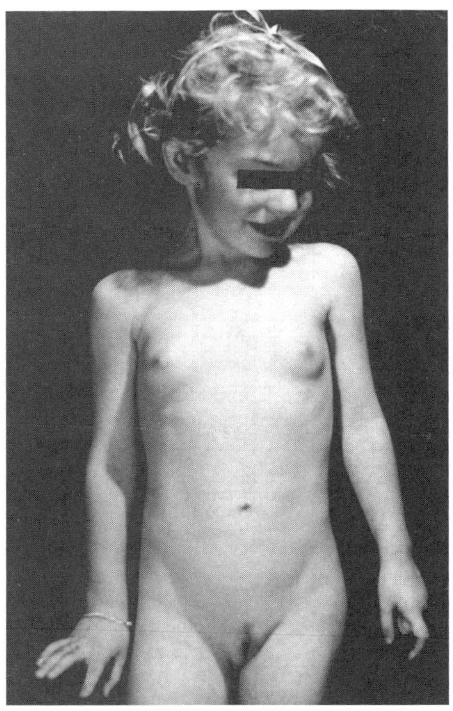

A

FIG. 1. Natural history of a girl with idiopathic precocious puberty before the advent of gonadotropin-releasing hormone (GnRH) therapy. She was first seen because of early development at the age of 3 2/12 years. Her menarche occurred at 5 6/12 years of age; she attained adult height at 10 years of age. **(A)** At age 3 6/12 years.

manner, it is often possible to carry out a thorough bimanual rectoabdominal examination. Ovarian masses, when present, are usually easily palpated. A vaginal pelvic exam is not necessary. Ultrasonography of the abdomen is a more sensitive tool for assessment of ovarian masses. Girls with true precocity frequently have mildly enlarged ovaries with multiple small follicular cysts similar to the ovaries seen in the adolescent with a normal age of puberty (32). A single large ovarian cyst may occur in isolation or with McCune-Albright syndrome.

The laboratory evaluation of the child depends on the initial clinical assessment. If the examination clearly shows an estrogen effect on the vaginal mucosa, and growth charts reveal an acceleration of linear growth, then more extensive testing is needed. If, on the other hand, the clinician suspects premature thelarche, the initial tests would include a radiograph film of the left hand and wrist for bone age and a vaginal smear for estrogen effect if one is tolerated. The radiograph for assessment of skeletal maturation is the single most useful test in the evaluation of the child with premature development. The bone age becomes significantly greater than the chronologic age and the height age in patients with true precocious puberty. A vaginal smear (maturational index) confirms estrogenization (see Chapter 1) and is useful both in confirming clinical impression and in following therapy. A typical smear in a patient with precocious puberty may show 35% superficial, 50% intermediate, and 15% parabasal cells. The

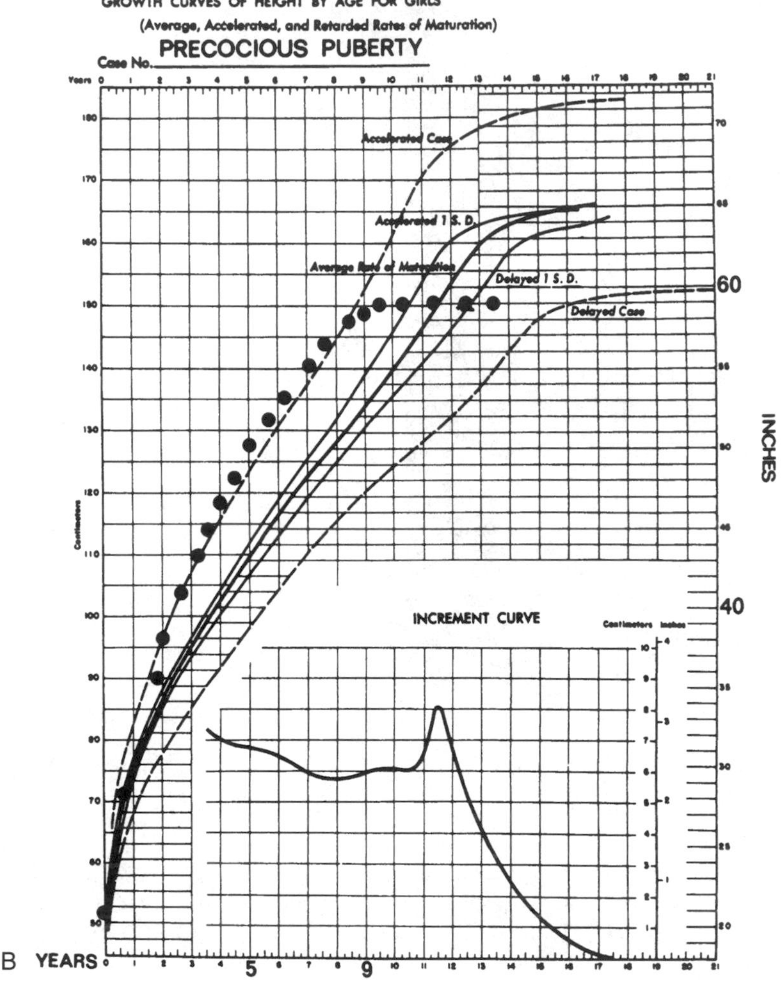

FIG. 1. *Continued.* **(B)** Height chart.

findings of estrogen excess (>40% superficial cells) should raise the suspicion of an estrogen-secreting lesion.

If the vagina shows little estrogen effect, and growth rate and bone age are normal, the patient can be monitored by her primary care physician at 3-month intervals to observe whether sexual development progresses or acceleration of linear growth occurs. Not uncommonly, a child has one or several transient episodes of breast budding and growth acceleration that resolve without therapy. Other children have very slow progression of precocity without rapid skeletal maturation. These children represent the "slowly progressive" variant of early

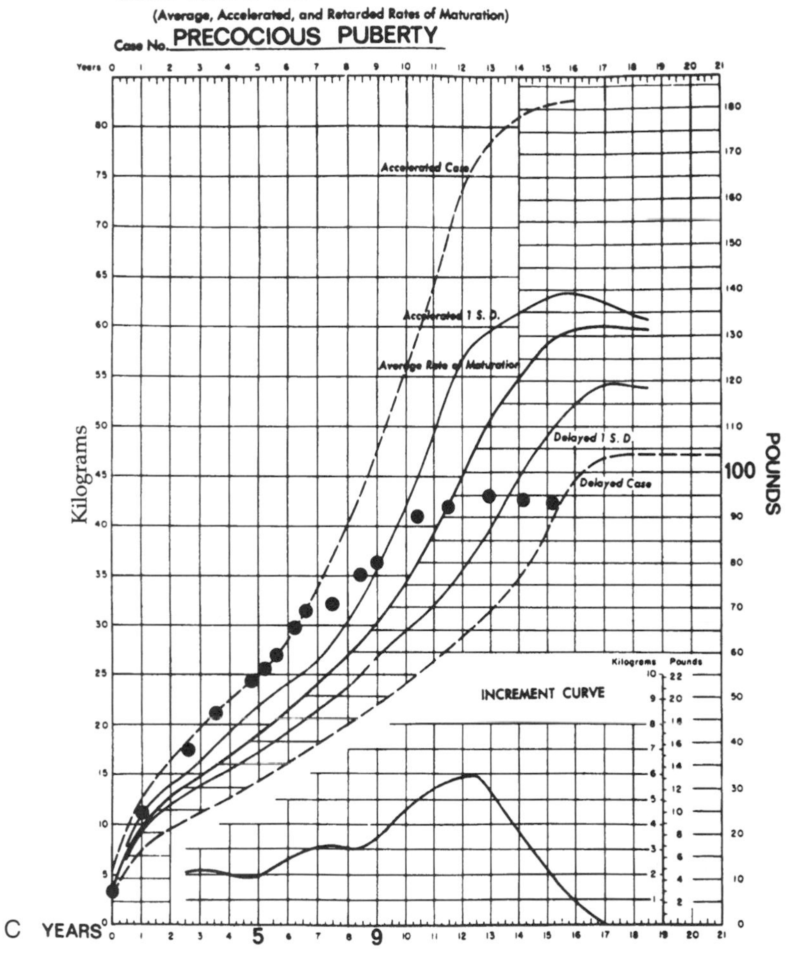

FIG. 1. *Continued.* **(C)** Weight chart.

puberty (33). They usually reach normal adult heights in the normal range without intervention.

If the girl has progressive sexual development, advancing bone age, acceleration of growth, or vaginal estrogenization, then consultation with a pediatric endocrinologist is indicated. In addition to determinations of bone age and maturational index (if tolerated), initial testing for the evaluation of suspected central precocious puberty usually includes serum levels of LH, FSH, estradiol, dehydroepiandrosterone sulfate (DHEAS), TSH, pelvic ultrasound for assessment of ovarian cysts and size and uterine size and configuration, and CT or MRI of the

CNS with contrast medium. Girls with precocious puberty between ages 6 and 8 years with height predictions in the normal range do not necessarily require further testing beyond a bone age. They should be followed, however, since height predictions may decline if bone age advances more rapidly than height age.

The interpretation of LH and FSH levels depends on which assay is used. Current commercially available assays include radioimmunoassays (RIA), and the newer and more sensitive immunoradiometric (IRMA), immunochemiluminometric, and immunofluorimetric assays (34–36,57). Since LH and FSH secretion is associated with sleep in early puberty, the random daytime serum LH and FSH values may not be helpful in differentiating among premature thelarche, pseudoprecocity, and early central precocious puberty. Random LH and FSH levels in the prepubertal range are usually seen in the early stages of true precocity; however, random LH levels in the pubertal range suggest advanced central precocity (Tanner breast stage 3). Thus, random daytime LH levels may be of value in confirming the clinical impression of active central puberty but will probably be in the prepubertal range both in early central puberty and in premature thelarche. Random FSH levels are less useful, since they are generally in the same range in premature thelarche and in precocious puberty. The IRMA and other sensitive assays provide better differentiation between precocious puberty and prepubertal states than older RIA assays.

The GnRH stimulation test (see Chapter 4) can help in the differential diagnosis of premature thelarche, gonadotropin-independent precocity, and true central precocity. Patients with true precocity exhibit nocturnal pulses of LH and FSH and a pubertal, LH-predominant response to the GnRH test, whereas girls with premature thelarche have a prepubertal FSH-predominant response, and those with gonadotropin-independent precocity or ovarian secreting cysts or tumors have a suppressed response to GnRH. The finding of a high estradiol level (100 to 200 pg/ml), low gonadotropin levels, and a suppressed response to GnRH should raise the possibility of an estrogen-secreting tumor or cyst, although this diagnosis should be apparent on ultrasound (see Chapter 15). The GnRH stimulation test is especially useful in tracking the response of the girl to GnRH analog therapy to ensure complete suppression of puberty (34) (Fig. 2).

The level of DHEAS is a marker of adrenal androgen production (see Chapter 7). Most girls with precocious puberty have age-appropriate DHEAS levels, although a few have premature adrenarche as well. Patients with precocity between 6 and 8 years of age have mean DHEAS levels similar to those of normal children with the same bone age (37).

In patients with excessive androgen effect, testosterone, DHEAS, and early-morning 17-hydroxyprogesterone (to detect 21-hydroxylase deficiency) and DHEA may be obtained. An adrenocorticotropic hormone (ACTH) stimulation test may be required to diagnose mild forms of congenital adrenal hyperplasia in the patient with premature pubarche. The child who has clitoromegaly, progressive virilization, or skeletal age advanced by more than 1 year certainly deserves a thorough evaluation.

Treatment and Followup

Treatment and followup depend on the diagnosis. Ovarian tumors should be managed as outlined in Chapter 15. Successful treatment of a tumor can be monitored by the demonstration of decreasing estrogen effects. Removal of an ovarian cyst will not result in permanent regression of puberty in girls with true precocity or McCune-Albright syndrome; thus, normal follicular cysts accompanying true precocity should not be removed. Severe cases of ovarian hyperstimulation resulting in precocious puberty may require aspiration (17). The ovarian cysts associated with central precocity should be observed because they are likely to regress with suppression of gonadotropins (see Chapter 15).

Although Depo-Provera and cyproterone acetate were used in the past to treat central precocious puberty, pubertal suppression was incomplete, and therapy did not improve the adult height (39–40). Suppression of puberty with GnRH analog agonists was initially pioneered by Crowley and associates, and these agents have become the treatment of choice for central precocious puberty (5,6,41–50). Continuous exposure to GnRH agonist analogs results in desensitization of pituitary gonadotropin-secreting cells. Currently, three GnRH analogs—histrelin, leuprolide, and nafarelin—are approved in the United States for the treatment of precocious puberty. In girls with central precocity, the advantages of a GnRH agonist are the selective and reversible suppression of LH and FSH, the return of estradiol to the prepubertal range, and the regression (or lack of progression) of breast development and the cessation of menses (Figs. 2 and 3). Growth velocity and skeletal maturation slow during GnRH analog suppression of puberty (Fig. 4). Since bone age advancement is slowed more than height age, predicted adult height is increased by this therapy (46,50) (Fig. 5). Several series of patients have shown modest to marked improvements in final height with GnRH analog agonist therapy (39,51,52). It is important for patients to be closely monitored during therapy to ensure that suppression of puberty is as complete as possible to maximize final height gain.

After GnRH analog therapy, menarche generally occurs within 1 to 2 years in patients with bone ages in the pubertal range, and menstrual cycles are similar to those in normal adolescent girls (53,54). Bone density, initially increased for age in patients with precocious puberty, declines during GnRH analog treatment but remains in the normal range (55).

Therapy with GnRH analogs is expensive and requires monthly injections of depot formulations or daily subcutaneous injections and regular monitoring of indices of pubertal suppression. Nasal analogs generally give less complete suppression. GnRH agonists are also effective in suppressing puberty in girls with precocity secondary to hypothalamic hamartomas and optic nerve gliomas associated with neurofibromatosis (11,14). During treatment with a GnRH analog, normal age-appropriate progression of adrenarche as determined by measurement of DHEAS occurs (37). Insulin growth factor-1 (also termed somatomedin-C) levels and nocturnal growth hormone secretion decrease dur-

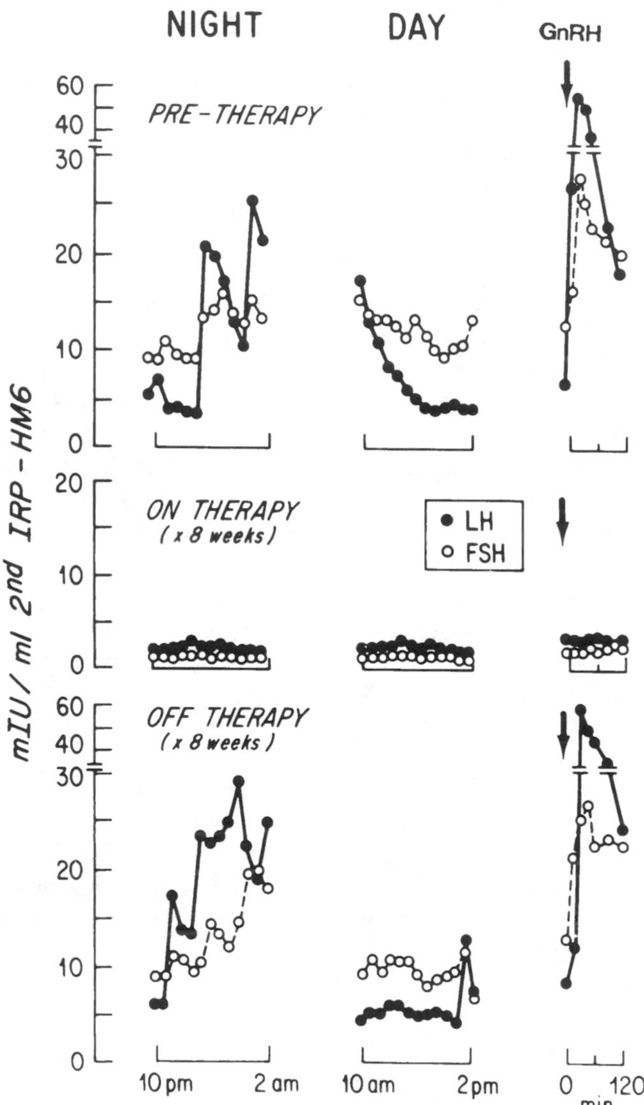

FIG. 2. Spontaneous night and daytime gonadotropin secretion and response to exogenous gonadotropin-releasing hormone (GnRH) administration in a 2-year-old with central precocious puberty before, during, and after discontinuation of GnRH analog therapy. LH, luteinizing hormone; FSH, follicle-stimulating hormone. (From Crowley WF, Comite F, Vale W, et al. Therapeutic use for pituitary desensitization with a long-acting LHRH agonist: a potential new treatment for idiopathic precocious puberty. *J Clin Endocrinol Metab* 1981;52:370; with permission.)

ing GnRH analog therapy, providing one of many lines of evidence that sex steroids augment growth hormone secretion during puberty (56).

Although a girl with precocious puberty may appear tall at the initial evaluation, she may eventually have a short final height because of premature epiphyseal closure. Several series have given final height estimates for girls with pre-

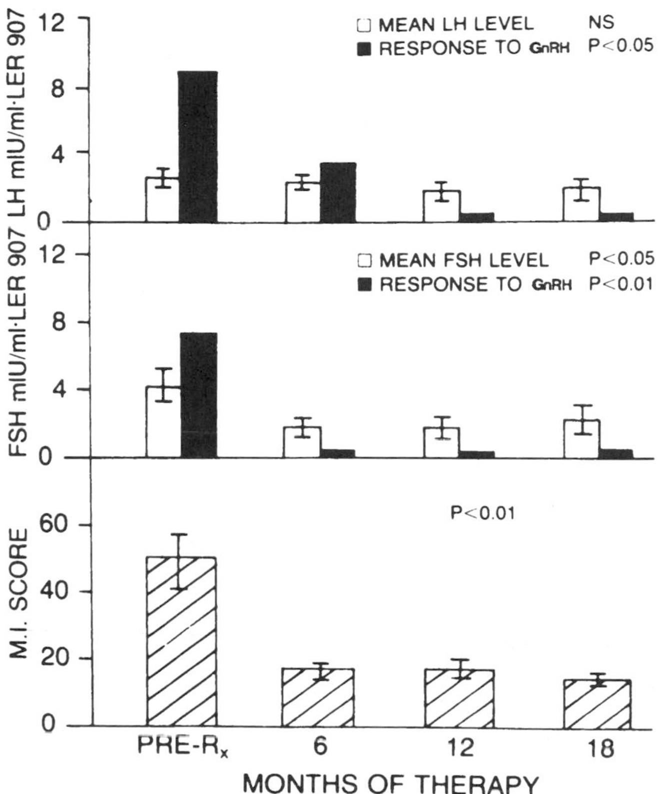

FIG. 3. Luteinizing hormone (LH) and follicle-stimulating hormone (FSH) (at baseline and in response to exogenous gonadotropin-releasing hormone [GnRH]), and maturation index (MI) score of vaginal cytology in nine girls with central precocious puberty before and during long-term therapy with GnRH analog. (From Mansfield MJ, Beardsworth DE, Loughlin J, et al. Long-term treatment of central precocious puberty with a long-acting analog of luteinizing hormone-releasing hormone. *N Engl J Med* 1983;309:1286; with permission.)

cocious puberty at 151 to 155 cm (18,19,38,39); however, recent small series of untreated patients have recorded final heights averaging within 1 standard deviation of normal (39,51). The final heights depended on the age of the children in the study and the rate of progression of their precocity. Children who develop progressive precocious puberty at young ages usually have more height deficit as adults. The majority of children who develop precocious puberty at the age of 6 to 8 years have acceptable final heights. Rosenfield (37) has suggested a useful algorithm for deciding when to initiate treatment for central precocity. If the child is 6 to 8 years old and has an acceptable initial predicted adult height >152 cm, she may be observed. If skeletal maturation progresses rapidly and predicted height declines to <152 cm or declines by ≥5 cm, treatment should be initiated. The psychosocial well-being of the patient and her family needs to be considered as well as the final height. In some patients, suppression of puberty is indicated

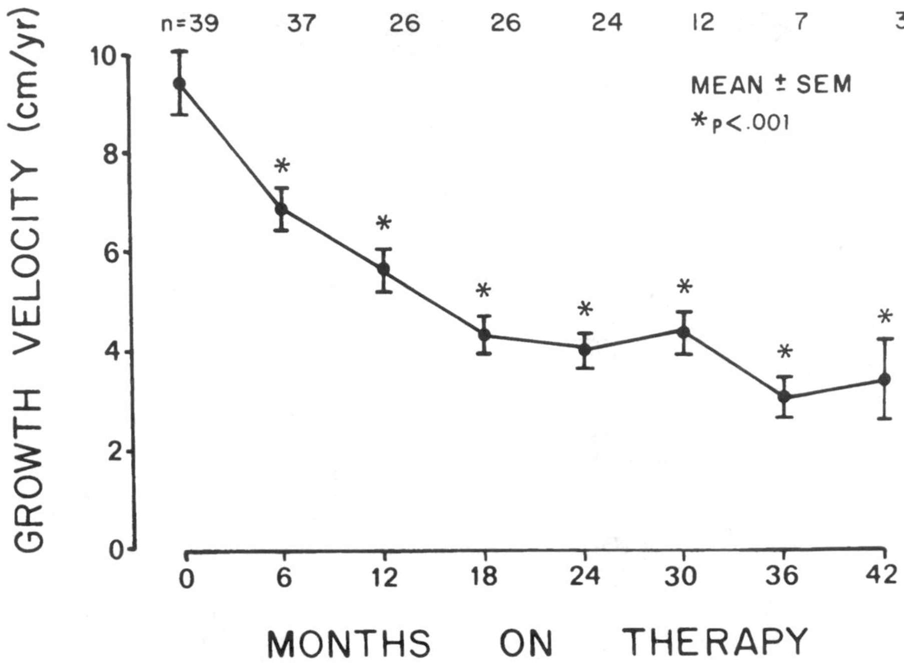

FIG. 4. Growth velocity before and during gonadotropin-releasing hormone (GnRH) analog therapy in 32 girls and 7 boys treated between 6 and 42 months. (From Boepple PA, Mansfield MJ, Wierman ME, et al. Use of a potent, long-acting agonist of gonadotropin-releasing hormone in the treatment of precocious puberty. *Endocr Rev* 1986;7:24; with permission.)

for psychosocial reasons despite a normal height prediction. In some patients in whom puberty is slowly progressive or intermittent, the endocrinologist may elect to withhold treatment and monitor the patient closely. Depo-Provera is occasionally used to stop menses when complete suppression of puberty is not required.

Important insights have also been gained on behavioral changes associated with gonadarche. Children with sexual precocity do not automatically manifest intellectual or psychosocial maturity. The degree of psychological maturity of a young girl is more likely to be related to her life experiences and her interactions with her peer group, siblings, and parents. Nevertheless, parents and investigators have noted that girls with sexual precocity sometimes have mood swings and impulsiveness, which resolve with the suppression of puberty during GnRH agonist therapy (58,59). Children with sexual precocity are at special risk for sexual abuse, and one study suggests that they tend to begin sexual relations at a slightly earlier age than their peers. It is important to reassure the young girl with precocious puberty and her parents that her growth and development are "early" but normal and that, if necessary, she can receive medicine to delay her development to a later age. Psychological consultation for the child

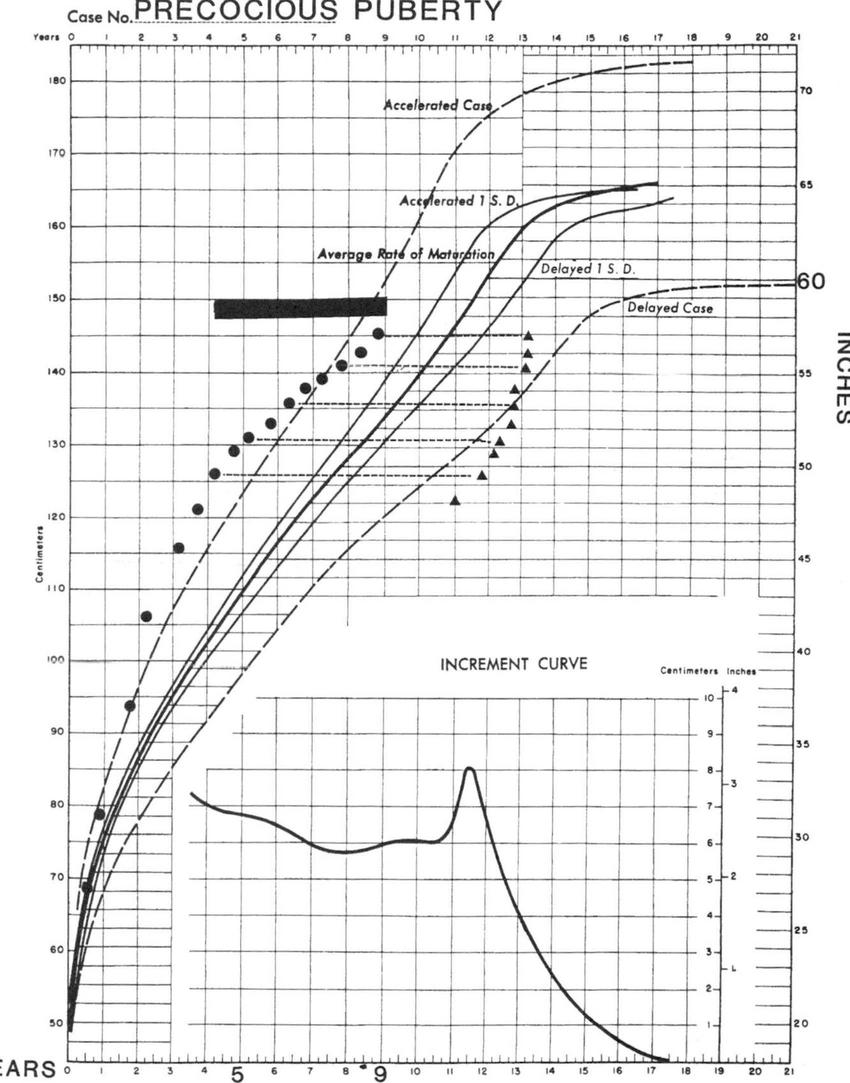

FIG. 5. Growth chart of a girl with true isosexual precocious puberty. Her onset of breast development occurred at 10 months and her menarche at 1 1/12 years. Note the acceleration of growth velocity and bone age. The patient began receiving gonadotropin-releasing hormone (GnRH) analog therapy (*bar*) at 4 2/12 years, and her growth decelerated. Bone age, which is shown with ▲ on the horizontal line to the right of the height measurement, was significantly advanced at the beginning of therapy (just under 12 years) but advanced only minimally over the next 4 1/2 years (slightly over 13 years). (Growth chart courtesy of Dr. M.J. Mansfield.)

and family may be indicated to help them with the stress of coping with early development.

Followup for the child with precocious puberty depends on the diagnosis and the treatment undertaken. Girls being treated with GnRH analog therapy need to be seen frequently for assessment of compliance with medication, height and weight monitoring, and physical examination. A GnRH stimulation test and determination of estradiol level are usually done within the first 1 to 3 months after the beginning of treatment to establish suppression, and repeated at 6- to 12-month intervals, since the dose may need to be increased. Bone age is determined at 6-month intervals. Vaginal cytology for maturation index may provide additional evidence of suppression. Ultrasound can be used to determine regression of uterine size. It is important to monitor these patients closely, since incomplete suppression of estrogen by GnRH analog may actually result in a further decrease in final height. The growth chart of a patient treated with an analog is shown in Fig. 5.

In girls with McCune-Albright syndrome with gonadotropin-independent puberty and cyclic gonadal steroid production, GnRH agonist therapy does not cause a decrease in estradiol or regression of pubertal changes (21,24). Feuillan and colleagues (22) reported some success with testolactone, an aromatase inhibitor that blocks the synthesis of estrogens, in five girls with McCune-Albright syndrome; however, the effectiveness of this treatment decreases with time in some patients.

CONTRASEXUAL PRECOCIOUS PUBERTY

Contrasexual precocity arises from excess androgen production from an adrenal or ovarian source, which results in acne, hirsutism, and virilization. The differential diagnosis includes (a) CAH, (b) Cushing's syndrome with tumor-related androgen excess, (c) adrenal tumors, and (d) androgen-secreting ovarian tumors such as lipoid cell and arrhenoblastomas.

Patient Assessment

The patient should have a careful physical examination, with emphasis on noting evidence of hirsutism, acne, or clitoral enlargement, and an adequate abdominal and bimanual rectal examination to exclude an ovarian mass. Ovarian tumors are usually palpable.

Laboratory tests to be considered include serum levels of LH, FSH, estradiol, testosterone, DHEAS, dehydroepiandrosterone (DHEA), 17-hydroxyprogesterone, androstenedione, and 11 deoxycortisol (see Fig. 6 in Chapter 2 for pathways of steroid biosynthesis). Blood for the baseline 17-hydroxyprogesterone level is best drawn between 7 and 8 AM, since the diurnal variation of adrenal hormones brings about a normal level in the afternoon in patients with mild deficiencies of 21-hydroxylase. In girls with suspected CAH, a 1-hour ACTH stimulation test (see Chapter 7) is useful in detecting a block in the adrenal pathways. Adrenal tumors are usually associated with elevated serum DHEA, DHEAS, and androstenedione and are not suppressible by dexamethasone. Serum testosterone may be elevated because of direct secretion by the tumor or because of peripheral conversion. Cushing's syndrome is usually accompanied by signs of excess cortisol production and poor linear growth. A 24-hour urine collection for determination of free cortisol is useful if Cushing's syndrome or cortisol resistance are under consideration. Thus, the diagnosis is made by careful hormone studies with ACTH testing in cases of suspected CAH, abdominal and bimanual rectoabdominal palpation, ultrasonography, CT or MRI scanning for visualizing the adrenals, and resection of identified tumors.

Treatment and Followup

Ovarian and adrenal tumors should be surgically excised if possible. Patients with CAH should receive glucocorticoid replacement (e.g., hydrocortisone, 13 to 25 mg/m^2/day divided in three daily doses) and be monitored every 3 months. If the bone age is not too advanced, breast development may regress when CAH is treated. As noted earlier, some patients may develop secondary central precocity and be candidates for GnRH analog therapy.

PREMATURE THELARCHE

Premature thelarche is defined as breast development without any other signs of puberty and is most commonly seen among young girls under 2 years of age. Occasionally, neonatal breast hypertrophy fails to regress within 10 months after birth; this persistent breast development is also characterized as premature thelarche. The child with typical premature thelarche has bilateral breast buds of 2 to 4 cm with little or no change in the nipple or areola. The breast tissue feels granular and may be slightly tender. In some cases, development is quite asymmetric; one side may develop 6 to 12 months before the other. Growth is not accelerated, and the bone age is normal for height age. No other evidence of puberty appears; the labia often remain prepubertal without obvious evidence of estrogen effect. A vaginal smear for maturation index may show atrophy or may show slight evidence of estrogenization. Similarly, the serum estradiol may be slightly elevated in some patients (60,61).

Occasionally, patients who initally present with premature thelarche eventually develop true central precocious puberty (62). In girls with premature thelarche, basal and post-GnRH serum levels of LH and FSH are generally in the prepubertal range, although Ilicki and colleagues (61) have found that basal levels of FSH and the response to GnRH were higher than in prepubertal control subjects. They have postulated that premature thelarche is due to a derangement in maturation of the hypothalamic–pituitary–gonadal axis, with higher than normal FSH secretion and increased peripheral sensitivity to the sex hormones. This hypothesis would explain the occurrence of this problem principally in 1- to 4-year-old girls. Premature thelarche is also seen more commonly in very-low-birthweight infants (63). Thus, peripheral sensitivity may play a partial role, but increasing evidence points toward the importance of transient ovarian secretion of estrogen under hypothalamic–pituitary control. The usual clinical course of regression, or at least lack of progression, of breast development would then correlate with the waning of the estrogen levels as the ovarian follicles become atretic.

Patient Assessment

The assessment of a patient with premature breast development includes a careful review of medications and creams recently used. Occasionally it is discovered that a package of the mother's or sister's oral contraceptive pills has been ingested by the child. Premarin cream applied to the vulva nightly for >2 to 3 weeks may result in breast changes. The physical examination should include notation of the appearance of the vaginal mucosa and of the size of the breasts, and a rectoabdominal examination to exclude an ovarian cyst. The uterus should not be enlarged in patients with premature thelarche. Growth charts should be updated and assessed to see whether the patient is continuing to grow at her previously established percentile of height and weight. Laboratory tests include a radiogram of the left hand and wrist for bone age, a maturational index and, in some cases, a GnRH stimulation test, determination of estradiol level, and ultrasonography of the pelvis.

Treatment and Followup

Treatment consists mainly of reassurance and careful followup to confirm that the breast development does not represent the first sign of precocious puberty (65). A thorough physical examination should be done at each visit. Linear growth and bone age should be monitored. Biopsy of the breast tissue is not indicated, because removal of the breast bud prevents normal development. Although in most cases of premature thelarche, breast development regresses or stabilizes, some children do develop central precocious puberty. These patients cannot be distinguished clinically at initial presentation, so that followup is appropriate. Parents should be reassured that this is usually a self-limited process and pubertal development will occur at the normal adolescent age.

PREMATURE MENARCHE

Premature menarche most likely represents a similar but less common response than premature thelarche to the transient production of estrogen by the ovary. Prepubertal girls may have uterine bleeding lasting 1 to 5 days, once or in cycles for several months, without other evidence of estrogen effect. Blanco-Garcia and coworkers (29) found estradiol levels to be significantly above the normal prepubertal range and a seasonal increase in isolated menses between September and January. Before the clinician can make this diagnosis, other causes of vaginal bleeding, including infection, trauma, foreign body, and tumors, need to be excluded (see Chapter 3).

PREMATURE ADRENARCHE

Premature adrenarche is defined as the isolated appearance of pubic and, occasionally, axillary hair before the age of 8 years without evidence of estrogenization or virilization. Patients usually also have axillary odor. The terminology is sometimes confusing, but premature pubarche refers to the clinical manifestations of early pubic (and/or axillary) hair and premature adrenarche to the early maturation of adrenal androgen secretion. In common usage, the terms are often interchanged. Most patients have an increase in urinary 17-ketosteroid production and increased plasma levels of DHEA and DHEAS, which suggests that hormone biosynthesis in the adrenal gland undergoes maturation prematurely to a pubertal pattern (64). Although production of these androgens is suppressible by dexamethasone and therefore dependent on ACTH, the mediator for the change at puberty and in premature adrenarche is unknown. Levels of DHEAS are similar to those in girls with stage 2 pubic hair (Fig. 6). Bone age is usually normal or 1 year advanced (appropriate for height age).

The cause of premature adrenarche is not yet known. The condition appears to be more common in black and Hispanic girls and obese boys and girls. In some medical centers, including ours, some adolescents with androgen excess and polycystic ovary syndrome have been observed to have a history of premature adrenarche (66,67) (see Chapter 7). Some girls with premature adrenarche do have evidence of a partial deficiency of 21-hydroxylase and possibly 3β-hydroxysteroid dehydrogenase or are heterozygotes for 21-hydroxylase deficiency (3,68–71). In a referred population with a predominance of ethnic groups known to have a high incidence of nonclassical 21-hydroxylase deficiency (Ashkenazi Jewish, Hispanic, and Italian), Temeck and colleagues (69) found that among girls with premature adrenarche between the ages of 2 and 7 years, 5 of 19 (26%) had 21-hydroxylase deficiency. In a study of 127 Italian children with premature pubarche who underwent ACTH testing, 12% had mild errors in steroidogenesis (71). These studies need to be repeated in ethnic populations with a lower incidence of these disorders, especially among American black chil-

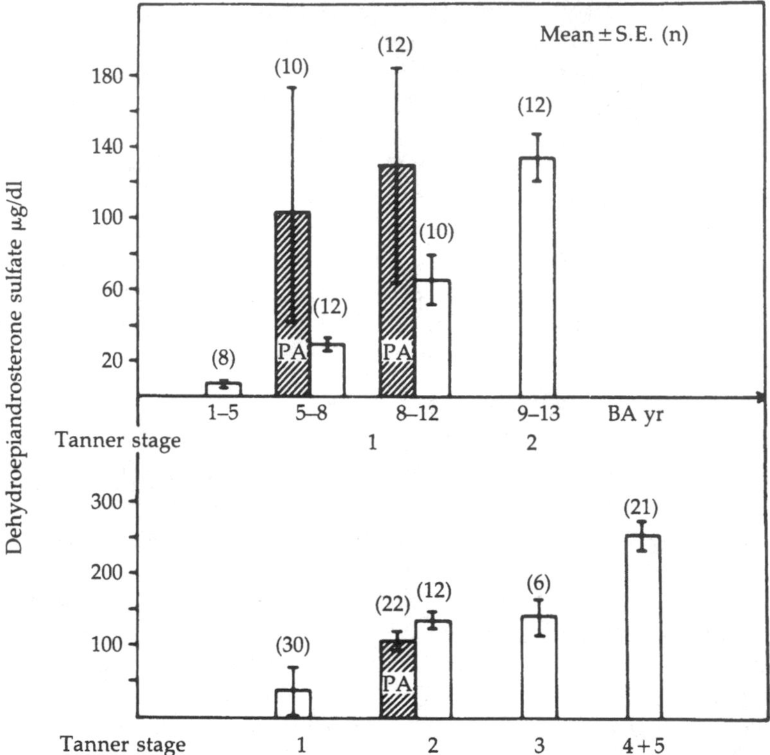

FIG. 6. Dehydroepiandrosterone sulfate (DHEAS) levels in girls with precocious adrenarche (PA) compared with normal girls of various bone ages (BA) and stages of pubic hair development (Tanner stages 1 to 4/5). DHEAS levels are appropriate for the Tanner stage of pubic hair but are elevated for the bone age. S.E., standard error; n, number. (From Korth-Schutz S, Levine LS, New MI. Dehydroepiandrosterone sulfate (DS) levels, a rapid test for abnormal adrenal androgen secretion. *J Clin Endocrinol Metab* 1076;42:1005; with permission.)

dren, since premature adrenarche is so common in these girls between the ages of 5 and 8 years (2). Thus, the exact percentage of children with adrenal enzyme deficiencies, the natural history, and the benefits of intervention need to be defined better, since doing a 1-hour ACTH test in all girls with premature adrenarche would add substantially to the expense of the evaluation. A 1-hour ACTH test is indicated in all girls with elevated baseline (7 to 8 AM) 17-hydroxyprogesterone, those whose bone age is advanced >1 year, those with increased linear growth, and those with any signs of clitoromegaly or virilization. Even in the absence of these indications, white girls, especially those from the ethnic groups with an increased risk of nonclassical 21-hydroxylase deficiency, should be screened with a DHEAS level and an early-morning 17-hydroxyprogesterone determination as a minimum.

Patient Assessment

The assessment of the patient with premature adrenarche is similar to that for contrasexual precocious puberty. The important findings on physical examination are the presence of pubic hair and axillary odor and the *absence* of breast development, estrogenization of the labia and vagina, and virilization (clitoromegaly).

The laboratory tests include determination of bone age, serum DHEAS, and early-morning (7 to 8 AM) 17-hydroxyprogesterone. As noted earlier, the criteria for ACTH testing need further refinement. However, in many medical centers, this test is performed on all patients to detect enzyme deficiencies and better define the potential causes of this condition. The differential diagnosis must exclude precocious puberty, CAH, and an adrenal or ovarian tumor. Sometimes, the diagnosis of adrenarche is made only in retrospect when further evidence of precocious puberty does not occur. It should be recalled that most patients with precocious puberty have an advanced bone age, growth spurt, and evidence of estrogenization on vaginal smear. Patients with tumors and some patients with CAH have evidence of virilization.

Treatment and Followup

The treatment of premature adrenarche is reassurance and followup. The child should be examined every 3 to 6 months initially to confirm the original diagnostic impression; evidence of virilization or early estrogen effect points to a different diagnosis. Growth data should be carefully plotted. It is hoped that treatment of late-onset 21-hydroxylase deficiency with corticosteroids will prevent the development of polycystic ovary syndrome in early adolescence. In general, pubertal development at adolescence can be expected to be normal. Some patients will have hirsutism and irregular menses as adolescents (66).

REFERENCES

1. Tanner JM. Trend towards earlier menarche in London, Oslo, Copenhagen, the Netherlands, and Hungary. *Nature* 1973;243:95.
2. Herman-Giddens ME, Slora EJ, Wasserman RC, et al. Secondary sexual characteristics and menses in young girls seen in office practice: a study from the pediatric research in office settings network. *Pediatrics* 1997;99:505.
3. Rosenfield RL. Normal and almost normal precocious variations in pubertal development premature pubarche and premature thelarche revisited. *Horm Res* 1994;41(suppl 2):7.
4. Pescovitz OH. Precocious puberty. *Pediatr Rev* 1990;11:116.
5. Hardin DS, Pescovitz OH. Central precocious puberty and its treatment with long-acting GnRH analogs. *Endocrinologist* 1991;1:163.
6. Wheeler MD, Styne DM. Diagnosis and management of precocious puberty. *Pediatr Clin North Am* 1990;37:1255.
7. Bridges NA, Christopher JA, Hindmarsh PC, Brook CGD. Sexual precocity: sex incidence and aetiology. *Arch Dis Child* 1994;70:116.

8. Hochman HI, Judge DM, Reichlin S. Precocious puberty and hypothalamic hamartoma. *Pediatrics* 1981;67:236.
9. Cacciari E, Frejaville E, Cicognani A, et al. How many cases of true precocious puberty in girls are idiopathic? *J Pediatr* 1983;102:357.
10. Judge DM, Kulin HE, Pagea R, et al. Hypothalamic hamartoma and luteinizing-hormone release in precocious puberty. *N Engl J Med* 1977;296:7.
11. Mahachoklertwattana P, Kaplan S, Grumbach M. The luteinizing hormone-releasing hormone-secreting hypothalamic hamartoma is a congenital malformation: natural history. *J Clin Endocrinol Metab* 1993;77:118.
12. Balagura S, Shulman K, Sobel EH. Precocious puberty of cerebral origin. *Surg Neurol* 1979;11:315.
13. Leiper AD, Stanhope R, Kiching P, et al. Precocious and premature puberty associated with treatment of acute lymphoblastic leukaemia. *Arch Dis Child* 1987;62:1107.
14. Laue L, Comite F, Hench K, et al. Precocious puberty associated with neurofibromatosis and optic gliomas. *Am J Dis Child* 1985;139:1097.
15. Pringle PJ, Stanhope R, Hindmarsh P, Brook CG. Abnormal pubertal development in primary hypothyroidism. *Clin Endocrinol* 1988;28(5):479.
16. Anasti JN, Flack MR, Froehlich J, et al. A potential novel mechanism for precocious puberty in juvenile hypothyroidism. *J Clin Endocrinol Metab* 1995;80:276.
17. Gordon CM, Austin DJ, Radovick S, Laufer MR. Primary hypothroidism presenting as severe vaginal bleeding in a premenarchal girl. *J Pediatr Adolesc Gynecol* 1997;10:35.
18. Sigurjonsdottir TJ, Hayles AB. Precocious puberty: a report of 96 cases. *Am J Dis Child* 1968; 115:309.
19. Thamdrup E. Precocious sexual development. *Dan Med Bull* 1961;8:140.
20. Pescovitz OH, Hench K, Green O, et al. Central precocious puberty complicating a virilizing adrenal tumor: treatment with a long-acting LHRH analog. *J Pediatr* 1985;106:612.
21. Wierman ME, Beardsworth DE, Mansfield MJ, et al. Puberty with gonadotropins: a unique mechanism of sexual development. *N Engl J Med* 1985;312:65.
22. Feuillan PP, Foster CM, Pescovitz OH, et al. Treatment of precocious puberty in the McCune-Albright syndrome with the aromatase inhibitor testolactone. *N Engl J Med* 1986;315:1115.
23. Foster CM, Feuillan P, Padmanabhan V, et al. Ovarian function in girls with McCune-Albright syndrome. *Pediatr Res* 1986;20:859.
24. Comite F, Shawker TH, Prescovitz OH, et al. Cyclical ovarian function resistant to treatment with an analogue of luteinizing hormone releasing hormone in McCune-Albright syndrome. *N Engl J Med* 1984;311:1032.
25. Lee PA, VanDop C, Migeon C. McCune-Albright syndrome: longterm follow up. *JAMA* 1986;256: 2980.
26. Weinstein LS, Shenker A, Gejman PV, et al. Activating mutations of the stimulatory G protein in the McCune Albright syndrome. *N Engl J Med* 1991;325:1688.
27. Freni-Titulaer LW, Cordero JF, Haddock L, et al. Premature thelarche in Puerto Rico. *Am J Dis Child* 1986;140:1263.
28. Bourguignon JP, Gerard A, Alvarez Gonzalez ML, et al. Effects of changes in nutritional conditions on timing of puberty: clinical evidence from adopted children and experimental studies in the male rat. *Horm Res* 1992;32(suppl 1):97.
29. Blanco-Garcia M, Evain-Brion D, Roger M, et al. Isolated menses in prepubertal girls. *Pediatrics* 1985;76:43.
30. Saggese G, Ghirri P, Del Vecchio A, et al. Gonadotropin pulsatile secretion in girls with premature menarche. *Horm Res* 1990;33:5.
31. Sane K, Pescovitz OH. The clitoral index: a determination of clitoral size in normal girls and in girls with abnormal sexual development. *J Pediatr* 1992;120:264.
32. Stanhope R, Adams J, Jacobs HS, Brook CGD. Ovarian ultrasound assessment in normal children, idiopathic precocious puberty, and during low dose pulsatile gonadotrophin releasing hormone treatment of hypogonadotropic hypogonadism. *Arch Dis Child* 1985;60:116.
33. Fontoura M, Brauner R, Prevot C, et al. Precocious puberty in girls: early diagnosis of a slowly progressing variant. *Arch Dis Child* 1989;64:1170.
34. Lee PA. Laboratory monitoring of children with precocious puberty. *Arch Pediatr Adolesc Med* 1994;148:369.
35. Neely EK, Wilson DM, Lee PA, et al. Spontaneous serum gonadotropin concentrations in the evaluation of precocious puberty. *J Pediatr* 1995;127:47.

36. Garibaldi LR, Picco P, Magier S, et al. Serum luteinizing hormone concentrations, as measured by a sensitive immunoradiometric assay, in children with normal, precocious or delayed pubertal development. *J Clin Endocrinol Metab* 1991;72:888.
37. Rosenfield RL. Selection of children with precocious puberty for treatment with gonadotropin releasing hormone analogs. *J Pediatr* 1993;124:989.
38. Bar A, Linder B, Sobel EH, et al. Bayley-Pinneau method of height prediction in girls with central precocious puberty: correlation with adult height. *J Pediatr* 1995;126:955.
39. Kletter GB, Kelch RP. Effects of gonadotropin-releasing hormone analog therapy on adult stature in precocious puberty. *J Clin Endocrinol Metab* 1994;79:331.
40. Shoevaart CE, Drop SLS, Otten BJ, et al. Growth analysis up to final height and psychosocial adjustment of treated and untreated patients with precocious puberty. *Horm Res* 1990;34:197.
41. Crowley WF, Comite F, Vale W, et al. Therapeutic use for pituitary desensitization with a long-acting LHRH agonist: a potential new treatment for idiopathic precocious puberty. *J Clin Endocrinol Metab* 1981;52:370.
42. Comite F, Cutler GB, Rivier J, et al. Short-term treatment of idiopathic precocious puberty with a long-acting analogue of luteinizing hormone releasing hormone. *N Engl J Med* 1981;305:1539.
43. Kreiter M, Burstein S. Rosenfield RL, et al. Preserving adult height potential in girls with idiopathic precocious puberty. *J Pediatr* 1990;117:364.
44. Kappy MS, Stuart T, Perelman A. Efficacy of leuprolide therapy in children with central precocious puberty. *Am J Dis Child* 1988;142:1061.
45. Comite F, Cassorla F, Barnes KM, et al. Luteinizing hormone releasing hormone analogue therapy for central precocious puberty. *JAMA* 1986;255:2613.
46. Mansfield MJ, Beardsworth DE, Loughlin JS, et al. Long-term treatment of central precocious puberty with a long-acting analogue of luteinizing hormone-releasing hormone. *N Engl J Med* 1983;309:1286.
47. Manasco PK, Pescovitz OH, Hill SC, et al. Six-year results of luteinizing hormone releasing hormone (LHRH) agonist treatment in children with LHRH-dependent precocious puberty. *J Pediatr* 1989:115:105.
48. Boepple PA, Mansfield MJ, Link K, et al. Impact of sex steroids and their suppression on skeletal growth and maturation. *Am J Physiol* 1988;255:E559.
49. Lee PA, Page JG, Leuprolide Study Group. Effects of leuprolide in the treatment of central precocious puberty. *J Pediatr* 1989;114:321.
50. Boepple PA, Mansfield MJ, Weirman ME, et al. Use of a potent, long acting agonist of gonadotropin-releasing hormone in the treatment of precocious puberty. *Endocrinol Rev* 1986;7:24.
51. Brauner R, Adan L, Malandry F, Zantleifer D. Adult height in girls with idiopathic true precocious puberty. *J Clin Endocrinol Metab* 1994;79:415.
52. Oerter KE, Manasco P, Barnes KM, et al. Adult height in precocious puberty after long-term treatment with deslorelin. *J Clin Endocrinol Metab* 1991;73:1235.
53. Jay N, Mansfield MJ, Blizzard RM, et al. Ovulation and menstrual function of adolescent girls with central precocious puberty after therapy with gonadotropin-releasing hormone agonists. *J Clin Endocrinol Metab* 1992:75;890.
54. Manasco PK, Pescovitz OH, Feuillan PP, et al. Resumption of puberty after long term luteinizing hormone-releasing hormone agonist treatment of central precocious puberty. *J Clin Endocrinol Metab* 1988;67:368.
55. Saggese G, Bertelloni S, Baroncelli GI, et al. Reduction of bone density: an effect of gonadotropin releasing hormone analogue treatment in central precocious puberty. *Eur J Pediatr* 1993;152:717.
56. Weirman ME, Beardsworth DE, Crawford JD, et al. Adrenarche and skeletal maturation during luteinizing hormone releasing hormone analogue suppression of gonadarche. *J Clin Invest* 1986;77:121.
57. Mansfield MJ, Rudlin CR, Crigler JF Jr, et al. Changes in growth and serum growth hormone and plasma somatomedin-C levels during suppression of gonadal sex steroid secretion in girls with central precocious puberty. *J Clin Endocrinol Metab* 1988;66:3.
58. Sonis WA, Comite F, Glue J, et al. Behavior problems and social competence in girls with true precocious puberty. *J Pediatr* 1985;106:156.
59. Ehrhart AA, Meyer-Bahlburg HFL, Bell JJ, et al. Idiopathic precocious puberty in girls: psychiatric follow-up in adolescence. *J Am Acad Child Psychiatry* 1984;23:23.
60. Escobar ME, Rivarola MA, Bergada C. Plasma concentration of oestradiol-17β in premature thelarche and in different types of sexual precocity. *Acta Endocrinol* (Copenh) 1976;81:351.

61. Ilicki A, Lewin RP, Kauli R, et al. Premature thelarche—natural history and sex hormone secretion in 68 girls. *Acta Paediatr Scand* 1984;73:756.
62. Pasquino AM, Pucarelli I, Passeri F, et al. Progression of premature thelarche to precocious puberty. *J Pediatr* 1995;126:11.
63. Nelson KG. Premature thelarche in children born prematurely. *J Pediatr* 1983;103:756.
64. Korth-Schultz S, Levine LS, New M. Dehydroepiandrosterone sulfate (DS) levels, a rapid test for abnormal adrenal androgen secretion. *J Clin Endocrinol Metab* 1976;42:1005.
65. Van Winter JT, Noller KL, Zimmerman D, Melton LJ. Natural history of premature thelarche in Olmsted County Minnesota, 1940–1984. *J Pediatr* 1990;116:278.
66. Ibanez L, Potau N, Virdis R, et al. Postpubertal outcome in girls diagnosed of premature pubarche during childhood: increased frequency of functional ovarian hyperandrogenism. *J Clin Endocrinol Metab* 1993;76:1599.
67. Miller DP, Emans SJ, Kohane I. A follow-up study of adolescent girls with a history of premature adrenarche. *J Adolesc Health* 1996;18.
68. Kaplowitz PB, Cockrell JL, Young RB. Premature adrenarche. *Clin Pediatr* 1986;25:28.
69. Temeck JW, Pang S, Nelson C, et al. Genetic defects of steroidogenesis in premature pubarche. *J Clin Endocrinol Metab* 1987;64:609
70. Granoff AB, Chasalow FI, Blethen SL. 17-Hydroxyprogesterone responses to adrenocorticotropin in children with premature adrenarche. *J Clin Endocrinol Metab* 1985;60:409.
71. Balducci R, Boscherini B, Mangiantini A, et al. Isolated precocious pubarche: an approach. *J Clin Endocrinol Metab* 1994;79:582.

6

Delayed Puberty and Menstrual Irregularities

This chapter presents a practical approach to delayed sexual development, amenorrhea, and dysfunctional uterine bleeding in young women. Chapters 1 and 4 should be mastered before an evaluation of any of these problems is undertaken. (Gonadal development and embryogenesis are reviewed in Chapters 2 and 8.) The goal in evaluating menstrual irregularities is to rule out the rare tumor or systemic disease and to make a diagnosis in order to present a discussion and treatment plan to the teenage girl and her parents.

Pubertal and menstrual problems of adolescents include (a) delayed sexual development, (b) delayed menarche with some pubertal development, (c) delayed menarche plus virilization, (d) secondary amenorrhea, (e) oligomenorrhea, and (f) dysfunctional uterine bleeding. The distinction between many of these entities is somewhat artificial because many of the problems that cause pubertal delay can also cause primary or secondary amenorrhea. For example, the patient with 45,X/46,XX (Turner's mosaic) or the patient with anorexia nervosa may present to the clinician with no sexual development, or primary or secondary amenorrhea. It is thus helpful for the clinician to think about a general approach to define the source of the hypothalamic–pituitary–ovarian axis abnormality and to determine whether a genital anomaly is present.

After the history and physical examination, the differential diagnosis can usually be divided on the basis of follicle-stimulating hormone (FSH) levels into categories of hypergonadotropic hypogonadism (ovarian failure) and hypogonadotropic hypogonadism (hypothalamic or pituitary dysfunction). Patients who appear to be well estrogenized but have amenorrhea may have a genital anomaly or polycystic ovary syndrome. These distinctions allow the clinician to focus on the causes and diagnostic tests that would be useful in formulating a treatment plan.

A careful history and physical examination are essential whenever the patient expresses concern about her physical development. A girl who has not experienced any pubertal development by the age of 13 years is more than 2 standard deviations beyond the normal age of initiating puberty and deserves a medical evaluation. For the exceptional girl who is known to have a debilitating chronic disease or who is involved in ballet or a competitive, endurance sport such as track or gymnastics that may be associated with a delay in development, the diagnostic work-up can be postponed until age 14 years. Absence of menarche by age 16 years is usually termed delayed menarche. No menarche by 18 years (some authors use 16 years) is termed primary amenorrhea. Only 3 in 1,000 girls will experience menarche after 15 1/2 years. In assessing the individual patient, the clinician needs to keep in mind the normal stages of puberty. For example, if the 15-year-old began her sexual development at the age of 14 years, she can usually be reassured that she can expect her menarche by the age of 16 or 17 years, 2 to 3 years after the onset of secondary sexual characteristics. The patient should be observed for a reassuring steady progression of growth and development. A halt in maturation signifies the need to do a thorough endocrine evaluation. Likewise, the girl who started her development at age 11 and has not had her menarche by age 15 years deserves an evaluation to determine the cause, including a careful pelvic examination to exclude a genital anomaly (see Chapter 8) before serum hormone levels are obtained.

The definition of secondary amenorrhea, and thus guidelines for timing of the evaluation, are problematic in the adolescent, since pregnancy is such a frequent cause of this complaint. Denial of intercourse is common among teenagers. Young adolescents may not understand their anatomy well enough to answer questions accurately or may have become pregnant by rape or incest. Thus, a pregnancy test should be done whenever an adolescent expresses concern about a menstrual period being late, even if only by 2 or 3 weeks. Such concern should prompt the physician to explore with the teenager a history of unprotected intercourse. Adolescents who are not sexually active are less likely to contact their physicians about mildly irregular or late menses. Nevertheless, a pregnancy test should be obtained promptly in adolescents with late menses, even if sexual activity is denied. Hormone tests and further evaluation of amenorrhea are usually reserved for adolescents who have had 3 to 6 months of amenorrhea without an obvious cause (such as dieting) and those with persistent oligomenorrhea, estrogen deficiency, or androgen excess (hirsutism, acne). Several illustrative case histories are included at the end of each section of this chapter.

The pertinent past history depends in part on the presenting complaint and may include the following:

1. Family history: heights of all family members; age of menarche and fertility of sisters, mother, grandmothers, and aunts (familial disorders include delayed menarche, androgen insensitivity, congenital adrenal hyperplasia, and some forms of gonadal dysgenesis); history of ovarian tumors (e.g., gonadoblastomas in intersex disorders); and history of endocrine (autoimmune) disorders such as thyroiditis and Addison's disease.

2. Neonatal history: maternal ingestion of hormones such as androgens or high-dose progestins that can cause clitoromegaly, maternal history of miscarriages, birth weight, congenital anomalies, lymphedema (Turner's syndrome), and neonatal problems suggestive of hypopituitarism such as hypoglycemia.
3. Previous surgery, irradiation, or chemotherapy.
4. Review of systems with special emphasis on a history of chronic disease, abdominal pain, diarrhea, headaches, neurologic symptoms, ability to smell, weight changes, eating disorders, sexual activity, medications, substance abuse, emotional stresses, competitive athletics, and hirsutism.
5. Age of initiation of pubertal development, if any, and rate of development.
6. Growth data plotted on charts, such as those illustrated in Chapter 4.

The physical examination involves a general assessment including height and weight (plotted on growth charts), blood pressure, palpation of the thyroid gland, and Tanner (Sexual Maturity Rating [SMR]) staging of breast development and pubic hair. The breasts should be compressed gently to examine for the presence of galactorrhea, since patients frequently do not report this abnormality. An evaluation should also be made for congenital anomalies, especially midline facial defects that may be associated with hypothalamic-pituitary dysfunction and the somatic stigmata of Turner's syndrome. Renal and vertebral anomalies and hernias may be associated with müllerian malformations. A neurologic examination is important in patients with delayed or interrupted puberty and should include an assessment of the ability to smell, fundoscopic examination, and screening visual field tests by confrontation (formal visual field tests are indicated if a pituitary tumor is diagnosed).

In the initial examination of the adolescent with no pubertal development, the gynecologic examination usually involves inspection of the external genitalia in a search for clitoromegaly, estrogen effect, and a normal hymen. Since the cause of the delay is likely an ovarian or hypothalamic-pituitary problem, visualizing the cervix is much less crucial in a girl with no pubertal maturation than in one with normal breast development but delayed menarche. However, in the nonobese prepubertal teenager, a simple rectoabdominal examination will often allow palpation of the cervix and the uterus. If needed to assess internal genital structures in the unestrogenized adolescent suspected to have a congenital abnormality such as absence of the uterus, the knee-chest position (see Chapter 1) can be used, just as in the prepubertal child, to visualize the vagina and the cervix. For the adolescent with pubertal development and delayed menarche, it is crucial to exclude a genital anomaly. Techniques for examining the adolescent girl are in Chapter 1. The girl with secondary amenorrhea, oligomenorrhea, and abnormal vaginal bleeding needs a gynecologic assessment, which usually involves a speculum examination or at minimum a bimanual rectoabdominal examination. Occasionally, external genital examination and ultrasonography are all the patient will allow.

The degree of estrogenization noted at the time of the initial examination can often help the clinician decide the extent of the workup indicated. The finding of a reddened, thin vaginal mucosa is consistent with estrogen deficiency and is more worrisome than the finding of an estrogenized, pink, moist vaginal mucosa. Obtaining a sample for vaginal smear for maturation index at the time of the examination can confirm and aid the clinical assessment of the degree of estrogen effect (see Chapter 1). After confirming that the patient is not pregnant, the clinician can prescribe a progestin challenge with oral medroxyprogesterone (5 or 10 mg once a day for 5 or 10 days) to determine whether the endometrium is primed with estrogen. Some clinicians prefer to use intramuscular progesterone-in-oil 50 to 100 mg or micronized progesterone. The response to progestin challenge tends to correlate with estradiol level. Kletzky and colleagues (1) reported that the mean estradiol concentration was 60 pg/ml in 63 women who had withdrawal bleeding versus a mean value of 18 pg/ml in 27 women who had no withdrawal response. Among a group of women with a screening estradiol of >50 pg/ml, Shangold and colleagues (2) found that a 10-day course of micronized progesterone, 300 mg, induced withdrawal bleeding in 90%. Micronized progesterone has the advantage of being safe during pregnancy, but pharmaceutical preparations are not widely available. The absorption of micronized progesterone appears to be enhanced by the presence of food, and the bioavailibility is approximately 10% compared with intramuscular progesterone (3). Bleeding typically tends to occur 2 to 3 days after the progestin dose but may occur up to 10 days later. The progestin withdrawal test is not indicated in the patient with delayed development or in the patient who clearly appears estrogen deficient on clinical examination, as bleeding will not occur.

Ultrasonography is not a routine part of the evaluation of menstrual disorders but can be extremely useful to confirm uterine agenesis, müllerian anomalies, or adnexal masses in an adolescent and to assess the adolescent who cannot be examined by rectoabdominal or vaginal abdominal palpation. The clinician should be cautious in the interpretation of the pelvic ultrasound in the adolescent with no puberty (no estrogenization) because the uterus may not be well visualized and thus may be assumed to be absent. If questions are raised at the time of the initial evaluation, the ultrasound can be repeated in a pediatric center accustomed to the appearance of the prepubertal uterus or after a course of estrogen therapy.

In adolescents, assessment of the pattern of growth can yield valuable information to contribute to a diagnosis. Failure of statural growth for several years may occur with Crohn's disease or an acquired endocrine disorder, or it may indicate that the adolescent has reached a bone age of 15 years and her epiphyses have fused. In conditions associated with poor nutrition, such as anorexia nervosa, celiac disease, and inflammatory bowel disease, weight is typically affected more than height. The patient is thus underweight for her height. In contrast, patients with acquired hypothyroidism, cortisol excess (iatrogenic or Cushing's syndrome), and Turner's syndrome are typically overweight for height.

Obtaining a radiograph of the wrist and hand for bone age can be helpful in assessing patients with delayed development to estimate final height (see Appendix 7). For example, hypothyroidism tends to delay bone age more than height age. (Height age is the age at which the patient's height would be on the 50th percentile on a growth chart.) With constitutional delay, both bone age and height age are similarly delayed. Menarche is more closely linked to bone age than to chronologic age.

Assessment of the percentage of body fat may also help in explaining to the patient the relationship of amenorrhea to the body composition. A low percentage of body fat has been associated with delayed puberty and amenorrhea in athletes and in patients with eating disorders. Although the relationship is an association and not necessarily causative, the determination may aid in setting realistic goals for the future. Methodologic issues abound in determining the best way to estimate percentage body fat. All office methods have problems, but the clinician rarely has available more accurate methods such as total body electrical conductivity (TOBEC) (4), magnetic resonance imaging (MRI) (5), optical techniques using a near infrared light beam, or underwater weighing techniques. A clinical *estimate* of percentage body fat can be obtained by measuring four sites of skinfold thickness (triceps, biceps, subscapular, and supraliac), using calipers and comparing the results with tables and equations given in Appendix 6 (6,7). Oppliger and Cassady have suggested that women athletes maintain a percentage body fat >12% to 14% (8); however, optimal ranges for adolescents that take growth, development, and menses into account have not been determined.

Initial laboratory screening tests for menstrual problems include a complete blood count (CBC) and serum levels of thyroid-stimulating hormone (TSH), follicle-stimulating hormone (FSH), and luteinizing hormone (LH). Serum prolactin level and T_4 may also be determined initially if a central cause of the delayed puberty or amenorrhea is suspected. In patients suspected to have a gonadal disorder because of significant short stature, determination of the prolactin level can be delayed until the result of the FSH level is known. In girls with delayed puberty or symptoms of chronic illness, a sedimentation rate is often obtained in addition to creatinine level and other chemistry determinations. An elevated sedimentation rate may be a clue to a diagnosis such as Crohn's disease, although a normal erythrocyte sedimentation rate does not exclude this diagnosis. It should be noted that many clinicians order both an LH and an FSH level in girls with menstrual abnormalities; others use only the FSH level to differentiate ovarian failure from other causes of amenorrhea. Unless a high FSH level is expected because of prior radiation therapy, a single high FSH should be repeated before a definitive statement about ovarian failure is made to the patient and family. Low to normal levels of FSH (and LH) imply a central nervous system (CNS) cause, for example, hypothalamic dysfunction, which may be primary or secondary to a chronic disease, stress, or an eating disorder or, rarely, a CNS tumor. Occasionally, blood sampling for the LH

TABLE 1. *Etiologic breakdown of pubertal abnormalities in 252 patients*

Abnormality[a]	Group total	No.	%
Hypergonadotropic hypogonadism			
CIOF	69		27
CCOF	40		16
46,XX		34	14
46,XY		6	2
Total	109		43
Hypogonadotropic hypogonadism			
Reversible	48		19
Physiologic delay		35	14
Weight loss/anorexia nervosa		6	2
Primary hypothyroidism		3	1
Congenital adrenal hyperplasia		3	1
Cushing's syndrome		1	0.5
Irreversible	29		12
Congenital deficiency syndromes			
Isolated GnRH deficiency		13	5
Forms of hypopituitarism		6	2
Congenital CNS defects		2	1
Acquired anatomic lesions			
Prolactin-secreting adenoma		3	1
Unclassified pituitary adenoma		2	1
Craniopharyngioma		1	0.5
Unclassified malignant pituitary tumor		1	0.5
Postsurgical hypopituitarism (craniopharyngioma)		1	0.5
Total	77		31
Eugonadism			
Anatomic	46		18
Rokitansky's syndrome		37	15
Transverse vaginal septum		7	3
Imperforate hymen		2	1
Inappropriate positive feedback	17		7
Androgen insensitivity syndrome	3		1
Total	66		26

[a]CIOF, chromosomally incompetent ovarian failure; CCOF, chromosomally competent ovarian failure; GnRF, gonadotropin releasing factor; CNS, central nervous system.

(From Reindollar RH, Byrd JR, McDonough PG. Delayed sexual development: a study of 252 patients. *Am J Obstet Gynecol* 1981;140:371; with permission.)

determination occurs during the midcycle LH surge, and the levels can be three times normal baseline levels. Thus, in the oligomenorrheic patient it is important to make sure that she did not have menstrual bleeding 2 weeks after the sample was drawn so that the results can be correctly interpreted. Occasionally, patients with normal FSH levels have subtle disorders of ovarian function, which have been evaluated in adult women with the clomiphene challenge test (9).

It is important to remember that although constitutional delayed puberty is common in boys, it is less common in girls. A definitive diagnosis is likely in the girl with delayed or interrupted puberty. The spectrum of disorders that were seen in a study of 252 patients evaluated between 1960 and 1980 in the

Reproductive Unit of the Medical College of Georgia is shown in Table 1 (10). It should be remembered, however, that this series was based on a referral population, and a different balance of diagnoses is likely to be seen by the primary care clinician.

HYPERGONADOTROPIC HYPOGONADISM

High FSH and LH Levels

Adolescents with elevated gonadotropins may have an abnormal karyotype (such as Turner's syndrome or, rarely, 46,XY gonadal dysgenesis) or a normal karyotype (such as autoimmune oophoritis, 46,XX premature ovarian failure, or ovarian failure associated with radiation or chemotherapy). In addition, some patients with chromosomal abnormalities of the autosomes may have ovarian failure. These patients typically present with delayed development but may have primary or secondary amenorrhea after undergoing some—or even complete—pubertal maturation. In the adolescent population, most patients with ovarian failure have gonadal dysgenesis or premature oocyte loss; in contrast, a higher percentage of patients in the adult population has autoimmune ovarian failure as a cause of premature menopause. It is important to remember that some patients with premature menopause may have fluctuating levels of gonadotropins and estradiol for months to years and may recover menstrual function spontaneously with the rare possibility of fertility. Although Alper and coworkers (11) reported that 6 of 80 (7.5%) women conceived after the diagnosis of premature ovarian failure, patients with elevated gonadotropins during adolescence are less likely to have a reversal of the hypogonadism. In addition, patients with autoimmune ovarian failure may develop adrenal insufficiency or other autoimmune endocrinopathies; thus, long-term followup is essential.

Initial evaluation of the adolescent with elevated FSH levels in the absence of a history of radiation therapy or chemotherapy includes a karyotype determination. In patients with 46,XX ovarian failure, further studies include assessment for autoimmune ovarian failure. In the hypertensive patient with elevated FSH and delayed puberty, serum levels of progesterone (and 11-deoxycorticosterone and corticosterone) are obtained in a search for the rare case of 17α-hydroxylase deficiency. Laparoscopy or laparotomy with gonadal biopsy is rarely indicated.

Gonadal Dysgenesis

Turner's syndrome occurs in approximately 1 of 2,000 live-born girls and in 1 of 15 spontaneous abortions (12). Slightly over one-half of patients with gonadal dysgenesis have the classic 45,X karyotype (Turner's syndrome). The stigmata of Turner's syndrome include short stature, broad chest, webbed neck, low hairline, short fourth or fifth metacarpals, cubitus valgus, genu valgum, ptosis, low-set ears, narrow high-arched palate, micrognathia, lymphedema, and multiple pigmented nevi. Some anomalies such as the webbed neck, low hairline, rotated auricle, puffy hands and feet, and nail dysplasia appear to be secondary to lymphatic obstruction (13). The mean final heights of girls with Turner's syndrome not treated with growth hormone have been reported to be 142 to 146.8 cm (56 to 58 inches) with two large studies giving a mean of 143 cm (14). A positive correlation has been found between the height standard deviation scores of mosaic patients and the frequency of normal chromosome constitution and a negative correlation of height with the frequency of cells with 45,X (15). Associated problems include cardiac anomalies in one-third (bicuspid aortic valve, coarctation of the aorta, mitral valve prolapse, dissecting aneurysms); renal anomalies in 35% to 70% (horseshoe kidneys, unilateral pelvic kidney, rotational abnormalities, duplicated collecting systems, and rarely ureteral pelvic obstruction and hydronephrosis); hearing impairment, otitis media, and mastoiditis in one-third; and an increased incidence of hypertension, achlorhydria, glucose intolerance, osteopenia, diabetes mellitus, and Hashimoto's thyroiditis (12–14,16–28). Gastrointestinal diagnoses include vascular malformations, which may present with bleeding and possibly an increased incidence of inflammatory bowel disease. Intelligence appears to be normal in most studies of patients with Turner's syndrome, although there can be specific deficits in spatiotemporal processing, visual motor coordination, and specific learning skills (12,29). A high incidence of mental retardation has been reported in girls carrying a small ring chromosome X (12). Girls may be held back in school because of immaturity and short stature, and parents and teachers may expect less of them (14). Clinicians should also ask about potential teasing at school and have counselors address these issues.

A young adolescent with Turner's syndrome has prepubertal female genitalia, bilateral streak gonads, and a normal uterus and vagina capable of responding to exogenous hormones; she may have sparse or absent pubic and axillary hair in spite of levels of dehydroepiandrosterone sulfate (DHEAS) that correspond to pubic hair stages 2 to 3. The growth chart of a Turner's syndrome patient is shown in Fig. 1; the height data are plotted on a special growth chart with percentiles for Turner's syndrome (these charts can be obtained from Genentech).* The older adolescent (15 or 16 years old) with undiagnosed or untreated Turner's syndrome usually has pubic and axillary hair, but no breast development or estrogenization of the vaginal mucosa (no ovarian function).

Forty to 50 percent of patients with gonadal dysgenesis have a mosaic karyotype (e.g., 46,XX/45,X) or a structural abnormality of the second X chromosome (e.g., deletion of part of the short arm [p-] or long arm [q-] of the X, ring chromosome, or isochromosome) (30,31). In a study of 478 patients with Turner's syndrome, 52.1% were 45,X; 10.9% were 45,X/46,XX; 4.6% were 45,X/47,XXX or another "superfemale" cell line; 16.1% had isochromosomes;

*Genentech, Inc., 460 Pt. Bruno Blvd., San Francisco CA 94080.

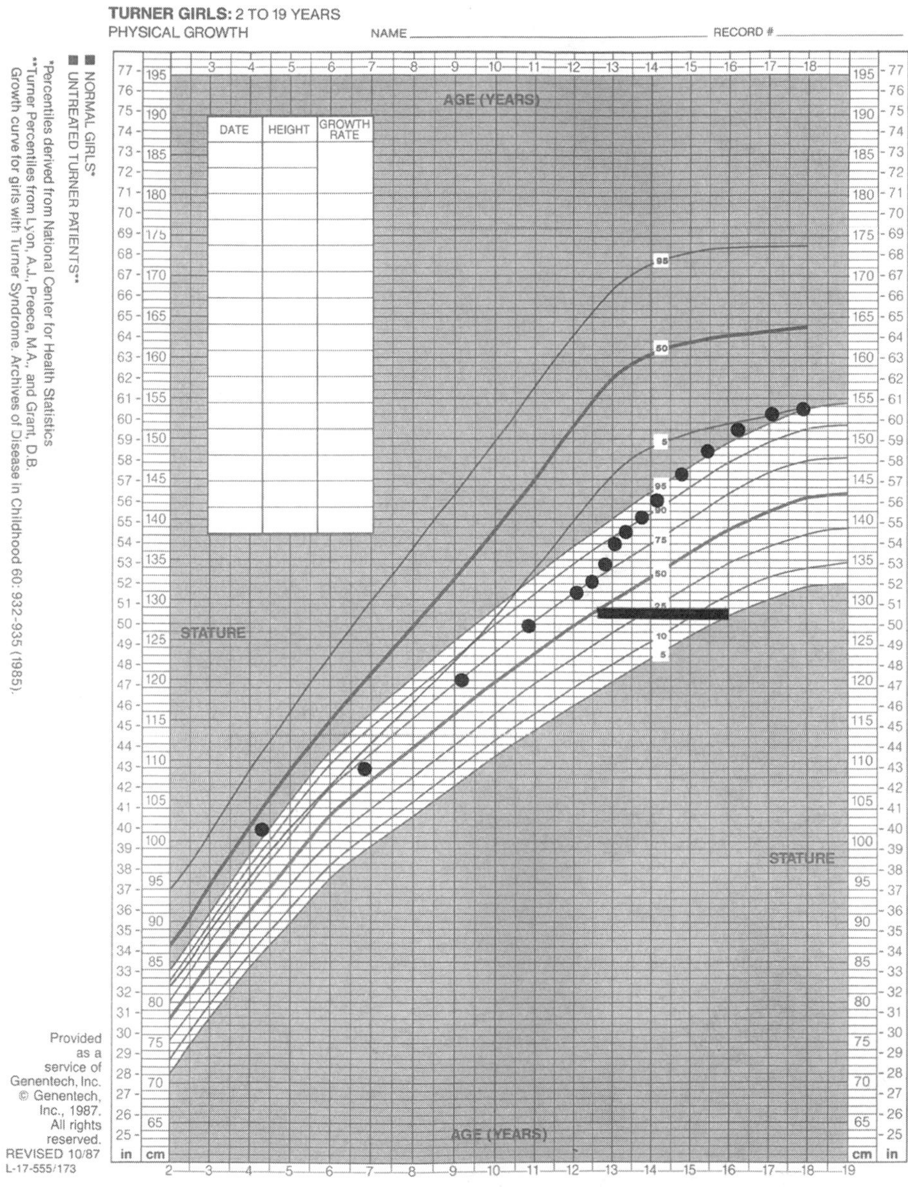

FIG. 1. Height chart of a girl with Turner's syndrome, treated with growth hormone (*bar*) and subsequently with estrogen-progestin replacement therapy.

4% had ring chromosomes; 7.7% had other structural abnormality of the X chromosome; and 4% were mosaic 45,X/46,XY (30). Such patients may show none or all of the classic stigmata of Turner's syndrome. "Critical" regions on both the long arm and the short arm of the X chromosome are essential for ovarian function. Deletions in proximal Xq13 and proximal Xq21 are associated with primary amenorrhea, whereas girls with deletions of Xq25–27 develop premature ovarian failure and secondary amenorrhea (13,32). Complete deletion of Xp also results in dysgenetic gonads. Absence or deletion of a portion of Xp (Xp21–Xpter) correlates with the physical stigmata of Turner's syndrome; deletion of Xq is likely to produce short stature (Fig. 2).

Thus, patients with Turner's mosaic may have (a) sexual infantilism, (b) some sexual development and primary amenorrhea, (c) secondary amenorrhea or irregular menses and short stature, or (d) regular menses and normal stature. It is estimated that 5% to 15% of patients with Turner's syndrome may have spontaneous thelarche. Girls with mosaic blood karyotypes, especially involving only the loss of the short arm of the X chromosome, are more likely to have pubertal maturation (6% in 45,X; 25% in mosaic patients; and 33% with isolated Xp deletions) (32). These girls may not have increased FSH, and thus Turner's syndrome should be considered in the adolescent with pubertal development and significantly short stature (in the absence of a family history of short stature). In the majority of girls with Turner's syndrome, FSH is usually elevated at birth, is suppressed during childhood, and rises to menopausal levels at the normal pubertal age (9 to 10 years) in those with gonadal failure.

Rarely, spontaneous pregnancies have been reported among patients with 45,X and mosaic blood karyotypes, even among some with elevated gonadotropin levels. The outcome of the reported pregnancies has been poor, with an increased risk of abortion, stillbirth, and chromosomally abnormal

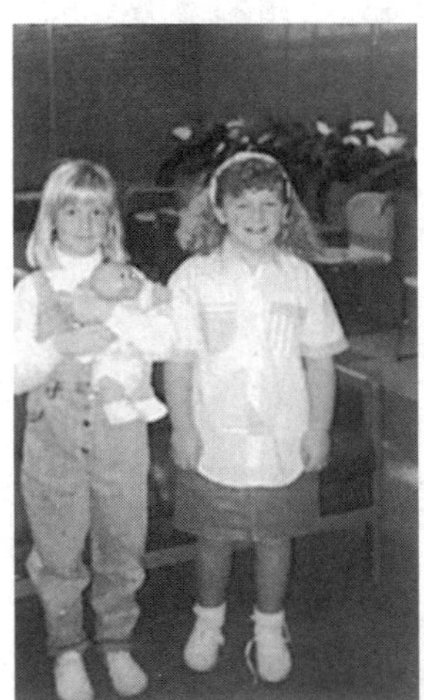

FIG. 2. Turner's syndrome. A 12-year-old girl with Turner's syndrome (*right*) is no taller than her 7-year-old sister. Other signs of the disorder are apparent only on closer inspection. (From Jackson DB, Saunders RB. *Child health nursing: a comprehensive approach to the care of children and their families.* Philadelphia: JB Lippincott, 1993; with permission.)

babies (Turner's syndrome and Down's syndrome) (33–35). Genetic counseling and prenatal diagnosis should be recommended to all fertile Turner's patients.

Followup of the patient diagnosed with Turner's syndrome should include ultrasound examination of the kidneys, cardiac assessment, and monitoring for hypertension, glucose intolerance, and thyroid dysfunction (those with isochromosome of the long arm of X are especially at risk of Hashimoto's thyroiditis) (19,20,22,36,37). Aggressive treatment of otitis media and audiometry are indicated. Careful attention should be given to subtle hearing loss and speech defects (14) in all patients with gonadal dysgenesis. Patients who are untreated and who have persistently high gonadotropin levels may show enlarged pituitary fossae, which suggests hyperplasia of the pituitary gland (38). After finding evidence of increased aortic root diameters in patients with Turner's syndrome, Allen and colleagues (19) have suggested that these patients should undergo periodic cardiac evaluation and echocardiography to monitor aortic root diameter as well as to detect bicuspid aortic valve, coarctation of the aorta, and hypertension. Although the American Academy of Pediatrics Committee on Genetics has recommended echocardiograms every 2 years (20), every 3–5 years may be sufficient. Further studies are needed to establish cost-effective guidelines for screening.

Data on long-term followup of patients with Turner's syndrome are beginning to emerge. In a study of middle-aged women with Turner's syndrome, nearly two-thirds were married, 16% had adopted children, and all were or had been employed (39). Nearly half of the 20 women with 45,X karyotype had had fractures, and many were not taking hormone replacement. Cardiac complications were rare, and hearing loss was reported in 61%. Thus, the periodicity of followup for each complication requires ongoing assessment and research (18). Support groups have been extremely important for providing support and education to patients, their families, and their clinicians. The Turner's Syndrome Society of the United States has booklets for families and for physicians.†

Patients with a 45,X karyotype may rarely have undetected Y DNA. With the increasing application of polymerase chain reaction technology, the detection of sex-determining region of the Y chromosome sequences or Y-chromosomal DNA can alert the clinician to the possible risk of virilization at puberty or a gonadal tumor. Occult Y material was identified in 1 of 40 Turner's patients (40). In older adolescents and adults without Y sequences, an annual pelvic examination is recommended. Some have suggested that if a pelvic examination is difficult, annual radiographs to detect pelvic calcification, or ultrasonography of the pelvis to detect gonadal tumors, should be considered. Hormonal therapy is discussed in a later section.

The term *pure gonadal dysgenesis* refers to patients with normal or tall stature and the gonadal abnormality of Turner's syndrome. Breast development

†Turner's Syndrome Society of the United States, 1313 SE Fifth Street, Suite 327, Minneapolis, MN 55414 (phone (612) 379-3607, (800) 365-9944; e-mail tesch005@tc.umn.edu; http://www.turner-syndrome-us.org). See reference 14 and further reading for publications.

is absent or poor; gonadotropin levels are high. The proportions are usually eunuchoid; the karyotype is usually 46,XX or 46,XY. The girl with a 46,XY karyotype, streak gonads, normal müllerian system, and lack of sexual development has Swyer's syndrome. The streak gonads do not produce androgens or antimüllerian hormone (also termed müllerian inhibiting substance) (see Chapters 2 and 8). Because of the presence of the Y chromosome, these patients are at increased risk of gonadal tumors and thus require removal of the gonads. Girls with the 47,XXX karyotype may also have ovarian failure and may have impairment on neuropsychological tests (although preselection bias may play a role in the reported findings) (29).

Patients with 46,XX ovarian failure may have a family history of premature menopause. Krauss and colleagues (41) have reported a family whose members had a deletion on the long arm X chromosome in the area responsible for follicular maintenance.

Ovarian Failure Secondary to Radiation or Chemotherapy

As more young women are surviving their childhood malignancies and living into adulthood, the effects of radiation and chemotherapy on gonadal function have become particularly relevant. These effects are discussed extensively in Chapter 19. A history of a malignancy treated with radiation to the pelvis or abdomen and/or chemotherapy suggests a diagnosis of ovarian failure. The likelihood of ovarian failure in relation to radiation is both dose- and age-related; the higher the dose and the older the patient, the greater the possibility of ovarian damage. In addition to ovarian failure, an adolescent who received pelvic radiation therapy before puberty often has a very small cervix and uterus despite estrogen therapy. Chemotherapeutic agents have also been associated with premature ovarian failure. Children and adolescents appear to be more resistant to the deleterious effects of these agents than adults. Adolescents may experience amenorrhea and elevated gonadotropins while receiving chemotherapy; subsequently, their menstrual function and hormone levels may return to normal some months to several years after completion of the course.

Autoimmune Oophoritis

The possibility of autoimmune oophoritis needs to be considered in any patient with normal karyotype and ovarian failure, because she may subsequently develop other endocrinopathies. In studies of adults with premature ovarian failure evaluated in medical centers, 18% to 50% have been reported to have evidence of autoimmune disease (10,42–44). Associated diseases have included thyroid disorders, Addison's disease, hypoparathyroidism, myasthenia gravis, diabetes mellitus, pernicious anemia, and vitiligo. Among women with premature ovarian failure, antithyroglobulin and antithyroid microsomal antibodies are commonly present; antibodies to smooth muscle, gastric parietal cells, mitochondria, cell nucleus, pancreatic islet cells, and the adrenals have also been reported (45). Antibodies against theca interna and corpus luteum cells, FSH receptors, and specific enzymes in the adrenals and ovaries have been described (42–47). Localization of staining for the presence of ovarian antibodies has been reported in the primary oocytes and in the granulosa cells of large secondary follicles (43). Patients may not have positive antiovarian antibody tests because the right antigens may not be included in the assay, the antibody may be only transiently present, or the pathogenesis of the ovarian failure may involve cell-mediated immunity.

Patients with autoimmune oophoritis may have a variable course with spontaneous remissions and the resumption of normal ovarian function (11,48). Amenorrhea and infertility persist in most patients. Whether corticosteroids, combined estrogen progestin therapy, or other therapies lead to any better prognosis is unclear, since controlled studies have not been performed. It has been postulated that estrogen therapy shifts the FSH to a more bioactive FSH. For most patients, assisted reproductive technologies with donor oocytes offer the best possibility for a pregnancy.

At the initial assessment of the patient with suspected autoimmune ovarian failure, baseline thyroid function tests, complete blood count, calcium and phosphorus and morning cortisol should be obtained. Serum can be sent for antibodies to thyroid, adrenal, ovary, islet cells, and parietal cells if these tests are available. The best way to assess the risk of adrenal insufficiency has not been rigorously evaluated. Some advocate an adrenocorticotropic hormone (ACTH) test with measurement of cortisol levels at 0 and 30 or 60 minutes as an appropriate screening test, with repeat measurements done annually to determine adrenal reserve. Others advocate monitoring DHEAS, ACTH, and morning cortisol levels annually or doing more extensive testing only in those with antiadrenal antibodies.

Resistant Ovary Syndrome

In resistant ovary syndrome, a rare condition, the ovaries appear normal at laparoscopy. Biopsy specimens reveal numerous primordial follicles (49). Ovarian follicular activity can be identified in some patients with the use of transvaginal ultrasonography. The ovaries may lack a receptor for gonadotropin function. During an infertility evaluation, a trial of exogenous human gonadotropin may be indicated to exclude the remote possibility that the patient has produced biologically inactive FSH and LH. The condition is rare and may not be a unique entity; many hypergonadotropic women have follicles that are intermittently demonstrable by ultrasound.

17α-Hydroxylase and Aromatase Deficiencies

The extremely rare disorder 17α-hydroxylase deficiency (P450c17) is not true gonadal failure but rather an enzyme deficiency that results in adrenal insufficiency, hypertension, and lack of gonadal sex steroids, including androgens and estrogens. Patients with a 46,XX karyotope have a female phenotype but no secondary sexual characteristics or sexual hair. Patients with a 46,XY karyotype may have a female phenotype, vaginal agenesis, and lack of müllerian structures but, unlike patients with androgen insensitivity (testicular feminization), do not have pubertal breast development. Progesterone levels are elevated.

A single case of an adolescent girl with a diagnosis of aromatase deficiency (P450arom), the inability to convert testosterone to estrogen, has been reported (50). The patient had masculinization of the external genitalia at birth but normal female internal genital structures; at the age of 14 years she had absence of breast development, mild virilization (clitoromegaly), multicystic ovaries, elevated testosterone and gonadotropin levels, and delayed bone age.

Other Causes of Ovarian Failure

Ovarian failure also occurs in patients with galactosemia, even those treated from infancy (51); myotonia dystrophica; trisomy 21 (52); sarcoidosis; and ataxia telangiectasia. Ovarian destruction has followed mumps oophoritis, gonococcal salpingitis (rarely), ovarian infiltrative processes (tuberculosis and mucopolysaccharidosis), and ovarian hemorrhage.

HYPOGONADOTROPIC HYPOGONADISM

Low to Normal FSH and LH Levels

Hypogonadotropic hypogonadism is the general term used for the diagnosis in patients with a delay in sexual development or menses associated with low to normal levels of gonadotropins. This may include patients with a central cause of the disorder such as chronic disease or undernutrition, a hypothalamic cause such as Kallmann's syndrome or a tumor, or a pituitary cause such as a microadenoma or infiltrative disease. A normal physiologic delay in puberty or menarche is a diagnosis of exclusion and requires a careful medical evaluation before watchful waiting or hormonal therapy is undertaken.

One of the most common causes of delayed puberty is poor nutrition. Poor intake, malabsorption, and increased caloric requirements commonly occur in such chronic diseases as cystic fibrosis, sickle cell disease, human immunodeficiency virus disease, renal disease, celiac disease, and Crohn's disease (53–56). The diagnosis is frequently evident before puberty, but especially in the case of Crohn's disease, it may have a subtle presentation with growth failure alone in the teenage years. On careful history, most, but not all, patients with Crohn's disease have a history of intermittent crampy abdominal pain, diarrhea, or constipation. The sedimentation rate is usually, but not invariably, elevated, and mild anemia and hypoalbuminemia may be present as clues. When the diagnosis is in doubt, gastrointestinal evaluation and screening tests such as antiendomysial and antigliadin antibodies (for celiac disease) may be indicated before it is assumed that low caloric intake is responsible for the problem. Renal problems associated with impaired growth include renal tubular acidosis, glomerular diseases treated with corticosteroids, and end-stage renal failure.

Self-imposed caloric restriction and intermittent dieting are common among adolescent girls, many of whom view themselves as overweight. Society's preoccupation with a thin physique may lead parents and children to restrict the diet inappropriately, causing weight loss or growth failure. Although anorexia nervosa is typically associated with secondary and, less commonly, primary amenorrhea, fear of obesity can cause significant growth failure even in prepubertal children (57). Because of the rarity of this presentation, however, it behooves the clinician to exclude a hypothalamic tumor, a malabsorptive state, and chronic disease in the prepubertal child with apparent eating disorder. Children may also have inadequate access to food because of family psychosocial problems, alcoholism, drug abuse, lack of financial resources, or homelessness.

Girls who are involved in ballet or competitive endurance sports such as track and gymnastics frequently have a delay in pubertal development and irregular menses (58,59) and gymnasts may eventually be short in stature. Delayed puberty may also be caused by endocrinopathies, including hypothyroidism, diabetes mellitus, and Cushing's syndrome. Acquired hypothyroidism may have a subtle onset that may be missed except for the slowing of statural growth. Girls with poorly controlled diabetes mellitus may have short stature and delayed puberty as well as irregular menstruation (60). The use of pharmacologic doses of corticosteroids to treat many medical diseases frequently causes an iatrogenic picture of Cushing's syndrome. Substance abuse and psychological problems such as severe depression may also be associated with an interruption of the pubertal process.

Hypothalamic dysfunction may be caused by a congenital defect such as Kallmann's syndrome, in which there is a lack of pulsatile release of gonadotropin-releasing hormone (GnRH), often associated with midline craniofacial defects or anosmia. Hypoplastic or absent olfactory sulci in the rhinencephalon can be detected by MRI. Distinguishing isolated GnRH deficiency from delayed puberty may be difficult if the patient with delayed puberty has not begun to show a normal postpubertal response to GnRH or GnRH analogs. Investigators have also tried to use shortened GnRH stimulation tests and leuprolide acetate challenges (61,62). Rosenfield (63) has suggested that gonadotropin deficiency is probable in a prepubertal teen girl with normal or low FSH if bone age is >13 years, anosmia or panhypopituitarism is present, there is no sleep-associated increase in LH, and GnRH tests show a flat response (see Fig. 8 in Chapter 4).

Patients with delayed puberty or menarche frequently have other members of the family who have experienced a significant delay. This history alone, however, should not prevent an evaluation of girls with delayed development, since other conditions can be present. Central lesions that need to be considered include tumors, hydrocephalus, brain abscesses, and infiltrative lesions such as tuberculosis, sarcoidosis, eosinophilic granuloma, Wegener's granulomatosis, lymphocytic hypophysitis, and CNS leukemia (64). Followup is critical to make sure that normal puberty occurs, since one of these conditions may become apparent later.

Craniopharyngiomas typically present between the ages of 6 and 14 years and cause headaches, poor growth, delayed development, and diabetes insipidus. Children who have received cranial radiation for leukemia therapy may have abnormalities of growth hormone secretion and may lack pulsatile GnRH secretion as well (65,66). Iron deposition from hemochromatosis and iron overload associated with transfusion therapy in thalassemia major can result in pubertal delay. Iron deposition in the thalassemic patient may also cause hypothyroidism, hypoparathyroidism, diabetes, cardiac failure, and/or pituitary dysfunction (67,68). Desferoxime can also affect growth. Hypogonadotropic hypogonadism is also associated with the Laurence-Moon-Biedl and Prader-Willi syndromes. Medications and illicit drugs such as cocaine can cause hyperprolactinemia.

Pituitary causes of interrupted development and irregular menses include hypopituitarism, either congenital or acquired, and tumors. Acquired hypopituitarism can result from head trauma (69), postpartum shock and necrosis (Sheehan's syndrome), pituitary infarction from conditions such as sickle cell disease, and, rarely, an autoimmune process (70). An entity known as empty sella can occur in children as well as adults and may be associated with hypothalamic pituitary dysfunction; in one series of children with multiple pituitary deficiencies, one-third had an empty sella (71). A normal-sized sella that is empty may be associated with pituitary hypoplasia, an unrecognized pituitary insult, dysfunction of the hypothalamus or higher centers resulting in diminished pituitary growth, or herniation of cerebrospinal fluid through a congenitally incomplete sellar diaphragm (72).

The most common, but still rare, pituitary tumor in adolescence is a prolactinoma, which typically causes primary or secondary amenorrhea rather than complete absence of pubertal development (see section on Hyperprolactinemia). Determination of serum prolactin level is a simple screening test and is indicated in patients with low or normal FSH and LH levels and interrupted puberty or amenorrhea. Pituitary adenomas that are not prolactinomas are not usually associated with amenorrhea and thus tend to be diagnosed at the time an imaging study is done for some other reason, such as headaches, or because tumor growth causes headaches or visual disturbances. These rare tumors may secrete FSH, LH, or high levels of the α-subunit of the glycopeptide hormones (73). Therapy with a GnRH agonist does not cause downregulation of mildly elevated FSH levels. These patients may have modest elevation of serum prolactin levels. Patients found to have these tumors should have further neuroendocrine evaluation in a search for abnormalities of ACTH production and growth hormone secretion. For non-prolactin-secreting lesions, asymptomatic microadenomas (<10 mm) are often observed; macroadenomas are usually treated with surgery and sometimes adjunctive radiation.

Thus, the evaluation of the adolescent with low to normal FSH and LH levels needs to focus on exclusion of a systemic disease, poor nutrition, CNS disorder, or endocrinopathy. This may include careful assessment of the growth charts, neurologic examination, CBC, sedimentation rate, thyroid function tests including TSH level, prolactin tests, and hand and wrist radiograph for bone age. Caloric counts of food diaries and gastrointestinal evaluation are indicated in those with poor nutrition. Evidence of other chronic diseases such as cystic fibrosis, renal failure, diabetes, or liver disease should be assessed. A skull radiograph with a cone-down view of the sella is useful only if calcification is present (e.g., from a craniopharyngioma) or the sella is enlarged or eroded. If a hypothalamic or pituitary tumor is under consideration or if the significantly delayed puberty has no apparent cause, then evaluation should include computed tomography (CT) scan or, preferably, MRI. Further neuroendocrine studies are important in the evaluation of patients with evidence of panhypopituitarism and some patients with tumors. Patients with a history of CNS radiation for leukemia should have their growth monitored carefully and neuroendocrine testing done if linear growth is abnormal. Formal visual field testing should be done in patients with pituitary tumors.

Eating Disorders

Eating disorders are prevalent in contemporary society. Some adolescents pursue thinness to the extreme of causing delayed development, delayed menarche, and secondary amenorrhea. Even simple weight loss in the adolescent may result in delayed menses or several months of amenorrhea. Adolescents with bulimia and normal weight for height may have regular or irregular menses. Two peaks of presentation of anorexia occur, at age 13 years and at 18 years, the first associated with pubertal maturation and body image concerns, and the second with separation and choices about jobs and college. Young women with other medical problems such as Turner's syndrome or diabetes mellitus may also have eating disorders. The criteria for the diagnosis of anorexia nervosa are summarized from *The Diagnostic and Statistical Manual of Mental Disorders IV* (DSM-IV) in Table 2 (74). Treating patients early in the course of the illness, even before these guidelines have been strictly met, may yield a better prognosis. These girls are often preoccupied with thoughts of food; some may restrict intake to several hundred calories per day and may feel inadequate and a pervasive lack of control. Other adolescents may binge and then purge by self-induced vomiting or by abuse of laxatives. Since these girls are frequently secretive about

TABLE 2. *Criteria for diagnosing eating disorders in adolescents*

Anorexia nervosa

Refusal to maintain body weight over a minimal normal weight for age and height (body weight <85% of that expected), or failure to make expected weight gain during period of growth.

Intense fear of gaining weight or becoming fat, even though underweight.

Disturbance in the way the patient experiences body weight, or denial of the seriousness of the current low body weight.

In postmenarcheal females, amenorrhea of at least three consecutive menstrual cycles.

Bulimia nervosa

Recurrent episodes of binge eating, characterized by eating, in a discrete period of time, an amount of food that is definitely larger than most people would eat during a similar period of time, *and* a sense of lack of control over eating during the episode.

Recurrent inappropriate compensatory behaviors in order to prevent weight gain, such as self-induced vomiting; misuse of laxatives, diuretics, enemas, or fasting; or excessive exercise.

Occurrence of binge eating and compensatory behaviors at least twice a week for 3 months, on average.

Self-evaluation unduly influenced by body shape and weight.

Disturbance does not occur exclusively during episodes of anorexia nervosa.

Eating disorders that do not meet the criteria for a specific eating disorder

Criteria for anorexia nervosa are met, but the individual has regular menses.

Criteria for anorexia nervosa are met except that the individual's current weight is in the normal range despite significant weight loss.

The criteria for bulimia nervosa are met, but the binge eating and compensatory mechanisms occur at a frequency of those specified for bulimia nervosa.

Regular use of inappropriate compensatory behavior by an individual of normal body weight after eating a small amount of food.

Repeatedly chewing and spitting out, but not swallowing, large amounts of food.

(Adapted from American Psychiatric Association. *DSM-IV. Diagnostic and statistical manual of mental disorders,* 4th ed. Washington, DC: American Psychiatric Association, 1994; with permission.)

their eating patterns, it is useful for the clinician to develop some techniques for eliciting an accurate history, such as saying, "Where would you like your weight to be? Do you have difficulty keeping your weight where you want it to be? Have you ever used vomiting or medicines to control your weight?"

Several medical problems have been associated with anorexia and bulimia, including dehydration and electrolyte imbalance. Vital signs are usually depressed in girls with anorexia nervosa, with low temperature, blood pressure, and pulse rate. Other signs include dry skin, lanugo, bruises, edema (during refeeding), murmurs, abdominal bloating, constipation, cold intolerance, and stress fractures. The differential diagnosis includes inflammatory bowel disease, celiac disease, Addison's disease, hyperthyroidism, malignancy, diabetes mellitus, depression, and CNS tumors.

Laboratory studies are tailored to the presentation and the likelihood of other medical illnesses. Initial screening tests usually include a CBC, urinalysis, and determination of sedimentation rate, blood urea nitrogen (BUN), creatinine, and electrolytes. In patients with amenorrhea, the gynecologic assessment should be individualized. For the girl with amenorrhea who has never been sexually active, the assessment includes an external genital examination and, usually, rectoabdominal palpation. Serum tests for FSH, prolactin, and TSH are helpful in establishing the diagnosis of hypothalamic amenorrhea. In girls with anorexia nervosa, serum levels of FSH and LH are low (75). Levels of TSH and T_4 are usually normal, but T_3 is often low and the inactive metabolite, reverse T_3, high. Even a girl with Turner's syndrome and severe anorexia nervosa may have suppression of gonadotropin levels. Cranial MRI scanning is indicated in patients, especially prepubertal girls, with neurologic symptoms, headaches, and atypical presentations. Substantial deficits in bone density may occur and may be irreversible and associated with low weight, estrogen deficiency, hypercortisalism, and insulin-like growth factor-1 (IGF-1) deficiency (76–78).

Frisch and McArthur (79,80) have proposed a chart for examining the relationships between height/weight and menstrual function. It should be noted that the critical weight or percentage body fat hypothesis has been challenged, that individual patients clearly show variation in the recovery of menstrual function at a particular weight, and that the tenth percentile of the weight/height chart may not hold for different ages during adolescence. However, the guidelines are useful in counseling patients to develop target weights and to give families general concepts about weight and height relationships. For example, using Fig. 3, a 13-year-old adolescent who is 5′5″ tall would be expected to weigh a minimum of 44 kg (97 lbs) or a *calculated* body fat percentage of 17% at the time of menarche, but if she later lost weight at age 16 to 18 years and developed secondary amenorrhea, she would need to achieve a weight of 49 kg (108 lbs) or a *calculated* body fat percentage of 22% to regain her menses. Given the normal weight gain of 10 pounds between the ages of 13 and 18 years, the clinician needs to consider both the patient's age and whether the patient has primary or secondary amenorrhea in utilizing the charts. A weight estimate for a 16- to 18-year-old with primary amenorrhea and anorexia nervosa is better determined from the weight for height charts associated with secondary amenorrhea than from the line for primary amenorrhea weights, because otherwise the expected weight will likely be set too low; statural growth has often been nearly completed because of exposure to low amounts of estrogen and adrenal androgens.

Another method of determining a normal target weight is to determine height age and then find the corresponding weight for that height age on the National Growth Charts or use the Percentiles for Weight and Height (National Center for Health Statistics, Height and Weight of Youths 12–17 years, United States). Patients benefit from being given a range (goal plus 10 lbs) of weights, not a single number. Patients who regain a normal weight for height but persist with amenorrhea frequently continue to have abnormal eating patterns and preoccupation with food. For those with either primary or secondary amenorrhea, Kreipe and colleagues (81,82) have found that patients have a mean of 92 ± 7% of ideal body weight (IBW) at the return of menses. In a study of 100 adolescents with anorexia nervosa, Golden and colleagues (83) found that menses

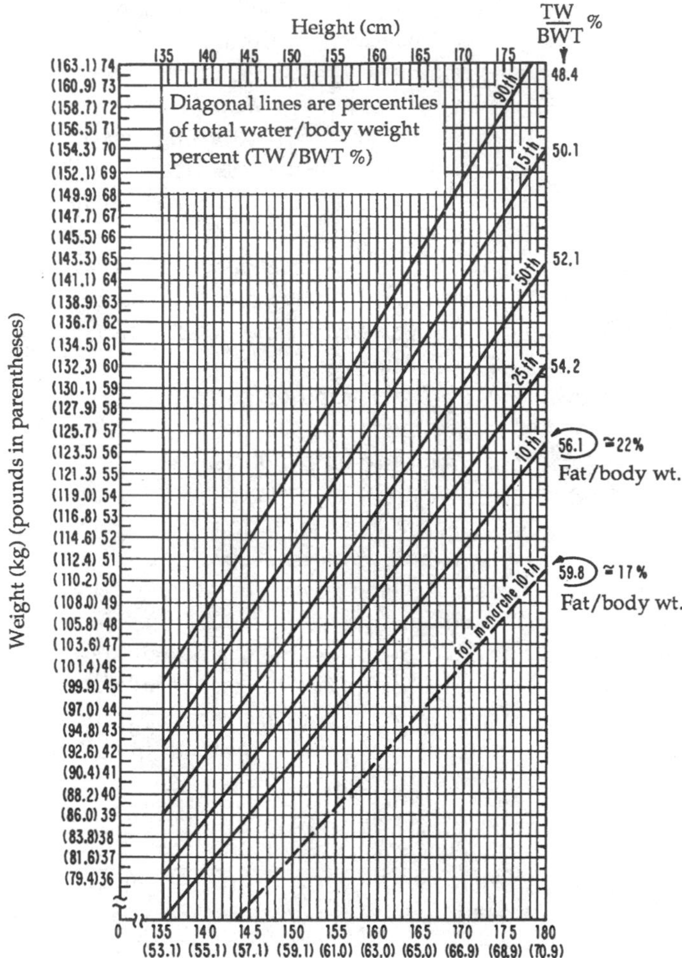

FIG. 3. Nomogram indicating the minimal weight a female of a given height should weigh to be likely to have normal menses. The lowest diagonal line is the 10th percentile of total water/body fat for menarche. The second lowest diagonal line is the 10th percentile for 18-year-old adolescents; this diagonal often corresponds to the weight needed for restoration of menses in an adolescent with weight loss and secondary amenorrhea. (From Frisch RE, McArthur JW. Menstrual cycles: fatness as determinant of minimum weight for height necessary for their maintenance or onset. *Science* 1974;185:949; with permission of the American Association for the Advancement of Science and Dr. Rose Frisch. Figure provided by Dr. Rose Frisch, Center for Population Studies, Cambridge, MA.)

resumed at a weight 2.05 kg more than the weight at which menses were lost and that the mean percent of standard body weight was 91.6% ± 9.1%; 86% of patients resumed menses within 6 months of achieving this weight.

The Female Athlete Triad: Disordered Eating, Amenorrhea, and Osteoporosis

In the past few years as more young women have participated in sports, the term *female athlete triad* has been coined to characterize the interrelatedness of disordered eating, amenorrhea, and osteoporosis. The triad is particularly likely to develop in girls who participate in sports in which the theme of achieving or maintaining an ideal body weight or optimal percentage of body fat is a common focus and scoring is partly subjective (84–86). Coaching strategies such as daily weigh-ins and strict weight standards may predispose young women to the triad. A highly structured life, social isolation, lack of a support system, and a family history of disordered eating are also frequently associated with this presentation. Although not all young women athletes with amenorrhea have all elements of the triad, consideration of each is important in evaluation of these patients in the office.

Exercise clearly has benefits, including improved cardiovascular fitness, socialization, involvement in peer groups, a sense of well-being, weight control, lowering of blood pressure, and improved lipid profile. A lower rate of cancers of the reproductive system and breast cancer has been reported in one study of former athletes (87). However, a progressive increase in exercise may lead to problems that have potential lifelong consequences, and thus they call for understanding, research, and appropriate counseling of athletes, families, and coaches.

For the past 15 years, amenorrhea in athletes has received considerable attention (84–86,88–96). The incidence of amenorrhea in particular sports has been unclear, in part because of the varying definitions used for secondary amenorrhea (usually 3 to 6 months of amenorrhea). In contrast to an expected incidence of 2% to 5% of amenorrhea in adult women, the incidence in athletes has been reported at 3% to 66%. For example, in a group of 250 premenopausal women runners, the prevalence of amenorrhea increased from 1% in normally active women to 11% in elite runners (90). Irregular menses in athletes have been associated with many factors, shown in Table 3 (84–101). Endurance activities, such as gymnastics, ballet, and running, are particularly likely to be associated with menstrual problems. Even swimmers who have more body fat than runners may experience menstrual dysfunction, most commonly short luteal phases. However, adolescents involved in normal after-school sports programs do not appear to be at increased risk of disrupted menstrual cycles (102), although the possibility of more subtle changes in GnRH pulsations or anovulation has not been examined in this population. Lowered salivary progesterone levels have been noted in recreational runners (average 12.5 miles/week) (103). Thus, athletes

TABLE 3. *Factors associated with irregular menses in athletes*

Low weight and weight loss
Low body fat (?sport related)
Eating disorders
Delayed menarche
Prior menstrual irregularity
Adolescent age group
Nonparous
Stress (associated with exercise)
Type of sport
Highest in running
Lower in swimming and cycling
High level of training
Diet (low calorie, vegetarian, high fiber)
Hereditary? metabolic?

with seemingly regular menses may in fact have anovulatory cycles or short luteal phases.

Pubertal development and menarche are often delayed in thin athletes, especially ballet dancers, gymnasts, and runners (6,100,101). Ballet dancers often have delayed thelarche and menarche with a normal age of adrenarche; they may also have irregular menses, a low percentage of body fat, high energy output, and decreased caloric intake with episodes of binging (59,104). Malina (105) has proposed that some of the delay in pubertal development in athletes may be attributed to the preselection of girls who have a thin body type and familial late development and who also excel in athletic endeavors. Some of the delay, however, likely also results from the girls' commitment to the sport. Particularly worrisome is the observation by Theintz and colleagues (106) that the growth spurt in gymnasts may be suboptimal and result in short stature. Although familial short stature and body type may be contributing factors in the observed results, it is likely that training and inadequate nutrition have an impact on growth velocity curves (Fig. 4). Frisch and coworkers (107) have previously reported that athletes who began their training premenarcheally experienced a delay in menarche and a higher incidence of amenorrhea than did athletes who began their training postmenarcheally. Each year of training before menarche was associated with a delay of menarche by 5 months.

The intensity of the exercise and the age of the athlete also appear to be contributing factors to amenorrhea. In most studies, a greater number of miles run per week is associated with a higher incidence of amenorrhea. In a survey of college runners, the incidence of amenorrhea was 20% for women running 20 miles/week and 43% for those running 60 to 80 miles/week (108). A lower incidence of amenorrhea (19%) was found in the runners participating in the marathon trials of the 1984 Olympics (109). Young runners and nulliparous runners are more likely to experience irregular cycles.

Diet may be suboptimal in many adolescent athletes, especially those participating in sports in which thinness is perceived as an advantage. In an attempt to

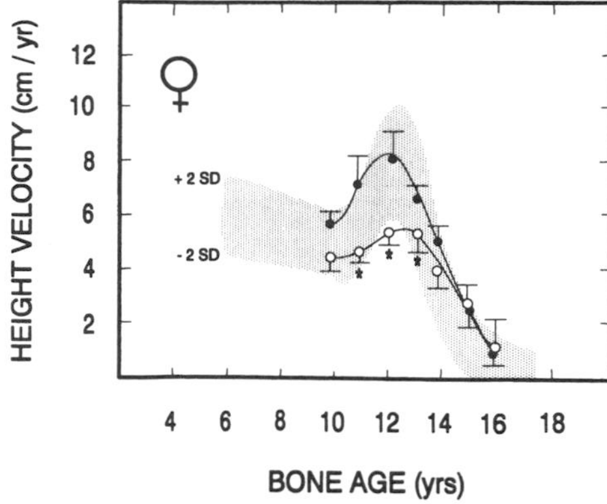

FIG. 4. Mean (± SEM) growth velocity as a function of bone age (RUS score) in gymnasts (*clear circles*) and swimmers (*dark circles*); asterisks indicate significance (at $p < 0.05$) as a function of chronologic age for normal children. (From Theintz GE, Howald H, Weiss U, Sizonenko PC. Evidence for a reduction of growth potential in adolescent female gymnasts. *J Pediatr* 1993;122:306–313; with permission.)

separate weight loss from strenuous exercise as causative factors, Bullen and colleagues (98) carried out a prospective study of menstrual cycles, assigning one group to weight maintenance and the other to weight loss. They found that exercise, especially if accompanied by weight loss, could reversibly disturb menstrual function. Those in the weight loss group experienced more delayed menses, and a higher percentage of patients had loss of the LH surge. Diets low in calories, fat, and red meat and high in carotene have been associated with amenorrhea (96,110–113). Weight loss in girls consuming a vegetarian diet appears to be more likely to induce menstrual dysfunction than a nonvegetarian diet (113).

Gadpaille and colleagues (114) reported an association between athletic amenorrhea, eating disorders, and a family history of major affective disorders. Disordered eating as part of the athletic triad can include anorexia nervosa, bulimia, purging, binging, and fasting. Preoccupations with food, dissatisfaction with body image, and fear of becoming fat are part of disordered eating patterns that may not reach the level of the DSM-IV criteria. Disordered eating has been reported in 15% to 62% of young female athletes (84,86). It is important to remember that girls with anorexia nervosa may have joined the track team and be exercising compulsively (often beyond the expectation of the coach) to lose additional weight.

The mechanism of exercise-related menstrual changes is unclear, but there are changes in prolactin, ACTH, gonadotropins, endorphins, catecholamines, thyroid hormone, insulin levels and sensitivity, growth hormone, and growth hormone binding protein (110,115–121). A normal LH response to GnRH in most runners suggests that the defect is at the level of the hypothalamus. Stress associated with the athletic endeavor also appears to increase the incidence of amenorrhea. Both athletes and young women with eating disorders may have hypercortisolism, blunted dexamethasone suppressibility, and reduced ACTH responses to corticotropin-releasing hormone (63,119).

Studies over the past decade have elucidated much of the pathophysiology in relation to bone mass gains in adolescence and the potential consequences of hypoestrogenic amenorrhea. A person's skeletal status is determined by the amount of bone at skeletal maturity and the rate of ongoing bone loss. Various studies have estimated that 33% to 60% of adult bone mass is acquired during the adolescent growth spurt (4,106,122–130). Bone mass is determined by factors such as inheritance, race, muscle strength, physical activity, circulating estrogen and androgens, tobacco use, weight, and dietary calcium (85,126). Bone density increases in both black and white girls during puberty, but the magnitude of the increase is greater in black girls, who eventually have a higher vertebral bone density at the end of puberty and a higher weight than white girls (126). Bonjour et al (123) and Theintz et al (124) reported marked acceleration of bone mass acquisition during early adolescence (age 11 to 14 years in girls) (Figs. 5 and 6). In their study, little bone mass accumulated after 15 years (Tanner stage 5). Rubin et al (128) have similarly noted accelerated bone mass acquisition during puberty, beginning at the age of 10 years in girls, and observed a positive impact of physical activity and calcium intake. Skeletal mineralization at puberty appears to be particularly dependent on the site, with marked gains in areas with a predominance of trabecular bone (e.g., lumbar spine). Weight

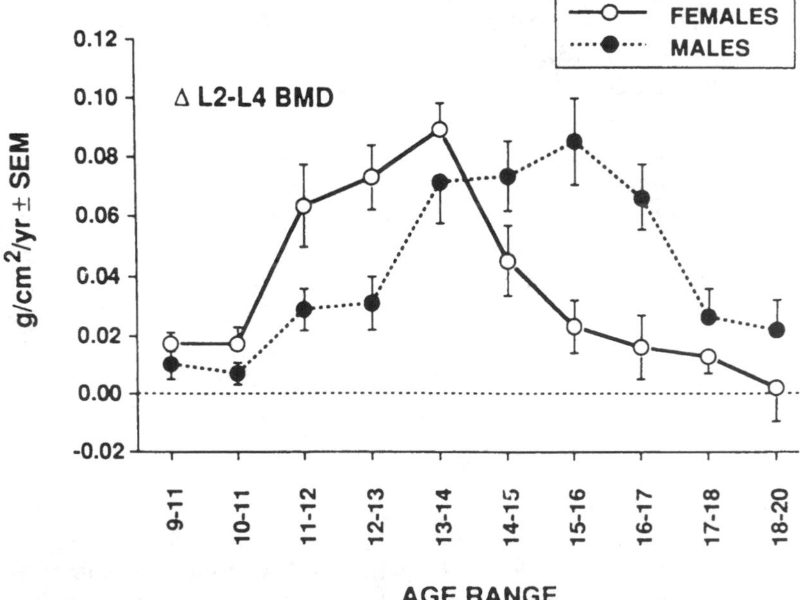

FIG. 5. Bone mass gain at lumbar spine during adolescence. Yearly increase in lumbar bone mineral density (BMD) [L2–L4 BMD]. Results are mean ± SEM. (From Theintz G, Buchs B, Rizzoli, R, et al. Longitudinal monitoring of bone mass accumulation in a healthy adolescent: evidence for a marked reduction after 16 years of age at the levels of lumbar spine and femoral neck in female subjects. *J Clin Endocrinol Metab* 1992;75:1060–1065; with permission.)

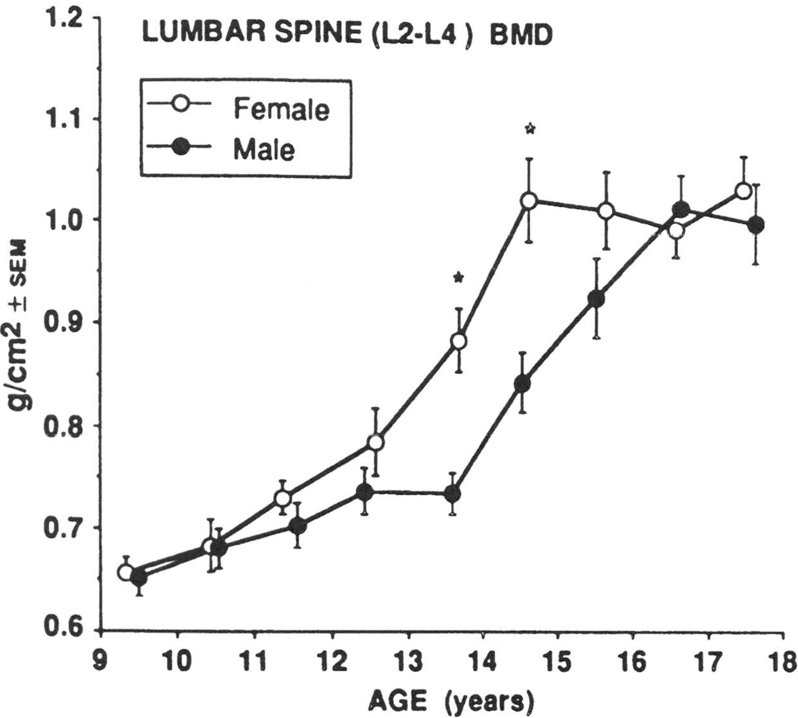

FIG. 6. Sex differences in age-related increment in bone mineral density (BMD) at the level of the lumbar spine (L2–L4) by age. (From Bonjour J, Theintz G, Buchs B, et al. Critical years and stages of puberty for spinal and femoral bone mass accumulation during adolescence. *J Clin Endocrinol Metab* 1991;73:555–563; with permission.)

changes correlate with trabecular mineralization, and height more strongly correlates with cortical bone changes (125).

Although the preponderance of evidence points to the acquisition of most bone mass during early adolescence, Recker et al (129) reported some gains even later. In a study of 156 college-age women attending professional schools, they observed that 6.8% of lumbar bone mineral density and 12.5% of total body bone mass was achieved in the third decade of life. The rate of bone density gain correlated positively with calcium/protein intake and physical activity and negatively with age. Oral contraceptive use was associated with a greater gain in total body bone mass.

Given the newer data on bone density and bone mass, studies have also focused on the potential consequences of athletic participation and estrogen deficiency on bone mass (130–139). Using CT of the vertebral trabecular bone, Cann's group (131) found osteopenia in young adult women with exercise-related amenorrhea.

Marcus and coworkers (132) found that while eumenorrheic runners had better bone density than sedentary eumenorrheic women, amenorrheic runners had decreased bone density by CT. Hetland (90) found that amenorrheic runners had significant reductions in estradiol levels and a 10% reduction in bone density compared with normally menstruating runners (oligomenorrheic runners were midway between) but that bone turnover appeared to be similar. Young runners 17 to 21 years of age who had started training early after menarche were particularly likely to have impressively low bone mineral density (BMD), using quantitative CT (QCT) of the lumbar spine (135).

In a study of 67 elite athletes 18 to 31 years old, Wolman and colleagues (136) found that the QCT lumbar spine measurements were substantially lower in the 25 amenorrheic women (≤1 menses/6 months) than the 27 eumenorrheic women and the 15 women taking oral contraceptive pills (168 vs. 211 vs. 215 mg/cm^3). Weight and height were also lower in the amenorrheic athletes. Increased calcium intake was associated with increased bone density in all groups. In a study of 43 girls 13 to 20 years old, of whom 28 were dancers, girls with low estrogen exposure scores had lower spine bone mineral density (measured by dual photon absorptiometry [DPA]) than girls with moderate or high estrogen scores (103). Spine BMD was also correlated with weight, weight/height, and testosterone levels. In a study of 97 female athletes 18 to 38 years old, Drinkwater and colleagues (137) found that women who had always had regular menstrual cycles had higher lumbar densities (measured by DPA) (1.27 g/cm^2) than those with a history of oligomenorrhea interspersed with regular cycles (1.18 g/cm^2) and than those who had never had regular cycles (1.05 g/cm^2). Weight appeared to have a more significant impact with increasing menstrual irregularity. The combination of body weight and menstrual pattern predicted 43% of the total variation in lumbar density. These researchers suggested that the effect of irregular menses may leave a residual impact on lumbar bone density. Another study found that body weight combined with months of amenorrhea and age of menarche predicted the bone mineral density at the lumbar spine of amenorrheic athletes ($R^2 = 0.71$) (139). At other sites, BMD was also predicted by duration of amenorrhea and weight. Several studies have raised the question of whether particular sites in the skeleton might be protected because of selective stresses on those bones. The data so far have yielded mixed results (138–143).

The proposed risk factors for osteoporosis in female athletes include the factors shown in Table 4 (84–86,104,144). Each of these issues needs to be assessed and addressed in the comprehensive evaluation of the adolescent who has amenorrhea and/or who participates in athletics.

The consequences of low bone density can be both long-term and short-term; an increased risk of stress fractures has been observed in many studies. In two surveys of ballet dancers, Warren and associates (101,142) found that the incidence of stress fractures rose with increasing age of menarche and that the incidence of secondary amenorrhea was twice as high among dancers with stress fractures as those without. In a study of 25 athletes with confirmed stress frac-

TABLE 4. *Factors associated with low bone density in athletes*

Low weight
Low percentage of body fat
Low estrogen
Delayed puberty
Duration of amenorrhea (present and past history)
Low use of oral contraceptives and other estrogens
Low androgen levels
Low calcium intake
Low protein intake
High fiber intake
Increased cortisol levels and increased increment during exercise
Eating disorders
Family history of osteoporosis
Lack of mechanical load

tures and matched control athletes, Myburgh and colleagues (145) reported that control subjects were more likely to have used oral contraceptive pills, were less likely to have oligomenorrhea or irregular menses, consumed more servings of calcium each day, and had higher BMD of the spine and hip than women with stress fractures. In a study of 2312 women on active duty (mean age 26.1 ± 5.8 years), Friedl (146) reported that a history of stress fracture ranged from 31.6% in non-black smokers with episodes of amenorrhea and a family history of osteoporosis to 8% for a black nonsmoker with normal menses and a negative family history. The odds ratios of a stress fracture for women ≤25 years old were 2.24 for a history of 6 months of amenorrhea, 1.96 for smokers, 1.78 for white or Asian ethnicity, and 1.66 for a family history of osteoporosis.

The lower bone density appears to be at least partially reversible in girls who begin to menstruate normally (133,137,147,148). Runners who regained their menses after a mean of 40 months of amenorrhea (associated with a decrease in training mileage and increase in body weight) experienced an increase in bone density in the 14-month followup; the two runners who remained amenorrheic had further decreases in bone density (147). However, Drinkwater et al (133,137,147) have observed that even though there is an increase in bone density initially in the first 2 years following resumption of menses, the increase ceased over the next 2 years and bone density remained below the average for their age group 4 years after resumption of menses.

Prevention efforts should involve safe training techniques for adolescents; educational efforts with athletes, parents, and coaches; promotion of positive and realistic images of women; screening and evaluation of athletes; and research. These adolescents often benefit from advice about weight gain and loss through exercise and diet (150). Adolescent athletes with amenorrhea deserve a medical and gynecologic evaluation, including assessment of estrogenization. The possibility of pregnancy should always be excluded. With the improvement in technology to measure spine and hip bone density (149), athletes at risk of osteoporosis due to estrogen deficiency may benefit from early diagnosis and monitoring during treatment, which may consist of a decrease in exercise, a gain in weight, and estrogen replacement.

Hyperprolactinemia

The spectrum of prolactin-secreting pituitary tumors, the natural history of prolactinomas, and the outcome of surgically and medically treated patients has become clearer in the past decade (151–162). The normal serum prolactin level in women ranges from 1 to 20 ng/ml with a mean of 8.9 ng/ml, although laboratories vary in reported values (156). Prolactin is secreted episodically, it has a half-life of about 20 minutes, and peak secretion occurs during sleep. In patients with pituitary tumors, often the sleep-related rhythm is abolished and prolactin values are elevated night and day.

Unlike most pituitary hormones, prolactin is regulated primarily by inhibition from the hypothalamus through secretion of a prolactin-inhibiting factor, dopamine. Dopamine and dopaminergic drugs, such as bromocriptine, lower serum prolactin levels. Drugs such as phenothiazines and other tranquilizers that block dopamine receptors, and agents such as reserpine and α-methyldopa that cause dopamine depletion in tuberoinfundibular neurons, raise prolactin levels.

The relative importance of other inhibiting factors and prolactin releasers such as estrogens, thyrotropin-releasing hormone (TRH), and serotonin is not fully elucidated. Estrogens stimulate prolactin release and result in an increase in the size and number of lactotropes. Prolactin secretion is increased during pregnancy, with prolactin levels peaking at term (100 to 300 ng/ml). Prolactin levels rise with each episode of nursing during the initial postpartum period, but by 4 to 6 months, prolactin levels are normal and the prolactin response to suckling no longer occurs. Although some patients taking or discontinuing oral contraceptives develop galactorrhea, studies have not shown an association between oral contraceptives and the development of prolactinomas. Hypothyroidism (with elevated TRH and TSH levels) is often associated with elevated prolactin levels.

Prolactin secretion is also affected by breast stimulation in some nonpregnant women and can increase following a large high-protein meal or during major stress (such as general anesthesia for surgery), orgasm, hypoglycemia, and marathon running (164,165). Optimally, therefore, the sample for serum prolactin determination should not be drawn after a large meal, strenuous exercise, or breast examination.

Hyperprolactinemia can occur because of various conditions, such as physiologic stimuli (pregnancy, exercise, stress), drugs, hypothyroidism, renal failure (decreased clearance of prolactin), hyperplasia of lactotropes (functional hyperprolactinemia), or a pituitary tumor (Table 5). The presenting complaint in the adolescent may be galactorrhea, interrupted pubertal development, or primary or secondary amenorrhea. The absence of galactorrhea is not unusual in the

TABLE 5. *Differential diagnosis of hyperprolactinemia and/or galactorrhea*

Pregnancy, postpartum, and postabortion
Pituitary tumor
Hypothalamic diseases and tumors: craniopharyngioma, sarcoidosis, eosinophilic granuloma, encephalitis, Chiari-Frommel syndrome, pituitary stalk section or compression, metastatic disease
Hypothyroidism
Drug-induced: phenothiazines, reserpine, prostaglandins, methyldopa, amitriptylene, cimetidine, benzodiazepines, haloperidol, cocaine, metoclopramide
Chronic renal failure
Local factors: chest wall surgery, trauma, nipple stimulation, herpes zoster, atopic dermatitis, thoracic burns
Tumors: bronchogenic or renal carcinoma
Other: stress, sleep-induced, hypoglycemia
Idiopathic

adolescent with hyperprolactinemia, especially in the girl with primary amenorrhea. One-half to two-thirds of adolescents with secondary amenorrhea and hyperprolactinemia have galactorrhea. Amenorrheic patients with low to normal FSH and LH, including those who have withdrawal flow to progestin, should have their serum prolactin measured as part of the initial evaluation. However, galactorrhea with normal menses and normal serum prolactin virtually excludes a tumor, although galactorrhea is unusual in this setting if the patient has never been pregnant (166).

The evaluation of the adolescent with hyperprolactinemia should include a menstrual history and a history of pregnancies and abortions, medications and illicit drugs, hirsutism or acne, symptoms of thyroid dysfunction, visual changes, and headaches. The physical examination should include a careful neurologic assessment, including fundoscopic examination, screening visual field test by confrontation, palpation of the thyroid gland, notation of vital signs, a careful breast examination, and evaluation of androgen excess and estrogenization by vaginal examination.

Pregnancy, hypothyroidism, renal and hepatic disease, polycystic ovary syndrome, and ingestion of drugs (including cocaine) should be ruled out in the patient with hyperprolactinemia. In most of these conditions, prolactin values are elevated to only 30 to 100 ng/ml. Repeat serum prolactin values should be measured under optimal conditions: with the patient in the fasting, nonexercised state with no breast stimulation. The TSH level also should be measured. Anteroposterior and lateral cone-down views of the sella are useful only in detecting calcification or lesions large enough to cause erosion or enlargement of the sella. The detection of small lesions and the anatomic definition of larger lesions require MRI scanning.

A prolactin level >100 ng/ml is suggestive of a prolactin-secreting tumor. The level of prolactin usually correlates with the size of the tumor (163). However, a tumor can be seen with only a minimal elevation of prolactin, especially in the case of nonfunctioning tumors that cause stalk compression. For example, patients with craniopharyngiomas, somatotropic tumors causing acromegaly, cysts (suprasellar arachnoid cysts and Rathke's cleft cyst), and nonfunctioning tumors may have elevated prolactin values (typically <200 ng/ml). Prolactinomas are classified as microadenomas (<10 mm) and macroadenomas (>10 mm). Patients classified as having functional hyperprolactinemia represent a spectrum of findings from mild hyperplasia of lactotropes to small pituitary microadenomas not visualized on imaging. Stimulation tests, suppression tests, and other neuroendocrine tests are usually reserved for patients with macroadenomas, preoperative evaluation, or patients with clinical signs or symptoms of hypopituitarism.

It is essential to assess estrogen status in these young women by serum estradiol level, vaginal smear, and progestin challenge because of the risk of low bone density (167–170). Klibanski and associates (167) have found reduced bone density in young women with hyperprolactinemia and serum estradiol levels <20 pg/ml. Bone density improved with therapy (168) but did not return to normal in all women. Biller and colleagues (169) monitored trabecular bone by CT prospectively in 52 hyperprolactinemic women and found further decreases in mean bone density in amenorrheic women. After the restoration of menses, bone density did improve in a subset of women, but a sustained period of amenorrhea may lead to permanent losses. A higher initial percent of ideal body weight and final serum androgen levels (testosterone and DHEAS) positively correlated with the slope of the bone density curve.

Once the diagnosis of a prolactin-secreting pituitary tumor has been made, the clinician needs to consider the size of the tumor, the estrogen status, the presence of troublesome galactorrhea, the need for contraception, and the young woman's desire for fertility. For patients with microadenomas or functional hyperprolactinemia with normal estrogen status and normal menses, and therefore not at increased risk for osteoporosis, observation is one option. In a study of 59 patients with idiopathic hyperprolactinemia, there was a high tendency to spontaneous cure, and progression to pituitary prolactinoma did not occur (171). In a study of 30 patients (age 16 to 38 years) with hyperprolactinemia followed up for 3 to 20 years (mean 5.2 years) with prolactin levels and tomograms or CT studies, only two patients had evidence of progression at 4 and 6 years. Four patients with initially normal radiographs developed signs of a tumor, but in none was there progression to a macroadenoma. Several patients had spontaneous resolution of amenorrhea and galactorrhea, and one-third of those with abnormal CT or tomograms initially had no evidence of tumor at their last followup study (172). Other studies of the natural history of these lesions have reported similar findings; many lesions will stay the same size or regress, with lowering of serum prolactin and reestablishment of menses over time (158,160,173,174). If observation is elected, close monitoring with both MRI and serum prolactin determinations is warranted (the observation of low prolactin levels alone does not provide adequate followup).

Most adolescents with microadenomas are estrogen deficient and therefore in need of therapy. They are at risk of bone loss and, most important, of not attaining normal peak bone mass. Treatment with bromocriptine restores menses and fertility in most patients and improves their estrogen levels. Patients thus need to be counseled to use effective barriers or low-dose oral contraceptives if they become sexually active. Published studies and our own experience suggest that after 2 years of bromocriptine therapy, some patients have normal prolactin levels and normal menses following discontinuation of the medication (157,161). It is not known, however, how many of these patients might have experienced a spontaneous recovery. Recurrent hyperprolactinemia can occur after even 4 to 8 years of treatment with reductions in dosage or discontinuation. Small numbers of patients with idiopathic hyperprolactinemia or nonprogressive microadenomas who are estrogen deficient have also been treated with cyclic conjugated estrogens (Premarin 0.625 mg) and medroxyprogesterone for a mean of 4 years, or low-dose (30- to 35-µg) oral contraceptives for a mean of 2.9 years with little if any effect on the long-term prognosis and at lower cost (175,176). Careful followup is indicated.

Transphenoidal surgery is rarely suggested for the treatment of microadenomas. Although success rates have been in the 90% range in the immediate postoperative period (177–180), it has been found on long-term followup that 17% to 50% of patients have recurrent hyperprolactinemia, even though a lesion may not be demonstrable on CT scan (158,162,179,180). A normal prolactin value 6 months after surgery indicates that a cure is likely to have occurred.

Macroadenomas do require therapy because if they are untreated, patients may experience further tumor growth, visual impairment, and hypopituitarism. Medical therapy with bromocriptine or a similar drug is the primary approach for the majority of patients. Bromocriptine can reduce prolactin levels substantially and cause shrinkage of the tumor over weeks to months (see Case 9 below) (181,182). The cytoplasmic volume of cells is decreased. Long-acting preparations of bromocriptine have yielded good success rates. In most patients, bromocriptine will have to be continued indefinitely, which is very expensive. The abrupt cessation of medication can result in increased tumor size. Tumor enlargement may occur in some patients despite bromocriptine therapy because of the presence of a nonfunctioning or non–prolactin-secreting tumor (183) or the occurrence of intrapituitary hemorrhage or tumor necrosis. Since prolactin levels may fall with bromocriptine therapy in spite of continued tumor enlargement, successful management must be monitored by prolactin levels, MRI, and clinical assessment, initially every 6 months. The indications for surgery include an inability to tolerate bromocriptine or other dopamine agonists in a patient who requires therapy, unresponsiveness to therapy (which usually indicates a cystic lesion), increasing tumor size despite therapy, persistent visual loss and chiasmal compression despite medical therapy, and pituitary apoplexy. With surgery, the recurrence risk for hyperprolactinemia is 20% to 80%. Radiation therapy has been advocated for large tumors that are refractory to medical and surgical management in patients who desire definitive therapy, but it may lead to hypopituitarism.

In young women desiring fertility, bromocriptine has been used effectively to lower prolactin levels. Discontinuation of bromocriptine therapy is recommended as soon as a pregnancy is diagnosed, although the European experience suggests that bromocriptine can be continued. Tumor-related complications, such as visual field defects, headaches, and diabetes insipidus, appear to occur in about 15% of bromocriptine-induced pregnancies but are uncommon in patients with microadenomas (<5%) (184,185). The risk of symptomatic tumor enlargement with macroadenomas is 15% to 35% for tumors previously treated with bromocriptine, compared with 4% to 7% for those previously treated with surgery and/or radiation therapy. The complications of tumor enlargement are usually reversible with the reinstitution of bromocriptine therapy for the remainder of the pregnancy. Prolactin levels fall after delivery, and there is no contraindication to breast-feeding.

Bromocriptine therapy is effective for treating estrogen deficiency, promoting fertility, and aiding in the cessation of lactation. The restoration of menses and ovulation occurs more rapidly and more reliably than does the cessation of galactorrhea. Bromocriptine is usually prescribed in slowly increasing dosages, starting with one-half of a 2.5-mg tablet at bedtime, followed a week later by one tablet at bedtime, followed in one week by half a tablet in the morning and one tablet at night, followed by one 2.5-mg tablet twice a day. A dosage of 5.0 to 7.5 mg/day is usually adequate in most patients with mild to moderate hyperprolactinemia, although some require a higher dose. Patients must be warned to be careful rising from bed in the morning because of the possibility of postural hypotension; some patients notice nausea, headache, dizziness, nasal congestion, and fatigue with bromocriptine therapy. In patients unable to tolerate oral bromocriptine because of nausea, Vermesh and coworkers (186) have reported that vaginal administration of this drug can result in detectable plasma bromocriptine levels and reduction of prolactin. Several new dopamine-agonist drugs have been developed, including quinogolide (CV 205–502) once-daily dose of 0.075 to 0.3 mg; pergolide; and the newly released cabergoline (Dostinex) 0.25 to 1.0 mg twice a week (187–189). The long-acting formulations of bromocriptine (both slow gastrointestinal release and injectable Parodel LAR) have had favorable effects on macroadenomas with more prolonged normoprolactinemia (190–192).

Long-term followup of patients is essential, whatever treatment option is chosen (observation, bromocriptine or cabergoline, surgery, and/or radiation) and includes monitoring of clinical status, determination of prolactin levels, formal testing of visual field, and imaging with MRI.

EUGONADISM

The term *eugonadism* has been used to include patients with normal estrogenization but failure to establish normal menstrual pattern. Patients with genital anomalies such as obstructed outflow and uterine agenesis are in this category (see Chapter 8). In addition, patients with polycystic ovary syndrome typically have normal to elevated levels of estrogens but oligomenorrhea and often evidence of androgen excess (see Chapter 7). Patients with many of the hypothalamic problems (e.g., stress and weight loss) may also fit midway between the categories of eugonadism and hypogonadotropic hypogonadism because their estrogen levels fall into the range seen in the follicular phase of the cycle but normal cyclicity does not occur.

TREATMENT GUIDELINES

Treatment is aimed at the cause of the problem, especially in patients with CNS tumors, Crohn's disease, or anorexia nervosa. For example, nutritional rehabilitation and corticosteroids or surgery may cause the teenager with Crohn's disease to begin spontaneous pubertal maturation. The girl with end-stage renal failure often experiences menarche following a successful renal transplant; in fact, ovulatory cycles may result in an unwanted pregnancy for the sexually active adolescent who has not previously used birth control. Girls with anorexia nervosa are treated by medical monitoring, including frequent weight checks, nutritional rehabilitation with slow weight gain, psychotherapy for the patient and family, and potentially estrogen replacement therapy.

Followup studies of adolescent patients with irregular cycles have been few. In a 10-year followup study of 46 adult women (mean age 24; range 18 to 32 years) with amenorrhea and normal prolactin levels, most women (6 of 9) with hypoestrogenic amenorrhea (weight loss, exercise) recovered normal cycles, but only 3 of 17 euestrogenic amenorrheic patients progressed to normal cycles (193). None of the patients with polycystic ovary syndrome or premature ovarian failure developed normal ovulatory cycles.

For many patients with irreversible estrogen deficiency or significant constitutional delay, estrogen replacement therapy is needed to bring about normal secondary sexual characteristics at an age commensurate with the peer group. Although few adolescents with ovarian failure experience vasomotor symptoms such as those seen in postmenopausal women or following oophorectomy, estrogen replacement reverses vaginal atrophy and decreases the risk of osteoporosis and fractures. In adults it lessens the risk of cardiovascular disease by 50% in observational studies (randomized trials are under way) and improves serum lipoprotein profiles (194–202).

The biggest worry for most patients and families is whether there is an increased risk of cancer, particularly cancer of the breast, which might offset some of the known benefits of estrogen replacement therapy. To date, there is conflicting evidence on the risk of breast cancer in postmenopausal women. Because similar studies have not been done on adolescents, conclusions must, unfortunately, be extrapolated from the data on adult women who use estrogens for menopausal therapy or for contraception. In the Nurses Health Study, Colditz and colleagues (203) found that the risk of breast cancer was increased among postmenopausal women using estrogen (relative risk [RR] 1.32, 95% confidence interval [CI]: 1.14, 1.54) and those using estrogen and progestin (relative risk 1.41, 95% CI: 1.15, 1.74) versus those who had never taken estrogen. The RR for women taking 5 to 9 years of therapy was 1.45 (95% CI: 1.22, 1.74). In contrast, in a study of women in the Seattle-Puget Sound Surveillance, Stanford and colleagues (204) did not find any increased risk in those who had taken estrogen (RR 0.9, 95% CI: 0.7, 1.3), and the risk was reduced in those who had had 8 or more years of hormone replacement therapy (RR 0.4, CI: 0.2, 1.0). (See Chapter 17 for studies in oral contraceptive users.)

Since many girls with gonadal dysgenesis, premature ovarian failure, or Kallmann's syndrome do not come to medical attention until they are 13 to 16 years old, therapy is undertaken at that time. The goals of therapy are to induce normal breast development and menses, increase growth velocity, and promote normal bone mass. In adolescents and young adults, the risk of low bone density appears to be especially related to the lack of spontaneous development, low weight, and exposure to radiation therapy (24). Patients who are known to have undergone chemotherapy and, especially, radiation therapy should have bone age and ovarian status evaluated at a chronologic age of 10 to 12 years and should be considered for replacement therapy when the diagnosis of ovarian failure has been established.

The optimal age for treating patients with a delay in sexual development because of competitive athletic participation or anorexia nervosa is unknown. In general, it seems preferable for patients to "earn" their estrogenization, pubertal development, and menses by making the necessary changes in lifestyle, especially by improving their nutrition. Coaches, parents, and athletes should be counseled about the optimal diet to establish normal growth and development and acquire normal bone mass. In girls with no development, the age of optimal estrogen replacement has not been determined. We believe that estrogen should be offered at least when the girl is 14 to 15 years old, taking into account predicted height (see Appendix 7) and the age when breast development and menses are desired by the teen.

In girls who experienced pubertal development and estrogenization at the normal age, followed later by amenorrhea and estrogen deficiency, a reasonable approach is to provide medical treatment and counseling in an attempt to bring about a change in lifestyle for 6 to 12 months before estrogen replacement is offered (89,205). Others prefer not to institute estrogen therapy in athletes within 3 years of menarche or before they are 16 years old, but scientific studies have not been done with regard to the advantages or disadvantages of this pattern of replacement therapy in terms of ultimate bone mass and the occurrence of stress fractures. Delayed menarche is a risk factor for low lumbar bone density in athletes (139). It is clear that in adult women, bone mass is lost rapidly in the first few years of estrogen deficiency, and irreversible bone loss has occurred by 3 years of nontreatment. Some girls will reduce the amount of exercise in order to allow puberty to progress; others may find their training schedule important for optimal performance, or they may be in a compulsive pattern associated with an eating disorder. Weight, height, estimated percentage of body fat (if possible), and diet should be monitored. Previously, patients were often allowed to remain estrogen deficient for years, which increased their risk of osteopenia. Although some anorexic and athletic patients refuse medical intervention, the potential problems of estrogen deficiency should be discussed with the patient and her family. Dual energy photon absorptiometry (DEXA) or dual photon absorptiometry of the lumbar spine (and hip) can be used to provide a baseline measurement and to impress the patient with the need to take the potential medical complication of bone loss seriously.

Calcium replacement alone does not substitute for estrogen replacement, but all adolescents should have adequate calcium intake. The average adolescent intake of calcium is about 900 mg/day (206). An intake of 1200 to 1500 mg of calcium is recommended by diet (see Appendix 8 for handout) or supplemental calcium; bone density can is improved in normal girls by increasing daily calcium intake from 80% to 110% of the RDA or by supplementing the intake with dairy products that furnish up to 1200 mg/day of calcium for 18 months to 3 years of treatment (137,207,222). Whether this leads to long-term gains if intake is reduced is less clear. Hypoestrogenic women require at least 1500 mg/day, but calcium intake should be considered an adjunct, not a replacement for estrogen. Adequate intake of Vitamin D is important. Trials of drugs (alendronate, calcitonin) and other hormones and growth factors used to treat osteoporosis in adult women have not been undertaken in adolescents. Exercise is also important for adolescents with hypoestrogenism to promote normal bone mass and cardiovascular fitness.

In an adolescent girl with an intact uterus, hormone replacement therapy requires the use of both estrogen and progestin in varying doses (14,28, 208–220). The goals of the estrogen component should be considered in three phases: (a) induction of breast development, (b) establishment of normal menses and, it is hoped, acquisition of normal bone mineralization, and (c) long-term maintenance of a normal estrogen state. A patient may need planning for all three phases of estrogen replacement or only the last phase, and the selection of the appropriate doses and the method of cycling depends on her individual needs. If progestins are prescribed, the timing of introducing treatment and the appropriate dose are dependent on the amount of breast development that the patient has achieved and whether the progestin is to be used only to give a progestin challenge, to be administered for several cycles to treat amenorrhea or dysfunctional uterine bleeding (DUB), or to be prescribed as part of long-term hormone replacement therapy.

For the induction of breast development in the girl with no secondary sexual characteristics (phase 1), several estrogen preparations and dosages have been used. Generally, a low dose of estrogen, such as 0.3 mg of conjugated estrogens

(Premarin), 0.3 mg estrone sulfate (Estratab), or 5 to 10 μg of ethinyl estradiol, is selected to induce initial breast development for 6 to 12 months.‡ The sequential administration of estradiol patches of 5, 10, and 25 μg/day over 12 to 24 months has also been suggested, but the lowest dose available commercially is 25 μg (28). The relative potencies of estrogens are summarized in Table 6. Oral contraceptives are not recommended for initial therapy because they contain progestin throughout the cycle, which is not a physiologic approach to the induction of normal breast development. During normal puberty, there is a long period of unopposed low levels of estrogen until ovulatory cycles begin (see Chapter 4). There has been speculation that particular doses of progestin or estrogen may be more likely to lead to tubular breasts, but a randomized study has not been done.

To further enhance breast development and to induce menses (phase 2), the estrogen dose is increased from 0.3 to 0.625 mg of conjugated estrogens. The timing of this change needs to be adjusted to the bone age, the predicted height, and the desire of the patient for rapid breast development. For example, in the girl who is short and initially had no pubertal development, the transition is likely to occur in 12 months. For the girl with ovarian failure who had already started her breast development, has achieved a normal height, and is eager for more breast development, the dose may be increased in 3 to 6 months. The timing of the introduction of progestin varies among centers. Although in the past some girls received unopposed estrogen daily until breakthrough bleeding occurred, we believe that this method should be discouraged because adolescents benefit from a predictable onset of menses, and many girls experience significant dysfunctional bleeding that may require intervention. We suggest the addition of a short course of progestin (5 or 10 mg of medroxyprogesterone) to the continuous conjugated estrogens within 2 to 3 months of the increase in dose to 0.625 mg.

In phase 2, if conjugated estrogens are prescribed, either of two dosing regimens can be selected:

Conjugated estrogens 0.625 mg daily *plus*
medroxyprogesterone 10 mg each day for the first 5 days of each month
OR
Conjugated estrogens 0.625 mg for days 1 to 25 *plus*
medroxyprogesterone 10 mg each day for days 21 to 25 each month

This dose of progestin is used only until breast development is completed over the next 6 months and then the dose of progestin is increased to 10 days and ultimately to 14 days for optimal protection of the endometrium if long-term hormone replacement is planned.

Long-term maintenance (phase 3) includes both an estrogen and a progestin. The estrogen is generally given daily or in cycles of 25 days each month and the progestin for 12–14 days each month.

---

‡The lowest dose of ethinyl estradiol commercially available is 20 μg.

TABLE 6. *Comparative effects of estrogen preparations on suppression of follicle-stimulating hormone (FSH) level, liver proteins, and bone density*

Estrogen	FSH levels	Liver proteins	Bone density
Conjugated estrogens (Premarin)	1.0 mg	0.625 mg	0.625 mg
Ethinyl estradiol (Estinyl)	5.0 μg	2–10 μg	5–10 μg
Transdermal estradiol (Estraderm)	—	—	50 μg
Piperazine estrone sulfate (Ogen)	1.0 mg	2.0 mg	0.625 mg
Micronized estradiol (Estrace)	1.0 mg	1.0 mg	1.0 mg

(From Speroff L, Glass RH, Kase NG. *Clinical gynecologic endocrinology and infertility,* 5th ed. Baltimore: Williams & Wilkins, 1994, Chapter 18; with permission. Sources of table: Genant HK, Cann CE, Ettinger B, et al. Quantitative computed tomography of vertebral spongiosa: a sensitive method for detecting early bone loss after oophorectomy. *Ann Intern Med* 1982;97:699. Marshchak CA, Lobo RA, Dozono-Takana R, et al. Comparison of pharmacodynamic properties of various estrogen formulations. *Am J Obstet Gynecol* 1982;144:511. Horsman A, Jones M, Francis R, et al. The effect of estrogen dose on postmenopausal bone loss. *N Engl J Med* 1983;309:1405. Field CS, Ory SJ, Wahner HW, et al. Preventive effects of transdermal 17β-estradiol on osteoporotic changes after surgical menopause: a two-year placebo controlled trial. *Am J Obstet Gynecol* 1993;168:114; with permission.)

For example, if conjugated estrogens are chosen, replacement therapy could be:

Conjugated estrogens 0.625 mg daily *plus*

medroxyprogesterone 10 mg each day for the first 14 days of each month

OR

Conjugated estrogens 0.625 mg for days 1–25 *plus*

medroxyprogesterone 10 mg each day for days 12–25 each month

Other estrogens may be used in place of conjugated estrogens including ethinyl estradiol 20 μg, transdermal estradiol 0.05 mg given continuously (patches changed twice a week), esterified estrogens (Estratab), micronized estradiol (Estrace), and piperazine estrone sulfate. Doses of transdermal estradiol range from 0.025 mg to 0.1 mg, and patches are changed once or twice a week depending on the product. Some adolescents tolerate the estradiol patches well and find changing them preferable to daily oral medication (oral progestin is still necessary). However, other adolescents complain of the patch falling off, have allergic reactions to the adhesive, or do not like the idea of having a potentially visible acknowledgment of a medical problem. Counseling needs to take these issues into account in the choice of therapy. Sequential hormonal regimens are also available with new packaging (PremPhase–14 days of Premarin 0.625 mg and 14 days of Premarin 0.625 mg and medroxyprogesterone 5 mg in a dial-pak) to assist the patient in taking her hormones correctly. Many clinicians prescribe oral contraceptives with 20 to 35 μg of ethinyl estradiol for replacement therapy, particularly in college students who prefer to be taking the same dosing as many of their friends. Elevated gonadotropin levels usually only partially suppress, even with what appears to be adequate doses, and thus monitoring levels is not helpful in determining estrogen doses.

Although all of the above doses will give the patient normal menses, the relative amounts of estrogen provided are quite different. Doses that are used for adolescents are based chiefly on the maintenance doses used for postmenopausal women (0.625 mg of conjugated estrogens, 0.3 mg of conjugated estrogens plus calcium, 20 to 25 μg of ethinyl estradiol, and 0.5 to 2.0 mg micronized estradiol) (195,196,216–220) to provide protection from bone loss. These doses, however, may not be applicable to the adolescent patient who needs to increase bone mass, not just maintain bone density. Our studies of adolescents with estrogen deficiency states treated with conjugated estrogens, 0.625 mg for 21 days of the month, found that a regimen started at a mean age of 16 years prevented further bone loss but did not result in normal bone mass (24), because either the dosage or the duration was inadequate, or other factors presently unstudied played a role. Higher doses of estrogen that have been suggested for aiding in bone acquisition include conjugated estrogens (Premarin) 0.9 to 1.25 mg, transdermal β-estradiol patches (Estraderm) 0.1 mg, ethinyl estradiol 30 to 35 μg, micronized estradiol (Estrace) 2 mg, all given in cycles (along with 14 days of progestin), or oral contraceptives but none of these has been subjected to clinical studies in teens.

As mentioned above, progestin doses are determined by medical indications (223–228). Doses of medroxyprogesterone vary from 2.5 to 10 mg and can be given in cycles or continuously. The goal of the progestin challenge in the diagnosis of amenorrhea is to establish that the endometrium is primed with estrogen, and thus 5 to 10 days of 10 mg of medroxyprogesterone are adequate for the test. In the therapy of delayed puberty after estrogen doses are increased, we often prescribe progestin 5 days per month for 6 months and 10 days for an additional 6 months before changing to maintenance therapy of 14 days. For the patient who requires short-term treatment for DUB, a duration of 10 to 14 days can be used, with 14 days prescribed for patients who will require ongoing management. Several studies suggest that protection of the endometrium from endometrial hyperplasia in postmenopausal women is optimal with 14 days of medroxyprogesterone. In a study of more than 1700 women treated with four different regimens of estrogen and progestin (conjugated estrogens 0.625 mg plus medroxyprogesterone with 2.5 or 5.0 mg daily or 5 or 10 mg for 14 days of a 28-day cycle), endometrial hyperplasia occurred in $<1\%$ (226); there were only five cases among women using the two lower-dose regimens, 2.5 mg continuously and 5 mg sequentially. Padwick and colleagues (214) have observed that women given continuous estrogen and cyclic progestin for 12 days have a predominantly proliferative endometrium if bleeding occurs on or before day 10 and a wholly or predominantly secretory endometrium with bleeding on day 11 or later. Cyclic medroxyprogesterone alone has also been reported to increase lumbar bone density in 21- to 45-year-old women (230).

The optimal progestin type and dosage have not been determined in teens. The most commonly used progestin is medroxyprogesterone, 10 mg; as noted above, doses as low as 5 mg are sufficient to protect the endometrium from endometrial hyperplasia in the vast majority of patients. Used sequentially in the postmenopausal woman, the progestins norethindrone and norgestrel may be more likely to lower high-density lipoprotein (HDL) cholesterol (227) unless used in small doses. Natural progesterone appears to be more effective than synthetic progestins in promoting the beneficial effects of estrogen on lipids (217) and is available as Prometrium (given 12–14 days/cycle). Further evaluation (ultrasound, endometrial biopsy, or dilation and curettage) is indicated in women taking long-term estrogen/progestin replacement therapy who develop persistent irregular bleeding with no obvious cause such as missed pills or pelvic infection.

Most adolescents prefer monthly menses and thus progestin cycles are prescribed monthly. Some adolescents (often athletes and girls with anorexia nervosa), however, prefer a minimum number of withdrawal menses and can be offered daily estrogen cycled every 60 or 90 days with progestin for 14 days or continuous estrogen/progestin. A study of postmenopausal women found that quarterly medroxyprogesterone (10 mg/day for 14 days) gave a similar rate of endometrial hyperplasia, but their menses were longer, often heavier, and more often unscheduled than when progestin was used monthly (221). Oral contraceptives have been prescribed similarly, with 9 weeks of 30 μg ethinyl estradiol and 150 μg desogestrel pill followed by one week off; breakthough bleeding and spotting were more common than in the usual cyclic regimens (222). Another option, frequently used in postmenopausal women but uncommonly in teens, is continuous conjugated estrogen 0.625 mg and medroxyprogesterone 2.5 mg daily (also available as PremPro); patients typically will experience irregular bleeding for the first 3 to 6 months and then amenorrhea.

A question that has been debated for some time is whether estrogen replacement therapy in the absence of weight gain and the establishment of normal cycles can bring about normal bone mass acquisition in young women with anorexia nervosa (223–225). In a large randomized trial of estrogen therapy in women with anorexia nervosa, Klibanski and colleagues (224) studied 48 amenorrheic women (mean age 24.9; range 16 to 42 years) who had had amenorrhea for a mean of 3.3 years in the estrogen group and 4.6 years in the control group (range 0.5 to 17.3 years). The estrogen replacement therapy used was either conjugated estrogens 0.625 mg on days 1 to 25 and medroxyprogesterone 5 mg on days 16 to 25, or oral contraceptive therapy (35-μg pill). The patients were monitored for an average of 1.5 years, and their spinal bone density was measured by dual energy techniques using CT. Although there was no statistical difference between the treated (+2.8 ± 11.0%) and the controls (-5.4 ± 22.6%), there was a difference between estrogen-treated patients and controls when patients who regained their menses spontaneously were excluded from the analysis (+2.2 ± 11.1% vs. −13.3 ± 17.8%; $p = 0.004$). For those who weighed <70% of their ideal body weight, the difference was particularly striking between the treated patients and the controls (+4.0 ± 8.8% vs. −20.1 ± 16.2%). In a nonrandomized study of patients with anorexia nervosa treated with oral contraceptive pills, an increase in total body bone mass and lumbar spine bone mineral density was observed (225).

In choosing estrogen replacement therapy for the adolescent with anorexia nervosa or athletic amenorrhea, who is often reluctant to use such therapy, we usually prescribe a low dose (such as 0.3 mg) of conjugated estrogens for 2 to 3 months to assure her that she can tolerate the medication, and then increase it to 0.625 to 0.9 mg with 14 days of progestin. Oral contraceptive pills provide higher doses of estrogen and contraception, if the medication is tolerated. Sexually active patients should receive oral contraceptives for hormone replacement.

The optimal age for estrogen replacement therapy of girls with Turner's syndrome is based on several factors. Because such a girl is short, therapy with growth hormone to enhance her final adult height needs to be considered and discussed with the patient and her family before estrogen therapy is begun. Delaying epiphyseal closure by postponing the use of estrogen is indicated, although the potential impact on ultimate bone mass has been debated. Some studies suggest that Turner's syndrome is associated with evidence of demineralization at the wrist and other sites from an early age (18,23,226). Mora and colleagues (226) found that girls who started estrogen therapy before the age of 12 years had better mineralization (measured by single photon densitometry of the wrist) than those who started after the age of 12, but the bone mineral content remained low. Others, however, have suggested that lumbar spine and whole body measurements using dual photon absorptiometry in girls receiving growth hormone alone are normal when pubertal status and age are controlled for in the study (23). Of interest, girls with normal estrogenization and Turner's syndrome have normal bone density (24). These two competing aims present a dilemma for the clinician in designing optimal therapy for these girls. Instituting growth hormone early so that estrogen therapy does not have to be delayed to late adolescence is a reasonable approach.

At some centers in the past, androgens, including oxandrolone, were given to patients with Turner's syndrome during late childhood and early adolescence in an attempt to promote growth. Although these hormones did result in significantly increased growth velocity during the first year of treatment, the final adult heights did not appear to be improved. The observation that low-dose estrogen promoted bone growth led to several trials of ethinyl estradiol at 100 ng/kg/day starting in late childhood (230–232). A significant growth acceleration occurred in most Turner's patients treated for 6 to 12 months, but at our center and others, it has been found that bone age increased and final height did not appear to be increased. The low-dose estrogen therapy did, however, result in increased IGF-1 (somatomedin-C) levels and psychological gains with the height spurt. Although the institution of estrogen therapy in midadolescence might be expected to cause shorter stature than institution in late adolescence because of closure of epiphyses, in fact we could not find any difference in final height between those treated at a mean age of 14.3 years and those treated at a mean age of 17.2 years (233) in the era before the availability of growth hormone. Most, but not all studies, have found that the stature of the Turner's patients is related to midparental height (229,233).

Therapy for Turner's patients usually includes synthetic growth hormone (234–236). In the first year of therapy of patients with Turner's syndrome, Rosenfield and associates (234) found that the mean growth rate for controls was 3.8 cm/year, for human growth hormone (met-HGH) 6.6 cm/year, for oxandrolone 7.9 cm/year, and for combination therapy with human growth hormone and oxandrolone 9.8 cm/year. The control and oxandrolone-alone groups were excluded from the study after the first year. Although height velocity did dccrcasc aftcr thc first ycar, Roscnfcld and collcagues (236) found sustained increases for at least 6 years in a 3- to 6-year followup of girls with Turner's syndrome. They reported that 14 of 17 (82%) of girls receiving HGH alone (changed during the study to seven times a week with a total dose of 0.375 mg/kg/week) and 41 of 45 (95%) of girls receiving combination therapy with oxandrolone and HGH exceeded their expected adult height. The 30 girls who had completed treatment had a mean height of 151.9 cm, in comparison with a projected mean height of 143.8 cm. The study criteria for cessation of therapy were a bone age $\geq$14 years and a growth rate $<$2.5 cm in the past year. (See Fig. 1 of a girl with Turner's syndrome treated with growth hormone at our hospital.) The mean final height in European girls treated at $>$10 years of age was 150.7 cm (238). The addition of estrogen to growth hormone treatment does not appear to be efficacious; in a study of 40 patients with Turner's syndrome, no statistical difference in the first-year growth rate during growth hormone treatment alone (7.5 $\pm$ 1.3 cm/yr) compared with growth hormone plus ethinyl estradiol (25 ng/kg/day) (8.1 $\pm$ 1.6 cm/yr), and minor breast development occurred more often in the estrogen-treated group (237). Similar results were noted with a dose of 100 ng/kg/day of ethinyl estradiol (239). Thus, treatment with estrogen is generally initiated at about the age of 14 or 15 (or after cessation of growth hormone therapy). If needed earlier and if growth issues have been addressed, low-dose ethinyl estradiol at 50 ng/kg/day can be given to a 12- to 14-year-old girl to give some breast development (12). Patients and parents need to be counseled about the benefits, costs, and potential risks of growth hormone treatment.

Treatment of adolescents with oligomenorrhea and anovulatory cycles is aimed at establishing normal menstrual flow and protection of the endometrium from hyperplasia. Progestins such as medroxyprogesterone, 10 mg, can be prescribed for 14 days each month (or every 2 months in patients with scant withdrawal flow). Patients with chronic anovulatory states, such as those with polycystic ovary syndrome, have an increased risk of endometrial carcinoma and should receive long-term progestin therapy or oral contraceptives (see Chapter 7).

Even though considerations of fertility are beyond the scope of this book, it is useful to be able to provide some information to teenagers with estrogen deficiency states. Many patients with irreversible ovarian failure, such as those with Turner's syndrome, who desire to have children will choose adoption; however, advances in technology have now shown that oocyte donation and in vitro fertilization are possible in women with ovarian failure (32,240–242). Current assisted-reproduction technologies include in vitro fertilization (IVF), gamete intrafallopian transfer (GIFT), and zygote intrafallopian transfer (ZIFT). Rarely, patients with autoimmune oophoritis and resistant ovary syndrome have been reported to have pregnancies spontaneously (because of the waxing and waning nature of the disorder) and have also had successful pregnancies after treatment with estrogens, corticosteroids (for autoimmune disease), gonadotropins, or clomiphene (243–246). Patients with GnRH deficiency can be induced to ovulate with gonadotropins or pulsatile GnRH. Although GnRH can also be used to induce pubertal development, oral estrogens are clearly easier and less expensive for this purpose. Patients with hypothalamic dysfunction and infertility need to have the issue of weight, exercise, and stress addressed and then, depending on the etiology, may be treated with clomiphene citrate, gonadotropins, or pulsatile GnRH. Ovulation can usually be induced in patients with hyperprolactinemia by the use of bromocriptine.

The most important part of the therapy undertaken by the physician is the ability to listen to questions and respond in a straightforward fashion. The adolescent needs to know that her parents are not keeping secrets from her about her medical condition. Drawings that underscore how normal she is and that illustrate current and potential technologies are extremely meaningful. The positive aspects of her condition and her ability to function as a normal woman should be emphasized. She may cope better with the issue of infertility if she receives information in response to her own questions. The girl with ovarian failure can be told about the many other young patients with infertility; she may know a couple who has spent years in infertility treatments. The fact that she can make plans that are right for her from the beginning of her marriage can help her think about the future. Acceptance of estrogen therapy is generally the easier part of the counseling, given the widespread lay information on osteoporosis, although families and patients often have questions about long-term risks.

Groups are available in many metropolitan centers for counseling patients (e.g., Turner's Society groups). Young adolescents may resist going to meetings, but parents, older adolescents, and young adults often find the support and education helpful. Teenagers also often discover the benefits of meeting one-on-one with another woman who has the same condition. For example, before surgery for reconstruction for vaginal agenesis, a girl may find it useful to meet a young woman who has already been through the experience. A girl is often relieved to discuss her diagnosis openly, since before the initial medical visit she may have feared that worse problems, such as cancer, have impaired her development or menses. Grief and mourning over the lack of function is normal, and frequent visits can help the patient come to terms with the problem. Denial of the diagnosis between visits is common, and the same questions may arise at each visit. The clinician frequently needs to do much of the talking during these appointments, with statements such as "I have other girls in my practice with this problem, and I find they worry about . . . ." Sometimes, a young patient will request to be excused from physical education class so that her lack of development will not be the subject of peer discussion; this request should be honored. The empathic health care provider can greatly aid the patient in accepting the medical diagnosis and the treatment plan.

DELAYED SEXUAL DEVELOPMENT

The absence of breast budding by the age of 13 years is 2 standard deviations beyond normal and requires an evaluation. If the teenager is a thin competitive athlete, then hormonal testing can be delayed until she is 14 years old. The stigmata of Turner's syndrome, especially short stature, or a falloff in height and weight gain, suggestive of malnutrition or a systemic disease, may prompt an earlier diagnosis. History and physical examination, along with evaluation of growth records, are essential. The chief complaint may be "no development," and yet evidence of breast budding and a growth spurt may indicate that development has indeed occurred and that observation of the patient is indicated. Pubic hair may imply that the patient is about to begin thelarche as well, but it should be remembered that girls with ovarian failure develop some pubic hair because of the rise of adrenal androgens. The aspects of the physical examination and assessment of the external genital examination are noted in Chapter 1.

Initial studies in the evaluation of delayed development include radiography of the wrist and hand for bone age, CBC, and determinations of sedimentation rate and levels of TSH, FSH, LH (see discussion in Chapter 5 of the types of gonadotropin assays). In the absence of short stature suggesting gonadal dysgenesis, determinations of the serum prolactin level and T_4 are often part of the initial work-up. The differential diagnosis is made by distinguishing hypergonadotropic hypogonadism from hypogonadotropic hypogonadism (Fig. 7). A patient with elevated gonadotropins has ovarian failure and needs to have her karyotype determined; a patient with a normal 46,XX karyotype and ovarian failure should be assessed for autoimmune disease. Adolescents with low or normal gonadotropin levels require evaluation for a systemic disease or a CNS disorder. Studies may include determinations of prolactin and IGF-1 (somatomedin-C) levels, skull radiograph, MRI scan, GnRH stimulation testing, and other neuroendocrine tests (e.g., growth hormone stimulation tests, cortisol response). MRI scans are preferred for CNS imaging over CT scans; sometimes, however, obtaining an MRI is problematic because of lack of cooperation or the presence of metal orthodontic braces or other hardware that impair the study. Formal visual field testing is indicated in the presence of a pituitary lesion. Other tests for systemic disease, depending on clinical suspicion, may include an evaluation for malabsorption and determinations of sweat chloride, antiendomysial and antigliadin antibodies, BUN, creatinine, electrolytes, calcium, phosphorus, and urinary osmolality and electrolytes. Patients thought to have a constitutional delay of puberty should be kept under surveillance for the possibility of an initially undetected CNS tumor or systemic disease.

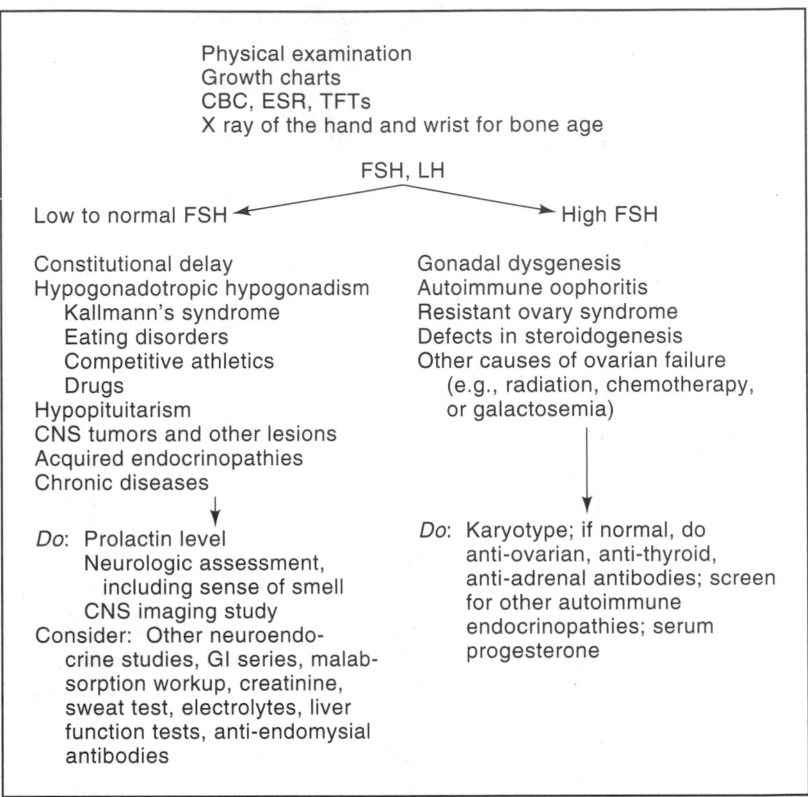

FIG. 7. Differential diagnosis of delayed development.

In patients with ovarian failure, therapy (as outlined in the section on Treatment Guidelines) should be undertaken as soon as the diagnosis is made in early adolescence. In patients with a constitutional delay, reassurance may be all that is necessary; however, many girls by the age of 14 to 15 years will elect to take exogenous hormones to promote normal breast development. Therapy can be stopped after the attainment of secondary sexual characteristics and menses to reassess whether the patient has a normal delay or hypothalamic dysfunction. If spontaneous development does not continue, then estrogen can be reinstituted for courses of 6 to 12 months with periodic discontinuation of therapy. Many patients begin to grow pubic hair after receiving estrogen replacement therapy; however, girls who have had CNS tumors and those with panhypopituitarism often have adrenal insufficiency and thus have absent or only scant pubic and axillary hair development.

Case 1

S. T. was evaluated at the age of 15 years because of "no development." She had always been the shortest member of her class. Physical examination revealed short stature and many of the stigmata of Turner's syndrome (low hairline, webbed neck, ptosis, increased carrying angle, and short fourth metacarpals). Her height was 54″ and her weight 105 lbs, her blood pressure was 125/80 mm Hg, and her pulse rate was 78 beats/min. Breast development was stage 1; no pubic or axillary hair was present.

Pertinent laboratory tests showed an FSH level of 143 mIU/ml, an LH level of 135 mIU/ml, and a karyotype of 45,X (Turner's syndrome). (See Treatment Guidelines for therapy.)

Case 2

C. O. was referred at the age of 15 10/12 because of delayed development. Her developmental milestones were normal; however, she had always been the shortest member of her class (she was an A student in the tenth grade). A review of systems was noncontributory. The family history revealed that one of her father's sisters had experienced menarche at the age of 20 years. On physical examination (Fig. 8), she was short and healthy-appearing with a height of 55 3/4″ and a weight of 86 lbs; her blood pressure was 105/70 mm Hg; and her pulse rate was 66 beats/min. The fundi were normal. Breast development was stage 1, although the areolae were slightly raised with a diameter of 2.4 cm. There was no pubic or axillary hair. The results of CBC, BUN determination, thyroid function tests, and urinalysis were normal; the FSH level was 7.7 mIU/ml and LH 6.3 mIU/ml. She had an extensive neuroendocrine evaluation, including CNS imaging and neuroendocrine studies, the results of which were normal.

The patient was then given conjugated estrogens (Premarin) 0.3 mg daily, and in a short time her breasts began to develop. Pubic hair appeared gradually. One year later, the estrogen dosage was increased to 0.625 mg given in cycles with 10 mg of medroxyprogesterone. The hormone therapy was discontinued after 18 months, and C. O. continued to have normal cyclic menses. One year later, she had an unplanned pregnancy, which she opted to terminate. She admitted that she had never thought she could get pregnant. Her cycles have remained normal, and she is currently using contraception.

Case 3

L. C. came to the clinic at the age of 16 6/12 years because of no sexual development. She recalled having been short since the age of 8 or 9 years. With her family, she had moved several times, and two of her grandparents had died when she was between the ages of 8 and 12 years. Otherwise, she had always been in good health and specifically denied having headaches, frequent infec-

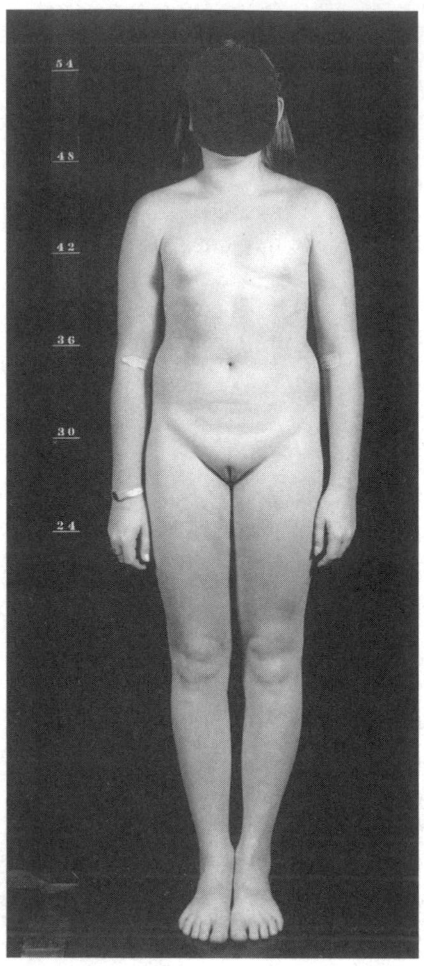

FIG. 8. Case 2: delayed puberty.

tions, eating disorders, and gastrointestinal symptoms. Her family members had not experienced any delays in pubertal development. Her father was 65″ tall; her mother was 62″ tall and had had menarche at the age of 13.

Physical examination showed her to be healthy with normal blood pressure and pulse rate. Her weight was 105 lbs and her height 58 1/4″. Breast development was Tanner stage 1, and pubic hair was stage 2. No axillary hair was present. The external genitalia were normal but unestrogenized, and a small uterus was palpable on rectoabdominal examination. The results of neurologic examination, including her sense of smell, were normal. Growth charts (Fig. 9) showed the patient to be slightly overweight for height; her bone age was 10 9/12 years and her height age 11 6/12 years. The LH level was 2.2 mIU/ml, the FSH level was <2.0 mIU/ml, the estradiol level was <20 pg/ml, the DHEAS level was 109

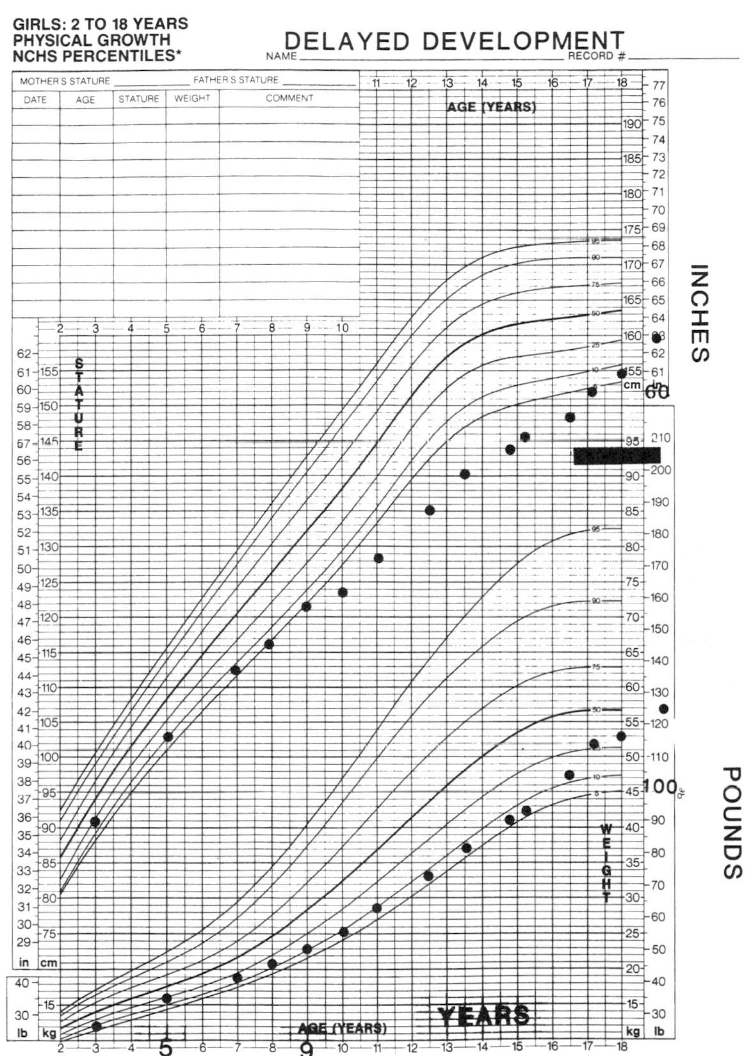

FIG. 9. Case 3: growth chart of patient with delayed development treated with estrogen/progestin therapy (bar).

μg/dl, and the prolactin level was 2.2 ng/ml. The results of thyroid function tests, urinalysis, CBC, and determination of creatinine level and sedimentation rate were normal. Because of the low levels of gonadotropins, further tests of the CNS were undertaken. The results of CNS imaging studies were normal. An overnight study of gonadotropin levels showed no detectable pulsations of LH or FSH (all values <2.0 mIU/ml), and GnRH stimulation testing showed a prepubertal pattern of LH and FSH. Cortisol and growth hormone responses were normal overnight and with insulin testing.

A diagnosis of hypogonadotropic hypogonadism was made, and estrogen therapy was begun: initially 0.3 mg of conjugated estrogens, which was subsequently increased to 0.625 mg with cyclic progestin and then to 1.25 mg. With 2 years of therapy, she developed pubertal breasts, with the areola measuring 2.5 cm and glandular tissue 6 × 6 cm, and pubic hair stage 3. Bone age was 13 years at a chronologic age of 18 years, and she had a significant growth spurt (Fig. 1). She currently takes oral contraceptives for estrogen replacement, and becomes estrogen deficient when her therapy is stopped for 2 to 3 months.

Case 4

M. C. was referred to the adolescent clinic by the renal clinic at the age of 15 6/12 because of delayed development. She had been diagnosed with immune complex nephritis at the age of 8 years and had begun dialysis for end-stage renal disease at the age of 11, the time when she recalled having begun to develop pubic hair. She had undergone a successful renal transplant at age 13 years. At the time of her clinic visit, her serum creatinine level was normal, and she was taking prednisone, 15 mg every other day, and azathioprine, 100 mg daily. She was concerned because she had never menstruated and her breasts had not developed.

Physical examination showed her to be short and overweight. Her height was 59 1/2″ and her weight 131 lbs (Fig. 10). Her blood pressure and pulse were normal. Breast development was Tanner stage 1, and pubic hair scant stage 2 to 3; no axillary hair was present. The abdominal examination revealed several large scars and a palpable kidney in the right lower quadrant. Pelvic examination revealed a prepubertal unestrogenized hymen; examination with the patient in the knee-chest position showed a normal vagina and cervix. Rectoabdominal examination showed a small, palpable cervix. Although the initial thought was that M. C.'s delay in puberty was likely to have been caused by her chronic illness, the fact that she had started to develop pubic hair at age 11 and not progressed to a normal puberty, in spite of the establishment of normal renal function following the transplant, suggested other diagnoses. Her bone age was 10 6/12 years. The results of thyroid function tests were normal, but surprisingly, gonadotropin levels were elevated: LH was 216 mIU/ml, and FSH was 297 mIU/ml. Her karyotype was 46,XY. With the diagnosis of 46,XY (Swyer's syndrome), M. C. underwent surgery to remove the intraabdominal gonads. The histopathology and staging procedure revealed bilateral gonadoblastomas with early invasive dysgerminoma. She has had no recurrence of tumor. M. C. was treated with estrogen replacement therapy and developed only small breasts in spite of the onset of menses. She later underwent an elective breast augmentation with satisfactory results.

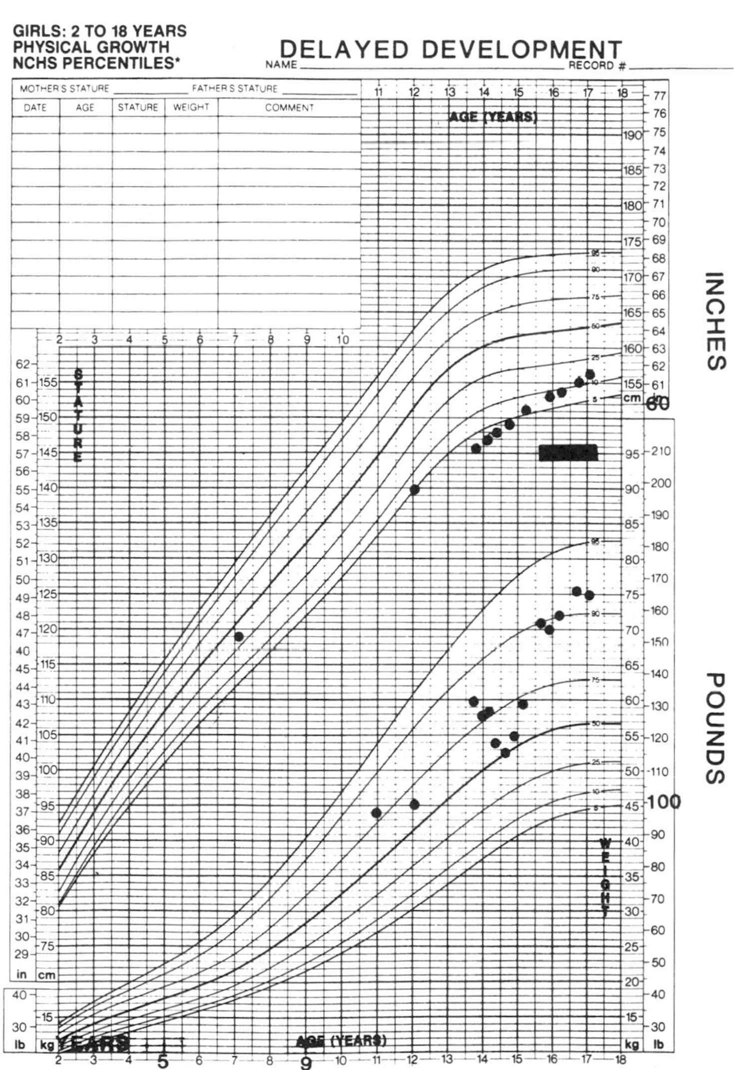

FIG. 10. Case 4: growth chart of patient with delayed development, renal transplant, and 46,XY gonadal dysgenesis.

DELAYED MENARCHE WITH SOME PUBERTAL DEVELOPMENT

The adolescent evaluated for a delay in the onset of menarche needs assessment not only for many of the disorders covered in the previous sections but also for the possibility of a genital anomaly, such as uterine agenesis (see Chapter 8). The lack of menses by age 15 to 16 years requires thoughtful consideration of the differential diagnosis (Figs. 11 and 12). The timing and tempo of the patient's previous pubertal growth and development are important. Bone age is more closely related to the onset of menses than is chronologic age. Although most girls have the onset of menses within 2 to 2 1/2 years of the beginning of breast development, the range is considerable, and menarche may not occur in

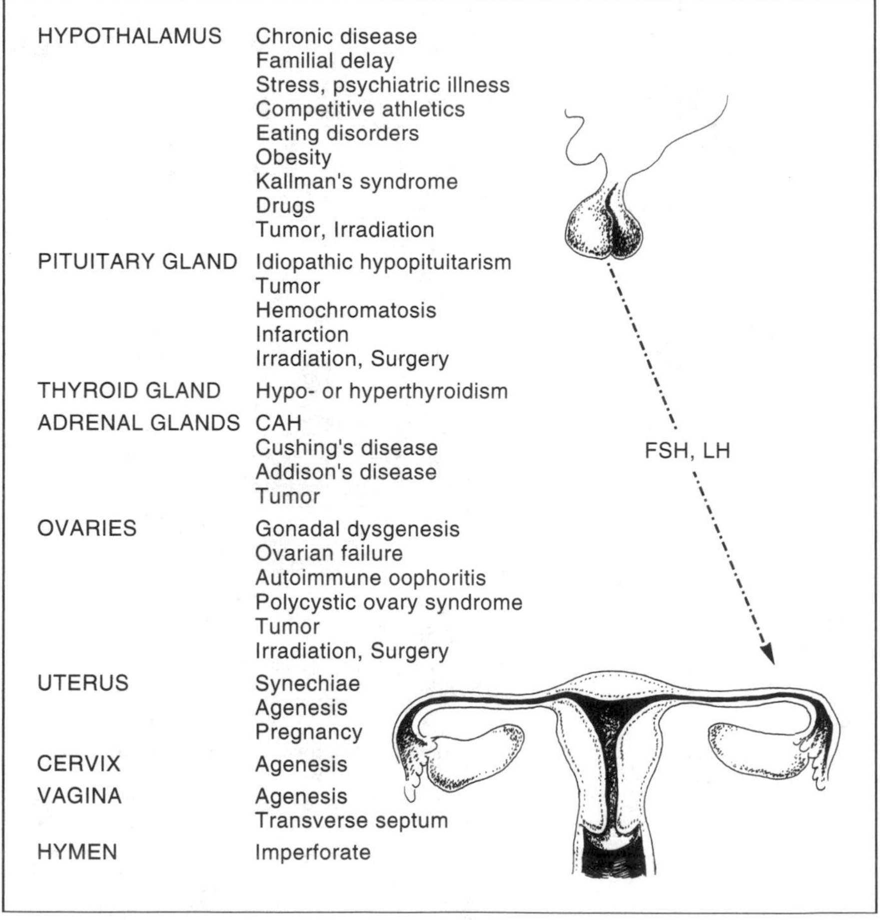

HYPOTHALAMUS
Chronic disease
Familial delay
Stress, psychiatric illness
Competitive athletics
Eating disorders
Obesity
Kallman's syndrome
Drugs
Tumor, Irradiation
PITUITARY GLAND
Idiopathic hypopituitarism
Tumor
Hemochromatosis
Infarction
Irradiation, Surgery
THYROID GLAND
Hypo- or hyperthyroidism
ADRENAL GLANDS
CAH
Cushing's disease
Addison's disease
Tumor
OVARIES
Gonadal dysgenesis
Ovarian failure
Autoimmune oophoritis
Polycystic ovary syndrome
Tumor
Irradiation, Surgery
UTERUS
Synechiae
Agenesis
Pregnancy
CERVIX
Agenesis
VAGINA
Agenesis
Transverse septum
HYMEN
Imperforate
FSH, LH

FIG. 11. Etiology of primary amenorrhea. CAH, congenital adrenocortical hyperplasia; FSH, follicle-stimulating hormone; LH, luteinizing hormone.

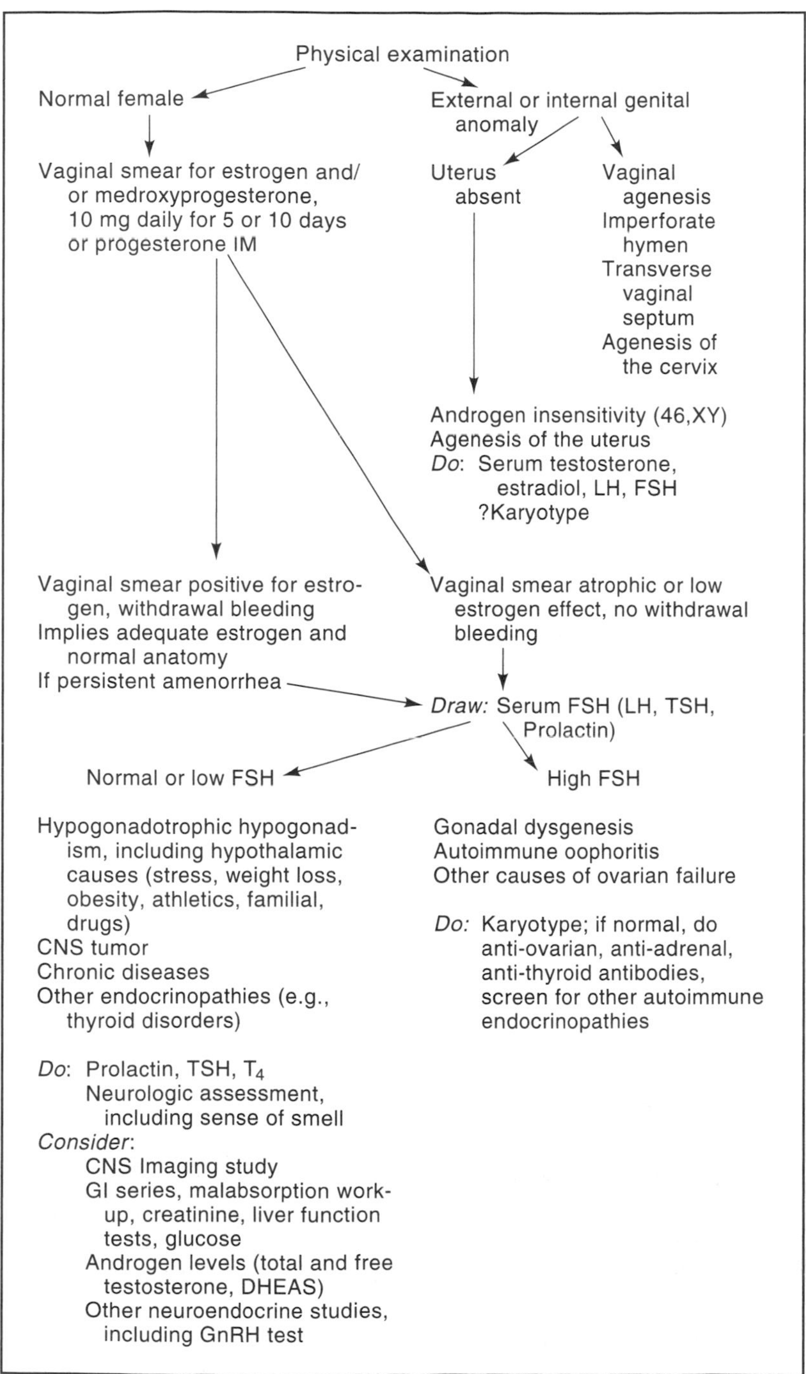

FIG. 12. Evaluation of delayed menarche in girls with some pubertal development.

an individual girl for 4 years. An interruption in the pattern of normal puberty should alert the physician to the possibility of a hypothalamic–pituitary–ovarian disorder, and thus, evidence of estrogenization is essential in determining the extent of evaluation. A girl with delayed menarche who has a late onset of normal puberty and a family history of delayed development causes less worry than a girl who began her development at the age of 11 and still has no menses at the age of 16.

A careful physical examination gives an excellent indication of endogenous hormone levels. Normal breast development and an estrogenized vagina imply that the patient is making estrogen. The genital examination is crucial in the patient with delayed menarche (see Chapters 1 and 8). Although an imperforate hymen should have been detected in the newborn nursery or during early childhood, it is sometimes not diagnosed until the patient is an adolescent. A bulging bluish-tinged hymen may be noted in the adolescent with an imperforate hymen and blood-filled vagina (hematocolpos). The patient with a transverse vaginal septum or vaginal and uterine agenesis has normal-appearing external genitalia, and her condition is therefore usually not detected until a pelvic examination is done for primary amenorrhea or pelvic pain.

If the hymenal opening appears to be adequate for a digital examination, then a gentle one-finger examination of the vagina will establish vaginal patency and allow palpation of the cervix and uterus by bimanual vaginal-abdominal examination. Visualization of the cervix and assessment of estrogenization of the cervical mucus and vagina are usually possible with a small Huffman speculum. If the clinician is unsure whether the opening is large enough for comfortable examination, a saline-moistened cotton-tipped applicator or urethral catheter can be used to make sure the vagina is patent and of normal length. Usually, in a patient with vaginal agenesis, a cotton-tipped applicator can be inserted only 1 to 2 cm. The uterus and adnexa can be palpated by rectoabdominal palpation with the patient in the lithotomy position. Ultrasonography can be used for confirmation of the findings. An MRI is important if anatomic detail is needed to define an obstructed genital tract or other congenital anomaly (see Chapter 8). During the physical examination and history, it is important to look for signs of androgen excess, including evidence of progressive hirsutism, clitoromegaly, and severe acne (see Chapter 7). Very rarely, pregnancy will occur without menarche.

If the genital examination is normal, assessment of estrogen effect by vaginal smear and progesterone withdrawal allows the clinician to think about diagnoses associated with eugonadism (normal estrogen levels), such as polycystic ovary syndrome, and those associated with estrogen deficiency, such as ovarian failure and hypothalamic disorders. After pregnancy has been excluded, a progestin challenge can be given to verify that the uterus is present and that the endometrium has been sufficiently stimulated with estrogen to cause withdrawal flow. Although a withdrawal flow in response to progesterone is generally reassuring, patients with prolactinomas and those in the early years of ovarian failure may have a normal response. A single serum level of estradiol is less helpful in assessing estrogenization than a progesterone withdrawal test or a vaginal smear for maturation index. However, it can be helpful in confirming the clinical impression of the degree of estrogenization. In general, unless the clinician can find factors such as undernutrition or profound stress to account for the lack of cycles, simple screening tests, including CBC, urinalysis, and determination of sedimentation rate and levels of FSH, LH, TSH, and prolactin, should be ordered. A radiograph of the hand and wrist to determine bone age is useful in girls who have not completed skeletal maturation.

Low to normal levels of gonadotropins imply that the evaluation should focus on the hypothalamic–pituitary axis; elevated gonadotropins imply ovarian failure. Further tests are similar to those indicated in the previous sections and in Figs. 7 and 12.

In the apparently estrogenized patient with normal gonadotropin levels and failure to have withdrawal bleeding from progesterone, the presence of a normal endometrium can be established by giving estrogen and progestin (e.g., conjugated estrogens 0.625 to 1.25 mg on days 1 to 25 and medroxyprogesterone 10 mg on days 21 to 25) for two to three cycles. However, a diagnosis of uterine synechiae (Asherman's syndrome) is sufficiently rare in the absence of a history of infections or abortion that this part of the evaluation can be delayed until other diagnoses are considered.

Menstrual cycles can be induced by the administration of medroxyprogesterone, 10 mg orally for 14 days (every 2 to 3 months). Although a withdrawal flow from progesterone is generally reassuring about the continuing presence of normal circulating levels of estrogen and a normal hypothalamic–pituitary axis, persistence of amenorrhea, any signs of headache, visual symptoms, galactorrhea, or an interruption in the tempo of the pubertal process necessitate further tests (Fig. 12).

A dilemma for the clinician may be whether to obtain radiographic studies of the CNS in the patient with normal serum gonadotropin and prolactin values. A lateral skull radiograph with a cone-down view of the sella can exclude calcification and an enlarged sella but will miss small lesions detectable by cranial MRI scan. There are no absolute guidelines; however, most pituitary tumors associated with primary or secondary amenorrhea in this age group secrete prolactin, interrupt normal prolactin inhibition sufficiently to cause a mild to moderate elevation of prolactin, or are associated with other signs or symptoms. Given the likelihood that most adolescents with hypothalamic amenorrhea have that condition because of stress, athletics, or weight changes, and nonfunctioning tumors that cause amenorrhea are extremely rare, an MRI scan is generally reserved for the evaluation of the patient with interrupted puberty, elevated prolactin level, abnormal sella seen on a radiograph of the skull (or cone-down view of the sella), and/or neurologic signs or symptoms. An MRI may also be indicated in the evaluation of the older adolescent or young adult woman who has persistent amenorrhea with no obvious etiology for the amenorrhea.

If possible, therapy should be directed at the underlying cause of hypogonadotropism. For example, weight loss due to depression should be treated with psychiatric therapies and dietary counseling. Athletic training schedules may need to be modified to allow the patient to go through the normal pubertal process. Achieving better glucose control in the young diabetic or decreased disease activity in Crohn's disease will often bring about menarche.

Estrogen replacement therapy is outlined in the section on Treatment Guidelines. If skeletal age is mature and no further growth can be anticipated, the dose of estrogen can be increased rapidly. Therapy should be discontinued intermittently (e.g., once a year for 2 to 3 months) to determine whether the hypothalamic–pituitary axis has begun to function more normally.

External or Internal Genital Anomalies

Imperforate Hymen and Transverse Vaginal Septum

The diagnosis of imperforate hymen should be made early in a child's life, but occasionally a patient reaches adolescence before the diagnosis is made. The patient may have a history of cyclic abdominal pain, often for several years, or may be asymptomatic. A bluish, bulging hymen and distention of the vagina with blood are found on genital inspection and rectoabdominal palpation. The repair of imperforate hymen can be accomplished in infancy, childhood, or adolescence when the diagnosis is made (see Chapter 8 for discussion of genital anomalies).

The rare complete transverse vaginal septum may be low or high in the vagina, but the external genitalia appear normal. The vagina appears short, and a mass is palpable above the examining finger and on rectoabdominal palpation. Obstruction by a high transverse septum results in hematometra and endometriosis. It should be noted that a transverse vaginal septum usually has a central small perforation but still may present with hematocolpos in the adolescent, mucocolpos in the child, or pyohematocolpos because of ascending infection.

Agenesis of the Vagina/Cervix/Uterus

Vaginal agenesis is usually accompanied by uterine agenesis, although infrequently a patient has a normal but obstructed uterus or rudimentary uterus with functional endometrium (244). Patients with Mayer-Rokitansky-Küster-Hauser syndrome have a 46,XX karyotype and normal ovaries and hormonal patterns, but the uterus and fallopian tubes are absent or rudimentary, and the upper two-thirds of the vagina is absent. The presence of normal breast and pubic hair development and normal female serum testosterone and pubertal estradiol levels makes this syndrome the likely diagnosis. Ultrasonography, which should be done to assess renal status, can confirm normal ovaries and the lack of a uterus. Diagnostic and surgical approaches are discussed in Chapter 8. Although chromosome studies may not be necessary for all well-estrogenized girls, an elevated testosterone level, lack of breast development, absent pubic hair, or virilization mandate further studies for an intersex state.

Androgen Insensitivity

The patient with androgen insensitivity (testicular feminization), a form of male pseudohermaphroditism, has good breast development with pale areola, and very sparse or absent pubic and axillary hair. The vagina is short, and the uterus and cervix are absent. More than 50% of these patients have an inguinal hernia. The karyotype is 46,XY. The gonads, which may be intraabdominal or in the inguinal rings, are testes; thus, the serum testosterone level is in the same range as in the pubertal male. Because of insensitivity to androgens and enhanced estrogen production, the patient develops a female habitus and external genitalia. The lack of pubic and axillary hair is the result of end-organ failure to respond to adrenal and testicular androgens (247–249) (see Chapters 2 and 8). Support groups are available.[§]

Case 5

E. B. presented with primary amenorrhea at the age of 16 years. Breast and pubic hair development had started when she was 11 or 12 years old. She had noted a slight whitish vaginal discharge for several years. Physical examination showed her to be healthy, with a height of 64″ and a weight of 125 lbs. Breast development was stage 5, and pubic hair development was stage 4. Pelvic examination revealed a well-estrogenized vagina and a normal cervix and uterus. Urine hCG level was negative. A vaginal smear showed 20% superficial and 80% intermediate cells (maturation index = [80 × 0.5] + [20 × 1.0] = 60). Following 10 days of medroxyprogesterone, she had a 4-day menstrual period. She began spontaneous menses 2 months later and has continued to have normal menstrual cycles.

Case 6

P. M. presented with primary amenorrhea at the age of 18 years. Breast development had occurred when she was 13 years old, but pubic and axillary hair had not appeared. She had recently gained 70 pounds, seemingly because of anxiety over her lack of periods. Physical examination showed her to be attractive but overweight, with a height of 64″ and a weight of 187 lbs. Her blood pres-

---

§Androgen Insensitivity Syndrome (AIS) Support Group, U.S. Representative, Ms. Sherri Groveman, 4297 Mt. Herbert Avenue, San Diego, CA 92117 (phone 619-569-5254).

sure was 140/80 mm Hg, and her pulse rate was 80 beats/min. Her breasts were stage 5 and pendulous. No axillary or pubic hair was present. Pelvic examination revealed a short vagina and no cervix or uterus. Laboratory tests showed a karyotype of 46,XY. The serum testosterone level was 281 ng/dl (normal female level, <55 ng/dl). A diagnosis of androgen insensitivity was made. After surgery to remove the intraabdominal testes, P. M. was given conjugated estrogens. She required extensive counseling about the issue of her femininity, sexual function, the creation of a longer vagina, and her inability to bear children. She subsequently lost 35 pounds by dieting.

Case 7

R. L. sought medical attention at the age of 18 years because of "no periods." Her breast and pubic hair development had started at the age of 12 years. She had always been the shortest member of her class, and she had worn bilateral hearing aids since the age of 11. Physical examination (Fig. 13) showed her to be short and overweight, with a height of 51″ and a weight of 105 lbs. She had hypertelorism, ptosis, a low hairline, an increased carrying angle, and short fourth metacarpals. Breast development was stage 5; pubic hair was stage 4. Pelvic examination revealed a poorly estrogenized vagina with a small

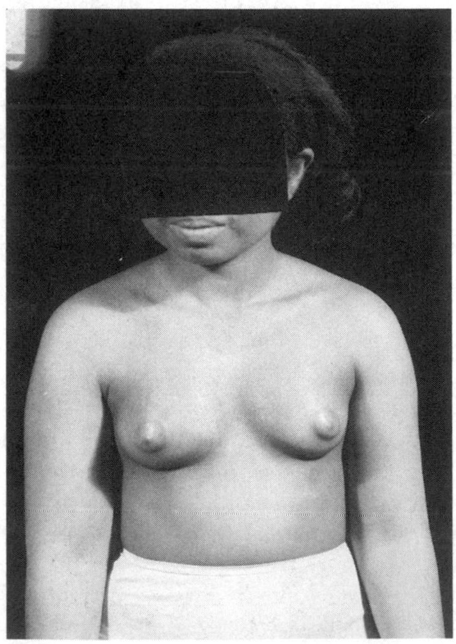

FIG. 13. Case 7: gonadal dysgenesis, karyotype 46,X,i(Xq).

cervix and uterus. Vaginal smear showed no evidence of estrogenization. Laboratory tests revealed a serum FSH level of 258 mIU/ml and an LH level of 173 mIU/ml, indicative of ovarian failure. Her karyotype was 46,X,i(Xq). The patient was given cyclic doses of conjugated estrogens and medroxyprogesterone and had a normal withdrawal flow each month. Subsequently, her treatment was changed to cyclic low-dose oral contraceptives.

Case 8

N. K. was referred at the age of 17 for primary amenorrhea. She was an "A" student in her senior year of high school and was involved in athletics. Her breast and pubic hair development had started at the age of 10 but subsequently stopped when she was 12. Her menses had never begun. She had had significant headaches for 4 years, which seemed to increase during the school year. Physical examination showed her to be pleasant and bright, with a height of 64″ and a weight of 111 lbs. Her blood pressure and pulse were normal. The breasts were Tanner stage 3 with small areolae, 1.7 cm on the right and 2.0 cm on the left, and glandular tissue 4 × 4 cm on the right and 5 × 6 cm on the left. No galactorrhea was present. Pubic hair was stage 3 to 4; the vagina was poorly estrogenized. The vagina was normal in length, and rectoabdominal examination revealed a cervix and a uterus. The results of neurologic examination, including fundoscopic examination, visual fields by confrontation, and sense of smell, were normal. The growth chart (Fig. 14) showed no increase in height since the age of 12 6/12 years. The history and examination suggested normal initiation of puberty followed by growth arrest and regression of estrogenization. Laboratory tests showed a bone age of 14 years, normal results of CBC and thyroid function tests, low gonadotropin levels (LH 5.2 mIU/ml and FSH <2.0 mIU/ml), undetectable estradiol, and markedly elevated prolactin of 13,000 ng/ml (normal <25 ng/ml). A radiograph of the skull showed an enlarged sella turcica, and cranial CT demonstrated a large pituitary and suprasellar mass (Fig. 15A). The result of formal visual field testing was normal. Neuroendocrine studies revealed prepubertal LH and FSH responses to GnRH, growth hormone deficiency, flat prolactin response to TRH, and normal cortisol levels.

After neurosurgical consultation, N. K. was given bromocriptine therapy. The dosage was gradually increased on a weekly basis; the prolactin levels fell progressively, and the tumor showed significant reduction in size (Fig. 15B and C). Her headaches disappeared. The estradiol levels ranged between 53 and 283 pg/ml, and breast development and vaginal estrogenization progressed. N. K. had normal withdrawal flow when medroxyprogesterone was given 1 year after she had started taking bromocriptine. Her first spontaneous menses occurred 2 months later. She will require long-term surveillance and therapy.

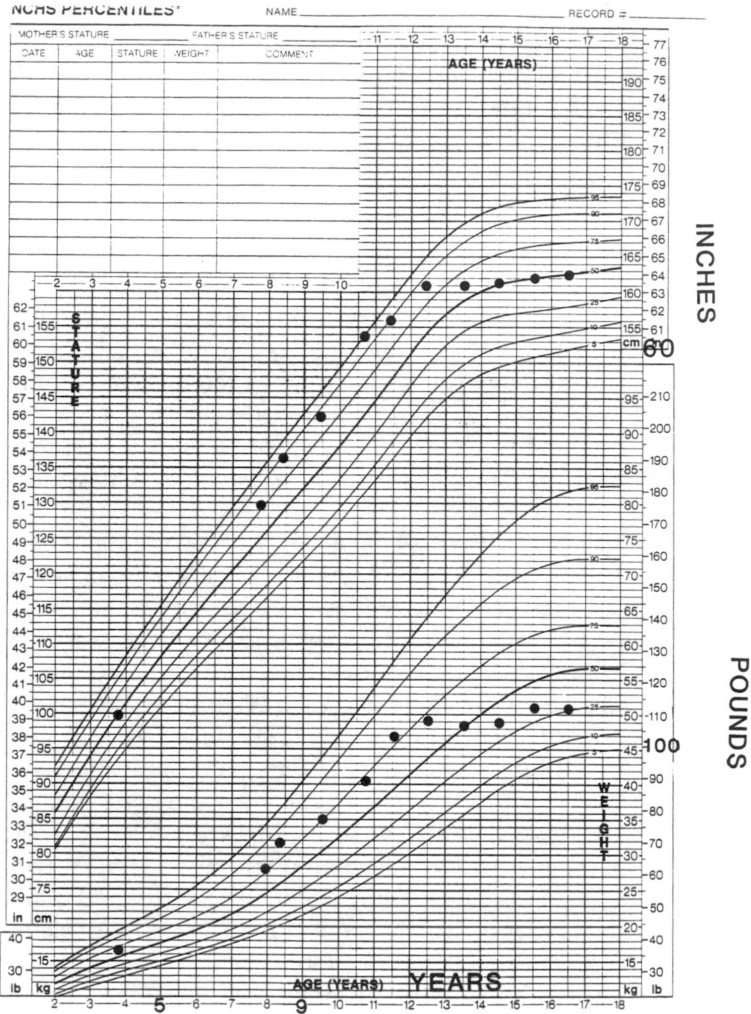

FIG. 14. Case 9: growth chart of patient with primary amenorrhea and a prolactinoma.

Case 9

C. E., a 16 4/12 year old girl, was referred for primary amenorrhea and tall stature. Her breast and pubic hair development had begun when she was between the ages of 13 and 14 years. She was active in sports (tennis) and thin. Her father was 6′4″ and her mother 5′11″ (midparental height, 5′11″). She had increasingly become concerned about being too tall and did not wish to be taller than her mother. On physical examination, she was 5′10 1/2″ (>95%) with a weight of 99 pounds (10%) (Fig. 16). Her breast development was Tanner stage

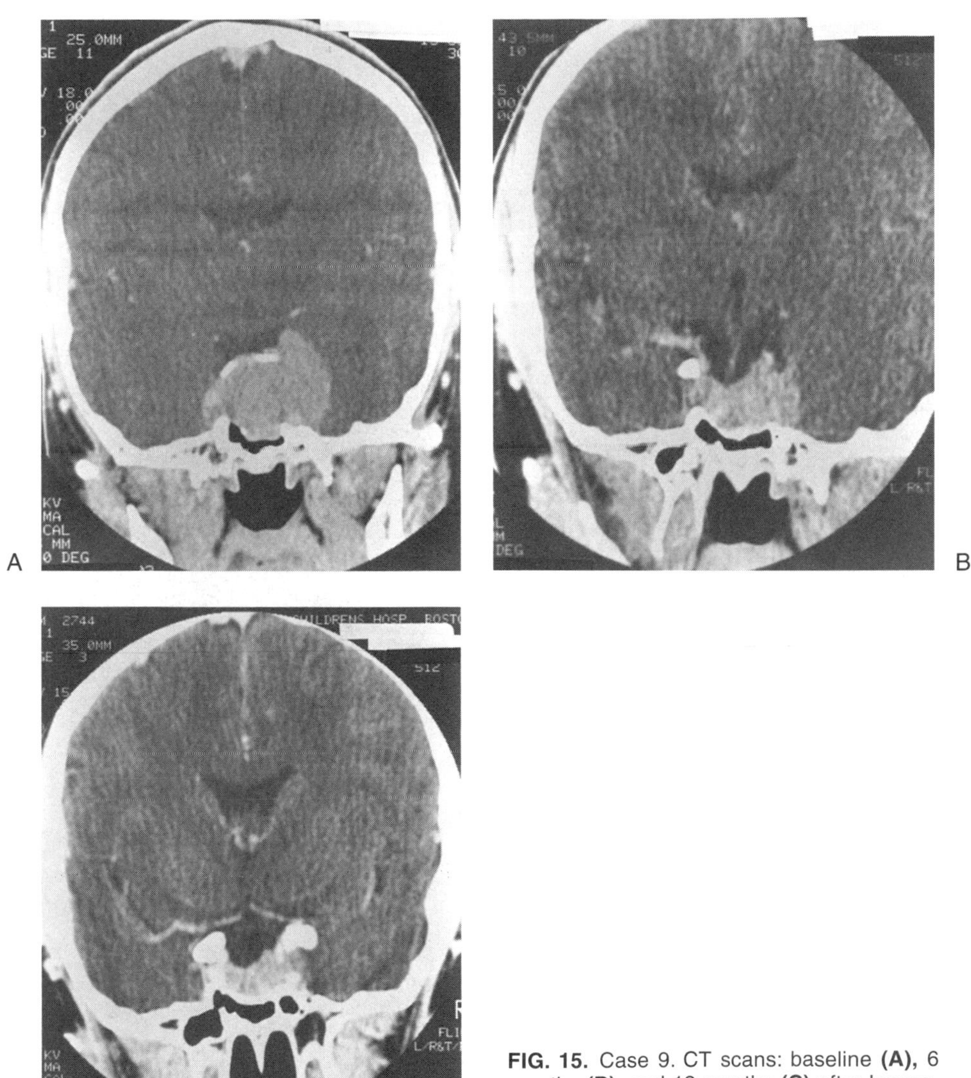

FIG. 15. Case 9. CT scans: baseline **(A),** 6 months **(B),** and 12 months **(C)** after bromocriptine therapy was begun.

3 to 4, and her pubic hair development was Tanner stage 4. Her external genitalia were normal, and a pelvic examination revealed an estrogenized vagina with a normal cervix and uterus. Her laboratory tests showed a FSH level of 5.4 mIU/ml, a LH level of 2.6 mIU/ml, a prolactin level of 3.7 ng/ml, and a normal TSH level. Her bone age was between 12 and 12 1/2, giving a predicted height of 6′2″ to 6′3.″ The benefits and risks of estrogen treatment, including thrombosis and hypertension, were discussed with C. E. and her family, and she

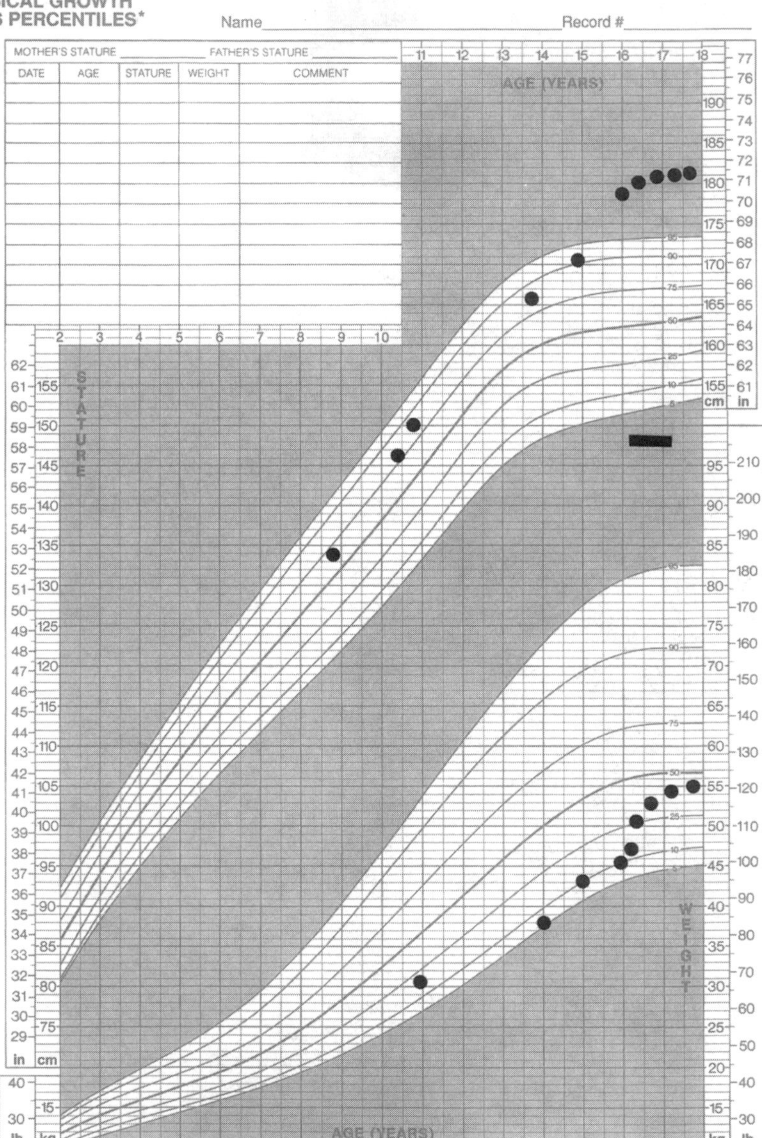

FIG. 16. Case 10: growth chart. Bar denotes estrogen-progestin therapy.

elected to take ethinyl estradiol 150 μg/day (increased slowly over a month from 20 μg/day) plus cyclic medroxyprogesterone each month for 1 year to accelerate skeletal maturation. She had normal menses, did not experience nausea or other problems, and was pleased with her final height and weight gain. She has continued to have normal menses while off medication.

It should be noted that the optimal dose of estrogen has not been defined for the treatment of tall stature, but doses of 100 to 250 μg of ethinyl estradiol have been used (250–252) to reduce height by 4 to 6 cm from that predicted. Oral contraceptives (20 to 35 μg/day) have not been shown to alter height unless the bone age is 9 to 10 years. Given the potential risks and controversial benefits, we believe high doses of estrogen should be offered only to patients who have a predicted height of over 6 feet, feel strongly about instituting therapy, understand the risks, and are under the care of an experienced physician.

DELAYED MENARCHE WITH VIRILIZATION/HIRSUTISM

Progressive hirsutism and/or virilization in association with delayed menarche is uncommon. Patients with amenorrhea and hirsutism usually have polycystic ovary syndrome or late-onset congenital adrenocortical hyperplasia (CAH). An abrupt onset of the hirsutism may signal a tumor. Patients with true virilization are rarer and may have polycystic ovary syndrome (PCO), late-onset CAH, an ovarian or adrenal tumor, mixed gonadal dysgenesis, an incomplete form of androgen insensitivity, 5α-reductase deficiency, gonadal dysgenesis (with virilization), or true hermaphroditism (see Chapters 2, 7, and 8). The diagnosis, laboratory evaluation, and treatment of PCO syndrome, adrenal and ovarian tumors, and late-onset CAH are discussed in Chapter 7. A physical examination is critical to establish the presence of breast development and a normal female genital tract.

Classic CAH usually presents as the virilization of the female newborn with or without a salt-losing tendency (see Chapter 2). Some patients, however, may have a mild block of adrenal steroid synthesis (21-hydroxylase, 3β-hydroxysteroid dehydrogenase, or 11β-hydroxylase deficiency) and may manifest clitoromegaly or hirsutism at puberty. Patients may present to the clinician with premature pubarche, delayed menarche, oligomenorrhea, or hirsutism. Those with 11β-hydroxylase deficiency may have associated hypertension.

Many patients who have classical CAH, even though they have been observed and treated since infancy, have menstrual irregularities, including delayed menarche. Many older adolescents with CAH and irregular menses do not take medication regularly; many younger adolescents have not had their dosage of medication changed to keep up with their accelerated growth. During the adolescent years, dosages need to be regulated by monitoring height and weight and measuring levels of serum 17-hydroxyprogesterone and androgens (testosterone, Δ^4-androstenedione and DHEAS), and plasma renin activity. In adolescents who have achieved full growth, continuous adrenal suppression and improved menstrual regularity can often be achieved by twice-a-day prednisone or once-a-day dexamethasone. Fertility is possible for the majority of patients with non-salt-losing CAH, although some have persistent anovulatory cycles and develop enlarged polycystic-like ovaries. In a study two decades ago, Money and Schwartz (253) noted a delay in the dating age and first romance, difficulty in establishing friendships, and inhibition of erotic arousal and expression in some patients with early-onset CAH.

A patient may have virilization from either an ovarian or an adrenal tumor, both before and after the onset of puberty or menarche. A serum testosterone value >150 to 200 ng/dl, androstenedione >500 ng/dl, *or* DHEAS >700 μg/dl should make the clinician suspicious of a tumor (see Chapter 7).

Chromosomal abnormalities may cause delayed menarche and virilization. At puberty, patients with mixed gonadal dysgenesis (MGD) show virilization (without evidence of estrogen effect) because the functioning intraabdominal testis produces testosterone. The reported chromosome patterns of patients with MGD have included 46,XY; 45,X/46,XY; 45,X/46,XX/46,XY; and 45,X (some likely have a missed second line). Essential is mosaicism with a 45,X stem and a stem with a Y (fragment) (254) to make the diagnosis of MGD (see Chapter 2). With a uterus present, patients should be given cyclic estrogen-progestin therapy to produce menses and referred to centers with assisted reproductive technologies and oocyte transfer, if desired. Because a dysgenetic intraabdominal testis has a high incidence of malignant transformation, it should be removed.

Patients with incomplete androgen insensitivity have a 46,XY karyotype, agenesis of the uterus, hirsutism, clitoral enlargement, and absence of breast development (248).

Rarely, patients with gonadal dysgenesis may show virilization at puberty. The streak gonads may contain Leydig-like cells that presumably secrete androgens. The possibility of a tumor should be excluded, as well as the presence of Y fragments.

A true hermaphrodite has ovarian and testicular tissue (see Chapter 2). Some appear to be almost normal females who develop mild to moderate virilization at puberty, depending on the balance of ovarian and testicular function. Gonadotropin concentrations may be normal or high (255).

SECONDARY AMENORRHEA

Patient Evaluation

Many of the causes of delayed menarche are also responsible for secondary amenorrhea; however, the two most common causes of missed periods in the adolescent are pregnancy and stress. A period that is 2 to 3 weeks overdue should be investigated to rule out pregnancy (see Chapter 1 for a review of pregnancy tests). The clinician should never assume that the adolescent is not pregnant simply because she denies a history of sexual intercourse. Many older teenagers are still fearful of admitting to having had intercourse; a girl aged 11 or 12 may not understand her own anatomy well enough to answer the questions accurately.

TABLE 7. *Percent of adolescent girls who reported missing three consecutive menses during the past year (n = 2156)*

Chronologic age	%
13	10.8
14	7.8
15	9.4
16	7.9
17	8.1
18	9.8
Gynecologic age[a]	**%**
0	12.5
1	13.5
2	9.7
3	9.6
4	6.1
5	8.5
6	5.3
7	5.4

[a]Gynecologic age is chronologic age minus the age of menarche.
(From Johnson J, Whitaker AH. Adolescent smoking, weight changes, and binge purge behaviors: associations with secondary amenorrhea. *Am J Public Health* 1992;82:47–54; with permission.)

Stress, changes in environment, weight changes, and eating disorders are responsible for most cases of missed periods in adolescents who are not pregnant. In a survey of eight high schools (94% of the students white, and ages evenly distributed from 14 to 17 years [2.5% ≤13, 5.5% ≥18]), Johnson and Whitaker (256) found that abnormal eating patterns were the most important risk factor for missing three consecutive menses in the previous year. The percentage of teens missing three cycles is shown is Table 7 by chronologic and gynecologic age (chronologic age minus age of menarche), and the odds ratios for risk factors are shown in Table 8.

TABLE 8. *Risk factors for secondary amenorrhea (missing three consecutive menses in past year)*

Risk factors for secondary amenorrhea	Odds ratio
Frequent binging and purging	4.17
Weight loss ≥4.5 kg	1.45
Weight gain ≥4.5 kg	1.71
Both weight loss and gain	2.59
Smoking ≥1 packs/day	1.96
First year post menarche	1.74

(From Johnson J, Whitaker AH. Adolescent smoking, weight changes, and binge purge behaviors: associations with secondary amenorrhea. *Am J Public Health* 1992;82:47–54; with permission.)

The magnitude of the weight loss in teens is sometimes evident only after a careful history and weight and height charts have been obtained. A young woman with depression may rapidly gain weight and become amenorrheic, and may then inaccurately view the weight gain as secondary to the loss of periods and retention of blood. Young women also often have irregular menses with illnesses, emotional upset, and changes in environment such as going away to summer camp, boarding school, or college. The involvement of increasing numbers of young adolescents in competitive athletics has been accompanied by increasing reports of menstrual irregularities (see section on the Female Athlete Triad). Patients with chronic diseases frequently benefit from an explanation of the cause of their menstrual irregularity. Failure to use contraceptives may result in an unwanted pregnancy if they do not understand that they are potentially fertile.

Given that teenagers may have irregular periods or amenorrhea for 3 to 6 months in the first 1 to 2 years after menarche, the clinician needs to decide which patients to evaluate. Generally, the abrupt cessation of menses for 4 months after regular cycles have begun, or persistent oligomenorrhea 2 years after menarche, should be taken as an indication for an evaluation. Clearly, many patients will not visit the clinician until 2, 3, or 8 months after amenorrhea occurs. Since the evaluation is simple (a physical examination, pregnancy test, progesterone challenge test, and endocrine laboratory studies), there is no need to wait an arbitrary length of time. For patients whose cycles were normal prior to the use of hormonal contraception, an evaluation (in addition to a physical examination and a pregnancy test) is generally recommended after 6 months in a teen who has discontinued oral contraceptives and 12 months in a teen who has discontinued DepoProvera.

The history in the patient with secondary amenorrhea should focus on issues of stress, recent changes in the environment, weight change, eating disorders, and involvement in competitive athletics. The review of systems should include questions about headaches, visual changes, galactorrhea, hirsutism, acne, chronic disease, and any medications or illicit drug use. Amenorrhea following childbirth may be due to pregnancy, or much more rarely Sheehan postpartum pituitary necrosis or Asherman's syndrome. Recent sexual activity and contraceptive use should also be assessed. The general physical examination should include a fundoscopic examination and a screen of visual fields by confrontation. The thyroid gland should be palpated, and the blood pressure and pulse rate noted. The areolae should be gently compressed to determine whether galactorrhea, usually not noted by the patient, is present. The physician should also search for evidence of androgen excess, including progressive hirsutism, clitoromegaly, or severe acne, and note the presence of acanthosis nigricans or ovarian enlargement (although the latter may prove difficult in the obese or poorly relaxed adolescent patient). The evaluation of the patient with androgen excess is considered in Chapter 7.

A sensitive pregnancy test and physical examination are the first steps in the evaluation. Assessment of the estrogen status allows the physician to divide

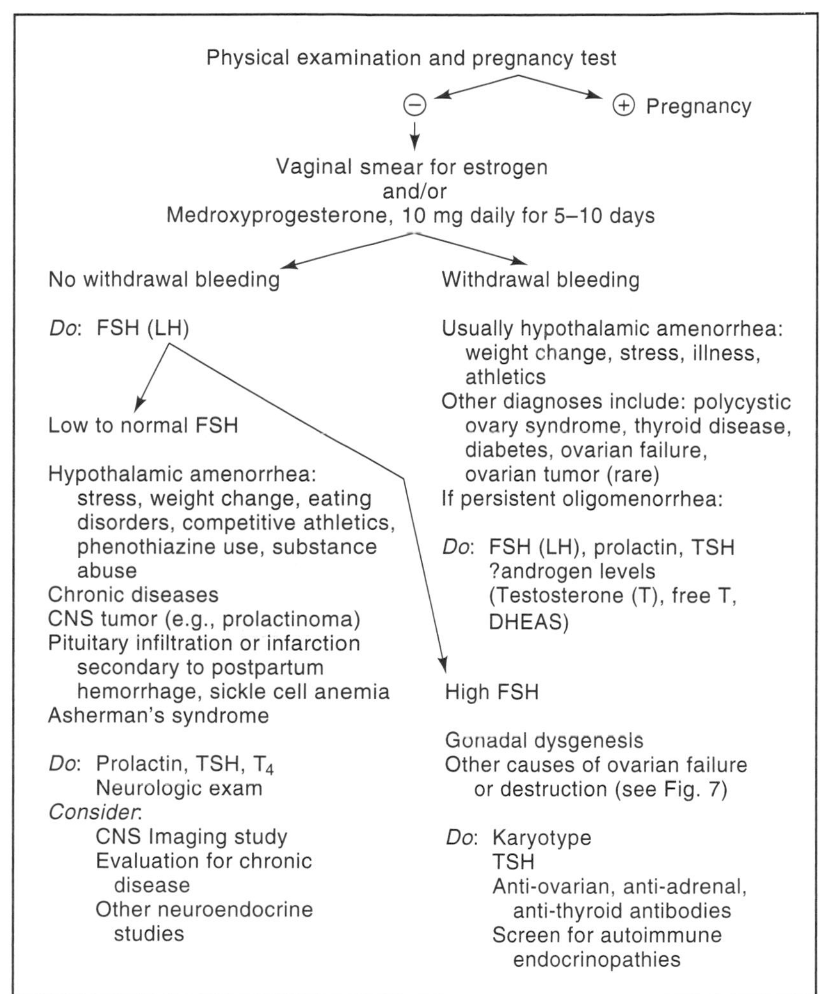

FIG. 17. Evaluation of secondary amenorrhea.

patients into two large categories (Fig. 17). If pregnancy has been excluded (negative pregnancy test after 2 weeks of abstinence), oral medroxyprogesterone (10 mg a day for 5 or 10 days) is usually selected for progestin challenge in sexually active patients. Some clinicians prefer to use progesterone-in-oil, 50 to 100 mg IM, or oral micronized progesterone. Generally, progesterone will not induce menses in a patient who has hypopituitarism due to a tumor; profound hypothalamic suppression from anorexia nervosa or massive weight gain; or ovarian failure because the endometrium is not primed with estrogen. These patients deserve an evaluation with laboratory tests to determine the cause of the estrogen deficiency.

Unless the patient has a history suggestive of Asherman's syndrome (uterine scarring and synechiae, usually secondary to a dilatation and curettage following postpartum or postabortal endometritis), most adolescents are not given a combined estrogen-progestin challenge as part of the initial evaluation until laboratory studies have been obtained. Vaginal examination and vaginal smear will show the patient with Asherman's syndrome to be estrogenized, but she will not have withdrawal bleeding from either progestin alone or combined estrogen-progestin therapy. Other rare causes of disruption of the endometrium include tuberculosis and uterine schistosomiasis. Before undertaking an extensive evaluation of the uterus of the adolescent who fails to withdraw from estrogen-progestin, the clinician should administer a higher dose of estrogen for several months and ensure compliance by counting the pills. In addition, it should be remembered that adolescents using low-dose birth control pills (which may have been provided confidentially by another clinic) may have scant or absent withdrawal flow.

Most patients who do have withdrawal bleeding from progesterone are normal; however, disorders such as polycystic ovary syndrome (PCO), ovarian tumors, Cushing's syndrome, thyroid disease, and diabetes should be excluded by physical examination, history, and the appropriate laboratory tests. Even in patients with a positive result of progesterone challenge test, prolonged amenorrhea (>6 months) or persistent oligomenorrhea without an explanation should be evaluated by measurement of serum TSH, FSH (and LH), and prolactin levels. In a study of adult women presenting with amenorrhea of 3 months' duration, 10% had an abnormal FSH level, 7.5% had a abnormal prolactin level, and 4.2% had a abnormal TSH level (257). Although some favor selective thyroid testing in adult women, we have noted that adolescents with hypothyroidism may have few clinical symptoms or signs to allow early diagnosis of thyroid disease, and therapy is inexpensive and effective.

If an LH level is obtained with the initial FSH level, an elevated LH and normal FSH may suggest the diagnosis of PCO and the need to measure androgen levels (free and total testosterone, DHEAS) even in the absence of obvious androgen excess. Patients with ovarian failure may continue to have sporadic menses in spite of elevated FSH. The management of teenage pregnancy and the diagnosis of ectopic pregnancy are discussed in Chapter 18.

In most patients who have abundant, watery cervical mucus, a positive vaginal smear for estrogen, or a normal response to progesterone, menses usually return spontaneously without treatment. Medroxyprogesterone, 10 mg orally for 14 days, is usually prescribed every 6 weeks to 3 months to prevent endometrial hyperplasia resulting from prolonged estrogen stimulation and to reassure the clinician that the patient is continuing to make estrogen. Birth control pills are appropriate to induce menstrual periods in girls who are sexually active and need contraception or in girls who are estrogen deficient.

Polycystic ovary syndrome is a common cause of secondary amenorrhea in both adolescents and older women (see Chapter 7). Adolescents who have oligomenorrhea, persistently elevated serum LH, low to normal FSH levels, and normal free testosterone levels probably represent one end of a spectrum of disturbed feedback. In some patients, the elevated LH with anovulation is a stress-induced phenomenon; in others, it appears to be secondary to PCO. Although serum androgen levels may be normal at the initial evaluation, later in adolescence some of these patients may have elevated testosterone levels.

High FSH and LH levels indicate ovarian failure. In rare cases, ovarian destruction has followed a severe gonococcal infection.

Case 10

A. N., aged 15, came to the clinic because of fatigue. Further questioning revealed that her last menstrual period had occurred 2 months previously. Her menarche was at the age of 12 years, and she had had regular cycles until the missed period. Although she initially denied the possibility of pregnancy, the urine pregnancy test result was positive, and her uterus was 8-week size.

Case 11

P. A., 14 1/2 years old, was referred for irregular menses. Her breasts and pubic hair had begun to develop when she was 10 to 11 years old, and menarche occurred at 13 2/12 years. She had had only five menstrual periods over the past 16 months, and her last menstrual period had been 1 month before the visit. She had been short for many years; her father was 5′10″ and her mother 5′3/4″ (midparental height 5′2 7/8″). Physical examination showed her to have short stature, with a height of 4′9″ (<5%) and weight of 108 lbs (30%) (Fig. 18). Her blood pressure was 106/70 mm Hg; her breast development was Tanner stage 5 and her pubic hair Tanner stage 4. The results of external genital examination and pelvic examination were normal. She had no stigmata of Turner's syndrome. Her bone age was 14 years; FSH level was 96.5 mIU/ml, and LH level was 34.8 mIU/ml; the TSH level was normal. Her karyotype was 45,X/46,X,i(Xq). She took growth hormone for 4 months at another hospital and then discontinued therapy. She then had several additional spontaneous menses, but had no withdrawal flow in response to medroxyprogesterone at age 15 1/2 years and was given oral contraceptives for estrogen replacement. At age 19, she discontinued the oral contraceptives on her own and continued for 4 months to have normal regular cycles. Her FSH level was 7.7 mIU/ml. She has been counseled about the need to use birth control if she desires to avoid the risk of unintended pregnancy.

Case 12

B. T., a 17-year-old boarding school student, had had amenorrhea for 3 years. Menarche had occurred when she was 12 years, followed by regular menses for

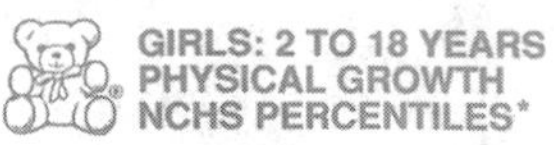

GIRLS: 2 TO 18 YEARS
PHYSICAL GROWTH
NCHS PERCENTILES*

Name________________ Record #________________

MOTHER'S STATURE ________ FATHER'S STATURE ________

DATE	AGE	STATURE	WEIGHT	COMMENT

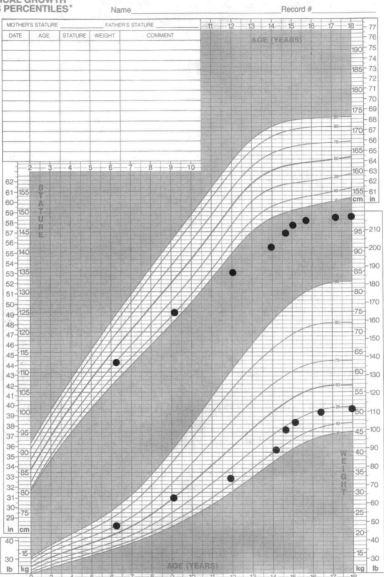

FIG. 18. Case 11: growth chart.

2 years until she became amenorrheic. The amenorrhea had been attributed to the stress of boarding school.

Physical examination showed her to be healthy, with a height of 63″ and a weight of 119 lbs. Vaginal examination showed poor estrogenization. Laboratory tests showed elevated gonadotropin levels: FSH, 63.9 and >100 mIU/ml; LH, 60.8 and 94.5 mIU/ml. Her karyotype was 46,XX, antiovarian antibodies were negative, and the results of thyroid tests were normal. With a diagnosis of premature ovarian failure, she needs to be observed for potential autoimmune endocrinopathies despite negative antibody studies. She initiated estrogen replacement therapy.

Case 13

K. M. was evaluated at the age of 12 6/12 years for amenorrhea. She had started her breast and pubic hair development at age 10 6/12 years and had her menarche at age 11 9/12 years. She subsequently had two monthly cycles and then amenorrhea for 9 months. She recalled having been short for some time, and had been treated with iron for anemia. She denied constipation, fatigue, intolerance to heat or cold, or school problems. Her mother was 60″ tall and her father 67 1/2″ tall; her 17-year-old brother was 69″ tall. Physical examination showed her height to be 55 1/2″ and her weight to be 84 lbs. Her blood pressure was 112/70 mm Hg, and her pulse was 66 beats/min. Her breast and pubic hair development were both Tanner stage 4. The vagina was well estrogenized, and rectal examination showed a normal-size uterus. Although the history of irregular menses was not particularly unusual in an early adolescent, the growth chart (Fig. 19) was a clue to the diagnosis. The patient had had little increase in height between the ages of 8 1/2 and 10 1/2 years but then had experienced the growth spurt of pubertal development. Her bone age was 11 years (delayed for a postmenarcheal adolescent), and indeed, thyroid function tests showed hypothyroidism with a T_4 of 1.8 μg/dl, thyroid-binding globulin index (TBGI) of 0.75, total T_3 of 54 ng/dl, and TSH of 990 μU/ml. Gonadotropin levels were normal (LH, 3.6 mIU/ml; FSH, 9.0 mIU/ml). She was given levothyroxine and experienced some behavioral problems at school as she converted from a placid child to a rebellious adolescent. Her menses resumed after 2 months of thyroid replacement, and she is currently on a dose of 0.125 mg levothyroxine daily. School performance and adolescent adjustment gradually improved over the following years.

Case 14

N. T., 16 years old, was referred for evaluation of amenorrhea that had lasted 2 years. She had normal breast and pubic hair development at the age of 11 and had menarche at the age of 12 11/12. Her menses were regular for about 6 months until she lost weight, going from about 125 lbs to 104 lbs on a “healthy

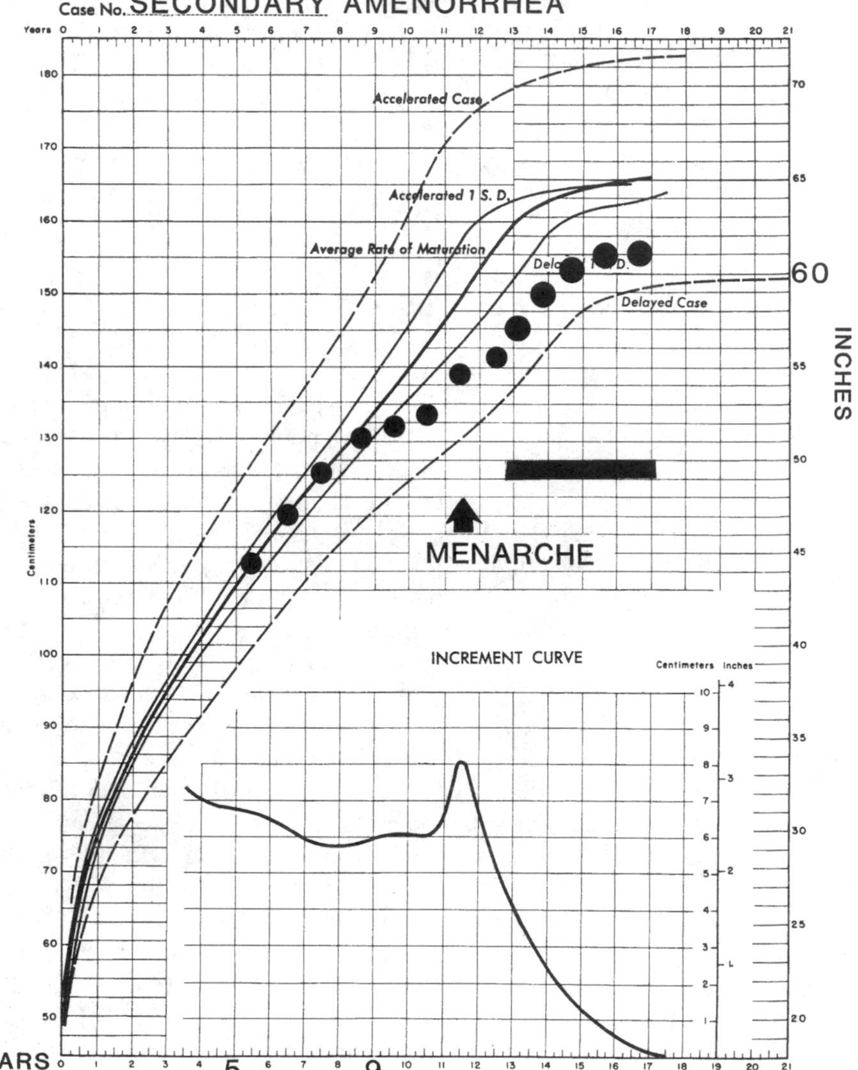

FIG. 19. Case 13: growth charts. **(A)** Height. **(B)** Weight. The bar and the larger dots represent therapy with thyroid replacement.

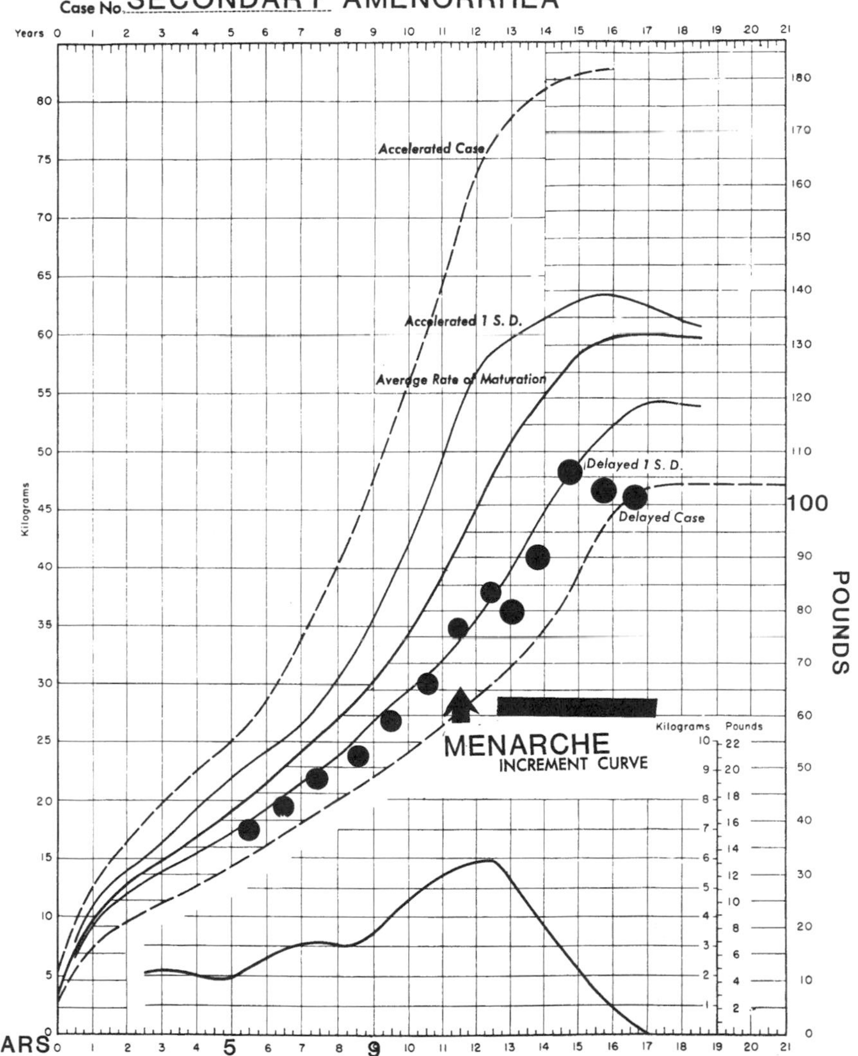

FIG. 19. (*Continued.*)

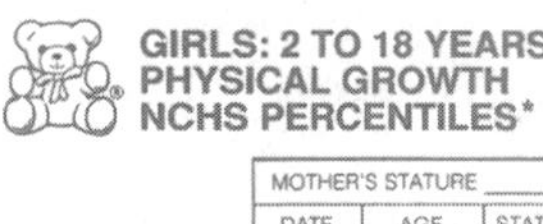

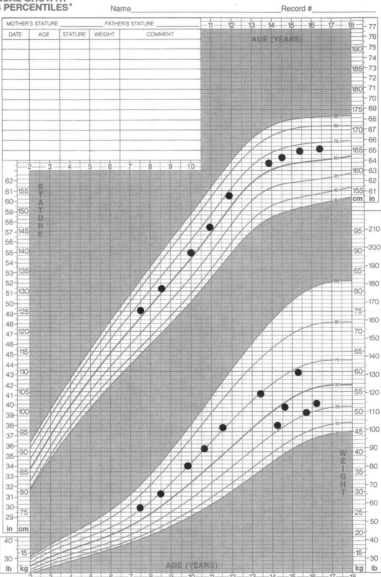

FIG. 20. Case 14: growth chart.

diet" by avoiding sweets, bread, and fats (Fig. 20). She subsequently gained weight to 135 pounds. She lost weight again, but was gaining again at the time of the visit. She was conscious of trying to maintain a "normal" weight, and she ate no red meat. She was active in after-school sports.

Physical examination showed a healthy appearance, a height of 5′5″, and a weight of 114 lbs. The results of the general physical examination and pelvic examination were normal except for a slightly diminished estrogen effect apparent on the vaginal mucosa. Her estimated percentage of body fat (using calipers) was 21%. The result of a urine pregnancy test was negative. Laboratory tests revealed an FSH level of 6.4 mIU/ml and normal prolactin and TSH levels. A vaginal smear showed 10% parabasal cells, 90% intermediate cells (maturation index [MI] = 45). She had only a very scant withdrawal flow in response to medroxyprogesterone taken orally for 10 days. The options were discussed with her, and she decided to take estrogen replacement for one year, to increase her calcium intake, and to stabilize her weight. She subsequently had normal menses.

Case 15

Identical twins M. R. and S. R. presented at the age of 20 years with amenorrhea of 2 years' duration. Both had experienced menarche between the ages of 13 and 14 years and had had regular monthly menses until they were 18, when they both increased their level of training in preparation for college athletics. M. R. lost 20 lbs and S. R. lost 15 lbs. Both had subsequently maintained stable weights between 112 and 120 lbs for the past 2 years, and were 66″ tall. Both continued to be active in competitive sports throughout the year. Physical examination of both patients revealed Tanner stage 5 breast and pubic hair development with markedly diminished estrogenization on vaginal examination. Otherwise, the results of pelvic examination and general assessments were normal. Laboratory values for the two girls were remarkably similar: the LH level was 4.6 mIU/ml for S. R. and 4.7 mIU/ml for M. R.; the FSH level was 10.6 mIU/ml for S. R. and 11.3 mIU/ml for M. R.; the prolactin level was 3.1 ng/ml for S. R. and 3.7 ng/ml for M. R.; the estradiol level was 27 pg/ml for S. R. and 28 pg/ml for M. R. Vaginal smears were slightly different, with S. R., who had lost less weight, having a better maturation index: 15% superficial, 85% intermediate cells (MI = 58) for S. R. versus 16% superficial, 53% intermediate, and 31% parabasal cells (MI = 43) for M. R. The options of weight gain, decreased activity level, improved calcium intake, and estrogen replacement were discussed with the two young women. They both elected to increase dietary calcium and to use transdermal estradiol patches and medroxyprogesterone (14 days/month) for 9 months. Withdrawal flow was normal; however, they discontinued the medication because of concerns about bloating. Six months later they began to decrease their athletic activity in preparation for graduation from college. Spontaneous menses returned.

SECONDARY AMENORRHEA WITH HIRSUTISM OR VIRILIZATION

The differential diagnosis of secondary amenorrhea with hirsutism and/or virilization includes PCO, congenital (or late-onset) adrenocortical hyperplasia, Cushing's syndrome, and ovarian and adrenal tumors (see Chapter 7).

OLIGOMENORRHEA

Teenagers with menses every 2 to 3 months often consult the clinician. They may feel different from their friends who are having regular monthly cycles. These menses may or may not be ovulatory. Premenstrual symptoms, dysmenorrhea, and a shift in the basal body temperature curve (see Chapter 1) that is confirmed by a rise in serum progesterone level suggest ovulation. Scant, irregular menses without cramps are most likely anovulatory and may characterize the early teenage years.

Adolescents who have evidence of androgen excess at any age, those who have persistent oligomenorrhea 2 to 3 years after menarche, and those with 4 to 6 months of amenorrhea deserve the same consideration as patients with secondary amenorrhea. The causes of oligomenorrhea are essentially the same as those shown earlier in Fig. 17. Fluctuating weight with rapid gain followed by crash dieting and eating disorders may disturb the hypothalamic–pituitary function in the adolescent and result in irregular periods. Ballet dancers and competitive athletes, such as runners and gymnasts, may have oligomenorrhea, especially those who started training in the prepubertal years. In addition, it should be remembered that the sexually active patient with a history of irregular menses who is not using contraception may have an unplanned pregnancy despite any number of negative pregnancy test results in the past.

The importance of evaluating cases of persistent oligomenorrhea was noted in a review at Children's Hospital in Boston many years ago. The charts of all adolescents who had been evaluated for oligomenorrhea not associated with weight loss, and who had been assessed over a 2-year period, were reviewed (258). Among the 42 adolescents (mean age 17.3, range 15 to 20 years), 19 had evidence of androgen excess (hirsutism, clitoromegaly, and/or severe acne) consistent with PCO or adrenal androgen excess, and 23 patients had no evidence of androgen excess. In the second group, 4 patients had persistently elevated LH levels that ranged from 34.5 to 41.0 mIU/ml, with normal FSH, DHEAS, and total and free testosterone levels; 15 had hypothalamic amenorrhea (and 6 of 15 returned to normal menses); 1 had hyperprolactinemia; and 3 had ovarian failure. Although the patients were seen in a referral center, the spectrum of potential diagnoses is representative.

Patients with hypothalamic suppression and normal results of physical examination and laboratory tests deserve reassurance and a careful explanation of menstrual cycles. The statement "You're normal; don't worry" is not sufficient.

Medroxyprogesterone acetate, 10 mg a day for 14 days each month, can be used to prevent endometrial hyperplasia; it is also especially useful to treat patients with a history of hypermenorrhea associated with irregular periods. Oral contraceptives (OCs) can be prescribed to the adolescent who needs contraception in that there is no evidence that hormonal therapy changes the long-term prognosis of patients for irregular cycles (see Chapter 17). It is important to make a diagnosis before the institution of OC therapy so that the patient knows that if she has PCO syndrome she is likely to return to oligomenorrhea following the discontinuance of OCs.

In older adolescents who have menses every 2 months with premenstrual symptoms and dysmenorrhea, the likelihood of ovulation is high, and no therapy is necessary. Basal body temperature charts can be useful in demonstrating ovulation; a luteal phase serum progesterone level can also document ovulation if needed.

ABNORMAL VAGINAL BLEEDING: DYSFUNCTIONAL UTERINE BLEEDING, POLYMENORRHEA, HYPERMENORRHEA

One of the most common problems reported by adolescents is irregular, profuse menstruation. Rarely, a teenager with her first period might even show a decrease of 10 to 20 percentage points in her hematocrit. More often, a teenager has irregular menses after menarche. Another teen may have had several years of regular cycles but begins to have periods every 2 weeks or prolonged bleeding for 14 to 20 days after 2 to 3 months of amenorrhea. A young adolescent is prone to anovulatory periods with incomplete shedding of a proliferative endometrium; the older adolescent may develop anovulatory cycles with stress or illness. A study of FSH/LH patterns in perimenarcheal girls with anovulatory bleeding suggests the prevalence of a maturation defect (259). The higher-than-normal levels of FSH in relation to LH may result in rapid follicular maturation and increased synthesis of estrogen, and absence of the midcycle surge of LH. Although dysfunctional uterine bleeding (DUB) may appear to be simply a defect in positive feedback and the lack of establishment of ovulatory cycles, most adolescents in fact are anovulatory during the first years following menarche and yet do not have DUB. Therefore, adolescents with DUB appear to have delayed maturation of normal negative feedback cyclicity; rising levels of estrogen do not cause a fall in FSH and subsequent suppression of estrogen secretion, and thus the endometrium becomes excessively thickened. In contrast, normal adolescents have an intact negative feedback mechanism that allows for orderly growth of the endometrium and withdrawal flow before the endometrium is excessively thickened. In addition, the occasional ovulatory cycle stabilizes endometrial growth and allows more complete shedding. Adolescents with conditions that cause sustained anovulation may also be likely to present with abnormal uterine bleeding; such problems include eating disorders, weight changes, athletic competition, chronic illnesses, stress, drug abuse, endocrine disorders, and most important, PCO. Interestingly, Apter (260) has observed that adolescents with late menarche have longer intervals until cycles become ovulatory than teens with early menarche.

In deciding whether the pattern of the adolescent is normal or abnormal, the clinician needs to be cognizant of normal variations. The adult menstrual cycle is 21 to 45 days, and an adult tends to have the same interval on a month-to-month basis (261). Although adolescents have a similar range of normal cycles, a given adolescent has more variability within this range than does the adult woman. A normal duration of flow is 3 to 7 days; a flow of >8 to 10 days is considered excessive. Normal blood loss is 30 to 40 ml (up to 80 ml) per menstrual period, which usually translates into 10 to 15 soaked tampons or pads per cycle. Unfortunately, however, self-reported estimation of blood loss by adolescents (and adult women) is inaccurate, unless the flow is very scant (262). Even counting the number of tampons or pads changed in a day cannot give the clinician an assessment of the likelihood of significant bleeding, defined as a blood loss of >80 ml per menstrual period—an amount that would result in iron deficiency anemia. Thus, the hematocrit should be measured in the girl who reports possible abnormal bleeding to determine the extent of blood loss.

The list of diagnoses to be considered in approaching the problem of abnormal vaginal bleeding in the adolescent is long but necessitates the careful consideration and examination of each patient. It is important to keep in mind that DUB connotes excessive, prolonged, unpatterned bleeding from the endometrium *unrelated to structural or systemic disease*, and thus other diagnoses must be excluded. Importantly, disorders of pregnancy and the possibility of pelvic infection must be appraised early in the evaluation. The differential diagnosis is shown in Table 9. A highly sensitive pregnancy test should be performed in the initial evaluation; ectopic pregnancy should be a consideration, especially in the adolescent with a previous history of pelvic inflammatory disease (PID) or sexually transmitted diseases (see Chapter 12). Adolescents with PID and endometritis caused by *Neisseria gonorrhoeae* or *Chlamydia trachomatis* frequently present with heavy or irregular bleeding. The possibility of these infections (especially *Chlamydia*) needs to be considered in the adolescent taking oral contraceptives who develops new breakthrough bleeding. Thus, a crucial part of the evaluation in an adolescent who might ever have been sexually active (history notwithstanding) are tests for *N. gonorrhoeae* and *C. trachomatis*. The sedimentation rate should be determined if PID is a likely possibility.

Patients with blood dyscrasias usually have other signs of bleeding such as petechiae, ecchymoses, or epistaxis; however, the teenager with von Willebrand's disease may not have a prior history of injuries and thus may be diagnosed only because of profuse menstruation starting with her menarche. Acquired von Willebrand's disease can occur in girls with systemic lupus erythematosus with the production of anti-von Willebrand factor antibody (263). Likewise, the teenager with chronic thrombocytopenic purpura, or the cardiac patient on warfarin, may have heavy menstrual bleeding. Patients with significant liver disease or who have undergone liver transplantation may have coagulopathies.

Irregular, heavy menstruation may accompany endocrine disorders that are also associated with secondary amenorrhea and anovulation. Adrenal problems such as late-onset 21-hydroxylase deficiency, Cushing's syndrome, and Addison's disease can cause anovulation; Addison's disease is also often associated with ovarian failure. Patients with hyperprolactinemia usually have amenorrhea but may have irregular bleeding from anovulation or a shortened luteal phase. In our experience, adolescents with hypothyroidism are more likely to experience amenorrhea, and those with hyperthyroidism, polymenorrhea. Similarly, patients with ovarian failure from Turner's syndrome or chemotherapy and/or radiation therapy may have irregular bleeding before the onset of amenorrhea. The anovulation of PCO syndrome is present early in adolescence; 20% to 30% of patients with PCO syndrome experience DUB. This diagnosis needs to be considered in adolescents with persistent DUB and those who initially have evidence of androgen excess (hirsutism, acne) or acanthosis nigri-

TABLE 9. *Differential diagnosis of abnormal vaginal bleeding in the adolescent girl*

Anovulatory uterine bleeding

Pregnancy-related complications
- Threatened abortion
- Spontaneous, incomplete, or missed abortion
- Ectopic pregnancy
- Gestational trophoblastic disease
- Complications of termination procedures

Infection
- Pelvic inflammatory disease
- Endometritis
- Cervicitis
- Vaginitis

Blood dyscrasias
- Thrombocytopenia
  - (e.g., idiopathic thrombocytopenic purpura, leukemia, aplastic anemia, hypersplenism, chemotherapy)
- Clotting disorders
  - (e.g., von Willebrand's disease, other disorders of platelet function, liver dysfunction)

Endocrine disorders
- Hypo- or hyperthyroidism
- Adrenal disease
- Hyperprolactinemia
- Polycystic ovary syndrome
- Ovarian failure

Vaginal abnormalities
- Carcinoma
- Laceration

Cervical problems
- Cervicitis
- Polyp
- Hemangioma
- Carcinoma

Uterine problems
- Submucous myoma
- Congenital anomalies
- Polyp
- Carcinoma
- Use of intrauterine device
- Breakthrough bleeding associated with oral contraceptives or other hormonal contraceptives
- Ovulation bleeding

Ovarian problems
- Cyst
- Tumor (benign, malignant)

Endometriosis

Trauma

Foreign body (e.g., retained tampon)

Systemic diseases
- Diabetes mellitus
- Renal disease
- Systemic lupus erythematosus

Medications
- Hormonal contraceptives
- Anticoagulants
- Platelet inhibitors
- Androgens
- Spironolactone

cans, because these girls are at increased risk of endometrial hyperplasia and the early development of endometrial carcinoma (rarely in the teenage years). Thus, long-term therapy with progestins or oral contraceptives needs to be prescribed in these girls.

Uterine abnormalities manifested by irregular bleeding include submucous myomas, congenital anomalies, and intrauterine device (IUD) use. Breakthrough bleeding from combined oral contraceptives is common, and patients using progestin-only methods such as DepoProvera, Norplant, or progestin-only pills frequently have irregular cycles. Congenital anomalies are sometimes detected by the presence of regular red menstrual bleeding followed by brown or prune-colored spotting intermenstrually; the bloody fluid may have a foul odor if infected by anaerobes. The normal uterus empties in a cyclic pattern, and the obstructed uterus or vagina empties through a fistula slowly over the month (see Chapter 8). The possibility of breakthrough bleeding in the adolescent taking oral contraceptives needs to be kept in mind, since the adolescent may have obtained the pills confidentially from a clinic and yet be brought to another physician by her mother for irregular menses. Unless the girl is seen alone and asked specifically about the use of oral contraceptive pills, the history may not become apparent. An occasional patient may have slight vaginal bleeding for 1 or 2 days at midcycle because of a fall in estrogen levels at ovulation; we have seen this particularly in athletes who do extensive running at midcycle. The bleeding may be more apparent to the adolescent who is exercising vigorously that day because of more rapid emptying of the menstrual blood from the vagina. A carefully kept menstrual calendar helps make the diagnosis.

Carcinoma of the vagina is rare among teenagers. Cervical problems may also cause bleeding, especially with trauma or postcoitally. Sexually transmitted infections such as those caused by *Trichomonas* and *C. trachomatis* can be associated with bleeding from a friable cervix. Young women with cystic fibrosis often have a large cervical ectropion with chronic inflammation; the cervix may bleed easily with coitus or when a speculum is inserted. Hemangiomas rarely occur on the cervix and cause bleeding especially with trauma or coitus. Cervical cancer can rarely present during adolescence and thus must be kept in the differential diagnosis.

Endometriosis has been associated with irregular menses from anovulation and also with brown spotting in the premenstrual phase of the cycle (see Chapter 9). Ovarian abnormalities, including tumors and cysts, may cause hypermenorrhea (see Chapter 15).

Systemic diseases (see Chapter 19) may interfere with normal cyclicity because of an impact on ovulation, an interference with normal coagulation, or a local endometrial infection such as tuberculosis (a common cause in third-world countries but exceedingly rare in the United States). Patients undergoing renal dialysis frequently have either amenorrhea or excessive menstrual flow; the menorrhagia may increase the transfusion requirement of the patient and thus frequently requires ongoing management with progestins or oral contraceptives.

Trauma may occur because of acute falls, waterskiing injuries, foreign objects introduced for masturbation, or sexual assault. The most common foreign body is a retained tampon, sometimes left in the vagina for weeks to months. The young adolescent may have tried to use a tampon and not realized the need for removal, or she may have put two tampons in the vagina and forgotten to remove one. The bleeding from a retained tampon is usually accompanied by a foul-smelling discharge.

Medications such as anticoagulants and platelet inhibitors can be associated with excessive bleeding. Adolescent athletes taking anabolic steroids may develop masculinization and anovulatory cycles, with irregular bleeding or amenorrhea. Tricyclic antidepressants and valproate can also cause irregular menses.

Categorizing bleeding as *cyclic* or *acyclic* may help the clinician focus on the appropriate diagnosis. For example, an adolescent with normal cyclic intervals but very heavy bleeding at the time of each cycle may have a blood dyscrasia or a uterine problem (submucous myoma or IUD use). Interestingly, in adults with heavy cyclic bleeding (>80 ml/cycle), the plasma concentrations of LH, FSH, and estradiol and the salivary levels of progesterone are not different from those in women with normal blood loss (264).

An adolescent with normal cycles but superimposed abnormal bleeding at any time throughout the cycle may have a foreign body within the vagina, uterine polyp, vaginal malignancy, congenital malformation of the uterus with obstruction, infection, cervical abnormality, or endometriosis. Adolescents with no cyclicity apparent, or cycles of <21 days or >40 to 45 days, usually have anovulatory DUB with lack of normal negative feedback. However, the other disorders associated with anovulation need to be considered, including psychosocial problems, eating disorders, athletic competition, PCO syndrome, ovarian failure, ovarian tumors, and endocrinopathies.

Two series have been published in the past 15 years concerning the differential diagnosis of adolescents requiring hospitalization for treatment of menorrhagia. The conclusions are somewhat different between the first and the second study. Claesson (265,266) looked at 59 patients hospitalized from 1971 to 1980 and reported a primary coagulation disorder in 20% of girls: one-quarter of those with hemoglobin <10 g/dl, one-third of those requiring transfusion, and one-half of those presenting at menarche. The diagnoses included idiopathic thrombocytopenia (ITP) (four), von Willebrand's disease (three), Glanzmann's disease (two), thalassemia major (one), and Fanconi's syndrome (one); seven patients had other conditions, and 34% were treated with dilatation and curettage (D&C). A second study published in 1994 by Falcone (267) reported 61 patients hospitalized between 1981 and 1991. Only 3% had newly diagnosed coagulation disorders: ITP (one), acute promyelocytic leukemia (one). However, 28% had past histories of significant medical problems, including leukemia, ITP, Glanzmann's disease, hypothyroidism, mental retardation, and rheumatoid arthritis; 50% had a history of irregular menses (defined as <25 or >35 days apart). The mean hemoglobin was 8.9 g/dl (3 standard deviations), and 41% required blood transfusions. In contrast to the earlier series, 93% responded to medical management, and only 8% underwent D&C, similar to our experience at Boston Children's Hospital. They reported no difference in the response of patients treated with intravenous Premarin versus oral estrogen/progestin combinations in the initial hemoglobin, percentage of patients transfused, or days in the hospital (the patients were not randomized).

Patient Assessment

The history, physical examination, and initial laboratory tests are crucial in determining the likely diagnoses as well as the urgency for immediate treatment. Questions should focus on date of menarche; menstrual pattern; duration, quantity, and color of the flow; and the presence of dysmenorrhea. The dates of the last menstrual period and the previous menstrual period should be recorded. A menstrual calendar is invaluable. Information about the use of tampons, contraceptive sponges, or other foreign objects should be elicited. The patient should be asked whether she is sexually active (realizing that the history must be taken confidentially and the answers may not always be honest), whether the bleeding was postcoital, and whether she is using oral contraceptives, a progestin-only method (DepoProvera, Norplant, progestin-only pills), or IUD. The patient should also be queried about previous sexually transmitted diseases and recent exposure to a new partner or a partner with urethritis or other infection. A general review of systems, including recent stresses, weight changes, eating disorders, athletic competition, chronic diseases, bleeding disorders, medications, illicit drugs, syncope, visual changes, headaches, gastrointestinal symptoms, acne, hirsutism, and acanthosis nigricans, and a family history of PCO syndrome and bleeding disorders, is essential.

The physical examination should include a general assessment with attention to the height, weight, body type, and fat distribution (to detect Cushing's syndrome or Turner's syndrome), blood pressure (standing and lying), evidence of androgen excess (acne, hirsutism, clitoromegaly), acanthosis nigricans, thyroid palpation, breast examination to detect galactorrhea, other signs of bleeding such as petechiae or bruises, and a pelvic examination. In most virginal adolescents and all sexually active adolescents, a one-finger digital examination can be done initially to check for foreign bodies within the vagina and to palpate the cervix. A speculum appropriate for the size of the hymenal opening can then be chosen, usually a Huffman speculum in the virginal patient and a Pederson speculum for the sexually active adolescent. Generally, a virginal patient can cooperate fully if the need for the examination is carefully explained and the examiner obtains her help. Sometimes the application of a small amount of lubricating jelly or lidocaine jelly to the introitus can aid in the insertion of the speculum. In some girls who have never used tampons, the opening is too small to allow a digital or a speculum examination. In these cases, a rectoabdominal examination suffices. Sometimes only an external examination can be accomplished. If the patient does not respond to simple hormonal treatment, ultrasonography of the pelvis and/or examination with the patient under anesthesia may be needed. Clearly, many adolescents in the early months after menarche may have several closely spaced menses and then revert to a normal pattern, and they can be simply observed without a full pelvic examination. However, even a virginal girl with continuous spotting, cyclic bleeding with superimposed bleeding throughout the cycle, bleeding sufficient to cause anemia, or persistent DUB deserves a careful gynecologic assessment.

During the speculum examination, tests should be obtained for *N. gonorrhoeae* and *C. trachomatis* in any patient who gives a history of being sexually active and in any patient whom the clinician suspects may have had intercourse. In the absence of bleeding at the time of the examination, wet preps are done and a Papanicolaou smear can also be obtained. A bimanual examination should be done to assess tenderness and enlargement of the uterus and adnexal pain and masses. A soft mass along the anterior-lateral vaginal wall is possibly an obstruction of the genital tract (see Chapter 8).

Laboratory tests should include a sensitive urine pregnancy test and a CBC with differential and estimate of platelet count. In girls who give an impressive history of bleeding and yet have a normal or only slightly depressed hemoglobin, a reticulocyte count is helpful in assessing the amount of bleeding. A sedimentation rate is useful if pelvic infection is a consideration. Coagulation studies (e.g., prothrombin time, partial thromboplastin time, specific studies for von Willebrand factor, and possibly a bleeding time) and platelet count are indicated in patients with heavy cyclic bleeding from menarche and those with a significant drop in hemoglobin or a hemoglobin <10 g/dl at presentation. Blood typing and cross-matching should be done for girls with acute hemorrhage or low hemoglobin when transfusion may be necessary.

Other tests depend on the physical examination and the length of the history of the DUB. Probably the most common test is TSH determination as a screening test for hypo- or hyperthyroidism. Other potential studies for patients with a long history of DUB include determination of FSH (and LH), prolactin, and serum androgens (total and free testosterone, DHEAS), especially in those with hirsutism or acne. Screening tests for diabetes should be individualized. Basal body temperature charts and a progesterone level obtained during the presumed luteal phase of the cycle can aid in the evaluation of ovulatory versus anovulatory menses, if needed. Ultrasonography can be helpful when a pelvic mass is felt, a uterine anomaly is suspected, or bimanual examination cannot be accomplished in a young adolescent with significant bleeding. If a uterine anomaly is detected, MRI can help define the anatomy further. A submucous myoma or an endometrial polyp, both rare in adolescents, may require further evaluation with hysterosalpingogram and/or hysteroscopy.

Treatment

The goals of the assessment are to determine which adolescent needs medical treatment and which adolescent can be observed in the hope that further maturation of the hypothalamic–pituitary–ovarian axis will result in normal cycles. The objective of hormonal treatment is to give estrogens to heal the endometrial bleeding sites by causing further endometrial proliferation and to give progestins to induce endometrial stability. The evaluation and treatment plan should aim at stopping bleeding; preventing a recurrence; identifying underlying organic disease if present; diagnosing any psychosocial pathology causing and/or exacerbating any menstrual disorders; preventing the progression of acne, hirsutism, and obesity, which can be caused by hormonal imbalances such as PCO syndrome; and preventing long-term pathologic sequelae. Thus, long-term followup is essential.

Although opinions clearly vary about the best mode of therapy, various hormonal regimens have been successful (259,266,268–272). In addition, some conditions, such as bone marrow transplantation for malignancies, may be better addressed with prophylactic GnRH agonists (DepoLupron) to suppress menses before a problem develops. Preliminary data show a 100% induction of amenorrhea with the use of a GnRH agonist for women without underlying uterine pathology during bone marrow transplantation (275).

The following classification and treatment schedules have been helpful in our clinical practices.

Mild Dysfunctional Bleeding

Mild DUB is defined as menses that are longer than normal, or the cycle is shortened for ≥2 months. The flow is slightly to moderately increased; hemoglobin level is normal.

Observation and reassurance is usually adequate. The patient should be encouraged to keep a menstrual calendar so that the need for intervention in the future can be assessed. Iron supplements will prevent anemia (especially if dietary intake is borderline). Antiprostaglandin medications, such as ibuprofen or naproxen sodium, taken during menstruation have been reported to reduce blood loss in patients with menorrhagia (273).

Moderate Dysfunctional Bleeding

Moderate DUB is defined as menses that are moderately prolonged, or the cycle remains shortened with frequent menses (every 1 to 3 weeks). The flow is moderate to heavy; and hemoglobin level often shows mild anemia.

Treatment consists of oral contraceptive pills, medroxyprogesterone (Provera), or other progestin. Combined oral contraceptive pills are more effective at stopping dysfunctional bleeding that is in progress than medroxyprogesterone. However, if the patient is not bleeding at the time of the visit, the patient or parent dislikes the use of birth control pills, or there is a medical contraindication to the use of estrogen, medroxyprogesterone can be tried as initial therapy. For short-term treatment of DUB, medroxyprogesterone 10 mg can be given once a day for 10 to 12 days; for adolescents who require ongoing therapy for persistent DUB (especially associated with PCO syndrome), it is preferable to give 14 days of progestin each month.

The medroxyprogesterone can be prescribed according to the calendar month or in cycles based on the first day of menstrual bleeding. If the calendar month is used, the patient is given medroxyprogesterone 10 mg once a day for the first 10 to 14 days of each month; this dosing schedule is simple for most patients to follow. However, some patients begin bleeding before the next dose is to be taken and may then need a start date based on menstrual bleeding or may need to use an oral contraceptive instead. In using the menstrual cycle system, the patient is instructed to start the medroxyprogesterone 10 mg on the 14th day of the menstrual cycle (day 1 is the first day of the last period) or at the time of the visit. A negative pregnancy test result must be established, and the patient should not be sexually active, as medroxyprogesterone is not a form of contraception. After the patient has a withdrawal flow, she starts medroxyprogesterone on day 14 again (Fig. 21). The pattern is continued for 3 to 6 months. If the patient starts bleeding even before she gets to day 14 of her cycle, then start-

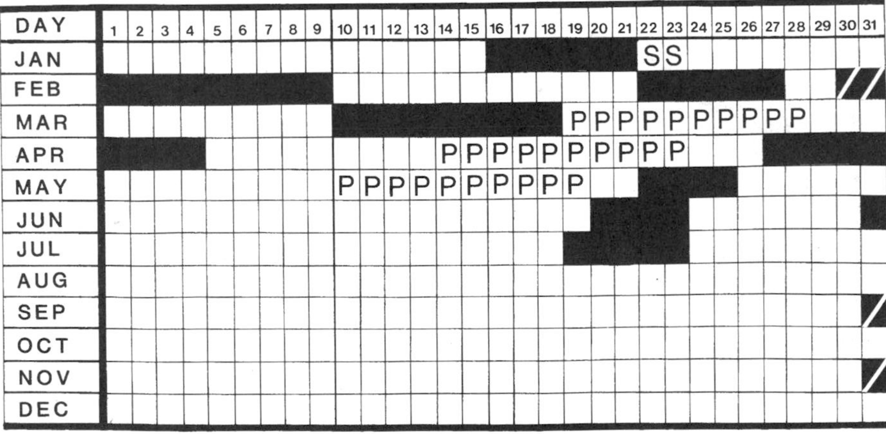

FIG. 21. A 14-year-old girl comes to the clinic on March 19 with a history of frequent periods (every 17—22 days). She is not bleeding at the time of her visit. The results of examination and laboratory studies are normal. She is treated with medroxyprogesterone (Provera), 10 mg daily for 10 days and then for 10 days from the 14th to the 23rd day of the two subsequent cycles. Her menses return to normal in June and July. *S*, spotting; *P*, Provera; *solid bars*, bleeding. On the normal menstrual calendar, the months without 30 or 31 days have slashed bars.

ing the medroxyprogesterone on day 10 or day 12 of the cycle for several cycles and extending the medroxyprogesterone to 14 days, or preferably switching to an oral contraceptive, will give better control of the cycle. Norethindrone acetate (Aygestin), 5 to 10 mg daily for 10 to 14 days, can be given instead of medroxyprogesterone, with 10 to 12 days acceptable for short-term use, and 14 days for long-term use.

For patients with heavy or prolonged dysfunctional bleeding, the initial use of an oral contraceptive, such as Lo/Ovral (Nordette, Levlen) for 21 days, is preferable to progestin-only methods. The patient can be told to take one Lo/Ovral twice a day for 3 or 4 days until the bleeding stops and then one a day to finish a 21-day cycle. The dose sometimes needs to be increased initially to three or four times a day to stop menstrual flow and then reduced to once a day. Norinyl (Ortho-Novum) 1/35 and other oral contraceptives have also been used successfully in some patients, given once or twice a day for 21 days. The clinician needs to keep in contact with the patient, since hormonal therapy can cause nausea and noncompliance, and adequate doses must be prescribed to prevent further bleeding.

The urgency of gaining control of the cycle is related to the amount of bleeding and the hematocrit; thus, in some adolescents with heavy bleeding and anemia, starting with Lo/Ovral four times a day may be necessary to stop bleeding within 24 to 36 hours. A useful regimen is: Lo/Ovral four times a day for 4 days, then three times a day for 3 days, then twice a day for 2 weeks.

DAY	1	2	3	4	5	6	7	8	9	10	11	12	13	14	15	16	17	18	19	20	21	22	23	24	25	26	27	28	29	30	31
JAN								S	S																					S	S
FEB																															
MAR							O	O	O	O	O	O	O	O	O	O	O	O	O	O	O	O	O	O	O	O					
APR						O	O	O	O	O	O	O	O	O	O	O	O	O	O	O	O	O	O	O	O						
MAY					O	O	O	O	O	O	O	O	O	O	O	O	O	O	O	O	O	O	O	O							
JUN																															
JUL																															
AUG																															
SEP																															
OCT																															
NOV																															
DEC																															

FIG. 22. A 14-year-old girl arrives at the emergency ward with profuse vaginal bleeding that followed markedly irregular cycles for the previous 3 months. The results of pelvic examination and clotting studies are normal; hematocrit is 28%. She is given Ovral q.i.d.; bleeding ceases the following day. She continues with Ovral for the remainder of the cycle and then is given cyclic Lo/Ovral or Ovral for 2 additional months. Lo/Ovral can also be used for initial therapy. *S*, spotting; *O*, Ovral; *solid bars*, bleeding. On the normal menstrual calendar, the months without 30 or 31 days have slashed bars.

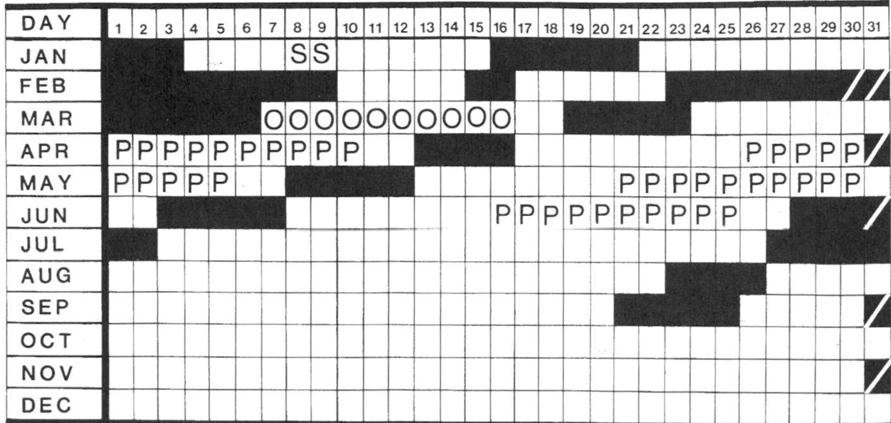

FIG. 23. The same case as illustrated in Fig. 22; however, the patient experiences moderate nausea and vomiting while receiving oral contraceptive therapy. The bleeding stops and the course is shortened to 10 days. Medroxyprogesterone (Provera), 10 mg daily, is given for 3 months from day 14 to 23 of each cycle. *S*, spotting; *O*, oral contraceptive; *P*, Provera.

With these doses of estrogen, antiemetics such as chlorpromazine, 5 to 10 mg, may need to be prescribed and taken by the patient 2 hours before each dose of OC to prevent nausea (see other options in Chapter 17). Ovral, other oral contraceptives, or norethindrone acetate (Aygestin) 5 mg may also be used similarly (Fig. 22).

Occasionally, patients experience excessive nausea with OCs in spite of using antiemetics; in these cases, the 21-day course of hormone can be shortened to 10 days, and medroxyprogesterone or norethindrone acetate can be given on a cyclic basis (Fig. 23). Failure to control bleeding with any of the above regimens should make the clinician consider a diagnosis other than anovulatory uterine bleeding.

A normal withdrawal flow will follow 2 to 4 days after the last hormone tablet has been taken. The OC is then discontinued for 7 days unless the withdrawal flow is abnormally heavy, in which case the pill-free interval can be shortened to 4 to 5 days. For significant bleeding, the patient usually continues to take OCs for 3 months. If a 50-μg pill (e.g., Ovral) or a twice-daily pill was used for the first cycle, the patient is usually given a lower-dose OC such as Lo/Ovral once a day for the next few cycles. The patient should receive careful instructions on 21-day versus 28-day pills; otherwise, confusion may result, and placebos may be used on hormone days or a 7-day withdrawal time not be observed. Oral contraceptives should be continued if birth control is needed. Otherwise, the patient can switch to cyclic medroxyprogesterone for an additional 3 to 6 months. A course of oral iron plus folic acid (1 mg daily) should also be prescribed to correct anemia.

Severe Dysfunctional Bleeding

Severe dysfunctional bleeding is defined as bleeding that is prolonged, with normal menstrual cycles disrupted. The flow is very heavy, and the hemoglobin level is reduced, often to <9 g/dl. Clinical signs of blood loss may be present.

The patient should be admitted to the hospital if initial hemoglobin is <7 g/dl, or if orthostatic signs are present, or if bleeding is heavy and hemoglobin is <10 g/dl. Transfusion should be considered if there are clinical signs of acute blood loss or the hemoglobin level is extremely low. Clotting studies should be done. If the hemoglobin is 8 to 10 g/dl and the patient and family are reliable and can maintain close telephone contact, the patient can be treated at home and monitored daily until bleeding ceases. For most patients, hospitalization is necessary.

An effective treatment is Lo/Ovral or Ovral every 4 hours until bleeding slows or stops (usually 4 to 8 tablets), then every 6 hours for 24 hours, every 8 hours for 48 hours, and then twice a day to complete a 21-day course of hormones. Alternatively, the Lo/Ovral or Ovral regimen can start with every 4 hours until bleeding is controlled and then can be tapered to one tablet four times a day for 4 days, three times a day for 3 days, and twice a day for 2 weeks; this schedule may be especially easy for emergency ward personnel to administer. Ortho-Novum 1/35 and other monophasic oral contraceptives have been used in similar doses, although the clinical experience has not been as vast. In acute severe hemorrhage, some physicians use conjugated estrogens (Premarin), 25 mg IV every 4 hours for two to three doses, whereas others use only combined oral contraceptives because of concern about possible thromboembolism and questionable efficacy of intravenous estrogens (274). Intravenous conjugated estrogens are particularly indicated when the patient may not be given anything by mouth or is unstable and may require critical care measures. Intravenous estrogen appears to increase clotting at the capillary level and thus is very rapidly effective. If intravenous estrogen is used, oral hormones such as Lo/Ovral or Ovral should be started at the same time to provide a progestin to stabilize the endometrium. Antiemetics are usually needed with any of the high-dose estrogen therapies. Transfusion needs are individualized on the basis of hemoglobin, blood loss, orthostatic symptoms, and the need to rapidly gain control of the bleeding.

If there is a contraindication to the use of estrogen, a trial of progestin such as norethindrone acetate (Aygestin), 5 to 10 mg, or medroxyprogesterone, 10 mg, can be given every 4 hours and then tapered to the regimen of four times a day for 4 days, three times a day for 3 days, and then twice a day for 2 weeks. Norethindrone appears to be more effective than medroxyprogesterone.

Occasionally, only very high doses of progestin (medroxyprogesterone, 40 to 80 mg/day; megestrol acetate (Megestrol) 80 mg twice a day; or DepoProvera, 100 mg IM daily for up to a week and then weekly to monthly) are effective to cause endometrial atrophy; breakthrough bleeding can be avoided by using a several-day course of estrogen (conjugated estrogens, 2.5 mg for 5 to 7 days, or an occasional transdermal estradiol patch). Patients may become cushingoid with these high doses, and injections are contraindicated in patients with bleeding disorders. More evaluation of the potential use of long-acting GnRH analogs is needed (273–277) (see Chapter 19).

If the regimen of hormone tablets every 4 hours fails to control bleeding within 24 to 36 hours, the possibility of pelvic pathology should be excluded by anesthesia examination and D&C. D&C may be needed earlier to treat a patient who cannot be given estrogen. Although this procedure can be both diagnostic and curative, the overwhelming majority of adolescents can be treated successfully with hormones alone. In addition, the adolescent with a long history of anovulation still needs followup care to prevent a recurrence of heavy bleeding.

A normal withdrawal flow occurs 2 to 4 days after the last hormone tablet. In patients with significant anemia, the placebo (off-pill) interval should be avoided, and OC given continuously until the hematocrit returns toward normal. If the hematocrit has increased, the patient can be cycled for 3 to 4 months (or longer) with an oral contraceptive (Lo/Ovral, Ovral, or, if tolerated without breakthrough bleeding, a pill such as Ortho-Novum 1/35). If necessary, the pill-free interval can be shortened to 4 to 5 days. Iron and folic acid therapy should be given along with hormone therapy as soon as the situation has stabilized (1 to 2 days).

The prophylaxis and management of adolescents with known coagulopathies is discussed in Chapter 19. Many girls with conditions such as von Willebrand's disease can be treated with DDAVP and/or oral contraceptives; others require GnRH agonists. A few centers have managed heavy menses in patients with marked difficulty handling menstrual hygiene with endometrial ablation (278).

Followup

Patients with a long history of anovulatory cycles and dysfunctional uterine bleeding have an increased risk of later infertility and endometrial carcinoma (279). This risk is especially a problem for patients with PCO syndrome. Thus, regular withdrawal with progestins (such as medroxyprogesterone, 14 days per month) or OCs are needed on a long-term basis in these high-risk girls. Careful followup is essential.

Case 16

A. N., 14 years old, was seen in the emergency ward with a history of pelvic pain and profuse vaginal bleeding for 4 days. Her menarche was at age 13 years, and she had normal cycles for 1 year. Her last regular menstrual period had occurred 2 weeks before the onset of this bleeding. She denied having ever

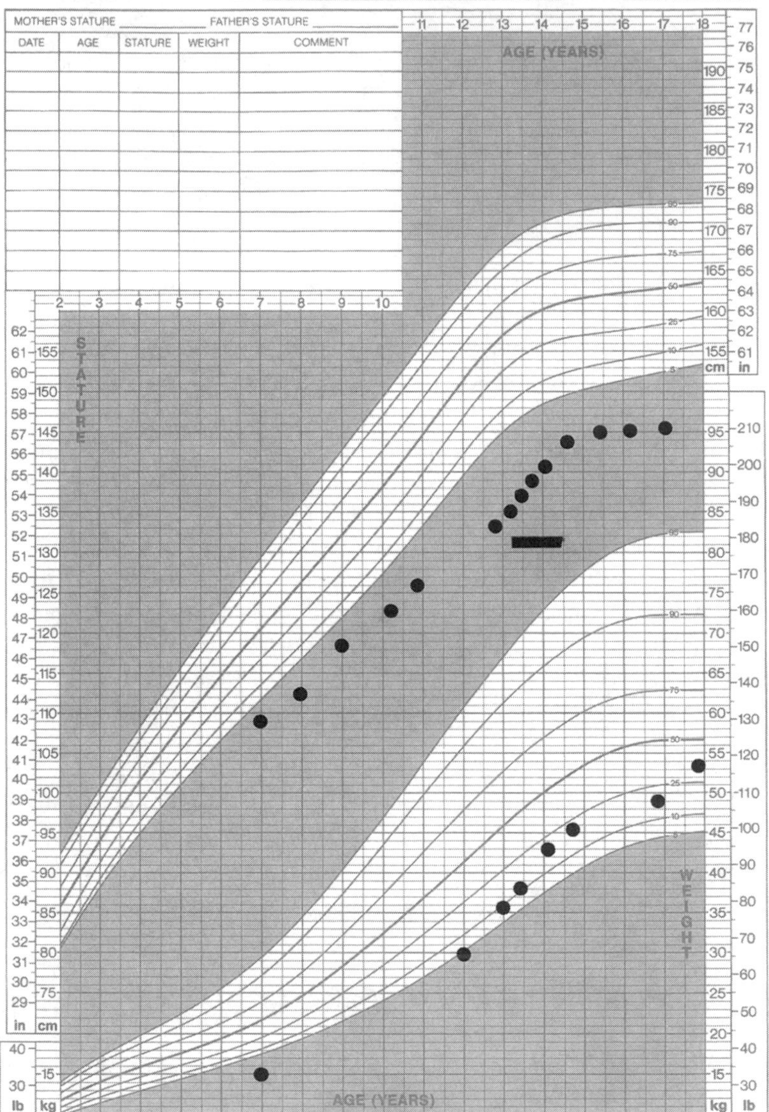

FIG. 24. Case 17: growth chart. Bar denotes growth hormone therapy.

been sexually active or having other bleeding problems. The result of general physical examination was normal, but her pelvic examination was difficult because of a small hymenal opening and discomfort on examination. The hematocrit was 28%. She was given Ovral four times a day and experienced some decrease in the amount of bleeding, but she had a moderate flow 3 days after hormonal therapy had begun. Ultrasonography revealed a mass in the right pelvis and the absence of the right kidney; she had a right uterine horn and an obstructed hemivagina. This case illustrates the need for more complete assessment and intervention in adolescents who do not respond promptly to estrogen/progestin therapy.

Case 17

O. N., 15 years old, was evaluated for irregular frequent menses every 14 to 62 days. She was first seen in the clinic at the age of 13 2/12 because of short stature. Breast and pubic hair development had begun when she was 11, and her menarche occurred when she was 12 11/12. Her father was 5′11″, and her mother was 5′3″. At the initial evaluation, she had a height of 136 cm and a weight of 37 kg (Fig. 24). She had Tanner stage 3 to 4 breast development and Tanner stage 4 pubic hair development. Her external genitalia were normal and estrogenized. Her bone age was 12 years. Because of the short stature, she had determinations of FSH (92.8 mIU/ml and 53.8 mIU/ml), thyroid function tests (normal results), and karyotype determination: 46 X,i(Xq). Despite her elevated gonadotropins, her ovaries appeared normal on ultrasound, and a 1-cm follicle was evident. She was treated with growth hormone until she had reached a bone age of 14 1/2 years. Her menses were irregular the first year of treatment, and then she began to have frequent menses every 16 to 20 days. She was initially treated with medroxyprogesterone, which did not result in normal cycles and was then given norethindrone acetate (Aygestin) 5 mg for 14 days each calendar month. She was subsequently prescribed OCs at age 16 to provide menstrual regulation, estrogen replacement, and contraception.

Case 18

A. J., 17 years old, presented for evaluation of heavy bleeding and pain. Her menarche had occurred when she was 13, and she had always had regular menses lasting 4 to 6 days, with mild dysmenorrhea. Her last menstrual period had begun 7 days before, and instead of decreasing by the sixth day, the flow had increased and was accompanied by moderately severe cramps. She denied ever having been sexually active.

Physical examination showed her to be afebrile and cooperative. Abdominal examination showed bilateral lower abdominal tenderness; pelvic examination showed a 2-cm hymenal opening, moderate vaginal bleeding, and cervical motion and adnexal tenderness. Samples were taken from the endocervix for *C. trachomatis* and *N. gonorrhoeae* cultures. Urine hCG was negative. Since the clinical impression was PID in spite of a negative history of sexual activity, a CBC and sedimentation rate were obtained, and the patient was treated for PID. In 2 days, she was markedly improved. Laboratory tests showed a hematocrit of 36%, white blood count (WBC) of 13,600/mm^3, and a sedimentation rate of 26 mm/hour. Endocervical cultures were positive for both *N. gon-*

orrhoeae and *C. trachomatis*. The patient finally admitted to having been sexually active, and her boyfriend was also treated. Oral contraceptives were prescribed for birth control. Even if a patient initially denies sexual activity, the clinician seeing adolescents needs to consider the possibility of PID in the evaluation of pelvic or abdominal pain or irregular bleeding.

Case 19

N. T., 19 years old, presented with a complaint of irregular menses and abdominal pain. Her menarche was at age 13 years, and she had a long history of irregular menses occurring every 3 to 8 weeks. She had previously been treated with OCs for dysfunctional uterine bleeding and had discontinued her pills 2 months prior to the appointment. Her last menstrual period had started 5 days before the visit, and she had experienced increasing bleeding and cramps. Her previous menstrual period had been 6 weeks earlier. Physical examination revealed bilateral lower abdominal tenderness and rebound. Pelvic examination revealed moderate bleeding and cervical motion and adnexal tenderness. Cultures were taken from the endocervix for *N. gonorrhoeae* and *C. trachomatis*. The result of urine hCG was positive, and quantitative hCG was 340 mIU/ml. Hematocrit was 35%, WBC 9000/mm^3, and sedimentation rate 36 mm/hour. The repeat hCG was unchanged, and the *Chlamydia* culture was positive. Laparoscopy revealed PID and an ectopic pregnancy. These two diagnoses are important considerations for the clinician seeing adolescents with vaginal bleeding.

Case 20

P. H., a 13-year-old asthmatic, was brought to the emergency ward because of a 1-week history of vomiting and headache and a 1-day history of bizarre behavior and hallucinations. She had been taking theophylline for many years, and the initial impression was that she might have taken a drug overdose. Her menarche had occurred at the age of 11, and she had had regular menses until 16 days before the visit, when heavy bleeding had begun. Physical examination showed pallor, disorientation, and heavy vaginal bleeding. The hymenal opening was small, and bimanual examination showed a normal uterus and adnexa. The hematocrit was 8.5%, WBC 6000/mm^3, and platelet count 14,000/mm^3. She was transfused with 6 units of blood, given 25 mg of conjugated estrogens intravenously, and given Ovral therapy every 4 hours. After the bleeding had slowed, the Ovral was tapered to one tablet every 6 hours for 2 days, then every 8 hours for 2 days, then twice daily for 2 1/2 months as maintenance until her platelet count was sufficient to allow menstrual flow. Bone marrow evaluation showed aplastic anemia. After her platelet count improved, her medication was switched to cyclic OCs.

REFERENCES

1. Kletzky OA, Davajan V, Nakamura RM, et al. Clinical categorization of patients with secondary amenorrhea using progesterone-induced uterine bleeding and measurement of serum gonadotropin levels. *Am J Obstet Gynecol* 1975;121:695.
2. Shangold MM, Tomai TP, Cook JD, et al. Factors associated with withdrawal bleeding after administration of oral micronized progesterone in women with secondary amenorrhea. *Fertil Steril* 1991;56:1040.
3. Simon JA, Robinson DE, Andrews MC, et al. The absorption of oral micronized progesterone: the effect of food, dose proportionality, and comparison with intramuscular progesterone. *Fertil Steril* 1993;60:26.
4. White CM, Hergenroeder AC, Klish WJ. Bone mineral density in 15- to 21-year-old eumenorrheic and amenorrheic subjects. *Am J Dis Child* 1992;146:31.
5. Frisch RE, Snow RC, Johnson LA, et al. Magnetic resonance imaging of overall and regional body fat, estrogen metabolism, and ovulation of athletes compared to controls. *J Clin Endocrinol Metab* 1993;77:471.
6. Duerenberg P, Pieters JJL, Hautvast JG. The assessment of the body fat percentage by skinfold thickness measurements in childhood and young adolescence. *Br J Nutr* 1990:63:293.
7. Pollock ML, Schmidt DH. Measurement of cardiorespiratory fitness and body composition in the clinical setting. *Compr Ther* 1980;6:12.
8. Oppliger RA, Cassady SL. Body composition assessment in women—special considerations for athletes. *Sports Med* 1994;17:353.
9. Scott RT, Leonardi MR, Hofmann GE, et al. A prospective evaluation of clomiphene citrate challenge test screening of the general infertility population. *Obstet Gynecol* 1993;82:539.
10. Reindollar RH, Byrd JR, McDonough PG. Delayed sexual development: a study of 252 patients. *Am J Obstet Gynecol* 1981;140:371.
11. Alper MM, Garner MB, Seibel MM. Premature ovarian failure: current concepts. *J Reprod Med* 1986;31:699.
12. Stratakis CA, Rennert OM. Turner's syndrome: molecular and cytogenetics, dysmorphology, endocrine, and other clinical manifestations and their management. *Endocrinologist* 1994;4:442.
13. Ogata T, Matsuo N. Turner's syndrome and female sex chromosome aberrations: deduction of the principal factors involved in the development of clinical features. *Hum Genet* 1995;95:607.
14. Rosenfeld RG. Turner's syndrome: a guide for physicians. The Turner's Syndrome Society. Gardiner-Caldwell Synermed, 1992.
15. Partsch CJ, Pankau R, Sippell WG, Tolksdorf M. Normal growth and normalization of hypergonadotropic hypogonadism in atypical Turner syndrome. *Eur J Pediatr* 1994;153:451.
16. Layman LC. An update on the treatment of hypogonadism, part 1: hypergonadotropic hypogonadism. *Adolesc Pediatr Gynecol* 1994;7:183.
17. Guvenc J, Turkbay D. Picture of the month. Denouement and discussion—Turner's syndrome. *Arch Pediatr Adolesc Med* 1994;148:1066.
18. Saenger P. Clinical review 48: the current status of diagnosis and therapeutic intervention in Turner's syndrome. *J Clin Endocrinol Metab* 1993;77:297.
19. Allen DB, Hendricks SA, Levy JM. Aortic dilation in Turner's syndrome. *J Pediatr* 1986;109:302.
20. AAP Committee on Genetics. Health supervision for children with Turner syndrome. *Pediatrics* 1995;96:1166.
21. Saenger P. Turner's syndrome. *N Engl J Med* 1996;335:1749.
22. Lippe B. Geffner ME, Dietrich RB, et al. Renal malformations in patients with Turner syndrome: imaging in 141 patients. *Pediatrics* 1988;82:852.
23. Neely EK, Marcus R, Rosenfeld RG, Bachrach LK. Turner syndrome adolescents receiving growth hormone are not osteopenic. *J Clin Endocrinol Metab* 1993;76:861.
24. Emans SJ, Grace E, Hoffer FA, et al. Estrogen deficiency in adolescents and young adults: impact on bone mineral content and effects of estrogen replacement therapy. *Obstet Gynecol* 1990;76:585.
25. Stepan JJ, Musilova J, Pacovsky V. Bone demineralization, biochemical indices of bone remodeling, and estrogen replacement therapy in adults with Turner's syndrome. *J Bone Miner Res* 1989;4:193.
26. Naeraa RW, Brixen K, Hansen RM, et al. Skeletal size and bone mineral content in Turner's syndrome: relation to karyotype, estrogen treatment, physical fitness, and bone turnover. *Calcif Tissue Int* 1991;49:77.
27. Rosenfield RG, Grumbach MM, eds. *Turner Syndrome*. New York: Marcel Dekker, 1990.

28. Lippe B. Turner syndrome. *Endocrinol Metab Clin North Am* 1991;20:121.
29. Bender BG, Linden MG, Robinson A. Neuropsychological impairment in 42 adolescents with sex chromosome abnormalities. *Am J Med Genet* 1993;48:169.
30. Kleczkowska A, Dmoch E, Kubien E, et al. Cytogenetic findings in a consecutive series of 478 patients with Turner syndrome. The Leuven experience 1965–1989. *Genet Counsel* 1990;1:227–233; Erratum *Genet Counsel* 1991;2:130.
31. Temtamy SA, Ghali I, Salam MA, et al. Karyotype/phenotype correlation in females with short stature. *Clin Genet* 1992;4l:147.
32. Heinze HJ. Ovarian function in adolescents with Turner syndrome. *Adolesc Pediatr Gynecol* 1994:7:3.
33. Groll M, Cooper M. Menstrual function in Turner's syndrome. *Obstet Gynecol* 1976;47:225.
34. Reyes FI, Koh KS, Faiman C. Fertility in women with gonadal dysgenesis. *Am J Obstet Gynecol* 1976;126:668.
35. Kaneko N, Kawagoe S, Hizoi M. 1990 Turner's syndrome—review of the literature with reference to a successful pregnancy outcome. *Gynecol Obstet Invest* 1990;29:81.
36. Gruneiro de Papendieck L, Lorcansky S, Coco R, et al. High incidence of thyroid disturbances in 49 children with Turner syndrome. *J Pediatr* 1987;111:258.
37. Miller MJ, Geffner ME, Lippe BM, et al. Echocardiography reveals a high incidence of bicuspid aortic valve in Turner syndrome. *J Pediatr* 1983;102:47.
38. Samaan NA, Stepanas AV, Danziger J, et al. Reactive pituitary abnormalities in patients with Klinefelter's and Turner's syndrome. *Arch Intern Med* 1979;139:198.
39. Sylven L, Hagenfeldt K, Brondum-Nielson K, et al. Middle-aged women with Turner's syndrome: medical status, hormonal treatment and social life. *Acta Endocrinol (Copenh)* 1991;125:359.
40. Medlej R, Lobaccaro JM, Berta P, et al. Screening for Y-derived sex determining Gene SRY in 40 patients with Turner syndrome. *J Clin Endocrinol Metab* 1992;75:1289.
41. Krauss CM, Turksoy RN, Atkins L, et al. Familial premature ovarian failure due to an interstitial deletion of the long arm of the X-chromosome. *N Engl J Med* 1987;317:125.
42. Alper MM, and Garner PR. Premature ovarian failure: its relationship to autoimmune disease. *Obstet Gynecol* 1985;66:27.
43. Damewood MD, Zacur HA, Hoffman GJ, et al. Circulating antiovarian antibodies in premature ovarian failure. *Obstet Gynecol* 1986;68:850.
44. Ahonen P, Miettinen A, Perheentupa J. Adrenal and steroidal cell antibodies in patients with autoimmune polyglandular disease type I and risk of adrenocortical and ovarian failure. *J Clin Endocrinol Metab* 1987;64:494.
45. Brelvisi L, Bombelli F, Sironi L, Doldi N. Organ-specific autoimmunity in patients with premature ovarian failure. *J Endocrinol Invest* 1993;16:889.
46. Smith BR, Furmaniak J. Adrenal and gonadal autoimmune diseases [Editorial]. *J Clin Endocrinol Metab* 1995;80:1502.
47. Betterle C, Rossi A, Pria SD, et al. Premature ovarian failure: autoimmunity and natural history. *J Clin Endocrinol Metab* 1993;39:35.
48. Rebar RW, Erickson GF, Yen SSC. Idiopathic premature ovarian failure: clinical and endocrine characteristics. *Fertil Steril* 1982;37:35.
49. Scully RE, ed. Case records of the Massachusetts General Hospital: case 46-1986. *N Engl J Med* 1986;315:1336.
50. Conte FA, Grumbach MM, Ito Y, et al. A syndrome of female pseudohermaphrodism, hypergonadotropic hypogonadism, and multicystic ovaries associated with missense mutations in the gene encoding aromatase (P450arom). *J Clin Endocrinol Metab* 1994;78:1287.
51. Kaufman FR, Kogut MD, Donnell GN, et al. Hypergonadotrophic hypogonadism in female patients with galactosemia. *N Engl J Med* 1981;304:994.
52. Hsiang YH, Berkovitz GD, Bland GL, et al. Gonadal function in patients with Down syndrome. *Am J Med Genet* 1987;27:449.
53. Finan AC, Elmer MA, Sasnow SR, et al. Nutritional factors and growth in children with sickle cell disease. *Am J Dis Child* 1988;142:237.
54. Platt OS, Rosenstock W, Espeland MA. Influence of sickle hemoglobinopathies on growth and development. *N Engl J Med* 1984;311:7.
55. Rosenbach Y, Dinari G, Zahavi I, et al. Short stature as the major manifestation of celiac disease in older children. *Clin Pediatr* 1986;25:13.
56. Weizman Z, Hamilton JR, Kopelman HR, et al. Treatment failure in celiac disease due to coexistent exocrine pancreatic insufficiency. *Pediatrics* 1987;80:924.

57. Pugliese MT, Lifshitz F, Grad G, et al. Fear of obesity: a cause of short stature and delayed puberty. *N Engl J Med* 1983;309:513.
58. Frisch RE, Gotz-Welbergen AV, McArthur JW, et al. Delayed menarche and amenorrhea of college athletes in relation to age of onset of training. *JAMA* 1981;246:1559.
59. Warren MP. The effects of exercise on pubertal progression and reproductive function in girls. *J Clin Endocrinol Metab* 1980;51:1150.
60. Djursing H. Hypothalamic-pituitary-gonadal function in insulin treated diabetic women with and without amenorrhea. *Dan Med Bull* 1987;34:139.
61. Cavallo A, Zhou XH. LHRH test in the assessment of puberty in normal children. *Horm Res* 1994;41:10.
62. Ibanez L, Potau N, Zampolli M, et al. Use of leuprolide acetate response patterns in the early diagnosis of pubertal disorders: comparison with the gonadotropin-releasing hormone test. *J Clin Endocrinol Metab* 1994;78:30.
63. Rosenfield RL. Puberty and its disorders in girls. *Endocrinol Metab Clin North Am* 1991;20:15.
64. Vance ML. Hypopituitarism. *N Engl J Med* 1994;330:1651.
65. Cicognani A, Cacciari E, Vecchi V, et al. Differential effects of 18- and 24-gy cranial irradiation on growth rate and growth hormone release in children with prolonged survival after acute lymphocytic leukemia. *Am J Dis Child* 1988;142:1199.
66. Costin G. Effect of low-dose cranial radiation on growth hormone secretory dynamics and hypothalamic-pituitary function. *Am J Dis Child* 1988;142:847.
67. Maurer HS, Lloyd-Still JD, Ingrisano C, et al. A prospective evaluation of iron chelation therapy in children with severe β-thalassemia. *Am J Dis Child* 1988;142:287.
68. Borgna-Pignatti C, DeStefano P, Zonta L, et al. Growth and sexual maturation in thalassemia major. *J Pediatr* 1985;106:150.
69. Miller WL, Kaplan SL, Grumbach MM. Child abuse as a cause of post-traumatic hypopituitarism. *N Engl J Med* 1980;302:724.
70. Barkan AL, Kelch RP, Marshall JC. Isolated gonadotrope failure in the polyglandular autoimmune syndrome. *N Engl J Med* 1985;312:1535.
71. Cacciari E, Zucchini S, Ambrosetto P, et al. Empty sella in children and adolescents with possible hypothalamic-pituitary disorders. *J Clin Endocrinol Metab* 1994;78:767.
72. Shulman DI, Martinez CR, Bercu BB, et al. Hypothalamic-pituitary dysfunction in primary empty sella syndrome in childhood. *J Pediatr* 1986;108:540.
73. Djerassi A, Coutifaris C, West VA, et al. Gonadotroph adenoma in a premenopausal woman secreting follicle-stimulating hormone and causing ovarian hyperstimulation. *J Clin Endocrinol Metab* 1995;80:591.
74. American Psychiatric Association. *DSM-IV*. Diagnostic and Statistical Manual of Mental Disorders, 4th ed. Washington, DC: American Psychiatric Association, 1994.
75. Boyar RM, Katz J, Finkelstein JW, et al. Anorexia nervosa: immaturity of the 24-hour luteinizing hormone secretory pattern. *N Engl J Med* 1974;291:861.
76. Rigotti NA, Neer RM, Skates SJ, et al. The clinical course of osteoporosis in anorexia nervosa: a longitudinal study of calcium and bone mass. *JAMA* 1991;265:1133.
77. Bachrach LK, Guido D, Katzman D, et al. Decreased bone density in adolescent girls with anorexia nervosa. *Pediatrics* 1990;86:440.
78. Kiriike N, Iketani T, Nakanishi S, et al. Reduced bone density and major hormones regulating calcium metabolism in anorexia nervosa. *Acta Psychiatr Scand* 1992:86:358.
79. Frisch RE, McArthur JW. Menstrual cycles: fatness as a determinant of minimum weight for height necessary for their maintenance or onset. *Science* 1974;185:949.
80. Frisch RE. Fatness and fertility. *Sci Am* March 1988;88.
81. Kreipe RE, Churchill BH, Strauss J. Long-term outcome of adolescents with anorexia nervosa. *Am J Dis Child* 1989;143:1322.
82. Shomento SH, Kreipe RE. Menstruation and fertility following anorexia nervosa. *Adolesc Pediatr Gynecol* 1994;7:142.
83. Golden NH, Jacobson MS, Schebendach J, et al. Resumption of menses in anorexia nervosa. *Arch Pediatr Adolesc Med* 1997;151:16.
84. Nattiv A, Agostini R, Drinkwater B, et al. The female athlete triad. *Clin Sports Med* 1994;13:405.
85. Yeager KK, Agostini R, Nattiv A, et al. The female athlete triad: disordered eating, amenorrhea, osteoporosis. *Med Sci Sports Exerc* 1993;25:775.
86. Putukian M. The female triad: eating disorders, amenorrhea, and osteoporosis. *Med Clin North Am* 1994;78:345.

87. Wyshak G, Frisch RE, Albright TE, et al. Bone fractures among former college athletes compared with nonathletes in the menopausal and postmenopausal years. *Obstet Gynecol* 1987; 69:121.
88. Bonen A. Exercise-induced menstrual cycle changes. *Sports Med* 1994;17:373.
89. Hergenroeder AC. Bone mineralization, hypothalamic amenorrhea, and sex steroid therapy in female adolescents and young adults. *J Pediatr* 1995;126:683.
90. Hetland ML, Haarbo J, Christiansen C. Running induces menstrual disturbances but bone mass is unaffected, except in amenorrheic women. *Am J Med* 1993;95:53.
91. Abraham SF, Beumont PJV, Fraser IS, et al. Body weight, exercise and menstrual status among ballet dancers in training. *Br J Obstet Gynecol* 1982;89:507.
92. Baker ER, Mathur RS, Kirk RF, et al. Female runners and secondary amenorrhea: correlation with age, parity, mileage, and plasma hormonal and sex-hormone-binding globulin concentrations. *Fertil Steril* 1981;36:183.
93. Snead DB, Stubbs CC, Weltman JY. Dietary patterns, eating behaviors, and bone mineral density in women runners. *Am J Clin Nutr* 1992;56:705.
94. Warren MP. Amenorrhea in endurance runners. *J Clin Endocrinol Metab* 1992;75:1393.
95. Yen SSC. Female hypogonatropic hypogonadism. *Endocrinol Metabol Clin North Am* 1993;22:29.
96. Baer JT, Taper LJ. Amenorrheic and eumenorrheic adolescent runners: dietary intake and exercise training status. *J Am Diet Assoc* 1992;92:89.
97. Bonen A, Belcastro AN, Ling WY, et al. Profiles of selected hormones during menstrual cycles of teenage athletes. *J Appl Physiol* 1981;50:545.
98. Bullen BA, Skrinar GS, Beitins IZ, et al. Induction of menstrual disorders by strenuous exercise in untrained women. *N Engl J Med* 1985;312:1349.
99. Schwartz B, Cumming DC, Riordan E, et al. Exercise-associated amenorrhea: a distinct entity? *Am J Obstet Gynecol* 1981;141:662.
100. Frisch RE, Wyshak G, Vincent L. Delayed menarche and amenorrhea in ballet dancers. *N Engl J Med* 1980;303:17.
101. Warren MP, Brooks Gunn J, Hamilton LH, et al. Scoliosis and fractures in young ballet dancers: relation to delayed menarche and secondary amenorrhea. *N Engl J Med* 1986;314:1348.
102. Wilson C, Emans SJ, Mansfield MJ, et al. The relationship of calculated percent body fat, sports participation, age, and place of residence on menstrual patterns in healthy adolescent girls at an independent New England high school. *J Adolesc Health Care* 1984;5:248.
103. Ellison PT, Lager C. Moderate recreational running is associated with lowered salivary progesterone profiles in women. *Am J Obstet Gynecol* 1986;154:1000.
104. Dhuper S, Warren MP, Brooks-Gunn J, Fox R. Effects of hormonal status on bone density in adolescent girls. *J Clin Endocrinol Metab* 1990;71:1083.
105. Malina RM. Menarche in athletes: a synthesis and hypothesis. *Ann Hum Biol* 1983;10:1.
106. Theintz GE, Howald H, Weiss U, et al. Evidence for a reduction of growth potential in adolescent female gymnasts. *J Pediatr* 1993;122:306.
107. Frisch RE, GotzWelbergen AV, McArthur JW, et al. Delayed menarche and amenorrhea of college athletes in relation to age of onset of training. *JAMA* 1981;246:1559.
108. Feicht CB, Johnson TS, Martin BJ, et al. Secondary amenorrhoea in athletes [Letter]. *Lancet* 1978; 2:1145.
109. Glass AR, Deuster PA, Kyle SB, et al. Amenorrhea in Olympic marathon runners. *Fertil Steril* 1987; 48:740.
110. Laughlin GA, Yen SS. Nutritional and endocrine-metabolic aberrations in amenorrheic athletes. *J Clin Endocrinol Metab* 1996;81:4301.
111. Kemmann E, Pasquale SA, Skaf R. Amenorrhea associated with carotenemia. *JAMA* 1983;249:926.
112. Deuster PA, Kyle SB, Moser PB, et al. Nutritional intakes and status of highly trained amenorrheic and eumenorrheic women runners. *Fertil Steril* 1986;46:636.
113. Pirke KM, Schweiger U, Laessle R, et al. Dieting influences the menstrual cycle: vegetarian versus nonvegetarian diet. *Fertil Steril* 1986;46:1083.
114. Gadpaille WJ, Sanborn CF, Wagner WW. Athletic amenorrhea, major affective disorders, and eating disorders. *Am J Psychiatry* 1987;144:939.
115. Baker E, Demers L. Menstrual status in female athletes: correlation with reproductive hormones and bone density. *Obstet Gynecol* 1988;72:683.
116. Hale RW, Kosasa T, Krieger J, et al. A marathon: the immediate effect on female runners' luteinizing hormone, follicle-stimulating hormone, prolactin, testosterone, and cortisol levels. *Am J Obstet Gynecol* 1983;146:550.

117. Shangold MM, Gatz ML, Thysen B. Acute effects of exercise on plasma concentration of prolactin and testosterone in recreational women runners. *Fertil Steril* 1981;35:699.
118. Chin WN, Chang FE, Doods WG, et al. Acute effects of exercise on plasma catecholamines in sedentary and athletic women with normal and abnormal menses. *Am J Obstet Gynecol* 1987;157:938.
119. Loucks AB, Mortola JF, Girton L, et al. Alternations in the hypothalamic-pituitary-ovarian and the hypothalamic-pituitary-adrenal axes in athletic women. *J Clin Endocrinol Metab* 1989:68:402.
120. Loucks AB, Laughlin GA, Mortola JF, et al. Hypothalamic-pituitary-thyroidal function in eumenorrheic and amenorrheic athletes. *J Clin Endocrinol Metab* 1992;75:514.
121. Kanaley JA, Boileau RA, Bahr JM, et al. Cortisol levels during prolonged exercise: the influence of menstrual phase and menstrual status. *Int J Sports Med* 1992;13:332.
122. Mansfield MJ, Emans SJ. Growth in female gymnasts: should training decrease during puberty? *J Pediatr* 1993;122:237.
123. Bonjour J, Theintz G, Buchs B, et al. Critical years and stages of puberty for spinal and femoral bone mass accumulation during adolescence. *J Clin Endocrinol Metab* 1991;73:555.
124. Theintz G, Buchs B, Rizzoli R, et al. Longitudinal monitoring of bone mass accumulation in healthy adolescent: evidence for a marked reduction after 16 years of age at the levels of lumbar spine and femoral neck in female subjects. *J Clin Endocrinol Metab* 1992;75:1060.
125. Slemenda CW, Reister TK, Hui SL, et al. Influences on skeletal mineralization in children and adolescents: evidence for varying effects of sexual maturation and physical activity. *J Pediatr* 1994;125: 210.
126. Gilsanz V, Roe TF, Mora S, et al. Changes in vertebral bone density in black girls and white girls during childhood and puberty. *N Engl J Med* 1991;325:1597.
127. Lloyd T, Andon MB, Rollings N, et al. Calcium supplementation and bone mineral density in adolescent girls. *JAMA* 1993;270:841.
128. Rubin K, Schirduan V, Gendreau P, et al. Predictors of axial and peripheral bone mineral density in healthy children and adolescents, with special attention to the role of puberty. *J Pediatr* 1993;123: 863.
129. Recker RR, Davies KM, Hinders SM. Bone gain in young adult women. *JAMA* 1992;268:2403.
130. Suominen H. Bone mineral density and long term exercise. *Sports Med* 1993;16:316.
131. Cann CE, Martin MC, Genant HK, et al. Decreased spinal mineral content in amenorrheic women. *JAMA* 1984;251:626.
132. Marcus R, Cann C, Madvig P, et al. Menstrual function and bone mass in elite women distance runners: endocrine and metabolic features. *Ann Intern Med* 1985;102:158.
133. Drinkwater BL, Nilson K, Chesnut CH, et al. Bone mineral content of amenorrheic and eumenorrheic athletes. *N Engl J Med* 1984;311:277.
134. Myerson M, Gutin B, Warren MP, et al. Total body bone density in amenorrheic runners. *Obstet Gynecol* 1992;79:973.
135. Louis O, Demeirleir K, Kalender W, et al. Low vertebral bone density values in young non-elite female runners. *Int J Sports Med* 1991;12:214.
136. Wolman RL, Clark P, McNally E, et al. Dietary calcium as a statistical determinant of spinal trabecular bone density in amenorrhoeic and oestrogen-replete athletes. *Bone Miner* 1992;17:415.
137. Drinkwater BL, Bruemner B, Chesnut CH. Menstrual history as a determinant of current bone density in young athletes. *JAMA* 1990:263:545.
138. Slemenda CW, Johnston CC. High intensity activities in young women: site specific bone mass effects among female figure skaters. *Bone Miner* 1993;20:125.
139. Rencken ML, Chesnut CH, Drinkwater BL. Bone density at multiple skeletal sites in amenorrheic athletes. *JAMA* 1996;276:238.
140. Wolman RL, Clark P, McNally E, et al. Menstrual state and exercise as determinants of spinal trabecular bone density in female athletes. *BMJ* 1990;301:516.
141. Young N, Formica C, Szmukler G, et al. Bone density at weight-bearing and nonweight-bearing sites in ballet dancers: the effects of exercise, hypogonadism, and body weight. *J Clin Endocrinol Metab* 1994;78:449.
142. Warren MP, Gunn J, Fox RP, Lancelot C, et al. Lack of bone accretion and amenorrhea: evidence for a relative osteopenia in weight-bearing bones. *J Clin Endocrinol Metab* 1991;72:847.
143. Myburgh KH, Bachrach LK, Lewis B, et al. Low bone mineral density at axial and appendicular sites in amenorrheic athletes. *Med Sci Sports Exerc* 1993;25:1197.
144. Constantini NW. Clinical consequences of athletic amenorrhoea. *Sports Med* 1994;17:213.
145. Myburgh KH, Hutchins J, Fataar AB, et al. Low bone density is an etiologic factor for stress fractures in athletes. *Ann Intern Med* 1990;113:754.

146. Friedl KE, Nuovo JA. Factors associated with stress fractures in young Army women: indications for further research. *Mil Med* 1992;157:334.
147. Drinkwater BL, Nilson K, Ott S, et al. Bone mineral density after resumption of menses in amenorrheic athletes. *JAMA* 1986;256:380.
148. Jonnavithula S, Warren MP, Fox RP, Lazaro MI. Bone density is compromised in amenorrheic women despite return of menses: a 2-year study. *Obstet Gynecol* 1993:81:669.
149. Thomas KA, Cook SD, Bennett JT, et al. Femoral neck and lumbar spine bone mineral densities in a normal population 3–20 years of age. *J Pediatr Orthop* 1990;11:48.
150. Hergenroeder AC, Phillips S. Advising teenagers and young adults about weight gain and loss through exercise and diet: practical advice for the physician. In: Shenker IR, ed. *Adolescent medicine*. Chur, Switzerland: Harwood Academic Publishers, 1994.
151. Chang RJ, Keye WR, Young JR. Detection, evaluation, and treatment of pituitary microadenomas in patients with galactorrhea and amenorrhea. *Am J Obstet Gynecol* 1977;128:356.
152. Cowden EA, Thomson JA, Doyle D, et al. Tests of prolactin secretion in diagnosis of prolactinomas. *Lancet* 1979;1:1156.
153. Forsbach G, Soria J, Canales E, et al. Gonadotropic responsiveness to clomiphene, LH, estradiol, and bromocriptine in galactorrheic women. *Obstet Gynecol* 1977;50:139.
154. Reichlin S. The prolactinoma problem. *N Engl J Med* 1979;300:313.
155. Weibe RH, Hammond CB, Handwerger S. Prolactin-secreting pituitary microadenoma: detection and evaluation. *Fertil Steril* 1978;29:282.
156. Kleinberg DL, Noel GL, Frantz AG. Galactorrhea: a study of 235 cases, including 48 with pituitary tumors. *N Engl J Med* 1977;296:589.
157. Blackwell RE, Younger JB. Long-term medical therapy and follow-up of pediatric-adolescent patients with prolactin-secreting macroadenomas. *Fertil Steril* 1986;45:713.
158. Schlechte JA, Sherman BM, Chapler FK, et al. Long-term follow-up of women with surgically treated prolactin-secreting pituitary tumors. *J Clin Endocrinol Metab* 1986;62:1296.
159. Pereira MC, Sobrinho LG, Afonso AM, et al. Is idiopathic hyperprolactinemia a transitional stage toward prolactinoma? *Obstet Gynecol* 1987;70:305.
160. Sisam DA, Sheehan JP, Sheeler LR. The natural history of untreated microprolactinomas. *Fertil Steril* 1987;48:67.
161. Rasmussen C, Bergh T, Wide L. Prolactin secretion and menstrual function after longterm bromocriptine treatment. *Fertil Steril* 1987;48:550.
162. Serri O. Progress in the management of hyperprolactinemia. *N Engl J Med* 1994;331:942.
163. Kane LA, Leinung MC, Scheithauer BW, et al. Pituitary adenomas in childhood and adolescence. *J Clin Endocrinol Metab* 1994;79:1135.
164. Dessypris A, Karonen SL, Adlercreutz H. Marathon run effects on plasma prolactin and growth hormone. *Acta Endocrinol (Copenh) (Suppl)* 1979;255:187.
165. Noel GL, Suh HK, Stone JG, et al. Human prolactin and growth hormone release during surgery and other conditions of stress. *J Clin Endocrinol Metab* 1972;35:840.
166. Dawajan V, Kletsky O, March CM. The significance of galactorrhea in patients with normal menses, oligomenorrhea, and secondary amenorrhea. *Am J Obstet Gynecol* 1978;130:894.
167. Klibanski A, Neer RM, Beitins IZ, et al. Decreased bone density in hyperprolactinemic women. *N Engl J Med* 1980;303:1511.
168. Klibanski A, Greenspan SL. Increase in bone mass after treatment of hyperprolactinemia amenorrhea. *N Engl J Med* 1986;315:542.
169. Biller BMK, Baum HBA, Rosenthal DI, et al. Progressive trabecular osteopenia in women with hyperprolactinemic amenorrhea. *J Clin Endocrinol Metab* 1992;75:692.
170. Schlecte J, Walkner L, Kathol M. A longitudinal analysis of premenopausal bone loss in healthy women and women with hyperprolactinemia. *J Clin Endocrinol Metab* 1992;75:698.
171. Sluijmer AV, Lappohn RE. Clinical history and outcome of 59 patients with idiopathic hyperprolactinemia. *Fertil Steril* 1992;58:72.
172. Schlechte J, Dolan K, Sherman B, et al. The natural history of untreated hyperprolactinemia: a prospective analysis. *J Clin Endocrinol Metab* 1989;68:412.
173. Koppelman MCS, Jaffe MJ, Rieth KG, et al. Hyperprolactinemia, amenorrhea, and galactorrhea: a retrospective assessment of twenty-five cases. *Ann Intern Med* 1984;100:115.
174. Jeffcoate WJ, Pound N, Sturrock ND, et al. Long-term followup of patients with hyperprolactinemia. *Clin Endocrinol* 1996;45:299.
175. Loriaux DL, Wild RA. Contraceptive choices for women with endocrine complications. *Am J Obstet Gynecol* 1993;168:2021.

176. Corenblum B, Donovan L. The safety of physiological estrogen plus progestin replacement therapy and with oral contraceptive therapy in women with pathological hyperprolactinemia. *Fertil Steril* 1993;59:671.
177. Post KD, Biller BJ, Adelman LS. Selective transphenoidal adenomectomy in women with galactorrhea-amenorrhea. *JAMA* 1979;242:158.
178. Keye WR, Chang RT, Monroe SE, et al. Prolactin-secreting pituitary adenomas in women: II. Menstrual function, pituitary reserves, and prolactin production following microsurgical removal. *Am J Obstet Gynecol* 1979;134:360.
179. Serri O, Rasio E, Beauregard H, et al. Recurrence of hyperprolactinemia after selective transphenoidal adenomectomy in women with prolactinoma. *N Engl J Med* 1983;309:280.
180. Maira G, Anile C, DeMarinis L, et al. Prolactin-secreting adenomas—surgical results. *Can J Neurol Sci* 1990;17:67.
181. Thorner MO, Martin WH, Rogol AD, et al. Rapid regression of pituitary prolactinomas during bromocriptine treatment. *J Clin Endocrinol Metab* 1980;51:438.
182. Tyson D, Reggiardo D, Sklar C, et al. Prolactin-secreting macroadenomas in adolescents. Response to bromocriptine therapy. *Am J Dis Child* 1993;147:1057.
183. Horvath E, Kovacs K, Smyth HS, et al. A novel type of pituitary adenoma: morphological features and clinical correlations. *J Clin Endocrinol Metab* 1988;66:1111.
184. Shewchuk AB, Adamson GD, Lessard P, et al. The effect of pregnancy on suspected pituitary adenomas after conservative management of ovulation defects associated with galactorrhea. *Am J Obstet Gynecol* 1980;136:659.
185. Griffith RW, Turkalj I, Braun P. Outcome of pregnancy in mothers given bromocriptine. *Br J Clin Pharmacol* 1978;5:227.
186. Vermesh M, Fossum GT, Kletzky OA. Vaginal bromocriptine: pharmacology and effect on serum prolactin in normal women. *Obstet Gynecol* 1988;72:693.
187. Ciccarelli E, Touzel R, Besser M, et al. Terguride—a new dopamine agonist drug: a comparison of its neuroendocrine and side effect profile with bromocriptine. *Fertil Steril* 1988;49:589.
188. Webster J, Piscitelli G, Polli A, et al. A comparison of cabergoline and bromocriptine in the treatment of hyperprolactinemic amenorrhea. *N Engl J Med* 1994;331:904.
189. Verlaat JW, Croughs JM, Brownell J. Treatment of macroprolactinomas with a new non-ergot, long-acting dopaminergic drug, CV 205-502. *Clin Endocrinol* 1990;33:619.
190. Lengyuel AM, Mussio W, Imamura P, et al. Long-acting injectable bromocriptine (Parlodel LAR) in the chronic treatment of prolactin-secreting macroadenomas. *Fertil Steril* 1993;59:980.
191. Haase R, Jaspers C, Schulte HM, et al. Control of prolactin-secreting macroadenomas with parenteral, long-acting bromocriptine in 30 patients treated for up to 3 years. *Clin Endocrinol* 1993;38:165.
192. Ciccarelli E, Grottoli, Miola C, et al. Double blind randomized study using oral or injectable bromocriptine in patients with hyperprolactinaemia. *Clin Endocrinol* 1994;40:193.
193. Davajan V, Kletzky O, Vermesh M, Anderson DJ. Ten-year follow-up of patients with secondary amenorrhea and normal prolactin. *Am J Obstet Gynecol* 1991;164:1666.
194. Weiss NS, Ure CL, Ballard JH, et al. Decreased risk of fractures of the hip and lower forearm and postmenopausal use of estrogen. *N Engl J Med* 1980;303:1195.
195. Lindsay R. Estrogen therapy in the prevention and management of osteoporosis. *Am J Obstet Gynecol* 1987;156:1347.
196. Ettinger B, Genant HK, Cann CE. Long-term estrogen replacement therapy prevents bone loss and fractures. *Ann Intern Med* 1985;102:319.
197. The Writing Group for the PEPI Trial. Effect of hormone therapy on bone mineral density. *JAMA* 1996;276:1389.
198. Johansen BW, Kaij L, Kullander S, et al. On some late effects of bilateral oophorectomy in the age range 15–30 years. *Acta Obstet Gynecol Scand* 1975;54:449.
199. Lobo RA, Pickar JH, Wild RA, et al. Metabolic impact of adding medroxyprogesterone acetate to conjugated estrogen therapy in postmenopausal women. *Obstet Gynecol* 1994;84:987.
200. Weighing the risks and benefits of hormone replacement therapy after menopause. *The Contraception Report* 1995;VI:1.
201. Davidson NE. Hormone-replacement therapy-breast versus heart versus bone [Editorial]. *N Engl J Med* 1995;332:1638.
202. Whitcroft SI, Crook D, Marsh MS, et al. Long-term effects of oral and transdermal hormone replacement therapies on serum lipid and lipoprotein concentrations. *Obstet Gynecol* 1994;84:222.
203. Colditz GA, Hankinson SE, Hunter DJ, et al. The use of estrogens and progestins and the risk of breast cancer in postmenopausal women. *N Engl J Med* 1995;332:1589.

204. Stanford JL, Weiss NS, Voight LF, et al. Combined estrogen and progestin hormone replacement therapy in relation to risk of breast cancer in middle-aged women. *JAMA* 1995;274:137.
205. Shangold M, Rebar RW, Wentz AC, Schiff I. Evaluation and management of menstrual dysfunction in athletes. *JAMA* 1990;263:1665.
206. NIH Consensus Development Panel. Optimal calcium intake. *JAMA* 1994;272:1942.
207. Chan GM, Hoffman K, McMurry M. Effects of dairy products on bone and body composition in pubertal girls. *J Pediatr* 1995;126:551.
208. Benjamin I, Block RE. Endometrial response to estrogen and progesterone therapy in patients with gonadal dysgenesis. *Obstet Gynecol* 1977;50:136.
209. Van Campenhout J, Choquette P, Vauclair R. Endometrial pattern in patients with primary hypoestrogenic amenorrhea receiving estrogen replacement therapy. *Obstet Gynecol* 1980;56:349.
210. Ross AH, Boyd ME, Colgan TJ, et al. Comparison of transdermal and oral sequential gestagen in combination with transdermal estradiol: effects on bleeding patterns and endometrial histology. *Obstet Gynecol* 1993;82:773.
211. Woodruff JD, Pickar JH. Incidence of endometrial hyperplasia in postmenopausal women taking conjugated estrogens (Premarin) with medroxyprogesterone acetate or conjugated estrogens alone. *Am J Obstet Gynecol* 1994;170:1213.
212. Hirvonen E, Malkonen M, Manninen V. Effects of different progestogens on lipoproteins during postmenopausal replacement therapy. *N Engl J Med* 1981;340:560.
213. The Writing Group for the PEPI Trial. Effects of estrogen or estrogen/progestin regimens on heart disease risk factors in postmenopausal women. The Postmenopausal Estrogen/Progestin Interventions (PEPI) trial. *JAMA* 1995;273:199.
214. Padwick ML, Pryse-Davies J, Whitehead MI. A simple method for determining the optimal dosage of progestin in postmenopausal women receiving estrogens. *N Engl J Med* 1986;315:930.
215. Prior JC, Vigna YM, Barr SI, et al. Cyclic medroxyprogesterone treatment increase bone density. *Am J Med* 1994;96:521.
216. Riggs BL, Wahner HW, Dunn WL, et al. Differential changes in bone mineral density of the appendicular and axial skeleton with aging: relationship to spinal osteoporosis. *J Clin Invest* 1981;67:328.
217. Horsman A, Jones M, Francis R, et al. The effect of estrogen dose on postmenopausal bone loss. *N Engl J Med* 1983;309:1405.
218. Quigley ME, Martin PL, Burnier AM, et al. Estrogen therapy arrests bone loss in elderly women. *Am J Obstet Gynecol* 1987;156:1516.
219. Lindsay R, Hart DM, Clark DM. The minimum effective dose of estrogen for prevention of postmenopausal bone loss. *Obstet Gynecol* 1984;63:759.
220. Ettinger B, Genant HK, Steiger P, Madvig P. Low-dosage micronized 17 β-estradiol prevents bone loss in postmenopausal women. *J Obstet Gynecol* 1992;166:479.
221. Ettinger B, Selby J, Citron JT, et al. Cyclic hormone replacement therapy using quarterly progestin. *Obstet Gynecol* 1994;83:693.
222. Cachrimanidow A-C, Hellber D, Nilsson S, et al. Long-interval treatment regimen with a desogestrel-containing oral contraceptive. *Contraception* 1993;48:205.
223. Bachrach LK, Katzman DK, Litt IF, et al. Recovery from osteopenia in adolescent girls with anorexia nervosa. *J Clin Endocrinol Metab* 1991;72:602.
224. Klibanski A, Biller BM, Schoenfeld DA, et al. The effects of estrogen administration on trabecular bone loss in young women with anorexia nervosa. *J Clin Endocrinol Metab* 1995;80:898.
225. Seeman E, Szmukler GI, Formica C, et al. Osteoporosis in anorexia nervosa: the influence of peak bone density, bone loss, oral contraceptive use, and exercise. *J Bone Miner Res* 1992:7:1467.
226. Mora S, Wever G, Guarneri MP, et al. Effect of estrogen replacement therapy on bone mineral content in girls with Turner syndrome. *Obstet Gynecol* 1992;79:747.
227. Rosenbloom AL, Frias JL. Oxandrolone for growth promotion in Turner's syndrome. *Am J Dis Child* 1973;125:385.
228. Urban MD, Lee PA, Dorst JP, et al. Oxandrolone therapy in patients with Turner's syndrome. *J Pediatr* 1979;94:823.
229. Sybert VP. Adult height in Turner syndrome with and without androgen therapy. *J Pediatr* 1984;104:365.
230. Ross JL, Cassorla FG, Skerda MC, et al. A preliminary study of the effect of estrogen dose on growth in Turner's syndrome. *N Engl J Med* 1983;309:1104.
231. Ross JL, Long LM, Skerda M, et al. Effect of low doses of estradiol on 6-month growth rates and predicted height in patients with Turner syndrome. *J Pediatr* 1986;109:950.

232. Martinez A, Heinrich JJ, Domene H, et al. Growth in Turner's syndrome: long-term treatment with low dose ethinyl estradiol. *J Clin Endocrinol Metab* 1987;65:253.
233. Demetriou E, Emans SJ, Crigler JF, Jr. Final height in estrogen treated patients with Turner syndrome. *Obstet Gynecol* 1984;64:459.
234. Rosenfeld RG, Hintz RL, Johanson AJ, et al. Three year results of a randomized prospective trial of methionyl human growth hormone and oxandrolone in Turner syndrome. *J Pediatr* 1988;113:393.
235. Raiti S, Moore WV, Van Vliet G, et al. Growth-stimulating effects human growth hormone therapy in patients with Turner syndrome. *J Pediatr* 1986;109:944.
236. Rosenfeld RG, Frane J, Attie KM, et al. Six-year results of a randomized, prospective trial of human growth hormone and oxandrolone in Turner syndrome. *J Pediatr* 1992;121:49.
237. Vandershueren-Lodeweyckx MV, Massa AG, et al. Growth-promoting effect of growth hormone and low dose ethinyl estradiol in girls with Turner's syndrome. *J Clin Endocrinol Metab* 1990; 70:122.
238. Van den Broeck J, Massa GG, Attanasio A, et al. Final height after long-term growth hormone treatment in Turner syndrome. *J Pediatr* 1995;127:729.
239. Massa G, Maes M, Heinrichs C, et al. Influence of spontaneous or induced puberty on the growth promoting effect of treatment with growth hormone in girls with Turner's syndrome. *Clin Endocrinol* 1993;38:253.
240. Navot D, Laufer N, Kopolovic J, et al. Artificially induced endometrial cycles and establishment of pregnancies in the absence of ovaries. *N Engl J Med* 1986;314:806.
241. Seibel MM. A new era in reproductive technology: in vitro fertilization, gamete intrafallopian transfer, and donated gametes and embryos. *N Engl J Med* 1988;316:828.
242. Asch RH, Balmaceda JP, Ord T, et al. Oocyte donation and gamete intrafallopian transfer in premature ovarian failure. *Fertil Steril* 1988;49:263.
243. Alper MM, Jolly EE, Garner PR. Pregnancies after premature ovarian failure. *Obstet Gynecol* 1986;67:59S.
244. Kreiner D, Droesch K, Navot D, et al. Spontaneous and pharmacologically induced remissions in patients with premature ovarian failure. *Obstet Gynecol* 1988;72:926.
245. Corenblum B, Rowe T, Taylor PJ. High-dose, short-term glucocorticoids for the treatment of infertility resulting from premature ovarian failure. *Fertil Steril* 1993;59:988.
246. Kim HH, Laufer MR. Developmental abnormalities of the female reproductive tract. *Curr Opin Obstet Gynecol* 1994;6:518.
247. Rutgers JL, Scully RE. The androgen insensitivity syndrome (testicular feminization): a clinicopathologic study of 43 cases. *Int J Gynecol Pathol* 1991;10:126.
248. Griffin JE. Androgen resistance: the clinical and molecular spectrum. *N Engl J Med* 1992;326:611.
249. Siegel SF. Molecular genetics of androgen insensitivity. *Adolesc Pediatr Gynecol* 1995;8:3.
250. Normann EK, Trystad O, Larsen S, et al. Height reduction in 539 tall girls treated with three different dosages of ethinylestradiol. *Arch Dis Child* 1991;66:1275.
251. Bailey JD, Park E, Cowell C. Estrogen treatment of girls with constitutional tall statute. *Pediatr Clin North Am* 1981;28:501.
252. Werder EA, Waibel P, Sege D, et al. Severe thrombosis during oestrogen treatment for tall stature. *Eur J Pediatr* 1990;149:389.
253. Money J, Schwartz M. Dating, romantic and nonromantic friendships, and sexuality in 17 early treated adrenogenital females, age 16–25. In: Lee PA, Plotnick LP, Kowarski AA, et al, eds. *Congenital adrenal hyperplasia.* Baltimore: University Press, 1977.
254. Federman D. *Abnormal sexual development.* Philadelphia: WB Saunders, 1968.
255. Hadjiathanasiou CG, Brauner R, Lortat-Jacob S, et al. True hermaphroditism: genetic variants and clinical management. *J Pediatr* 1994:125:738.
256. Johnson J, Whitaker AH. Adolescent smoking, weight changes, and binge purge behaviors: associations with secondary amenorrhea. *Am J Public Health* 1992;82:47.
257. Laufer MR, Floor AE, Parsons KE, et al. Hormone testing in women with adult-onset amenorrhea. *Gynecol Obstet Invest* 1995;40:200.
258. Emans SJ, Grace E, Goldstein DP. Oligomenorrhea in adolescent girls. *J Pediatr* 1980;97:815.
259. Ansel S, Jones G. Etiology and treatment of dysfunctional uterine bleeding. *Obstet Gynecol* 1974;44:1.
260. Apter D, Vihko R. Early menarche, a risk factor for breast cancer, indicated early onset of ovulatory cycles. *J Clin Endocrinol Metab* 1983:57:82.
261. Treloar AE, Boynton RE, Behn BG, et al. Variation in the human menstrual cycle through preproductive life. *Int J Fertil* 1970;12:77.

262. Fraser IS, McCarron G, Markham R. A preliminary study of factors influencing perception of menstrual blood loss volume. *Am J Obstet Gynecol* 1984;149:788.
263. Soff GA, Green D. Autoantibody to von Willebrand factor in systemic lupus erythematosus. *J Lab Clin Med* 1993;121:424.
264. Eldred JM, Thomas EJ. Pituitary and ovarian hormone levels in unexplained menorrhagia. *Obstet Gynecol* 1994;84:774.
265. Claessens EA, Cowell CA. Acute adolescent menorrhagia. *Am Obstet Gynecol* 1981;139:277.
266. Claessens EA, Cowell CA. Dysfunctional uterine bleeding in the adolescent. *Pediatr Clin North Am* 1981,28:369.
267. Falcone T, Desjardins C, Bourque J, et al. Dysfunctional uterine bleeding in adolescent. *J Reprod Med* 1994;39:761.
268. Altchek A. Dysfunctional uterine bleeding in adolescence. *Clin Obstet Gynecol* 1977;20:633.
269. Bayer SR, DeCherney AH. Clinical manifestations and treatment of dysfunctional uterine bleeding. *JAMA* 1993;269:1823.
270. Hillard PA. Abnormal uterine bleeding in adolescents. *Contemp Pediatr* 1995;12:79.
271. Athen PI, Henderson MC, Witz CA. Abnormal uterine bleeding. *Med Clin North Am* 1995;79:329.
272. Cowan BD, Morrison JC. Management of abnormal genital bleeding in girls and women. *N Engl J Med* 1991;324:1710.
273. Fraser IS, Pearse C, Shearman RP, et al. Efficacy of mefenamic acid in patients with a complaint of menorrhagia. *Obstet Gynecol* 1981;58:543.
274. Devore GR, Owens O, Kase N. Use of intravenous premarin in the treatment of dysfunctional uterine bleeding—a double-blind randomized control study. *Obstet Gynecol* 1982;59:285.
275. Laufer MR, Townsend NL, Parsons KE, et al. The use of leuprolide acetate for the induction of amenorrhea in women undergoing bone marrow transplantation (BMT): a pilot study. *J Reprod Med* 1997;42:(in press).
276. Laufer MR, Rein MS. Treatment of abnormal uterine bleeding with gonadotropin-releasing hormone analogues. *Clin Obstet Gynecol* 1993;36:668.
277. Ghalie R, Porter C, Radwanska E, et al. Prevention of hypermenorrhea with leuprolide in premenopausal women undergoing bone marrow transplantation. *Am J Hematol* 1993;42:350.
278. Wingfield M, McClure N, Mamers PM, et al. Endometrial ablation: an option for the management of menstrual problems in the intellectually disabled. *Med J Aust* 1994;160:533.
279. Southam AL, Richart RM. The prognosis for adolescents with menstrual abnormalities. *Am J Obstet Gynecol* 1966;94:637.

FURTHER READING

Rieser PA, Underwood LE. Turner's syndrome: a guide for families. Turner Society, 1992.

Rosenfeld RG. Turner's syndrome: a guide for physicians. The Turner's Syndrome Society. Gardiner-Caldwell Synermed, 1992.

7

Endocrine Abnormalities Associated with Hirsutism

Signs of androgen excess, especially hirsutism and acne, can be a troubling problem for the adolescent and young adult woman. Although the degree of hirsutism may be related to familial, racial, or ethnic factors that determine the capacity of the hair follicle to respond to androgens, in most cases excess androgen production from the ovaries and/or adrenal glands is responsible for the clinical problem of hirsutism. Oligomenorrhea or anovulatory dysfunctional uterine bleeding accompanying the signs of androgen excess should especially alert the clinician to the possibility of polycystic ovary syndrome (PCO). Whatever the cause of the hirsutism, the patient will benefit from a careful explanation of the etiology, diagnosis, and therapy, since acne and hirsutism may have a negative impact on the self-image of the maturing adolescent.

DEFINING HIRSUTISM

Two types of hair are found on the human body: terminal hair (>0.5 cm long, coarse, and usually pigmented) and vellus or lanugo hair (downy, fine, and light-colored). Terminal hairs undergo several phases, including a growing phase (anagen), an involutional phase (catagen), and a resting phase (telogen). The initiation of anagen is influenced by hormonal factors. The distribution and number of the pilosebaceous units (sebaceous gland and hair follicle) are largely determined by genetic factors but are influenced by endocrinologic factors such as the rate and amount of androgen secretion, the concentration of sex hormone–binding globulin (SHBG), the peripheral conversion of weak androgens to potent androgens, and the sensitivity of the pilosebaceous unit to androgens (1) (Fig. 1).

An increase in the distribution and quantity of terminal hair may bring the patient to the physician with the complaint of hirsutism. Hirsutism may also be noted by the physician during a routine physical examination or during an eval-

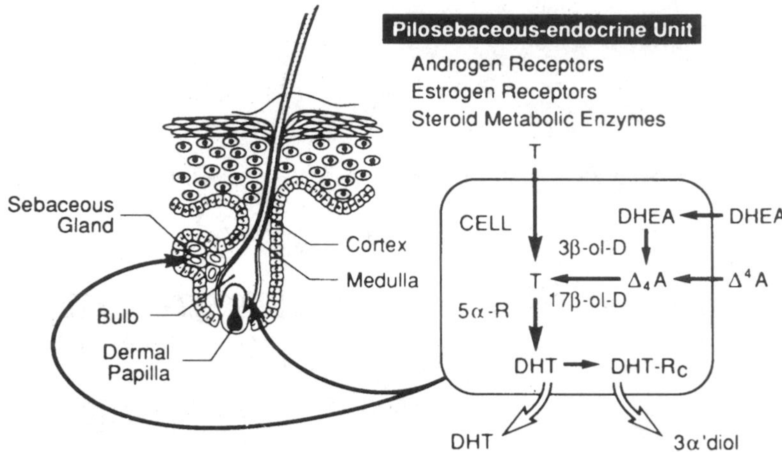

FIG. 1. Endocrinology of the pilosebaceous unit—a diagram of the pilosebaceous unit as an endocrine target as well as local modulation of endocrine microenvironments via enzymatic conversion of androgens to more potent androgen and to estrogens. Both dehydroepiandrosterone (DHEA) and Δ^4–A'dione (Δ^4–A) can be converted to testosterone (T) within the hair follicle. 3β–ol–D, 3β-hydroxysteroid dehydrogenase; 5α–R, 5α–reductase; DHT–R_C, dihydrotestesterone receptors. (Yen SSC. Chronic anovulation caused by peripheral disorders. In: Yen SSC, Jaffe RB, eds. *Reproductive endocrinology: physiology, pathophysiology, and clinical management,* 3rd ed. Philadelphia: WB Saunders, 1991:589; with permission.)

uation of irregular menses. Excessive downy hair is usually referred to as *hypertrichosis* and occurs, for example, in adolescents with anorexia nervosa.

The clinician may encounter difficulty in establishing whether the amount of hair is excessive, since the spectrum of "normal" is at best ill-defined. In a study of 400 young women in Wales, McKnight (2) reported that 84% of women had terminal hair on the lower arm and leg, 70% also had terminal hair on the upper arm and leg, and 26% had terminal hair on the face, usually on the upper lip. In 10% of the women, the facial hair was noticeable, and in 4%, it was characterized as a true disfigurement. Seventeen percent of women had hair on the chest or breast, usually periareolar; 35% had hair on the abdomen, usually along the linea alba up to the umbilicus; 16% had hair in the lumbosacral area; and 3% had hair on the upper back. Nine percent had considerable hair on most or all of these areas and were therefore considered hirsute. The appreciation of the degree of hirsutism is partially subjective and related to a comparison of the degree of hirsutism in the patient to that noted in other female family members. For this reason, scoring systems (see below) that are reproducible for different patients and followup visits are helpful (3,4).

ETIOLOGY OF HIRSUTISM

The differential diagnosis of hirsutism is listed in Table 1. Many patients with mild hirsutism and regular menses have a familial or ethnic predisposition.

TABLE 1. *Causes of hirsutism in adolescents*

Ovarian disorders
Polycystic ovary syndrome (PCO)
Hyperthecosis
Tumors
Enzyme deficiency (e.g., 17-ketosteroid reductase deficiency)
Adrenal disorders
Congenital adrenal hyperplasia (21-hydroxylase, 11β-hydroxylase, 3β-hydroxysteroid dehydrogenase deficiencies)
Cushing's disease
Tumors
Idiopathic hirsutism
Drugs (phenytoin, danazol, diazoxide, minoxidil, glucocorticoid excess, androgens, valproate)
Pregnancy
Hypothyroidism
Central nervous system injury
Hyperprolactinemia
Stress
Anorexia nervosa, malnutrition
Peripheral tissue
?Excessive activity of 5α-reductase and/or 17-ketosteroid reductase
Male pseudohermaphroditism, mixed gonadal dysgenesis

Drugs such as phenytoin, corticosteroids, danazol, diazoxide, minoxidil, anabolic steroids, and androgens cause hirsutism. In one study, 80% of women treated with valproate before the age of 20 years had PCO or hyperandrogenism (5). Pregnancy, hypothyroidism, anorexia nervosa, malnutrition, and chronic central nervous system disorders (e.g., mental and motor retardation) can be accompanied by excess hair growth.

Most cases of significant hirsutism result from the overproduction of androgens or their precursors from an ovarian and/or adrenal source (6–17). Most women with hirsutism have increased testosterone production rates, and increased levels of free testosterone are detectable in 80% to 85% of hirsute women. In cases in which hyperandrogenism is not detected, hirsutism may be due to an increased sensitivity of the follicle to low levels of androgen, increased conversion of testosterone to dihydrotestosterone (DHT), an androgen other than testosterone and androstenedione, an elevated level not detected because of the normal fluctuation of secretion, or the presence of more numerous hair follicles. Hirsutism in women with normal menses and normal testosterone levels appears to be related to increased 5α-reductase activity in the skin (18). In a study of women with PCO from the United States, Italy, and Japan, similar levels of luteinizing hormone (LH), testosterone, and estradiol were found, but levels of 3α-androstanediol (a reflection of utilization of androgens by target tissues) were high in women from Italy and the United States and normal in Japanese women, who had much less hirsutism (19). Testosterone induces the production of enzymes in the hair follicle, and thus once a terminal hair begins to grow, less androgen is required to stimulate its continued growth. This factor probably accounts, in part, for the fact that a less than optimal response is frequently achieved by hormone suppression therapy, which by biochemical parameters (lowering of free testosterone) should be successful.

Occasionally, stress may precipitate excess secretion of LH and increased production of androgens from the theca cells; the abnormal hormone production reverses when the acute stress is over. With her immature hypothalamic–pituitary–ovarian axis, an adolescent may be particularly prone to this type of disorder. In addition, adolescents with oligomenorrhea in the first few years after menarche may have mild elevations of androgens and a PCO-like picture. With time, most of these girls manifest the typical PCO picture, but some appear to progress to normal ovulatory cycles, having experienced a transient hyperandrogenism (20).

Hyperprolactinemia may be accompanied by increased secretion of adrenal androgens, especially dehydroepiandrosterone sulfate (DHEAS), because of prolactin receptors in the adrenal glands, and may also be associated with PCO. Hirsutism is mild, as the peripheral action of the androgens is limited because prolactin has a blocking action on the conversion of testosterone to DHT (1). The rare occurrence of male pseudohermaphroditism or mixed gonadal dysgenesis may be manifested by virilization at puberty. Any signs of rapid progression of hirsutism or the presence of virilization (clitoromegaly, temporal hair recession, deepening of the voice, changes in muscle pattern) should prompt an immediate assessment of hormone status to exclude the possibility of an androgen-producing tumor or male gonad.

Production of Androgens

The rate of testosterone production in adult women correlates most closely with the degree of hirsutism/virilization. Mildly increased facial hair; increased facial hair and menstrual disturbances; and facial hair, menstrual disturbances, and clitoromegaly represent a spectrum of hirsutism that corresponds to stepwise levels of increased testosterone production (21,22). Free or unbound testosterone levels correlate better than *total* testosterone levels with the clinical signs of hirsutism and testosterone production rate. All but a small fraction of serum testosterone is bound: tightly to SHBG, also termed testosterone-estradiol binding globulin (TEBG), and more weakly bound to albumin. Free and albumin-bound testosterone are the biologically active forms (12). Although normal adult women have twice the SHBG concentration of normal men, hirsute women with elevated androgen levels have SHBG levels lower than those of normal women.

The sources of androgens are noted in Fig. 2. The relative contributions vary during the menstrual cycle and with the time of day (18,23). The major adrenal androgens are dehydroepiandrosterone (DHEA) and its sulfate, DHEAS; androstenedione; and testosterone. The stroma and theca interna of the ovaries secrete primarily testosterone and androstenedione. In normal women, approximately 80% to 90% of DHEA is secreted by the adrenal glands and 10% to 20%

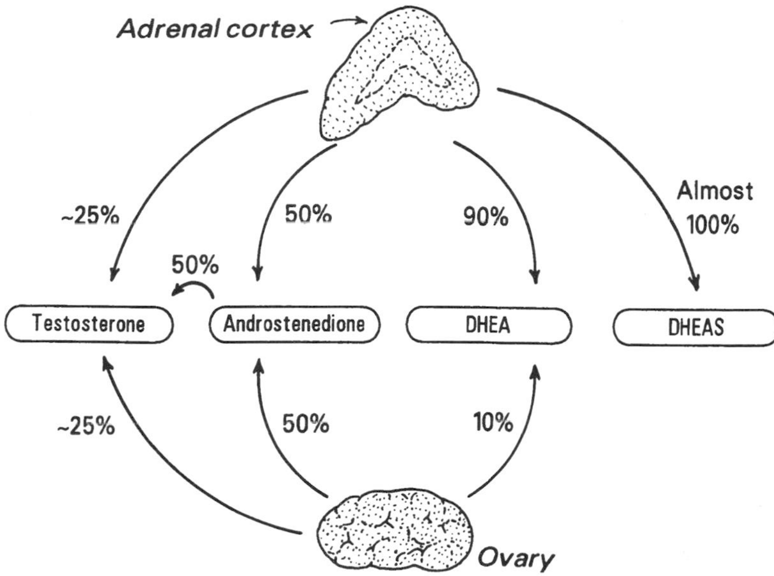

FIG. 2. Source of androgens in adult women. DHEA, dehydroepiandrosterone; DHEAS, DHEA sulfate.

by the ovaries. More than 90% of DHEAS is secreted by the adrenal glands. The diurnal variation of DHEA is similar to that of cortisol, with peak levels in the early morning. DHEAS has a long half-life, with less fluctuation in levels, and thus, measurement of DHEAS is more easily interpreted in the evaluation of hirsute patients. Androstenedione is secreted equally by the adrenal glands and the ovaries in normal women.

The source of testosterone is variable: 0% to 30% comes from the adrenal glands, 5% to 25% from the ovaries, and 50% to 60% is produced by the peripheral conversion of precursors, such as DHEA and androstenedione. In hirsute women with PCO, the ovaries are responsible for a much greater percentage of the testosterone production. Virtually all DHT comes from peripheral conversion of testosterone through the enzymatic action of 5α-reductase; it is the DHT that is the biologically active and potent androgen at the level of the hair follicle. The DHT from the pilosebaceous unit does not reenter the circulation as DHT but rather as 3α-androstanediol glucuronide.

Polycystic Ovary Syndrome

Polycystic ovary (PCO) syndrome, sometimes termed functional ovarian hyperandrogenism, is the cause of hirsutism in most adolescent patients. *Polycystic ovary syndrome* is not a single, well-defined entity but rather a spectrum of clinical disorders associated with increased androgen production from the ovaries and frequently the adrenal glands as well, often with abnormal gonadotropin secretion and insulin resistance (11–15,18,19,24–28). Clinical presentations may vary and include hirsutism, obesity, oligomenorrhea, anovulation, and infertility. Adolescents with PCO usually have a normal age of menarche, although occasionally PCO may cause delayed menarche and hirsutism or virilization. Most, but certainly not all, adolescents with PCO are overweight for height. The majority of patients have irregular menses from the time of menarche and often have hirsutism and/or acne beginning either before or around the time of menarche. The abnormal gonadotropin secretory patterns associated with PCO are apparent very early in adolescence, which suggests a central defect (29,30). Recent interest has also focused on the possible relationship between premature adrenarche and the later development of PCO in some adolescents. Patients identified as having mild defects in cortisol synthesis and those with adrenal hyperresponsiveness (exaggerated adrenarche) appear to be more likely to progress to PCO in adolescence than other girls (31–33). Emotional stress at puberty could perhaps cause increased adrenocorticotropic hormone (ACTH) production, adrenal sensitivity, or both. Since the percent conversion of androstenedione to estrone is related to body weight, obesity at the time of puberty and during adolescence and the normal insulin resistance that occurs with puberty could be additive factors (18,34,35). Obesity is also associated with lower levels of SHBG and higher levels of unbound testosterone (36). Only rarely have specific abnormalities in ovarian steroidogenesis (e.g., 17-ketosteroid reductase deficiency) been reported (37). There is a familial incidence of PCO, but the inheritance patterns have not been defined and are likely to reflect the heterogeneity of patterns of PCO.

A major feature of PCO is chronic anovulation. The pituitary gland has heightened sensitivity to gonadotropin-releasing hormone (GnRH) and exaggerated pulsatile release of LH with increased pulse frequency and amplitude. The LH levels are often tonically elevated, and the LH/FSH ratio may be elevated. The high LH levels stimulate the ovary to secrete increased amounts of androgen from the stromal tissue; the androgens are converted peripherally to estrone and estradiol. Estrogens, which are secreted tonically rather than cyclically, are hypothesized to augment pituitary sensitivity to GnRH (38–40) (Figs. 3 and 4). Under long-term LH stimulation, the polycystic ovaries secrete excess androstenedione and testosterone (10,11). The action of testosterone is further augmented because androgens decrease SHBG and thereby increase the level of free testosterone. In contrast, estrogen increases SHBG. Thus, sex steroids tend to amplify their own effects. In addition, nutritional factors and insulin also play important roles in determining the production of SHBG. In hirsute women, the low SHBG level facilitates the rapid uptake of free androgens and their peripheral conversion to estrogen. Peripheral conversion of androgens to estrogens takes place in muscle and adipose tissue, the latter being increased in many PCO patients, thus increasing estrogen production. With low levels of SHBG, PCO patients have free estrogen levels that are higher than in normal women in the

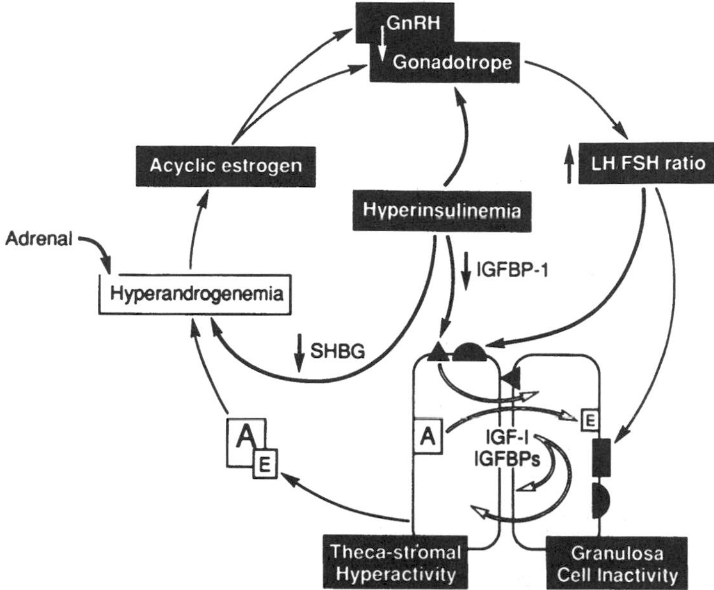

FIG. 3. Diagrammatic depiction of the interdependent events of an increased LH/FSH ratio, hyperinsulinemia, intraovarian autocrine and paracrine actions of insulin and insulin-like growth factors (IGFs), and IGF-binding proteins (BPs) in the development of hyperandrogenism and acyclic extraglandular estrogen formation that sustains the hyperactivity of the theca cells and inactivity of the granulosa cells in patients with polycystic ovarian syndrome. Adrenal contribution to the androgen pool may be an important clue to the pathogenesis of this syndrome. SHBG, sex hormone-binding globulin; GnRH, gonadotropin-releasing hormone; LH, luteinizing hormone; FSH, follicle-stimulating hormone; A, androgens; E, estrogens; ▲, insulin or IGF receptors; ◗, LH receptors; ■, FSH receptors. (Yen SSC. Chronic anovulation caused by peripheral endocrine disorders. In: Yen SSC, Jaffe RB, eds. *Reproductive endocrinology: physiology, pathophysiology, and clinical management,* 3rd Ed. Philadelphia: WB Saunders, 1991:602; with permission.)

midfollicular phase of the cycle (39). The constant, acyclic levels of estradiol cause abnormal feedback to the pituitary and hypothalamus, and prolonged unopposed stimulation of the endometrium by estradiol and estrone places the PCO patient at a higher risk of developing uterine cancer (41,42).

In contrast to the high LH levels in many patients with PCO, FSH levels are low to normal. The low levels may result from (a) the inhibitory feedback of estrogen on FSH, (b) the relative insensitivity of FSH secretion to GnRH, and (c) the production of inhibin from the polycystic ovaries that could inhibit the release of FSH (38,39). Estradiol may cause decreased dopamine secretion at the hypothalamic level that leads to increased GnRH pulses, which in turn may selectively increase LH secretion and LH bioactivity and decrease FSH secretion. In the ovary, a relative aromatase defect secondary to FSH deficiency and high intraovarian androgen levels impairs follicular maturation and cyclic production of estradiol and induces follicular atresia.

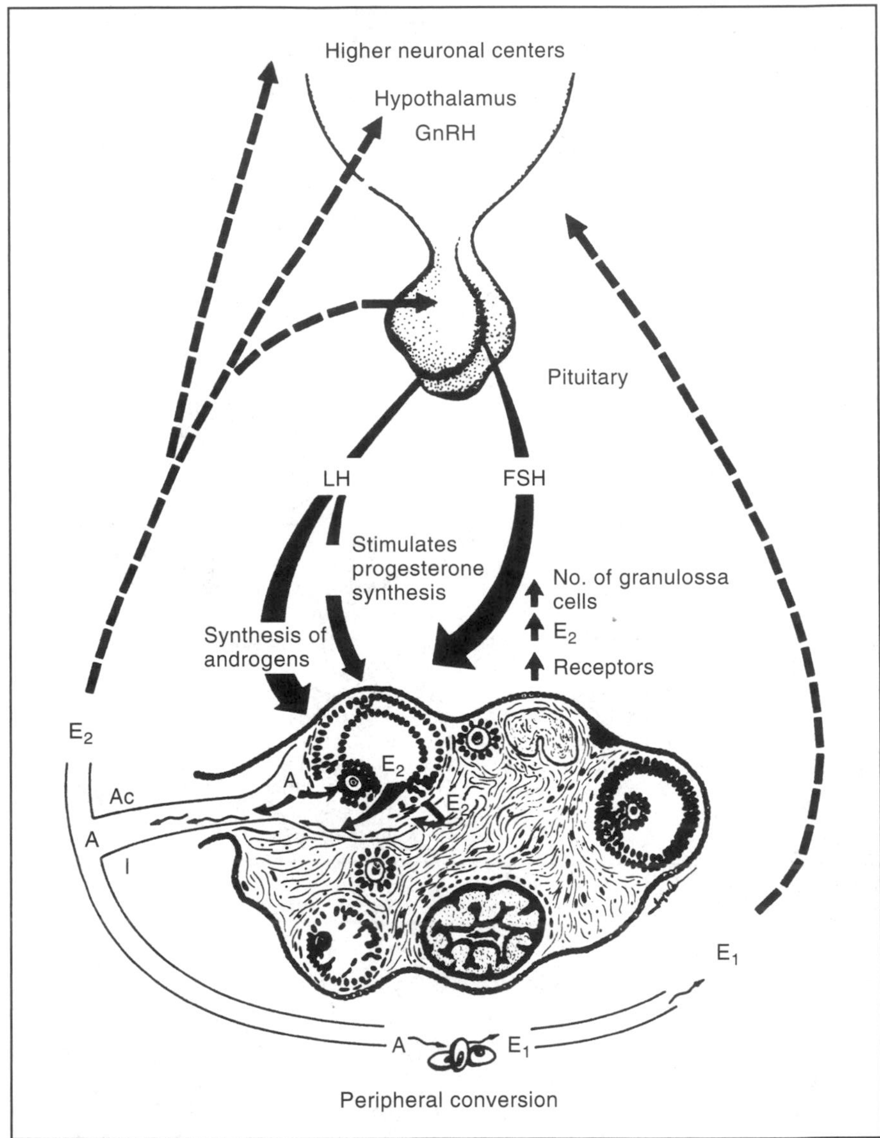

FIG. 4. Hypothalamic–pituitary–ovarian interaction in the regulation of follicular maturation and steroid biosynthesis. GnRH, gonadotropid-releasing hormone; LH, luteinizing hormone; FSH, follicle-stimulating hormone; E_2, estradiol; A, androstenedione; E_1, estrone; Ac, activin; I, inhibin. The ovary shows the various stages of growth of the follicle and the formation and regression of the corpus luteum.

Hyperinsulinemia is evident in many PCO patients in both the fasting and the glucose-stimulated states (10,43,44). The presence of acanthosis nigricans (velvety, verrucous, hyperpigmented skin often over the nape of the neck, in the axillae, beneath the breasts, and in the vulva and other body folds) (Fig. 5) has been associated with insulin resistance (44,45). Acanthosis nigricans (AN) consists of hyperkeratosis, epidermal papillomatosis, and hyperpigmentation. Growth factors thought to be responsible for the appearance of acanthosis nigricans include insulin, insulin-like growth factor-I (IGF-I), epidermal growth factor, and testosterone. If not associated with malignancy (unlikely in the young woman), AN is a relatively specific but not very sensitive marker for insulin resistance (IR). Barbieri and others (17) have suggested that the patient with AN should be considered to have or be at risk for the development of severe insulin resistance, ovarian stromal hyperthecosis, major lipid abnormalities including hypercholesterolemia, non–insulin-dependent diabetes mellitus (NIDDM) (44), and essential hypertension.

In 1983, Barbieri and Ryan (45) proposed a hypothesis linking hyperandrogenism (HA), insulin resistance (IR), and acanthosis nigricans (AN) as the HAIR-AN syndrome. The insulin resistance is probably due to post-binding defects in the insulin action pathway (10,45–47). Barbieri and associates (10) suggested that if women with significant ovarian androgen excess (serum testosterone >100 ng/dl) are studied, approximately 50% will have insulin resistance

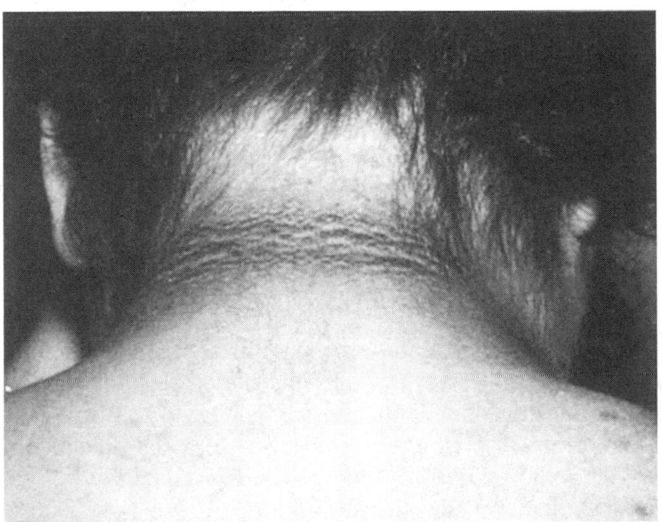

FIG. 5. Acanthosis nigricans. (From Yen SSC. Chronic anovulation caused by peripheral endocrine disorders. In: Yen SSC, Jaffe RB, eds. *Reproductive endocrinology: physiology, pathophysiology, and clinical management*, 3rd ed. Philadelphia: WB Saunders, 1991;576; with permission.)

and compensatory hyperinsulinemia. A positive correlation has been noted between fasting insulin levels and circulating testosterone and androstenedione levels (26). Caribbean Hispanic women have twice the prevalence of PCO of other ethnic groups and have an increased prevalence of insulin resistance (18,46). It is possible that the association of hyperandrogenism and insulin resistance in PCO syndrome represents a genetic linkage (45–47).

Barbieri and associates (10) have postulated that hyperinsulinemia and insulin resistance are not just associated with androgen excess but may play a role in causing the abnormalities in PCO. They have proposed that both insulin and LH regulate ovarian stromal and thecal androgen production. In support of the theory are in vitro studies that have shown that insulin and insulin-like growth factors (IGFs) can stimulate androgen accumulation in incubations of ovarian stroma obtained from hyperandrogenic women (48) and can regulate thecal and stromal responsiveness to gonadotropins (17). IGFs are associated with binding proteins (BP), which modulate their bioavailability (49). Even though tissues are insulin resistant, high levels of insulin may be able to stimulate ovarian androgen production by interacting with IGF-I receptors or by acting through a "nonclassic insulin receptor–intracellular messenger pathway" (17). Insulin also appears to inhibit the production of SHBG (47,50,51). Lowering androgen levels to the normal range in women with PCO using long-acting GnRH analogs, cyproterone acetate, or bilateral oophorectomy does not improve the insulin resistance, and thus the insulin resistance can be considered part of the syndrome (52). Of interest, a short-term glucose load can produce a large rise in insulin and increases in circulating androgens (androstenedione, testosterone, and dihydrotestosterone) in women with the HA-IR syndrome but not in control subjects or hyperandrogenic non-insulin-resistant women (53). However, the transient physiologic hyperinsulinemia produced by an oral glucose load (such as might occur with a normal meal) appears to be insufficient to produce hyperandrogenism (50). Obese women with PCO develop a greater degree of insulin resistance as body mass increases than do eumenorrheic controls (54).

Evidence is accumulating that improvement of insulin function may lead to improvement in some features of PCO. A small number of PCO patients treated with metformin, a biguanide drug that improves the action of insulin at the cellular level, showed an improvement in insulin sensitivity and a decrease in androgen levels and in some a return of menstrual cycles and three spontaneous pregnancies (55). Nestler and Jukubowicz (56) found that obese women with PCO given metformin showed a reduction in insulin and evidence of reduction of ovarian cytochrome p450c17α activity (decreased 17-hydroxyprogesterone (17-OHP) before and after leuprolide stimulation), decreased LH and free testosterone, and increased SHBG. Similar data are emerging on troglitazone, a new drug that decreases insulin resistance. In a study of 25 women with PCO, troglitazone improved insulin and reduced androgens and two women had ovulatory menses (57). The relationship between adrenal androgen secretion and insulin resistance continues to be elucidated (54,58).

Several other metabolic abnormalities have also been noted in women with PCO. In comparison with control subjects, women with PCO may have higher levels of triglycerides and very-low-density lipoprotein cholesterol and lower levels of high-density lipoprotein cholesterol, secondary to the obesity but also potentially related to the androgen excess (36,59,60). The risk of cardiovascular disease independent of the risk conferred by obesity is unknown. Twenty percent of obese PCO women have impaired glucose tolerance or frank NIDDM by their third to fourth decade of life (45).

Ovarian morphology in PCO is variable and ranges from normal-appearing ovaries to enlarged ovaries with a thickened glistening capsule ("oyster shell"), multiple small peripheral cysts, and increased stroma or hyperthecosis. The number of growing and atretic follicles is doubled in PCO patients to 20 to 100 cystic follicles.

The spectrum of ovarian pathology in ovarian androgen excess is mirrored in the ultrasound findings (13,61–66). The ovaries may appear normal on ultrasound, although more commonly the ovaries appear enlarged, with multiple (≥10 follicular cysts 2 to 8 mm in diameter) tiny cysts in a peripheral pattern underneath the cortex of the ovary, giving a "string of pearls" configuration (62). Ovarian stromal hyperechogenicity and increased cross-sectional area are common in PCO (17). In contrast, multicystic or multifollicular ovaries with the small cysts distributed throughout the ovary are more typical of early pubertal or perimenarcheal adolescents who are anovulatory. However, the distinction can be difficult, and Stanhope et al (63) have documented the progression from multicystic to polycystic in one adolescent with delayed menarche. Women with hirsutism and regular menses (idiopathic hirsutism) frequently have "polycystic ovaries" as demonstrated by ultrasound (65). "PCO-like" ovaries can occur in patients who have other sources of androgen excess, such as untreated or undiagnosed congenital adrenocortical hyperplasia (CAH) and adrenal adenomas or carcinomas, or in women who have conditions associated with chronic anovulation (including Cushing's disease, acromegaly, hypothyroidism, and hyperprolactinemia). Color flow Doppler ultrasound is also being explored. Ultrasound can help in defining the likely pathogenesis in some patients and in excluding some ovarian lesions, but it cannot be used to definitely rule out or in the diagnosis of PCO.

Barbieri and colleagues (10) have proposed two basic subgroupings of ovarian hyperandrogenism. Patients in one subgroup, HA-IR, have hyperandrogenism, marked insulin resistance, chronic hyperinsulinemia, normal or slightly elevated LH, and normal prolactin, often associated with ovarian stromal hyperthecosis. Ovarian hyperthecosis is characterized by the presence of islands of luteinized thecal cells in the ovarian stroma at a distance from the follicles (18). Testosterone levels are often markedly elevated. Patients in the second subgroup,

HA–non-IR, have hyperandrogenism, minimal insulin resistance, markedly elevated LH, and often slightly elevated prolactin.

Although only rarely is a true enzymatic deficiency in the ovaries demonstrable, Barnes and colleagues (67) have suggested that women with PCO have both pituitary and ovarian responses to the GnRH agonist nafarelin similar to those seen in normal men. They have hypothesized that regulation of cytochrome p450c17 (17-hydroxylase and C-17, 20-lyase) is abnormal and that this enzyme is overstimulated because of excessive levels of LH or because of an intrinsic defect within the thecal interstitial cells. Others have suggested that there is dysregulation of 11β-hydroxysteroid dehydrogenase in PCO (68). Thus, the ovaries may play more of a role than was originally suggested.

The role of the adrenal glands in the pathogenesis of PCO is controversial. Although many patients (up to 60%) with PCO have mildly to moderately elevated DHEAS levels (300 to 600 μg/dl) and evidence of hyperresponsive adrenal glands on ACTH testing and adrenal scintiscans (69,70), most adolescents with androgen excess do not have specific adrenal enzyme deficiencies. Lucky and colleagues (71) have hypothesized that some patients have an exaggerated adrenarche. New evidence has begun to shed some light on the etiology of the heightened adrenal sensitivity (14,72,73). Patients with PCO syndrome and elevated DHEAS produced more androgens in response to ACTH stimulation than did control women before, but not after, 2 months of ovarian suppression with GnRH agonists. Carmina et al (73) also documented a blunted response to ACTH with 6 months of ovarian suppression. The relative hyperestrogenic state of PCO syndrome may be an important factor in enhancing adrenal sensitivity. Insulin may also modulate adrenal androgen production (14).

Adrenal Enzyme Deficiencies

Depending on the population studied (ethnic origin and referral versus primary care practice), late-onset 21-hydroxylase deficiency, also termed nonclassic CAH, is found in 1% to 10% of adult women with hirsutism (32,74–83). Overall, the severe form of congenital adrenal hyperplasia with 21-hydroxylase deficiency is found in 1 of 12,000 and the mild or nonclassical form in 1 of 100 to 1 of 1000, depending on the population (3% among Ashkenazi Jews) (82,83). We reported 21-hydroxylase deficiency in 2 of 22 adolescent girls and young women with hirsutism (79), and Ibanez et al (32) found this deficiency in only 1 of 42. In 100 consecutive women with the classic features of PCO, Benjamin and colleagues (80) reported that 4% of women had homozygous CAH and 15% had heterozygous CAH.

New and colleagues (84,85) have been in the forefront of tracing much of the family pedigrees and genetics of patients with nonclassic 21-hydroxylase CAH. The enzyme 21-hydroxylase is a specific microsomal cytochrome P-450 (cytochrome p450c21). Nonclassic CAH is an autosomal recessive disorder with a gene located on chromosome 6, in proximity to the HLA locus. The association of this disorder with HLA-B14;DR1 has been a useful marker in distinguishing nonclassic from classic CAH, which is associated with HLA-Bw47;DR7 (84,85). Several mutations of the 21-hydroxylase gene have been associated with adrenal hyperplasia (12,86). Patients with nonclassic CAH have a spectrum of clinical presentations: some have severe hirsutism and menstrual irregularity; others are asymptomatic. Asymptomatic patients with nonclassic CAH and abnormal hormone levels are termed "cryptic." Speiser and New (84) have also identified a group of patients termed compound heterozygotes with one severe (classic) and one mild (nonclassic) 21-hydroxylase allele; these patients have a higher 17-hydroxyprogesterone response to ACTH than do homozygous nonclassical patients but are no more likely to have signs of androgen excess.

ACTH testing with measurement of 17-hydroxyprogesterone levels at baseline and 60 minutes later has been the cornerstone of diagnosis of 21-hydroxylase deficiency (78,79,87), although overlap between heterozygotes and normal subjects and heterozygotes and homozygotes for nonclassical CAH does occur. The use of early morning levels (7 to 8 AM) of serum (or salivary) 17-hydroxyprogesterone is a useful screening test for this disorder (88,89) (see section on Laboratory Studies). Although some have argued that diagnosis is not essential, since treatment of adult women with nonclassic 21-hydroxylase deficiency is adequate without the use of corticosteroids, we believe that an adolescent with 21-hydroxylase deficiency should be appropriately diagnosed and treated with corticosteroids to ascertain whether the long-term androgenic sequelae and PCO can be prevented with early intervention.

Controversy continues to surround the prevalence of 3β-hydroxysteroid dehydrogenase deficiency (3β-HSD) as a cause of hirsutism in the general population. Unlike other enzymes involved in the pathway from cholesterol to cortisol synthesis, 3β-HSD is not a cytochrome P450, and the deficiency is not HLA-linked (90). Patients originally reported to have this deficiency had elevations primarily of DHEAS, not of testosterone. In a referral population in New York, Pang and coworkers (78) suggested that 17 of 116 hirsute women had evidence of a "partial" 3β-HSD block on ACTH testing. Others have suggested that many of the patients with "mild" or "partial" defects had these changes secondary to extrinsic factors, such as ovarian and adrenal androgens and estrogen. Azziz and colleagues (91) argued that responses of DHEA and 17-hydroxypregnenolone follow in a continuum and that patients diagnosed with 3β-HSD deficiency were merely above the 95% percentile but not clearly a distinct population. Using the stringent criteria of requiring patients to have responses that are three times the upper control limit for either steroid response, they found that no patients among 86 women with hirsutism and hyperandrogenic oligomenorrhea met this standard. Three women (2.3%) did have 21-hydroxylase deficiency. The women with exaggerated DHEA and 17-OH pregnenolone responses had higher DHEAS values than their less responsive counterparts, but similar total and free

T, SHBG, LH, FSH, DHEA/androstenedione, and 17-OH pregnenolone/17-OH progesterone levels. Mathieson and associates (92) similarly reported isolated increases in 17-OH pregnenolone and DHEA but felt that none of the 78 patients had 3β-HSD deficiency.

The recent discovery of the two 3β-HSD genes (type I and type II) is likely to increase further understanding of these disorders. The type II gene expression occurs in the adrenals and gonads. Patients with salt-wasting 3β-HSD have a homozygous or compound heterozygous mutation involving an altered gene structure or amino acid residue. The non-salt-wasting form of severe 3β-HSD deficiency involves amino acid substitution mutations. However, the few girls with premature pubarche and those with hirsutism tested for these genes have not been found to have altered gene sequences, which suggests that the etiology of the decreased 3β-HSD activity is unknown (93). More data are needed in adolescents.

Deficiencies of 11β-hydroxylase and 17-ketosteroid reductase are quite rare (12,37,94,95). The 11-hydroxylase deficiency is not HLA linked (85); the structural gene for cytochrome p450c11 enzyme (for 11-hydroxylation, 18-hydroxylation, and 18-oxidation) is located on chromosome 8. Lee and colleagues (96) have reported a familial hypersecretion of adrenal androgens transmitted as a dominant non–HLA-linked trait; the affected family members had premature adrenarche, hirsutism, and amenorrhea.

Other Diagnoses

Other rare diagnoses to be considered in the patient with hirsutism are Cushing's disease, ovarian or adrenal tumors, and intersex states. Cushing's disease should be considered in the hypertensive obese adolescent with irregular menses and hirsutism, particularly if other stigmata of Cushing's syndrome are present (weakness, spontaneous ecchymoses, purple striae larger than 1 cm, hypokalemia, osteoporosis) (12).

Androgen-producing ovarian and adrenal tumors should be considered in patients with virilization, rapid onset of hirsutism, or markedly elevated baseline androgen levels (97–99,101) (see below). Adrenal carcinomas are usually palpable at the time of diagnosis; these lesions typically secrete DHEA and androstenedione, which are converted to testosterone in the periphery. Some secrete testosterone directly. Since some lesions lack the ability to convert DHEA to DHEAS, both these hormones need to be measured in the patient suspected of having a tumor. Adrenal adenomas can be quite small at presentation in spite of high levels of androgens. Ovarian tumors may cause hirsutism (see Chapter 15) and, with the exception of luteomas, are usually palpable on bimanual examination or detectable by ultrasound. Occasional small ovarian tumors are suppressible by estrogen-progestin therapy.

PATIENT EVALUATION

The initial history should focus on (a) recent changes in the amount of hair, (b) the location of new hair, (c) the relation of hair development to the onset of puberty and menses, (d) acne, (e) drug intake (including anabolic steroid use in athletes), (f) stress, (g) changes in weight, voice pitch, and scalp hair distribution (including evidence of balding), (h) the onset of skin changes suggestive of acanthosis nigricans (AN) (45–47) (see Fig. 5), (i) any family history of hirsutism, PCO, adrenal enzyme deficiencies, diabetes, hyperinsulinism, or infertility, and (j) ethnic background. Increased terminal hair over the face (especially the chin), sternum, upper abdomen, or back is usually a sign of significant hirsutism. Hirsutism associated with menstrual irregularity deserves careful attention. Acne that has a very early or late age of onset, is persistent or recalcitrant, or relapses after isotretinoin (Accutane) should be evaluated with hormone levels whether or not hirsutism is also present (100). A history of virilization or an abrupt onset of hirsutism should raise the suspicion of a tumor or intersex state.

The physical examination should include a search for signs of thyroid disorders, galactorrhea, acne, AN, stigmata of Cushing's disease, and abdominal and pelvic masses. Typically, AN is associated with hyperinsulinemia, PCO, and/or hyperthecosis. The distribution and quantity of the hair should be noted. Hirsutism should be scored to enable assessment of the degree of the problem and to provide baseline data for followup. Bardin and Lipsett (3) have suggested a criteria of 1+ for each portion of the face involved (upper lip, chin, sideburns) and 4+ for the entire chin, neck and face. A more time-consuming but preferable method is the use of the Ferriman and Gallwey scoring system (4) (Fig. 6). In a study of 430 women aged 15 to 74 years, a score above 7 was found in 4.3% of women and a score above 10 in 1.2%. The appearance of the patient can be circled on a flow sheet in the chart and the total score recorded. Mild temporal alopecia may occur in androgenic states.

A lower skinfold dimension has been observed for the dorsum of the hand at the midpoint of the second and third proximal phalanges in adult women with Cushing's disease (1.5 ± 0.2 mm, range 1.0 to 1.8 mm) compared with adult women with either PCO (2.8 ± 0.5, range 2.0 to 4.0 mm) or HAIR-AN (mean 4.4 ± 0.5, range 4.0 to 5.0 mm) (97). This finding needs to be validated in adolescents. Any signs of virilization—significant temporal balding, deepening of the voice, clitoral enlargement (Fig. 7), or changes in body fat or muscle distribution—should prompt an assessment to exclude hyperthecosis, an adrenal or ovarian tumor, adrenal enzyme deficiency, or intersex disorder. The width of the clitoral glans should be measured; a normal width is considered to be <5 mm (see Chapter 1). If the patient has hirsutism, signs of virilization, and/or irregular menses, a vaginal or rectal bimanual examination should be done to assess ovarian size.

(Grade 0 at all sites indicates absence of terminal hair.)

Site	Grade	Definition
1. Upper Lip	1	A few hairs at outer margin.
	2	A small moustache at outer margin.
	3	A moustache extending halfway from outer margin.
	4	A moustache extending to mid-line.
2. Chin	1	A few scattered hairs.
	2	Scattered hairs with small concentrations.
	3 & 4	Complete cover, light and heavy.
3. Chest	1	Circumareolar hairs.
	2	With mid-line hair in addition.
	3	Fusion of these areas, with three-quarter cover.
	4	Complete cover.
4. Upper back	1	A few scattered hairs.
	2	Rather more, still scattered.
	3 & 4	Complete cover, light and heavy.
5. Lower back	1	A sacral tuft of hair.
	2	With some lateral extension.
	3	Three-quarter cover.
	4	Complete cover.
6. Upper abdomen	1	A few mid-line hairs.
	2	Rather more, still mid-line.
	3 & 4	Half and full cover.
7. Lower abdomen	1	A few mid-line hairs.
	2	A mid-line streak of hair.
	3	A mid-line band of hair.
	4	An inverted V-shaped growth.
8. Arm	1	Sparse growth affecting not more than a quarter of the limb surface.
	2	More than this; cover still incomplete.
	3 & 4	Complete cover, light and heavy.
9. Forearm	1, 2, 3, 4	Complete cover of dorsal surface; 2 grades of light and 2 of heavy growth.
10. Thigh	1, 2, 3, 4	As for arm.
11. Leg	1, 2, 3, 4	As for arm.

A

FIG. 6. (A),(B). Hirsutism scoring sheet. The Ferriman and Gallwey system for scoring hirsutism. A score of 8 or more indicates hirsutism. (From Hatch R, Rosenfield RL, Kim MH, et al. Hirsutism: implications, etiology, and management. *Am J Obstet Gynecol* 1981;149:815. Adapted from Ferriman D, Gallwey JD. Clinical assessment of body hair growth in women. *J Clin Endocrinol Metab* 1961;21:1440; with permission.)

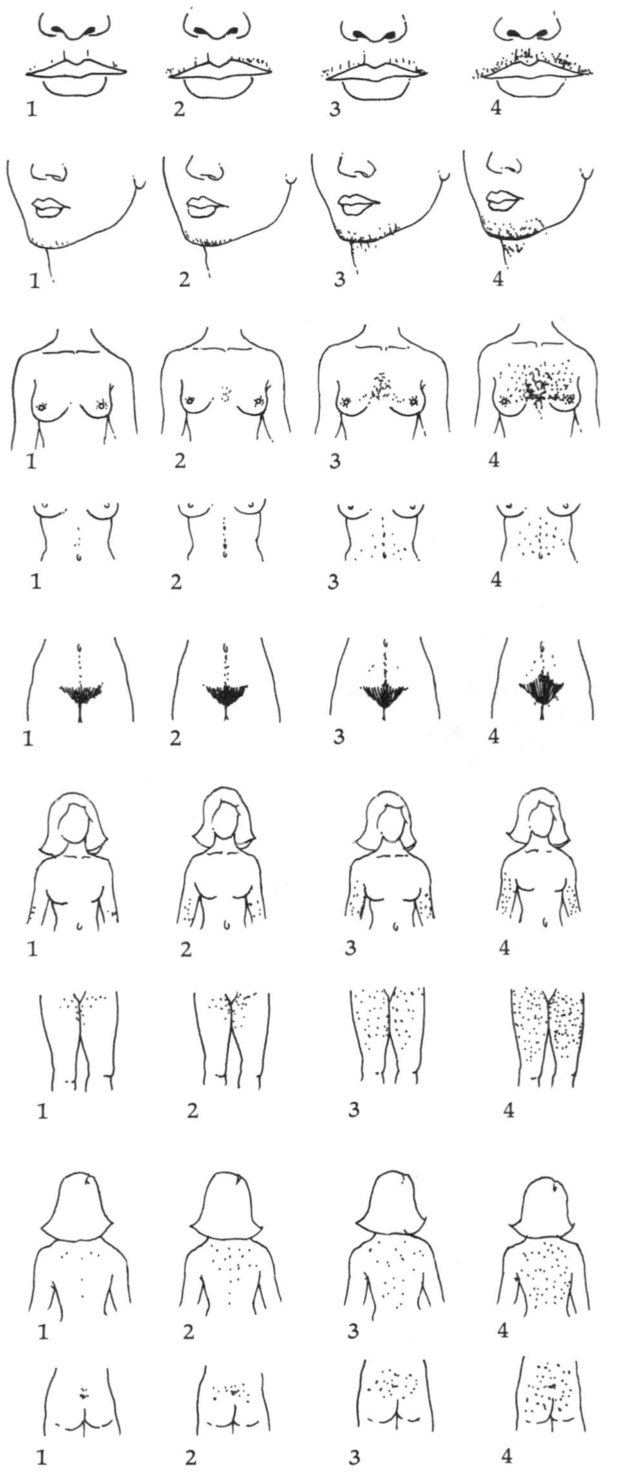

FIG. 6. *Continued*

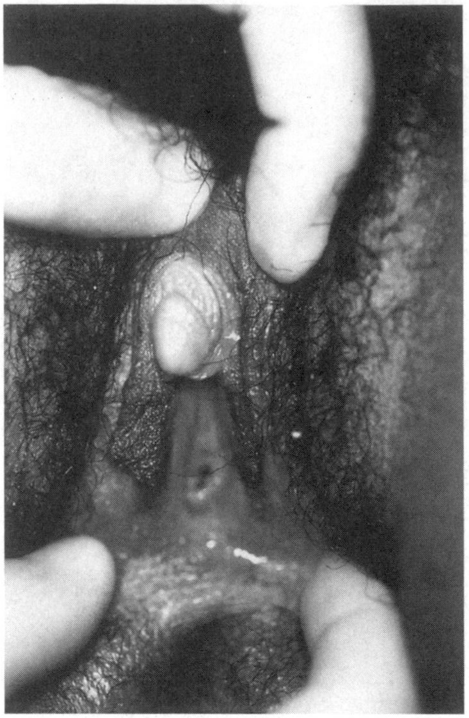

FIG. 7. Clitoral enlargement.

LABORATORY STUDIES

The aim of laboratory tests is to assist in determining the cause of the patient's hirsutism. In most cases of oligomenorrhea and hirsutism, PCO is the cause of the symptom complex, and thus, laboratory tests should be based on the clinical presentation and potential other diagnoses that need to be considered. If the evolution of symptoms such as progressive hirsutism has occurred over 6 to 12 months, or if virilization is present, more extensive studies are necessary to rule out a possible androgen-producing tumor.

Levels of serum androgens need to be determined at a qualified laboratory, and normal standards at the individual lab must be reported. Since hormonal levels vary throughout the day, morning sampling is preferred. Because hormone tests are expensive, some endocrinologists prefer to draw two or three samples (either 20 minutes apart or on subsequent days at 8 AM), pool equal aliquots of serum from each of the samples, and then obtain a single determination. Others use a single sample initially, and if androgen levels are all normal on the random sample in a hirsute patient, the determinations are repeated or several aliquots are pooled if further diagnostic information is needed. In the adult patient, the clinician has the advantage of 10 or more years of menstrual history, which increases the likelihood that the hirsute, oligomenorrheic woman indeed has PCO, which can be diagnosed with a minimum of laboratory tests. In dealing with the adolescent patient, the clinician is often in much more of a quandary about the differential diagnosis because menstrual cycles may be irregular for several years in normal adolescents, hirsutism is often much less striking in the young teen with PCO, and transient hyperandrogenism has been reported to occur during the pubertal process. Additionally, in patients with mild hirsutism, apparent skin sensitivity to androgens and the level of serum free testosterone seem to contribute equally; thus, about half of patients with mild hirsutism may have normal free testosterone levels (102). Even women with moderate to severe hirsutism, normal ovarian function, and normal menses can have normal screening serum androgen levels.

Although recommendations vary depending on the clinical presentation, the initial laboratory evaluation of a case of significant or progressive hirsutism usually includes serum levels of testosterone, free testosterone, and DHEAS. If amenorrhea, oligomenorrhea, or chronic anovulation is present, LH, FSH, and prolactin are measured. The TSH level is also usually determined, because the subtle signs and symptoms of hypothyroidism in adolescents are easy to miss, and treatment is simple. Serum levels of FSH are important to exclude gonadal failure in the amenorrheic adolescent; LH levels, if elevated, may help suggest the clinical diagnosis of PCO in the young adolescent. In the adult woman, LH levels may be less frequently determined because the clinical history is usually more conclusive. Because the samples are drawn at one point in time, elevated LH levels may be found in normal adolescents at ovulation, those under stress, and those with PCO. Adolescents with PCO may have normal or elevated LH levels. LH-to-FSH ratios are 2.5:1 to 3:1 in some, but not all, patients with PCO. Samples for serum hormone levels should not be drawn immediately following the withdrawal flow to a progestin challenge, since hormone levels may be altered (103).

Although at some centers only the *total* testosterone level is determined in hirsute adult women with the aim of using the test primarily to exclude a tumor, we have found that adding a *free* testosterone level is helpful because adolescents may have only mild hirsutism and irregular menses at the initial presentation of PCO. The presence of an abnormal free testosterone level is useful in establishing a likely diagnosis and outlining therapy and followup for the adolescent and her family. If virilization is present or a tumor is under consideration, serum levels of DHEA and androstenedione are added.

A testosterone level above 150 to 200 ng/dl (depending on the laboratory normal values), DHEAS above 700 μg/dl, or androstenedione above 500 ng/dl should raise the suspicion of a tumor or intersex disorder. Testosterone levels between 100 and 200 ng/dl have rarely been associated with tumors. Testosterone levels may be quite elevated (150 to 220 ng/dl) in girls with hyperthecosis. Because of the need for extensive and expensive tests to exclude a tumor, it is critical that a markedly elevated testosterone be verified in a specialized endocrine laboratory; commercial laboratories may use less specific assays that include cross-reacting substances and thus falsely elevate the total testosterone value. Derksen and colleagues (104) have reported that benign ovarian and adrenal disorders can be differentiated from adrenal carcinoma by a dexamethasone test (3 mg/day for 5 days with DHEAS normally suppressed and cortisol <3.3 μg/dl in patients without tumor); however, the clinical presentation of the patients diagnosed with tumors was suggestive of the need for further evaluation (105). Determination of the karyotype is reserved for adolescents with significant virilization (especially associated with vaginal/uterine agenesis), a serum testosterone level in the male range, or elevated FSH and is helpful in detecting mixed gonadal dysgenesis or male pseudohermaphroditism.

The need to do ACTH testing in patients with hirsutism is controversial. Since testing is expensive, our current approach is to suggest that ACTH testing for 21-hydroxylase deficiency be done on girls with clitoromegaly, markedly elevated DHEAS, a history of premature adrenarche, a family history of CAH, an ethnic history of a high prevalence of CAH, and, most important, a high baseline early-morning level of 17-OHP. Girls with what appears to be "typical PCO" can have 17-OHP measured between 7 and 8 AM in the follicular phase of the menstrual cycle. Girls with PCO may have minor elevations of 17-OHP. If the 17-OHP level is >200 ng/dl, ACTH testing can be obtained unless the baseline level is >1000 ng/dl, in which case the diagnosis of 21-hydroxylase deficiency can be made without further testing. Azziz and Zacur (89) found that a basal 17-OHP level >200 ng/dl had a positive predictive value of 80% (95% CI: 28%, 99%) and a negative predictive value of 100% (95% CI: 97%, 100%). The likelihood of a 21-hydroxylase deficiency is increased if the baseline level of 17-OHP is >400 ng/dl. Some clinicians prefer to perform a modified ACTH test on all patients with significant hirsutism, measuring 17-OHP at baseline and 60 minutes after giving 0.25 mg of ACTH. The rise seen with late-onset CAH is typically >6.5 ng/dl/min with levels >1000 ng/dl (usually >1500 ng/dl) at 60 minutes. Pang and colleagues (78) reported that women with nonclassic CAH had 60-minute stimulated levels of 17-OHP of 5404 ± 3234 ng/dl (normal, 334 ± 194 ng/dl) with a markedly abnormal ratio of 17-hydroxypregnenolone to 17-OHP of 0.4 ± 0.2 (normal, 3.4 ± 1.5). In heterozygotes for nonclassic CAH, the rise in 17-OHP may be intermediate between the normal range and the homozygous response. The pathways of steroid biosynthesis and the standards for the 1-hour ACTH test are in Figs. 8–10.

Decreased 3β-HSD activity has been found to be an important cause of hirsutism by some groups (78,81,106,107), although as noted earlier, the etiology of this change appears not to be genetically linked in most. The changes may be secondary to the estrogen and androgen milieu. Patients with decreased 3β-HSD activity usually have elevated DHEAS and not a marked increase in testosterone. Multiple hormone levels at baseline and 60 minutes later should be measured, and the results of the ratios compared to the standards developed by Pang and colleagues (78); stimulated 17-hydroxypregnenolone rose to 2276 ± 669 ng/dl

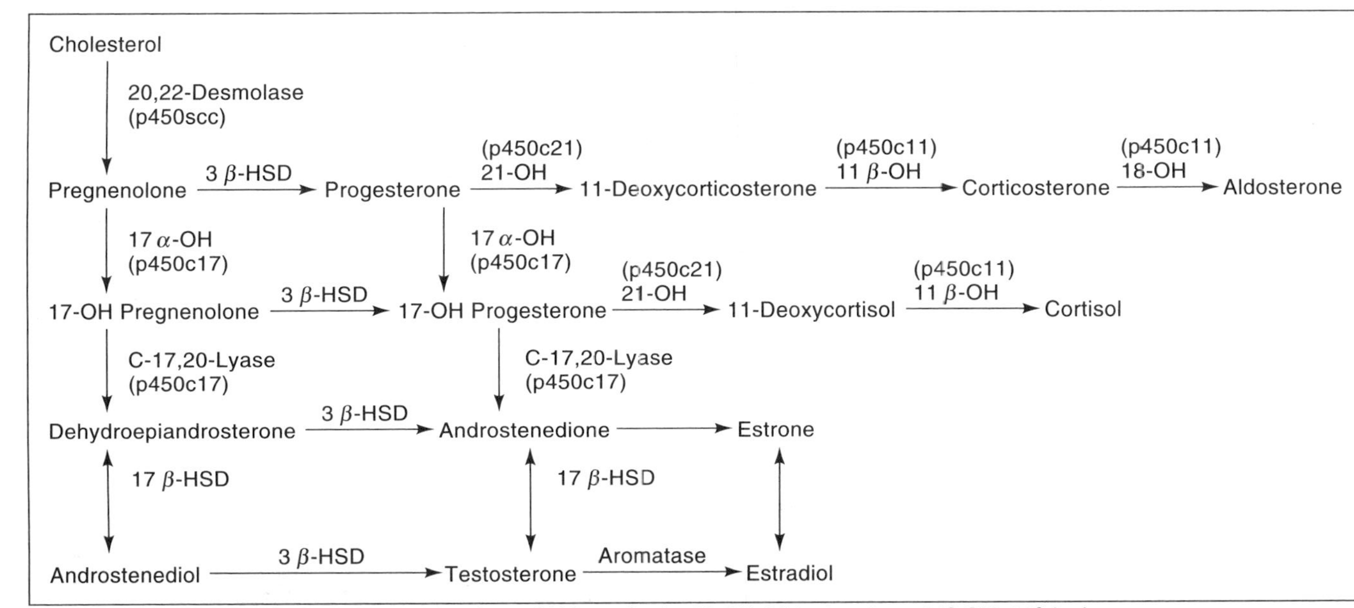

FIG. 8. Major pathways of steroid biosynthesis. 21-OH, 21-hydroxylase; 11β-OH, 11β-hydroxylase; 18-OH, 18-hydroxylase; 3β-HSD, 3β-hydroxysteroid dehydrogenase; 17β-HSD, 17β-hydroxysteroid dehydrogenase (17-ketosteroid reductase); 17α-OH, 17α-hydroxylase; C-17, 20-Lyase also termed 17,20 desmolase.

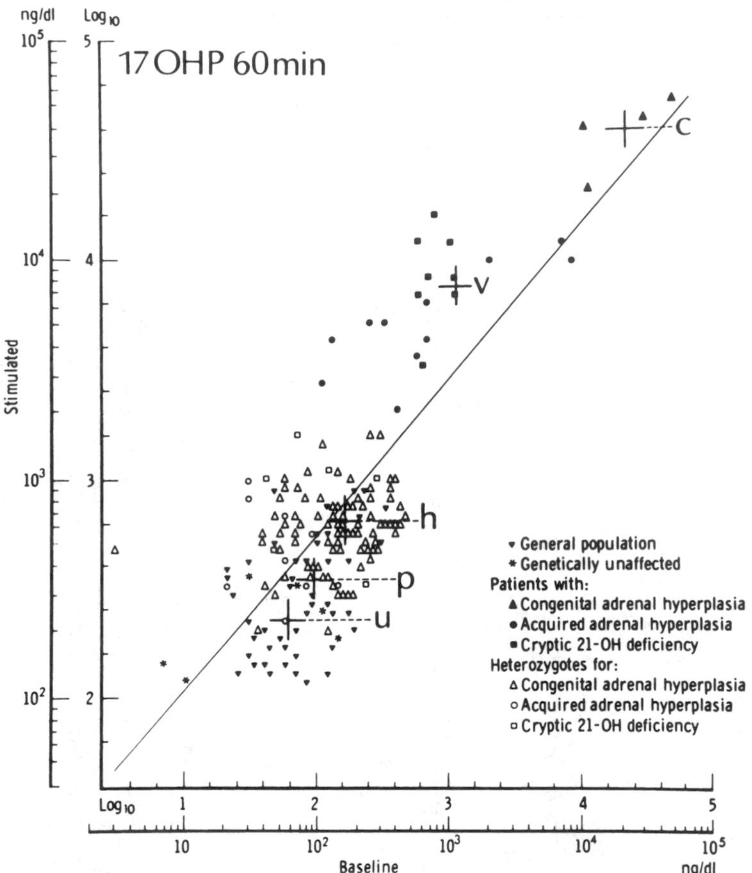

FIG. 9. Nomogram relating baseline to ACTH-stimulated serum concentrations of 17-hydroxyprogesterone. The scales are logarithmic. A regression line for all data points is shown. The mean for each group is indicated by a large cross and adjacent letter: c, classic 21-hydroxylase deficiency; v, variant or nonclassic 21 hydroxylase deficiency (combined mean of values in patients with cryptic and late-onset disease); h, heterozygotes for all forms of 21-hydroxylase deficiency; p, general population; u, persons known to be unaffected (e.g., siblings of patients with 21-hydroxylase deficiency who carry neither affected parental haplotype as determined by HLS typing); OH, hydroxyl. (From White PC, New MI, DuPont B. Congenital adrenal hyperplasia. Parts I and II. *N Engl J Med* 1987;316:1519 and 1580; with permission.)

(normal, 985 ± 327 ng/dl) and DHEA to 2787 ± 386 ng/dl (normal, 1050 ± 384 ng/dl) with increased stimulated ratios of 17-hydroxypregnenolone to 17-OHP (11 ± 2.0) and DHEA to androstenedione (7.5 ± 2.3; normal, 4.6 ± 1.5). This group has suggested using four criteria 60 minutes after ACTH stimulation to establish a diagnosis: 17-hydroxypregnenolone levels ≥1693 ng/dl, DHEA ≥1818 ng/dl, 17-hydroxypregnenolone/17-OHP ratio ≥64, and 17-hydroxypregnenolone/cortisol ratio >52 (108) (Fig. 10). We have used a markedly elevated early morning DHEA as a screening test before ordering an ACTH stimulation test, but the sensitivity and specificity of this test have not been studied in adolescents.

If the stigmata of Cushing's disease are present, a 24-hour urine sample should be collected for determination of urinary free cortisol and creatinine. An 8 AM cortisol level after a bedtime (11 PM) dose of 1 mg of dexamethasone is also frequently measured. If the serum level of cortisol is not well suppressed (<5 μg/dl), or if the level of urinary free cortisol is abnormal, formal dexamethasone suppression testing is done. A pituitary adenoma should be excluded in hyperandrogenic adolescents with hyperprolactinemia.

A few centers, but not most, have reported that androstanediol glucuronide levels are helpful in examining the etiology of hirsutism in adult women, since an increased level reflects utilization of androgens by target tissue (109,110). Androstanediol glucuronide, although not an androgen itself, is a metabolite of the pathway of testosterone to dihydrotestosterone, which is an important step in androgen expression. Levels of this metabolite appear to correlate with the clinical response to spironolactone therapy in patients with idiopathic hirsutism (110). Rittmaster and Thompson (111) have suggested that androstanediol glucuronide may be a better marker for adrenal androgen secretion than DHEAS.

The utility of routine dexamethasone testing is disputed in the evaluation of girls who have hirsutism, but are not being evaluated for Cushing's disease or a tumor. Ehrmann and Rosenfield (15) have suggested that the test can be useful in distinguishing between adrenal and ovarian causes of hirsutism. A 5-day course of dexamethasone (longer in patients who are obese or who have relatively high DHEAS levels) is given, and the levels of free testosterone, DHEAS, and cortisol used to separate diagnostic categories. Normal suppression of free testosterone in their laboratory is a level <8 pg/ml; normal suppression of DHEAS and cortisol is considered a level below the adult control range. Subnormal suppression of free testosterone with normal adrenal suppression rules out CAH and usually is indicative of PCO (rarely a tumor). Inadequate suppression of cortisol indicates Cushing's syndrome or noncompliance with the dexamethasone. Normal suppression of androgens is considered an indication for an ACTH test. The dexamethasone test has never been used widely, in part because of the added expense but also because free testosterone levels are not standardized in many laboratories. Others also argue that screening procedures should rely heavily on clinical evaluation (104), that most, if not all, patients can be treated with oral contraceptives, and that determining the exact etiology of the hirsutism thus becomes less important. In our clinic, we use dexamethasone tests occasionally; we will give a 5-day dexamethasone test following an ACTH stimulation test for patients with markedly elevated DHEA and DHEAS to ensure that suppression is normal, and we use an overnight test to aid in the exclusion of Cushing's syndrome. For the 5-day dexamethasone test, testosterone, free testosterone, DHEA, DHEAS, androstenedione, and cortisol can be measured at

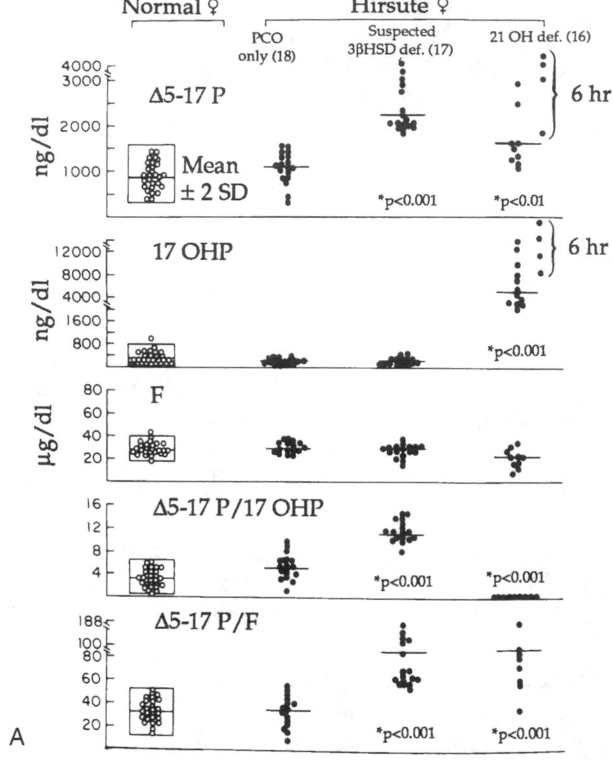

FIG. 10. (A) Serum hormone responses to ACTH stimulation 60 minutes after 0.25 mg given intravenously to normal women and women with hirsutism. Polycystic ovary syndrome (PCO), suspected 3β-hydroxysteroid deficiency (PCO usually heightened adrenal sensitivity), and 21-hydroxylase deficiency. (From Pang S, Lerner A, Stoner E, et al. Late-onset adrenal steroid 3β-hydroxysteroid dehydrogenase deficiency. I. A cause of hirsutism in pubertal and postpubertal women. *J Clin Endrocrinol Metab* 1985;60:428; with permission.)

baseline and on the morning of the fifth day of dexamethasone (0.5 mg four times a day). In patients with PCO, DHEA and DHEAS typically suppress to <80% and 50%, respectively, with a dexamethasone test. Even if the free testosterone falls into the normal range, the level typically rises on maintenance doses (0.1 to 0.5 mg/day), clinical improvement is unlikely, and side effects are common (75). Ehrmann and colleagues (112) have also found that a nafarelin (GnRH agonist) test demonstrated supranormal responses of 17-OHP levels (>259 ng/dl) in women with PCO and a close correlation with the results of the 5-day dexamethasone test, but this test has not been used in clinical practice.

Because of the evolving information on the metabolic abnormalities associated with PCO, clinicians should assess the lipid profile of these young women. With the increased risk of gestational diabetes and NIDDM in obese women

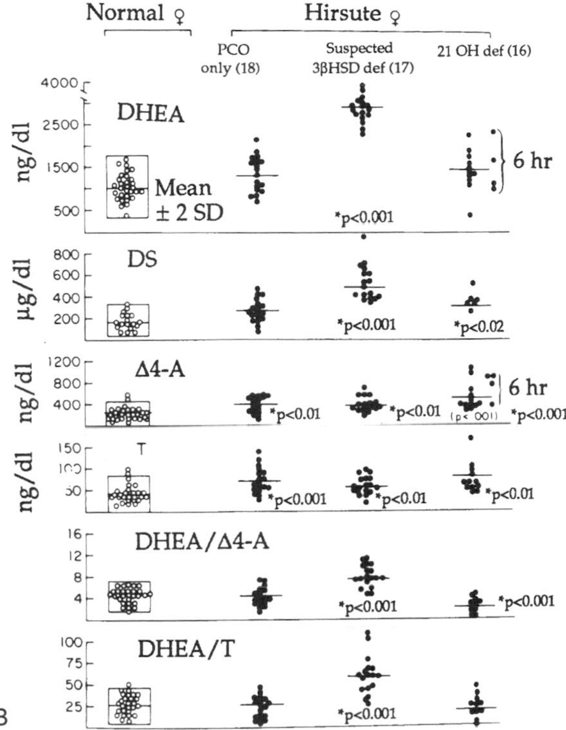

FIG. 10 *Continued.* **(B)** Serum androgen levels 60 minutes after ACTH stimulation in normal women and women with hirsutism. 3β-HSD def, suspected 3β-hydroxysteroid dehydrogenase deficiency (or heightened adrenal sensitivity); 21 OH def, 21-hyroxylase deficiency; Δ5-17P, 17-hydroxypregnenolone; 17 OHP, 17-hydroxyprogesterone; F, cortisol; DHEA, dehydroepiandrosterone; DS, dehydroepiandrosterone sulfate; Δ4-A, androstenedione; T, testosterone. (From Pang S, Lerner A, Stoner E, et al. Late-onset adrenal steroid 3β-hydroxysteroid dehydrogenase deficiency. I. A cause of hirsutism in pubertal and postpubertal women. *J Clin Endrocrinol Metab* 1985;60:428; with permission.)

with PCO, an assessment of carbohydrate tolerance should be considered at baseline and at followup. Fasting glucose and insulin levels can give some estimate of hyperinsulinism and insulin resistance. The best screening test for glucose intolerance in teens has not been determined; a fasting or 2-hour postprandial glucose is preferable to a glycosylated hemoglobin as an initial screen.

Ultrasonography can be helpful in assessing the ovaries of obese and poorly relaxed adolescents but should be performed selectively. Transvaginal ultrasonography has given better detail for ovarian morphology in these patients and can also be used to evaluate the thickness of the endometrium. The adrenal glands can also be visualized by ultrasonography, but computed tomography or magnetic resonance imaging should be ordered if an adrenal tumor is suspected. Laparoscopy is not indicated in making the diagnosis of PCO in adolescents.

The diagnosis of PCO in adolescents can be made by the typical clinical history, the exclusion of other clinical entities, and the finding of elevated free testosterone in the setting of anovulatory cycles and androgen excess (hirsutism, acne). The total testosterone level is also often elevated. Typically, but not always, the LH levels are high (may be >30 mIU/ml with radioimmunoassay) and/or the ratio of LH/FSH is >2.5 (LH and FSH should be assayed against the same reference standard). It should be remembered that an increased LH/FSH ratio may be associated with androgen excess per se, as with ovarian tumors or CAH. Intermittent sampling may also miss the abnormal gonadotropin ratio. An increased LH/FSH ratio in the absence of elevated free testosterone does not make a diagnosis of PCO, although the patient may later develop the more evident clinical and laboratory signs. In some clinical research centers, further confirmatory studies of PCO are done, such as looking for an exaggerated LH response with normal FSH response to GnRH and increased androstenedione and/or testosterone response to human chorionic gonadotropin (hCG) stimulation. Suppression-stimulation testing, however, cannot be used to exclude a neoplasm definitively in the patient with markedly elevated testosterone.

TREATMENT

Treatment of hirsutism is aimed at the cause, if possible. The sooner a diagnosis is made in the adolescent, the more likely it is that further progression of hirsutism can be arrested. The majority of patients with progressive hirsutism and menstrual irregularities have PCO. The potential aims of therapy should be discussed with each patient and a therapeutic decision made. The aims may deal with any or all of the four potential problems: (a) protecting the endometrium from continuous stimulation with estrogen (and dysfunctional uterine bleeding) and lessening the likelihood of endometrial cancer, (b) managing the irregular menses, (c) lessening the hirsutism, or at least preventing further new hair growth, and (d) addressing the consequences of infertility. In addition, the clinician needs to be involved in long-term surveillance of the patient for NIDDM and cardiovascular disease; there is also some preliminary evidence of an increased risk of breast cancer (12).

In the adolescent who is not sexually active and does not have significant or progressive hirsutism, the first two problems can be managed by the use of progestin withdrawal (12 to 14 days of 10 mg medroxyprogesterone every 4 to 6 weeks). The patient should understand that much of the abnormal physiology, such as increased free testosterone, is not altered over the long term by this therapy. For the adolescent with significant hirsutism, with enlarged ovaries, or in need of contraception, oral contraceptives are generally well tolerated. The oral contraceptive suppresses the hypothalamic–pituitary–ovarian axis, lowers ovarian secretion of steroids through alterations in IGF-1 and IGF-BP-1 (6,17), usually lowers adrenal androgen secretion (decreases DHEAS), and provides protection to the endometrium (113–116). In addition, the estrogen increases SHBG and thereby decreases free testosterone. Although few comparative studies have been done that use different oral contraceptive pill formulations, we have preferred to start with low-dose 30- to 35-μg pills, such as Brevicon/Modicon, Desogen, OrthoCept, Ortho-Cyclen, OrthoTri-Cyclen, or Demulen 1/35. Other pills such as 1 mg norethindrone/35 μg ethinyl estradiol, Tri-Norinyl, Ortho-Novum 7/7/7, or Triphasil can also be used, provided that acne improves during therapy. In general, oral contraceptives with high doses of norgestrel should be avoided in these young women. Very rarely, a pill with 50 μg ethinyl estradiol is needed for a few cycles, especially in patients with markedly elevated free testosterone and hyperthecosis; the dosage can be lowered in several months to a 30- to 35-μg pill once the free testosterone levels decrease. Continuous pills for 3 to 4 months (followed by 7 days off) also may help to lessen the increase in LH and testosterone during the placebo pills in patients with very high levels of these hormones (117) or inadequate response. In patients who develop hypertension or nausea on the pill, even a pill with 20 μg of ethinyl estradiol can be used to decrease free testosterone levels. In adolescents who will be taking the pills for many years, we often measure the free testosterone in the second or third week of the second cycle after the patient begins taking hormones to make sure that adequate suppression has occurred. It is also important to consider early intervention with oral contraceptives in adolescents taking valproate so that the full spectrum of PCO can potentially be prevented.

Hirsutism improves in 50% to 70% of hirsute women treated with oral contraceptive pill suppression. The adolescent girl needs to understand that the goal is to prevent the growth of new hairs while she uses cosmetic measures such as electrolysis to treat preexisting hair follicles. It is important to consider the rare tumor in adolescents with a pretreatment serum testosterone >150 to 200 ng/dl (done in a reliable laboratory) even if suppression occurs, because tumors can be suppressed by oral contraceptives, norethindrone, and GnRH analogs.

Spironolactone has been used successfully in adult women and adolescents for the treatment of hirsutism. Spironolactone is an aldosterone antagonist with antiandrogenic effects; this drug competes at the androgen receptor level and inhibits 5α-reductase activity to decrease conversion of testosterone to DHT, thus lessening hair growth, midshaft diameter, and sebum production. This drug is particularly useful with idiopathic hirsutism (Fig. 11). The drug has been administered in several regimens, usually at 100 to 200 mg/day in two divided doses (118,119). In patients not also taking oral contraceptives, the cyclic administration on days 4 to 22 of the cycle may reduce the occurrence of irregular menses. The dosage of 100 mg/day (given as 50 mg twice daily) is less likely to be associated with metrorrhagia than the higher 200 mg/day (120). Side effects (which include polyuria, polydipsia, dizziness, breast pain, and headache) are usually transient and disappear without any intervention (121). The possible long-term problems have not been fully defined. Adolescents should not use this drug if they are at risk of pregnancy because the drug can

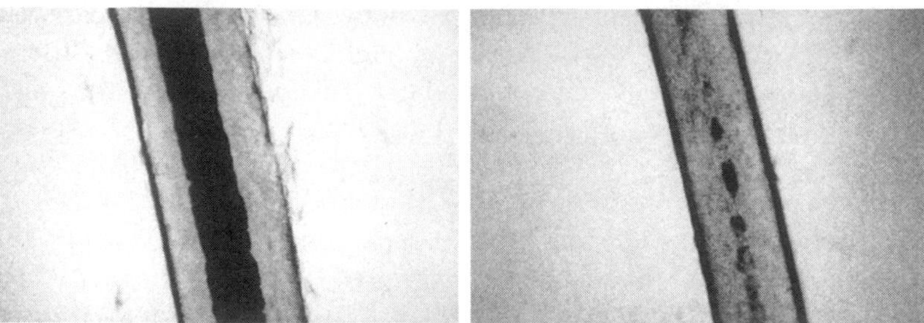

FIG. 11. Hair plucked from the facial area of a woman with hirsutism before (*left panel*) and after (*right panel*) treatment for 6 months with spironolactone plus oral contraceptives. Notice the decrease in the medullary diameter of the hair. (From O'Brien RC, Cooper ME, Murray RM, et al. Comparison of sequential cyproterone acetate/estrogen versus spironolactone/oral contraceptive in the treatment of hirsutism. *J Clin Endocrinol Metab* 1991;72:1008; with permission.)

potentially prevent normal masculinization of the male fetus. Thus, for most adolescents with moderate to severe hirsutism, spironolactone should be given along with oral contraceptives for therapy. Some clinicians prefer to give oral contraceptives for 1 to 6 months alone first, and then the spironolactone is added so that side effects related to either drug are not confused. Others begin both medications at the same time. It must be stressed to the adolescent that a noticable difference may not be appreciated for 3 to 6 months and the existing hair will not disappear.

Cyproterone acetate along with low-dose estrogen replacement, available in Europe, has yielded comparable or better results than spironolactone plus oral contraceptives in reducing total hair diameter and medullary diameter (the part with the pigment) (122). It is a competitive inhibitor of DHT, binding to its specific receptors; it reduces 5α-reductase in the skin and lowers ovarian androgen secretion by inhibiting gonadotropin release (18). Finasteride, a specific competitive inhibitor of 5α-reductase, appears to have a clinical effect similar to spironolactone; both treatments result in a decrease in anagen hair diameters and in Ferriman-Gallwey scores (123). Flutamide, an antiandrogen, both alone and in combination with oral contraceptives, appears efficacious in reducing hirsutism score, hair diameter, and acne with an efficacy similar to that of spironolactone (124–128), but the potential for unexpected hepatotoxicity during treatment with the drug has limited its use (129). Several other antiandrogens, such as ketoconazole, which is an inhibitor for P-450 steroidogenic enzymes and blocks synthesis of androgens, have also been tried but can be associated with adverse side effects (121).

GnRH analogs have been promising for lessening the hirsutism score and the hair shaft diameter in patients with PCO in most, but not all, studies (130–138). Therapy is generally reserved for severe cases not responding to oral contraceptives and spironolactone. Estrogen-progestin therapy needs to be administered in addition to the GnRH analogs to prevent the long-term consequences of estrogen deficiency. Leuprolide acetate plus oral contraceptives and spironolactone can also lead to clinical improvement in women when previous therapy has failed. In a small study, Rittmaster and Thompson (111) reported that GnRH analogs appeared to be marginally more efficacious in women with PCO than in those with idiopathic hirsutism.

Bromocriptine has been prescribed in women with both hyperprolactinemic PCO and normoprolactinemic PCO (139–141), but the efficacy in treating androgen excess is questionable. The use of somatostatin analogs (octreotide) and growth hormone may be another approach to improving ovarian function in women (142). Insulin sensitizing agents such as metformin and troglitazone are useful in elucidating the pathophysiology of PCO, and studies are underway to examine their indications for therapy. Topical antiandrogens are under investigation and may hold promise for the treatment of this frustrating disorder.

Weight loss is an important adjunct to hormonal intervention, because fat cells appear to be responsible for some of the peripheral conversion of the prehormone androstenedione (143–147). Obesity per se is associated with increases in total and free testosterone and DHEAS in adults as well as adolescent girls. In addition, hyperinsulinism, which may drive up the androgen levels, may improve with weight loss. Guzick and colleagues (147) reported that an average weight loss of 16.2 kg in 12 hyperandrogenic, anovulatory women resulted in an increase of SHBG, a decline in free testosterone, and a decline in fasting insulin levels. Four of six women resumed ovulation. Diets that are high in fiber and complex carbohydrates may lower insulin secretion, but controlled studies are needed to determine whether any specific diets beyond one for weight loss are helpful (8). Cessation of smoking is another useful adjunct to therapy, since cigarette smoking can be associated with elevated androstenedione levels, likely of adrenal origin.

Although some studies in adult women have suggested both short-term and long-term benefits of dexamethasone in the reduction of high androgen levels and the establishment of normal menses (108), our experience in treating adolescents with PCO and hirsutism with corticosteroids and the experience of other investigators treating adults have not found this to be efficacious for most patients (28,113,148). Many patients with PCO do have elevated adrenal androgen levels (without an adrenal enzyme deficiency) and will experience lowering of serum androgen levels during a dexamethasone test, but few adolescents have clinical improvement in hirsutism or regularity of menses with long-term corticosteroid suppression. In our studies and those of others, it is necessary to lower free testosterone level to the normal range with *both* the 5-day dexamethasone test (0.5 mg four times a day) and a maintenance dose of once-daily dexamethasone (113,149). If dexamethasone is selected, the maintenance dose should be started slowly in 0.1-mg increments (dose is 0.1 to 0.5 mg, with the usual dose 0.25 mg/day). Adrenal androgens suppress at lower doses than cortisol (150) but still may not remain in the normal range once the high-dose dexamethasone is discontinued (113). In our experience, daily doses of 0.5 mg of dexamethasone often resulted in overtreatment, weight gain, and striae. Shorter-acting prednisone (e.g., 5 mg once daily, or occasionally 2.5 mg once or twice daily) or methyl prednisolone (4 mg daily) is preferable to dexamethasone in the rare adolescent with PCO and hyperresponsiveness of the adrenal glands, who appears to benefit from adrenal suppression. Others have prescribed cortisone acetate (12.5 mg in the morning, 25 mg at night for 1 month, and then 25 mg at night). The morning cortisol level should remain above 2 μg/dl. The results of a study of 14 girls with adrenal androgen excess (Fig. 12) show the difficulty of suppressing free testosterone in hirsute girls with dexamethasone therapy, especially in contrast to the excellent results achieved with oral contraceptive therapy. Occasional patients with both PCO and late-onset CAH have benefited from a course of both oral contraceptives and corticosteroids to lessen androgen excess. Girls treated with corticosteroids need to wear MediAlert bracelets and be cautioned about the short-term and long-term consequences of adrenal suppression.

Patients with late-onset 21-hydroxylase deficiency CAH have traditionally been treated with glucocorticoid therapy, such as low-dose dexamethasone or prednisone. As overtreatment is more common with dexamethasone, we prefer to prescribe prednisone 5 mg at bedtime. Some investigators have argued that

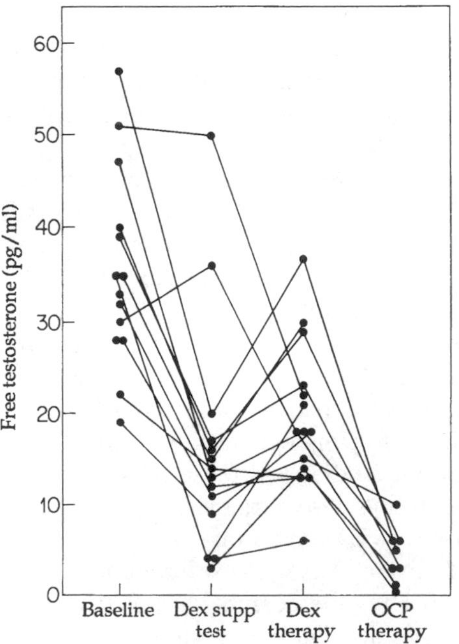

FIG. 12. Free testosterone levels before therapy, after 4-day dexamethasone suppression test, and during long-term dexamethasone therapy in 14 hirsute adolescent patients (without 21-hydroxylase deficiency) and in 8 patients receiving oral contraceptive therapy. In this study, the normal range of free testosterone was 3.3 to 15 pg/ml. Dex, dexamethasone; OCP, oral contraceptive pill. (From Emans SJ, Grace E, Woods ER, et al. Treatment with dexamethasone of androgen excess in adolescent patients. *J Pediatr* 1988;112: 821; with permission.)

other forms of treatment without glucocorticoids are as efficacious as corticosteroids, or more so, in these women. Carmina and Lobo (151) found that suppression of the ovary with a GnRH analog was beneficial for patients with demonstrated late-onset 21-hydroxylase deficiency and that the decrease in hirsutism was greater than during the previous 6-month treatment with dexamethasone. Spritzer and colleagues (152) also reported that cyproterone acetate therapy was more effective in reducing the hirsutism score (but not the serum testosterone or androstenedione levels) than hydrocortisone (20 mg/day) therapy for women with late-onset CAH. Because we generally diagnose patients with late-onset CAH in early to mid-adolescence at our center, we have been prescribing corticosteroid therapy to try to avoid the long-term consequences of the development of PCO. Whether this approach will be successful in the prevention of hirsutism and PCO is unknown at present. Patients with ovarian or adrenal tumors are treated surgically (see Chapter 15).

Regardless of the therapy chosen, the patient also needs help in achieving good cosmetic results. Bleaching of the fine hair, especially on the face, can be accomplished with 6% hydrogen peroxide or commercial preparations of facial bleaches. The addition of 10 drops of ammonia per 30 ml of peroxide just before use will activate the peroxide and increase bleaching. Depilatories, shaving, and wax epilation remove hair temporarily. Electrolysis, if done by an experienced person, permanently destroys the hair bulb and, in most cases, avoids pitlike scars and regrowth of incompletely destroyed hairs. A patient should have her own individual electrolysis needle and should also be given the option of using EMLA cream (lidocaine 2.5% and prilocaine 2.5%) for 1 hour before the electrolysis to lessen the discomfort (153). Laser epilation appears to be promising in selected patients (the currently used particles require light skin). The AN may improve with weight loss; topical therapy with lachydrin 12% or tretinoin cream (Retin A) have also been used with variable success.

The induction of ovulation in infertile PCO patients is beyond the scope of this book, but approximately 80% of patients will have anovulatory infertility, which is not usually difficult to treat. However, spontaneous pregnancies do occur, and adolescents may mistakenly believe that they are infertile. Because of oligomenorrhea, they may present quite late in pregnancy. Infertility treatments may involve adrenal suppression, clomiphene citrate, exogenous gonadotropins and hCG, isolated FSH, pulsatile GnRH, and GnRH analogs followed by exogenous gonadotropins (12–14). Although wedge resection of the ovaries was frequently used in the past, it is not a first-line therapy and should not be used for the treatment of androgen excess in adolescents because of the risk of subsequent pelvic adhesions. Newer surgical approaches are laparoscopic diathermy or laser "drilling" to decrease the stromal ovarian component that is producing the androgens (154). This therapy is generally successful, but limited, in that the increased stroma will return. The disadvantages have included intraabdominal adhesions, the need for surgery and general anesthesia, and in one case ovarian atrophy (14,155–157).

Case 1

K. T. presented at the age of 15 years with a history of irregular menses and increasing hirsutism. She had started her pubic hair development at age 11 and her breast development at age 12. Her menarche occurred at age 13 10/12 years, and she had a second menstrual period 7 months later. She was otherwise in good health, and her increments in height and weight had been normal. On physical examination, she appeared to be healthy and to have moderate facial hirsutism and mild acne. Her height was 156.5 cm (10th percentile) and her weight 46 kg (10th percentile). She had increased hirsutism on the upper lip, chin, and sideburns, and the Ferriman-Gallwey score was 25. Otherwise, the results of her general examination and pelvic examination were normal. Initial laboratory tests revealed an LH of 42.5 mIU/ml, FSH of 13.5 mIU/ml, DHEAS of 198 μg/dl (normal <335 μg/dl), testosterone of 63 ng/dl (normal <55 ng/dl), free testosterone, 8.8 pg/ml (normal <6.3 pg/ml). An ACTH stimulation test showed that her 17-OHP increased from 1352 ng/dl at baseline to 7849 ng/dl at 60 minutes, consistent with late-onset 21-hydroxylase deficiency. She was given prednisone 5 mg at bedtime. As she remained amenorrheic with significant hirsutism, oral contraceptives were begun, initially norethindrone 0.5 mg/ethinyl estradiol 35 μg and then changed to Loestrin 1/20 because of nausea. Her acne resolved, and she underwent electrolysis. She had good cosmetic results and has chosen to continue taking oral contraceptives. Her younger sister had a rise in 17-OHP from 68 ng/dl at baseline to 1349 ng/dl at 60 minutes in response to ACTH and has no hirsutism; she has been shown to be a heterozygote (76).

The ACTH test was performed on K. T. because of her early and progressive hirsutism in spite of an increased LH/FSH ratio and normal DHEAS; however, the diagnosis could have been made by determination of a single early-morning 17-OHP.

Case 2

L. K., 15 years old, presented because of irregular menses. Her menarche occurred at the age of 11, and she had had irregular menses every 2 to 4 months. Her LMP had been 4 months earlier. She had been overweight since childhood and had gained 60 pounds in the past 2 years. She had been sexually active once, 2 years before the office visit. She had a family history of obesity and diabetes mellitus. On physical examination she was obese with a height of 164.7 cm (60%) and weight 116.2 kg (>95%). Her blood pressure was 112/74 mm Hg. She had moderate acne on her face and back with hyperpigmented velvety skin on the back of her neck and in her axilla (acanthosis nigricans). She had mild striae on her abdomen. Her breast and pubic hair development was Tanner stage 5. Her Ferriman and Gallwey score was 15. Her pelvic examination was normal, and she did not have clitoromegaly. Laboratory evaluation revealed negative urine hCG, LH 11.3 mIU/ml, FSH 4.9 mIU/ml, testosterone 62 ng/dl (normal <55 ng/dl), free testosterone 12.0 pg/ml (normal <6.3 pg/ml), DHEAS 251 μg/dl (normal, <335 μg/dl), normal TSH and prolactin levels, elevated fasting insulin of 40 uU/ml, normal fasting glucose of 83 mg/dl, and elevated cholesterol of 239 mg/dl. She was diagnosed with hyperandrogenism, insulin resistance, and acanthosis nigricans (HAIR-AN). She was treated with medroxyprogesterone to give normal withdrawal flow and started on oral contraceptives. She made several visits to the nutritionist and managed to lose some weight.

REFERENCES

1. ACOG. Evaluation and treatment of hirsute women. *Tech Bull* 1995;203:1.
2. McKnight E. The prevalence of "hirsutism" in young women. *Lancet* 1964;1:410.
3. Bardin CW, Lipsett MB. Testosterone and androstenedione blood production rates in normal women and women with idiopathic hirsutism or PCO. *J Clin Invest* 1967;46:891.
4. Ferriman D, Gallwey JD. Clinical assessment of body hair growth in women. *J Clin Endocrinol Metab* 1961;21:1440.
5. Isojarvi JIT, Laatikainen TJ, Pakarinen AJ, et al. Polycystic ovaries and hyperandrogenism in women taking valproate for epilepsy. *N Engl J Med* 1993;329:1383.
6. Barbieri RL. Hyperandrogenism: new insights into etiology, diagnosis, and therapy. *Curr Opin Obstet Gynecol* 1992;4:372.
7. Hatch R, Rosenfield RL, Kim MH, et al. Hirsutism: implications, etiology and management. *Am J Gynecol* 1981;140:815.
8. Rosenfield RL, Ehrlich EN, Cleary RE. Adrenal and ovarian contributions to the elevated free plasma and androgen levels in hirsute women. *J Clin Endocrinol* Metab 1972;34:92.
9. Yen SSC. The polycystic ovary syndrome. *Clin Endocrinol* 1980;12:177.
10. Barbieri RL, Smith S, Ryan KJ. The role of hyperinsulinemia in the pathogenesis of ovarian hyperandrogenism. *Fertil Steril* 1988;50:197.
11. McKenna TJ. Pathogenesis and treatment of polycystic ovary syndrome. *N Engl J Med* 1988; 318:558.
12. ACOG. Hyperandrogenic chronic anovulation. *Tech Bull* 1995;202:1.
13. Franks S. Polycystic ovary syndrome. *N Engl J Med* 1995;333:853.
14. Udoff LC, Adashi EY. Polycystic ovarian disease: current insights into an old problem. *Adolesc Pediatr Gynecol* 1996;9:3.
15. Ehrmann DA, Rosenfield RL. An endocrinologic approach to the patient with hirsutism. *J Clin Endocrinol Metab* 1990;71:1.
16. Udoff L, Adashi E. Polycystic ovarian disease: a new look at an old subject. *Curr Opin Obstet Gynecol* 1995:7:340.
17. Barbieri RL. Hyperandrogenism, insulin resistance and acanthosis nigricans. 10 years of progress. *J Reprod Med* 1994;39:327.
18. Yen SC. Chronic anovulation caused by peripheral endocrine disorders. In: Yen SSC, Jaffe RB, eds. *Reproductive endocrinology: physiology, pathophysiology, and clinical management*, 3rd ed. Philadelphia: W.B. Saunders, 1991:576.
19. Carmina E, Koyama T, Chang L, et al. Does ethnicity influence the prevalence of adrenal hyperandrogenism and insulin resistance in polycystic ovary syndrome? *Am J Obstet Gynecol* 1992;167: 1807.
20. Siegberg R, Nilsson CG, Stenman UH, et al. Endocrinologic features of oligomenorrheic adolescent girls. *Fertil Steril* 1986;46:852.
21. Rosenfield RL. Relationship of androgens to female hirsutism and infertility. *J Reprod Med* 1973; 11:87.
22. Rosenfield RL. Studies of the relation of plasma androgen levels to androgen action in women. *J Steroid Biochem* 1975;6:695.
23. Speroff L, Glass RH, Kase NG. *Clinical gynecologic endocrinology and infertility,* 5th ed. Baltimore: Williams & Wilkins, 1994.

24. Coney P. Polycystic ovarian disease: current concepts of pathophysiology and therapy. *Fertil Steril* 1984;42:667.
25. Lobo RA, Goebelsmann U. Effect of androgen excess on inappropriate gonadotropin secretion as found in the polycystic ovary syndrome. *Am J Obstet Gynecol* 1982;142:394.
26. Burghen GA, Givens JR, Kitabchi AE. Correlation of hyperandrogenism with hyperinsulinism in polycystic ovary disease. *J Clin Endocrinol Metab* 1980;50:113.
27. Shoupe D, Kumar DO, Lobo RA. Insulin resistance in polycystic ovary syndrome. *Am J Obstet Gynecol* 1983;147:588.
28. Loughlin T, Cunningham S, Moore A, et al. Adrenal abnormalities in polycystic ovary syndrome. *J Clin Endocrinol Metab* 1986;62:142.
29. Zumoff B, Freeman R, Coupey S, et al. A chronobiologic abnormality in luteinizing hormone secretion in teenage girls with the polycystic-ovary syndrome. *N Engl J Med* 1983;309:1206.
30. Apter D, Butzow T, Laughlin GA, Yen SSC. Accelerated 24 h luteinizing hormone pulsatile activity in adolescent girls with ovarian hyperandrogenism: relevance to the developmental phase polycystic ovarian disease. *J Clin Endocrinol Metab* 1994;79:119.
31. Temeck J, Pang S, Nelson C, et al. Genetic defect of steroidogenesis in premature pubarche. *J Clin Endocrinol Metab* 1987;64:609.
32. Ibanez L, Potau N, Zampolli M, et al. Source localization of androgen excess in adolescent girls. *J Clin Endocrinol Metab* 1994;79:1778.
33. Miller D, Emans SJ, Kohane I. A followup study of adolescent girls with a history of premature pubarche. *J Adolesc Health* 1996;18:301.
34. Siiteri PK, MacDonald PC. Role of extraglandular estrogen in human endocrinology. In: Greep RO, Astood E, eds. *Handbook of physiology: endocrinology*. Washington: American Physiological Society, 1973;2(part 1):615.
35. Reid RL, Van Vugt DA. Weight-related changes in reproductive function. *Fertil Steril* 1987;48:905.
36. Wild RA, Alaupovic P, Givens JR, Parker IJ. Lipoprotein abnormalities in hirsute women. *Am J Obstet Gynecol* 1992;167:1813.
37. Pang S, Softness B, Sweeney WJ, et al. Hirsutism, polycystic ovarian disease, and ovarian 17-ketosteroid reductase deficiency. *N Engl J Med* 1987;316:1295.
38. Rebar R, Judd HL, Yen SSC, et al. Characterization of the inappropriate gonadotropin secretion in polycystic ovary syndrome. *J Clin Invest* 1976;57:1320.
39. Waldstreicher J, Santoro NF, Hall JE, et al. Hyperfunction of the hypothalamic-pituitary axis in women with polycystic ovarian disease: indirect evidence for partial gonadotrophic desensitization. *J Clin Endocrinol Metab* 1988;66:165.
40. Dunaif A. Do androgens directly regulate gonadotropin secretion in the polycystic ovary syndrome? *J Clin Endocrinol Metab* 1986;63:215.
41. Farhi DC, Nosanchuk J, Silverberg SG. Endometrial adenocarcinoma in women under 25 years of age. *Obstet Gynecol* 1986;68:741.
42. Coulam CB, Annegers JF, Kranz JS. Chronic anovulation syndrome and associated neoplasia. *Obstet Gynecol* 1983;61:403.
43. Moller DE, Flier JS. Detection of an alteration in the insulin-receptor gene in a patient with insulin resistance, acanthosis nigricans, and the polycystic ovary syndrome (type A insulin resistance). *N Engl J Med* 1988;319:1526.
44. Grasinger CC, Wild RA, Parker IJ. Vulvar acanthosis nigricans: a marker for insulin resistance in hirsute women. *Fertil Steril* 1993;59:583.
45. Barbieri RL, Ryan KJ. Hyperandrogenism, insulin resistance, acanthosis nigricans: a common endocrinopathy with unique pathophysiologic features. *Am J Obstet Gynecol* 1983;147:90.
46. Dunaif A. Insulin resistance and ovarian hyperandrogenism. *Endocrinologist* 1992;2:248.
47. Poretsky L, Piper B. Insulin resistance, hypersecretion of LH, and a dual-defect hypothesis for the pathogenesis of polycystic ovary syndrome. *Obstet Gynecol* 1994;84:613.
48. Barbieri RL, Makris A, Randall RW, et al. Insulin stimulates androgen accumulation in incubations of ovarian stroma obtained from women with hyperandrogenism. *J Clin Endocrinol Metab* 1986;62:905.
49. Morales AJ, Laughlin GA, Butzow T, et al. Insulin, somatotropic, and luteinizing hormone axes in lean and obese women with polycystic ovary syndrome: common and distinct features. *J Clin Endocrinol Metab* 1996;81:2854.
50. Fox JH, Licholai T, Green G, Dunaif A. Differential effects of oral glucose-mediated versus intravenous hyperinsulinemia on circulating androgen levels in women. *Fertil Steril* 1993;60:994.

51. Buyalos RP, Geffner ME, Watanabe RM, et al. The influence of luteinizing hormone and insulin on sex steroids and sex hormone-binding globulin in the polycystic ovarian syndrome. *Fertil Steril* 1993;60:626.
52. Geffner ME, Kaplan SA, Bersch N, et al. Persistence of insulin resistance in polycystic ovarian disease after inhibition of ovarian steroid secretion. *Fertil Steril* 1986;45:327.
53. Smith S, Ravnikar VA, Barbieri RL. Androgen and insulin response to an oral glucose challenge in hyperandrogenic women. *Fertil Steril* 1987;48:72.
54. Rittmaster RS, Deshwal N, Lehman L. The role of adrenal hyperandrogenism, insulin resistance, and obesity in the pathogenesis of polycystic ovarian syndrome. *J Clin Endocrinol Metab* 1993;76:1295.
55. Velazquez EM, Mendoza S, Maner T, et al. Metformin therapy in polycystic ovary syndrome reduces hyperinsulinemia, insulin resistance, hyperandrogenemia, and systolic blood pressure, while facilitating normal menses and pregnancy. *Metabolism* 1994;43:647.
56. Nestler JE, Jukubowicz DJ. Decreases in ovarian cytochrome P450c17α activity and serum free testosterone after reduction of insulin secretion in polycystic ovary syndrome. *N Engl J Med* 1996;3335:617.
57. Dunaif A, Scott D, Finegood D, et al. The insulin sensitizing agent troglitazone: a novel therapy for polycystic ovary syndrome. *J Clin Endocrinol Metab* 1996;81:3299.
58. Speiser PW, Serrat J, New MI, Gertner JM. Insulin insensitivity in adrenal hyperplasia due to nonclassical steroid 21-hydroxylase deficiency. *J Clin Endocrinol Metab* 1992;75:1421.
59. Mattsson L, Cullberg G, Hamgerber L, et al. Lipid metabolism in women with polycystic ovary syndrome: possible implications for an increased risk of coronary heart disease. *Fertil Steril* 1984;42:579.
60. Wild RA, Bartholomew MJ. The influence of body weight on lipoprotein lipids in patients with polycystic ovary syndrome. *Am J Obstet Gynecol* 1988;159:423.
61. Adams J, Polson DW, Franks S. Prevalence of polycystic ovaries in women with anovulation and idiopathic hirsutism. *Br Med J* 1986;293;355.
62. Brook C, Jacob H, Stanhope R. Polycystic ovaries in childhood. *Br Med J* 1988;296:878.
63. Stanhope R, Adams J, Brook C. Evolution of polycystic ovaries in a girl with delayed menarche. *J Reprod Med* 1988;33:482.
64. Franks S. Polycystic ovary syndrome: a changing perspective. *Clin Endocrinol* (Oxf) 1989;31:87.
65. Franks BH, Polson DW, Adams J, et al. Polycystic ovaries—a common finding in normal women. *Lancet* 1988:1:870.
66. Conway GS, Honour JW, Jacobs HS. Heterogeneity of the polycystic ovary syndrome: clinical, endocrine, and ultrasound features in 556 patients. *Clin Endocrinol* (Oxf) 1989;30:459.
67. Barnes RB, Rosenfield RL, Burstein S, et al. Pituitary-ovary responses to Nafarelin testing in the polycystic ovary syndrome. *N Engl J Med* 1989;320:559.
68. Rodin A, Thakkar K, Taylor N, et al. Hyperandrogenism in polycystic ovary syndrome: evidence of dysregulation of 11 β-hydroxysteroid dehydrogenase. *N Engl J Med* 1994;330:460.
69. Givens J, Andersen R, Ragland J, et al. Adrenal function in hirsutism: I. Diurnal change and response of plasma androstenedione, testosterone, 17-hydroxyprogesterone, cortisol, LH and FSH to dexamethasone and 1/2 unit ACTH. *J Clin Endocrinol Metab* 1975;40:988.
70. Gross MD, Wortsman J, Shapiro B, et al. Scintigraphic evidence of adrenal cortical dysfunction in polycystic ovary syndrome. *J Clin Endocrinol Metab* 1986;62:197.
71. Lucky AN, Rosenfield RL, McGuire J, et al. Adrenal androgen hyperresponsiveness to adrenocorticotropin in women with acne and/or hirsutism: adrenal enzyme defects and exaggerated adrenarche. *J Clin Endocrinol Metab* 1986;62:840.
72. Ditkoff EC, Fruzzetti F, Chang L, et al. The impact of estrogen on adrenal androgen sensitivity and secretion in polycystic ovary syndrome. *J Clin Endocrinol Metab* 1995;80:603.
73. Carmina E, Gonzalez F, Chang L, et al. Reassessment of adrenal androgen secretion in women with polycystic ovary syndrome. *Obstet Gynecol* 1995;85:971.
74. Blankenstein J, Faiman C, Reyes F, et al. Adult onset familial adrenal hyperplasia due to incomplete 21-hydroxylase deficiency. *Am J Med* 1980;68:441.
75. Lobo RA, Goeblesmann U. Adult manifestation of congenital adrenal hyperplasia due to incomplete 21-hydroxylase deficiency mimicking polycystic ovary disease. *Am J Obstet Gynecol* 1980;138:720.
76. Migeon CJ, Rosewaks Z, Lee P, et al. The attenuated form of 21-hydroxylase deficiency as an allelic form of 21-hydroxylase deficiency. *J Clin Endocrinol Metab* 1980;51:647.
77. Kohn B, Levine LS, Pollack MS, et al. Late-onset steroid 21-hydroxylase deficiency: a variant of classical congenital adrenal hyperplasia. *J Clin Endocrinol Metab* 1982;55:817.

78. Pang S, Lerner A, Stoner E, et al. Late-onset adrenal steroid 3β-hydroxysteroid dehydrogenase deficiency. I. A cause of hirsutism in pubertal and postpubertal women. *J Clin Endocrinol Metab* 1985;60:428.
79. Emans SJ, Grace E, Fleischnick E, et al. Detection of late-onset 21-hydroxylase deficiency congenital adrenal hyperplasia in adolescents. *Pediatrics* 1983;72:690.
80. Benjamin F, Deutsch S, Saperstein H, et al. Prevalence of and markers for the attenuated form of congenital adrenal hyperplasia and hyperprolactinemia masquerading as polycystic ovarian disease. *Fertil Steril* 1986;46:215.
81. Eldar-Geva T, Hurwitz A, Vecsei P, et al. Secondary biosynthetic defects in women with late-onset congenital adrenal hyperplasia. *N Engl J Med* 1990;323:855.
82. White PC, New MI, DuPont B. Congenital adrenal hyperplasia. Parts I and II. *N Engl J Med* 1987;316:1519 and 1580.
83. Miller WL. Genetics, diagnosis, and management of 21-hydroxylase deficiency. *J Clin Endocrinol Metab* 1994;78:241.
84. Speiser PW, New MI. Genotype and hormonal phenotype in nonclassical 21-hydroxylase deficiency. *J Clin Endocrinol Metab* 1987;64:86.
85. Speiser PW, New MI, White PC. Molecular genetic analysis of nonclassic steroid 21-hydroxylase deficiency associated with HLA-B14, DR1. *N Engl J Med* 1988;319:19.
86. Siegel SF, Lee PA, Rudert WA, et al. Phenotype/genotype correlation in 21-hydroxylase deficiency. *Adolesc Pediatr Gynecol* 1995;8:9.
87. New MI, Franzieska L, Lerner AJ, et al. Genotyping steroid 21-hydroxylase deficiency: hormonal reference data. *J Clin Endocrinol Metab* 1983;57:320.
88. Zerah M, Pang S, New MI. Morning salivary 17-hydroxyprogesterone is useful screening test for nonclassical 21-hydroxylase deficiency. *J Clin Endocrinol Metab* 1987;65:227.
89. Azziz R, Zacur HA. 21-hydroxylase deficiency in female hyperandrogenism: screening and diagnosis. *J Clin Endocrinol Metab* 1989;69:577.
90. Globerman H, Rosler A, Theodor R, et al. An inherited defect in aldosterone biosynthesis caused by a mutation in or near the gene for steroid 11-hydroxylase. *N Engl J Med* 1988;319:1193.
91. Azziz R, Bradley EL Jr, Potter HD, Boots LR. 3β-hydroxysteroid dehydrogenase deficiency in hyperandrogenism. *Am J Obstet Gynecol* 1993;168:889.
92. Mathieson J, Couzinet B, Wekstein-Noel S, et al. The incidence of late-onset congenital adrenal hyperplasia due to 3 β-hydroxysteroid dehydrogenase deficiency among hirsute women. *Clin Endocrinol* 1992;36:383.
93. Pang S. Genetics of 3β-hydroxysteroid dehydrogenase deficiency disorder. *GGH* 1996;12:5.
94. Fiet J, Gueux B, Gourmelen M, et al. Comparison of basal and adrenocorticotropin-stimulated plasma 21-deoxycortisol and 17-hydroxyprogesterone values as biological markers of late-onset adrenal hyperplasia. *J Clin Endocrinol Metab* 1988;66:659.
95. Cathelineau G, Brerault JL, Fiet J, et al. Adrenocortical 11α-hydroxylation defect in adult women with postmenarchial onset of symptoms. *J Clin Endocrinol Metab* 1980;51:345.
96. Lee PA, Migeon CJ, Bias WB, et al. Familial hypersecretion of adrenal androgens transmitted as a dominant, non-HLA linked trait. *Obstet Gynecol* 1987;69:259.
97. Corenblum B, Kwan T, Gee S, Wong NC. Bedside assessment of skin-fold thickness: a useful measurement for distinguishing Cushing's disease from other causes of hirsutism and oligomenorrhea. *Arch Intern Med* 1994;154:777.
98. Kamilaris TC, DeBold R, Manolas KJ, et al. Testosterone-secreting adrenal adenoma in a peripubertal girl. *JAMA* 1987;258:2558.
99. Lee PDK, Winter RJ, Green OC. Virilizing adrenocortical tumors in childhood: eight cases and a review of the literature. *Pediatrics* 1985;76:437.
100. Lucky AW, Biro FM, Simbarti LA, et al. Predictors of severity of acne vulgaris in young adolescent girls: results of a five year longitudinal study. *J Pediatr* 1997;130:30.
101. Chetkowski RJ, Judd HL, Jagger PI, et al. Autonomous cortisol secretion by a lipoid cell tumor of the ovary. *JAMA* 1985;254:2628.
102. Reingold SB, Rosenfield RL. The relationship of mild hirsutism or acne in women to androgens. *Arch Dermatol* 1987;123:209.
103. Anttila L, Koskinen P, Kaihola H-L, et al. Serum androgen and gonadotropin levels decline after progestogen-induced withdrawal bleeding in oligomenorrheic women with or without polycystic ovaries. *Fertil Steril* 1992;58:697.
104. Derksen J, Nagesser SK, Meinders AE, et al. Identification of virilizing adrenal tumors in hirsute women. *N Engl J Med* 1994;331:968.

105. McKenna TJ. Screening for the sinister causes of hirsutism [Editorial]. *N Engl J Med* 1994;331;1015.
106. Bongiovanni AM. Acquired adrenal hyperplasia: with special reference to 3β-hydroxysteroid dehydrogenase. *Fertil Steril* 1981;35:599.
107. Lobo RA, Goebelsmann U. Evidence for reduced 3β-hydroxysteroid dehydrogenase activity in some hirsute women thought to have polycystic ovary syndrome. *J Clin Endocrinol Metab* 1981;53:394.
108. Zerah M, Schram P, New MI. The diagnosis and treatment of nonclassical 3β-HSD deficiency. *Endocrinology* 1991:1:75.
109. Paulson RJ, Scrafini PC, Catalino JA, et al. Measurements of 3α, 17β-androstanediol glucuronide in serum and urine and the correlation with skin 5α-reductase activity. *Fertil Steril* 1986;46:222.
110. Kirschner MA, Samojlik E, Szmal E. Clinical usefulness of plasma androstanediol glucuronide measurements in women with idiopathic hirsutism. *J Clin Endocrinol Metab* 1987;65:597.
111. Rittmaster RS, Thompson DL. Effect of leuprolide and dexamethasone on hair growth and hormone levels in hirsute women: the relative importance of the ovary and the adrenal in the pathogenesis of hirsutism. *J Clin Endocrinol Metab* 1990;70:1096.
112. Ehrmann DA, Rosenfield RL, Barnes RB, et al. Detection of functional ovarian hyperandrogenism in women with androgen excess. *N Engl J Med* 1992;327:157.
113. Emans SJ, Grace E, Woods ER, et al. Treatment with dexamethasone of androgen excess in adolescent patients. *J Pediatr* 1988;112:821.
114. Nappi C, Farace MJ, Leone F, et al. Effect of a combination of ethinyl estradiol and desogestrel in adolescent with oligomenorrhea and ovarian hyperandrogenism. *Eur J Obstet Gynecol Reprod Biol* 1987;25:209.
115. Jung-Hoffmann C, Kuhl H. Divergent effects of two low-dose oral contraceptives on sex hormone-binding globulin and free testosterone. *Am J Obstet Gynecol* 1987;156:199.
116. Wiebe RH, Morris CV. Effect of an oral contraceptive on adrenal and ovarian androgenic steroids. *Obstet Gynecol* 1984;63:12.
117. Ruchhoft EA, Elkind-Hirsch KE, and Malinak R. Pituitary function is altered during the same cycle in women with polycystic ovary syndrome treated with continuous or cyclic oral contraceptives or a gonadotropin-releasing hormone agonist. *Fertil Steril* 1996;66:54.
118. Shapiro G, Evron S. A novel use of spironolactone: treatment of hirsutism. *J Clin Endocrinol Metab* 1980;51:429.
119. Cumming DC, Yang JC, Rebar RW, et al. Treatment of hirsutism with spironolactone. *JAMA* 1982;247:1295.
120. Helfer EL, Miller JL, Rose LI. Side-effects of spironolactone therapy in the hirsute woman. *J Clin Endocrinol Metab* 1988;66:208.
121. Knochenhauer ES, Azziz R. Advances in the diagnosis and treatment of the hirsute patient. *Curr Opin Obstet Gynecol* 1995;7:344.
122. O'Brien RC, Cooper ME, Murray RM, et al. Comparison of sequential cyproterone acetate/estrogen versus spironolactone/oral contraceptive in the treatment of hirsutism. *J Clin Endocrinol Metab* 1991;72:1008.
123. Wong IL, Morris RS, Ghang L, et al. A prospective randomized trial comparing finasteride to spironolactone in the treatment of hirsute women. *J Clin Endocrinol Metab* 1995;80:233.
124. Erenus M, Gurbuz O, Durmusoglu F, et al. Comparison of the efficacy of spironolactone versus flutamide in the treatment of hirsutism. *Fertil Steril* 1994;61:613.
125. Ciotta L, Cianci A, Marletta E, et al. Treatment of hirsutism with flutamide and a low-dosage oral contraceptive in polycystic ovarian disease patients. *Fertil Steril* 1994;62:1129.
126. Cusan L, Dupont A, Gomez JL, et al. Comparison of flutamide and spironolactone in the treatment of hirsutism: A randomized controlled trial. *Fertil Steril* 1994;61:281.
127. Fruzzette F, DeLorenzo D, Ricci C, et al. Clinical and endocrine effects of flutamide in hyperandrogenic women. *Fertil Steril* 1993;60:806.
128. Couzinet B, Pholsena M, Young J, et al. The impact of a pure anti-androgen (flutamide) on LH, FSH, androgens and clinical status in idiopathic hirsutism. *Clin Endocrinol* 1993;39:157.
129. Wysowski DK, Fireman, Tourtelot JB, et al. Fatal and nonfatal hepatotoxicity associated with flutamide. *Ann Intern Med* 1993;118:860.
130. Steingold K, DeZiegler D, Cedars M, et al. Clinical and hormonal effects of chronic gonadotropin-releasing hormone agonist treatment in polycystic ovarian disease. *J Clin Endocrinol Metab* 1987;65:773.
131. Couznet B, LeStrat N, Brailly S, et al. Comparative effects of cyproterone acetate or a long-acting

gonadotropin-releasing hormone agonist in polycystic ovarian disease. *J Clin Endocrinol Metab* 1986;63:1031.
132. Steingold KA, Judd HL, Nieberg RK, et al. Treatment of severe androgen excess due to ovarian hyperthecosis with a long-acting gonadotropin-releasing hormone agonist. *Am J Obstet Gynecol* 1986;154:1241.
133. Andreyko JL, Monroe SE, Jaffe RB. Treatment of hirsutism with a gonadotropin-releasing hormone agonist (Nafarelin). *J Clin Endocrinol Metab* 1986;63:854.
134. Carr BR, Breslau NA, Givens C, et al. Oral contraceptive pills, gonadotropin-releasing hormone agonists, or use in combination for treatment of hirsutism: a clinical research center study. *J Clin Endocrinol Metab* 1995;80:1169.
135. Falsetti L, Pasinetti E. Treatment of moderate and severe hirsutism by gonadotropin-releasing hormone agonists in women with polycystic ovary syndrome and idiopathic hirsutism. *Fertil Steril* 1994;61:817.
136. Morcos RN, Abdul-Malak ME, Shikora E. Treatment of hirsutism with a gonadotropin-releasing hormone agonist and estrogen replacement therapy. *Fertil Steril* 1994;61:427.
137. Carmina E, Janni A, Lobo RA. Physiological estrogen replacement may enhance the effectiveness of the gonadotropin-releasing hormone agonist in the treatment of hirsutism. *J Clin Endocrinol Metab* 1994;78:126.
138. Elkind-Hirsch KE, Anania C, Mack M, et al. Combination gonadotropin-releasing hormone agonist and oral contraceptive therapy improves treatment of hirsute women with ovarian hyperandrogenism. *Fertil Steril* 1995;63:970.
139. El Tabbakh GH, Loutfi IA, Azab I, et al. Bromocriptine in polycystic ovarian disease: a controlled clinical trial. *Obstet Gynecol* 1988;71:301.
140. Steingold KA, Lobo RA, Judd HL, et al. The effect of bromocriptine on gonadotropin and steroid secretion in polycystic ovarian disease. *J Clin Endocrinol Metab* 1986;62:1048.
141. Seibel MM, Oskowitz S, Kamrava M. Bromocriptine response in normoprolactinemic patients with polycystic ovary disease: a preliminary report. *Obstet Gynecol* 1984;64:213.
142. Piaditis GP, Hatziionanidis AH, Trovas GP, et al. The effect of sequential administration of octreotide alone and octreotide/growth hormone simultaneously on buserelin stimulated ovarian steriod secretion in women with polycystic ovary syndrome. *Clin Endocrinol* 1996;45:595.
143. Glass AR, Dahms WT, Abraham GE. Secondary amenorrhea in obesity: etiologic role of weight related androgen excess. *Fertil Steril* 1978;30:243.
144. Harlass FE, Playmate SR, Fariss BL. Weight loss is associated with correction of gonadotropin and sex steroid abnormalities in the obese anovulatory female. *Fertil Steril* 1984;42:649.
145. Hosseinian AH, Kim MH, Rosenfield C. Obesity and oligomenorrhea are associated with hyperandrogenism independent of hirsutism. *J Clin Endocrinol Metab* 1976;42:765.
146. Pasquali R, Antenucci D, Casimirri F, et al. Clinical and hormonal characteristics of obese and amenorrheic hyperandrogenic women before and after weight loss. *J Clin Endocrinol Metab* 1989:68:173.
147. Guzick DS, Wing R, Smith D, et al. Endocrine consequences of weight loss in obese, hyperandrogenic, anovulatory women. *Fertil Steril* 1994;61:598.
148. Abraham G, Chakmakjian ZH, Buster JE, et al. Ovarian and adrenal contributions to peripheral androgens in hirsute women. *Obstet Gynecol* 1975;46:169.
149. Moll GW, Rosenfield RL. Plasma free testosterone in the diagnosis of adolescent polycystic ovary syndrome. *J Pediatr* 1983;102:461.
150. Rittmaster R, Loriaux DL, Cutler GB. Sensitivity of cortisol and adrenal androgens to dexamethasone suppression in hirsute women. *J Clin Endocrinol Metab* 1985;61:462.
151. Carmina E, Lobo RA. Ovarian suppression reduces clinical and endocrine expression of late-onset congenital adrenal hyperplasia due to 21-hydroxylase deficiency. *Fertil Steril* 1994;62:738.
152. Spritzer P, Billaud L, Thalabard J-C, et al. Cyproterone acetate versus hydrocortisone treatment in late-onset adrenal hyperplasia. *J Clin Endocrinol Metab* 1990;70:642.
153. Wagner RF Jr, Flores CA, Argo LF. A double blind placebo controlled study of a 5% lidocaine/prilocaine cream (EMLA) for topical anesthesia during thermolysis. *J Dermatol Surg Oncol* 1994;20:148.
154. Armar NA, McGarrigle HH, Honour J, et al. Laparascopic ovarian diathermy in the management of anovulatory infertility in women with polycystic ovaries: endocrine and clinical outcome. *Fertil Steril* 1990;53:45.
155. Donesky BW, Adashi EY. Surgically induced ovulation in the polycystic ovary syndrome: wedge resection revisited in the age of laparoscopy. *Fertil Steril* 1995;63:439.
156. Heylen SM, Puttermans PJ, Brosens IA. Polycystic ovarian disease treated by laparoscopic organ

laser capsule drilling: comparison of vaporization versus perforation technique. *Hum Report* 1994:9:1038.

157. Balen AH, Jacobs HS. A prospective study comparing unilateral and bilateral laparoscopic ovarian diathermy in women with polycystic ovary syndrome. *Fertil Steril* 1994:62:921.

FURTHER READING

Haseltine FP, Redmond GP, Wentz AC, et al. An NICHD Conference on androgens and women's health. *Am J Med* 1996;98:1S.

8

Structural Abnormalities of the Female Reproductive Tract

The development of the female reproductive tract is a complex process that involves cellular differentiation, migration, fusion, and canalization with probable apoptosis (programmed cell death). This integrated series of events brings about numerous possibilities for abnormal development and anomalies. Structural anomalies of the female reproductive tract become apparent at varying chronologic times during life, and the diagnosis and treatment may not be straightforward. Most anomalies involving the external genitalia are apparent at birth (see Chapter 2), while obstructive and nonobstructive anomalies of the reproductive tract can be apparent at birth, during childhood, at puberty, at menarche, during adolescence, or later in adult life.

In this chapter, the normal embryologic development of the female reproductive tract will be presented, followed by anatomic and clinical descriptions of developmental anomalies of lateral and vertical fusion of the urogenital sinus and müllerian duct systems. In addition, the diagnosis, management, and treatment of developmental and acquired structural disorders of the labia and vulva, such as labial hypertrophy and ritual female "circumcision"/mutilation, will be discussed.

The diagnosis, management, and surgical treatments of all female reproductive tract anomalies have changed with improvements in diagnostic imaging techniques, surgical and nonsurgical techniques and instrumentation, and the rapidly expanding field of reproductive medicine and assisted reproductive technologies. Long-term followup of the differing structural anomalies will be presented in relation to body image, patient satisfaction, and sexual and reproductive function.

NORMAL DEVELOPMENTAL EMBRYOLOGY OF THE REPRODUCTIVE TRACT

The development of the female genital tract begins at 3 weeks of embryogenesis and continues into the second trimester of pregnancy. During the first 3 months of embryonic life, the primordia of both the male and the female reproductive tracts are present and develop together. Gonadal development results from the migration of primordial germ cells to the genital ridge (see Chapter 2), whereas the genital tract itself results from the formation and reshaping of the müllerian ducts (paramesonephric ducts), urogenital sinus, and vaginal plate.

The cell layers involved in the formation of the female reproductive tract are the mesoderm, the endoderm, and the ectoderm.

The *mesoderm* is divided into (a) paraxial mesoderm, which breaks up into segmental blocks (somites), forming the sclerotome (spinal cord, bone), dermatome (dermis), and myotome (musculature); (b) the intermediate mesoderm, which connects the paraxial and lateral plate as it differentiates into nephrogenic cord, forming the three kidney systems [pronephros (degenerates), mesonephros (only the wolffian system remains), metanephros (develops into the true kidney)]; and (c) the lateral plate, which forms mesothelial or serous membranes of the peritoneal and pericardial cavities. In the peritoneum, the mesoderm provides primordium for the müllerian system and gonads. A defect or insult at any given somite or its contiguous mesoderm may give rise to congenital defects of multiple systems, such as the kidneys, the gonads, and corresponding ducts.

The *endoderm* is the epithelial lining of the primitive gut, the intraembryonic portions of the allantois and vitelline duct, respiratory tract, tympanic cavity and eustachian tube, tonsils, thyroid, parathyroid, thymus, liver, pancreas, urinary bladder, and urethra. The urogenital sinus forms the urinary bladder, allantois, and the prostatic, membranous, and penile urethra in males. It forms the urethra and vestibule in females. Both the prostate in males and the urethral/paraurethral glands in females are outbuddings of the urethra.

The *ectoderm* forms the central nervous system, the peripheral nervous system, and the sensory epithelium of sense organs. Of note, the fusion of endoderm and ectoderm contributes to patency (opening) and canalization, and defects result in fusion failures or imperforate/obstruction defects.

During the indifferent stage of development, two pairs of genital ducts develop in both sexes: the mesonephric ducts and the paramesonephric ducts. Paired mesonephric or wolffian ducts connect the mesonephric kidney to the cloaca (Fig. 1A). The ureteric bud arises from the mesonephric duct at approximately the 5th week and induces differentiation of the metanephros, which later becomes the functional kidney; the mesonephric kidney degenerates at 10 weeks (Fig. 1B). The müllerian (paramesonephric) ducts are first identified in embryos of both sexes at the 10-mm stage (6th week) by the thickening of the anterior lateral coelomic epithelium covering the wolffian body; a slight groove lined with distinct epithelial cells is present, and a tube is subsequently formed by fusion of the lips of the groove. The elongating müllerian ducts lie lateral to the wolffian ducts until they reach the caudal end of the mesonephros, at which point they direct medially to nearly touch in the midline near the cloaca (Fig. 1C). The urorectal septum forms by the 7th week to separate the rectum from the urogenital sinus (Fig. 1D). By the 30-mm stage (9th week), the müllerian ducts progress

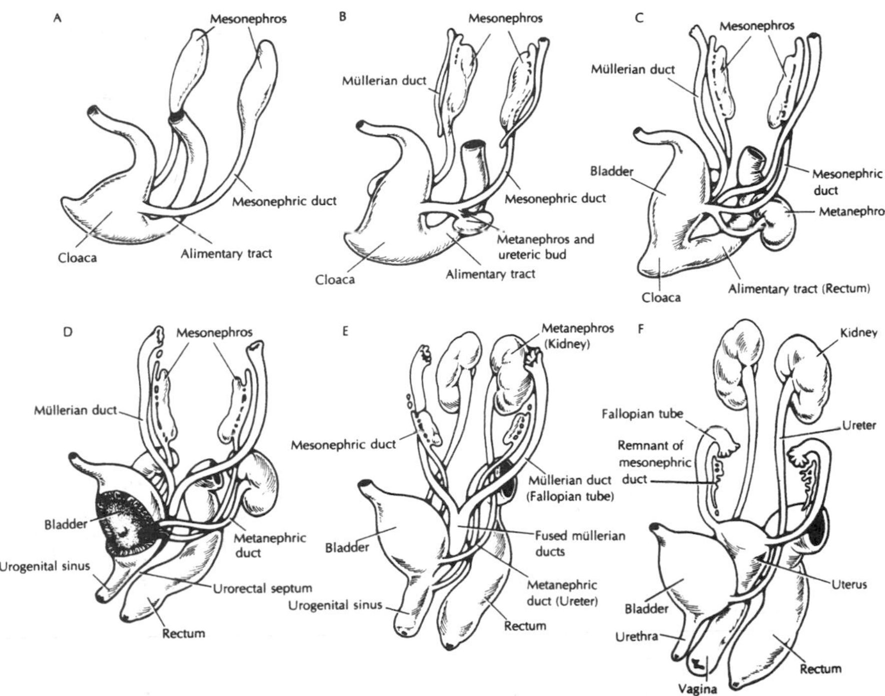

FIG. 1. Embryonic development of the female genitourinary tract. **(A)** Paired mesonephric or wolffian ducts connect the mesonephric kidneys to the cloaca. **(B)** The utereric bud arises from the mesonephric duct at approximately the 5th week and induces differentiation of the metanephros, which later becomes the functional kidney with degeneration of the mesonephric kidney at 10 weeks. **(C)** Paired müllerian ducts develop from invagination of the coelomic epithelium at approximately 6 weeks and grow alongside the mesonephric ducts to end near the cloaca. **(D)** The urorectal septum forms by the 7th week to separate the rectum from the urogenital sinus. **(E)** Adjacent sections of the distal müllerian ducts fuse to form the uterovaginal canal, which inserts into the urogenital sinus at Müller's tubercle. **(F)** The vaginal plate forms at Müller's tubercle and canalizes to form the vagina by the 5th month. (From Shatzkes DR, Haller JO, Velcek FT. Imaging of uterovaginal anomalies in the pediatric population. *Urol Radiol* 1991;13:58; and Markham SM, Waterhouse TB. Structural anomalies of the reproductive tract. *Curr Opin Obstet Gynecol* 1992;4:867; with permission.)

caudally and reach the urogenital sinus to form the uterovaginal canal, which inserts into the urogenital sinus at Müller's tubercle (Figs. 1E, 2A and 3A). By the 48-mm stage (12th week), the two ducts have completely fused into a single tube, the primitive uterovaginal canal, and two solid evaginations grow from the distal aspects of the müllerian tubercle: the sinovaginal bulbs (Figs. 2B and 1F). The sinovaginal bulbs are of urogenital sinus origin. Proximal to the sinovaginal bulbs, outgrowths from the müllerian ducts at Müller's tubercle result in the formation of the vaginal plate (Figs. 2B and 1F). The first and second portions of the müllerian ducts eventually form the fimbria and the fallopian tubes (Figs. 1F

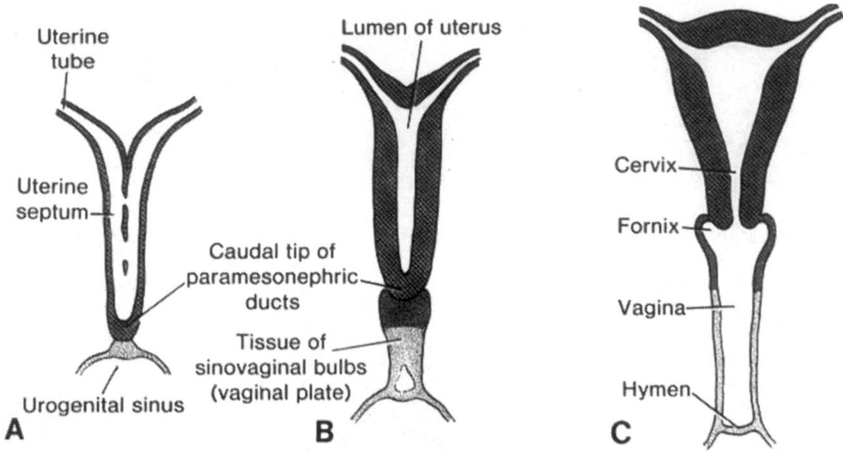

FIG. 2. Schematic drawing showing the formation of the uterus and vagina. **(A)** At 9 weeks. Notice the disappearance of the uterine septum. **(B)** At the end of the 3rd month. Notice the tissue of the sinovaginal bulbs. **(C)** Newborn. The upper portion of the vagina and the fornices are formed by vacuolization of the paramesonephric tissue and the lower portion by vacuolization of the sinovaginal bulbs. Prior to birth the hymen becomes perforate. (From Sadler TW. *Langman's medical embryology*, 6th ed. Baltimore: Williams & Wilkins, 1990; with permission.)

and 3B), while the distal segment forms the uterus and the upper vagina (Figs. 2C and 3B).

It is the growth of the vaginal plate in conjunction with the sinovaginal bulbs that results in the restructuring of the urogenital sinus from a long, narrow tube to a broad, flat vestibule. These changes result in the positioning of the female urethra down to the future perineum. Canalization of the vaginal plate begins caudally and continues in a cephalad direction, creating the lower vagina (Fig. 2B and C). Canalization is complete by the 5th month of gestation. The distal-most portions of the sinovaginal bulbs proliferate to from the hymenal tissue (Fig. 2C). The hymen becomes perforate before birth.

ABNORMALITIES OF THE FEMALE REPRODUCTIVE TRACT

External Genitalia

Ambiguous Genitalia

The diagnosis, evaluation, and medical management of ambiguous genitalia are presented in Chapter 2. The surgical management of these conditions is presented here by diagnosis.

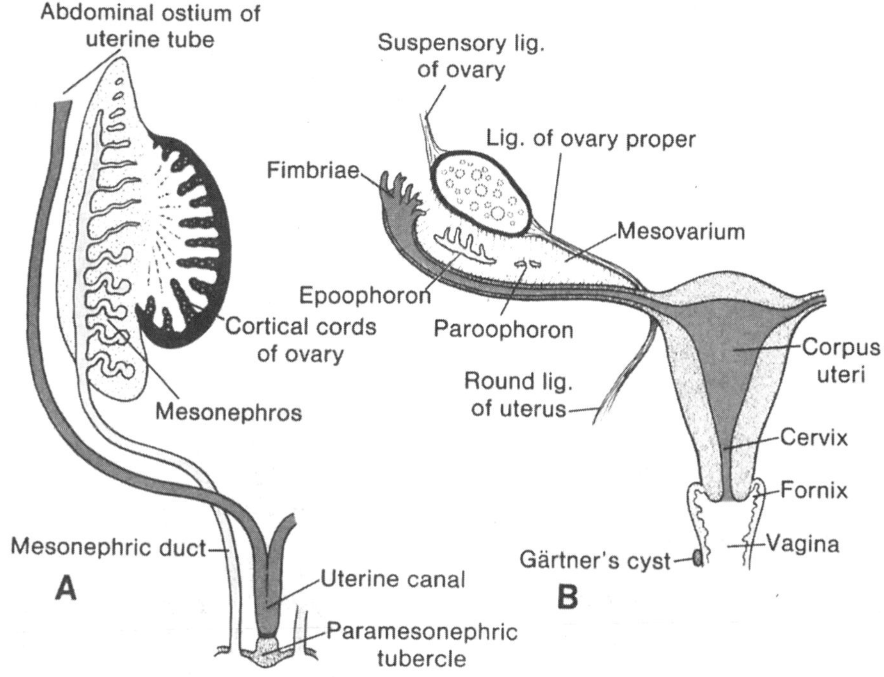

FIG. 3. (A) Schematic drawing of the female genital ducts at the end of the 2nd month of development. Noticc the paramesonephric or müllerian tubercle and the formation of the uterine canal. **(B)** The genital ducts after descent of the ovary. The only parts remaining of the mesonephric system are the epoophoron, the paroophoron, and Gärtner's cyst. Notice the suspensory ligament of the ovary, the ligament of the ovary proper, and the round ligament of the uterus. (From Sadler TW. *Langman's medical embryology*, 6th ed. Baltimore: Williams & Wilkins, 1990; with permission.)

Female Pseudohermaphrodites

It should be emphasized that female pseudohermaphrodites are females with ovaries and are potentially fertile. Thus, regardless of the appearance of the external genitalia, the sex assignment should be female. The majority of these individuals have masculinized external genitalia from congenital adrenal hyperplasia, but this can also result from maternal ingestion of exogenous androgens or from a maternal androgen-producing tumor. The type and extent of surgery depends on the degree of masculinization and the defined anatomy. Surgery may include clitoroplasty, labioplasty, and vaginoplasty (1–5). The buried clitoris may respond to high levels of androgens (which may occur with noncompliance of taking corticosteroids in adolescents with CAH) with painful erections; thus, clitoral recession is usually accompanied by partial corporectomy, preserving the neurovascular bundle, and reanastomosis and preservation of the glans. Historically, surgeons (pediatric general surgeons, urologists, and gynecologists) have performed the entire procedure (clitoroplasty, labioplasty, and vaginoplasty) in one, or at the most two, operations at 6 to 12 months of life. This technique may require an additional operation for revision of the vagina after puberty (6). Alternatively, vaginoplasty can sometimes be delayed until later in adolescence, as there is evidence that girls undergoing vaginoplasty in adolescence report a high level of satisfaction (7,8), whereas those undergoing vaginoplasty early in life have a low rate of compliance with dilators and less satisfaction with the long-term outcome (6,9).

Androgen Abnormality/Insensitivity

Androgen abnormality/insensitivity, a form of male pseudohermaphroditism, may result from a wide variety of syndromes as outlined in Table 1 of Chapter 2 (8–11). With complete androgen insensitivity (testicular feminization), the individual has normal breast development but has pale areola, absent or very sparse pubic and axillary hair, a short vaginal pouch, and absence of the uterus and cervix (12,13) (see Chapters 2 and 6). The gonads may be intraabdominal or in the inguinal rings; the serum testosterone level is in the range of the normal male. Because of insensitivity to androgens and enhanced estrogen production, the patient develops a female habitus and external genitalia. These patients have elevated levels of antimüllerian hormone, also called müllerian inhibitory substance, during the first year of life; normal values from age 1 to puberty; and elevated levels again after pubertal development begins (14).

Because the gonads in such patients have a high rate of malignant degeneration, they should be prophylactically removed after the patient has attained full height and breast development (see Chapter 15). Rarely, children have had malignant degeneration of 46,XY gonads during childhood; therefore, it is suggested that patients in whom the diagnosis is made before puberty be monitored with radiologic imaging for the development of a pelvic mass (15,16). Ultrasonography of the pelvis can be used to supplement rectoabdominal examination. Breast development is usually better in patients who have their gonads in place during adolescent development than in those who have undergone gonadectomy in childhood. After gonadectomy, the patient should receive estrogen replacement.

Before surgery is undertaken, the patient needs to understand her anatomy. The physician should stress the patient's femininity and her ability to have normal sexual relations; she must, however, ultimately accept the fact that she cannot have menses or bear children. Relating the patient's condition to genes or chromosomes can be helpful. Because of the openness of medical records to patients and families, the patient deserves a careful explanation about genetic patterns and assurance that although most people think that an XY individual is a male, in fact, there are women with this genetic pattern because of changes at the level of the DNA. The physician needs to answer questions honestly and at the same time emphasize that the patient's phenotype is female. The necessary surgery can be explained as removal of gonads, rather than testes; gonads can be viewed as organs that did not develop into either testes or ovaries because of the chromosomal problem. The risk of tumor should be openly discussed. Patients with androgen insensitivity syndromes usually have a blind vaginal pouch that, if needed, can be elongated with the use of vaginal dilators as described below.

Partial androgen insensitivity has also been reported but is less frequent than complete androgen insensitivity (see Table 1 of Chapter 2) (9,10). A typical reported patient may have a 46,XY karyotype, labial fusion, a blind vas deferens, and testes located in the labioscrotal folds. At puberty, the patient develops

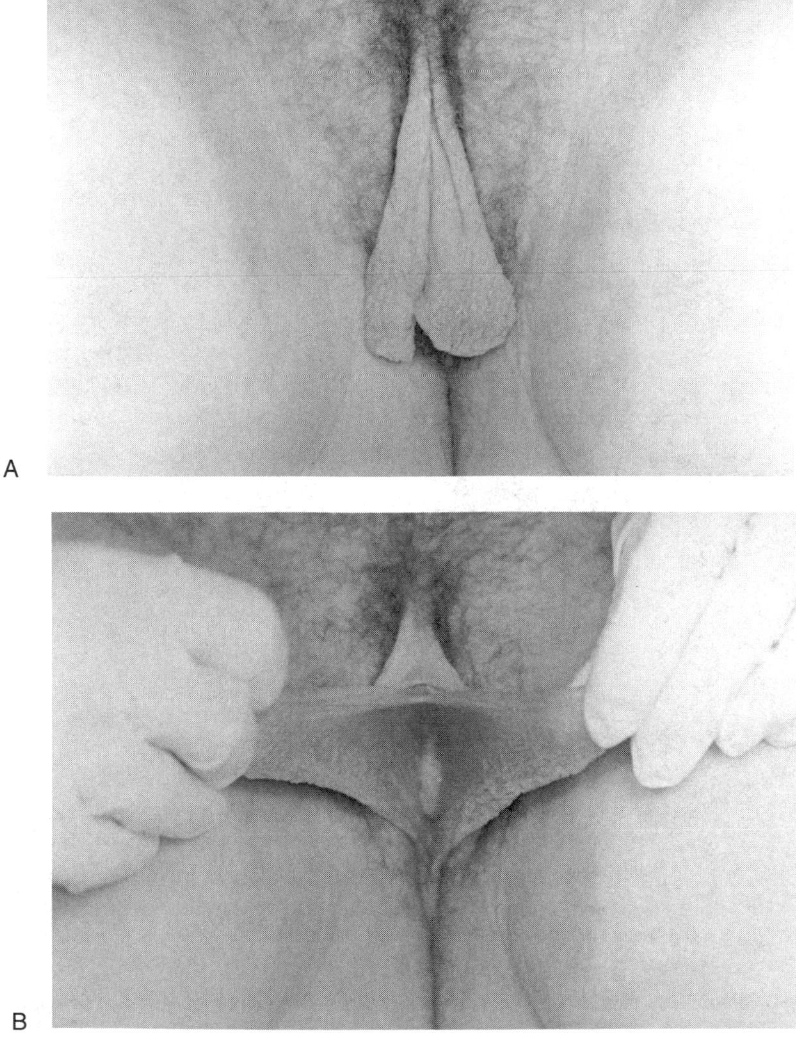

FIG. 4. **(A)** Bilateral labial hypertrophy. **(B)** Bilateral labial hypertrophy fully extended.

breasts and pubic and axillary hair. Because of the absence of the uterus, the patient usually seeks medical care for amenorrhea. Gonadal removal should not be delayed in adolescents with incomplete androgen insensitivity because of the potential for further virilization once the diagnosis has been made. In one series of 11 patients with incomplete androgen insensitivity, of whom 5 were prepubertal, 8 showed evidence of germ cell neoplasia (15).

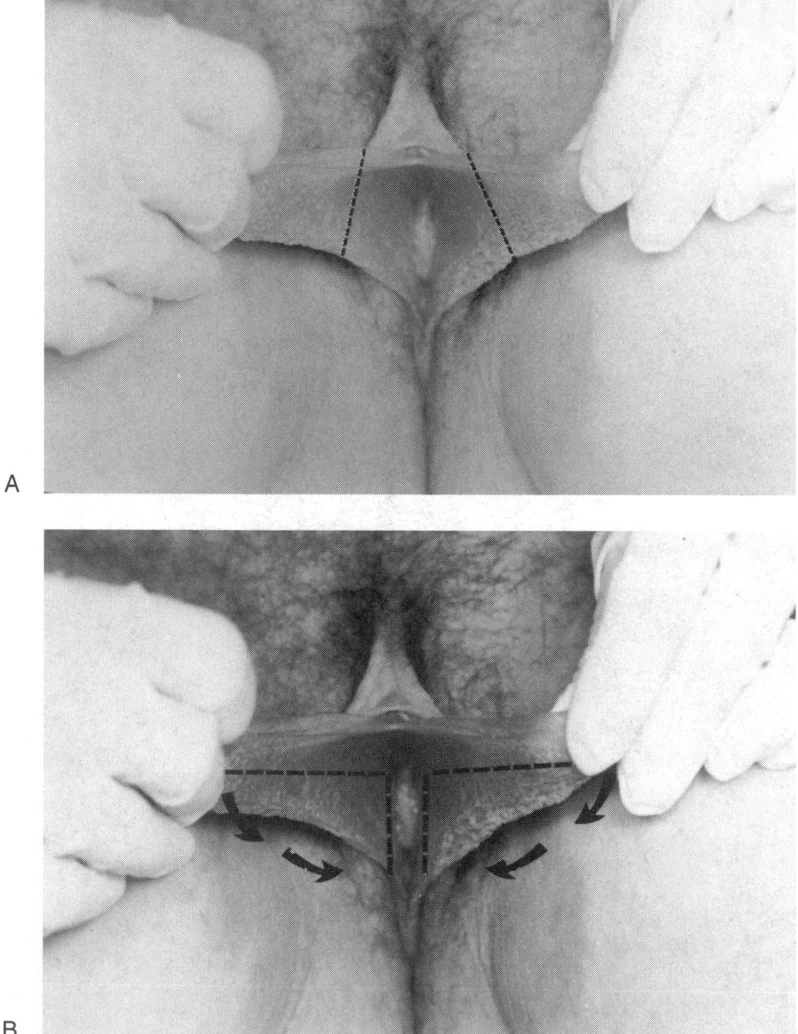

FIG. 5. (A) Resection of the excess labial tissue in a case of labial hypertrophy. **(B)** An alternative method for labioplasty. (From Laufer MR, Galvin WJ. Labial hypertrophy: a new surgical approach. *Adolesc Pediatr Gynecol* 1995;8:39; with permission.)

Patients with androgen abnormality/insensitivity syndromes or other gonadal abnormalities may present with ambiguous genitalia or infantile male genitalia. It may be determined that these individuals should be reared as female (see Chapter 2); thus, feminizing genital reconstruction will need to be performed (3,17). An inadequate phallus for urination in a standing position and sexual function is usually the sole basis for the decision to proceed with feminizing reconstruction. The procedure is performed with the goals of obtaining adequate clitoral sensation, properly positioned clitoris and labia, an adequate vagina (size, location, and consistency), satisfactory voiding in a seated position, and a normal-appearing vulva (3,17).

Labial Hypertrophy

Enlargement of one or both labia minora (Fig. 4A and B) can result in irritation and pain or can interfere with sexual activity or activity involving vulvar compression, such as horseback riding; in addition, the cosmetic deformity may result in psychosocial distress. Nonsymptomatic patients should be reassured that asymmetry or hypertrophy is not a serious developmental abnormality. Symptomatic labial hypertrophy can be addressed with counseling about hygiene and the avoidance of tight clothes; these measures are usually sufficient to relieve the discomfort. If symptoms persist, or if the appearance is troublesome to the young woman, then a surgical procedure for labioplasty can be recommended. The labioplasty can be accomplished by resection of the hypertrophic excess labial tissue and the creation of symmetrically reduced labia (Fig. 5A); we have recently described an alternative technique for labioplasty with wedge resection and reanastomosis in an attempt to decrease the exposed scar and improve outcome (Fig. 5B) (8,18). During the postoperative period, patients should protect the vulvar area from friction by the thighs when walking and strive to keep the area clean and dry to improve healing. Protection of the vulvar area during the postoperative healing period can be aided by a plastic athletic support cup worn inside the patient's underwear; this allows for normal activity without the risk of friction from the thighs against the suture area (18).

Female Genital Mutilation

Female "circumcision" is practiced in approximately 26 African countries, in the Middle East, and in Muslim populations of Indonesia and Malaysia (19,20). In these countries, the prevalence rates range from 5% to 99% (19); it is estimated that 80 to 110 million women worldwide are affected (20). According to the World Health Organization, "Female circumcision is significantly associated with poverty, illiteracy and low status of women, with communities in which people face hunger, ill health, overwork, and lack of clean water" (21). Female mutilation procedures present a health hazard and have short- and long-term physical, psychological, sexual, and reproductive effects.

The procedure is usually performed between the ages of 4 and 10 years, most commonly at the age of 7 years (19,20). The procedure varies according to ritual and has been classified by Toubia (19) according to the degree of tissue removal/destruction as follows:

Type I (clitoridectomy). Removal of a part of the clitoris or the whole organ.

Type II (clitoridectomy). Excision of the clitoris and part of the labia minora.

Type III (modified infibulation). Removal of the clitoris and the labia minora, with incision of the labia majora to create raw surfaces. The anterior two-thirds of the labia majora are reapproximated to cover the urethra and introitus, leaving an opening of the lower third for the passage of urine and menstrual blood.

Type IV (total infibulation). Removal of the clitoris and the labia minora, with incision of the labia majora to create raw surfaces. The labia majora are reapproximated to cover the urethra and introitus, leaving a very small opening for the passage of urine and menstrual blood.

The procedure is usually performed without anesthesia by a midwife or village woman and usually involves ritual and ceremony as a rite of passage into the adult village society (20). The reapproximation of the raw labial surfaces described in types III and IV is accomplished with sutures of silk or catgut or by thorns or twigs (20). The legs of the girl are then bound from the hip to the ankles for up to 40 days so that scar tissue will form (20).

The immediate risks from the procedure include pain, hemorrhage, damage to the urethra and/or anus, local infection, shock, sepsis, and death (19,20). The long-term risks include transmission of blood-borne pathogens from unsterilized instruments [hepatitis, human immunodeficiency virus (HIV)], chronic pain, recurrent urinary tract infections, chronic vaginitis and/or endometritis, dysuria, dysmenorrhea, dyspareunia, apareunia, the need for "surgical" revision prior to intercourse, and possible further revision prior to vaginal delivery (19,20,22).

Health care providers must be cognizant of the existence of ritual female "circumcision," its long-term side effects, and the physical appearance of the perineum after the procedure has been done (see Color Plate 21). A woman may request a revision or a deinfibulation procedure. Extreme sensitivity is essential so that the woman can identify exactly what area of the genital region she wants revised. We usually have the patient demonstrate with a hand-held mirror the exact areas that she wants revised, and we also use drawings to specifically illustrate the appearance of the external genitalia before and after the procedure. With this level of detailed informed consent, the patient's cultural, sexual, and reproductive wishes can be respected. In addition, with the patient dictating the final result, she is retaking control of the genital area that was mutilated by the direction of adults at a time when she was not in control. Figure 6 shows a schematic drawing of the revision procedure, and Color Plate 22 shows the result of the revision in the patient shown in Color Plate 21.

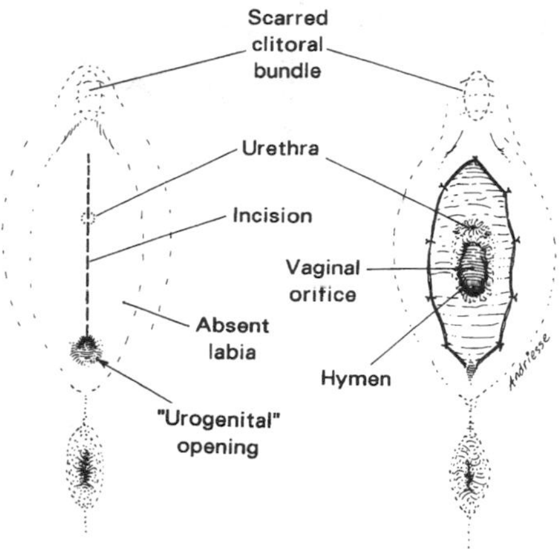

FIG. 6. Schematic diagram after female mutilation (Color Plate 21), and re-creation of the introitus (Color Plate 22). [From Goldstein DP, Laufer MR, Davis AJ. *Gynecologic surgery in children and adolescents: a text atlas.* New York: Springer-Verlag (in preparation); with permission.]

Disorders of Mesonephric Remnants

Persistent wolffian duct derivatives are commonly found in normal females (23,24). These remnants can result in pain or pelvic masses as follows:

A *hydatid of Morgagni cyst* itself does not usually cause pain (Fig. 7), although torsion of the cyst can result in colicky, lower abdominal/pelvic pain with or without nausea and vomiting. Once torsion has occurred, the cyst may become gangrenous. Intermittent torsion of the cyst can also occur, resulting in intermittent symptoms. These cysts can be removed laparoscopically; the fallopian tube can be salvaged and not compromised.

Cysts of the broad ligament can result in large simple cystic pelvic masses (Fig. 8). Patients may present with pain and/or abdominal distension, or the cysts may be identified on routine examination. The cysts are usually simple in appearance on ultrasound. Surgery may be indicated if there is pain or abdominal distension; resection is not mandatory for asymptomatic broad ligament cysts, as they are benign embryologic remnants. If surgery is undertaken, care must be taken to identify the cyst as arising from the broad ligament, with appropriate identification of the fallopian tube (Fig. 9), as the fallopian tube may be distended and stretched over the surface of the cyst (Fig. 8). After removal of the cyst, the distended fallopian tube and redundant peritoneum are left to regress to normal size (Fig. 10).

Gartner's canal (duct) may retain a ureteral connection and form an ectopic ureter, which may communicate with the perineum (see Fig. 1 of Chapter 3). In addition, remnants of Gartner's ducts can result in cystic formations of the cervix or vaginal walls. These embryologic remnants do not need to be resected unless they cause pain or interfere with sexual activity or the use of tampons.

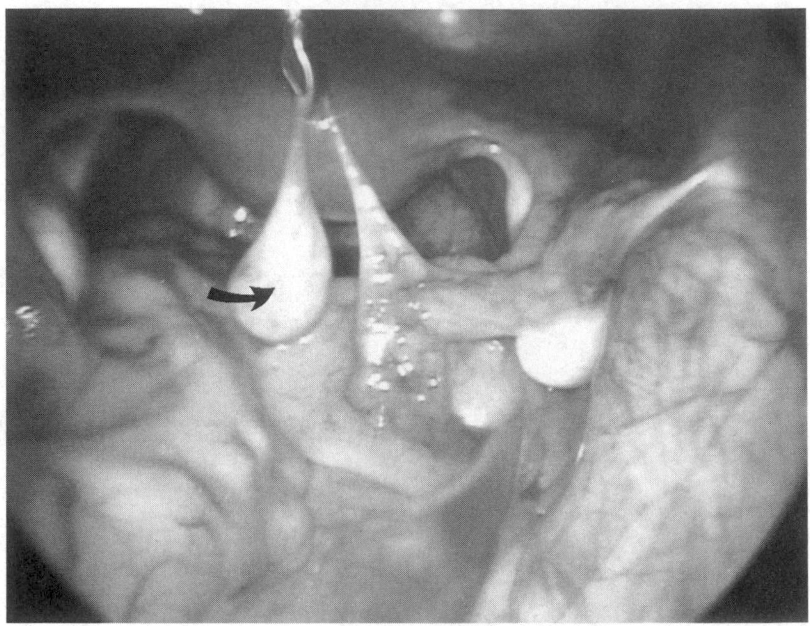

FIG. 7. A hydatid of Morgagni cyst (*arrow*) seen laparoscopically.

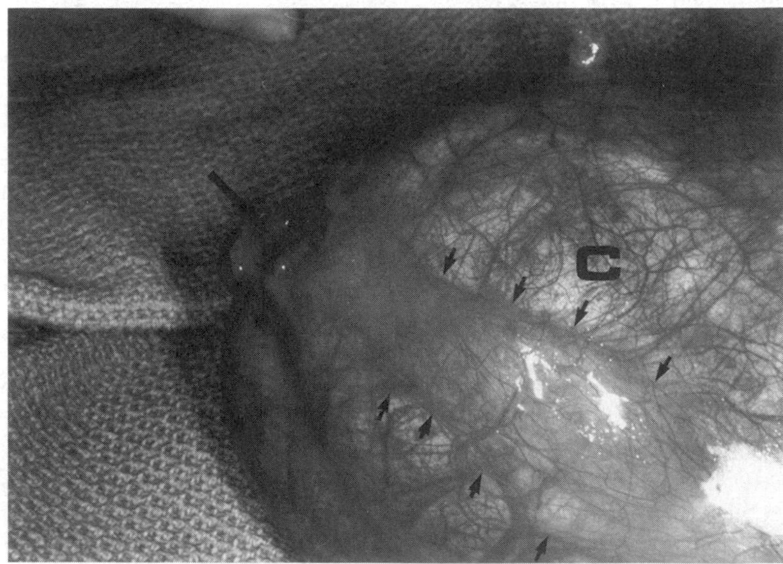

FIG. 8. Distorted, stretched left fallopian tube over the left broad ligament cyst. C, cyst, *small arrows* pointing to edges of stretched fallopian tube, *large arrow* pointing to fimbriated end of tube.

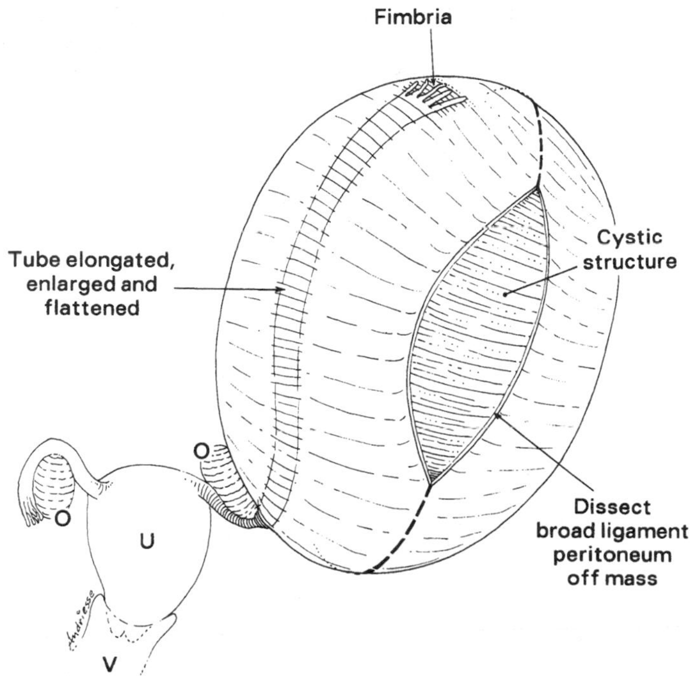

FIG. 9. Schematic diagram of broad ligament cyst with demonstration of incision for preservation of fallopian tube. O, ovary; U, uterus; V, vagina. [From Goldstein DP, Laufer MR, Davis AJ. *Gynecologic surgery in children and adolescents: a text atlas*. New York: Springer-Verlag (in preparation); with permission.]

Introital Abnormalities

Masses

Introital masses are common in the neonate and young child and include developmental and nondevelopmental abnormalities (see Chapter 3). The differential diagnosis includes urethral prolapse (see Fig. 8 of Chapter 3), ectopic ureter (see Fig. 1 of Chapter 3), prolapsed ureterocele (see Fig. 10 of Chapter 3), hymeneal skin tag (see Fig. 17 of Chapter 1), rhabdomyosarcoma (see Color Plate 7), condyloma (see Color Plate 8 and Fig. 4 of Chapter 13), paraurethral cyst (see Fig. 9 of Chapter 3), vaginal cyst, obstructed hemivagina (Fig. 11), or imperforate hymen (see Fig. 14 of Chapter 1). The patient should be examined in order to determine the origin of the mass. In a neonate or child, the "pull-down" traction maneuver for visualizing the introitus should be utilized (see Fig. 6 of Chapter 1) to visualize the entire vestibule and distal vagina.

In the adolescent, the above-mentioned abnormalities may exist, and in addition Bartholin's duct cysts, or abscess may occur. Bartholin's duct cysts do

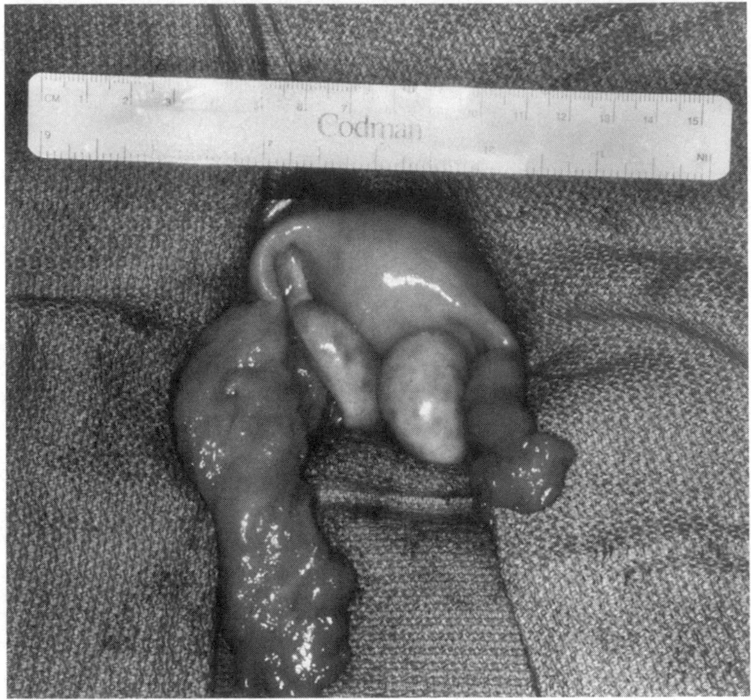

FIG. 10. Fallopian tubes, ovaries, and uterus seen after resection of broad ligament cyst. Notice distorted enlarged left fallopian tube.

not need to be removed unless the patient is symptomatic. If the Bartholin's duct becomes infected and an abscess forms, it must be drained (see Chapter 12).

Ectopic Ureter

An ectopic ureter (see Fig. 1 of Chapter 3) that communicates with the perineum can cause chronic vaginal irritation, vulvar/vaginal "wetness," or pain (see Chapter 3) (25). Ultrasound may be utilized to assist in the diagnosis, and an intravenous pyelogram is confirmatory. According to the Weigert-Meyer rule, the ectopic ureter communicates with the upper pole of the duplex kidney; the greater the distance of the ectopic location from the orthotopic ureteral orifice, the more dysplastic is the upper pole of the duplex kidney (26). A pediatric urologist should be consulted for corrective surgery to appropriately ligate/implant the ectopic ureter and/or to perform an upper pole nephrectomy (27).

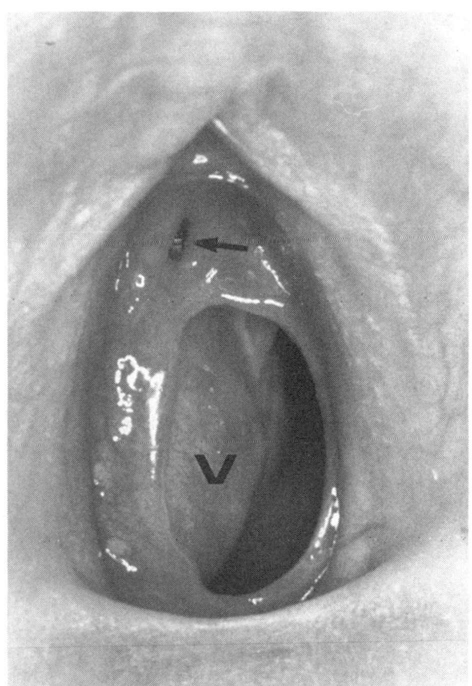

FIG. 11. Obstructed left hemivagina with mucocolpos in a 6-year-old. *Arrow* shows urethra; V, wall of obstructed hemivagina seen as a lateral sidewall bulge.

Prolapsed Ureterocele

When the duplex collecting system has a ureter that ends in a ureterocele, the ectopic ureter with ureterocele also arises from the upper collecting system in the duplex kidney. The ureterocele may present as an introital mass if it prolapses though the urethra (see Fig. 10 of Chapter 3). The prolapsed ureterocele is managed by marsupialization of the obstructed end to relieve the obstruction, and then the nonobstructed duplex ureter prolapse is reduced into the bladder; additional urologic procedures of the ectopic ureter, bladder, or upper pole of the kidney may be required (27–29).

Introital Cysts

Hymeneal, periurethral, and vaginal cysts are usually of the epidermal inclusion variety. Most of these cysts will resolve spontaneously within 3 months. If the cyst does not resolve and is symptomatic, then the cyst should be marsupialized. Prior to surgical intervention, a transperineal ultrasound is helpful to confirm the diagnosis. In addition, cystoscopy should be performed at the time of marsupialization to rule out a urethral diverticulum.

Hymenal Skin Tags

Hymenal skin tags (see Fig. 17 of Chapter 1) are common findings. They usually regress, but if a lesion is symptomatic with inflammation or bleeding, it should be excised to make sure that there is no malignancy, and to relieve the symptoms.

Congenital Hymenal Abnormalities

Congenital variations of the hymen are demonstrated in Fig. 10 of Chapter 1. An adolescent's abnormal hymen that results in a small orifice should be corrected surgically if she is unable to use tampons, douche, insert vaginal cream or suppositories, or have vaginal intercourse. The cribriform, septate, or microperforate hymen can be revised with resection of the "excess" hymenal tissue to create a functional hymenal ring.

Bladder Exstrosphy

Exstrophy of the urinary bladder is an uncommon anomaly that requires timed reconstruction in a series of stages (27). The anal orifice is usually close to the vagina. Years after repair, adolescents may complain of introital stenosis or of the structural abnormality of the mons and/or clitoris. The upper reproductive tract is usually normal. Individuals with this condition have a bifid clitoris (Fig. 12).

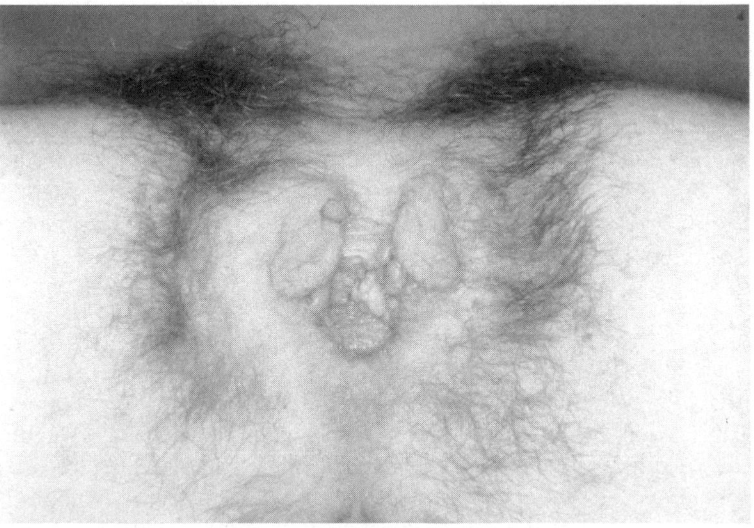

FIG. 12. Gynecologic features in an adolescent with a history of bladder exstrophy following successful bladder repair; notice bifid clitoris and pubic hair.

It is not uncommon for women with a history of bladder exstrophy to develop cervical/uterine prolapse. Surgery can alleviate the prolapse and its associated symptoms of pain, irritation, vaginal discharge/bleeding, or difficulty with sexual activity. The repair usually requires a monsplasty, a Williams vulvovaginoplasty, and a Manchester-Fothergill procedure in a one-stage operation. The result is usually excellent, and patients have full sexual and reproductive function. Pregnancy can occur without complication; delivery can be achieved by either a vaginal or an abdominal route (30).

Cloacal Anomalies

A cloaca is a common canal involving the gastrointestinal, urinary, and genital tracts. A wide range of anatomic variation can occur with the interruption of the normal differentiation of these three organ systems (31–33). The abnormality usually results in a failure of the normal fusion of the müllerian ducts with subsequent duplication of the uterus and proximal vagina (Fig. 13A). The sinovaginal bulbs do not form, and the vaginal plate does not develop normally. The urogenital sinus persists, and the urethra enters high on the anterior wall; the hymen and lower vagina do not form appropriately. The examination reveals a "blank" perineum (Fig. 13B). Before corrective surgery is performed, the patient needs to have the existing anatomy clearly defined with radiologic and endo-

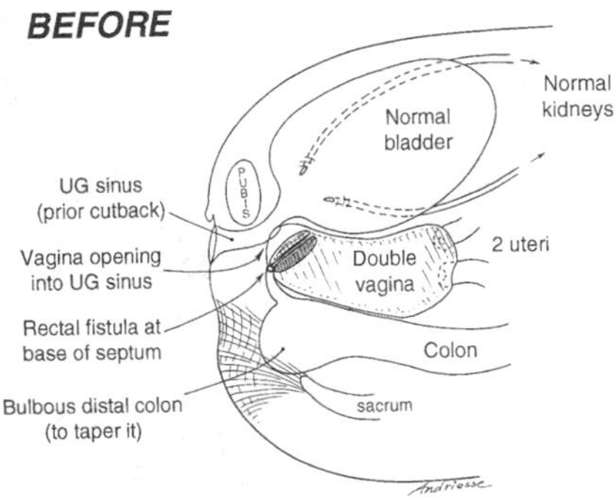

A

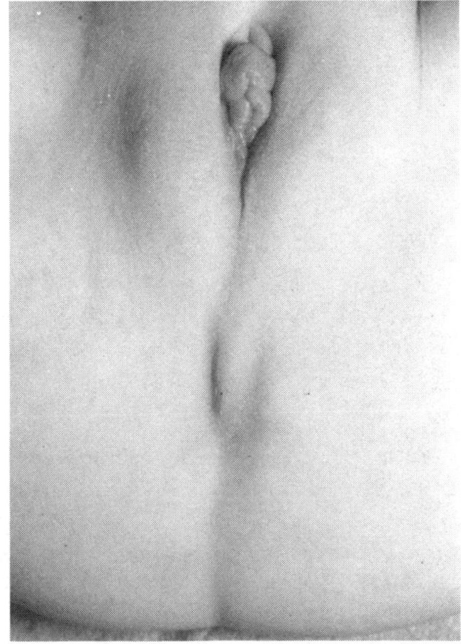

B

FIG. 13. (A) Cloacal anomaly before reconstruction. UG, urogenital. (From Hendren WH. Urogenital sinus and cloacal malformations. *Semin Pediatr Surg* 1996;5:72; with permission.) **(B)** The "blank" perineum of the cloacal anomaly. (From Hendren WH. Urogenital sinus and cloacal malformations. *J Pelvic Surg* 1995;1:149; with permission.)

scopic evaluations (32,34). According to W. Hardy Hendren's reports of 35 years of extensive experience with 133 patients, surgical repair for a primary cloaca is usually done when the patient is between the ages of 9 and 18 months (32). Surgical construction for individuals with a cloacal abnormality is performed by a pediatric surgeon or by a team consisting of a pediatric surgeon, a pediatric urologist, and a pediatric gynecologist. Through extensive procedures, separate functional urinary, gastrointestinal, and reproductive tracts are created (Fig. 14A). As shown in Fig. 14B, there is a perineal body between the new anus and the pull-through vagina. The new urethra lies just beneath the somewhat enlarged clitoris. When the patient is older, the labial tissue can be moved more posteriorly to surround the vaginal opening (35). Multiple revisions of the surgery may be required to create a satisfactory result for all affected functional systems. Full sexual and reproductive function is possible; pregnancy has been reported but requires abdominal delivery (32).

Anomalies of the Uterus and Vagina

In general, anomalies of the female reproductive tract result from abnormalities of agenesis/hypoplasia, vertical fusion (canalization abnormalities resulting from abnormal contact with the urogenital sinus), lateral fusion (duplica-

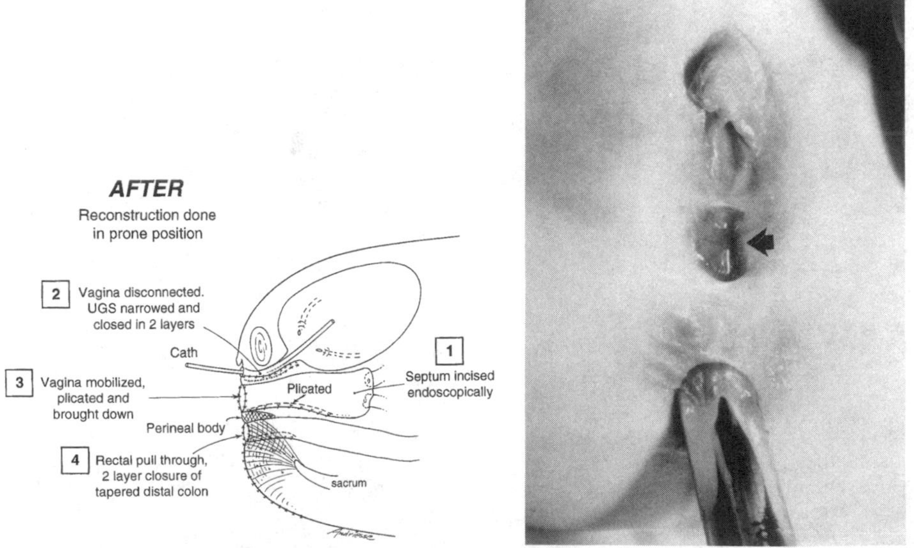

FIG. 14. (A) Cloacal anomaly after reconstruction. **(B)** Three months after reconstruction of patient in Fig. 13 with arrow at constructed vaginal orifice, and a dilator in the anorectal canal. UGS, urogenital sinus. (From Hendren WH. Urogenital sinus and cloacal malformations. *Semin Pediatr Surg* 1996;5:72; with permission.)

tion), or resorption (septum). Each of these abnormalities create an individual scenario of complaints and symptoms, physical findings, evaluation, and therapy. Uterine and vaginal malformations may be identified by the clinician incidentally on physical examination or when a patient experiences primary amenorrhea, acute and/or chronic pelvic pain, abnormal vaginal bleeding, or a foul-smelling vaginal discharge (often worsen at the time of menses). Patients with anomalies that result in obstruction of a functional reproductive tract usually have complaints that differ from those without an obstructive anomaly. Combined uterine and vaginal obstructions may be difficult to diagnose and treat. Although rare, these entities are challenging and are frequently missed in the early adolescent years because the pelvic pain, irregular bleeding, or vaginal discharge may be attributed to functional disturbances (36). Ultrasonography, magnetic resonance imaging (MRI), laparoscopy, examination with the patient under anesthesia, and/or intraoperative hysterosalpingograms may be useful in defining the anatomy in these patients so that the appropriate management options can be presented and reconstruction, if needed, can be performed. Obstructive anomalies will require immediate intervention to relieve the obstruction, whereas nonobstructive anomalies do not require surgical intervention unless the patient has reached reproductive age and has been shown to be adversely affected by the anomaly.

The basic classification of anomalies of the müllerian tract include agenesis/hypoplasia, vertical fusion (canalization) defects, and lateral fusion (duplication) defects. In 1983, Buttram (35,37) classified müllerian anomalies into six subgroups as outlined in Table 1. The American Fertility Society (AFS) (now the American Society for Reproductive Medicine) has adopted a similar classification system (38). The AFS system is based on the degree of failure of normal development and separates the anomalies into groups with similar clinical manifestations and prognoses for fetal salvage upon treatment. These different subtypes of anomalies based on reproductive function were proposed to allow for long-term studies of the reproductive outcomes of each type of anomaly in order to provide better information for health care providers who counsel affected individuals.

The AFS classification system does not include vaginal anomalies but allows for the inclusion of a description of associated vaginal, tubal, or urinary anomalies. Figures 15 to 45 demonstrate schematic diagrams of variations of defects of the female genital tract adapted from the AFS classification system, which we have expanded and revised to include and demonstrate uterine, cervical, tubal, vaginal, and renal abnormalities (38,39).

The etiology of anatomic defects of the female genital tract is not fully understood. Most forms of isolated müllerian duct and urogenital sinus malformations are inherited in a polygenic/multifactorial fashion, although some mendelian forms of inheritance exist and may be a component of a mendelian multiple malformation syndrome (40–43). Table 2 lists heritable disorders associated with müllerian anomalies (42).

TABLE 1. *Classification of müllerian anomalies according to the American Society for Reproductive Medicine (formerly the American Fertility Society) classification system*

Type I: "Müllerian" agenesis or hypoplasia
- A. Vaginal (uterus may be normal or exhibit a variety of malformations)
- B. Cervical
- C. Fundal
- D. Tubal
- E. Combined

Type II: Unicornuate uterus
- A1a. Communicating (endometrial cavity present)
- A1b. Noncommunicating (endometrial cavity present)
- A2. Horn without endometrial cavity
- B. No rudimentary horn

Type III: Uterus didelphys

Type IV: Uterus bicornuate
- A. Complete (division down to internal os)
- B. Partial
- C. Arcuate

Type V: Septate uterus
- A. Complete (septum to internal os)
- B. Partial

Type VI: Diethylstilbestrol-related anomalies
- A. T-shaped uterus
- B. T-shaped with dilated horns
- C. T-shaped

(Adapted from Buttram VC, Jr. Müllerian anomalies and their management. *Fertil Steril* 1983;40:159. Buttram VC Jr, Gibbons WE. Mullerian anomalies: a proposed classification (an analysis of 144 cases). *Fertil Steril* 1979;32:40. The American Fertility Society. The American Fertility Society classifications of adnexal adhesions, distal tubal occlusion, tubal occlusion secondary to tubal ligation, tubal pregnancies, Müllerian anomalies, and intrauterine adhesions. *Fertil Steril* 1988;49:944; with permission.)

FIGS. 15–45. Anomalies of the upper female reproductive tract, as adapted from the American Fertility Society's classification system and expanded with the addition of vaginal and renal anomalies. [Adapted from Goldstein DP, Laufer MR, Davis AJ. *Gynecologic surgery in children and adolescents: a text atlas.* New York: Springer-Verlag (in preparation); with permission; and American Fertility Society. The American Fertility Society classifications of adnexal adhesions, distal tubal occlusion, tubal occlusion secondary to tubal ligation, tubal pregnancies, müllerian anomalies, and intrauterine adhesions. *Fertil Steril* 1988;49:944; with permission.]

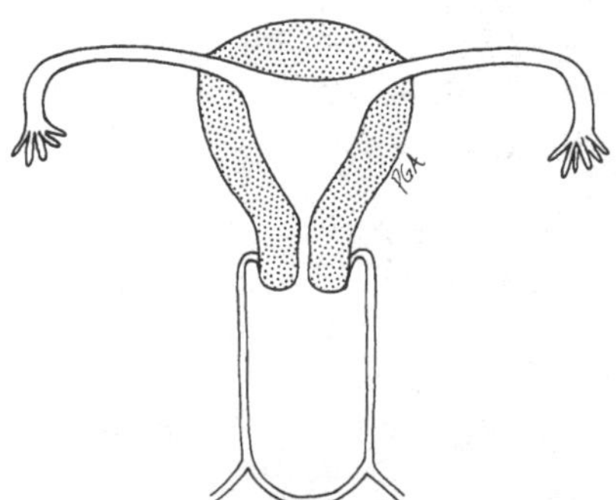

FIG. 15. Imperforate hymen.

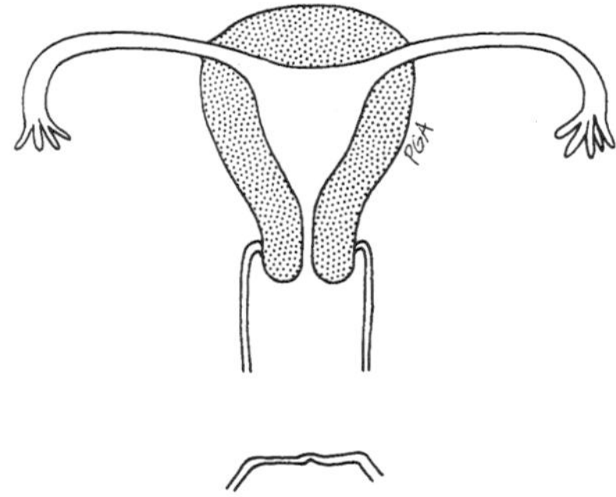

FIG. 16. Agenesis (atresia) of the lower vagina.

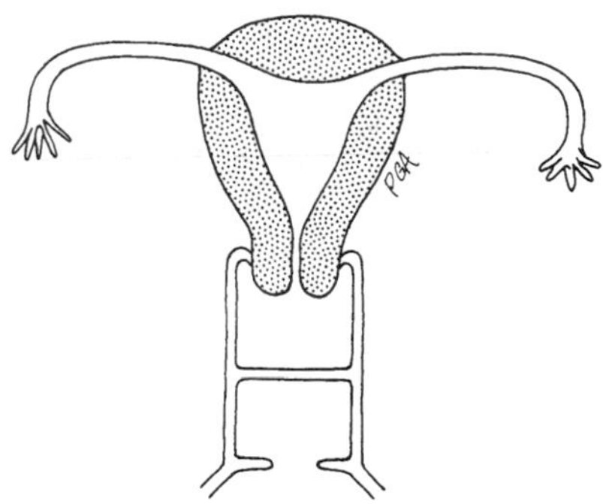

FIG. 17. Transverse vaginal septum.

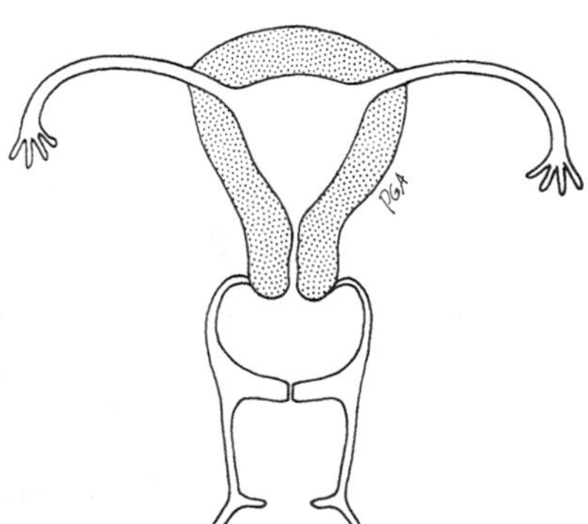

FIG. 18. Transverse vaginal septum with microperforation.

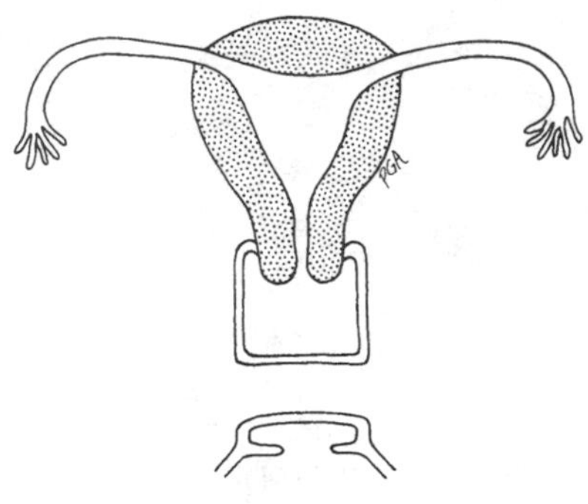

FIG. 19. Agenesis (atresia) of the lower vagina, or thick transverse vaginal septum.

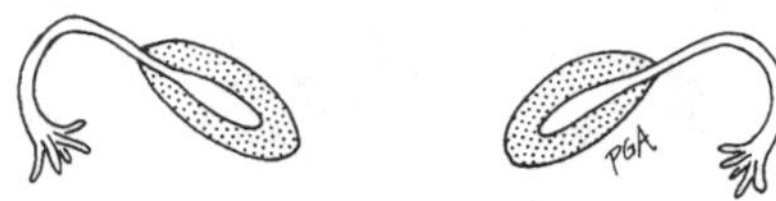

FIG. 20. Vaginal agenesis with rudimentary uterine horns (of note, in cases of vaginal agenesis the uterus may be normal or exhibit a variety of malformations).

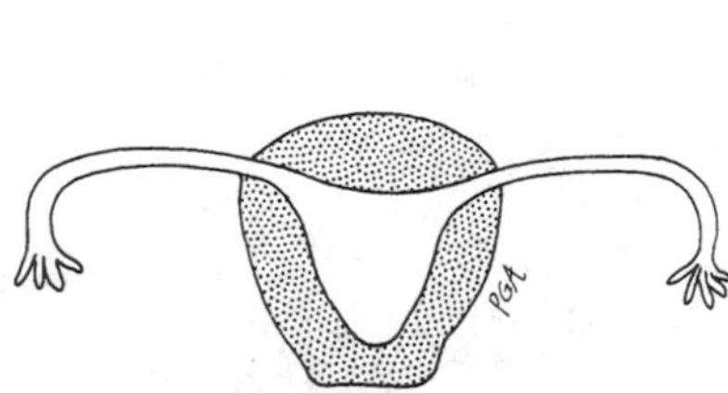

FIG. 21. Vaginal agenesis with agenesis of the cervix.

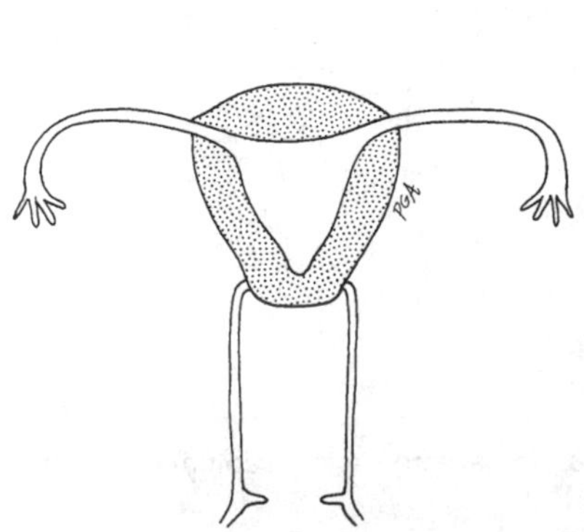

FIG. 22. Cervical agenesis with the presence of a vagina.

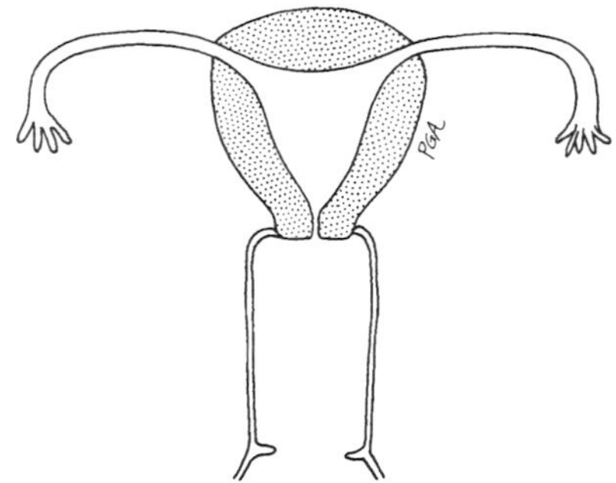

FIG. 23. Cervical hypoplasia with the presence of a vagina.

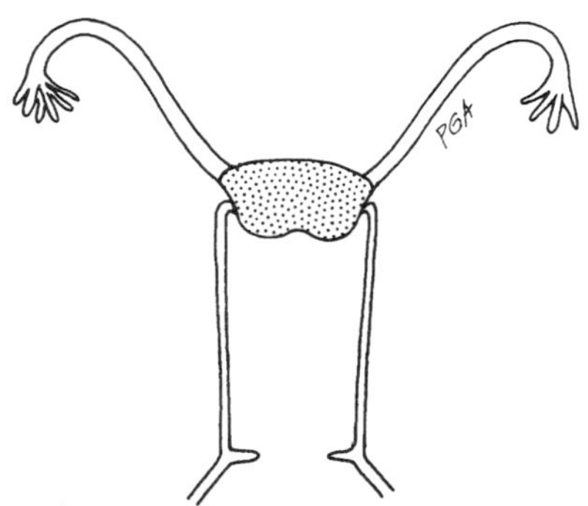

FIG. 24. Uterine/cervical hypoplasia.

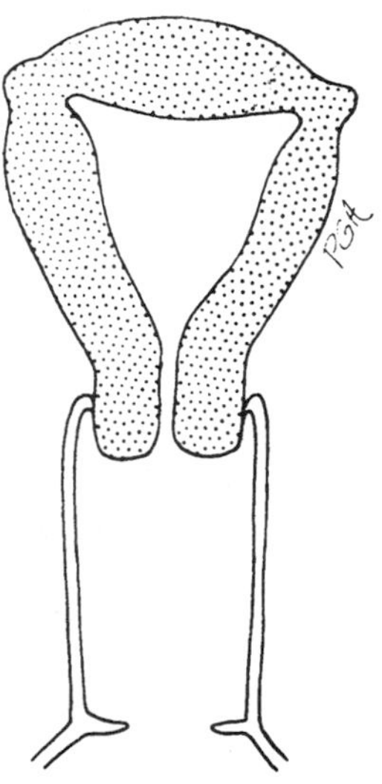

FIG. 25. Fallopian tube agenesis.

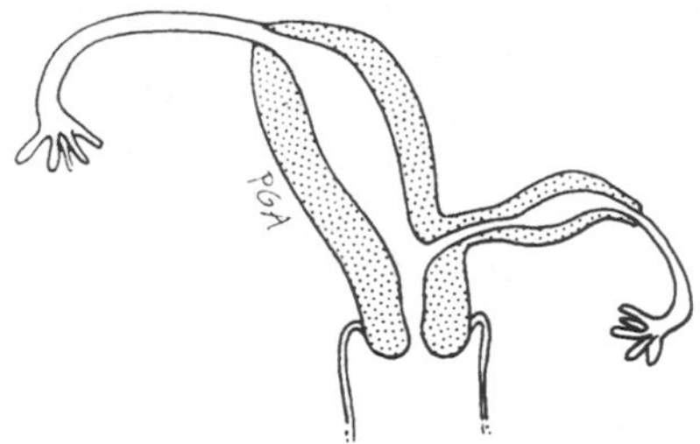

FIG. 26. Unicornuate uterus with communicating uterine horn.

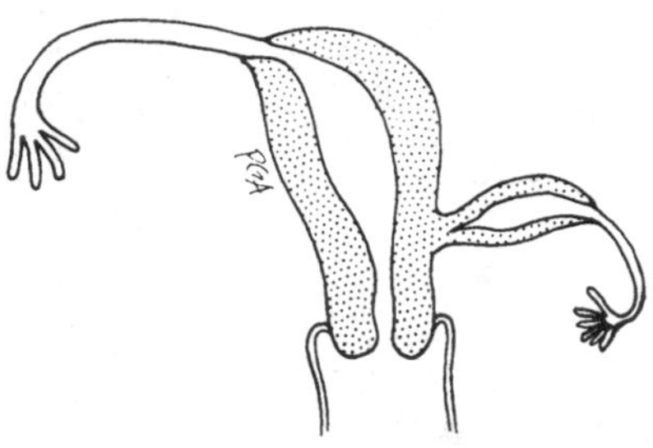

FIG. 27. Unicornuate uterus with noncommunicating uterine horn (containing an endometrial cavity) fused to unicornuate uterus.

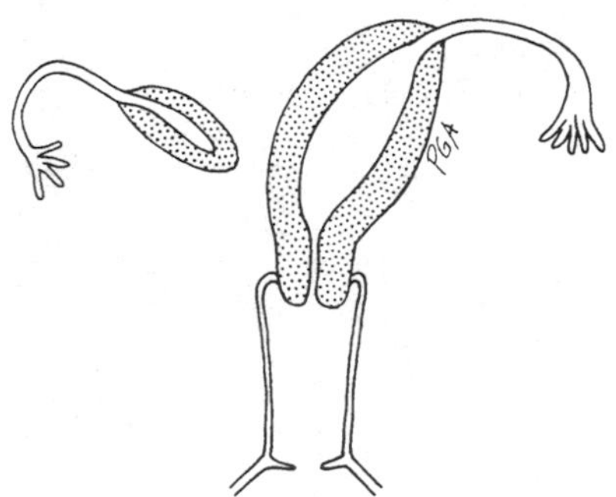

FIG. 28. Unicornuate uterus with noncommunicating uterine horn (containing an endometrial cavity) not fused to unicornuate uterus.

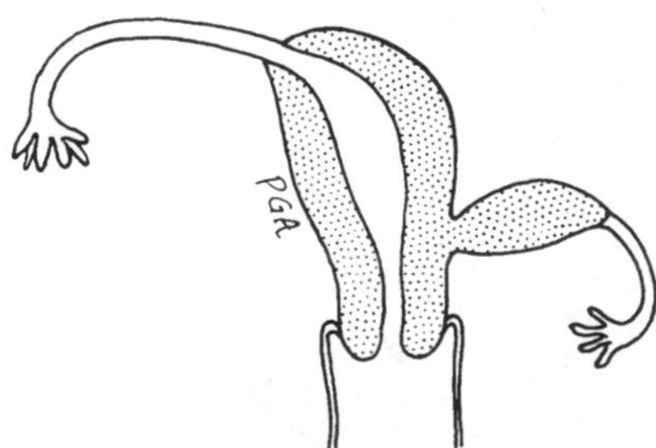

FIG. 29. Unicornuate uterus with uterine horn (not containing an endometrial cavity) fused to unicornuate uterus.

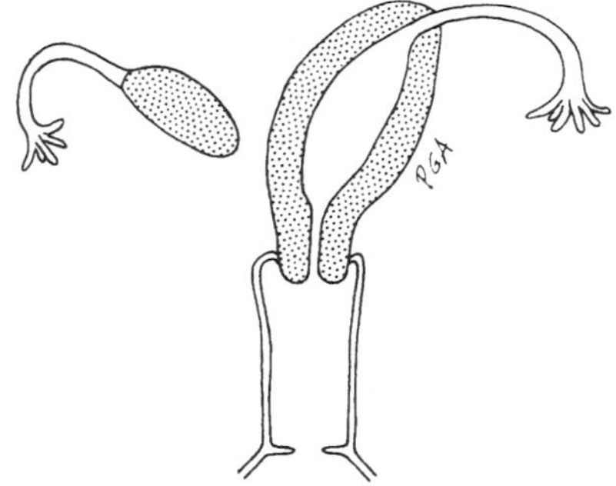

FIG. 30. Unicornuate uterus with uterine horn (not containing an endometrial cavity) not fused to unicornuate uterus.

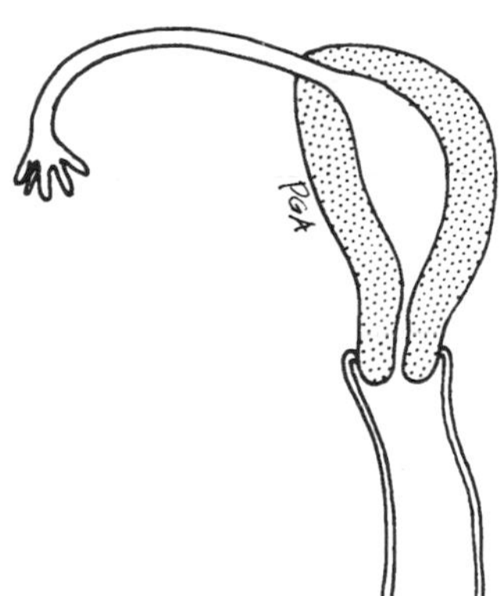

FIG. 31. Unicornuate uterus.

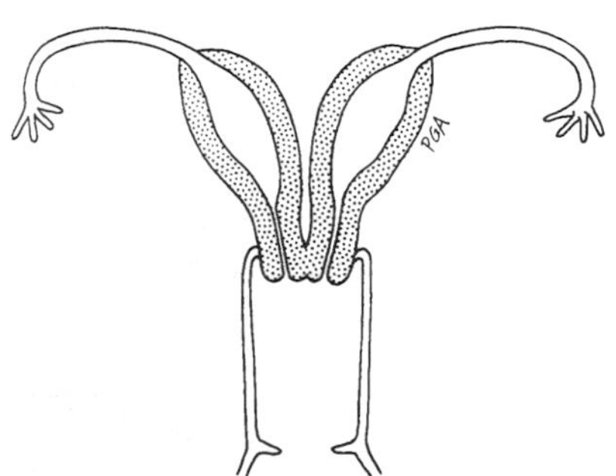

FIG. 32. Uterus didelphys, bicollis, with normal vagina.

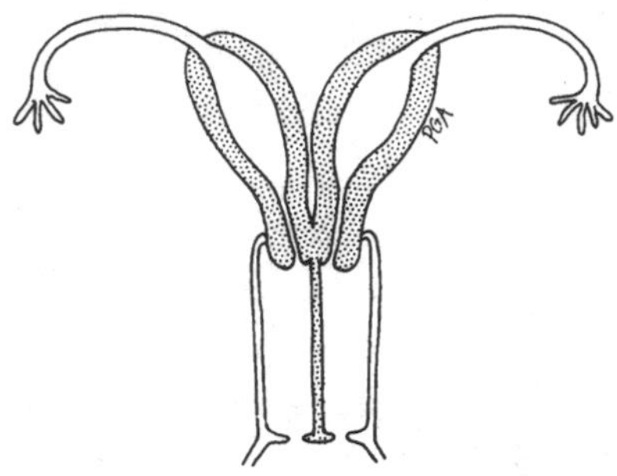

FIG. 33. Uterus didelphys, bicollis, with complete vaginal septum.

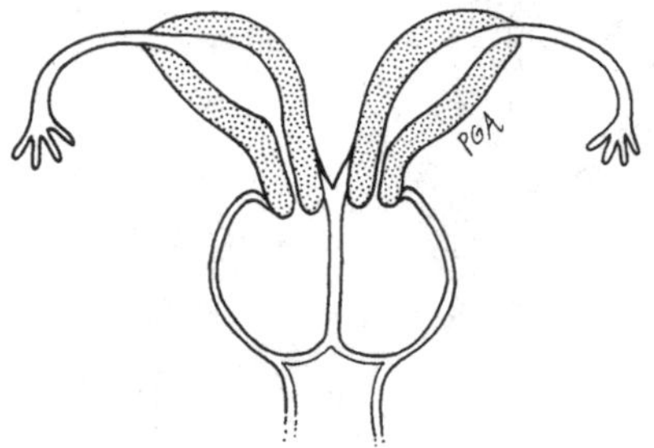

FIG. 34. Uterus didelphys, bicollis, with complete upper vaginal septum with bilateral obstruction.

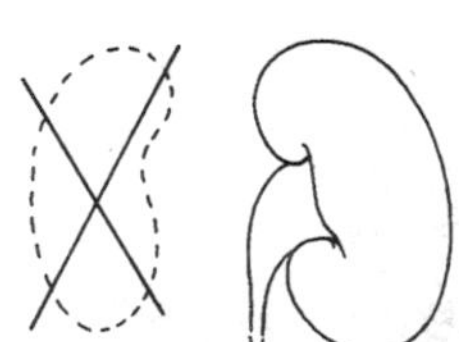

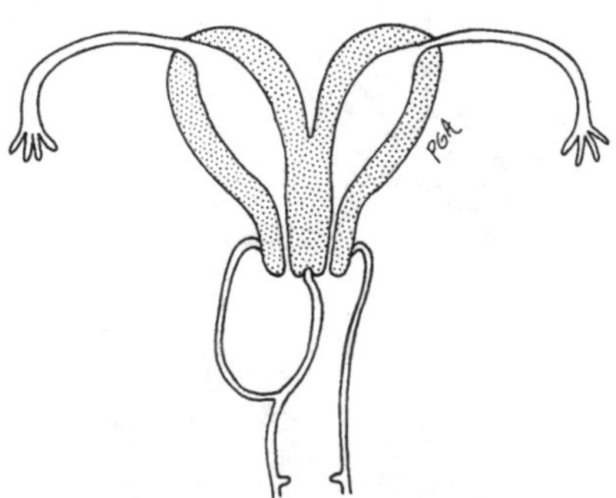

FIG. 35. Uterus didelphys with obstructed hemi-vagina with ipsolateral renal agenesis.

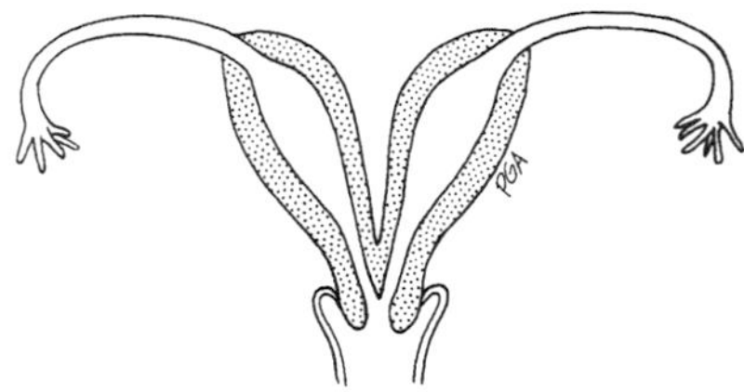

FIG. 36. Uterus bicornuate: complete (division down to internal os).

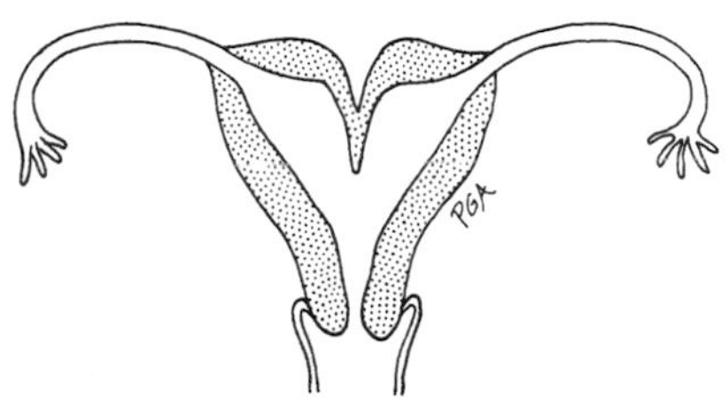

FIG. 37. Uterus bicornuate: partial.

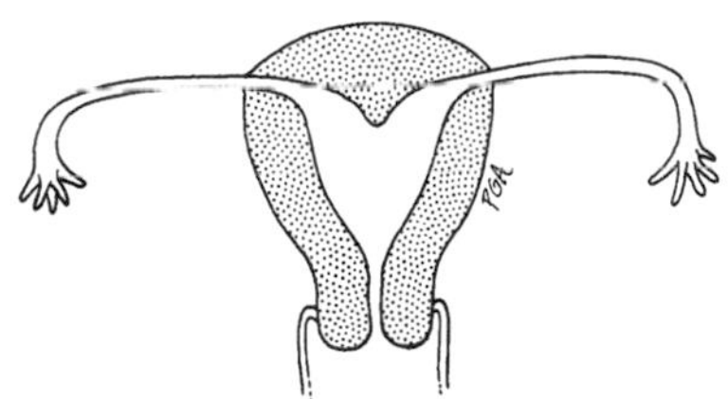

FIG. 38. Uterus bicornuate: arcuate.

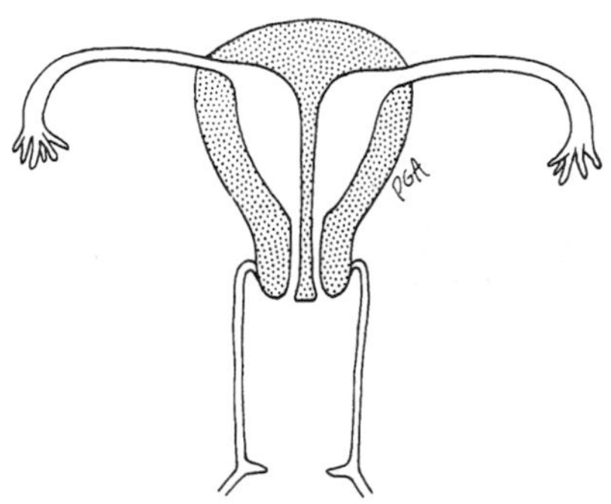

FIG. 39. Septate uterus: complete (septum to external os).

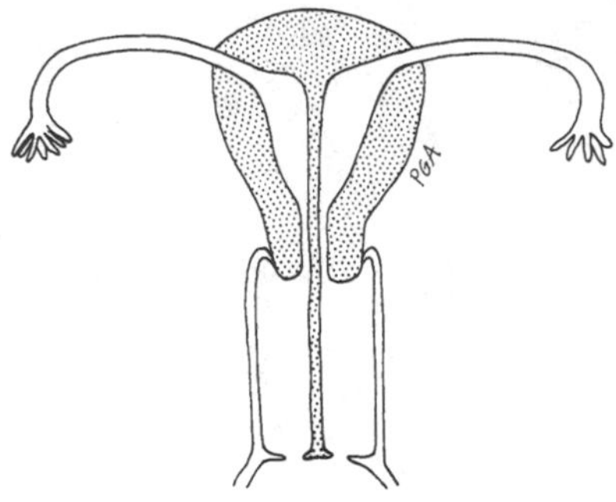

FIG. 40. Septate uterus: complete with associated vaginal septum.

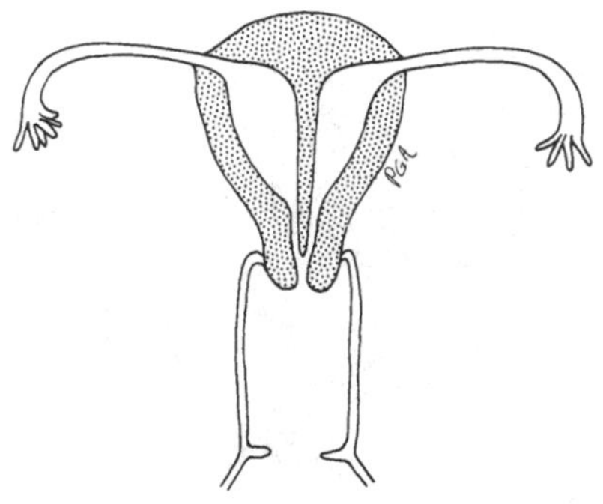

FIG. 41. Septate uterus: complete (septum to internal os).

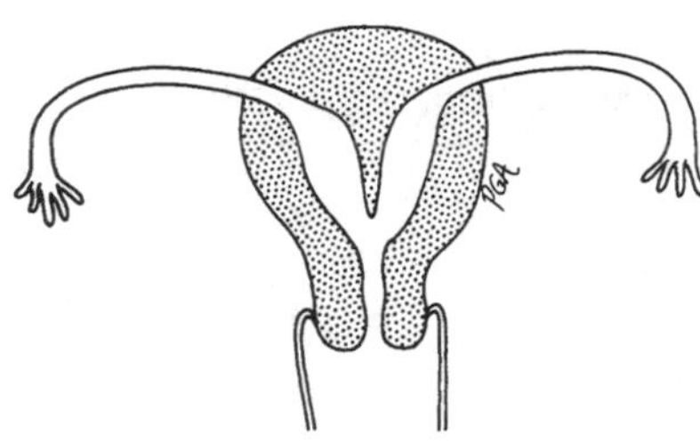

FIG. 42. Septate uterus: partial.

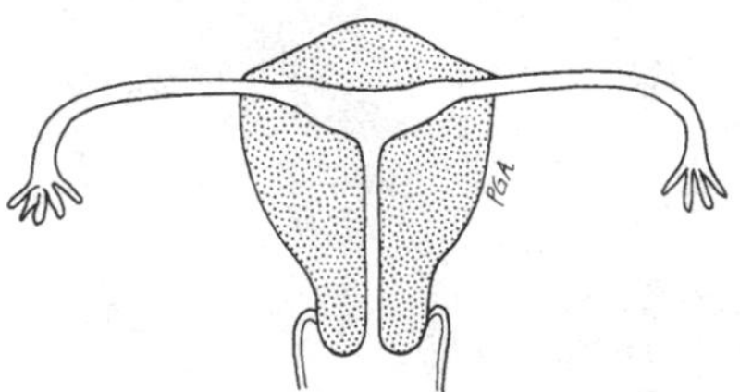

FIG. 43. Diethylstilbestrol-related anomalies: T-shaped uterus.

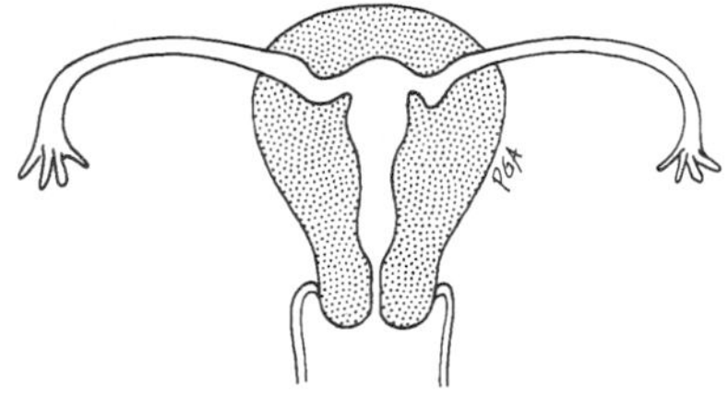

FIG. 44. Diethylstilbestrol-related anomalies: T-shaped with dilated horns.

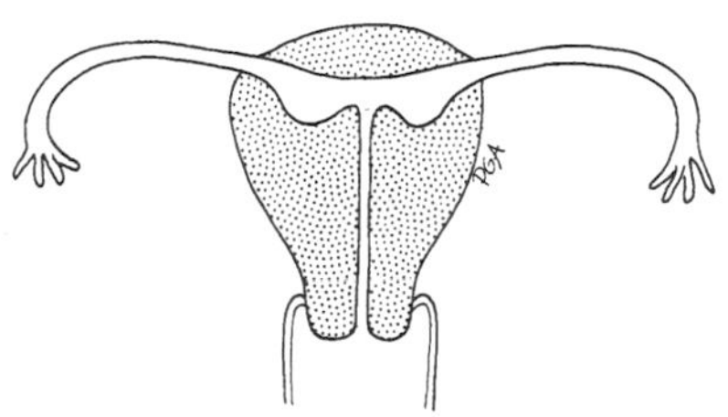

FIG. 45. Diethylstilbestrol-related anomalies: T-shaped variation.

The true incidence of müllerian duct anomalies is not known. Different reports have described a wide range of incidence, depending on whether a general population is evaluated at the time of obstetric delivery, or one with a history of infertility or habitual miscarriage (44–46). In a study of fertile women who were evaluated for müllerian duct anomalies at the time of tubal ligation, an incidence of 3.2% was identified (46). Many women may have an underlying asymptomatic müllerian duct anomaly; since they have no pain, pelvic mass,

TABLE 2. *Heritable disorders associated with müllerian anomalies*

Mode of inheritance	Disorder (MIM no.[a])	Associated müllerian defect
Autosomal dominant	Camptobrachydactyly (11415)	Longitudinal vaginal septa
	Hand-Food-Genital (14000)	Incomplete müllerian fusion
Autosomal recessive	Kaufman-McCusick (23670)	Transverse vaginal septa
	Johanson-Blizzard (24380)	Longitudinal vaginal septa
	Renal/genital/middle ear anomalies (26740)	Vaginal atresia
	Fraser syndrome (21900)	Incomplete müllerian fusion
	? Uterine hernia syndrome (26155)	Persistent müllerian duct derivatives
Polygenic/multifactorial	Mayer-Rokitansky-Küster-Hauser syndrome (27700)	Müllerian aplasia
X-linked	? Uterine hernia syndrome (26155)	Persistent Müllerian duct derivatives

[a]MIM no., listing in McCusick VA. *Mendelian inheritance in man*, 8th ed. Baltimore: The Johns Hopkins Press, 1988. (From Shulman LP, Elias S. Developmental abnormalities of the female reproductive tract: pathogenesis and nosology. *Adolesc Pediatr Gynecol* 1988;1:230; with permission.)

infertility, or reproductive compromise, they may not come to diagnosis. Because familial occurrences of anomalies of the female reproductive tract have been reported, families should be screened by history for the possibility that female relatives have also been affected (47).

Most uterine abnormalities are asymptomatic but may be diagnosed after habitual abortions, menstrual abnormalities, or infertility. Patients with segmental agenesis/hypoplasia usually present with primary amenorrhea if there is no functioning endometrium in a remnant/rudimentary obstructed uterus, or with cyclic or chronic pelvic pain if there is a vaginal, cervical, or uterine obstruction but a normally functioning endometrium. As the ovaries form from the genital ridge they usually have normal structure and function. In cases of vaginal agenesis, cervical and/or uterine structures may or may not be present. If the cervix and uterus are absent, the ovaries and distal fallopian tubes are present, as they are not of müllerian origin. Patients with a totally obstructed genital tract usually have a mucocolpos at birth or a hematocolpos at the time of menarche.

The diagnosis of a structural defect of the female genital tract is usually based on symptoms, history, and physical examination. The genital exam may reveal an imperforate hymen (see Fig. 14 of Chapter 1 and Fig. 46), or a vaginal dimple with vaginal agenesis (see Color Plate 20). Alternatively, the exam may reveal a "blind" vaginal pouch with only the lower vagina present (Fig. 47).

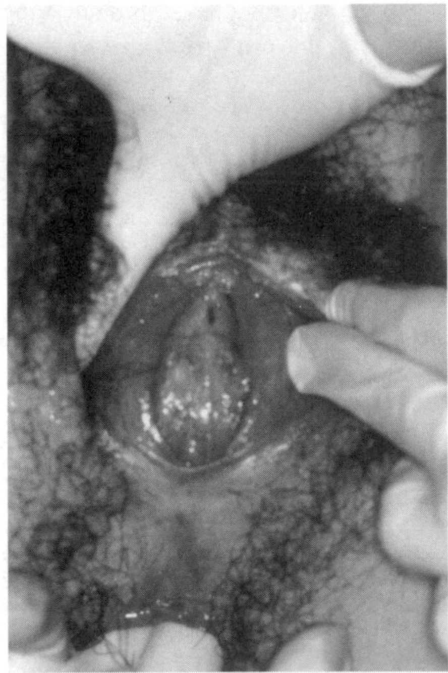

FIG. 46. Hymen with hematocolpos.

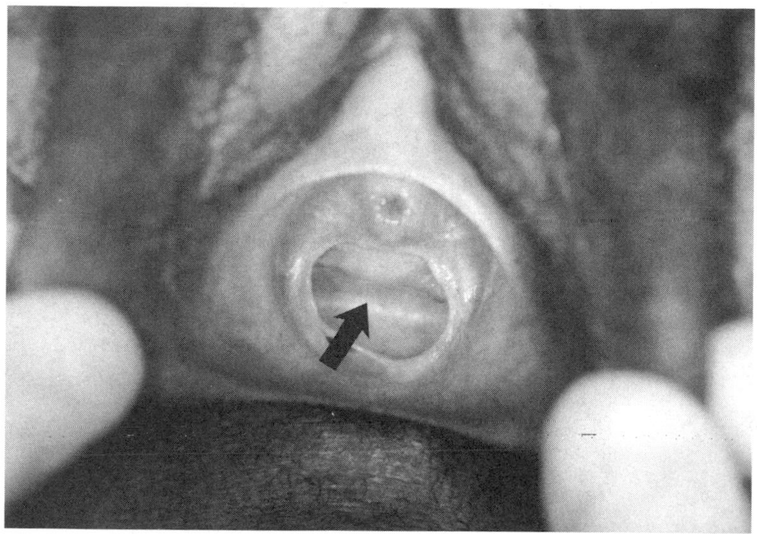

FIG. 47. "Blind" vaginal pouch, with transverse vaginal septum at *arrow.*

Diagnostic imaging of abnormalities of the female reproductive tract can assist in determining the correct diagnosis with delineation of the anatomy and guidance in the formation of a surgical plan for correction of the anomaly. As a result of the obstructive anomaly, patients may have a grossly enlarged blood-filled vagina (hematocolpos) (Fig. 48), uterus (hematometra), and/or fallopian tubes (hematosalpinix). Ultrasound is helpful in identifying the anatomy in all cases of reproductive tract anomalies (48–53) and can be used in a transabdominal, transvaginal, or transperineal approach (48–51,53). MRI can be helpful in determining the anatomy in cases of complicated obstructive anomalies, and many consider it the "gold standard" for imaging of anomalies of the reproductive tract (54–57). It is especially useful in determining the presence or absence of the cervix in complex anomalies, or the presence of functioning endometrium in cases of a noncommunicating obstructed rudimentary uterine horn. A hysterosalpingogram, performed on an outpatient basis with the use of fluoroscopy, can be helpful in determining the patency and possible complex communications in cases of genital tract anomalies (56). In cases of complicated müllerian anomalies, additional information may also be obtained by examination with the patient under anesthesia, vaginoscopy, laparoscopy, and/or hysteroscopy, although with radiologic advances these procedures are now required less frequently (56,58).

Urinary tract anomalies are the most common abnormality associated with congenital anomalies of the female reproductive tract, as the development of a normal müllerian duct is unlikely without the normal development of the mesonephric duct (48,59). Urinary tract abnormalities in patients with müllerian

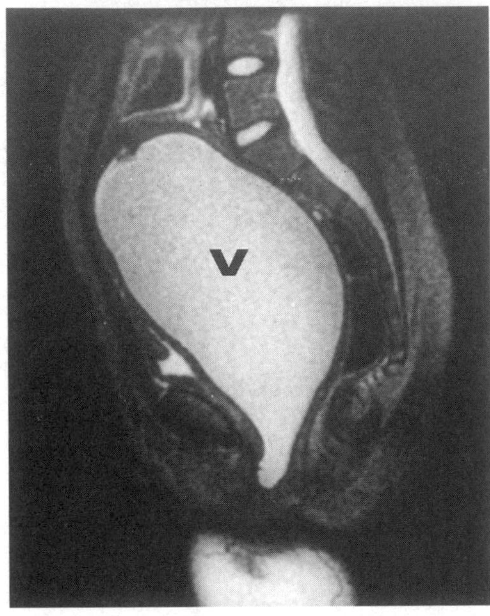

FIG. 48. Magnetic resonance imaging of atresia of the lower vagina resulting in a large hematocolpos. V, obstructed blood-filled vagina. (Courtesy of Carol Barnewolt, M.D., Children's Hospital, Boston.)

duct anomalies include ipsilateral renal agenesis, duplex collecting systems, renal duplication, and horseshoe-shaped kidneys. In the general population, the incidence of unilateral renal agenesis has been estimated to be between 1 in 600 to 1 in 1200, on the basis of autopsy studies (60,61). The incidence of associated genital abnormalities in female patients with renal anomalies is estimated to be between 25% and 89% (61,62).

Other extragenital malformations include congenital scoliosis, limb bud deformity, lacrimal duct stenosis, external auditory canal stenosis, congenital heart disease, inguinal hernia, imperforate anus, and malposition of the ovary (36,63,64). Patients with obstructive and nonobstructive anomalies have an increased incidence of endometriosis (see Chapter 9) and resultant extensive adhesions (65–67).

DIAGNOSIS AND TREATMENT OF SPECIFIC ANOMALIES OF THE FEMALE GENITAL TRACT

Imperforate Hymen

Imperforate hymen (Fig. 15) is probably the most common obstructive anomaly of the female reproductive tract. Familial occurrences of imperforate hymen have been reported; although most cases are isolated events, families should be screened by history for possibly affected female relatives (47). The diagnosis of imperforate hymen should be made at birth, as obstetricians and pediatricians should determine whether there is a patent hymen during the newborn period; many young women with an imperforate hymen may reach menarche before the diagnosis is made. At birth a bulge from the mucocolpos (see Fig. 11 of Chapter 3) may be evident, as there is an increase in vaginal secretions during the newborn period because of maternal estradiol stimulation. If the imperforate hymen is not diagnosed, the mucus will most likely resorb and the bulge will no longer be present. The thin membrane of the imperforate hymen can be visualized within the hymeneal ring.

The adolescent patient with an imperforate hymen may have a history of cyclic abdominal pelvic pain, often for several years, or she may be asymptomatic. A bluish, bulging hymen (Fig. 46) and a vagina distended with blood may be found on genital inspection and rectoabdominal palpation. In some cases, the vagina may be extremely large, and the condition may result in back pain, pain with defecation, nausea and vomiting, and/or difficulty with urination. In extreme cases, hydronephrosis due to mechanical obstruction of the ureters from the grossly enlarged vagina can occur.

The repair of an imperforate hymen can be accomplished in infancy, childhood, or adolescence, although the repair is facilitated when estrogen stimulation is present (early infancy or post pubertal). Bupivacaine hydrochloride 0.5% is injected into the area before the incision is made. One method utilizes a Bovie device (with the plastic shield cut back and placed on three-fourths of the tip to help prevent inadvertent injury to the surrounding tissues) to incise the membrane of the imperforate hymen close to the hymenal ring (Fig. 49). An incision is made, and the mucus, secretion (Fig. 50), or old blood (Fig. 51) is evacuated. Care must be taken, as the fluid within the obstructed vagina may be under considerable pressure; in addition, the "old blood" is usually very thick and may clog the suction tubing. We find it helpful to have more than one wall suction setup available. Once an initial incision has been made and the obstructed fluid drained, the hymeneal area is opened further to create an orifice of "normal" size and remove the excess hymeneal tissue. The vaginal mucosa is then sutured to the hymeneal ring so that the area does not adhere and result in a recurrence of the obstruction (Fig. 49). Additional bupivacaine hydrochloride 0.5% is injected into the repair area, or topical 2% lidocaine jelly can be placed at the conclusion of the procedure for additional postoperative analgesia. In treatment of the imperforate hymen, puncture of a mucocolpos or hematocolpos without definitive surgical repair should be avoided, since the viscous fluid may not drain adequately and the small perforations will allow ascension of bacteria and the possibility of infection, such as pelvic inflammatory disease or tuboovarian abscess.

Transverse Vaginal Septum

Transverse vaginal septa (Fig. 17) are believed to arise from a failure in fusion and/or canalization of the urogenital sinus and müllerian ducts. The complete transverse vaginal septum may be located at various levels (low, middle, or high)

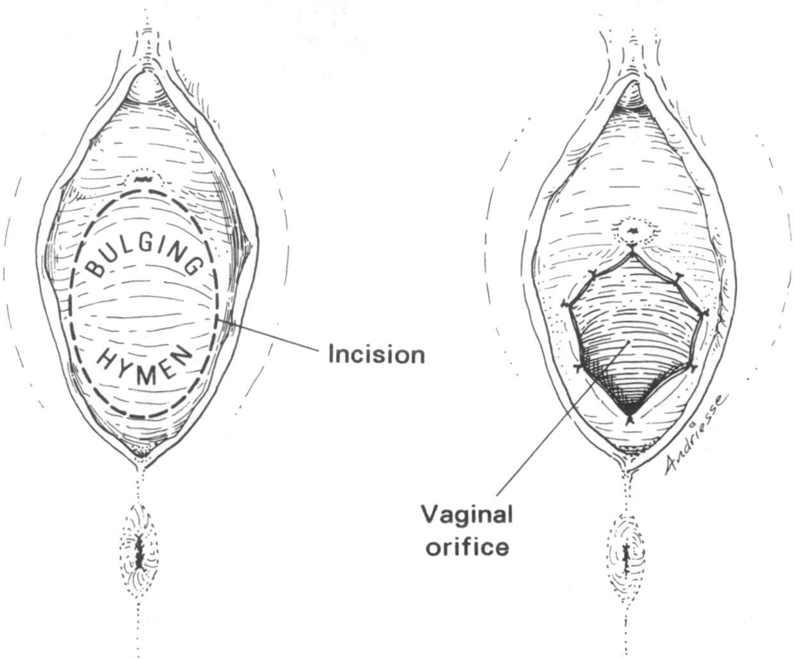

FIG. 49. Schematic drawing of the surgical correction of an imperforate hymen. [From Goldstein DP, Laufer MR, Davis AJ. *Gynecologic surgery in children and adolescents: a text atlas.* New York: Springer-Verlag (in preparation); with permission.]

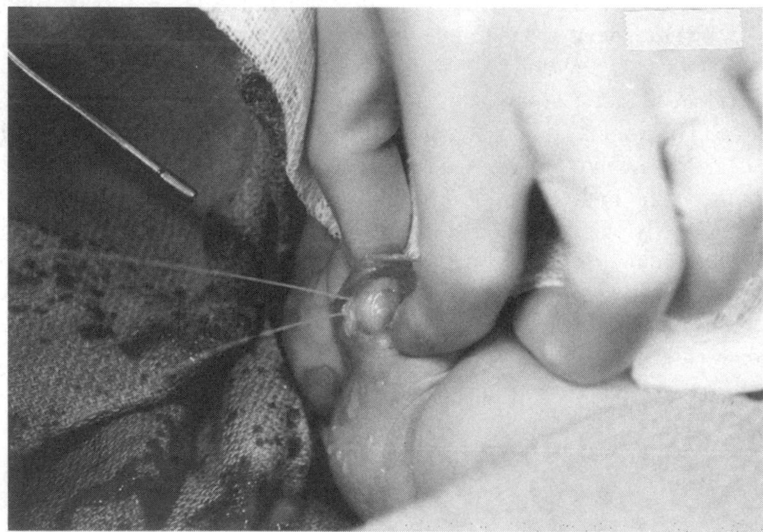

FIG. 50. Draining of a mucocolpos in a newborn with an imperforate hymen; predrainage image is shown in Fig. 11 of Chapter 3.

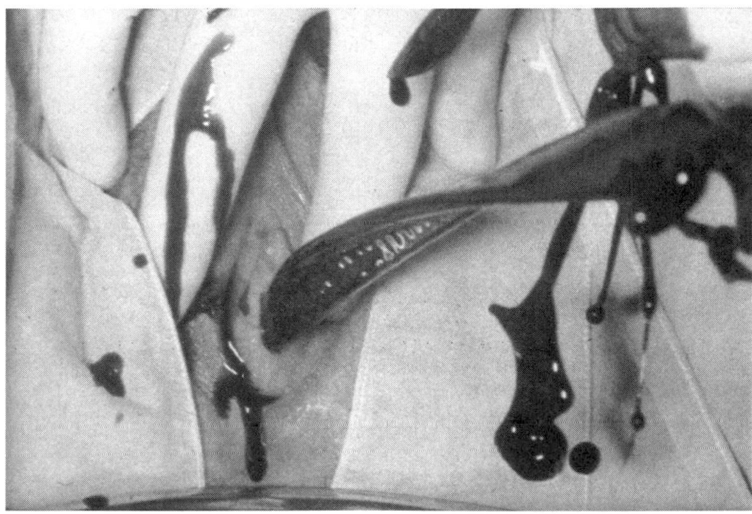

FIG. 51. Draining of a hematocolpos in an adolescent with an imperforate hymen.

in the vagina (Fig. 52); the external genitalia appear normal. Approximately 46% of vaginal septi occur in the upper vagina, 40% in the middle vagina, and 14% in the lower vagina (68). The vagina is short or appears as a "blind pouch" (Fig. 47). The septa are usually less than 1 cm thick and may completely or incompletely extend from one vaginal sidewall to the other. Transverse vaginal septa commonly have a small central (Fig. 18) or eccentric perforation (69) but still may present with hematocolpos in the adolescent, mucocolpos in the child,

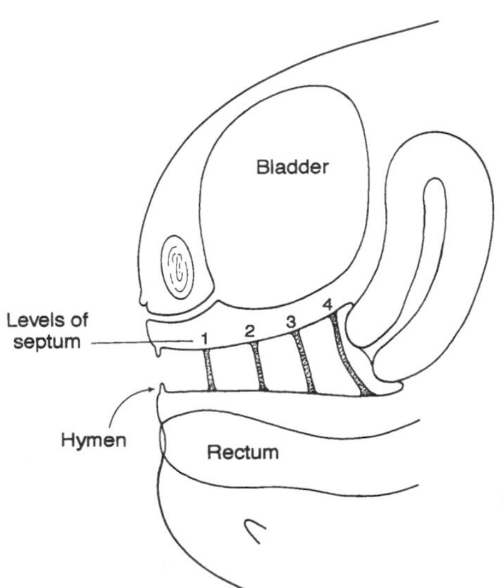

FIG. 52. Schematic drawing of locations of transverse septum. [From Goldstein DP, Laufer MR, Davis AJ. *Gynecologic surgery in children and adolescents: a text atlas.* New York: Springer-Verlag (in preparation); with permission.]

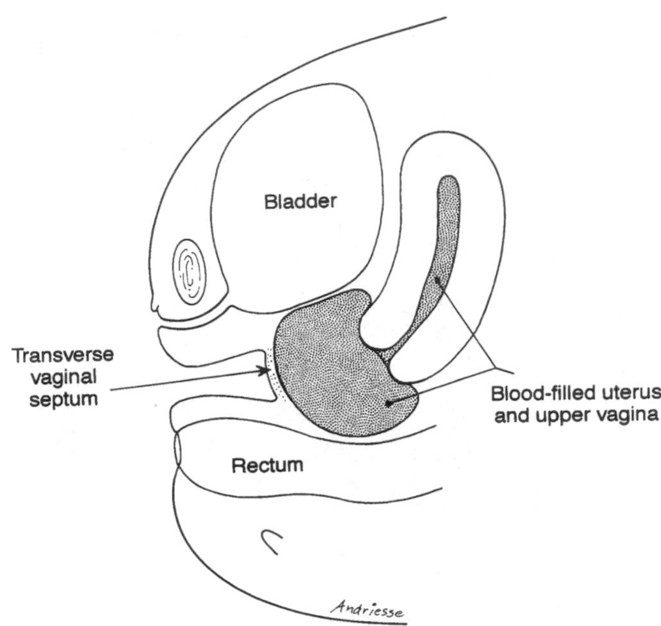

FIG. 53. Drawing of transverse vaginal septum with resulting hematocolpos and hematometra. [From Goldstein DP, Laufer MR, Davis AJ. *Gynecologic surgery in children and adolescents: a text atlas*. New York: Springer-Verlag (in preparation); with permission.]

and/or pyohematocolpos caused by ascending infection through the small perforation. If there is no perforation in the transverse septum, there is a resultant obstruction with hematocolpos during menses; a mass is palpable above the examining finger and on rectoabdominal palpation (Fig. 53). An obstruction with a high transverse septum resulting in hematometra may lead to endometriosis (70).

Ultrasound or MRI may help define the septum and its thickness preoperatively (Fig. 54). Knowing the thickness of the septum can be helpful at the time of surgery. It is also extremely important to identify a cervix on ultrasound or MRI in order to differentiate between a high septum and congenital absence of the cervix (see below).

Surgical approaches depend on the septal thickness and the possible need for vaginoplasty to create a patent tract. The surgical procedure involves incision of small septa with resection of the septal tissue, and end-to-end anastomosis of the upper and lower vaginal mucosa (Fig. 55). Preoperative dilatation of the transverse septum with hard vaginal dilators may decrease the thickness of the vaginal septum and facilitate the reanastomosis of the upper and lower vaginal mucosa. We find that it is best to perform this procedure when the patient has an upper vagina distended with menstrual blood products, as this acts as a natural tissue expander to increase the amount of upper vaginal tissue available to be reanastomosed to the lower vagina, and also thins the septal tissue. A Z-plasty technique may help pre-

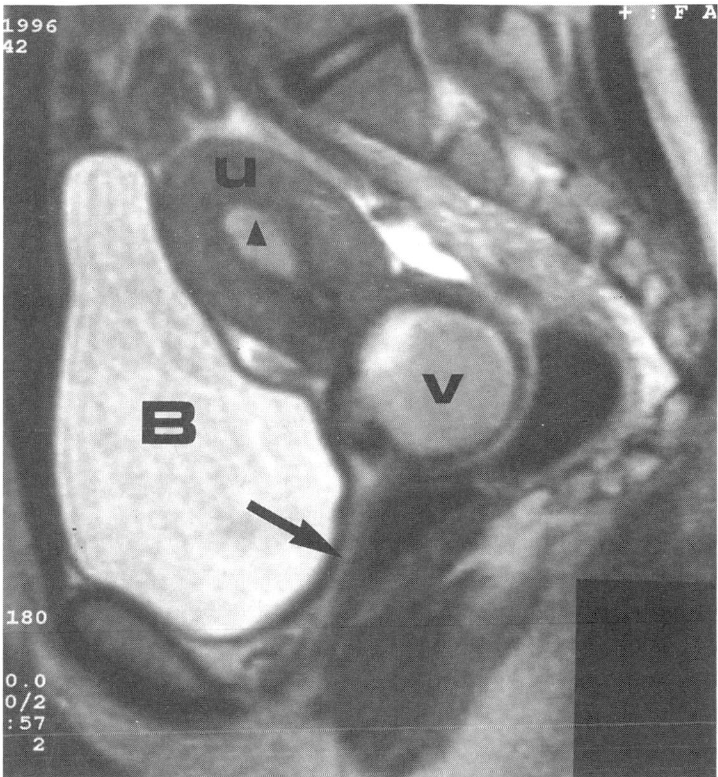

FIG. 54. Magnetic resonance imaging of transverse vaginal septum with resulting blood-filled upper vagina (V) and uterus (U) with hematometra (▲). B, bladder, *arrow* at lower vagina. (Courtesy of Carol Barnewolt, M.D., Children's Hospital, Boston).

vent circumferential scar formation perpendicular to the vaginal axis in a case of thicker septum (Fig. 56). To prevent injuries to the urethra or rectum, a urinary catheter and a finger in the rectum can guide surgery. If necessary, a probe can be passed transfundally through the uterus, down through the endocervical canal, and into the upper vagina so as to tent up the septum and aid in the resection. If the suture line is under tension, a large (No. 24 French) Malecot catheter can be left in place to avoid stricture and reobstruction of the vaginal tract. If there is not enough vaginal mucosa to accomplish a pull-through procedure and reanastomosis of the vaginal mucosa, a skin graft may be necessary to create a patent vaginal tract.

Vaginal Atresia

Vaginal atresia (Figs. 16, 20, and 21) occurs when the urogenital sinus fails to contribute to the lower portion of the vagina. The uterus, cervix, and upper vagina are normal, and the absent lower vagina is replaced by fibrous tissue.

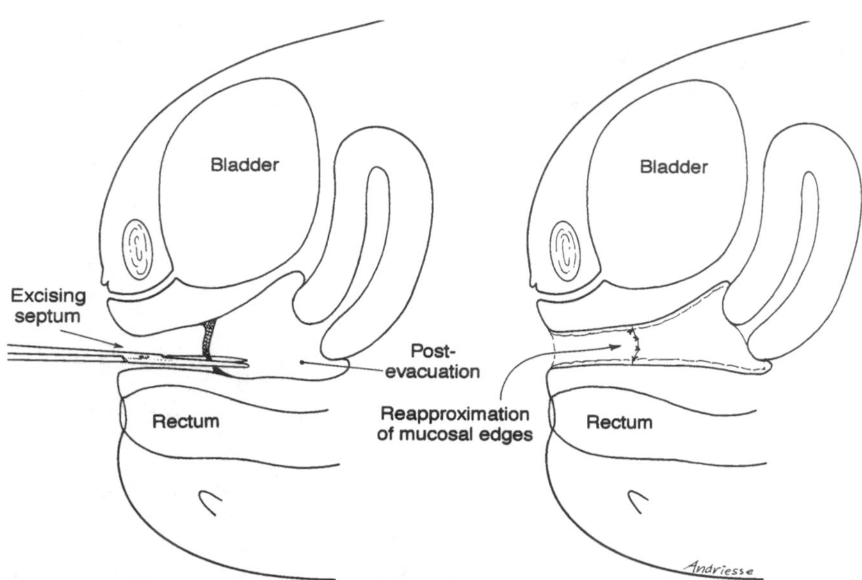

FIG. 55. Drawing of resection of transverse septum with reapproximation of the mucosal edges. [From Goldstein DP, Laufer MR, Davis AJ. *Gynecologic surgery in children and adolescents: a text atlas.* New York: Springer-Verlag (in preparation); with permission.]

These patients usually present with primary amenorrhea, and with menarche may develop cyclic or chronic pain and a pelvic or abdominal mass as the upper vagina fills with obstructed blood and secretions (Fig. 57).

Physical examination reveals normal secondary sexual characteristics; the introital examination reveals a vaginal dimple, as seen in Color Plate 20. A rectoabdominal exam is helpful to palpate possible midline structures (upper vagina, cervix, and/or uterus).

Ultrasonography, which should be done to assess renal status, can confirm normal ovaries, the presence of an obstructed upper vagina, and the presence of a normal cervix and uterus (50). Also, MRI (Fig. 48) may be helpful in the evaluation of these patients, especially to determine whether a cervix is present and to exclude the diagnosis of cervical agenesis (see below) and if functional endometrium is present in a normal uterus or rudimentary uterine horn.

In individuals with agenesis or atresia of the lower vagina, an obstruction with a hematocolpos of the upper vagina will result at the time of menarche and requires a surgical procedure to relieve the obstruction when the hematocolpos is diagnosed. The surgery is best performed when a large hematocolpos is present (Fig. 57). A transverse incision is made in the area where the hymenal ring should be located. Dissection is carried out through the fibrous area of the absent lower vagina, until the bulging upper vagina is reached. The obstruction is then drained and the vaginal mucosa identified. It is then possible to do a pull-

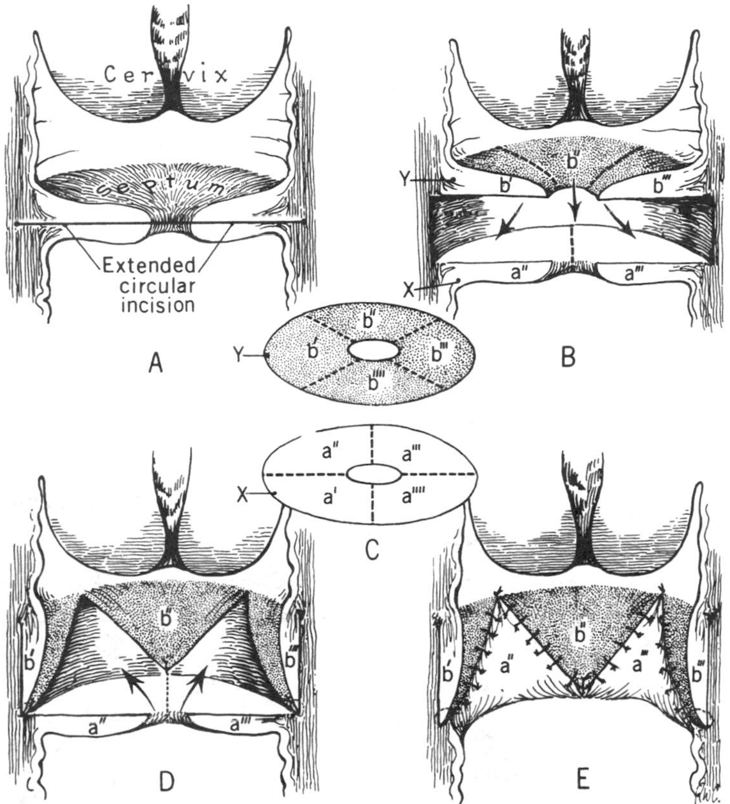

FIG. 56. Z-plasty technique for thick vaginal septum. (From Garcia RF. Z-plasty correction for congenital transverse vaginal septum. *Am J Obstet Gynecol* 1967;99:1164; with permission.)

through procedure to bring the distended upper vaginal tissue down to the introitus (Fig. 58). The upper vaginal tissue is held in place and sutured (with interrupted sutures) to the hymenal ring, as shown in Fig. 59. After the pull-through procedure has been performed, patients have normal sexual and reproductive function.

Vaginal Agenesis (Müllerian Aplasia)

Vaginal agenesis, müllerian aplasia (Mayer-von Rokitansky-Küster-Hauser syndrome), is the congenital absence or hypoplasia of the fallopian tubes, uterine corpus, uterine cervix, and proximal portion of the vagina (71–74). Vaginal agenesis is usually accompanied by cervical and uterine agenesis, although approximately 7% to 10% of patients have a normal but obstructed uterus or a rudimentary uterus with functional endometrium (75–78) (Figs. 20 and 21 and see Color Plates 20, 25, and 26). Vaginal agenesis must be differentiated from

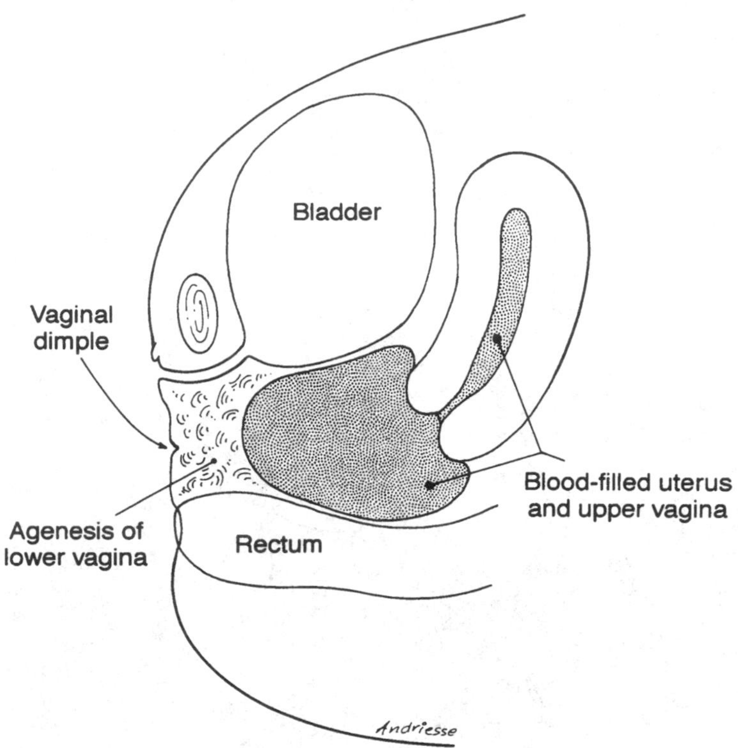

FIG. 57. Diagram of agenesis of the lower vagina with normal uterus and cervix, and resulting blood-filled upper vagina. [From Goldstein DP, Laufer MR, Davis AJ. *Gynecologic surgery in children and adolescents: a text atlas.* New York: Springer-Verlag (in preparation); with permission.]

vaginal atresia (Fig. 16). Another variant is the presence of a uterus but agenesis of the vagina and cervix (Fig. 21).

Müllerian aplasia is estimated to occur in about 1 in 1000 to 1 in 83,000 female births, but the most widely cited incidence is approximately 1 in 5000 female births (79). Mayer-von Rokitansky-Küster-Hauser syndrome is second only to gonadal dysgenesis as a pathologic cause of primary amenorrhea in a referral center (see Table 1 of Chapter 6). These individuals have a normal female 46, XX karyotype and normal ovarian hormonal/oocyte function. Ovarian sex steroid production is normal in these women, and thus puberty and the development of secondary sexual characteristics progress normally except that menstrual flow is absent. The presence of normal breast and pubic hair development, and normal female serum testosterone and pubertal estradiol levels, make this syndrome the likely diagnosis. Although chromosomal studies are not necessary for all of these individuals, an elevated testosterone level, lack of breast development, absent pubic hair, or virilization mandate further stud-

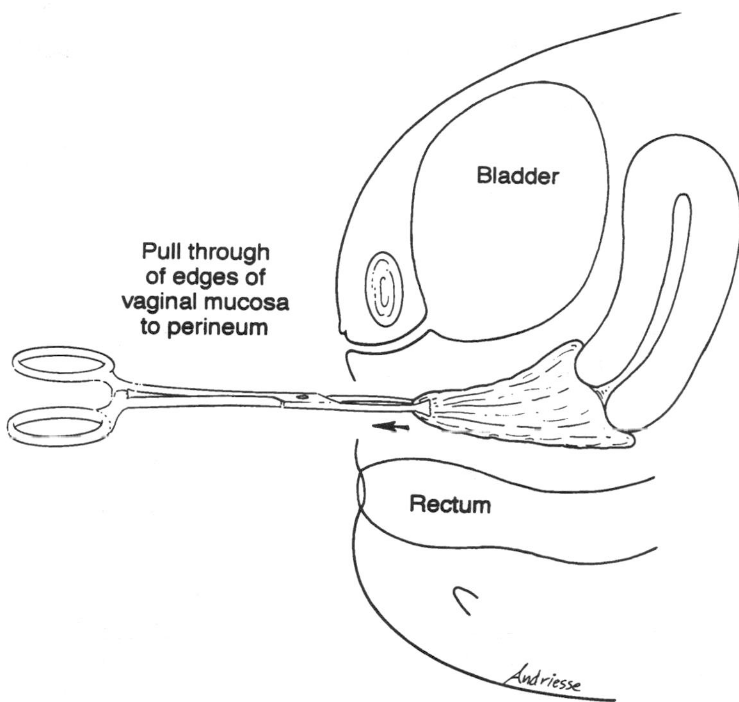

FIG. 58. After drainage of obstructed lower vagina, the normal upper vaginal tissue is pulled through to the perineum to create a normal vagina. [From Goldstein DP, Laufer MR, Davis AJ. *Gynecologic surgery in children and adolescents: a text atlas*. New York: Springer-Verlag (in preparation); with permission.]

ies for an intersex state (see Chapters 2 and 6). The average age at the time of diagnosis has been reported to be between 15 and 18 years. Müllerian aplasia has also been associated with maternal deficiency of galactose-1-phosphate uridyl transferase (80). A high percentage of individuals with Müllerian aplasia exhibit renal and skeletal abnormalities. An association has been demonstrated between Mayer-von Rokitansky-Küster-Hauser and Klippel-Feil (congenital fusion of the cervical spine, short neck, low posterior hair line, and painless limitations of cervical movement) syndromes (81). In addition the MURCS association has been described, which includes: müllerian duct aplasia, renal aplasia, and cervicothoracic somite dysplasia (82).

Physical examination reveals normal secondary sexual development, normal perineum, and a vaginal dimple/small pouch (see Color Plate 20). The hymenal fringe is usually present along with the small vaginal pouch, as they are both derived embryologically from the urogenital sinus. A rectoabdominal exam is helpful to determine whether the midline structures (upper vagina, cervix, and/or uterus) are present.

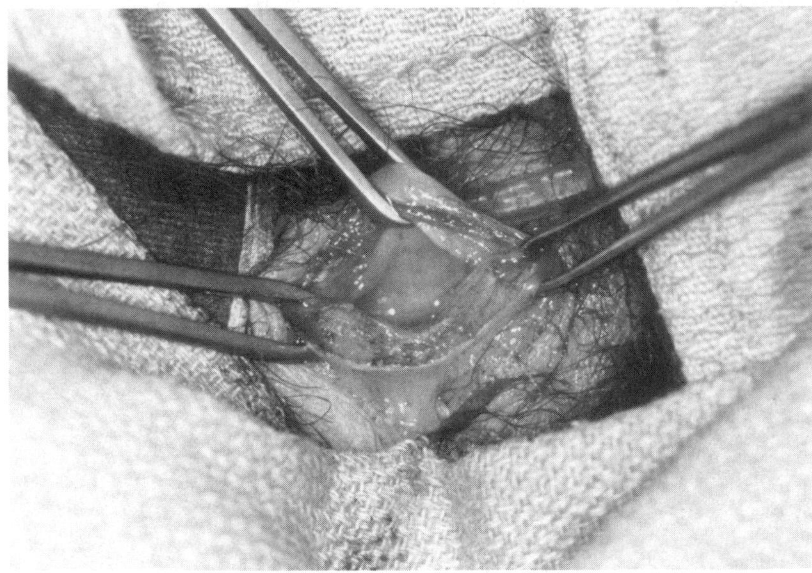

FIG. 59. After drainage of obstructed lower vagina, the normal upper vaginal tissue is pulled through to the perineum; the upper vaginal mucosa is stitched to the created introitus with interrupted sutures to create a normal patent vagina. (Notice that the clamps are approximating the upper and lower tissue to be stitched together).

Ultrasonography, which should be done to assess renal status, can confirm normal ovaries and the lack of a uterus. Remnants of uterine structures may be present (see Color Plates 25 and 26) and may cause cyclic or chronic abdominal/pelvic pain and require surgical excision if endometrium is present in a noncommunicating rudimentary horn. MRI may be helpful in the evaluation of vaginal agenesis, especially to determine whether functional endometrium is present in a normal uterus or rudimentary uterine horn (83).

Laparotomy is almost never indicated in the diagnostic evaluation, and laparoscopy for cases of vaginal agenesis without pelvic pain is not necessary unless the anatomy cannot be defined by other modalities; alternatively, if cyclic or chronic pelvic pain develops, then an assessment and treatment of the pelvis for an obstructed uterine horn and possible endometriosis are indicated (see below).

The treatment of müllerian aplasia should be preceded by counseling of the young woman and her parents. Attention must be given to the psychosocial issues as well as to the correction of the anatomic abnormality. The patient's cooperation and positive attitude are vital to the ultimate success of the creation of a functional vagina (84). The timing for the nonsurgical or surgical creation of a vagina for those individuals with agenesis of the vagina, cervix, and uterus is elective. If surgery is needed, we recommend that adolescents wait until the middle to late teens so that they can be responsible for and comfortable with the therapy. Surgery is usually done in the summer or during a school vacation so that the patient has adequate time for recovery without having to miss school or answer embarrassing questions from her peers.

The nonoperative method of creating a functional vagina involves the use of pressure against the vaginal dimple in order to create a progressive invagination of the mucosa. The Frank (85) nonsurgical approach for creation of a vagina involves the use of graduated hard dilators. The smallest dilator (or a small pediatric blood drawing tube) is pressed firmly (until she feels mild discomfort, not pain) against the vaginal dimple (Fig. 60) daily for at least half an hour after a warm bath. The patient is instructed to insert the tube downward and inward in the line of the normal vaginal axis. We begin the dilatation process with the use of a pediatric blood drawing tube, and once an adequate vaginal dimple has been established we utilize Young's Dilators (F.E. Young & Co., Skokie, IL). Creation of a vagina has also been reported without the use of dilators but with repetitive coitus (86). The Ingram modification of the Frank method utilizes a bicycle seat mounted on a stool to facilitate vaginal dilatation (87). The method is simple and nonoperative and works best when a vaginal dimple/pouch is already present. The nonoperative methods of creating a vagina can achieve a functional vagina in 4 to 6 months, on the average.

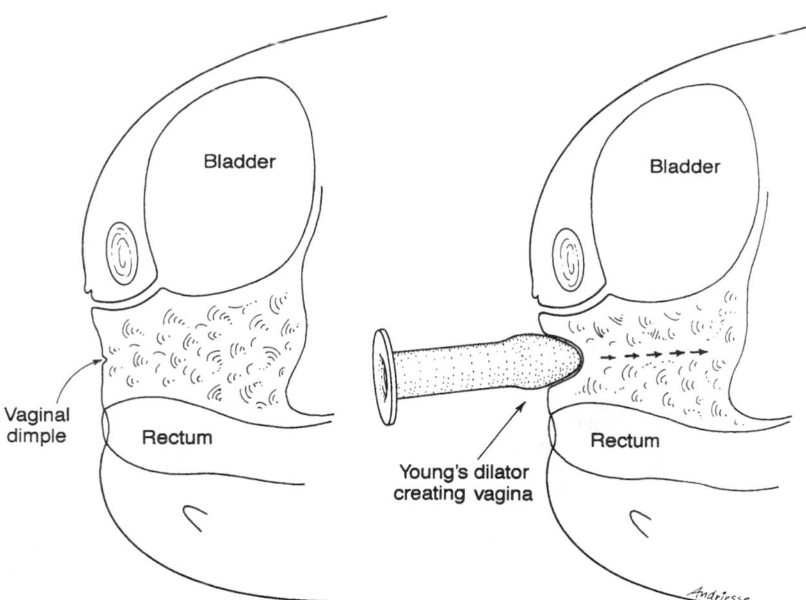

FIG. 60. Graduated hard dilator pressed against the perineum in the Frank nonsurgical approach for creation of a vagina. [From Goldstein DP, Laufer MR, Davis AJ. *Gynecologic surgery in children and adolescents: a text atlas.* New York: Springer-Verlag (in preparation); with permission.]

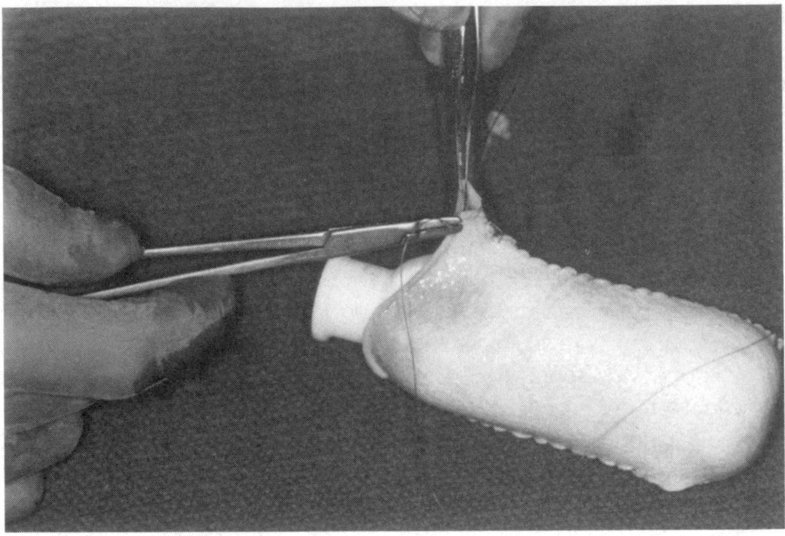

FIG. 61. The skin graft is sewn around a mold.

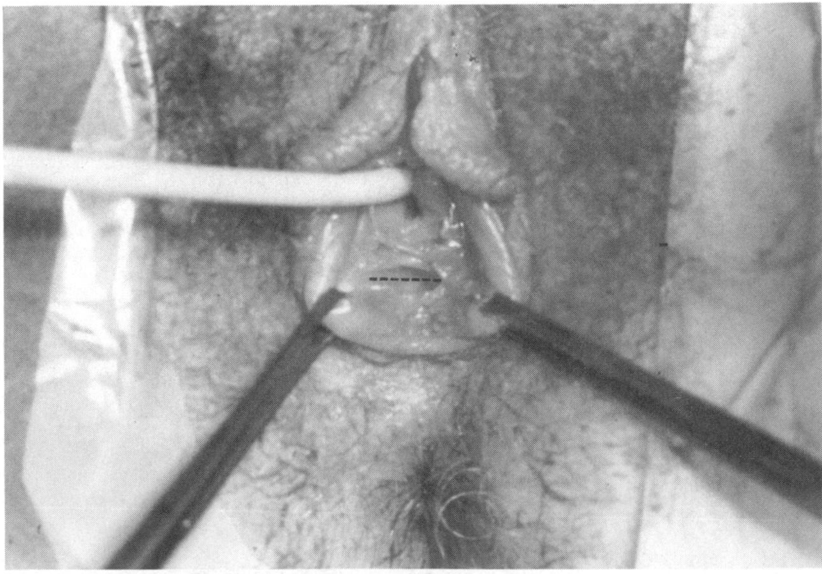

FIG. 62. Incision of the perineum (*dashed line*) followed by dissection of the fibrous tissue below the bladder, above the rectum, and to the level of the peritoneal reflection for creation of a neovagina.

If the use of dilators has been unsuccessful, or if the patient prefers surgery after a thorough discussion of the advantages and disadvantages, surgical creation of a vagina can be accomplished by one of several techniques (88–91). The McIndoe procedure (89,90), used commonly by gynecologists, utilizes a split-thickness skin graft (0.018 to 0.022 inches) taken from the buttocks. To make sure that the graft is aesthetic, the patient can use a magic marker to outline her bathing suit borders so that the graft site is not visible when she wears a bathing suit. The skin graft is placed over a stent, dermal side out (Counsellor technique) (Fig. 61). With the patient in the lithotomy position, a transverse incision is made at the vaginal dimple (see Color Plate 20 and Fig. 62), and a cavity is dissected to the level of the peritoneum (Fig. 63), meticulous hemostasis and asepsis being observed. The mold and skin graft are inserted, and the labia minora are secured around the stent to prevent expulsion. The Foley catheter inserted earlier is removed, and suprapubic bladder drainage is accomplished. After 7 days of strict bed rest and a low-residue diet, the stent is removed (Fig. 64) and the graft site revised. A dilator is needed to prevent contraction of the vaginal graft, and the

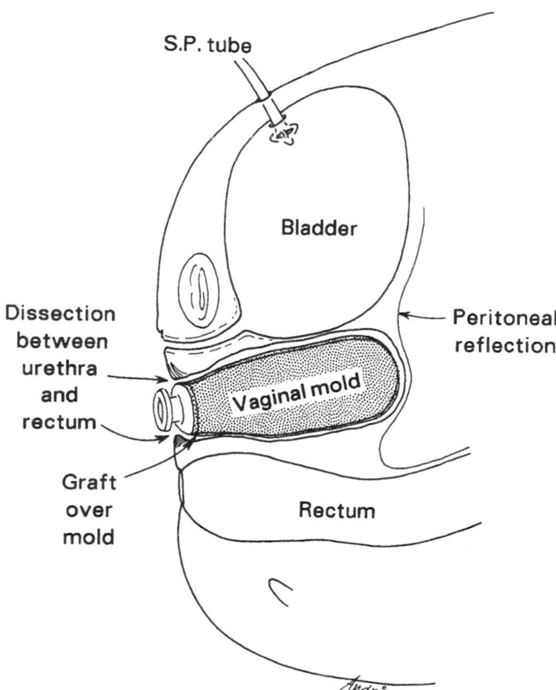

FIG. 63. Vaginal mold with skin graft in place; notice that the mold with the skin graft reaches the level of the peritoneal reflection. S. P., supra pubic. [From Goldstein DP, Laufer MR, Davis AJ. *Gynecologic surgery in children and adolescents: a text atlas.* New York: Springer-Verlag (in preparation); with permission.]

patient is instructed to wear the dilator continually for 3 months, removing it only during urination, defecation, showering, or sexual activity (which can be initiated 3 weeks postoperatively if the patient desires). The patient is seen for frequent followup visits to check the graft (Fig. 65). After the initial 3 months, the patient is instructed to wear the dilator at night for 6 months unless she has regular intercourse. Since failure to comply with followup treatment can lead to vaginal stenosis, surgery should not be contemplated until the patient understands the procedure and her involvement. Talking with another patient who has already had successful surgery is very helpful for many adolescents.

Long-term followup of patients who have had a McIndoe vaginoplasty has shown excellent function and patient satisfaction (6,7,92,93). A patient with a neovagina requires yearly examinations, as there have been cases of carcinoma involving the skin grafts (94,95).

The use of full-thickness skin grafts for the creation of a vagina has been described (96,97). Its proponents report that there is less graft stricture or stenosis than in the split-thickness technique.

The Williams vulvovaginoplasty (98) (Fig. 66) involves the creation of a vaginal pouch. A U-shaped incision is made, and full-thickness skin flaps from the labia majora are used to create a kangaroo-like pouch, horizontal to the perineum (Fig. 67A). A dilator is used daily for 3 to 4 weeks but is not necessary after that. The axis of the vagina is different for coitus, but difficulties can be overcome. Coitus and the use of a dilator assist in the creation of a functional vagina (Fig. 67B). The pelvic structures are not entered in this operation, and thus the risk of fistula formation is low. It is particularly useful in patients with a previously failed vaginoplasty and those who have had radical pelvic surgery or irradiation.

The use of bowel for the creation of a vagina is an option advocated primarily by pediatric surgeons (99–101). The procedure is accomplished via a laparotomy with the creation of a loop of bowel and preservation of its vascular pedicle (Fig. 68A). The bowel loop is them positioned so that one end is pulled down to the introitus for creation of a neovagina, and the distal end is closed to create the blind pouch (Fig. 68B). An end-to-end reanastomosis is then performed to recreate a patent gastrointestinal tract (Fig. 68C). The final result is shown in Fig. 69. Stenosis is believed to be more common when ileum is used than when colon is used (100), and thus, procedures have been proposed to reconfigure the small bowel to increase the diameter (101). This procedure has the advantage over a McIndoe procedure in that vaginal dilators are not required to maintain a patent vagina postoperatively. Also, the patient is not required to remain at bed rest for 7 days, as with the McIndoe procedure. Disadvantages have been reported. Patients complain of the need to wear a pad daily because of the chronic vaginal discharge from the bowel mucosa. In addition, some patients find that they need to douche daily to avoid a foul odor. Adenocarcinomas have developed in the large or small bowel intestinal grafts for the vaginal reconstruction (102). With the increasing risk of HIV transmission during adolescence and young adulthood (see Chapter 14) and the poor barrier effect of gastroin-

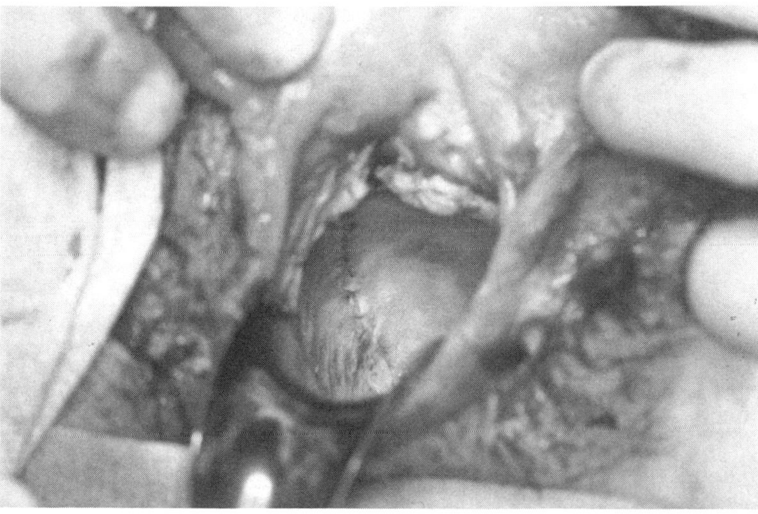

FIG. 64. After 7 days of strict bed rest and a low-residue diet, the stent is removed. Notice the suture line of the skin graft of the newly created vagina.

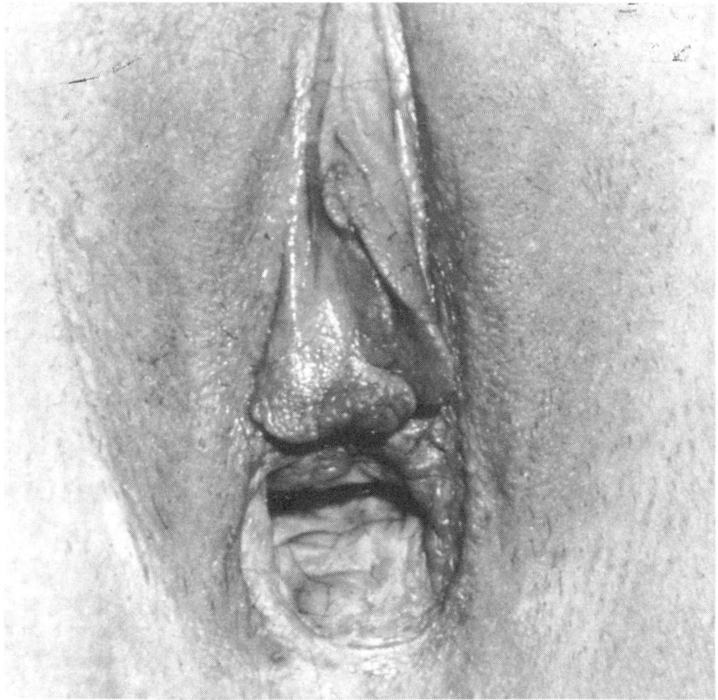

FIG. 65. Followup of vagina created with split-thickness skin graft.

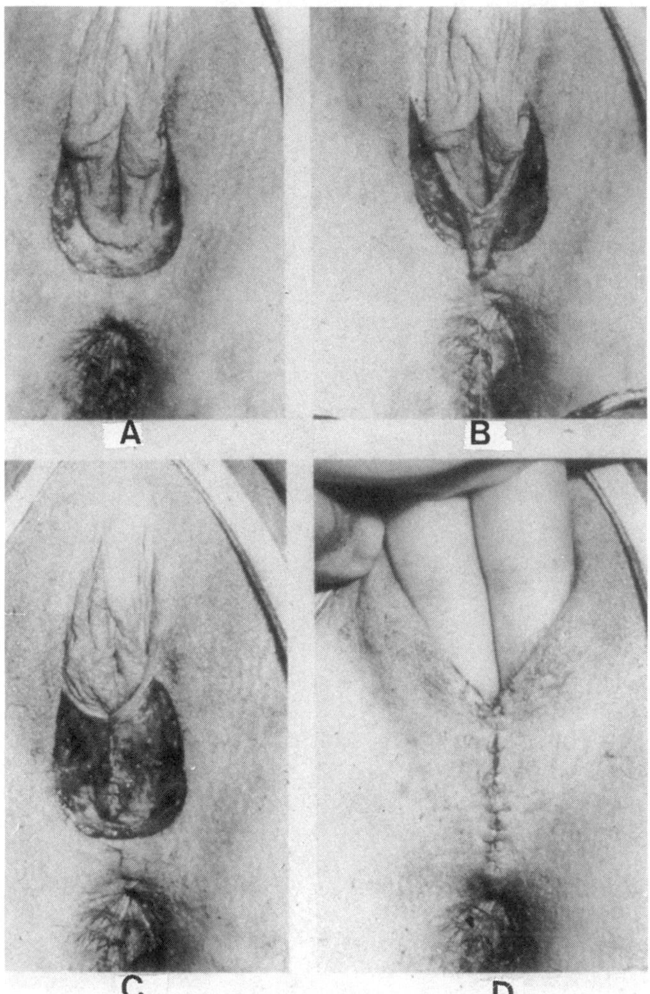

FIG. 66. Williams vulvovaginoplasty. **(A)** Initial incision. **(B)** The edges of the inner skin layer are brought together and sutured. **(C)** The edges of the inner layer are almost completely brought together. **(D)** The outer layer is sutured over the inner layer. Two fingers are inserted into the introitus of the new "vagina". (From Edmonds DK. *Dewhurst's practical paediatric and adolescent gynecology*, 2nd ed. London: Butterworth, 1989; with permission.)

testinal mucosa compared with skin, we prefer the McIndoe procedure for the creation of a vagina in cases of vaginal agenesis.

Other methods for creation of a functional vagina that use the pelvic peritoneum (103,104) or human amnion have been reported (105). The use of human amnion is not practical because of the risk of HIV transmission. In addition, the

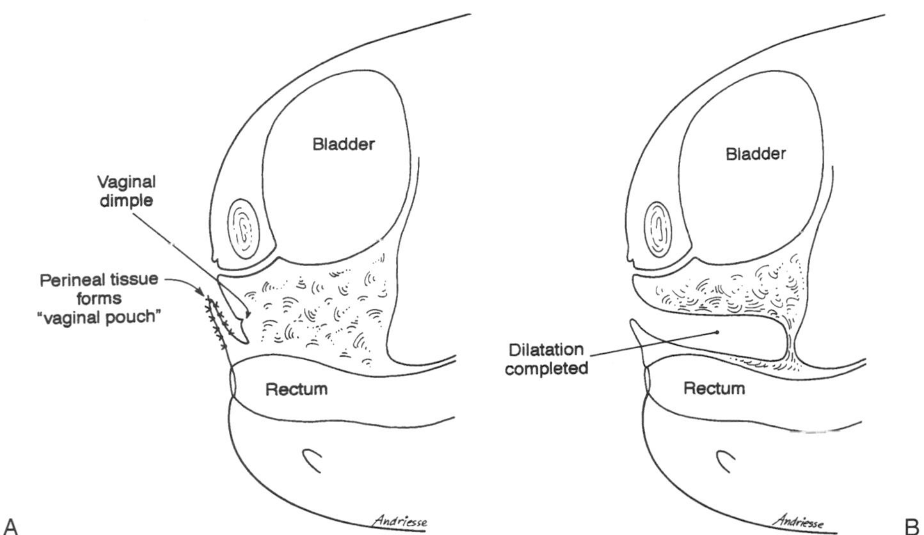

FIG. 67 (A) Schematic drawing at completion of Williams procedure. **(B)** Schematic drawing months after completion of Williams procedure with creation of a vagina with the use of dilators and vaginal intercourse. [From Goldstein DP, Laufer MR, Davis AJ. *Gynecologic surgery in children and adolescents: a text atlas.* New York: Springer-Verlag (in preparation); with permission.]

use of muscle and skin flaps for the creation of a vagina has been described (106–108).

Some procedures modify the Frank technique of perineal pressure for the creation of a vagina, utilizing the placement of a Plexiglas mold placed against the vaginal dimple. The Plexiglas mold has sutures attached to it, which are guided through the vesicorectal space into the peritoneal cavity and out through the abdominal wall (109–111). Tension is increasingly applied to the abdominal wall sutures that pull the Plexiglas mold resulting in the creation of a dilated vagina. After sufficient length of the new vagina has been achieved with serially increased tension the mold and sutures are removed. The patient continues to use hard vaginal dilators to create a functional length of the vagina.

Cervical Atresia/Hypogenesis

Cervical agenesis (Figs. 20–24) is rare (112–114) but is extremely important to diagnose correctly. The true diagnosis of cervical atresia requires the absence of the upper vagina, as embryologically the upper vagina does not develop in the absence of the cervix. Patients may present with primary amenorrhea, cyclic or chronic abdominal or pelvic pain, and/or a distended uterus. Ultrasonography and MRI can aid in defining anatomy (115).

If cervical agenesis is diagnosed, hysterectomy with removal of the obstructed uterus has usually been recommended, as this condition has not yet been particularly amenable to surgical attempts at reconstruction (114–117). However, the creation of an epithelialized "endocervical" tract and vagina, utilizing a specially created vaginal/cervical mold and both skin and mucosal grafts, has been reported (112,118,119). The creation of a "vaginal-uterine fistula tract" places

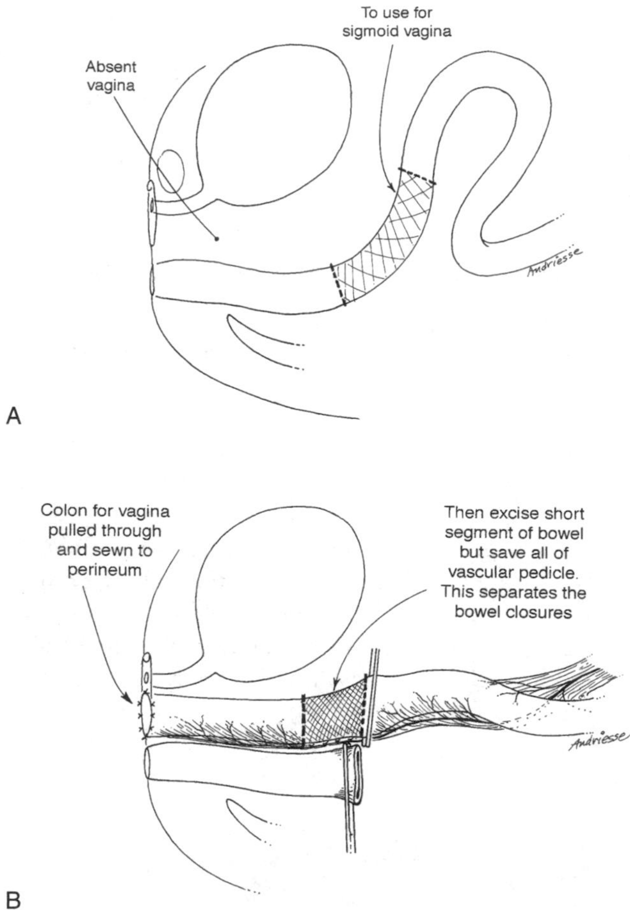

FIG. 68. Technique for sigmoid vaginoplasty. **(A)** Identification of distal sigmoid with blood supply that will reach to the perineum. The bowel segment should not be isolated and divided at both ends at this point, lest length of mesentery be misjudged. **(B)** Distal end of bowel segment is divided and pulled through to perineum and sewn there, which ensures that the bowel comes down with adequate slack and no tension on its mesentery. Only then is the upper end of the bowel segment divided, care being taken to preserve its adjacent blood supply. Removing the short segment of bowel above that will separate the rectosigmoid anastomosis from the closure of rhe upper end of the bowel used for the vagina to protect against fistula formation. (From Hendren WH, Atala A. Use of bowel for vaginal reconstruction. *J Urol* 1994;152:752; with permission.)

the patient at risk of an ascending infection, recurrent obstruction, sepsis, and possible septic death (36,113,120–122). However, successful pregnancies have followed these procedures (77,123,124), and a zygote intrafallopian tube transfer (ZIFT) in a patient with congenital cervical atresia following a fistulous drainage procedure has been reported (125).

Variations of cervical agenesis can occur with a single midline uterus, or with hemiuteri, as shown in Color Plates 25 and 26. If a patient with hemiuteri and cervical agenesis is not experiencing pain, then the uteri should not be removed to maintain reproductive potential; a successful pregnancy has occurred with the use of ZIFT in women with rudimentary uterine horns and cervical agenesis (125). If a patient develops pain, continuous oral contraceptives can be used to suppress retrograde menses so that reproductive function can be preserved.

Obstructed Uterine Rudimentary Horns: Diagnosis and Surgical Treatment

In women with müllerian aplasia and cyclic or chronic abdominal or pelvic pain, a noncommunicating uterine horn with functional endometrium should be suspected (Figs. 27 and 28). Ultrasound and/or MRI may be useful in identifying the noncommunicating uterine horn and determining whether an endometrial stripe is present. Laparoscopy may be needed to diagnose and remove the obstructed rudimentary noncommunicating uterine horn (see Color Plate 27). Figures 70 to 72 demonstrate the laparoscopic approach to the removal of the obstructed uterine horn seen in Color Plate 27 (126). Since patients with a unicornuate uterus have an increased risk of premature labor, metroplasty may improve reproductive outcome, although no controlled studies of excision of the

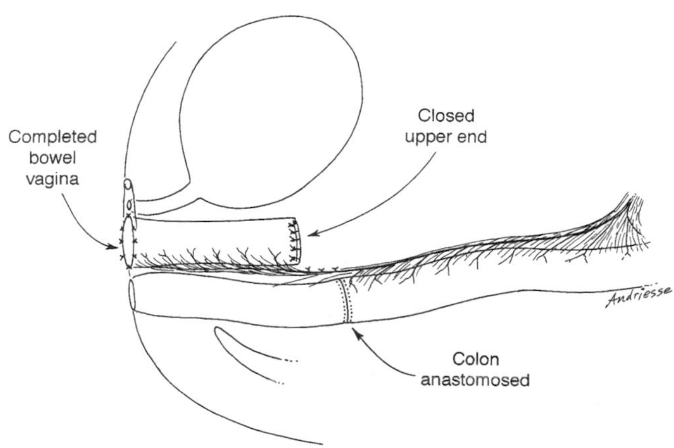

FIG. 68. (C) Completed sigmoid vagina. (From Hendren WH, Atala A. Use of bowel for vaginal reconstruction. *J Urol* 1994;152:752; with permission.)

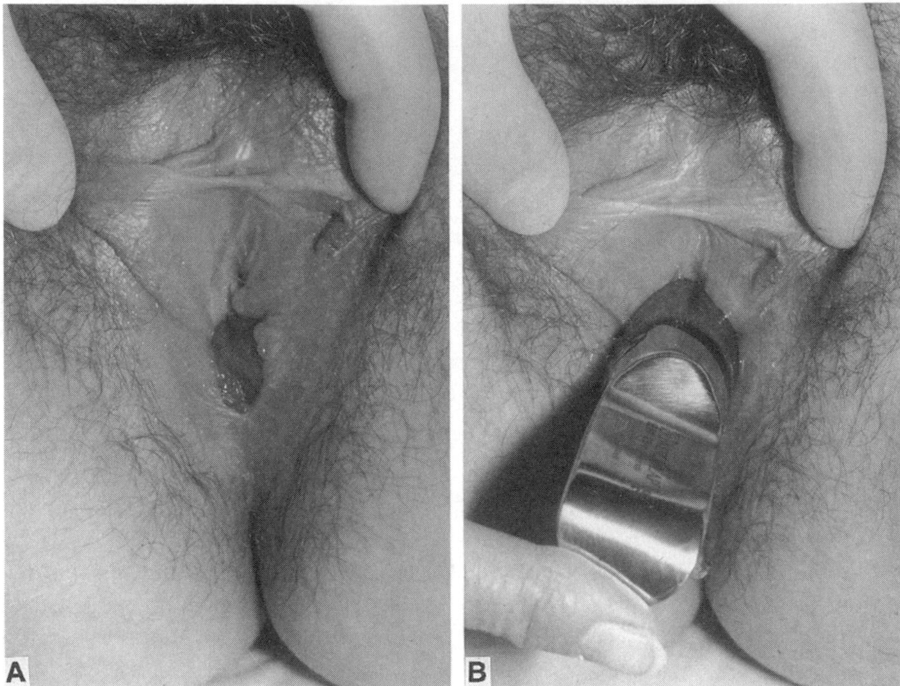

FIG. 69. (A) Postoperative view of the perineum with the sigmoid vagina anastomosed to vaginal introitus. **(B)** No. 26 Hegar dilator (6 inches long) reveals normal vaginal caliber and depth. Patients are advised to pass the dilator periodically to ensure continuation of adequate caliber. This procedure is not as important as it would be for a skin graft vagina, which will contract if not periodically dilated in this fashion or by coitus. (From Hendren WH, Atala A. Use of bowel for vaginal reconstruction. *J Urol* 1994;152:752; with permission.)

blind horn versus metroplasty have been done. Patients with an obstructed uterine horn are at increased risk of endometriosis, but the endometriosis is usually found to resolve after the correction of the obstruction (see Chapter 9). Excision of the obstructed rudimentary blind horn will prevent endometriosis by eliminating reflux. Spontaneous pregnancies in obstructed uterine horns have been reported (127).

True Duplication and Incomplete Fusion of the Müllerian Ducts

A true duplication of the uterus is rare (Figs. 32–36). This abnormality results from unilateral or bilateral duplication of the müllerian ducts and subsequent doubling of reproductive structures on one or both sides. These are not hemiuteri. True duplication may also result in the very rare occurrence of complete duplication of the vulva, bladder, urethra, vagina, and anus (Fig. 73).

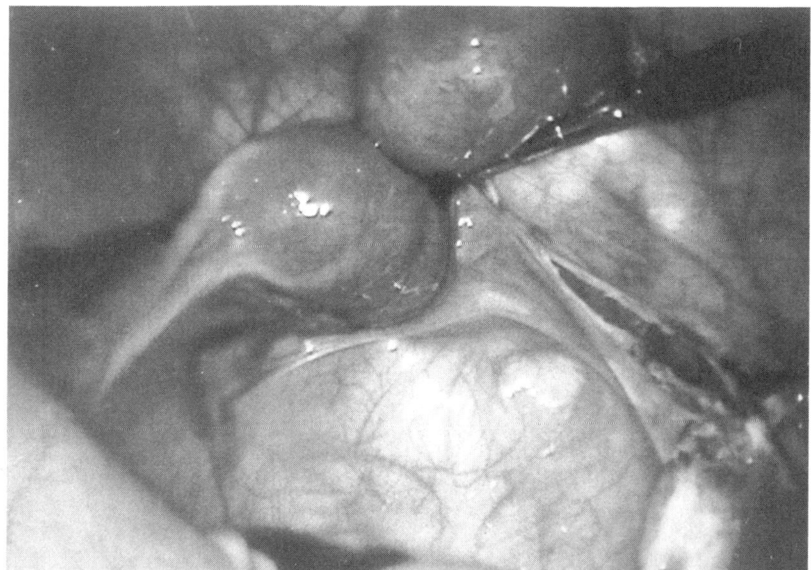

FIG. 70. Laparoscopic approach to removal of the obstructed right uterine horn shown in Color Plate 27.

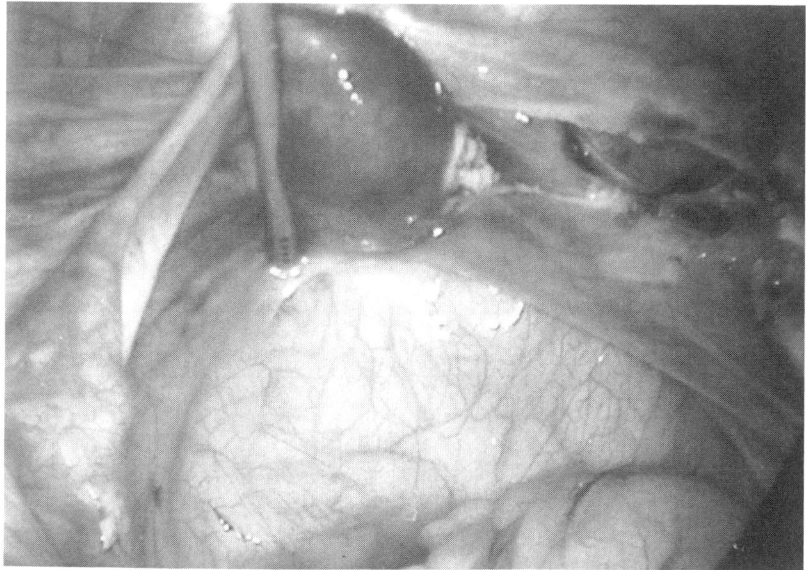

FIG. 71. Completion of laparoscopic resection of obstructed right uterine horn in Color Plate 27.

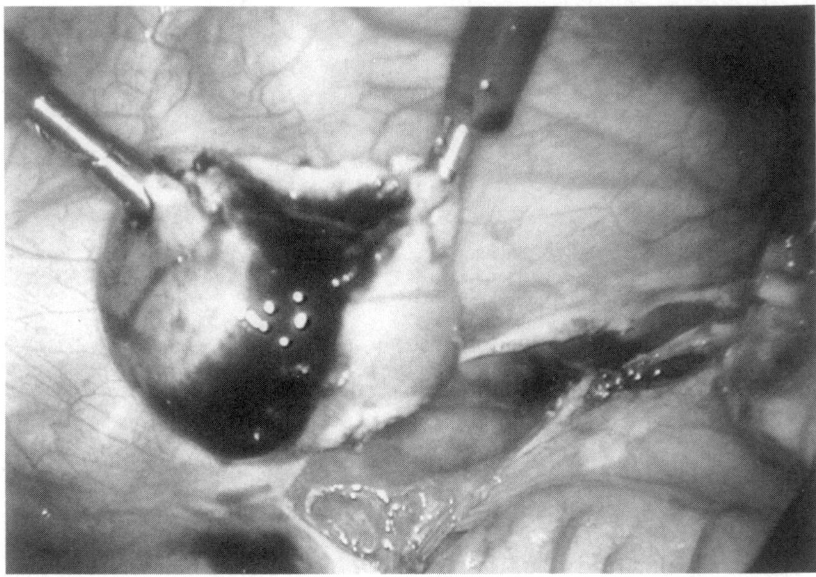

FIG. 72. Right uterine horn being morcellated to facilitate laparoscopic removal. Notice the dark old blood of the hematometra.

Septate uteri (Fig. 40) with a septate vagina can be associated with duplication of the colon, anus, urethra, bladder, vagina, and vulva. A uterus didelphys with bicollis has separate uterine cavities and two cervices (Fig. 32); in 75% of cases the vagina is septate (Figs. 33–35). Patients with a didelphic uterus usually have adequate reproductive outcomes, and thus metroplasty is contraindicated. The patient may experience difficulties from the vaginal septum, such as a need to use two tampons (one in each hemivagina), difficulty with sexual intercourse, or difficulty with vaginal delivery at childbirth. Resection of the vaginal septum, if needed, can be accomplished in an outpatient surgical setting. The vaginal septum is removed by "wedging" out the complete septum and then reapproximation of the normal vaginal mucosa. This technique removes all of the thickened septum so that no "ridge" remains.

Most uterine fusion/duplication abnormalities do not require surgical intervention (43). If patients experience pain, recurrent miscarriage, or premature labor, the abnormality should be repaired by either metroplasty or hysteroscopic removal of the uterine septum (128–130).

A variation of this abnormality is the obstructed hemivagina with ipsilateral renal agenesis (36,131–134) (Fig. 35). Patients with this condition have regular periods, as they have a nonobstructed hemivagina with associated cervix and hemiuterus. On physical exam, a mass is felt to bulge from the lateral wall of the vagina toward the midline (Fig. 14). Ultrasound is helpful in making the diagnosis. In addition, if unilateral renal agenesis is known to exist (Fig. 35), the pos-

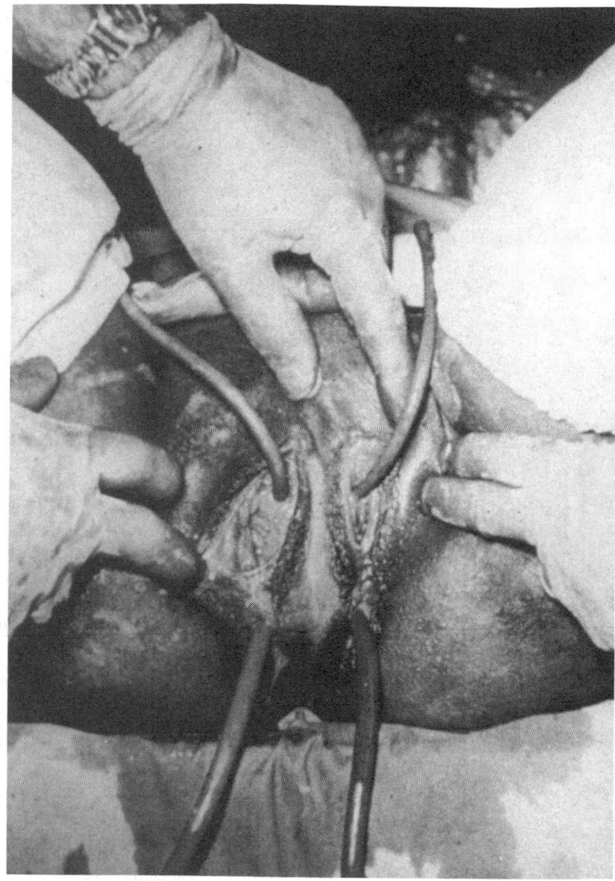

FIG. 73. Complete duplication of the vulva, bladder, urethra, vagina, and anus. (Courtesy of James L. Breen, M.D., Saint Barnabas Medical Center, Livingston, New Jersey.)

sibility of an obstructed hemivagina must be entertained. In cases of an obstructed hemivagina, the wall of the obstructed vagina must be resected to relieve the obstruction. Initially, a wide incision is made in the wall of the obstructed hemivagina to allow adequate drainage of the obstructed fluid. The remainder of the septal wall is then resected to create a single vaginal vault. If there is distorted anatomy from the marked dilatation of the obstructed hemivagina, then a second procedure to resect the remaining septal wall may be necessary. After resection of the septal wall of the obstructed hemivagina, the patient has normal function with a single vagina, two cervices, and two hemiuteri.

A unicornuate uterus (Fig. 31) is a single horned uterus that has a single round ligament and fallopian tube. The other hemiuterus, round ligament, and fallopian tube are usually absent. Variations of hemiuteri can occur with the existence of noncommunicating uterine horns with or without active endometrium (see Color Plate 27; Figs. 28 and 30). The single asymmetric uterus communicates with a single cervix and a normal vagina. Associated renal anomalies are common. Patients with a unicornuate uterus are at increased risk of infertility, endometriosis, premature labor, and breech presentation (135).

In the patient with a bicornuate uterus, the uterine fundus is deeply indented. The level of the indentation can be complete (Fig. 36), partial (Fig. 37) or arcuate (Fig. 38); the vagina is usually normal.

In cases of uterine septum, the external surface of the uterus appears to have a normal configuration, but there are two endometrial cavities (Figs. 39–42). In cases of recurrent pregnancy loss, the septum can be resected hysteroscopically (136–137).

Pregnancy Outcome in Women with Müllerian Duct Anomalies

Several studies have been made of the outcomes of pregnancies in women with müllerian duct abnormalities (139–142). In general, there is an increased rate of unexplained infertility, endometriosis, spontaneous abortion, breech presentation, and premature delivery. Women who have had lower vaginal agenesis corrected by the creation of a neovagina are able to conceive and to maintain a pregnancy if a normal cervix and uterus are present. In addition, pregnancy has been reported in a woman with vaginal agenesis and nonfused müllerian bulbs (74). The wider use of assisted reproductive technologies will also enhance the reproductive function of women with congenital abnormalities of the reproductive tract.

REFERENCES

1. Engert J. Surgical correction of virilized female external genitalia. *Prog Pediatr Surg* 1989;23:151.
2. Bailez MM, Gearhart JP, Migeon C, Rock J. Vaginal reconstruction after initial construction of the external genitalia in girls with salt-wasting adrenal hyperplasia. *J Urol* 1992;148:680.
3. Duckett JW, Baskin LS. Genitoplasty for intersex anomalies. *Eur J Pediatr* 1993;152:S80.
4. Donahoe PK, Gustafson ML. Early one-stage surgical reconstruction of the extremely high vagina in patients with congenital adrenal hyperplasia. *J Pediatr Surg* 1994;29:352.
5. Hendren WH, Atala A. Repair of the high vagina in girls with severely masculinized anatomy from the androgenital syndromes. *J Pediatr Surg* 1995;20:91.
6. Goerzen JL, Gidwani GP, et al. Outcome of surgical reconstructive procedures for the treatment of vaginal anomalies. *Adolesc Pediatr Gynecol* 1994;7:76.
7. Strickland JL, Cameron WJ, Krantz KE. Long-term satisfaction of adults undergoing McIndoe vaginoplasty as adolescents. *Adolesc Pediatr Gynecol* 1993;6:135.
8. Costa EMF, Mendonca BB, Inácío M, et al. Management of ambiguous gentalia in pseudohermaphrodites: new perspectives on vaginal dilation. *Fertil Steril* 1997;67:229.
9. Kim HH, Laufer MR. Developmental abnormalities of the female reproductive tract. *Curr Opin Obstet Gynecol* 1994;6:518.
10. Griffin JE. Androgen resistance: The clinical and molecular spectrum. *N Engl J Med* 1992;326:611.
11. Speroff L, Glass RH, Kase NG. Normal and abnormal sexual development. In: Mitchell C, ed. *Clinical gynecologic endocrinology and infertility*, 5th ed. Baltimore: Williams & Wilkins, 1994.

12. Shah R, Woolley MM, Costin G. Testicular feminization: the androgen insensitivity syndrome. *J Pediatr Surg* 1992;27:757.
13. Siegel SF. Molecular genetics of androgen insensitivity. *Adolesc Pediatr Gynecol* 1995;8:3.
14. Rey R, Mebarki F, Forest MG, et al. Anti-mullerian hormone in children with androgen insensitivity. *J Clin Endocrinol Metab* 1994;79:960.
15. Cassio A, Cacciari E, E'Errico A, et al. Incidence of intratubular germ cell neoplasia in androgen insensitivity syndrome. *Acta Endocrinol* (Copenh) 1990;123:416.
16. Rutgers JL, Scully RE. The androgen insensitivity syndrome (testicular feminization): a clinicopathologic study of 43 cases. *Int J Gynecol Pathol* 1991;10:126.
17. Kogan S. Feminizing genital reconstruction for male pseudohermaphroditism. *Eur J Pediatr* 1993; 152:S85.
18. Laufer MR, Galvin WJ. Labial hypertrophy: a new surgical approach. *Adolesc Pediatr Gynecol* 1995; 8:39.
19. Toubia N. Female circumcision as a public health issue. *N Engl J Med* 1994;331:712.
20. Council on Scientific Affairs, American Medical Association. Female genital mutilation. *JAMA* 1995; 274:1714.
21. World Health Organization, International Federation of Gynecology and Obstetrics. Female circumcision. *Eur J Obstet Gynecol Reprod Biol* 1992;45:153.
22. Aziz FA. Gynecologic and obstetric complications of female circumcision. *Int J Gynecol Obstet* 1980;17:560.
23. Gardner GH, Greene RR, Peckham BM. Normal and cystic structures of the broad ligament. *Am J Obstet Gynecol* 1948;55:917.
24. Bransilver BR, Ferenczy A, Richart RM. Female genital tract remnants. An ultrastructural comparison of hydatid of Morgagni and mesonephric ducts and tubules. *Arch Pathol* 1973;96:255.
25. See WA, Mayo M. Ectopic ureter: a rare cause of purulent vaginal discharge. *Obstet Gynecol* 1991; 78:552.
26. Meyer R. Normal and abnormal development of the ureter in the human embryo—a mechanistic consideration. *Anat Rec* 1946;96:355.
27. Hinman F. *Atlas of pediatric urologic surgery.* Philadelphia: WB. Saunders, 1994.
28. Hendren WH, Monfort GJ. Surgical correction of ureteroceles in childhood. *J Pediatr Surg* 1971;6:235.
29. Hendren WH, Mitchell ME. Surgical correction of ureteroceles. *J Urol* 1979;121:590.
30. Krisiloff M, Puchner PJ, et al. Pregnancy in women with bladder exstrophy. *J Urol* 1978;119:478.
31. Hendren WH. Cloacal malformations: experience with 105 cases. *J Pediatr Surg* 1992;27:890.
32. Hendren WH. Urogenital sinus and cloacal malformations. *J Pelvic Surg* 1995;1:149.
33. Hendren WH. Urogenital sinus and cloacal malformations. *Semin Pediatr Surg* 1996;5:72.
34. Jaramillo D, Lebowitz RL, Hendren WH. The cloacal malformation radiologic findings and imaging recommendations. *Radiology* 1990;177:441.
35. Buttram VC Jr. Müllerian anomalies and their management. *Fertil Steril* 1983;40:159.
36. Pinsonneault O, Goldstein DP. Obstructing malformations of the uterus and vagina. *Fertil Steril* 1985; 44:241.
37. Buttram VC Jr, Gibbons WE. Müllerian anomalies: a proposed classification (an analysis of 144 cases). *Fertil Steril* 1979;32:40.
38. The American Fertility Society. The American Fertility Society classifications of adnexal adhesions, distal tubal occlusion, tubal occlusion secondary to tubal ligation, tubal pregnancies, müllerian anomalies, and intrauterine adhesions. *Fertil Steril* 1988;49:944.
39. Goldstein DP, Laufer MR, Davis AJ. *Gynecologic surgery in children and adolescents: a text atlas.* New York: Springer-Verlag (in press).
40. Verp MS, Simpson JL, et al. Heritable aspects of uterine anomalies. I. Three familial aggregates with Müllerian fusion anomalies. *Fertil Steril* 1983;40:80.
41. Carson SA, Simpson JL, et al. Heritable aspects of uterine anomalies. II. Genetic analysis of müllerian aplasia. *Fertil Steril* 1983;40:86.
42. Shulman LP, Elias S. Developmental abnormalities of the female reproductive tract: pathogenesis and nosology. *Adolesc Pediatr Gynecol* 1988;1:230.
43. Petrozza JC, Gray MR, Davis AJ, Reindollar RH. Congenital absence of the uterus and vagina is not commonly transmitted as a dominant genetic trait: outcomes of surrogate pregnancies. *Fertil Steril* 1997;67:387.
44. Bennett MJ, Berry JVJ. Preterm labour and congenital malformations of the uterus. *Ultrasound Med Biol* 1979;5:83.

45. Stray-Petersen B, Stray-Petersen S. Etiologic factors and subsequent reproductive performance in 195 couples with a prior history of habitual abortion. *Am J Obstet Gynecol* 1984;148:140.
46. Simón C, Tortajada M, Martinez L, et al. Müllerian defects in women with normal reproductive outcome. *Fertil Steril* 1991;56:1192.
47. Usta IM, Awwad JT, et al. Imperforate hymen: report of an unusual familial occurrence. *Obstet Gynecol* 1993;82:655.
48. Shatzkes DR, Haller JO, Velcek FT. Imaging of uterovaginal anomalies in the pediatric population. *Urol Radiol* 1991;13:58.
49. Valdes C, Malini S, Malinak LR. Ultrasound evaluation of female genital tract anomalies: a review of 64 cases. *Am J Obstet Gynecol* 1984;149:285.
50. Scanlan KA, Pozniak MA, et al. Value of transperineal sonography in the assessment of vaginal atresia. *AJR* 1990;154:545.
51. Nussbaum Blask AR, Sanders RC, Gearhart JP. Obstructed uterovaginal anomalies: demonstration with sonography. Part I: neonates and infants. *Pediatr Radiol* 1991;179:79.
52. Nussbaum Blask AR, Sanders RC, Rock JA. Obstructed uterovaginal anomalies: demonstration with sonography. Part II: teenagers. *Pediatr Radiol* 1991;179:84.
53. Raga F, Bonilla-Musoles F, et al. Congenital müllerian anomalies: diagnostic accuracy of three-dimensional ultrasound. *Fertil Steril* 1996;65:523.
54. Markham SM, Huggins GR, et al. Cervical agenesis combined with vaginal agenesis diagnosed by magnetic resonance imaging. *Fertil Steril* 1987;48:143.
55. Fedele L, Dorta M, et al. Magnetic resonance imaging in Mayer-Rokitansky-Kuster-Hauser syndrome. *Obstet Gynecol* 1990;76:593.
56. Pellerito JS, McCarthy SM, et al. Diagnosis of uterine anomalies: relative accuracy of MR imaging, endovaginal sonography, and hysterosalpingography. *Radiology* 1992;183:795.
57. Bakri YN, Al-Sugair A, Hugosson C. Bicornuate nonfused rudimentary uterine horns with functioning endometria and complete cervical vaginal agenesis: Magnetic resonance diagnosis. *Fertil Steril* 1992; 58:620.
58. Markham SM, Waterhouse TB. Structural anomalies of the reproductive tract. *Curr Opin Obstet Gynecol* 1992;4:867.
59. Sadler TW. *Langman's medical embryology*, 6th ed. Philadelphia: Williams & Williams, 1990.
60. Fielding C. Obstetric studies in women with congenital solitary kidneys. *Acta Obstet Gynecol Scand* 1965;44:555.
61. Thompson DP, Lynn HB. Genital anomalies associated with solitary kidney. *Mayo Clin Proc* 1966;41: 538.
62. Erdogan E, Okan G, Daragenli O. Uterus didelphys with unilateral obstructed hemivagina and renal agenesis on the same side. *Acta Obstet Gynecol* Scand 1992;71:76.
63. Tran ATB, Arensman RM, Falterman KW. Diagnosis and management of hydrohematometrocolpos syndrome. *Am J Dis Child* 1987;141:632.
64. Golan A, Langer R, et al. Congenital anomalies of the müllerian system. *Fertil Steril* 1989;51:747.
65. Sanfilippo JS, Wakim NG, Schikler KN, Yussman MA. Endometriosis in association with uterine anomaly. *Am J Obstet Gynecol* 1986;154:39.
66. Olive DL, Henderson DY. Endometriosis and müllerian anomalies. *Obstet Gynecol* 1987;69:412.
67. Fedele L, Bianchi S, et al. Endometriosis and nonobstructive müllerian anomalies. *Obstet Gynecol* 1992;79:515.
68. Lodi A. Contributo clinico statistico sulle malformazioni della vagina osservate nella clinica ostetrica e ginecologica di Milano dal 1906 al 1950. *Ann Ostet Ginecol* 1951;73:1246.
69. Suidan FG, Azoury RS. The transverse vaginal septum: a clinicopathologic evaluation. *Obstet Gynecol* 1979;54:278.
70. Rock JA, Zacur HA, Dlugi AM, et al. Pregnancy success following surgical correction of imperforate hymen and complete transverse vaginal septum. *Obstet Gynecol* 1982;59:448.
71. Mayer CAJ. Über Verdoppelungen des Uterus und ihre Arten, nebst Bemerkungen über Hasenscharte ind Wolfsrachen. *J Chir Auger* 1829;13:525.
72. von Rokitansky KF. Über die sogenannten Verdoppelungen des Uterus. *Med Jb Öst Staat* 1938;26:39.
73. Küster H. Uterus bipartitus solidus rudimentarius cum vagina solida. *Z Geb Gyn* 1910;67:692.
74. Hauser GA, Schreiner WE. Das Mayer-Rokitansky-Küster syndrome. *Schweiz Med Wochenschr* 1961; 91:381.
75. Solomons E. Conception and delivery following construction of an artificial vagina: a report of a case. *Obstet Gynecol* 1956;7:329.
76. Murray J, Gambrell RD. Complete and partial vaginal agenesis. *J Reprod Med* 1979;22:101.

77. Singh J, Devi YL. Pregnancy following surgical correction of nonfused müllerian bulbs and absent vagina. *Obstet Gynecol* 1983;61:267.
78. Bates WG, Winfred WL. A technique for uterine conservation in adolescents with vaginal agenesis and a functional uterus. *Obstet Gynecol* 1985;66:290.
79. Evans TN, Poland ML, Boving RL. Vaginal malformations. *Am J Obstet Gynecol* 1981;141:910.
80. Cramer DW, Ravnikar VA, et al. Müllerian aplasia associated with maternal deficiency of galactose-1-phosphate uridyl transferase. *Fertil Steril* 1987;47:930.
81. Willemson WNP. Combination of Mayer-Rokitansky-Küster and Klippel-Feil syndromes. a case report and review of the literature. *Eur J Obstet Gynecol Reprod Biol* 1982;13:229.
82. Duncan PA, Shapiro LR, et al. The MURCS association of müllerian duct aplasia, renal aplasia, and cervicothoracic somite dysplasia. *J Pediatr* 1979;95:399.
83. Fedele L, Dorta M, Brioschi D. Magnetic resonance imaging in Mayer-Rokitansky-Kuster-Hauser syndrome. *Obstet Gynecol* 1990;76:593.
84. Coney PJ. Effects of vaginal agenesis on the adolescent: prognosis for normal sexual and psychological adjustment. *Adolesc Pediatr Gynecol* 1992;5:8.
85. Frank RT. The formation of an artificial vagina without operation. *Am J Obstet Gynecol* 1938;35:1053.
86. D Alberton A, Santi F. Formation of a neovagina by coitus. *Obstet Gynecol* 1972;40:763.
87. Ingram JM. The bicycle seat stool in the treatment of vaginal agenesis and stenosis: a preliminary report. *Am J Obstet Gynecol* 1981;140:867.
88. Abbé R. New method of creating a vagina in a case of congenital absence. *Med Rec* 1898;54:836.
89. McIndoe AH, Banister JB. An operation for the cure of congenital absence of the vagina. *J Obstet Gynaecol Br Commonw* 1938;45:490.
90. Cousellor VS. Congenital absence and traumatic obliteration of vagina and its treatment with inlaying Thiersch grafts. *Am J Obstet Gynecol* 1938;36:632.
91. McIndoe A. Treatment of congenital absence and obliterative conditions of the vagina. *Br J Plast Surg* 1950;2:254.
92. Buss JG, Lee RA. McIndoe procedure for vaginal agenesis: results and complications. *Mayo Clin Proc* 1989;64:758.
93. Martintez-Mora J, Isnard R, et al. Neovagina in vaginal agenesis: surgical methods and long-term results. *J Pediatr Surg* 1992;27:10.
94. Duckler L. Squamous cell carcinoma developing in an artificial vagina. *Obstet Gynecol* 1972;40:35.
95. Rotmensch J, Rosenshein N, et al. Carcinoma arising in the neovagina: case report and review of the literature. *Obstet Gynecol* 1983;61:534.
96. Sadove RC, Horton CE. Utilizing full-thickness skin grafts for vaginal reconstruction. *Clin Plast Surg* 1988;15:443.
97. Chen Y-BT, Cheng T-J, et al. Spatial W-plasty full-thickness skin graft for neovaginal reconstruction. *Plast Reconstr Surg* 1994;94:727.
98. Williams EA. Congenital absence of the vagina—a simple operation for its relief. *J Obstet Gynaecol Br Commonw* 1964;71:511.
99. Wesley JR, Coran AG. Intestinal vaginoplasty for congenital absence of the vagina. *J Pediatr Surg* 1992;27:885.
100. Hensle T, Dean G. Vaginal replacement in children. *J Urol* 1992;148:677.
101. Hendren WH, Atala A. Use of bowel for vaginal reconstruction. *J Urol* 1994;152:752.
102. Andryjowicz E, Qizilbash MB, et al. Adenocarcinoma in a cecal neovagina—complication of irradiation: Report of a case and review of the literature. *Gynecol Oncol* 1985;21:235.
103. Davydov SN, Zhvitiashvili OD. Formation of vagina from peritoneum of Douglas pouch. *Acta Chir Plast* 1974;16:35.
104. Tamaya T, Imai A. The use of peritoneum for vaginoplasty in 24 patients with congenital absence of the vagina. *Arch Gynecol Obstet* 1991;249:15.
105. Morton KE, Dewhurst CJ. Human amnion in the treatment of vaginal malformations. *Br J Obstet Gynaecol* 1986;93:50.
106. McGraw JB, Massey FM, et al. Vaginal reconstruction with gracilis myocutaneous flaps. *Plast Reconstr Surg* 1976;59:176.
107. Wang TN, Whetzel T, et al. A fasciocutaneous flap for vaginal and perineal reconstruction. *Plast Reconstr Surg* 1987;80:95.
108. Tobin GR, Day TG. Vaginal and pelvic reconstruction with distally based rectus abdominis myocutaneous flaps. *Plast Reconstr Surg* 1988;81:62.
109. Vecchietti G. Le neo-vagin dans le syndrome de Rokitansky-Kuster-Hauser. *Rev Med Suisse Romande* 1979;99:593.

110. Gauwerky JFH, Wallwiener D, Bastert G. An endoscopically assisted technique for construction of a neovagina. *Arch Gynecol Obstet* 1992;252:59.
111. Ghirardini G, Popp LW. New Approach to the Mayer-von-Rokitansky-Küster-Hauser syndrome. *Adolesc Pediatr Gynecol* 1994;7:41.
112. Farber M. Congenital atresia of the uterine cervix. *Semin Reprod Endocrinol* 1986; 4:33.
113. Niver DH, Barrette G, Jewelewicz R. Congenital atresia of the uterine cervix and vagina: three cases. *Fertil Steril* 1980;33:25.
114. Dillon WP, Mudalier N, Wingate M. Congenital atresia of the cervix. *Obstet Gynecol* 1979;54:126.
115. Markham SM, Parmley TH, Murphy AA, et al. Cervical agenesis combined with vaginal agenesis diagnosed by magnetic resonance imaging. *Fertil Steril* 1987;48:143.
116. Rock JA, Schlaff WD, et al. The clinical management of congenital absence of the uterine cervix. *Int J Gynaecol Obstet* 1984;22:231.
117. Regan L, Dewhurst J. Atresia of the cervix. *Pediatr Adolesc Gynecol* 1985;3:83.
118. Farber M, Marchant DJ. Reconstructive surgery for congenital atresia of the uterine cervix. *Fertil Steril* 1976;27:1277.
119. Cukier J, Batzofin JH, et al. Genital tract reconstruction in a patient with congenital absence of the vagina and hypoplasia of the cervix. *Obstet Gynecol* 1986;68:32S.
120. Geary LW, Weed JC. Congenital atresia of the uterine cervix. *Obstet Gynecol* 1973;42:213.
121. Baker ER, Horger EO, Williamson HO. Congenital atresia of the uterine cervix: two cases. *J Reprod Med* 1982;27;39.
122. Casey AC, Laufer MR. Cervical agenesis: septic death after surgery. *Obstet Gynecol* 1997;90:706.
123. Zarou GS, Espesito JM, Zarou DM. Pregnancy following surgical correction of congenital atresia of the cervix. *Int J Obstet Gynecol* 1973;11:143.
124. Hampton HL, Meeks GR, et al. Pregnancy after successful vaginoplasty and cervical stenting for partial atresia of the cervix. *Obstet Gynecol* 1990;76:900.
125. Thijssen RFA, Hollanders JMG, et al. Successful pregnancy after ZIFT in a patient with congenital cervical atresia. *Obstet Gynecol* 1990;76:902.
126. Laufer MR. Laparoscopic resection of obstructed hemi-uteri in a series of adolescents. Presented at the Annual meeting of the North American Society for Pediatric and Adolescent Gynecology, 1997.
127. Kirschner R, Löfstrand T, Mark J. Pregnancy in a non-communicating, rudimentary uterine horn. *Acta Obstet Gynecol Scand* 1979;58:499.
128. Jones HW, Rock JA. Reproductive impairment and the malformed uterus. *Fertil Steril* 1981;36:137.
129. Rock J, Schlaff W. The obstetric consequences of uterovaginal anomalies. *Fertil Steril* 1985;43:681.
130. Sanfilippo JS. Strassman procedure for correction of a class II Müllerian anomaly in an adolescent. *J Adolesc Health* 1991;12:63.
131. Constantian HM. Ureteral ectopia, hydrocolpos, and uterus didelphys. *JAMA* 1966;197:54.
132. Gilliland B, Dyck F. Uterus didelphys associated with unilateral imperforate vagina. *Obstet Gynecol* 1976;48:5S.
133. Stassart JP, Magel TC, et al. Uterus didelphys, obstructed hemivagina, and ipsilateral renal agenesis: the University of Minnesota experience. *Fertil Steril* 1992;57:756.
134. Tridenti G, Bruni V, et al. Double uterus with a blind hemivagina and ipsilateral renal agenesis: clinical variants in three adolescent women: case reports and literature review. *Adolesc Pediatr Gynecol* 1995;8:201.
135. Fedele L, Zamberletti D, et al. Reproductive performance of women with unicornuate uterus. *Fertil Steril* 1987;47:416.
136. Daly DC, Walter CA, et al. Hysteroscopic metroplasty: surgical technique and obstetric outcome. *Fertil Steril* 1983;39:623.
137. DeCherney AH, Russell JB, et al. Resectoscope management of müllerian fusion defects. *Fertil Steril* 1986;45:726.
138. Fayez JA. Comparison between abdominal and hysteroscopic metroplasty. *Obstet Gynecol* 1986;68: 399.
139. Stein AL, March CM. Pregnancy outcome in women with müllerian duct anomalies. *J Reprod Med* 1990;35:411.
140. Michalas SP. Outcome of pregnancy in women with uterine malformations: evaluation of 62 cases. *Int J Gynecol Obstet* 1991;35:215.
141. Makino T, Umeuchi M, et al. Incidence of congenital uterine anomalies in repeated reproductive wastage and prognosis for pregnancy after metroplasty. *Int J Fertil* 1992;37:167.
142. Kirk EP, Chuong CJ, et al. Pregnancy after metroplasty for uterine anomalies. *Fertil Steril* 1993;59: 1164.

9

Dysmenorrhea, Pelvic Pain, and the Premenstrual Syndrome

Pelvic pain is frequent in adolescent women and can be characterized as acute or chronic. Pain is the physiologic response to many pathophysiologic conditions such as distension, stretching, compression, irritation (chemical or infectious), ischemia, neuritis, and necrosis. Pelvic pain can also be referred from another anatomic site. Pelvic pain can arise from numerous causes, including diseases or conditions affecting the gastrointestinal (GI) tract, the urogenital tract, the reproductive tract, and the musculoskeletal system. An extensive listing of nongynecologic and gynecologic causes of acute and chronic pelvic pain is given in Table 1 (1,2). Stress and psychosocial issues may increase the intensity of the symptoms and affect the individual's response to pain and the ability to cope with it. This chapter discusses the approach, diagnosis, and treatment of the adolescent with acute and/or chronic pelvic pain, dysmenorrhea, endometriosis, and premenstrual syndrome.

ACUTE PELVIC PAIN

The adolescent girl with acute pelvic pain should receive aggressive evaluation and management, as the differential diagnosis includes life-threatening conditions. The gynecologic causes of acute pain include infections, ovarian cysts, endometriosis, ectopic pregnancy, and adnexal torsion. A genital tract obstruction (see Chapter 8) may cause acute symptoms at the time of menarche, although these anomalies can also result in chronic or cyclic pelvic pain. Symptoms associated with infection usually occur over several days. Pelvic inflammatory disease (PID) (see Chapter 12) is extremely important to consider in the differential diagnosis of acute pelvic pain in the sexually active adolescent; it has been identified as the most common gynecologic disorder leading to the hospitalization of reproductive-age women in the United States (3). The onset of pain associated with adnexal torsion, rupture of an ovarian cyst (see Chapter 15), or

TABLE 1. *Differential diagnosis of pelvic pain in adolescents*

- Nongynecologic
  - Gastrointestinal
    - Appendicitis
    - Intestinal obstruction
    - Perforation
    - Gastric ulcer
    - Gastritis
    - Abdominal angina
    - Cholecystitis/cholangitis
    - Diverticular disease
    - Gastroenteritis (bacterial, parasitic)
    - Irritable bowel disease
    - Ulcerative colitis
    - Crohn's disease (granulomatous colitis)
    - Meckel's diverticulum
    - Mesenteric adenitis
    - Pancreatitis
    - Hepatitis
    - Metabolic disease (steatorrhea, sprue, intermittent acute porphyria, lactase deficiency)
    - Obstruction (adhesions, hernias, irradiation, tumors, volvulus)
    - Psychogenic (anxiety)
    - Constipation
  - Genitourinary
    - Pyelonephritis/abscess
    - Cystourethritis
    - Interstitial cystitis
    - Calculi
    - Ureteral obstruction
    - Ureteral diverticulum/ polyp
  - Musculoskeletal
    - Congenital anomalies
    - Bone and joint inflammations/infections (spine, sacrum, ilium, femoral head)
    - Trauma
    - Tumors
  - Neurologic
    - Nerve entrapment
    - Neuroma
  - Psychological
    - History of physical/sexual abuse
    - History of trauma
    - Psychosomatic
  - Systemic
    - Systemic lupus erythematosus
    - Neurofibromatosis
    - Lymphoma

- Gynecologic
  - Acute
    - Pregnancy-related
      - Ectopic pregnancy (with/without rupture)
      - Threatened/spontaneous abortion
    - Ovarian
      - Cyst/mass (benign/malignant)
      - Mumps oophoritis
      - Torsion

TABLE 1. *(Continued)*

- Gynecologic (continued)
  - Acute (continued)
    - Fallopian tube
      - Hydrosalpinx
      - Torsion
    - Infection
      - Endometritis (posttherapeutic abortion, postpartum)
      - Pelvic inflammatory disease/tubo-ovarian abscess
      - Septic pelvic thrombophlebitis
    - Vaginitis/vulvitis
      - Contact dermatitis
      - Inflammatory/infection
      - Lichen sclerosis
      - Bartholin's cyst/abscess
  - Cyclic
    - Mittelschmerz
    - Dysmenorrhea
    - Endometriosis/adenomyosis
    - Leiomyomata (fibroids)
    - Obstructive müllerian anomalies
    - Premenstrual syndrome
    - Ovarian
      - Cyst/mass (benign/malignant)
      - Torsion
    - Fallopian tube
      - Hydrosalpinx
      - Torsion
  - Dyspareunia (pain with sexual intercourse)
    - Vaginismus
    - Inflammatory/infection
  - Chronic
    - Endometriosis/adenomyosis
    - Pelvic adhesions
    - Leiomyomata (fibroids)
    - Chronic infection
      - Endometritis (posttherapeutic abortion, postpartum)
      - Pelvic inflammatory disease/tubo-ovarian abscess
      - Septic pelvic thrombophlebitis
    - Obstructive müllerian anomalies
    - Premenstrual syndrome
    - Ovarian
      - Cyst/mass (benign/malignant)
      - Torsion
    - Fallopian tube
      - Hydrosalpinx
      - Torsion
    - Vaginitis/vulvitis
      - Chronic dermatitis
      - Inflammatory/infection
      - Lichen sclerosis
      - Bartholin's cyst/abscess

(Adapted from Rapkin AJ, Reading AE. Chronic pelvic pain. *Curr Probl Obstet Gynecol Fertil* 1991;14:101; and Laufer MR. Endometriosis in adolescents. *Curr Opin Pediatr* 1992;4:582; with permission.)

an ectopic pregnancy (see Chapter 18) is usually abrupt, sharp, and severe. Nausea and/or vomiting may occur with severe pain. However, intermittent or partial adnexal torsion, or an unruptured ectopic pregnancy, may produce crampy pain for several days to weeks prior to an acute episode of complete torsion with infarction of the fallopian tube and/or ovary, or rupture of the ectopic pregnancy.

In deciding whether the pain is gynecologic in origin, the health care provider must consider GI causes, such as appendicitis, intestinal obstruction or perforation, volvulus, inflammatory bowel disease, infections (e.g., *Giardia*, *Shigella*, *Salmonella*), lactose intolerance, irritable bowel syndrome, or constipation (Table 1). Urinary tract infections and calculi may result in acute pain. Orthopedic causes of pain are frequently forgotten and can be missed initially; the evaluation should include a complete history, an examination of the range of motion of the hips and spine, and tests of the sacroiliac joints.

A complete pain history must include its location, nature, intensity, and radiation; factors that relieve and exacerbate the pain such as walking, exercise, eating, urination, or bowel movements; the date of the last menstrual period; contraceptive and sexual history; associated symptoms such as fever, chills, diarrhea, vomiting, or dysuria; and previous pelvic pain and/or surgery. Infants and prepubertal girls (and adolescents less commonly) may have torsion of a normal adnexa (ovary and/or tube) (Fig. 1) (see Chapter 15); several weeks to years later, these same individuals may experience torsion of the other adnexa and if the second torsed ovary is not salvageable the individual is sterile (3–5). The psychosocial history should be elicited to assess whether stress, substance use, or sexual abuse might be contributing factors to any case of pelvic pain.

A complete physical examination should be undertaken, special attention being given to palpation of the abdomen, in a search for evidence of masses, tenderness, organomegaly, or peritoneal irritation. Depending on the age of the patient and the size of the hymenal opening, a bimanual vaginal–abdominal, rectoabdominal, or rectovaginal–abdominal examination should be done to assess the size of the uterus, the presence or absence of cervical motion tenderness, and/or ovarian/adnexal tenderness. A speculum examination to assess the vagina and cervix should be done in all sexually active patients and in virginal patients if the examination can be accomplished without trauma. Tests for *Chlamydia trachomatis* and *Neisseria gonorrhoeae* should be obtained in all patients who have ever had consenting or nonconsenting sexual activity. Lubricant should not be used for the digital vaginal or speculum examination unless cervical specimens have already been obtained.

Laboratory tests depend on the initial assessment and may include complete blood count (CBC) with differential, erythrocyte sedimentation rate (ESR), C-reactive protein (CRP), urinalysis, urine culture, cervical cultures, sensitive pregnancy test, and stool specimen for occult blood. A high leukocyte count (WBC) usually indicates infection or inflammation; the WBC may be slightly elevated or high in cases of ischemia, as may occur secondary to adnexal torsion

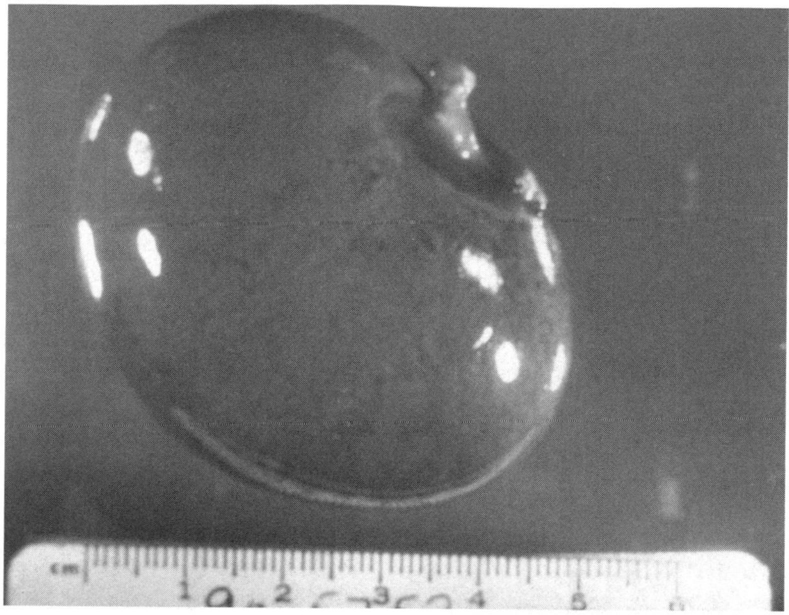

FIG. 1. Torsion of an ovary in a 6-week-old infant.

or bowel obstruction. In acute hemorrhage, the hematocrit may not reflect the extent of blood loss, as there may not have been time for intravascular equilibration to have taken place.

In children or adolescents in whom a pelvic or adnexal mass is palpated or an adequate pelvic examination is not possible, ultrasonography (transabdominal and/or vaginal probe) can be used to aid in the evaluation. It is important to remember that adolescents normally have 1- to 2-cm ovarian follicles, which, though often termed "simple cysts" on ultrasound evaluation, are normal findings. In addition, children can have numerous small simple ovarian cysts, which usually measure 1 to 5 mm. Endometriosis and PID cannot be excluded by a normal ultrasound.

Cul-de-sac free fluid is present with ruptured simple or hemorrhagic ovarian cysts and with leaking or ruptured ectopic pregnancies (see Color Plate 31). Determination of the type of free fluid can be made by culdocentesis. In culdocentesis, a speculum is placed into the vaginal vault, povidone-iodine is used to prep the vaginal vault, local anesthetic can be infiltrated with a spinal needle into the anterior lip of the cervix, a tenaculum is used to grasp the anterior lip of the cervix, and a spinal needle is used to aspirate fluid from the posterior cul-de-sac. Cul-de-sac free fluid from a ruptured simple cyst is clear or straw-colored, whereas that from a ruptured hemorrhagic cyst or ectopic pregnancy demonstrates free blood. If the blood does not clot, it most likely originates from an intraperitoneal process, whereas if it does clot, it is most likely the result of a misdirected intravascular aspiration. The utility of culdocentesis in the clinical setting of a sensitive and rapid pregnancy test and ultrasound has been questioned (6). At our institution we find this procedure rarely useful because of the availability of a sensitive pregnancy test and ultrasound, and also because of the severity of pain during the procedure.

A patient experiencing "waves" of acute pelvic pain with or without nausea may be experiencing complete or intermittent torsion of an ovary or fallopian tube (Fig. 2). Ultrasonography in a case of ovarian torsion may reveal an echogenic mass within the ovary. Ultrasound Doppler flow studies may be helpful in the assessment of ovarian torsion, although it is frequently difficult to determine the presence of Doppler flow in normal ovaries (4–10). The theory of the usefulness of Doppler flow is that at the site of the torsion, the diameter of the vessel proximal to the occlusion is increased, and thus the disruption of flow can be identified. Cost–benefit studies are still under investigation, and thus the value of color Doppler for screening for ovarian torsion is as yet unproved (11). Ovarian torsion is more common on the right side and may mimic acute appendicitis, with right lower quadrant pain, vomiting, rebound tenderness, and leukocytosis. For unclear reasons, girls in the 7- to 10-year-old range are especially prone to this problem. Reports have demonstrated that torsed ovaries can be "detorsed" laparoscopically with salvage of the ovary (12–14). Whether pexis of

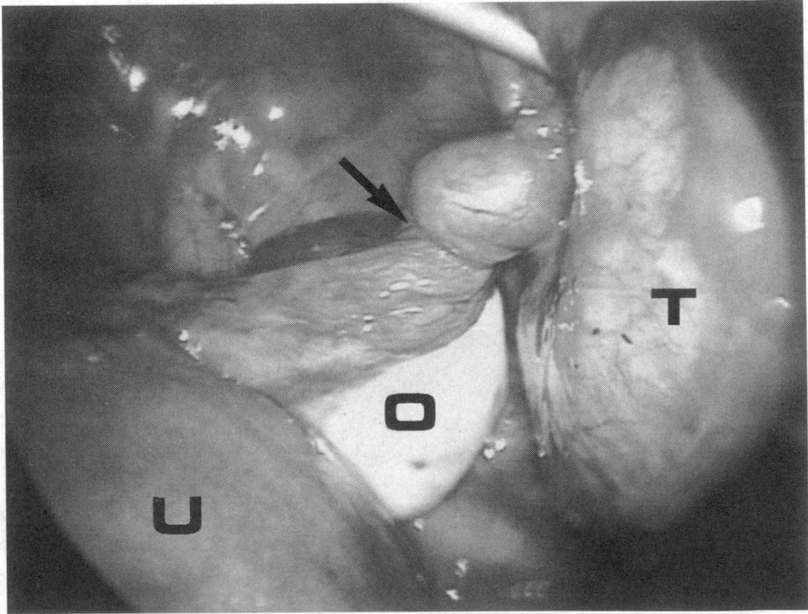

FIG. 2. Torsion of a fallopian tube (*arrow*). O, ovary; U, uterus; T, distal fallopian tube.

the contralateral ovary can be helpful in preventing a second episode of ovarian torsion of a normal ovary needs evaluation. If oophoropexy is elected, it can be safely accomplished by an operative laparoscopic approaches (15).

When evaluating pelvic pain, gastrointestinal and skeletal radiographs, bone scans, and other radiologic studies should be ordered as clinically indicated by the history and physical examination.

Depending on clinical and laboratory assessment, patients with pelvic pain will fall into one of several categories requiring further surgical evaluation, non-surgical evaluation, or discharge with followup (16). Some conditions such as acute hemoperitoneum, ruptured tubo-ovarian abscess, appendicitis, and other GI surgical emergencies require definitive surgery. Some conditions such as gastroenteritis, urinary tract infection, and PID require medical management; others (e.g., urinary calculi) require further investigation.

Not infrequently, the diagnosis remains in doubt, and diagnostic and/or operative laparoscopy may be invaluable for a definitive assessment. Laparoscopy is a safe means of evaluating the pelvis in adolescents and young adults and is also increasingly used in the management of general surgical, cardiovascular, and thoracic neurosurgical conditions in infants and children. At the time of laparoscopy, the appendix should be visualized to confirm that it is normal. Laparoscopy has been shown to be useful in the diagnosis of salpingitis (17–20), although its use for this diagnosis is not the current standard of care in the United States because of the risks of general anesthesia. When PID or appendicitis may exist, laparoscopy may help to define the underlying disease process. Visualization of a "normal pelvis" (see Color Plate 23) rules out the need for further surgical intervention and can help direct the subsequent evaluation and therapy. Often, in cases of ruptured ovarian cysts or hemorrhagic corpus luteum, free blood and clots (see Color Plate 31) can be aspirated and hemostasis ensured by fulguration of areas of bleeding via laparoscopy. Hemoperitoneum is not a contraindication to laparoscopy as long as the patient is not hypotensive. Laparoscopy can be implemented in a routine operating room fashion with the use of a 5-, 7-, or 10-mm laparoscope and general anesthesia, or with one of the newer 1.6-, 1.8-, or 2-mm laparoscopes and local anesthesia (21). We are currently investigating the use of these smaller laparoscopes (optical catheters) for determining the etiology of pelvic pain in adolescents (22). Others have explored the use of laparoscopy as an office or outpatient procedure in adult women (23,24).

The principal findings in 121 adolescent girls (11–17 years old) who underwent laparoscopy by the Gynecology Service of Children's Hospital, Boston, for acute pelvic pain between 1980 and 1986 are shown in Table 2. The most common diagnosis was a complication of an ovarian cyst. Interestingly, the causes of acute pelvic pain did not appear to be age related (Table 3).

Acute pain in the adolescent may also occur at menarche if there is an obstructive müllerian anomaly. This can result in hematometra or hematocolpos. The presentation, diagnosis, evaluation, and treatment of anomalies of the reproductive tract are discussed in Chapter 8.

TABLE 2. *Principal laparoscopic diagnoses in 121 adolescent patients 11 to 17 years old with acute pelvic pain (Children's Hospital, Boston, 1980–1986)*

Diagnosis	No.	(%)
Ovarian cyst	47	(39)
Acute pelvic inflammatory disease	21	(17)
Adnexal torsion	9	(8)
Endometriosis	6	(5)
Ectopic pregnancy	4	(3)
Appendicitis	13	(11)
No pathologic condition	21	(17)

Mittelschmerz

Mittelschmerz is the term applied to ovulatory pain. The patient typically experiences dull pain at the time of ovulation in one lower quadrant, lasting from a few minutes to 6 to 8 hours. In rare instances, the pain is severe and crampy and persists for 2 to 3 days. The cause of this pain is unknown, but the spillage of normal follicular fluid as the follicle cyst ruptures and expels the oocyte may irritate the peritoneum. Ultrasonography studies have detected small quantities of fluid at midcycle in 40% of normal women's cycles (25).

In most cases, the diagnosis of mittelschmerz is evident from the recurrent nature of the mild discomfort. Documentation of the midcycle occurrence of the pain by menstrual charts is helpful. If the patient is being examined for the first episode or for an exceptionally severe episode, other diagnoses must be excluded, including appendicitis, ovarian torsion, rupture of an ovarian cyst, and ectopic pregnancy.

Therapy for mittelschmerz should aim first at a careful explanation to the young woman and her family of the benign nature of the pain and its cause. A heating pad and analgesics such as prostaglandin inhibitors (ibuprofen, naproxen sodium) are helpful. If the pain becomes repetitive in an expected cyclic fashion, oral contraceptive pills (OCs) can be used to inhibit ovulation.

TABLE 3. *Age-related prevalence of principal laparoscopic findings in 121 adolescent patients 11 to 17 years old with acute pelvic pain (Children's Hospital, Boston, 1980–1986)*

	No. of patients (%)		
Diagnosis	Age 11–13	Age 14–15	Age 16–17
Ovarian cyst	12 (50)	16 (35)	19 (37)
Acute pelvic inflammatory disease	4 (17)	7 (16)	10 (19)
Adnexal torsion	0 (0)	7 (16)	2 (4)
Endometriosis	0 (0)	2 (4)	4 (7)
Ectopic pregnancy	0 (0)	3 (7)	1 (2)
Appendicitis	3 (13)	4 (9)	6 (12)
No pathologic condition	5 (20)	6 (13)	10 (19)
Total	24 (20)	45 (37)	52 (43)

DYSMENORRHEA

Dysmenorrhea, or pain with menses, is common in adolescents. Analyzing data from the National Health Examination Survey for 12- to 17-year-old girls, Klein and Litt (26) found that 59.7% of 2699 reported dysmenorrhea, and of those with dysmenorrhea, 14% frequently missed school because of cramps. In a survey of private school girls (mean age 15.5 ± 1.1 years) done by our faculty, dysmenorrhea was reported as mild by 32%, moderate by 15%, and severe by 6% (27). Most dysmenorrhea in adolescents is primary (or functional), but it may also be secondary to endometriosis (see below), obstructing müllerian anomalies (see Chapter 8), or other pelvic pathology.

Typically, the 14- or 15-year-old teenager, 1 to 3 years after menarche, begins to experience crampy lower abdominal pain with each menstrual period. Usually, the pains start within 1 to 4 hours of the onset of the menses and last for 24 to 48 hours. In some cases, the pain may start 1 to 2 days before the menses and continue for 2 to 4 days into the menses. Nausea and/or vomiting, diarrhea, lower backache, thigh pain, headache, fatigue, nervousness, dizziness, or rarely syncope may accompany the cramps.

Etiology

Historically, the etiology of primary dysmenorrhea was poorly understood, and many myths and hypotheses were promoted. Pickles (28) was the first to suggest that dysmenorrhea might be related to a "menstrual stimulant" found in human menstrual fluid that induced smooth muscle contractions. In later studies, he found that the substance was a mixture of prostaglandins $F_{2\alpha}$ ($PGF_{2\alpha}$) and E_2 (PGE_2) (29,30). Menstrual fluid prostaglandin levels were several times higher in ovulatory than in anovulatory cycles. Uterine jet washing, endometrial sampling, and collection of menstrual fluid have generally confirmed higher endometrial prostaglandin levels in women with primary dysmenorrhea than in those without symptoms (30,31).

In the uterus, phospholipids from the dead cell membranes are converted to arachidonic acid, which can be metabolized by at least two enzymes: lipoxygenase, which begins the production of leukotrienes, and cyclooxygenase, which leads to cyclic endoperoxides (PGG_2 and PGH_2). The cyclic endoperoxides are then converted by specific enzymes to prostacyclin, thromboxanes, and the prostaglandins PGD_2, PGE_2, and $PGF_{2\alpha}$. Prostaglandin $PGF_{2\alpha}$ mediates pain sensation and stimulates smooth muscle contraction, whereas PGE_2 potentiates platelet disaggregation and vasodilatation (32). Exogenously administered PGE_2 and $PGF_{2\alpha}$ can produce uterine contractions as well as systemic symptoms such as vomiting, diarrhea, and dizziness. Although plasma levels of prostaglandins are normal in dysmenorrheic women, increased sensitivity or generalized overproduction of prostaglandins may occur.

The prostaglandin hypothesis has been further strengthened by the observation that drugs that inhibit prostaglandin synthesis can relieve dysmenorrhea and the associated symptoms (32–37). Several clinical studies have found that nonsteroidal antiinflammatory drugs (NSAIDs) are effective in the relief of pain. NSAID agents are divided into two classes: carboxylic acids and enolic acids. Enolic acid agents (phenylbutazone and piroxicam) act by inhibition of the isomerase/reductase step in the production of PGE_2 and $PGF_{2\alpha}$. The carboxylates, most frequently used in the treatment of dysmenorrhea, can be divided into four categories: salicylic acids/esters (aspirin, diflunisal), acetic acids (indomethacin, sulindac, tolmetin), propionic acids (ibuprofen, naproxen, fenoprofen, ketoprofen, flurbiprofen), and fenamates (mefenamic acid, meclofenamate, tolfenamic acid, flufenamic acid) (32). The salicylic acids and esters appear to inhibit cyclooxygenase; but aspirin has little potency compared with some of the other NSAIDs in reducing prostaglandin synthesis, and it may increase menstrual flow (38). Thus, aspirin is used less often in the treatment of dysmenorrhea. Indomethacin is the best known drug of the acetic acid group for treating dysmenorrhea, but its side effects have prevented its use by most, if not all, patients. Thus the clinician selects chiefly from the two last groups, propionic acids and fenamates, for clinical treatment of dysmenorrhea.

Ibuprofen and naproxen have been most widely studied for the relief of pain in dysmenorrhea. For example, Chan and associates (34) correlated the relief of dysmenorrhea by ibuprofen with the reduction in menstrual prostaglandin release as measured by a method that can detect menstrual prostaglandin activity in tampon specimens. Total menstrual prostaglandin release per cycle fell from a control level of 59.8 ± 7.2 to 16.8 ± 2.3 (gram $PGF_{2\alpha}$ equivalents) with the use of ibuprofen (34). Numerous clinical studies have found these agents to be effective in both adult and adolescent women, giving pain relief in 67% to 86% of patients. The sodium salt of naproxen has a more rapid absorption than naproxen and can give very rapid relief of symptoms. The prostaglandin inhibitor flurbiprofen also appears to be very effective in the relief of dysmenorrhea (39).

The fenamates are potent inhibitors of prostaglandin synthesis and in addition can antagonize the action of already formed prostaglandins (37). This increased activity may give this class of drug a theoretic advantage in treatment. Clinical studies of meclofenamate have shown effectiveness (40,41); this drug also inhibits the activity of 5-lipoxygenase, but the clinical importance of the inhibition of leukotrienes is unknown.

OCs lessen dysmenorrhea, probably in part related to their antiovulatory actions as well as their ability to produce endometrial hypoplasia, less menstrual flow, and subsequently less prostaglandins (34).

With the advent of the research on prostaglandins as the cause of dysmenorrhea, the potential influence of psychological issues on dysmenorrhea has received little attention. However, in a study of adolescents treated for dysmenorrhea with naproxen sodium, DuRant and colleagues (42) made the interesting observation that girls with increased life crisis events experienced greater severity of symptoms in the first month of therapy than did other girls. It is possible that prostaglandins may increase in response to physical and psychological stress or that the patient may be more keenly aware of pain when distressed by other problems in her life. As therapy was continued, life stress ceased to have a significant influence on the severity of dysmenorrhea. Those with persistent symptoms, however, did have lower self-concept at followup, perhaps because of their initial high expectation of receiving relief.

Patient Assessment

In assessing the adolescent with dysmenorrhea, the physician needs to know her menstrual history and the timing of her cramps, pain, and/or premenstrual symptoms, as well as her response to them. The key questions are these: Is she missing school? If so, how many days? Does she miss other activities? Social events? Does she have nausea and vomiting, diarrhea, or dizziness? What medications has she used to treat the symptoms? What makes the pain better? Worse? What is the nature of the mother–daughter interaction? Does or did her mother or sister have cramps? Is there a family history of endometriosis? Young women whose cramps are disabling out of proportion to the apparent severity may have confounding factors contributing to their symptoms, such as a reluctance to attend school, a history of physical or sexual abuse, or significant psychosocial problems. The questions about previous medications are particularly crucial, because with the availability of over-the-counter NSAIDs, many adolescents have tried these medications in subtherapeutic doses and have subsequently discarded the concept of their usefulness.

For the virginal adolescent who has mild symptoms, a normal physical examination, including inspection of the genitalia to exclude an abnormality of the hymen, is reassuring. Adolescents with moderate or severe dysmenorrhea who are sexually active should have a speculum and bimanual pelvic examination. In the majority of adolescents who are carefully prepared, a vaginal examination is atraumatic. A rectoabdominal examination with the patient in the lithotomy position is all that is possible for some non-sexually active girls, and this exam will exclude adnexal tenderness and masses. A speculum examination is not necessary if it is not easily tolerated. If the pelvic anatomy needs to be further evaluated, and a rectoabdominal exam is noncontributory or not an option, ultrasonography may be necessary. Ultrasonography is useful in defining suspected uterine and vaginal anomalies with obstruction but will not detect abnormalities such as intraabdominal or pelvic adhesions or endometriosis.

Treatment

Treatment includes a careful explanation to the patient of the nature of the problem and a chance for her to ask questions regarding her anatomy. If the results of examination are normal, treatment should be directed at symptomatic relief. The most common approach is to prescribe one of the NSAID compounds: naproxen sodium (Aleve 220 mg or Anaprox 275 mg), two tablets given immediately and then one every 6 hours; naproxen sodium double-strength (Anaprox DS), 550 mg twice a day; naproxen (Naprosyn), 250 to 375 mg two to three times a day; ibuprofen, 400 to 800 mg (with a loading dose of 800 mg) every 4 to 6 hours; or mefenamic acid, 500 mg given immediately and then 250 mg every 6 hours. Alternatively, flurbiprofen (50 mg every 6 hours or 100 mg two to three times daily), or meclofenamate (100 mg initially, followed by 50 to 100 mg every 6 hours) can also be used to treat dysmenorrhea.

Most patients can obtain effective relief by starting the antiprostaglandin medicine at the onset of the menses and continuing for the first 1 to 2 days of the cycle, or for the usual duration of cramps. The patient should be told to begin taking the medicine as soon as she knows her menses are coming: "at the first sign of cramps or bleeding." A loading dose is important in patients with symptoms that are severe and occur rapidly. For such patients, a rapidly absorbed drug such as naproxen sodium would be preferable. Generally, giving the medicine at the onset of the menses prevents the inadvertent administration of the drug to a pregnant woman. However, a patient who is not sexually active and has severe cramps accompanied by early vomiting, and thus is unable to take medication, may often benefit from starting the drug 1 or 2 days before the onset of her menses. A patient may respond to a higher dose or to another NSAID. Since life stresses may lessen the pain relief in the first cycle, the determination of effectiveness in an individual patient should be based on the response in more than one cycle. Usually, medication is prescribed for two to three cycles before it is changed. In addition, a patient may have previously taken inadequate doses of a medicine, particularly ibuprofen, to obtain relief.

The NSAID compounds should be avoided in preoperative patients and patients with known or suspected ulcer disease, GI bleeding, clotting disorders, renal disease, allergies to aspirin or NSAIDs, or aspirin-induced asthma. All of the NSAIDs should be taken with food, even though some patients prefer only liquids on the first day of the cycle. The side effects of these drugs appear minimal in short-term use, but the possibility of allergy and GI irritation and bleeding should be explained to the patient. Some patients complain of fluid retention or fatigue with the use of these agents.

In some patients, NSAID drugs are contraindicated or produce undesirable side effects. In these adolescents, an alternative is tramadol hydrochloride tablets. Tramadol is a centrally acting analgesic that acts by binding to μ-opioid receptors and inhibiting the reuptake of norepinephrine and serotonin; it is not a member of either the NSAID or narcotic drug groups. It is indicated for moderate to severe pain, and it appears to be nonaddictive. Its efficacy is comparable to that of codeine (30 mg) and oxycodone (5 mg). It is prescribed as 50-mg pills that are taken as 50 to 100 mg every 6 hours; an individual should not take more than eight pills in 24 hours.

In addition to traditional Western medical therapies, patients should be encouraged to exercise, eat a well-balanced diet, and work to reduce stress in their lives. Some girls can continue to exercise or participate in competitive sports during their menses; others may find the discomfort to be too great. Some herbal teas, fruits, and vegetables have been reported to be beneficial to women with dysmenorrhea (43).

The adolescent should be seen initially every 3 or 4 months to evaluate the effectiveness of the therapies. Such visits also facilitate the rapport between health care provider and patient that is essential in the treatment of this problem. Only a few adolescents use their symptoms for secondary gains, such as an excuse to stay out of school or to gain sympathy from their parents. The vast majority of adolescents need to be encouraged to discuss their symptoms and should not be made to feel emotionally unstable because they complain of pain.

If the patient fails to respond to antiprostaglandin drugs and continues to have severe pain or vomiting, or if at the initial evaluation she needs birth control, a course of combination estrogen/progestin OCs (see Chapter 17) should be initiated. Cramps are usually substantially, if not completely, relieved with the anovulatory cycles and scantier flow. If severe cramps persist despite three cycles of ovulation suppression therapy, laparoscopy is indicated to exclude endometriosis or other organic causes (44).

If dysmenorrhea is relieved by OCs, medication is usually prescribed for 3 to 6 months and then discontinued (frequently during the summer, when school attendance will not be disrupted). Often, the patient will continue to have relief from cramps for several additional (commonly anovulatory) cycles before the more severe dysmenorrhea recurs. When the cramps recur, a trial of other antiprostaglandin drugs may again be attempted as the sole therapy before OCs are reinstituted. The adolescent with severe dysmenorrhea usually prefers to continue with long-term OCs. The return of increasingly severe dysmenorrhea in spite of continued use of OCs again raises the possibility of organic disease such as endometriosis and calls for a reevaluation and consideration of laparoscopy for definitive diagnosis.

CHRONIC PELVIC PAIN

Chronic pelvic pain is a common and serious health issue for women. A recent study found that although chronic pelvic pain occured in one of seven women in the United States between the ages of 18 and 50, only 49% of those with pain reported that the cause was known (45). The diagnosis of chronic pelvic pain in an adolescent is similar to that for acute pelvic pain except that the tempo of the investigation is usually not urgent. An accurate assessment of psychosocial issues and the impact of the pain on the life of the child or adolescent is essential. Chronic pain can be a significant source of frustration for the patient and her parents, and it is not unusual for them to search for multiple opinions from the medical community. Many of these teenagers will have missed many days of school and will be far behind in their schoolwork. If, for example, bowel spasm resulted in the initial symptoms of pain, reluctance to return to school may intensify the pain, causing further absences. Although short-term tutoring may be essential, the physician should work with the adolescent and her family to encourage her to return to normal social interaction and to school. Granting a request for long-term home tutoring is rarely in her best interests. On the other hand, a definitive diagnosis is extremely important because parents and patients are often concerned that cancer or some other life-threatening condition is present. The girl's complaints should be assessed thoroughly so that she feels that her symptoms are taken seriously by the health care provider. A recommendation "to see a counselor" may be interpreted by the adolescent as meaning "the pain is in your head." In addition, important diagnoses such as PID or endometriosis may be missed unless a complete assessment is undertaken in the patient with persistent pelvic pain. The physician needs to reassure the patient that efforts will be made to sort out her problem and that she will not be abandoned even if no diagnosis can be established.

The evaluation of the child or adolescent with chronic pelvic pain requires a history and physical examination similar to that just described for acute pelvic pain. The common problems included in the differential diagnosis are shown in Table 1. The history and assessment should take into account the possible gynecologic, GI, urologic, musculoskeletal, and psychosomatic causes. The patient can be asked to grade the pain on a scale of 1 to 10. This can be helpful in deciding on the long-term management of the chronic pain. A complete history must include questions relating to past or present sexual abuse, as sexual abuse and physical abuse have both been noted to be associated with chronic pelvic pain (46–49). A complete physical examination including abdominal palpation, musculoskeletal assessment for hernias, and pelvic examination should be performed. It is helpful to ask the patient during the examination to point with one finger to the location of the pain and then to ask her what factors (e.g., exercise, sexual activity, food, urination, bowel movement) relieve or exacerbate the pain. For example, girls with endometriosis may have a constellation of symptoms that include cyclic severe dysmenorrhea, rectal pressure and other bowel problems, and dyspareunia. Activity may increase the symptoms in patients with adhesions and with many of the musculoskeletal problems. Since constipation and other GI disorders (irritable bowel syndrome, lactose intolerance) are such common causes of pelvic discomfort in adolescents, a careful bowel history, dietary history (including information about gum chewing and carbonated beverages), and rectal examination are important. A trial of stool softeners, high-fiber diet, and increased fluid intake is often essential before other diagnoses are considered.

The practitioner performing the musculoskeletal examination should assess the range of motion of the hips and spine, check for normal results of the straight-leg raising test and the absence of symptoms with pelvic compression, and look for bone tenderness. Neoplasms of the pelvis and lower spine may be missed on plain radiographs and may require a bone scan for detection. Stress fractures of the pubic ramus and ischium can occur in runners, who may present with hip or groin pain, exacerbated by activity, and bone tenderness.

As noted previously, the pelvic examination should be performed with the patient in the lithotomy position so that the reproductive structures can be adequately assessed. A speculum examination is important to identify genital tract obstruction and anomalies and to obtain samples for *C. trachomatis* and *N. gonorrhoeae* tests and Papanicolaou smear, if the patient was ever or is possibly sexually active or is over 18. The bimanual palpation (rectoabdominal or rectovaginal–abdominal) should attempt to localize tender areas, and the posterior cul-de-sac should be assessed for pain.

The laboratory evaluation usually includes a CBC with differential, ESR or CRP, urinalysis and urine culture, cervical tests, and a sensitive test for pregnancy. As described above, pelvic ultrasonography can be used to assess a mass or a suspected genital tract malformation and to screen patients in whom a satisfactory pelvic examination is not possible. It is advisable to ask the radiologist to screen the kidneys by ultrasound to look for unilateral renal agenesis or other renal anomalies if a genital tract anomaly is suspected.

In our practice, we have evaluated several young adolescents in the earliest stages of pubertal development who have persistent pelvic discomfort and large tender multifollicular ovaries (Fig. 3); we have treated them symptomatically with analgesics and low doses of NSAIDs, and the symptoms have resolved with further pubertal development. As noted above, some investigators have suggested that transabdominal color Doppler ultrasound can be useful in the evaluation of a painful ovary in adolescents. When prepubertal ovaries are found to be enlarged and multicystic, an evaluation for thyroid disease is indicated. In many young girls or adolescents, multicystic ovaries are asymptomatic and are noted when ultrasonography is done for other indications. Operative evaluation should be avoided unless ovarian torsion or tumor is suspected. A full presentation of the diagnosis and management of ovarian masses is presented in Chapter 15.

Gastrointestinal series, urologic studies, bone scans, and consultations by specialists should be obtained as needed, not routinely in all adolescents with chronic pelvic pain.

For undiagnosed chronic pelvic pain in adolescents, laparoscopy has become an invaluable aid to diagnosis and therapy (16,44,50–54). Laparoscopy allows the physician to make or confirm a specific diagnosis, obtain samples for biopsy, lyse adhesions, and perform operative therapeutic procedures. Before the procedure, the gynecologist should discuss with the patient and her family the possibilities and limitations of operative surgery during the laparoscopy, and determine whether the patient desires a laparotomy if the needed procedure cannot safely be performed by laparoscopy. This preoperative counseling can avoid the need for a later second anesthetic for a laparotomy. Negative findings (see Color Plate 23) at laparoscopy can be equally valuable in reassuring the patient and her

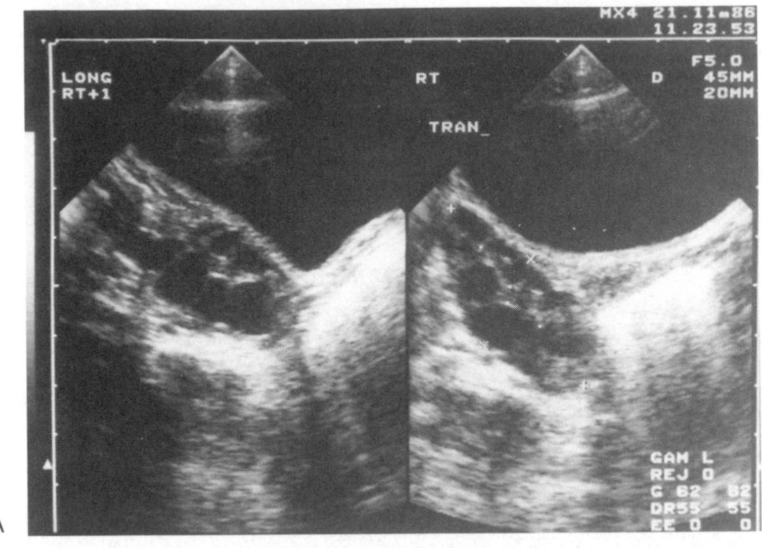

A

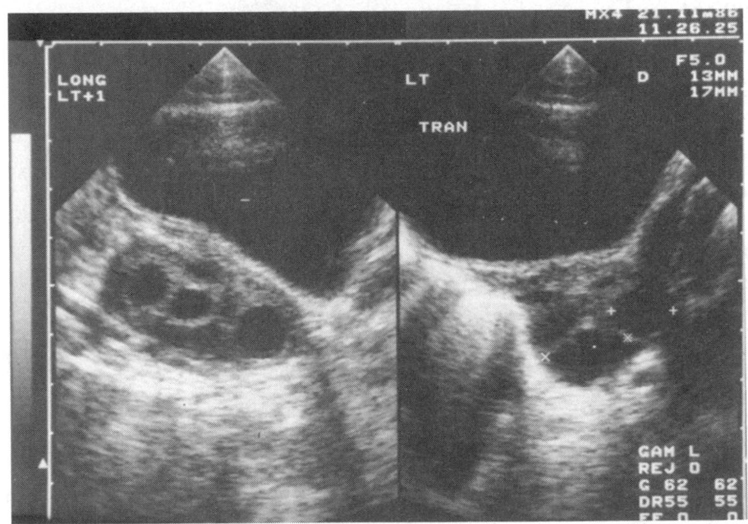

B

FIG. 3. Longitudinal and transverse ultrasound views of enlarged multicystic ovaries in an 11-year-old girl with chronic pelvic pain. **(A)** Right ovary. **(B)** Left ovary. Such ovaries are often asymptomatic in early pubertal girls.

family and in helping her accept the fact that she has a functional problem that is likely to respond to medical and psychological therapy.

At our institution, laparoscopy in the evaluation of the adolescent or young adult with chronic pelvic pain is indicated if the patient's pain is unresponsive to prostaglandin inhibitors and OCs over a 3- to 6-month interval. As previously noted, laparoscopy is useful for the confirmation or exclusion of clinically suspected endometriosis, chronic PID, ovarian cysts, or pelvic adhesions.

Laparoscopy for Chronic Pelvic Pain

At Children's Hospital, Boston, laparoscopy is performed with the patient under general endotracheal anesthesia, usually in the ambulatory surgery unit. A 2-, 5-, 7-, or 10-mm laparoscope is used through an umbilical vertical incision, and a second trocar site is established in the suprapubic area. A uterine mobilizer attached to the cervix to allow mobilization of the uterus can be placed in the sexually active patient, but is not necessary in all patients. If a uterine manipulator is used, the patient is placed in the dorsal lithotomy position, and if it is not used, the patient is placed in the dorsal supine position. In addition, a Foley catheter is placed in all patients, as it is unclear how long the surgical procedure will take, and if a catheter is used to empty the bladder and is then removed the bladder may refill to a point of obstructing the surgeon's view. An oral–gastric tube is helpful in emptying the stomach, and the patient's respirations are temporarily ceased during the moments of insertion of the insufflation needle and trocar.

The results of laparoscopy in the diagnosis of chronic pelvic pain at Children's Hospital, Boston, between July 1974 and December 1983 are shown in Table 4. It should be noted that patients suspected of having PID on the basis of history and elevated sedimentation rate were not included in this series, since the laparoscopy in these patients was performed largely to confirm the diagnosis and evaluate the severity of PID rather than to establish the diagnosis of chronic pelvic pain.

As noted in Table 4, three-quarters of the adolescents who underwent laparoscopy at Children's Hospital, Boston, for chronic pelvic pain had intrapelvic pathologic conditons; endometriosis was diagnosed most frequently. The age-related incidence of findings is shown in Table 5. As one would expect, the finding of endometriosis increases with age. The next most common finding was postoperative adhesions, usually associated with a history of appendectomy or ovarian

TABLE 4. *Postoperative diagnosis in 282 adolescent patients with chronic pelvic pain (Children's Hospital, Boston, 1974–1983)*

Diagnosis	No. of patients	(%)
Endometriosis	126	(45)
Postoperative adhesions	37	(13)
Serositis	15	(5)
Ovarian cyst	14	(5)
Uterine malformation	15	(5)
Other[a]	4	(2)
No pathologic condition	71	(25)

[a]Ileitis, infarcted hydatid of Morgagni, pelvic congestion.

TABLE 5. *Age-related incidence of laparoscopic findings in 129 adolescent patients with chronic pelvic pain (Children's Hospital, Boston, 1980–1983)*

	No. of patients (%)				
Diagnosis	Age 11–13	Age 14–15	Age 16–17	Age 18–19	Age 20–21
Endometriosis	2 (12)	9 (28)	21 (40)	17 (45)	7 (54)
Postoperative adhesions	1 (6)	4 (13)	7 (13)	5 (13)	2 (15)
Serositis	5 (29)	4 (13)	0 (0)	2 (5)	0 (0)
Ovarian cyst	2 (12)	2 (6)	3 (5)	2 (5)	0 (8)
Uterine malformation	1 (6)	0 (0)	1 (2)	0 (0)	1 (0)
Other	0 (0)	1 (3)	2 (4)	1 (3)	0 (0)
No pathologic condition	6 (35)	12 (37)	19 (36)	11 (29)	3 (23)

cystectomy. In most of these adolescents, the pain was acyclic, was often aggravated by physical activity or coitus, and was relieved by rest. The preoperative pelvic examination frequently revealed some adnexal thickening and cul-de-sac or adnexal tenderness and nodularity. Preoperative treatment was variable; predominantly, suppression of ovulation with OCs or antiprostaglandins was used. Because of the small number of patients, the natural history is unknown except that a few have subsequently developed endometriosis.

Other findings included PID (see Chapter 12), ovarian cysts (see Chapter 15), genital tract malformations with obstruction (see Chapter 8), and cases of ileitis, infarcted hydatid of Morgagni, inguinal defects (Fig. 4), and adhesions (Fig. 5). The pain in the patients with chronic PID was generally acyclic and not related

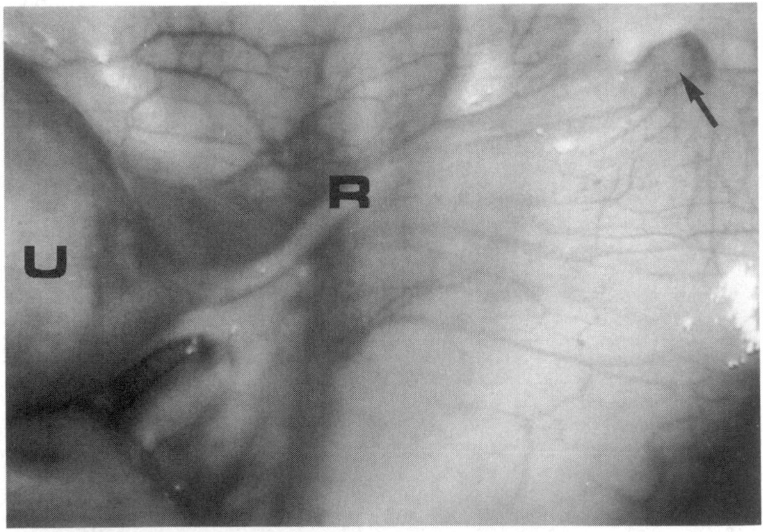

FIG. 4. Laparoscopic view of an enlarged right inguinal ring (*arrow*), a potential hernia site. R, round ligament; U, uterus.

to physical activity; pelvic examination revealed tender or nontender adnexal thickening in most of these girls.

No apparent gynecologic cause of the chronic pain was found in one-quarter of the patients; of those with negative findings, 74% felt that their symptoms were improved at followup. Whether the knowledge of normal anatomy contributed to the positive outcome is unknown, although several patients with a history of PID were considerably reassured. At other centers, a larger percentage of normal laparoscopic examination results has been reported. The much higher number of patients with early endometriosis in the Children's Hospital, Boston, series may reflect the difficulty of identifying very early endometriosis, thus underscoring the need for biopsy of hyperemic petechial lesions. The results of treatment of the first 140 patients in our earlier series are shown in Table 6.

In a more recent study at Children's Hospital, Boston, adolescent women aged 13 to 21 were evaluated when their pelvic pain had lasted longer than 3 months and had not responded to NSAIDs and OCs (44). Approximately 70% of them had endometriosis; the laparoscopic findings are shown in Table 7. The presenting symptoms of the patients with and without endometriosis are shown in Table 8.

Other series of laparoscopic findings in adolescents have found a higher proportion of patients having PID; this may reflect both the population studied (inner city vs. suburban), the inclusion–exclusion criteria, the ability to recognize very early or atypical endometriosis, and the distribution of the age of the study population. For example, in a study of 100 women between the ages of 15 and 19, Strickland and coworkers (51) found that 46 had a normal pelvis, 29 had evidence of PID, 12 had endometriosis, and 13 had other pathologic conditions of the pelvis, including paratubal cysts, multicystic ovaries, and adhesions.

TABLE 6. *Results of initial treatment in 140 adolescent patients with chronic pelvic pain*

Condition	No. of patients	Improved (%)	Recurrence (%)
Endometriosis alone	66	47 (71)	19 (29)
Postoperative adhesions	18	16 (89)	2 (11)
Uterine anomalies			
With endometriosis	8	8 (100)	0 (0)
Without endometriosis	4	4 (100)	0 (0)
Pelvic inflammatory disease	10	5 (50)	5 (50)
Hemoperitoneum	6	5 (83)	1 (17)
Functional ovarian cysts	5	4 (80)	1 (20)
Serositis	4	3 (75)	1 (25)
No pathologic condition seen	19	14 (74)	5 (26)
Total	140	106 (76)	34 (24)

(From Goldstein DP, deCholnoky C, Emans SJ, et al. Laparoscopy in the diagnosis and management of pelvic pain in adolescents. *J Reprod Med* 1980;24:254; with permission.)

TABLE 7. *Laparoscopic findings in adolescent patients with chronic pelvic pain not responding to oral contraceptives and nonsteroidal antiinflammatory drugs*

Laparoscopic findings	Number (%)
Visible endometriosis	31/46 (67.4)
Adhesions	11/46 (23.9)
Prior surgery	8
With endometriosis	3
Without endometriosis	5
No prior surgery	3
With endometriosis	3
Without endometriosis	0
Grossly normal pelvis	5/46 (10.9)
Functional cysts	4/46 (8.7)
Paratubal cysts	4/46 (8.7)
Müllerian anomalies	3/46 (6.5)
With endometriosis	1
Without endometriosis	2

(From Laufer MR, Goitein L, Bush M, Cramer DW, Emans SJ. Prevalence of endometriosis in adolescent women with chronic pelvic pain not responding to conventional therapy. *J Pediatr Adolesc Gynecol* 1997;10:199–202.)

TABLE 8. *Characteristics of subjects with and without endometriosis*

Characteristics	Patients with endometriosis (n = 32) Number (%)	Patients without endometriosis (n = 14) Number (%)
Age (years)		
≤14	7 (21.8)	1 (7.2)
15–17	20 (62.5)	10 (71.4)
≥18	5 (15.6)	3 (21.4)
Mean age (years) at menarche	12.3	12.3
Mean time (months) at menarche	3.7	3.9
Duration of oral contraceptives (months)		
≤3	17 (53.1)	5 (35.7)
4–11	9 (28.1)	6 (42.9)
≥12	6 (18.8)	3 (21.4)
Prior surgery	3 (9.4)	5 (35.7)
Presenting symptoms		
Acyclic and cyclic pain	20 (62.5)	8 (57.1)
Acyclic pain	9 (28.1)	3 (21.4)
Cyclic pain	3 (9.4)	3 (21.4)
Gastrointestinal pain	11 (34.3)	6 (42.9)
Urinary symptoms	4 (12.5)	4 (33.3)
Irregular menses	3 (9.4)	6 (42.9)*
Vaginal discharge	2 (6.3)	2 (14.3)

*$p < 0.05$.

(From Laufer MR, Goitein L, Bush M, Cramer DW, Emans SJ. Prevalence of endometriosis in adolescent women with chronic abdominal/pelvic pain not responding to conventional therapy. *J Pediatr Adolesc Gynecol* 1997;10:199–202.)

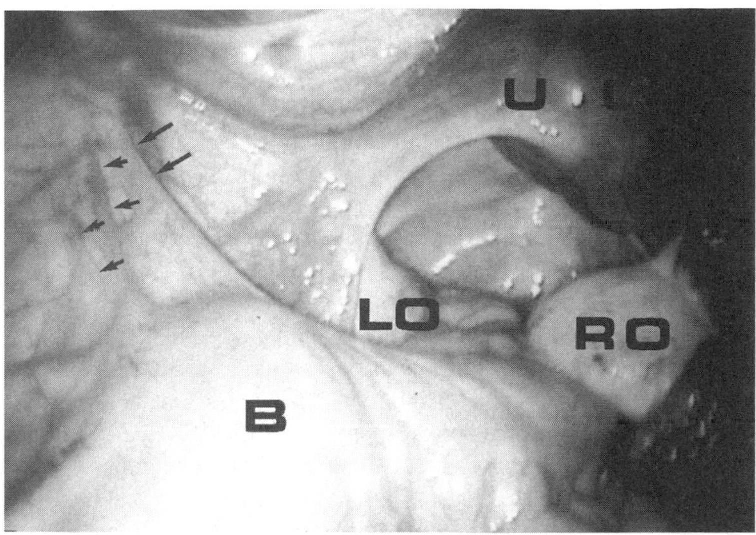

FIG. 5. Bowel adhesions (*arrows*) to sidewall. B, bowel; LO, left ovary; RO, right ovary; U, uterus.

An association between chronic pelvic pain and bowel-to-pelvic sidewall adhesions (Fig. 5) has been debated. The cause of adhesions is unknown, but it is believed to be the result of infection, previous surgery, or endometriosis. In women with chronic pelvic pain, a recent study found a higher rate of colon-to-sidewall adhesions than in controls (93.3% vs 13.3%) (55). These authors also found that adhesions may occur with or without the presence of endometriosis, but that those patients with chronic pelvic pain had a higher rate of endometriosis than controls (46.7% vs. 6.7%). Others have suggested that a causal relationship between adhesions and pelvic pain is unproved (56). At our institution, when bowel adhesions are identified in adolescents with chronic pelvic pain, a laparoscopic lysis of adhesions is undertaken, and then a cul-de-sac biopsy specimen is obtained for microscopic evaluation to rule out atypical endometriosis (see below). Our studies have shown a correlation of adhesions with endometriosis in patients with pelvic pain; as shown in Table 7, no cases of adhesions were identified in patients without a history of previous surgery or the existence of endometriosis (44). Patients who have undergone prior surgery may have adhesions as a result, or may have a herniation of bowel or omentum at the site of a previous laparoscopy incision.

The data collected at our institution and others reinforce the need to take the symptoms of chronic pelvic pain seriously. A careful history, pelvic examination, appropriate laboratory tests, and laparoscopy as indicated should be done in the pursuit of a diagnosis and treatment.

Endometriosis

Endometriosis is defined as the presence of endometrial glands and stroma outside the normal anatomic location of the lining of the uterus (see Color Plate 28). The etiology of endometriosis has not been determined, but many theories have been proposed. Endometriosis is believed to occur in 1% to 17% of menstruating women (57,58). Historically, endometriosis was considered a disease of women in the reproductive years, but it has been reported in women aged 10.5 (59) to 76 years (60). An accurate determination of the prevalence in the adolescent population is difficult because the definitive diagnosis requires a laparoscopic evaluation, which only occurs with a specific indication; a selection bias thus exists for determining the prevalence in the overall adolescent population. Most adult patients with endometriosis present with pain, a pelvic mass, or infertility. Adolescents usually present with pelvic pain, as endometriomas and infertility are rare in this patient population. The definitive diagnosis of endometriosis must be established by laparoscopy with or without pathologic identification of biopsy specimens. Treatment with endometriosis-specific drug therapy, as outlined below, should not be undertaken without a definitive diagnosis.

Proposed theories about the causes of endometriosis include the following:

1. Sampson's (61,62) theory of retrograde menstruation, which proposes that there is retrograde transport of viable fragments of endometrium through the fallopian tubes at the time of menstruation that leads to seeding of the peritoneal cavity. Factors such as shorter cycle lengths, longer duration of flow, and possibly heavier flow in women with endometriosis than in control women lend credence to the hypothesis that retrograde menstruation is primarily responsible for endometriosis (63).
2. Meyer's (64) theory of embryologically totipotent cells that undergo metaplastic transformation into functioning endometrium.
3. Halban's (65) theory of metastases of endometrial cells though vascular or lymphatic spread; this theory serves to explain the occurrences of endometriosis in the lung (66) or brain (67).
4. The theory of deficient cell-mediated immunity, with impaired "clearing" of endometriotic cells from aberrant locations (68,69).

There may be a genetic predisposition to, or etiology of, endometriosis. Ranney (70) first reported the familial occurrence of endometriosis in a retrospective study of 53 families. Simpson and associates (71) reported a 6.9% rate of endometriosis in first-degree relatives of women with the disease, compared with only 1% of control relatives; the most probable mode of inheritance being polygenic and multifactorial. As the general population and health care providers have become increasingly educated about the existence and prevalence of endometriosis, there is an increase in referrals for young women to undergo definitive diagnosis for chronic pelvic pain. It is our observation that this is especially true of mothers who suffered from chronic pelvic pain as adolescents but received diagnosis and treatment for endometriosis only as adults.

Studies of women undergoing laparoscopy (72,73) or peritoneal dialysis (74) have shown that retrograde menstruation occurs in 76% to 90% of all menstruating women. The extent of the reflux may be different or immunologic responses may be variable in women with endometriosis than in those free of the disease. Women with endometriosis are more likely to have a history of severe cramps; whether the greater uterine contractility predisposes them to endometriosis or whether the cramps are secondary to the early development of endometriosis is unanswered. The role of endogenous estrogens is also under study; smokers who began their habit before the age of 17 and smoke a pack or more a day have a lower risk of endometriosis, possibly because of lower estrogen levels (63).

In 1948, Meigs (75) reported that the incidence of endometriosis in all adolescents was 6%; others have also attempted to estimate the prevalence (53,76,77). The prevalence of endometriosis in adolescents with chronic pelvic pain has been determined to be approximately 45% to 65% (52,59,78,79). The prevalence rate in adolescents with chronic pelvic pain not responding to NSAID and OC therapy has been reported to be as high as 70% (74) and is presented in detail below. The key to the determination of endometriosis is to include it in the differential diagnosis and proceed with laparoscopy when indicated.

Endometriosis is the most common pathologic condition of the pelvis in adolescents with chronic pelvic pain (Tables 4–7). As noted in Table 5, endometriosis as a cause of chronic pelvic pain increases with age, from 12% in the 11- to 13-year old group to 54% in the 20- to 21-year-old group. The history usually reveals cyclic and/or acyclic pelvic pain. In one study from our institution, 64% of adolescents with endometriosis had cyclic pain and 36% acyclic pain (59). Our more recent study of adolescents with chronic pain not responding to NSAIDs and OCs showed that approximately 90% of the patients with endometriosis had some acyclic pain (Table 8). Some patients experience an increase in symptoms at midcycle and again with menses. The pain tends to increase in severity over time and may occur throughout the month. Although OCs and antiprostaglandin medications may give some initial relief, the pain usually persists, leading to laparoscopy for a definitive diagnosis and therapy as shown in Fig. 6 (84). Other presenting symptoms of adolescents with chronic pelvic pain not responding to NSAIDs and OCs are shown in Table 8, categorized according to those with and without endometriosis (44). Most adolescents with diagnosed endometriosis present with symptoms of pain, although adult women may be asymptomatic and the disease detected during an evaluation for infertility. The cause of the pain may be related to prostaglandin release, or swelling and bleeding within the endometriotic implants. Endometriosis pain may be incapacitating in patients with both minimal and extensive disease; no clear correlation has been established between the extent of disease and severity of pain (80–83). Cornillie and colleagues (80) found that it is the deeply infil-

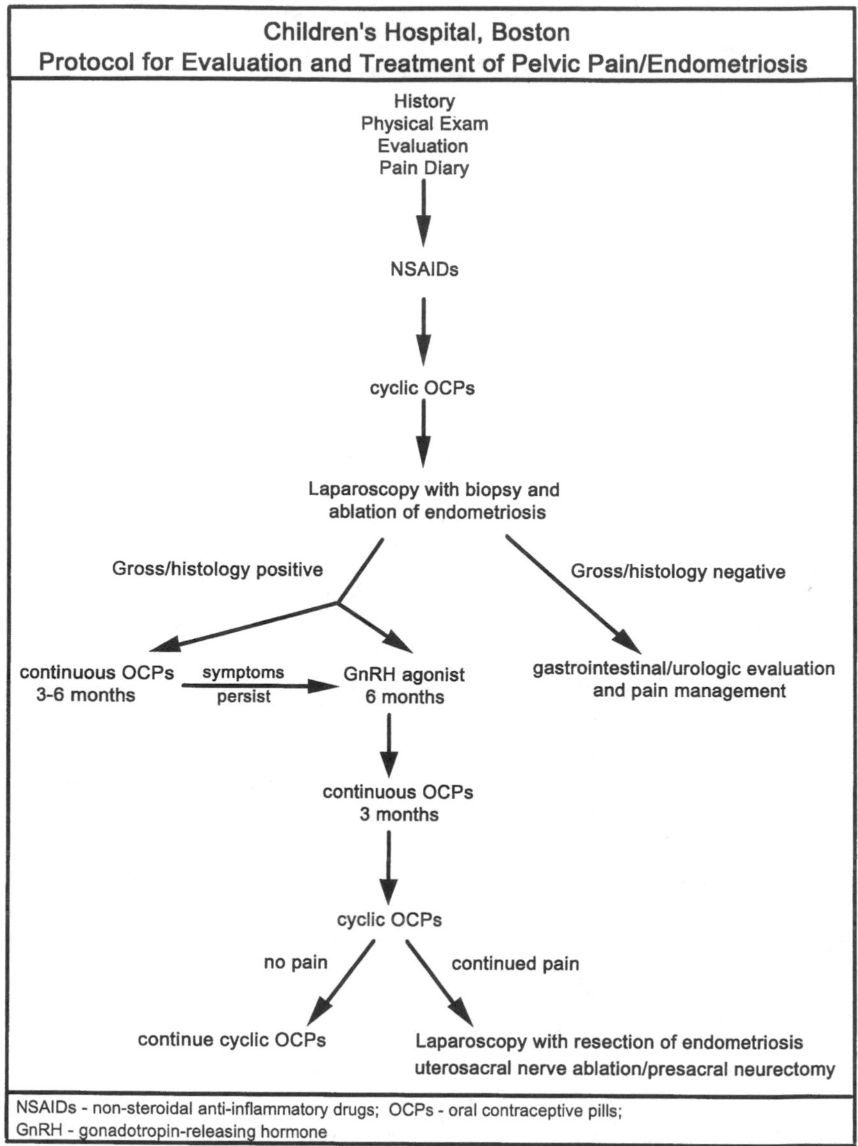

FIG. 6. Protocol for evaluation and treatment of pelvic pain/endometriosis. (Adapted from Bandera CA, Brown LR, Laufer MR. Adolescents and endometriosis. *Clin Consult Obstet Gynecol* 1995;7:200; with permission.)

trating endometriotic lesions that are most active and strongly correlate with pelvic pain, while Fedele and colleagues (81) found no relation between the severity of pain and stage of the disease or site of the endometriosis lesions.

Pelvic examination in the adult woman with endometriosis classically reveals tender nodules in the posterior vaginal fornix (cul-de-sac) and along the uterosacral ligaments. The ovary may be involved, with an endometrioma or dense periovarian adhesions, and the uterus may be fixed and retroverted. In contrast, the pelvic examination of adolescents with endometriosis often reveals mild to moderate tenderness rather than nodules or masses.

Endometriosis is staged according to the criteria of the American Society for Reproductive Medicine (formerly the American Fertility Society), which are based on a point system (Fig. 7) (84). Classic endometriosis has been described as blue/brown/gray "powder burns." Classic and "atypical" implants have been categorized on an expanded basis of morphologic appearance: "white" lesions; clear vesicular lesions; red, "flame," or petechial lesions; reddish-brown implants; and blue/brown/gray "powder burn" implants (85-90). The implants seen in adolescents may not be typical of the lesions seen in adult women; adolescents may have clear vesicles, pearly granular punctations (white implants), and/or small hemorrhagic or petechial spots of the pelvic peritoneum (see Color Plate 28). We have recently described a new technique of filling the pelvis with liquid to aid in the visualization of clear lesions of endometriosis (91). In earlier reports from our institution, adolescents with chronic pelvic pain were found to have a rate of endometriosis of 45% and a rate of serositis of 5% (Table 4). The cases of serositis may be what is now referred to as atypical clear lesions of endometriosis, thus giving an overall prevalence of 50% of adolescents with chronic pelvic pain having endometriosis. Some authors have suggested that the earliest signs of endometriosis are hemosiderin staining of the peritoneal surfaces in dependent areas of the pelvis (92). If atypical endometriosis is suspected, or if the gross appearance of the pelvis is normal in a patient with chronic pelvic pain, a pelvic peritoneal biopsy specimen from the cul-de-sac may help confirm a diagnosis of endometriosis (93,94). Nisolle and colleagues (93) found microscopic endometriosis in 6% of patients with a grossly visible pelvis. In our series, one of five patients (20%) with a visibly normal pelvis was found to have biopsy-proven endometriosis (44). Adult endometriosis is particularly common at the site of entry from the tubes into the peritoneal cavity (the fallopian tube ostia), in the adjacent structures (ovary and uterosacral ligament at the base of the broad ligament), and in fixed structures (92). In the ovary, large endometrial cysts can develop: so-called endometriomas or chocolate cysts, possibly at the site of the postovulatory corpus luteum (92). Endometriosis within the ovary (endometrioma) is much less common in adolescents and may represent disease progression.

There may be a natural progression of endometriosis, evolving from atypical lesions in adolescents to the classic lesions in adult women. Adolescent endometriosis may present with atypical lesions of the cul-de-sac and no other definable disease. Martin et al (87) reported a pattern of evolution of subtle

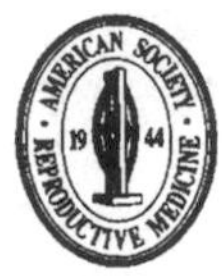

AMERICAN SOCIETY FOR REPRODUCTIVE MEDICINE
REVISED CLASSIFICATION OF ENDOMETRIOSIS

Patient's Name ______________________ Date ______________

Stage I (Minimal) - 1-5
Stage II (Mild) - 6-15
Stage III (Moderate) - 16-40
Stage IV (Severe) - >40
Total ______________

Laparoscopy ________ Laparotomy ________ Photography ________
Recommended Treatment ______________________

Prognosis ______________

PERITONEUM	**ENDOMETRIOSIS**	<1cm	1-3cm	>3cm
	Superficial	1	2	4
	Deep	2	4	6
OVARY	R Superficial	1	2	4
	Deep	4	16	20
	L Superficial	1	2	4
	Deep	4	16	20
	POSTERIOR CULDESAC OBLITERATION	Partial		Complete
		4		40
OVARY	**ADHESIONS**	<1/3 Enclosure	1/3-2/3 Enclosure	>2/3 Enclosure
	R Filmy	1	2	4
	Dense	4	8	16
	L Filmy	1	2	4
	Dense	4	8	16
TUBE	R Filmy	1	2	4
	Dense	4*	8*	16
	L Filmy	1	2	4
	Dense	4*	8*	16

*If the fimbriated end of the fallopian tube is completely enclosed, change the point assignment to 16.

Denote appearance of superficial implant types as red [(R), red, red-pink, flamelike, vesicular blobs, clear vesicles], white [(W), opacifications, peritoneal defects, yellow-brown], or black [(B) black, hemosiderin deposits, blue]. Denote percent of total described as R___%, W___% and B___%. Total should equal 100%.

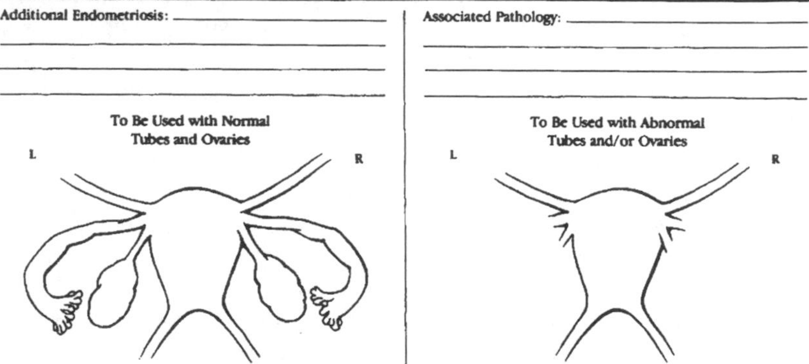

FIG. 7. Revised American Society for Reproductive Medicine classification of endometriosis:1996. (From American Society for Reproductive Medicine. Revised American Society for Reproductive Medicine Classification of Endometriosis: 1996. *Fertil Steril* 1997;67:817; with permission.)

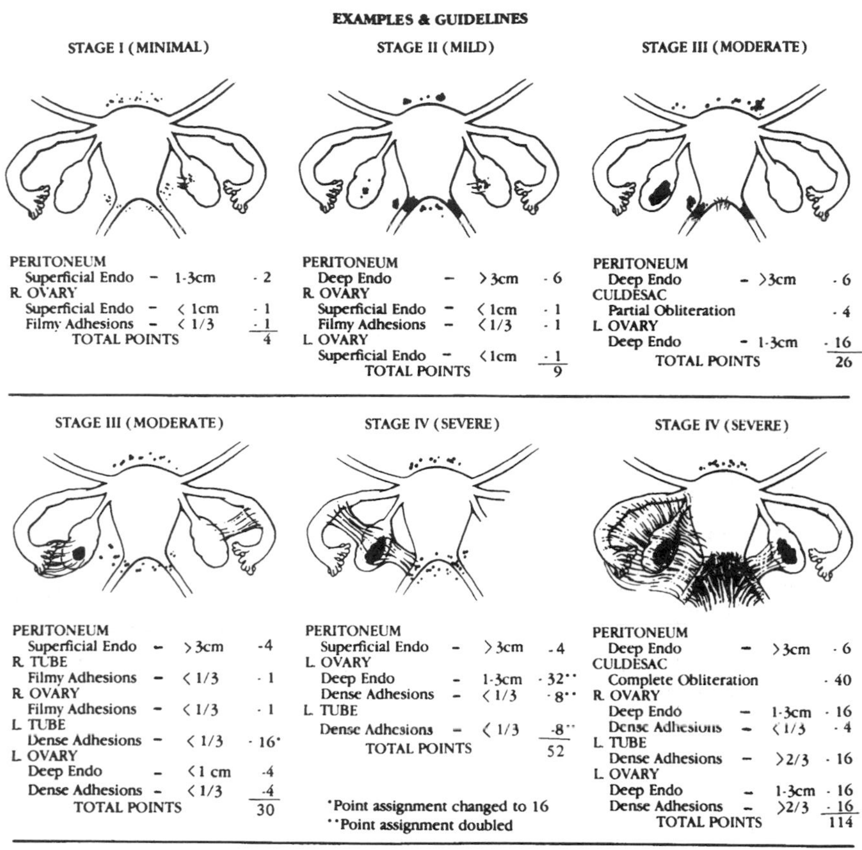

FIG. 7. *(Continued).*

lesions in adolescence and more classic disease a decade later. Redwine demonstrated that "clear" and "red" lesions occur at a mean age 10 years earlier than do "black" lesions (77). In our recent series, 77.4% of adolescents were found to present with stage I disease and 22.6% with stage II disease; no patients presented with stage III or IV disease (44). This finding is in contrast to those in adults showing a higher stage of endometriosis at the time of presentation (95), and it also argues for the possibility that the disease progresses with age.

The incidence of endometriosis is found to be greatly increased in patients with obstructive anomalies of the reproductive tract (see Chapter 8) (96). Schifrin and co-workers (97) concluded that müllerian tract anomalies predispose adolescents to endometriosis. Adolescents with congenital obstructing müllerian malformations often have severe endometriosis classified as stage III or IV, even in early adolescence. Endometriosis associated with obstructive anomalies has been reported to completely resolve after correction of the obstruction

(98). Congenital anomalies associated with endometriosis include imperforate hymen, vaginal septum, hematocolpos, hematometra, and uterine anomalies.

The importance of finding endometriosis early lies not only in the relief of symptoms but also, it is hoped, in the preservation of reproductive potential and suppression of possible natural disease progression (82,99). Infertility commonly results when endometriosis causes anatomic distortion of the pelvic organs and/or the fallopian tubes. Data from animal studies show a clear cause-and-effect relationship between endometriosis and infertility (100–102). The causes of infertility as they relate to endometriosis are beyond the scope of this book, but it is important for the health care provider to refer patients with chronic pain or diagnosed endometriosis to gynecologists who provide state-of-the-art therapies to treat the pelvic pain and, it is hoped, avoid the progression of the disease and its sequelae.

The optimal therapy for adolescents and adult women with endometriosis is still being debated. The patient needs to understand the pros and cons of each surgical and medical option and that recurrence of endometriosis is common. Surgery remains the initial treatment.

Treatment of endometriosis begins with surgical resection/destruction of visible lesions at the time of diagnosis (Fig. 8). A laparoscopy should never be performed only to diagnose endometriosis without advantage being taken of the opportunity for surgical therapy. Surgical therapy utilizes several techniques to maximally remove or destroy visible lesions of endometriosis; these techniques include gross resection, laser vaporization, endocoagulation, and electrocoagulation (unipolar or bipolar). Advances in operative laparoscopic techniques and

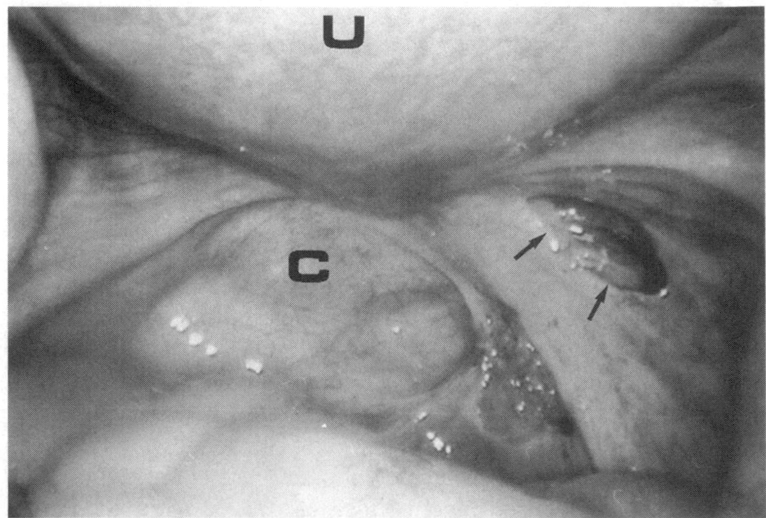

FIG. 8. Peritoneal "defects" (*arrows*) after resection of endometriosis. U, uterus; C, cul-de-sac.

instrumentation have increased the extent and degree of difficult surgical procedures that can be approached via laparoscopy. Whatever the surgical approach, the goal is removal and destruction of all visible endometriosis, lysis or resection of adhesions, restoration of normal pelvic anatomy, and maintenance of all reproductive organs. Resection or lysis of adhesions can be achieved with laparoscopic scissors, with or without cautery. In our institution, we favor the gross resection of endometriotic lesions and/or carbon dioxide (CO_2) laser vaporization. Regardless of the surgical approach to treating the endometriosis and/or adhesions, care must be taken to avoid damage to the bowel, bladder, ureters, and major blood vessels; the patient must be informed that these complications are a known risk of all operative laparoscopic procedures, and if an injury occurs it will be repaired by laparotomy when that injury is identified.

The use of laparotomy to treat endometriosis is decreasing as laparoscopic surgeons become more experienced. Although rare in adolescents, endometriomas that are encountered can be removed safely through the laparoscope. An endometrioma needs to be excised and its cyst wall resected.

Historically, it has been argued that laparotomy provides better depth perception and has the added advantage of allowing direct palpation of the diseased tissue. The relevance of these points is minimized with the improved skill of the laparoscopist and with improved instrumentation. Laparoscopy has the advantages of magnification. Laparotomy may be needed if there are extensive adhesions, or endometriotic implants that are not safely resectable via pelviscopy.

The success rate of surgery in resecting/ablating endometriotic lesions is believed to be high (103,104). Endometriotic implants reappear in 28% of patients within 18 months (105) and in 40% after 9 years of followup (106). Lysed adhesions re-form in 40% to 50% of patients (107). Long-term followup of pelvic pain after surgery has shown 70% to 100% rates of improvement immediately after surgery (106,107), and 82% 1 year later (108). Another study showed a 66% rate of pain reduction 5 years after surgery (109).

After the initial optimal surgical resection/vaporization of endometriosis, medical therapy can be prescribed (Fig. 6). Medical management can achieve two goals: pain control and hormonal suppression of the disease to avoid progression. In the selection of a medical therapy, it is important to consider the patient's age, the severity of symptoms, the duration of symptoms, and the extent of disease.

Endometrium and endometriotic implants contain receptors for estrogen, progesterone, and androgens (110–112). Estrogens stimulate the growth of endometriotic tissue, whereas androgens result in atrophy. Progesterone stimulates endometrial growth, while synthetic progestins inhibit endometrial growth through their androgenic properties. Thus, the basis of medical therapy for pain from endometriosis is to take advantage of the reliance of endometrial tissue on steroid hormones for growth and function. A complete listing of possible hormonal therapies and their side effects is given in Table 9.

TABLE 9. *Comparison of hormonal therapies for endometriosis*[a]

Therapy	Resultant hormone state			Side effects
	Acyclic	Hypoestrogenic	Hyperandrogenic	
NSAIDs	-	-	-	Inadequate pain control, gastrointestinal irritation
Noncyclic OCs	+	-	-	Nausea, breakthrough bleeding, other side effects listed for OCs
Progestins	+	+	-	Breakthrough bleeding, depression, bloating, decreased libido
Methyltestosterone	±	-	++	Virilization, masculinization of a female fetus
Danazol	+	+	++	Weight gain, acne, hirsutism, voice changes
GnRH agonist	+	++	-	Vasomotor symptoms (hot flushes), bone loss, vaginal dryness
GnRH agonist plus steroid add-back	+	?	-	Possible decreased vasomotor symptoms, bone loss,
(Premarin and Provera or OCs)	+	?	-	vaginal dryness
Mifepristone (RU 486)	+	±	-	Anorexia, nausea, dizziness, somnolence
Bilateral oophorectomy	++	++	-	Vasomotor symptoms, bone loss, vaginal dryness

[a]NSAIDs, nonsteroidal antiinflammatory drugs; OC, oral contraceptive; GnRH, gonadotropin-releasing hormone; ++, extremely effective; +, effective; ±, sporadically effective; -, not effective; ?, questionably effective.

(From Laufer MR. Endometriosis in adolescents. *Curr Opin Pediatr* 1992;4:582; with permission.)

NSAIDs are effective in the treatment of some cases of endometriosis, but many patients do not respond to this management. Naproxen sodium was proved to be significantly better than placebo in relieving the symptoms of dysmenorrhea in patients with endometriosis (113). Long-term narcotic use should be avoided, and if the patient is in such significant pain, further evaluation and treatment of the disease process are indicated. It is important to stress that hormonal therapy is suppressive and not curative. Hormonal therapy is usually continued for 3 to 6 months to allow for adequate regression of the disease.

The use of OCs for ovarian suppression has long been advocated for the treatment of endometriosis. Continuous OCs have been used to create a "pseudopregnancy" (114). This term is used because of the amenorrhea and decidualization of the endometrial tissue induced by the combined estrogen and progestin. The adolescent should be instructed that she may have irregular bleeding for up to 3 months before amenorrhea is induced. This form of treatment has been reported to relieve the pelvic pain associated with endometriosis in > 80% of patients, although the relief can be transient (115). A progestin-dominant pill such as Lo/Ovral can be initiated; the pill may be doubled or tripled or estrogen can be added if breakthrough bleeding occurs. Ortho-Novum 1/35 (Norinyl 1+35) and Loestrin 1/20 or 1.5/30 may be used similarly; triphasic agents are not usually as effective because of the change in progestin dose. The principal problems with the "pseudopregnancy" therapy are headaches, fluid retention, nausea, weight gain, emotional lability, and hypertension.

Progestins have been found to have varying effectiveness in the treatment of endometriosis (116,117). Commonly used regimens include medroxyprogesterone acetate 30 to 50 mg orally per day, or 150 mg intramuscularly every 1 to 3 months (59,117,118). High dosages are required for benefit, and side effects are not well tolerated. The principal complaints in adolescents are weight gain, bloating, acne, headaches, fluid retention, emotional lability, and irregular menses. This treatment modality is usually reserved for those individuals who cannot tolerate continuous OCs or have a contraindication to their use.

The creation of a high androgen state with exogenous androgens has been shown to produce atrophy of endometriotic implants and improve pelvic pain (119). Methyltestosterone can improve pelvic pain associated with endometriosis; its usual dosage is 5 to 10 mg given buccally every day (119). When this dosage is used, pain will be improved but ovulation is not usually inhibited. This therapy can result in the undesirable side effect of masculinization, and if ovulation is not inhibited and a conception results while the patient is receiving this therapy, a masculinized female fetus may result. In our institution, we do not utilize this therapy for adolescents with endometriosis because of the severe adverse effects such as weight gain, bloating, acne, headaches, fluid retention, emotional lability, irregular menses, and virilization.

Danazol, an isoxazole derivative of 17α-ethinyl testosterone, is effective in the treatment of pain associated with endometriosis, as it results in an acyclic hypoestrogenic-hyperandrogenic state by interrupting ovarian follicular development and thereby inhibiting the growth and function of the endometriotic tissue (120, 121). Although danazol appears to be very effective in the treatment of pelvic pain associated with endometriosis, we do not prescribe it for adolescents because of its unacceptable side effects, which include weight gain, edema, irregular menses, acne, oily skin, hirsutism, and a deep voice change. Some side effects, such as hirsutism and voice deepening, are not always reversible with discontinuation of the medication. The standard dosage is 800 mg/day in divided dosages. Danazol offers effective contraception at doses of 400 to 800 mg/day (120); sexually active patients treated with < 400 mg/day require additional methods of contraception. Pain from endometriosis treated with danazol has been reported to be relieved in 85% to 90% of patients (122). In the same study, pain returned to the majority of treated patients within 1 year after they stopped therapy. In another study, the recurrence rate of symptoms and physical findings in patients treated with danazol was approximately 5% to 20% per year (120). A prospective randomized study in adult women has failed to show that danazol was superior to placebo in improving pregnancy rates in women with minimal endometriosis (123), in agreement with a previous study (124). Other problems with this medication include decreased high-density lipoprotein cholesterol, a mild increase in insulin resistance, an alteration in liver proteins, and androgenic effects on the developing fetus if the adolescent becomes pregnant while taking the drug. The drug should therefore be avoided in patients with hepatic dysfunction, severe hypertension, congestive heart failure, and borderline renal function. Because of these side effects, other treatment modalities have replaced this therapy, and as mentioned above, we do not currently prescribe danazol to adolescents.

Currently, the first-line and most widely used therapy for endometriosis is the creation of an acyclic, low-estrogen environment to prevent bleeding in the implants and to prevent additional seeding of the pelvis during retrograde menstruation (120). This goal has been pursued by the use of gonadotropin-releasing hormone (GnRH) agonists such as nafarelin and leuprolide. Continuous GnRH stimulation results in downregulation of the pituitary and resultant hypoestrogenism. This reversible medical return to a prepubertal (hypoestrogenic, hypogonadotropic) state is very effective in creating a hypoestrogenic environment for the suppression of endometriosis. GnRH agonists are available in many formulations: nasal spray, subcutaneous injection, and intramuscular injection. In the adolescent population, compliance is a major issue, and thus the decision whether to use a twice-daily nasal spray or a monthly intramuscular injection is important. The nasal spray, if selected, is given as one puff twice daily in alternating nostrils (125). If depot-leuprolide (Lupron) is used, a dosage of 3.75 mg every 4 weeks will induce amenorrhea and hypoestrogenism in > 90% of women (126). Lupron is also available in an 11.25-mg dosage given every 3 months. If induction of amenorrhea is not achieved with these dosages, the dosage can be increased to 7.5 mg every 4 weeks, or 22.5 mg every 3 months.

Henzl and colleagues (127) examined the comparative effects of nafarelin and danazol in the treatment of endometriosis. They showed that GnRH was as effective as danazol in reducing endometriosis as demonstrated on second-look laparoscopy, and it was better tolerated. Other authors have reported similar results (125,126,128). Dlugi and colleagues (129) found that 3.75 mg of depot-leuprolide given intramuscularly every 4 weeks for six doses was effective in improving pelvic pain in 85% of patients, compared with improvement in 43% of patients receiving placebo.

The side effects of GnRH agonist therapy include hypoestrogenic symptoms such as hot flashes, vaginal dryness, and decreased libido (121,127). The most worrisome long-term side effect of GnRH analog therapy is decreased bone density, and thus the United States Food and Drug Administration (FDA) has not approved its prescription for courses of therapy lasting longer than 6 consecutive months (126,130,131). The prolonged hypoestrogenic state places the patient at risk for trabecular bone loss. Dawood et al (130) showed a 7% trabecular bone loss in individuals when GnRH agonists were used for 6 months. Reports differ about the reversibility of this bone loss, and its clinical significance is questionable (131). The use of GnRH agonist therapy in adolescents, however, may present the added risk of long-term effects on bone because of the importance of the adolescent years to acquisition of normal bone density. Once again, the risks, benefits, and alternatives of various therapies need to be openly discussed with all adolescents and their parents.

It is our current practice to offer all adolescents over age 16 with endometriosis a 6-month course of GnRH agonist therapy following surgical diagnosis and resection/vaporization. At the conclusion of this initial medical therapy, continuous OCs are prescribed for 3 months, followed by cyclic OCs. If patients do well with this therapy, they continue to take cyclic OCs until they desire fertility. If they have cyclic pain with the cyclic menses, they can return to the use of continuous OCs. For adolescents less than 16 years of age we utilize continuous OCs as first-line medical therapy so as to avoid possible adverse effects of GnRH agonists on bone formation. If these therapies do not succeed, then patients are offered additional surgery followed by additional medical therapy. It is important for the clinician to keep in mind other diagnoses in addition to the endometriosis, such as irritable bowel syndrome, lactose intolerance, or psychological issues in the adolescent with persistent pain.

Additional surgical options for patients with persistent pelvic pain include pelvic denervation procedures such as laser uterosacral nerve ablation (LUNA) (132,133) and presacral neurectomy (134–137). LUNA can safely be achieved with the use of a CO_2 laser through a laparoscope. It is important to know the surgical landmarks; we ablate the medial two-thirds of the uterosacral ligaments (which contain the uterosacral nerves) within 1 cm of the uterus so as to avoid damage to the ureters (Figs. 9 and 10). In a randomized trial comparing LUNA with sham surgery for dysmenorrhea, ablation was found to be more effective in relieving pain for the first 3 months after surgery; < 50% of women continued to

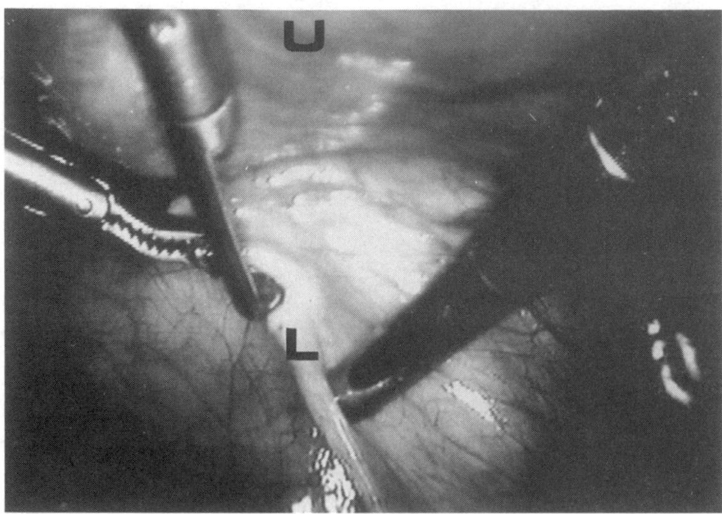

FIG. 9. Right laser uterosacral nerve ablation (LUNA) in progress. U, uterus; L, uterosacral ligament.

have relief 1 year later (132). A later study showed that LUNA benefited women with dysmenorrhea who had not responded to NSAIDs (133). Presacral neurectomy procedures have been performed for many years, with successful relief of dysmenorrhea and dyspareunia as great as 73% to 77% (134). Another evaluation of presacral neurectomy showed a high rate of relief of dysmenorrhea and central pelvic pain, but no improvement in lateral pain, back pain, or dyspareunia (135). Additional reports have shown that this procedure can be performed safely and effectively by either laparotomy or laparoscopy (136,137). Although it is *not* an appropriate treatment for adolescents and young adults, hysterectomy with bilateral salpingo-oophorectomy is believed to be the definitive surgical procedure for the treatment of endometriosis, with approximately 90% elimination of symptoms postoperatively (104). If one or both ovaries remain *in situ,* there is believed to be a 7% rate of recurrence of symptoms (138). If the disease is severe, as many as 33% of women experience recurrence of symptoms if bilateral oophorectomy is not performed (104).

Following additional surgery, or after initial medical therapy has failed, the only medical option may be the long-term use of GnRH agonists. Numerous studies have been undertaken in an attempt to alleviate the long-term side effects of the GnRH agonists. The goal of GnRH agonist therapy with "add-back" hormonal therapy is to reduce the deleterious side effects on bone and lipid metabolism. Studies of add-back regimens have examined the use of differing combinations of hormonal replacement. Surrey and others (139) reported on the effects of combining norethindrone with a GnRH agonist in the treatment of symptomatic endometriosis, while Cedars and colleagues (140) studied the use of GnRH

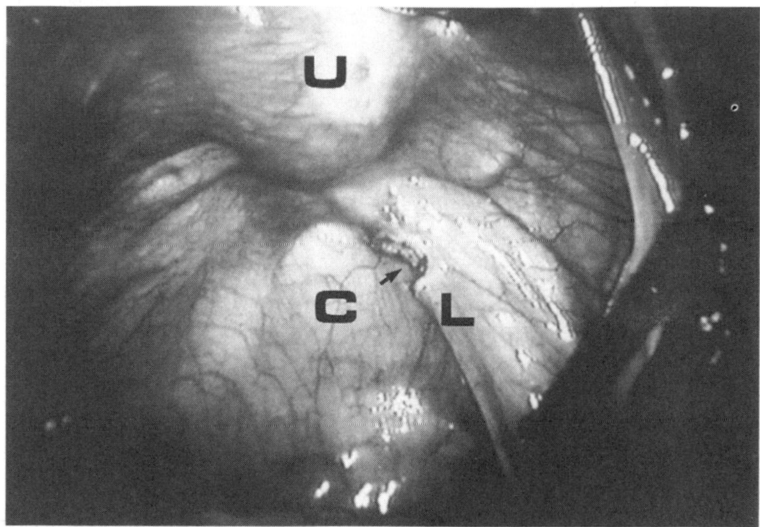

FIG. 10. Result of right laser uterosacral nerve ablation (LUNA) (*arrow*) in Fig. 9. U, uterus; L, uterosacral ligament; C, cul-de-sac.

agonist with medroxyprogesterone. Other studies have shown beneficial effects of the long-term use of GnRH agonists in combination with the use of progestin therapy in maintaining bone density (139,140–142,143). Studies have examined the use of GnRH agonist with estrogen add-back. Barbieri (141) has proposed an "estrogen threshold hypothesis" in the treatment of women with endometriosis. This theory proposes that there is an estrogen threshold for the reduction of endometriosis that is of a lesser degree of hypoestrogenism than the degree of hypoestrogenism resulting in bone resorption (Fig. 11). In addition to evaluating add-back with steroid hormones, others have studied the sole use or additional use of etidronate or parathyroid hormone to preserve bone density (144,145). Further studies of patients with symptomatic endometriosis and the possible long-term use of GnRH agonist with hormonal add-back therapy may be key to the safe long-term treatment of endometriosis in adolescents. When prescribing add-back therapy in adolescents, we currently use conjugated estrogens 0.625 mg/day and medroxyprogesterone 2.5 mg/day in a continuous fashion; calcium supplementation is also prescribed.

Theoretically, GnRH antagonists should be advantageous over GnRH agonists, as there is no initial stimulatory phase and they thus result in faster gonadal suppression. The many side effects of the antagonists have inhibited their approval by the FDA, including histamine release and anaphylaxis. Further studies and improvement of these drugs are needed before they can be approved and released.

RU 486 (mifepristone) is a synthetic steroid with both antiprogesterone and antiglucocorticoid activity. Numerous studies have shown that long-term treat-

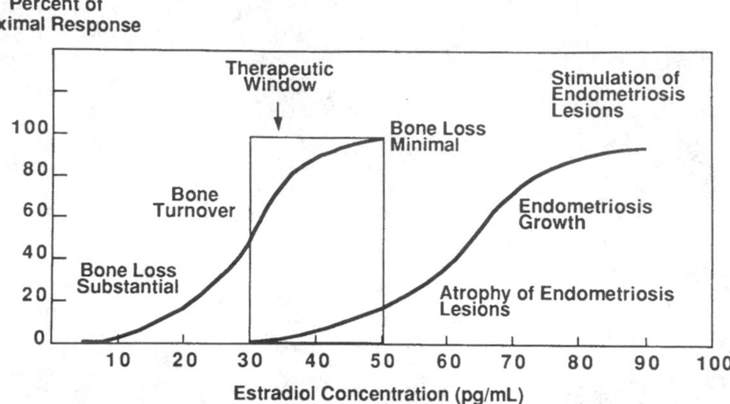

FIG. 11. Estradiol therapeutic window in the treatment of endometriosis. The concentration of estradiol required to cause growth of the lesions of endometriosis may be greater than the concentration required to stabilize bone mineral density. (From Barbieri RL. Hormone treatment of endometriosis: The estrogen threshold hypothesis. *Am J Obstet Gynecol* 1992;166:740; with permission.)

ment results in anovulation. Kettel et al (146) showed a decrease in pelvic pain in patients with endometriosis treated with 100 mg/day of RU 486, but no improvement in gross disease as seen at followup laparoscopy. Further double-blind studies are needed.

Future developments in the treatment of endometriosis may be able to take advantage of the protein growth factors that regulate the epithelial and stromal elements of the endometrium. Modulation of the immune system, which may possibly play a critical role in pain, scarring, and infertility, may offer another method of treating endometriosis. Some adult women with stage II, III, and IV endometriosis have elevated levels of serum CA 125, and this marker may provide a potential means for monitoring treatment (95,121,147). Studies have not been done in adolescents.

Therapy for adolescent pelvic pain associated with endometriosis clearly needs to be individualized because adolescents are very conscious of side effects and will become noncompliant. Frequent appointments, support, and careful listening and response to concerns and questions are an important part of the medical care. Diet and exercise are extremely important in assisting adolescents with endometriosis to cope with this chronic disease. In addition, adolescents with endometriosis find a support network with meetings, a newsletter, phone conversations, and "big sisters with endometriosis" helpful. We have collaborated to established such a group, the Teen Endometriosis Education Network (TEEN) in Boston within the structure of the Endometriosis Association's Boston chapter (148). The adolescents reported that the support group was beneficial in providing educational material and support to themselves, their families, and school systems. In addition, the Boston chapter of the Endometriosis Association and the Division of Gynecology at the Children's Hospital, Boston, are collaborating in the creation of an educational video on adolescent endometriosis for schools, health care providers, patients, and their families.

Endosalpingiosis

Endosalpingiosis is a pathologic condition that differs from endometriosis in that glands without stroma are present. Little is known of the clinical correlation with this pathologic entity. Only one published report describes a correlation with pelvic pain in three patients with endosalpingiosis (149). In a recent study, we reviewed the pathologic reports from women younger than 22 who had undergone peritoneal biopsy identified with endosalpingiosis; those with a pathologic diagnosis of endometriosis were excluded (150). The presenting symptoms included pelvic pain (100%), acyclic pain (36%), cyclic pain (9%), cyclic and acyclic pain (55%), irregular menses (45%), GI symptoms (55%), urinary symptoms (36%), and vaginal discharge (9%). Initial postoperative therapy included cyclic OCs (55%), continuous OCs (36%), and progestin-only pills (9%). Long-term follow-up was obtained for an average of 12.6 months. Subjects had pain when not taking medications, and all were maintained by medical management for endometriosis (OCs, danazol, or GnRH agonist). Thirty-three percent of the subjects required additional surgery 6, 10, or 12 months after the initial surgery, at which time all were found to have endometriosis. It is thus our conclusion that the clinical presentation of endosalpingiosis is one of pelvic pain, operative findings are varied, and the clinical course and response may be similar to that of endometriosis. Additional studies are required to better define the clinical disease of endosalpingiosis so that surgeons and patients confronted with this pathologic entity have a better understanding of its clinical course and possible treatment options.

Uterine and Vaginal Malformations with Obstruction

Obstructive müllerian anomalies can result in both acute or chronic pelvic pain. In addition, as mentioned above, there is a high rate of endometriosis in cases of obstructive müllerian anomalies (97). A complete description of the presentation, diagnosis, and treatment of these conditions is given in Chapter 8.

PREMENSTRUAL SYNDROME

Premenstrual syndrome (PMS) includes a cluster of symptoms that occur in a cyclic fashion beginning 1 to 2 weeks prior to menses and disappearing within a few days of the onset of menses. Premenstrual dysphoric syndrome was recently included in DSM-IV to allow better diagnostic criteria and enhanced therapeutic approaches (Table 10) (151). The PMS constellation of symptoms commonly reported by adolescents and adult women includes bloating, weight gain, breast soreness, hunger, thirst, fatigue, acne, constipation, hot flashes, chills, difficulty concentrating, and mood change (irritability or depression) (152–154). Adolescents and adults with migraine headaches may suffer an increase in headaches premenstrually and with menses; similarly, those with epilepsy may note an increase in the severity and/or frequency of seizures in the luteal phase of the cycle, premenstrually, or with the onset of menses. Cognitively challenged individuals may have behavior outbursts that are difficult for their caretakers to cope with, and psychotic patients may exhibit more uncontrollable actions in a cyclic fashion in the luteal phase of the cycle. Premenstrual exacerbation may occur in some rare medical conditions, such as hepatic porphyria (155). In addition, recent case reports have indicated that rare patients develop sensitivity to naturally produced progesterone and may have hives or even life-threatening allergic reactions during the luteal phase; these manifestations are reversed by GnRH agonists or oophorectomy (156,157).

Most adolescent girls are aware of some premenstrual symptoms, and active listening, reassurance, and improvement in diet and exercise are usually sufficient to manage them. Adolescents who experience severe symptoms often are under stress

TABLE 10. *Research criteria for premenstrual dysphoric disorder*[a]

A. In most menstrual cycles during the past year, five (or more) of the following symptoms were present for most of the time during the last week of the luteal phase, began to remit within a few days after the onset of the follicular phase, and were absent in the week postmenses, with at least one of the symptoms being either (1), (2), (3), or (4):
   (1) markedly depressed mood, feelings of hopelessness, or self-deprecating thoughts
   (2) marked anxiety, tension, feelings of being "keyed up," or "on edge"
   (3) marked affective lability (e.g., feeling suddenly sad or tearful or increased sensitivity to rejection)
   (4) persistent and marked anger or irritability or increased interpersonal conflicts
   (5) decreased interest in usual activities (e.g., work, school, friends, hobbies)
   (6) subjective sense of difficulty in concentrating
   (7) lethargy, easy fatigability, or marked lack of energy
   (8) marked change in appetite, overeating, or specific food cravings
   (9) hypersomnia or insomnia
   (10) a subjective sense of being overwhelmed or out of control
   (11) other physical symptoms, such as breast tenderness or swelling, headaches, joint or muscle pain, a sensation of "bloating," weight gain

B. The disturbance markedly interferes with work or school or with usual social activities and relationships with others (e.g., avoidance of social activities, decreased productivity and efficiency at work or school).

C. The disturbance is not merely an exacerbation of the symptoms of another disorder, such as Major Depressive Disorder, Panic Disorder, Dysthymic Disorder, or a Personality Disorder (although it may be superimposed on any of these disorders).

D. Criteria A, B, and C must be confirmed by prospective daily ratings during at least two consecutive symptomatic cycles. (The diagnosis may be made provisionally prior to this confirmation.)

[a]In menstruating females, the luteal phase corresponds to the period between ovulation and the onset of menses, and the follicular phase begins with menses. In nonmenstruating females (e.g., those who have had a hysterectomy), the timing of luteal and follicular phases may require measurement of circulating reproductive hormones.

(From American Psychiatric Association. DSM-IV. *Diagnostic and statistical manual of mental disorders,* 4th ed. Washington DC: American Psychiatric Association, 1994; with permission.)

and have other psychosocial issues that need to be addressed, not just by medical evaluation of the PMS but also by psychological counseling. About 20% to 40% of adult women of reproductive age have symptoms sufficiently bothersome to cause a temporary deterioration in interpersonal relationships or job effectiveness; fewer than 5% of adult women have severe symptoms (152,158).

The cause of PMS has been variously attributed to estrogen and progesterone because of the occurrence of these symptoms in the luteal phase of the cycle and the disappearance when ovulation (and the resultant rise in progesterone levels) is inhibited by GnRH agonists (160). Although several forms of progesterone have been prescribed for treatment, double-blind studies have not demonstrated the efficacy of this approach (161). In fact, it has been suggested that higher adverse premenstrual scores occur in menstrual cycles with high luteal-phase plasma progesterone and estradiol concentrations (162). Other studies have not detected a difference in hormone levels between women with a mood disorder of PMS and those without symptoms (163). In addition, one study has demonstrated that neither the timing nor the severity of PMS symptoms was altered by mifepristone-induced menses or luteolysis, which suggests that the endocrine events of the late luteal phase do not directly generate the symptoms of PMS (164).

Women with PMS appear to have symptoms consistent with exaggerated neurotransmitter responses to estrogen and progesterone fluctuations. The changes occur in the opioidergic system, the γ-aminobutyric system (GABA), and the serotonergic system. In 1981, Reid and Yen (165) proposed a hypothesis that endogenous opiates triggered the premenstrual symptoms. In an assessment of the pattern of symptoms, Reid (166) attributed the changes in the 2 weeks before menses—breast swelling and tenderness, lower abdominal bloating, and constipation—to the production of endogenous central, and perhaps peripheral, opiates. Since actual body weight may not increase in spite of bloating, changes that the patient notes may occur because of local fluid shifts and bowel wall edema. The release of the opiates may also increase the appetite and result in unusual food cravings as well as fatigue, depression, and emotional lability. Later in the cycle, the shift toward anxiety and irritability, vague abdominal cramps with loose bowel movements or diarrhea, headaches, chills, and sweats may result from withdrawal of endogenous opiates as hormone levels fall. In sensitive women, cyclic exposure to the neuropeptides, and subsequent withdrawal from their central effects, may result in a cascade of neuroendocrine changes that cause clinical symptoms. Support for this hypothesis has come from animal experiments, the observation of the effects of opiates on nonaddicts and the consequences of withdrawal in addicts, and the improvement in symptoms with the administration of the opiate antagonist (naltrexone) and with exercise (167). Support for the involvement of the GABA and serotonergic system in the pathogenesis of PMS comes from the positive therapeutic responses to alprazolam and the selective serotonin reuptake inhibitors (SSRIs) including fluoxetine, sertraline, and fluvoxamine (172,173,182–184).

Therapeutic approaches to PMS may be improved by increased understanding of its pathophysiology and the interaction of biologic and psychological factors.

Biologic factors that cause PMS may be influenced by personal psychological and social factors (154). Alteration of the ovulatory menstrual cycle can alleviate symptoms, and thus drug therapy may be considered in adolescents with significant symptoms that have not responded to nonpharmacologic management. The health care provider should realize that most drug trials are hampered by the definition of PMS, the sample size, and the strong placebo effect. In addition, adolescents are often at risk of unprotected intercourse and pregnancy, and many of the medications should not be prescribed to potentially pregnant adolescents. In most adolescents, premenstrual symptoms are mild, and the recognition that they are a real entity can be reassuring. For those troubled by their symptoms, the cyclic occurrence should be established by prospective recording symptoms on a special calendar for two to three cycles; many such calendars are in use by PMS clinics (159). Without documentation on a calendar, mood alterations and depression occurring throughout the cycle may be attributed to PMS, and adequate psychological intervention will not be undertaken. A calendar is also useful in deciding which symptoms are most troubling to the patient. Although no controlled studies have demonstrated the benefit of diet or exercise, most centers start with this approach because the lifestyle changes are healthy and undoubtedly give the adolescent a sense of control over her life. A program of aerobic exercise should be strongly encouraged as a first line of therapy. Patients are also instructed to avoid salty foods, alcohol, caffeine, chocolate, and concentrated sweets and to eat four to six smaller meals per day during the premenstrual period. A written sheet with foods to avoid (e.g., cola, coffee, hot dogs, canned foods, chips) and to add to the diet (e.g., unsalted popcorn, raw vegetables and fruits, skim milk, complex carbohydrates, high-fiber foods, low-fat meats) is helpful to the young woman. Additional dietary alternative therapies have been reported (43). Areas of stress should be identified. Stress-reduction programs such as biofeedback or self-hypnosis may be helpful. Many patients experience an increased sense of well-being and control with a program of improved nutrition, exercise, and stress management.

For adolescents who do not respond to lifestyle changes and have persistent and significant symptoms, pharmacologic therapies include NSAIDs, OCs, diuretics, SSRIs, and other options discussed below. Mefenamic acid (250 mg every 8 hours starting on day 16 of the cycle, increased to 500 mg on day 19 of the cycle) has been shown in one small study of 15 women with PMS to improve fatigue, headache, and general aches and pains; this medication may be especially useful in patients with severe dysmenorrhea as well (170). Other NSAIDs used in treating dysmenorrhea may be similarly useful, but none of them should be prescribed to the adolescent who is likely to become pregnant.

Although many patients complain of weight gain, actual daily measurements may reveal no change, rather, fluid shifts and bowel wall edema may result in the symptoms. For true edema and weight gain from fluid retention, a diuretic such as spironolactone can be given (168,169).

Although OCs have given variable results in adult women with PMS, many adolescents, especially those with premenstrual exacerbation of seizures or headaches, show striking improvement on OCs with 30 to 35 μg of estrogen and a medium dose of progestin. Oral contraceptives may thus be effective in adolescents and are especially useful if birth control is also needed.

SSRIs have been beneficial in the treatment of PMS (182,183). In a randomized trial of women with PMS, fluoxetine in dosages from 20 to 60 mg/day continuously was superior to placebo (183,184). In addition, the researchers determined that the 20-mg dosage reduced the potential for side effects while maximizing therapeutic efficacy. Many dosing regimens for fluoxetine have been reported, including a single dose in the early luteal phase (182), a continuous daily dosage throughout the cycle (183), and daily dose only during the late luteal phase (182). Daily sertaline and fluvoxamine in pilot studies have also been shown to be more effective than placebo in treating PMS. Alprazolam (0.25 mg 3 times daily from day 20 until the second day of menstruation and then tapered by one tablet/day) relieved premenstrual symptoms in a double-blind study of women with PMS (174), but concern about patients' becoming dependent on this drug and having withdrawal symptoms has made us reluctant to use alprazolam in adolescents.

The GnRH agonists can prevent the cyclic progesterone and estrogen production; however, this approach may be more useful as a probe in defining the cause of the problem than as a long-term treatment because of the potential for osteoporosis in estrogen-deficient patients. According to a hypothesis similar to Barbieri's estrogen threshold hypothesis (141), preventing ovulation and cyclic hormones but allowing some estrogen secretion might protect the bones from osteoporosis, treat PMS symptoms, and avoid the negative long-term effects of the GnRH agonists. More recently, many studies have shown a beneficial effect of the long-term use of a GnRH agonist with add-back therapy for the treatment of PMS (179–181). These therapies may be beneficial in the treatment of severe symptoms, but their unknown effects on adolescent bone density require caution for their use in the adolescent population.

A variety of other drugs have been used in adult women, but none of the studies has focused on adolescents. For example, low-dose danazol (200 to 400 mg/day) has appeared beneficial in a small study (171); however, reliable contraception is needed at doses of < 400 mg/day. Danazol may inhibit ovulation and thus decrease cyclic hormonal responses, but it is likely to have undesirable side effects in adolescents and should be avoided. Bromocriptine has been used in adult women to alleviate breast soreness, but this symptom is rarely a major complaint of adolescents. In adolescents with breast soreness, we prefer to suggest reducing caffeine consumption and to prescribe a small dose of NSAIDs. Despite the widespread popularity of progesterone and many anecdotal reports of its success, only two of the nearly dozen prospective randomized, placebo-controlled studies have shown a benefit significantly greater than that of a placebo (175,176), and one recent large double-blind, placebo-controlled study of progesterone failed to demonstrate any effect that was greater than that of placebo (177). Vitamin B_6 has been popular with some self-help groups. Studies of its efficacy have been conflicting. One recent placebo-controlled study of 150 mg of vitamin B_6 found that while some premenstrual symptoms such as dizziness and behavioral symptoms were improved, most patients still experienced significant symptoms (178). Other studies have not found a beneficial effect. In view of the concern about the toxic potential of this vitamin to cause sensory neuropathy, even in low doses, patients need to be cautioned about this risk.

The plethora of drugs shown to be effective in small studies shows that more data are clearly needed to document their efficacy before adolescents are exposed to their potential risks. In addition, adolescents need to be asked whether they are taking over-the-counter medications.

Much more needs to be learned about PMS and its causes; recent advances have improved the possibilities for drug therapy in the treatment of PMS in adolescents.

REFERENCES

1. Rapkin AJ, Reading AE. Chronic pelvic pain. *Curr Probl Obstet Gynecol Fertil* 1991;14:101.
2. Laufer MR. Endometriosis in adolescents. *Curr Opin Pediatr* 1992;4:582.
3. Velebil P, Wingo PA, Xia Z, et al. Rate of hospitalization for gynecologic disorders among reproductive-age women in the United States. *Obstet Gynecol* 1995;86:764.
4. Davis LG, Gerscovich EO, Anderson MW, Stading R. Ultrasound and Doppler in the diagnosis of ovarian torsion. *Eur J Radiol* 1995;20:133.
5. Davis AJ, Feins NR. Subsequent asynchronous torsion of normal adnexa in children. *J Pediatr Surg* 1990;25:687.
6. Vermesh M, Graczykowski JW, Sauer MV. Reevaluation of the role of culdocentesis in the management of ectopic pregnancy. *Am J Obstet Gynecol* 1990;162:411.
7. Quillin SP, Siegil MJ. Transabdominal color Doppler ultrasonography of the painful adolescent ovary. *J Ultrasound Med* 1994;13:549.
8. Tepper R, Lerner-Geva L, Zalel Y, et al. Adnexal torsion: the contribution of color Doppler sonography to diagnosis and post-operative follow-up. *Eur J Obstet Gynecol Reprod Biol* 1995;62:121.
9. Fleischer AC, Stein SM, Cullinan JA, Warner MA. Color Doppler sonography of adnexal torsion. *J Ultrasound Med* 1995;14:523.
10. Willms AB, Schlund JF, Meyer WR. Endovaginal Doppler ultrasound in ovarian torsion: a case series. *Ultrasound Obstet Gynecol* 1995;5:129.
11. American College of Obstetricians and Gynecologists (ACOG) Technical Bulletin. *Gynecologic ultrasonography.* 1995;215.
12. Shalev E, Mann S, Romano S, et al. Laparoscopic detorsion of adnexa in childhood: a case report. *J Pediatr Surg* 1991;26:1193.
13. Shalev E, Peleg D. Laparoscopic treatment of adnexal torsion. *Surg Gynecol Obstet* 1993;176:448.
14. Iwabe T, Harada T, Miura H, et al. Laparoscopic unwinding of adnexal torsion caused by ovarian hyperstimulation. *Hum Reprod* 1994;9:2350.
15. Laufer MR, Billett A, Diller L, et al. A new technique for laparoscopic prophylactic oophoropexy prior to craniospinal irradiation in children with medulloblastoma. *Adolesc Pediatr Gynecol* 1995;8:77.
16. Goldstein DP. Acute and chronic pelvic pain. *Pediatr Clin North Am* 1989;365:573.
17. Wølner-Hanssen P, Svensson L, Mårdh P-A, Weström L. Laparoscopic findings and contraceptive use in women with signs and symptoms suggestive of acute salpingitis. *Obstet Gynecol* 1985;66:233.
18. Heinonen PK, Miettinen A. Laparoscopic study on the microbiology and severity of acute pelvic inflammatory disease. *Eur J Obstet Gynecol Reprod Biol* 1994;57:85.
19. Bevan CD, Johal BJ, Mumtaz G, et al. Clinical, laparoscopic and microbiological findings in acute salpingitis: report on a United Kingdom cohort. *Br J Obstet Gynaecol* 1995;102:407.
20. Eschenbach DA, Wølner-Hanssen P, Hawes SE, et al. Acute pelvic inflammatory disease: association of clinical and laboratory findings with laparoscopic findings *Obstet Gynecol* 1997;89:184.
21. Faber BM, Coddington CC. Microlaparoscopy: a comparative study of diagnostic accuracy. *Fertil Steril* 1997;67:952.

22. Kahn JA, Chiang V, Shrier LA, Holder D, Emans SJ, DuRant R, Fishman SJ, Laufer MR. Microlaparoscopy with conscious sedation for the evaluation of suspected PID in adolescents: a preliminary report. *J Pediatr Adolesc Gynecol* 1997;10:163.
23. Feste JR. Outpatient diagnostic laparoscopy using the optical catheter. *Contemp Obstet Gynecol* 1995;8:54.
24. Palter SF, Olive DL. Office laparoscopy under local anesthesia for infertility: utility, acceptance, and cost-benefit/outcome analyses. Presented at the Fifty-first Annual Meeting of the American Society of Reproductive Medicine, 1995.
25. Hann LE, Hall DA, Black EB, et al. Mittelschmerz: sonograph demonstration. *JAMA* 1979;241:2731.
26. Klein JR, Litt IF. Epidemiology of adolescent dysmenorrhea. *Pediatrics* 1981;68:661.
27. Wilson C, Emans SJ, Mansfield J, et al. The relationship of calculated percent body fat, sports participation, age, and place of residence on menstrual patterns in healthy adolescent girls at an independent New England high school. *J Adolesc Health Care* 1984;5:248.
28. Pickles VR. A plain muscle stimulant in the menstruum. *Nature* 1957;180:1198.
29. Pickles VR, Cletheroe HJ. Further studies of the menstrual stimulant. *Lancet* 1960;2:959.
30. Pickles VR, Hall WJ, Best FA, et al. Prostaglandins in endometrium and menstrual fluid from normal and dysmenorrheic subjects. *Br J Obstet Gynaecol* 1965;72:185.
31. Halbert IR, Demers L, Fontana J, et al. Prostaglandin levels and endometrial jet wash specimens in patients with dysmenorrhea before and after indomethacin therapy. *Prostaglandins* 1975;10:1047.
32. Smith RP. Primary dysmenorrhea and the adolescent patient. *Adolesc Pediatr Gynecol* 1988;1:23.
33. Alvin PE, Litt IF. Current status of the etiology and management of dysmenorrhea in adolescence. *Pediatrics* 1982;70:516.
34. Chan WY, Dawood MY, Fuchs F. Prostaglandins in primary dysmenorrhea. Comparison of prophylactic and nonprophylactic treatment with ibuprofen and use of oral contraceptives. *Am J Med* 1981; 70:535.
35. Henzl MR, Buttram V, Segre EJ, et al. The treatment of dysmenorrhea with naproxen sodium. *Obstet Gynecol* 1977;127:818.
36. Larkin RM, Van Arden DE, Poulson AM. Dysmenorrhea: treatment with an antiprostaglandin. *Obstet Gynecol* 1979;54:456.
37. Budoff PW. Use of mefenamic acid in the treatment of primary dysmenorrhea. *JAMA* 1979;241:2713.
38. Klein JR, Litt IF, Rosenberg A, et al. The effect of aspirin on dysmenorrhea in adolescents. *J Pediatr* 1981;98:987.
39. DeLia JE, Emery MD, Taylor RH, et al. Flurbiprofen in dysmenorrhea. *Clin Pharmacol Ther* 1982; 32:76.
40. Smith RP, Powell JR. Simultaneous objective and subjective evaluation of meclofenamate sodium in the treatment of primary dysmenorrhea. *Am J Obstet Gynecol* 1987;157:611.
41. Smith RP. The dynamics of nonsteroidal anti-inflammatory therapy for primary dysmenorrhea. *Obstet Gynecol* 1987;70:785.
42. DuRant RH, Jay MS, Shoffitt T, et al. Factors influencing adolescents' responses to regimens of naproxen for dysmenorrhea. *Am J Dis Child* 1985;139:489.
43. Gladstar R. *Herbal healing for women*. New York: Simon & Schuster, 1993.
44. Laufer MR, Goitein L, Bush M, Cramer DW, Emans SJ. Prevalence of endometriosis in adolescent women with chronic pelvic pain not responding to conventional therapy. *J Pediatr Adolesc Gynecol* 1997:10:199.
45. Mathias SD, Kuppermann M, Liberman RF, et al. Chronic pelvic pain: prevalence, health-related quality of life, and economic correlates. *Obstet Gynecol* 1996;87:321.
46. Harrop-Griffiths J, Katon W, Walker E, et al. The association between chronic pelvic pain, psychiatric diagnoses, and childhood sexual abuse. *Obstet Gynecol* 1988;71:589.
47. Rapkin AJ, Kames LD, Darke LL, et al. History of physical and sexual abuse in women with chronic pelvic pain. *Obstet Gynecol* 1990;76:92.
48. Reiter RC, Shakerin LR, Gambone JC, et al. Correlation between sexual abuse and somatization in women with somatic and nonsomatic chronic pelvic pain. *Am J Obstet Gynecol* 1991;165:104.
49. Walling MK, Reiter RC, O'Hara MW, et al. Abuse history and chronic pain in women: I. prevalences of sexual abuse and physical abuse. *Obstet Gynecol* 1994;84:193.
50. Goldstein DP, deCholnoky C, Leventhal JM, Emans SJ. New insights into the old problem of chronic pelvic pain. *J Pediatr Surg* 1979;14:675.
51. Strickland DM, Hauth JC, Strickland KM. Laparoscopy for chronic pelvic pain in adolescent women. *Adolesc Pediatr Gynecol* 1988;1:31.

52. Goldstein DP, deCholnoky C, Emans SJ, et al. Laparoscopy in the diagnosis and management of pelvic pain in adolescents. *J Reprod Med* 1980;24:251.
53. Vercellini P, Fedele L, Arcaini L, et al. Laparoscopy in the diagnosis of chronic pelvic pain in adolescent women. *J Reprod Med* 1989;34:827.
54. Özaksit G, Cağlar T, Zorlu CG, et al. Chronic pelvic pain in adolescent women: diagnostic laparoscopy and ultrasonography. *J Reprod Med* 1995;40:500.
55. Keltz MD, Peck L, Liu S, et al. Large bowel-to-pelvic sidewall adhesions associated with chronic pelvic pain. *J Am Assoc Gynecol Lapar* 1995;3:55.
56. Alexander-Willimas J. Do adhesions cause pain? *Br Med J* 1987;294:659.
57. Ranney B. Etiology, prevention and inhibition of endometriosis. *Clin Obstet Gynecol* 1980;23:875.
58. Barbieri RL. Etiology and epidemiology of endometriosis. *Am J Obstet Gynecol* 1990;162:565.
59. Goldstein DP, deCholnoky C, Emans SJ. Adolescent endometriosis. *J Adolesc Health Care* 1980;1:37.
60. Houston D. Evidence for the risk of pelvic endometriosis by age, race, and socioeconomic status. *Epidemiol Rev* 1984;6:167.
61. Sampson JA. Peritoneal endometriosis due to the menstrual dissemination of endometrial tissue into the peritoneal cavity. *Am J Obstet Gynecol* 1927;14:422.
62. Sampson JA. The development of the implantation theory for the origin of peritoneal endometriosis. *Am J Obstet Gynecol* 1940;40:549.
63. Cramer DW, Wilson L, Stillman RJ, et al. The relationship of endometriosis to menstrual characteristics, smoking, and exercise. *JAMA* 1985;255:1904.
64. Meyer R. Uber entzundliche neterope epithelwucherungen im weiblichen Genetalg ebiet und uber eine bis in die Wurzel des Mesocolon ausgedehnte benigne Wucherung des Dar mepithel. *Virchows Arch Pathol Anat* 1909;195:487.
65. Halban J. Hysteroadenosis metastica. *Wien Klin Wochenschr* 1924;37:1205.
66. Foster DC, Stern JL, Buscema J, et al. Pleural and parenchymal pulmonary endometriosis. *Obstet Gynecol* 1981;58:552.
67. Thibodeau LL, Prioleau GR, Manuelidis EE, et al. Cerebral endometriosis: case report. *J Neurosurg* 1987;66:609.
68. Halme J, Becker S, Haskill S. Altered maturation and function of peritoneal macrophages: possible role in pathogenesis of endometriosis. *Am J Obstet Gynecol* 1987;156:783.
69. Dmowski W, Braun D, Gebel H. Endometriosis: genetic and immunologic aspects. *Prog Clin Biol Res* 1990;323:99.
70. Ranney B. Endometriosis. IV. Hereditary tendency. *Obstet Gynecol* 1971;37:734.
71. Simpson JL, Elias S, Malinak LR, et al. Heritable aspects of endometriosis: I. Genetic studies. *Am J Obstet Gynecol* 1980;137:327.
72. Halme J, Hammond MG, Hulka JF, et al. Retrograde menstruation in healthy women and in patients with endometriosis. *Obstet Gynecol* 1984;64:151.
73. Liu DTY, Hitchcock A. Endometriosis: its association with retrograde menstruation, dysmenorrhoea and tubal pathology. *Br J Obstet Gynaecol* 1986;93:859.
74. Blumenkrantz MJ, Gallagher N, Bashore RA, Tenckhoff H. Retrograde menstruation in women undergoing chronic peritoneal dialysis. *Obstet Gynecol* 1981;57:667.
75. Meigs J. Endometriosis. *Ann Surg* 1948;127:795.
76. Wolfman W, Kreutner K. Laparoscopy in children and adolescents. *J Adolesc Health Care* 1984;5:251.
77. Motashaw N. Endometriosis in young girls. *Contrib Gynecol Obstet* 1987;16:22.
78. Chatman D, Ward A. Endometriosis in adolescents. *J Reprod Med* 1982;27:156.
79. Bandera CA, Brown LR, Laufer MR. Adolescents and endometriosis. *Clin Consult Obstet Gynecol* 1995;7:200.
80. Cornillie FJ, Oosterlynck D, Lauweryns JM, Koninckx PR. Deeply infiltrating pelvic endometriosis: Histology and clinical significance. *Fertil Steril* 1990;53:978.
81. Fedele L, Parazzini F, Bianchi S, et al. Stage and localization of pelvic endometriosis and pain. *Fertil Steril* 1990;53:155.
82. Koninckx PR, Meuleman C, Demeyere S. Suggestive evidence that pelvic endometriosis is a progressive disease, whereas deeply infiltrating endometriosis is associated with pelvic pain. *Fertil Steril* 1991;55:759.
83. Fukaya T, Hoshiai H, Yajima A. Is pelvic endometriosis always associated with chronic pain? A retrospective study of 618 cases diagnosed by laparoscopy. *Am J Obstet Gynecol* 1993;169:719.
84. American Society for Reproductive Medicine. Revised American Society for Reproductive Medicine classification of endometriosis: 1996. *Fertil Steri*l 1997;67:817.

85. Redwine DB. Age-related evolution in color appearance of endometriosis. *Fertil Steril* 1987;48: 1062.
86. Stripling MC, Martin DC, Chatman DL, et al. Subtle appearances of pelvic endometriosis. *Fertil Steril* 1988;49:427.
87. Martin DC, Hubert GD, Vander Zwaag R, El-Zeky FA. Laparoscopic appearances of peritoneal endometriosis. *Fertil Steril* 1989;51:63.
88. Wiegerinck MAHM, Van Dop PA, Brosens IA. The staging of peritoneal endometriosis by the type of active lesion in addition to the revised American Fertility Society classification. *Fertil Steril* 1993; 60:461.
89. Redwine DB, Yocum LB. A serial section study of visually normal pelvic peritoneum in patients with endometriosis. *Fertil Steril* 1990;54:648.
90. Davis DD, Thillet E, Lindemann J. Clinical characteristics of adolescent endometriosis. *J Adolesc Health* 1993;14:362.
91. Laufer MR. Identification of clear vesicular lesions of atypical endometriosis: a new technique. *Fertil Steril* 1997;68:739.
92. Haney AF. Endometriosis. Pathogenesis and pathophysiology. In: Wilson EA, ed. *Endometriosis.* New York: Liss, 1987:23.
93. Nisolle M, Berliere M, Paindaveine B, et al. Histologic study of peritoneal endometriosis in infertile women. *Fertil Steril* 1990;53:984.
94. Murphy AA, Green WR, Bobbie D, et al. Unsuspected endometriosis documented by scanning electron microscopy in visually normal peritoneum. *Fertil Steril* 1986;46:522.
95. Olive DL, Henderson DY. Endometriosis and müllerian anomalies. *Obstet Gynecol* 1987;69:412.
96. Hornstein MD, Harlow BL, Thomas PP, Check JH. Use of a new CA 125 assay in the diagnosis of endometriosis. *Hum Reprod* 1995;10:932.
97. Schifrin BS, Erez S, Moore JG. Teen-age endometriosis. *Am J Obstet Gynecol* 1973;116:973.
98. Sanfilippo JS, Wakim NG, Schikler KN, Yussman MA. Endometriosis in association with uterine anomaly. *Am J Obstet Gynecol* 1986;154:39.
99. D'Hooghe TM, Bambra CS, Raeymaekers BM, Koninckx PR. Serial laparoscopies over 30 months show that endometriosis in captive baboons (*Papio anubis, Papio cynocephalus*) is a progressive diseasea. *Fertil Steril* 1996;65:645.
100. Schenken RS, Asch RH, Williams RF, Hodgen GD. Etiology of infertility in monkeys with endometriosis: luteinized unruptured follicles, luteal phase defects, pelvic adhesions, and spontaneous abortions. *Fertil Steril* 1984;41:122.
101. Schenken RS, Asch RH. Surgical induction of endometriosis in the rabbit: effects on fertility and concentrations of peritoneal fluid prostaglandins. *Fertil Steril* 1989;34:581.
102. Kaplan CR, Eddy CA, Olive DL, Schenken RS. Effects of ovarian endometriosis on ovulation in rabbits. *Am J Obstet Gynecol* 1989;160:40.
103. Redwine DB. Conservative laparoscopic excision of endometriosis by sharp dissection: life table analysis of reoperation and persistent or recurrent disease. *Fertil Steril* 1991;56:628.
104. Olive DL, Schwartz LB. Endometriosis. *N Engl J Med* 1993;328:1759.
105. Gordts S, Boeckx W, Brosens I. Microsurgery of endometriosis in infertile patients. *Fertil Steril* 1984;42:520.
106. Olive DL. Conservative surgery. In: Schenken RS, ed. *Endometriosis: contemporary concepts in clinical management.* Philadelphia: JB Lippincott, 1989:213.
107. Vancaillie T, Schenken RS. Endoscopic surgery. In: Schenken RS, ed. *Endometriosis: contemporary concepts in clinical management.* Philadelphia: JB Lippincott, 1989:249.
108. Nezhat C, Hood J, Winer W, et al. Videolaseroscopy and laser laparoscopy in gynaecology. *Br J Hosp Med* 1987;38:219.
109. Redwine DB. Treatment of endometriosis-associated pain. *Infertil Reprod Med Clin North Am* 1993; 3:697.
110. Tamaya T, Motoyama T, Ohono Y. Steroid receptor levels and histology of endometrium and adenomyosis. *Fertil Steril* 1979;31:396.
111. Janne O, Kauppila A, Kokko E. Estrogen and progestin receptors in endometriotic lesions: comparison with endometrial tissue. *Am J Obstet Gynecol* 1981;141:562.
112. Fujishita A, Nakane PK, Koji T, et al. Expression of estrogen and progesterone receptors in endometrium and peritoneal endometriosis: an immunohistochemical and in situ hybridization study. *Fertil Steril* 1997;67:856.
113. Kauppila A, Ronnberg L. Naproxen sodium in dysmenorrhea secondary to endometriosis. *Obstet Gynecol* 1985;65:379.

114. Kistner RW. The treatment of endometriosis by inducing pseudopregnancy with ovarian hormones: a report of 58 cases. *Fertil Steril* 1959;10:539.
115. Luciano AA, Pitkin RM. Endometriosis: approaches to diagnosis and treatment. *Surg Annu* 1984; 16:297.
116. Moghissi KS, Boyce CR. Management of endometriosis with oral medroxyprogesterone acetate. *Obstet Gynecol* 1976;47:265.
117. Luciano AA, Turksoy N, Carleo J. Evaluation of oral medroxyprogesterone acetate in the treatment of endometriosis. *Obstet Gynecol* 1988;72:323.
118. Vercellini P, De Giorgio, Oldani S, et al. Depot medroxyprogesterone acetate versus an oral contraceptive combined with very low-dose danazol for long-term treatment of pelvic pain associated with endometriosis. *Am J Obstet Gynecol* 1996;175:396.
119. Hammond MG, Hammond CB, Parker RT. Conservative treatment of endometriosis externa: the effects of methyltestosterone therapy. *Fertil Steril* 1978;29:651.
120. Barbieri RL, Hornstein MD. Medical therapy for endometriosis. In: Wilson EA, ed. *Endometriosis.* New York: Liss, 1987:111.
121. Barbieri RL. New therapy for endometriosis. *N Engl J Med* 1988;318:512.
122. Dmowski WP, Cohen MR. Antigonadotropin (danazol) in the treatment of endometriosis: evaluation of post-treatment fertility and three-year follow-up data. *Am J Obstet Gynecol* 1978;130:41.
123. Bayer SR, Seibel MM, Saffan DS, et al. Efficacy of danazol treatment for minimal endometriosis in infertile women. *J Reprod Med* 1988;33:179.
124. Hull ME, Moghissi KS, Magyar DF, et al. Comparison of different treatment modalities of endometriosis in infertile women. *Fertil Steril* 1987;47:40.
125. Burry KA. Nafarelin in the management of endometriosis: quality of life assessment. *Am J Obstet Gynecol* 1992;166:735.
126. Barbieri RL. Treatment of endometriosis with the GnRH agonists. In: Barbieri RL, Friedman AJ, eds. *Gonadotropin releasing hormone analogs: applications in gynecology.* New York: Elsevier, 1991:63.
127. Henzl MR, Corson SL, Moghissi K, et al. Administration of nasal nafarelin as compared with oral danazol for endometriosis. *N Engl J Med* 1988;318:485.
128. Kennedy SH, Williams IA, Brodribb J, et al. A comparison of nafarelin acetate and danazol in the treatment of endometriosis. *Fertil Steril* 1991;53:998.
129. Dlugi AM, Miller JD, Knittle J. Lupron depot (leuprolide acetate for depot suspension) in the treatment of endometriosis: a randomized, placebo-controlled, double-blind study. *Fertil Steril* 1990;54:427.
130. Dawood MY, Lewis V, Ramos J. Cortical and trabecular bone mineral content in women with endometriosis: effect of gonadotropin releasing hormone agonist and danazol. *Fertil Steril* 1989;52: 21.
131. Fogelman I. Gonadotropin-releasing hormone agonists and the skeleton. *Fertil Steril* 1992;57:715.
132. Lichten EM, Bombard J. Surgical treatment of primary dysmenorrhea with laparoscopic uterine nerve ablation. *J Reprod Med* 1987;32:37.
133. Gürgan T, Urman B, Aksu T, et al. Laparoscopic CO_2 laser uterine nerve ablation for treatment of drug resistant primary dysmenorrhea. *Fertil Steril* 1992;58:422.
134. Lee RB, Stone K, Magelssen D, et al. Presacral neurectomy for chronic pelvic pain. *Obstet Gynecol* 1986;68:517.
135. Tjaden B, Schlaff WD, Kimball A, Rock JA. The efficacy of presacral neurectomy for the relief of midline dysmenorrhea. *Obstet Gynecol* 1990;76:89.
136. Perez JJ. Laparoscopic presacral neurectomy. *J Reprod Med* 1990;35:625.
137. Candiani GB, Fedele L, Vercellini P, et al. Presacral neurectomy for treatment of pelvic pain associated with endometriosis: a controlled study. *Am J Obstet Gynecol* 1992;167:100.
138. Walters MD. Definitive surgery. In: Schenken RS, ed. *Endometriosis: contemporary concepts in clinical management.* Philadelphia: JB Lippincott, 1989:267.
139. Surrey ES, Gambone JC, Lu JKH, Judd HL. Effects of combining norethindrone with a gonadotropin-releasing hormone agonist in the treatment of symptomatic endometriosis. *Fertil Steril* 1990;53:620.
140. Cedars MI, Lu JKH, Meldrum DR, Judd HL. Treatment of endometriosis with a long-acting gonadotropin-releasing hormone agonist plus medroxyprogesterone acetate. *Obstet Gynecol* 1990; 75:641.
141. Barbieri RL. Hormone treatment of endometriosis: the estrogen threshold hypothesis. *Am J Obstet Gynecol* 1992;166:740.
142. Surrey ES, Judd HL. Reduction of vasomotor symptoms and bone mineral density loss with combined norethindrone and long-acting gonadotropin releasing hormone agonist therapy of symptomatic endometriosis: a prospective randomized trial. *J Clin Endocrinol Metab* 1992;75:558.

143. Ravn P, Bergqvist A, Hansen MA, et al. Treatment of endometriosis with the luteinizing hormone-releasing hormone agonist Nafarelin. Effects on bone turnover and bone mass. *Menopause* 1994;1:11.
144. Surrey ES, Fournet N, Voigt B, Judd H. Effects of sodium etidronate in combination with low-dose norethindrone in patients administered a long-acting GnRH agonist: a preliminary report. *Obstet Gynecol* 1993;81:581.
145. Finkelstein JS, Klibanski A, Schaefer EH, et al. Parathyroid hormone for the prevention of bone loss induced by estrogen deficiency. *N Engl J Med* 1994;331:1618.
146. Kettel LM, Liu JH, Murphy AA, et al. Endocrine responses to long-term administration of the antiprogesterone RU486 in patients with pelvic endometriosis. *Fertil Steril* 1991;56:402.
147. Barbieri RL. CA-125 in patients with endometriosis. *Fertil Steril* 1986;45:767.
148. Thomas PP, Higgins PH, Wolfe DH, Laufer MR. Development of a support network for adolescents with endometriosis. *J Pediatr Adolesc Gynecol* 1996;9:155.
149. Keltz MD, Kliman HJ, Arici AM, Olive DL. Endosalpingiosis found at laparoscopy for chronic pelvic pain. *Fertil Steril* 1995;64:482.
150. Laufer MR, Heerema AE, Parsons KE, Barbieri RL. Endosalpingiosis: description/classification of presentation and follow up. *Gynecol Obstet Invest* 1998;46:195.
151. American Psychiatric Association. *DSM-IV. Diagnostic and statistical manual of mental disorders*, 4th ed., Washington, DC, American Psychiatric Association, 1994.
152. American College of Obstetricians and Gynecologists (ACOG) Committee Opinion. Committee on Gynecologic Practice. *Premenstrual Syndrome*. 1989;66.
153. Fisher M, Trieller K, Napolitano B. Premenstrual symptoms in adolescents. *J Adolesc Health Care* 1989;10:369.
154. Keye W Jr, ed. *The premenstrual syndrome*. Philadelphia: WB Saunders, 1988.
155. Bargetzi MJ, Meyer UA, Birkhaeuser MH. Premenstrual exacerbations in hepatic porphyria: prevention by intermittent administration of an LH-RH agonist in combination with a gestagen. *JAMA* 1989;261:864.
156. Slater JE. Recurrent anaphylaxis in menstruating women: treatment with a luteinizing hormone-releasing hormone agonist: a preliminary report. *Obstet Gynecol* 1987;70:542.
157. Meggs WJ, Pescovitz OH, Metcalfe D, et al. Progesterone sensitivity as a cause of recurrent anaphylaxis. *N Engl J Med* 1984;311:1236.
158. Johnson SR, McChesney C, Bean JA. Epidemiology of premenstrual symptoms in a nonclinical sample: 1. Prevalence, natural history and help-seeking behavior. *J Reprod Med* 1988;33:340.
159. Mortola JF, Girton L, Beck L, Yen SSC. Diagnosis of premenstrual syndrome by a single, prospective and reliable instrument: the calendar of premenstrual experiences. *Obstet Gynecol* 1990;76:302.
160. Muse KN, Cetel NS, Futterman LA, et al. The premenstrual syndrome: effects of "medical ovariectomy." *N Engl J Med* 1984;311:1345.
161. Maddocks S, Hahn P, Moller F, et al. A double-blind placebo-controlled trial of progesterone vaginal suppositories in the treatment of premenstrual syndrome. *Am J Obstet Gynecol* 1986;154:573.
162. Hammerback S, Damber JE, Backstrom T. Relationship between symptom severity and hormone changes in women with premenstrual syndrome. *J Clin Endocrinol Metab* 1989;68:125.
163. Rubinow DR, et al. Changes in plasma hormones across the menstrual cycle in patients with menstrually related mood disorder and in control subjects. *Am J Obstet Gynecol* 1988;158:5.
164. Schmidt PJ, Nieman LK, Grover GN, et al. Lack of effect of induced menses on symptoms in women with premenstrual syndrome. *N Engl J Med* 1991;324:1174.
165. Reid RL, Yen SSC. Premenstrual syndrome. *Am J Obstet Gynecol* 1981;139:85.
166. Reid RL. Endogenous opiate peptides and premenstrual syndrome. *Semin Reprod Endocrinol* 1987;5:191.
167. Chuong CJ, Coulam CB, Bergstralh, et al. Clinical trial of naltrexone in premenstrual syndrome. *Obstet Gynecol* 1988;72:332.
168. Vellacott ID, Shroff NE, Pearce MY, et al. A double-blind, placebo-controlled evaluation of spironolactone in the premenstrual syndrome. *Curr Med Res Opin* 1987;10:450.
169. O'Brien PMS, Craven O, Selby C, et al. Treatment of premenstrual syndrome by spironolactone. *Br J Obstet Gynaecol* 1979;86:142.
170. Mira M, NcNeil D, Fraser IS, et al. Mefenamic acid in the treatment of premenstrual syndrome. *Obstet Gynecol* 1986;68:395.
171. Sarno AP, Miller EJ Jr, Lundblad EG. Premenstrual syndrome: beneficial effects of periodic, low-dose danazol. *Obstet Gynecol* 1987;70:33.
172. Yonkers KA, Halbreich U, Freeman E, et el. Sertraline in the treatment of premenstrual dysphoric disorder. *Psychopharmacol Bull* 1996;32:41.

173. Freeman EW, Rickels K, Sondheimer SJ. Fluvoxamine for premenstrual dysphoric disorder. a pilot study. *J Clin Psychiatry* 1996;57:56.
174. Smith S, Rinehart JS, Ruddock VE, et al. Treatment of premenstrual syndrome with alprazolam: results of a double-blind, placebo-controlled, randomized crossover clinical trial. *Obstet Gynecol* 1987;70:37.
175. Dennerstein L, Spencer-Gardner C, Gotts G, et al. Progesterone and the premenstrual syndrome: a double-blind crossover trial. *Br Med J* 1985;29:1617.
176. Baker ER, Best RG, Manfredi RL, et al. Efficacy of progesterone vaginal suppositories in alleviation of nervous symptoms in patients with premenstrual syndrome. *J Assist Reprod Genet* 1995;12:205.
177. Freeman EW, Richels K, Sondheimer SJ, et al. A double-blind trial of oral progesterone, alprazolam, and placebo in treatment of severe premenstrual syndrome. *JAMA* 1995;274:51.
178. Kendall KE, Schnurr PP. The effects of vitamin B6 supplementation on premenstrual symptoms. *Obstet Gynecol* 1987;70:145.
179. Mortola JF, Girton L, Fischer U. Successful treatment of severe premenstrual syndrome by combined use of gonadotropin-releasing hormone agonist and estrogen/progestin. *J Clin Endocrinol Metab* 1991;72:252A.
180. Leather AT, Studd JWW, Watson NR, et al. The prevention of bone loss in young women treated with GnRH analogues with "add-back" estrogen therapy. *Obstet Gynecol* 1993;81:104.
181. Mezrow G, Shoupe D, Spicer D, et al. Depot leuprolide acetate with estrogen and progestin add-back for long-term treatment of premenstrual syndrome. *Fertil Steril* 1994;62:932.
182. Daamen MJ, Brown WA. Single-dose fluoxetine in management of premenstrual syndrome. *J Clin Psychiatry* 1992;53:210.
183. Steiner M. Fluoxetine in the treatment of LLPDD: a multi-center, placebo-controlled, double-blind trail. *Int J Gynecol Obstet* 1994;46(suppl 2):122.
184. Steiner M, Steinberg S, Stewart D, et al. Fluoxetine in the treatment of premenstrual dysphoria. *N Engl J Med* 1995;332:1528.

10

Perioperative Considerations for Pediatric and Adolescent Gynecologic Surgery

Comprehensive preoperative preparation of patients undergoing surgical procedures is essential to ensure a positive experience for the patient and her family. Preoperative teaching serves to decrease anxiety and the fear of the unknown that surrounds impending surgical procedures. Decreasing anxiety can have a positive effect on the patient's emotional as well as physical state. In patients undergoing pediatric and adolescent gynecologic surgery, the developmental issues of childhood and adolescence and issues of sexuality increase the need for comprehensive and sensitive teaching.

A general knowledge of growth and development is necessary in caring for infants, children, and adolescents. It is also important for the health care provider to assess the child's cognitive level in order to select an accurate and effective preprocedural method of teaching. Age group classifications vary, as there are no clear definitions of boundaries and individuals develop at different rates.

In order to understand the communications of children and adolescents and the meaning of their behavior, health care providers must be familiar with the age-specific general thought process. This knowledge helps direct interventions and suggests ways of enhancing interactions and communications with children. Intervention through preparation and support of children and adolescents who are scheduled for surgery can acknowledge their fears and prevent short- and long-term problems related to the surgical experience.

PREOPERATIVE EDUCATION AND MANAGEMENT

The need for surgical preparation is predicated on the belief that hospitalization and surgery are stressful and anxiety-producing experiences that can lead to long-term psychological problems in some children (1). Children entering the hospital for surgery leave the familiar surroundings of their home and enter a strange environment. Melamed and Siegal (1) have noted that 10% to 35% of children exhibit immediate or sustained emotional and behavioral problems, night terrors, increased dependency, regression, eating disturbances, and increased fearfulness following hospitalization for surgery. When a child does not have knowledge of a situation, the sense of fear is increased. Anxiety in both children and parents has been found to influence the child's response to medical care. The preparation of a child for surgery reduces psychological upset after hospitalization (2). In a study of different models of psychological preparation and supportive care designed to increase the adjustment of children hospitalized for elective surgery, systematic preparation, rehearsal, and supportive care prior to each stressful procedure resulted in significantly less upset and thus more cooperation from the children (3).

Effective preoperative and perioperative teaching in the pediatric setting must always include consideration of the parents' needs and fears. Children are very adept at sensing their parents' feelings and level of stress. The child's ability to remain calm is enhanced when the parents are well prepared for upcoming events. Because parents report that their own anxiety and stress may prevent them from understanding or remembering all of the information provided before surgery, health care providers should recognize the need to reintroduce concepts and repeat information (4).

Procedures involving the reproductive organs, whether the patient is an infant, a child, or an adolescent, tend to create a higher level of anxiety than procedures involving other parts of the body. The social, cultural, and psychological effects of genital surgery can be significant and must be addressed preoperatively. Parental fears about the loss of a child's virginity during procedures such as a vaginal exam under anesthesia, and particularly repair of an imperforate hymen, are common. We have found parental and patient anxiety to be decreased if preoperative teaching is initiated when it is determined that a surgical procedure will be necessary. The details of the procedure, intraoperative care, and postoperative management are outlined. The risks and benefits of the surgery are discussed, and the patient and guardians are given ample opportunity to express their concerns and fears and to ask questions. This discussion should be conducted in a relaxed setting to allow for the opportunity to address all issues. If postoperative analgesics or narcotics will be needed, a prescription is given to the patient or family at this time to eliminate the need for a stop at a pharmacy immediately after discharge.

Preparation Modalities

Preparatory booklets, films, puppet shows, slide presentations, and tours of the operating rooms and hospital postoperative surgical recovery floors are some of the modalities that are effective, depending on age group, for preoperative preparation. Preparation is focused on factual information about the purpose and timing of events. The health care provider can also prepare a child for procedures and events by giving a verbal description of sensations she may experience. Content is geared to the child's cognitive level of development. The child is encouraged to communicate and express fears and to establish trust in and familiarity with the surgical staff. Fear can be alleviated with stories or by demonstrations with toys or stuffed animals.

In a study conducted by Ellerton and Merriam (5), children responded with decreased anxiety and were shown to cope positively with the perioperative course after watching a video depicting a child going through the preoperative and postoperative experience. In addition to videos, children respond well to modeling techniques such as puppet shows, cartoons, or dolls. Having the parents present during induction of anesthesia and allowing the child to bring a special toy into the operating room can also help to comfort many children (Fig. 1). Parents should be encouraged to participate in any preoperative program and/or tours offered by the hospital.

Play

Play is one way a child can manipulate or control a situation, and it can help in coping with stress and provide effective learning. Toddlers use play to translate feelings, drives, and fantasies into action. Play permits children to respond to challenge, influence the environment, initiate action, and observe results. Health care workers can structure play so that it has a therapeutic function. The use of toys,

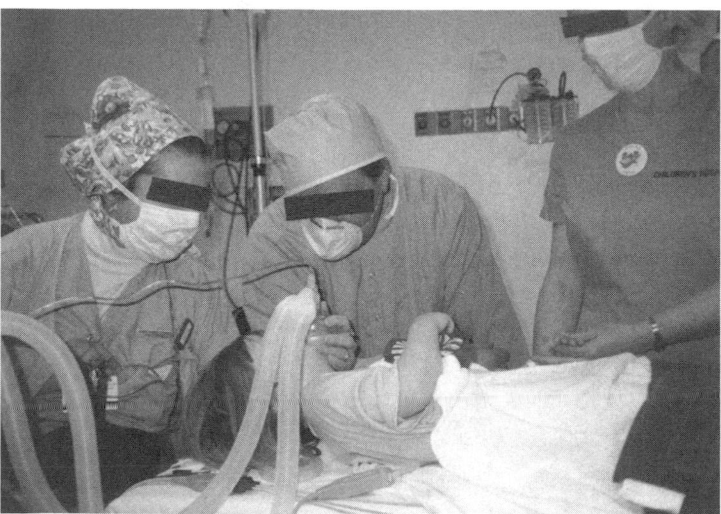

FIG. 1. A father's or mother's presence and a favorite toy help children cope during the induction of anesthesia.

games, books, and available medical equipment provides children opportunities to communicate with health care providers in a nonthreatening atmosphere (6).

Preoperative rehearsal play has been shown to reduce anxiety in children (7). When the child has limited verbal skills, play can be the most effective means of communication. Play sessions before surgery, involving hospital equipment such as blood pressure cuffs, stethoscopes, surgical masks, and surgical gloves, can help ease a child's fears of the highly technical surgical environment. Drawings, dolls, and puppets help children demonstrate their understanding of their health care. Dolls or stuffed animals can be used as "patients" to demonstrate blood drawing, stitches, bandages, and the use of thermometers.

More detailed and sophisticated age-appropriate medical teaching aids are becoming available to reassure and educate patients. Anatomically correct dolls help teach older children about body parts and how they will be treated. Organized board games are available to provide information about health care or hospitalization and are appealing to children from preschoolers through teenagers (8).

Drawing

Artwork can be a valuable assessment and communication tool for the health care provider preparing a child for surgery. Drawing is the universal language of children, and in the immediate preoperative period it can help younger children to express feelings, fears, and experiences they may not be able to verbalize (Fig. 2). Children of all ages can present invaluable information through drawing.

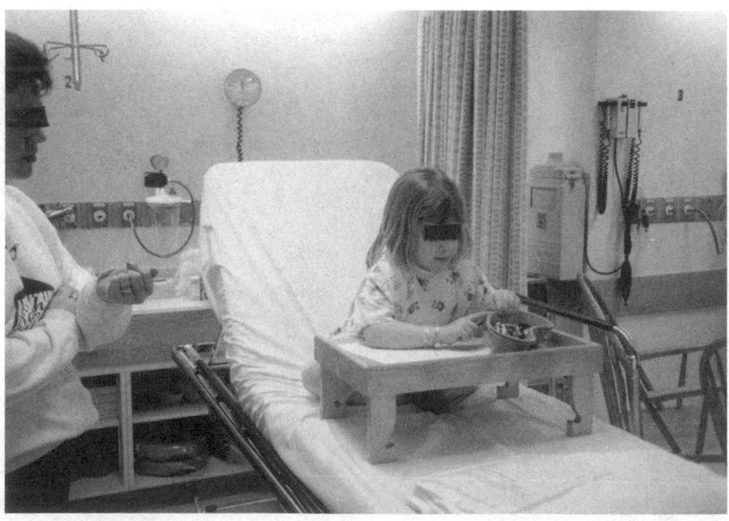

FIG. 2. Drawing during the immediate perioperative period can help younger children express feelings, fears, and experiences they may not be able to verbalize while providing a pleasant motor activity at a highly emotional time.

Drawings can also decrease children's anxiety by providing them with a motor activity at a highly emotional time (9). Children's drawings often reveal concerns about mutilation, body changes, and loss of self-control. By using drawing as an assessment tool to recognize the fears and fantasies of a child, the health care provider can intervene to dispel any misconceptions. Drawing of objects and rehearsal of procedures can help prevent serious misinterpretation and fears (9).

AGE GROUP AND DEVELOPMENTAL CONSIDERATIONS

Developmental or age-group stages may be defined somewhat differently from textbook to textbook. Mott and associates (10) describe five stages: infancy, early childhood, middle childhood, late childhood, and adolescence. These descriptions and key concepts of general age group/developmental stages and other considerations relating to gynecologic surgical procedures are summarized below (10–12).

Infancy

Infancy is usually described from the time of birth until the age of 1 year. The provision of comfort and security should be the primary focus in meeting the developmental needs of infants. Long periods of preoperative fasting are no longer believed to be necessary for infants and young children (13), and the guidelines for fasting are often modified for the very young infant to decrease upset due to hunger. For preoperative purposes, breast milk is considered a clear fluid. This allows a mother to breast-feed her child before surgery, decreasing stress to both the infant and the mother. Allowing the infant to use a pacifier and/or bring a security object into the operating room is also very effective in decreasing the stress of separation during the perioperative period (13).

Early Childhood

Early childhood constitutes the toddler period, which spans the years from late infancy until age 5, before entry into kindergarten. The toddler phase includes early language development and locomotion; toddlers have a limited ability to communicate and reason. They are threatened by changes in routine, and they are curious. The toddler may interpret separation from a parent as abandonment. She is often terrified by unfamiliar hospital staff dressed in unusual clothes or masks and may benefit from having a parent present as much as possible. A parent's presence in the postanesthesia care unit greatly reduces anxiety as the toddler emerges from the effects of anesthesia (Fig. 3).

The preschool period between toddler age and kindergarten is one of intellectual and emotional growth. The hospital-related fears of the toddler and

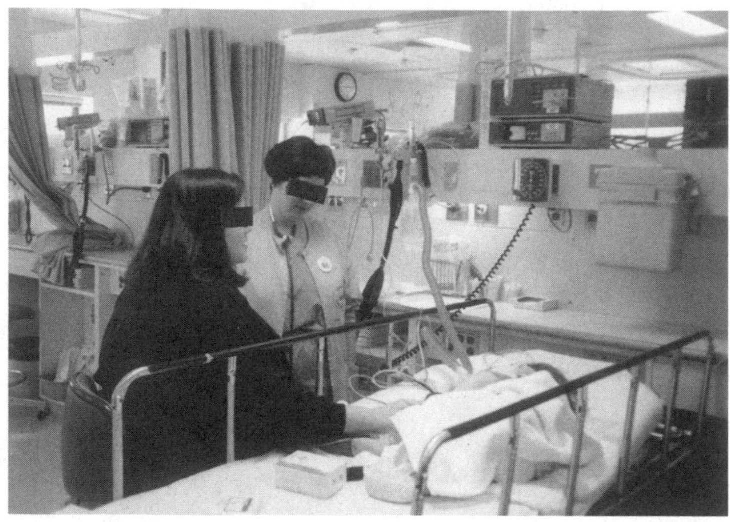

FIG. 3. A parent's presence in the postanesthesia care unit decreases the child's anxiety on emergence from the effects of anesthesia.

preschool child focus on being in a new environment, disruption of routines, body mutilation, abandonment, and separation. Readiness for a new experience must be assessed, as well as the need for continued physical and emotional support in the new environment. These children respond with anxiety to new sights and sounds and cannot distinguish between real and imagined dangers. Procedures that require entry into the body, such as injections or the withdrawal of body fluids, can be intrusive and threatening. It is important for adults to answer a child's questions. Children can become confused and anxious when large words are used and if the explanations are usually directed to the parent. Pretend play, in which the patient is "the doctor" can not only allay fears but bring the child's specific concerns to the forefront. In a study of preoperative preparation of children, Ellerton and Merriam (5) found that many children are quite anxious about removing all of their clothing before a surgical procedure. The simple practice of allowing a child to wear her underwear into the operating room and replacing it before she leaves the operating room can help allay some of her fears. During discussion of the surgical experience at the preoperative visit, visible relief can be observed in a child after she receives this information (5).

Preschoolers can often predict upcoming events by clues in the environment. Attempting to keep secrets from them only leads to misinterpretation and lack of trust in caregivers. Honesty is an important aspect of any preoperative preparation.

Middle Childhood

Middle childhood encompasses the time from kindergarten through the third or fourth grade. During this developmental stage, the child is less egocentric and develops relationships with adults outside the family through school activities. The child learns to adapt to new environments and experiences.

This child's concept of health is related to physical experience and capacity for activity. She usually has a good understanding of the external body but vague ideas about the structure and function of internal body parts. There is a dramatic increase in the child's vocabulary, articulation skills, correct use of grammar, and attention span. Fears are concerned with personal safety and unexpected experiences, and, at the end of middle childhood, with performance. Aggression and anger are best handled with consistency, clear limits, and avoidance of a power struggle. Children use coping strategies previously learned to deal with stress, and they may adopt new strategies as they struggle with multiple, and sometimes conflicting, requests and expectations.

During this stage, children are eager to learn about the world, to affirm their sexual identity, and to develop relationships with peers. They find new ways to solve problems and can accommodate better to a variety of new experiences. They are now capable of true cooperation. Fears are more related to reality than during the preschool stage. Separation fears are less predominant, but other fears related to injury, mutilation, or death are important (14). School-age children often want to be brave and courageous and display bravado in threatening situations, but in fact they may require support. Children may use rituals to defend themselves from anxiety, such as mumbling "magic words." During hospitalization or visits to a doctor, the school-age child may feel that her body is no longer in her possession.

Reading becomes easier for school-age children and books may give them relief from worries. Preparation booklets in a comic-book or other age-appropriate form may be utilized to stimulate the child's interest in the content while teaching her what to expect during the upcoming surgery. The school-age child becomes keenly interested in becoming a member of a group. Groups for admission preparation may emphasize that the child is not alone in the upcoming experience.

Late Childhood

Late childhood encompasses the time from third or fourth grade until adolescence. It is a time of increased independence as the child spends more time away from home at school, clubs, and play. The child's concept of health becomes more sophisticated. She gains an understanding of the human body and the physiologic functions of the internal organs. Play, at this stage, enables children to learn more about themselves, their interests, and abilities.

The child's longer attention span facilitates organization of information for later retrieval. Children can use and apply previously learned material more efficiently. During late childhood, children use language to express thought and to communicate new knowledge. Success is judged by self-satisfaction and the recognition received from others.

The physical changes of early puberty can trigger positive, negative, and/or ambivalent responses from young girls. Intense feelings of modesty and self-consciousness can be present. Once again, allowing a girl to keep her underwear on preoperatively and ensuring that it is replaced before she awakens, effectively decreases her anxiety level. A girl in this age group may have very specific questions about the effects of a surgical procedure on her virginity and future reproductive capabilities. Encouraging her to verbalize her concerns is important, since she may be too embarrassed to ask (15). A few simple statements from a nurse or doctor stating "what a lot of girls are concerned about" and how the staff will "take care of that" can be extremely effective in calming many fears.

Older children seem to benefit from preparation several days before the event so they have time to think about how they will respond and what actions or behaviors they can use to cope with and/or participate in the experience (1). Research by Wolfer and Visintainer (16) indicated that older children who used home preparatory materials 1 week before hospital admission showed better adjustment than those receiving routine care. Meng (17) demonstrated that older children experienced a reduction in anxiety following a preadmission program a week prior to surgery, while younger children experienced increased anxiety until admission.

Adolescence

The onset of puberty is a major transition, as the adolescent begins to formalize attitudes and beliefs about health. Learning is best achieved when the adolescent is an active participant in an environment conducive to her involvement. Motivation to learn is high when the adolescent is interested in the subject matter. Older adolescents have the ability to think abstractly, can consider hypotheses, and are not bound by what they can see and experience. They can follow an argument and consider several alternative ways to achieve goals.

Adolescence is further defined by a multitude of cultural, subcultural, community, and familial factors. The adolescent is struggling to move from childhood into an adulthood that is both desired and feared and into a new world of independent relationships. Adolescents may be secretive with parents and are not likely to express their fears and anxieties. Defensive behavior may mask fears and anxiety. Adolescents are determining values and ideals and developing sexual identity. Peer relations, body image, sexuality, and fertility become increasingly important. Gynecologic surgical procedures directly affect these issues. Sometimes, adolescent girls can and will verbally articulate their concerns. At other times, it is the health care provider's responsibility to initiate discussion of these issues.

Peer relations are paramount in the minds of most adolescents. Many adolescents feel it necessary to keep their physical ailments or "differences" secret from their friends for fear of rejection. The possibility of a visible scar on a young woman's breast or abdomen can be very disturbing. Opportunities must be given preoperatively for a girl to talk about body image issues and whether, how, and when she will tell her peers about the impending surgery. An increasing number of surgical procedures of the abdomen can be done through minimally invasive surgery (operative laparoscopy), decreasing the size of the visible scar and therefore minimizing changes in body image.

Repair of gynecologic congenital anomalies or surgical treatment of cervical dysplasia can heighten adolescent concerns about sexuality and fertility. Facts and reassurance given by the health care provider are necessary and helpful, but additional support in the form of peer group counseling and/or social services is often beneficial.

The emotional impact of some gynecologic conditions can be devastating to a patient and her family. Poland and Evans (18) observed young women with vaginal agenesis through the course of diagnosis, surgical repair, and subsequent life events. A wide range of concerns were voiced by these young women, including anger, depression, and fear of rejection because of their altered fertility and sexuality. Good relationships with parents and the ability to share feelings with family and friends seemed to be the best indicator of a good emotional outcome after diagnosis and vaginoplasty (18). However, the sensitive provision of options and contact with other young women with the same diagnosis and operative procedure has proved essential in the immediate and long-term emotional and social health of these young women in our institution. Health care providers can take an active role in guiding patients and parents to support programs.

Maintaining confidentiality when dealing with adolescents and their parents is essential. To ensure accurate answers to sensitive questions about sexuality and peer relations, a system must be in place whereby health care providers speak to adolescents and their parents both separately and together before surgery. The existence of a nonpregnant state must be verified before surgery can be performed. Careful preoperative teaching in the health care provider's office regarding the need for strict compliance with birth control methods must be stressed to the sexually active adolescent. Routine preoperative pregnancy testing on the day of surgery is important and helpful in the care of adolescents (19–21). Parents may react negatively to this testing in the belief that the health care provider or institution assumes that their daughter is sexually active. An explanation that this testing is hospital policy and not an assessment of sexual activity is necessary and usually quite effective. Policies and procedures surrounding confidentiality issues are further discussed in Chapter 21 and must be clearly defined by individual health care facilities.

Concerns about fertility, while present at every stage, are most commonly voiced by parents of adolescents having gynecologic surgery. Additionally, some parents may feel guilt and need reassurance that they are not responsible for their daughter's condition. Health care providers must provide ample opportunity for parents to speak separately about these and other concerns. Factual information within the laws and guidelines of confidentiality should be relayed.

PERIOPERATIVE EDUCATION AND MANAGEMENT

Almost any young child taken into an unfamiliar environment by strangers will be extremely frightened. A young child's hospital-related fears may focus on separation from parents. Traditionally, parents and children were separated during the immediate preoperative, intraoperative, and postoperative phases of care. Today, in many hospital settings, there are opportunities in each of these phases when a parent can and should be allowed and encouraged to stay with the child for support and to participate in care. All efforts should be made to minimize the amount of time during which children and parents are separated.

Allowing a parent to participate in the induction process helps alleviate some fear and anxiety associated with anesthesia (4). Parent-present induction, whereby a parent dons a surgical jumpsuit, escorts the child into the operating room, and stays with her until induction of anesthesia has taken place, can aid in keeping a small child calm just before surgery. Conversely, very anxious parents may only heighten the child's anxiety (22). Careful assessment of the child and parent is imperative to ensure a positive outcome of this technique. Selection of the appropriate person to accompany the child to the operating room is individually based on the parent's comfort with their prospective role and their ability to be supportive to the child (4). Separation anxiety in an older infant can be effectively managed with parent-present induction.

If the parent is present during induction of anesthesia and/or accompanies the child to the operating room, the parent is carefully prepared for the sights and sounds of the experience, including the child's response to the anesthetic agents. After the induction of anesthesia, the parent is escorted to a family waiting area, before the child undergoes positioning and surgical preparation.

POSTOPERATIVE EDUCATION AND MANAGEMENT

The patient and her family should be prepared for expected postoperative events before they leave the hospital. As mentioned above, postoperative analgesics or narcotics should be prescribed at the preoperative visit for the sake of convenience. The patient and her family should be educated about wound care, diet, activity, and patient management prior to discharge. In addition, they should be informed of the possible postoperative complications and of indications for concern and when to contact health care providers.

In summary, the anxiety associated with visits to the doctor, hospitalization, and surgery can become overwhelming and detrimental to physical and emotional recovery. Children, like adults, need help and information about impending anxiety-provoking procedures, whether in the form of written material, careful discussion, or other preprocedural or preoperative modalities. Information about the anxiety-provoking event can change feelings into definable fears. Special consideration must be given to the social, psychological, and developmental needs of patients and parents of patients undergoing gynecologic procedures in order to help ensure an excellent physical and emotional outcome.

REFERENCES

1. Melamed BG, Siegel L. Reduction of anxiety in children facing hospitalization for surgery. *J Consult Clin Psychol* 1975;43:511.
2. Bates T, Broome M. Preparation of children for hospitalization and surgery: a review of the literature. *J Pediatr Nurs* 1986;1:230.
3. Visintainer M, Wolfer J. Psychological preparation for surgical pediatric patients: the effect of children's and parents' stress responses and adjustments. *Pediatrics* 1975;56:187.
4. LaRosa PA, Murphy JA, Wade JA, Clasby LL. Implementing a parent present induction program. *AORN J* 1995;61:526.
5. Ellerton M, Merriam C. Preparing children and families psychologically for day surgery: an evaluation. *J Adv Nurs* 1994;19:1057.
6. Zieglar DB, Prior MM. Preparation for surgery and adjustment to hospitalization. *Pediatr Surg Nurs* 1994;29:655.
7. Burnstein S, Meichenbaum D. The work of worrying in children undergoing surgery. *J Abnorm Child Psychol* 1979;7:121.
8. Azarnoff P. Teaching materials for pediatric health professionals. *J Pediatr Health Care* 1990;4:282.
9. O'Malley ME, McNamara ST. Children's drawings: a preoperative assessment tool. *AORN J* 1993; 57:1074.
10. Mott SR, James SR, Sperhac AM. *Nursing care of children and families*, 2nd ed. Redwood City, CA: Addison-Wesley, 1990.
11. Petrillo M, Sanger S. *Emotional care of the hospitalized child*. Philadelphia: JB Lippincott, 1980.
12. Waechter EH, Blake FG. *Nursing care of children*, 9th ed. Philadelphia: JB Lippincott, 1976.
13. Frankville D. Preparing children for anesthesia and surgery. *West J Med* 1995;162:52.
14. Squires VL. Child-focused perioperative education: helping children understand and cope for surgery. *Semin Periop Nurs* 1995;4:80.
15. Lynch M. Preparing children for day surgery. *Child Health Care* 1994; 23:75.
16. Wolfer J, Visintainer M. Pre-hospital psychological preparation for tonsillectomy patients: effects on children's and parents' adjustment. *Pediatrics* 1979;64:646.
17. Meng A. Parents' and children's reaction toward impending hospitalization for surgery. *Maternal-Child Nurs J* 1980;9:83.
18. Poland ML, Evans TN. Psychological aspects of vaginal agenesis. *J Reprod Med* 1985;30:340.
19. Manley S, deKelaita G, et al. Preoperative pregnancy testing in ambulatory surgery. *Anesthesiology* 1995;83:690.
20. Azzam FJ, Padda GS, DeBoard JW, et al. Preoperative pregnancy testing in adolescents. *Anesth Analg* 1996;82:4.
21. Pierre N, Moy LK, Redd S, et al. Evaluation of a pregnancy testing protocol in adolescents undergoing surgery. *J Pediatr Adolesc Gynecol* 1998;11:139.
22. Horne DJ, Vatmanidis P, Careri A. Preparing patients for invasive medical and surgical procedures. 2: using psychological interventions with adults and children. *Behav Med* 1994;20:15.

11

Vulvovaginal Complaints in the Adolescent

Vaginitis represents a common gynecologic problem in the adolescent despite the fact that she has developed a more resistant, estrogenized vaginal epithelium; pubic hair; and labial fat pads. The striking difference between prepubertal and adolescent vaginitis is the shift in etiology. Vulvovaginitis in the prepubertal child is often nonspecific and results from poor perineal hygiene, whereas vaginitis in the adolescent usually has a specific cause, often related to sexual contact. Vaginal discharge may also be the presenting symptom in the adolescent with cervicitis secondary to *Neisseria gonorrhoeae*, *Chlamydia trachomatis*, or herpes simplex. In addition to these true infections, physiologic leukorrhea, a normal desquamation of epithelial cells secondary to estrogen effect, is probably the most common discharge in the pubescent girl.

This chapter includes a description of the various causes of vaginitis as well as of vulvar disease, toxic shock, and the urethral syndrome. Infections with *N. gonorrhoeae* and *C. trachomatis* are covered in Chapter 12 and human papillomavirus (HPV) in Chapter 13.

VAGINAL DISCHARGE

The evaluation of vaginal discharge in the adolescent should include a history of symptoms (pruritus, odor, quantity), other illnesses such as diabetes or human immunodeficiency virus (HIV) infection, recent oral medications such as broad-spectrum antibiotics or oral contraceptive pills (OCs), previous similar episodes of vulvovaginal symptoms, and treatments. A history of broad-spectrum antibiotics or poorly controlled diabetes mellitus is frequently a clue to the diagnosis of *Candida* vaginitis. Candida vaginitis and bacterial vaginosis often recur despite compliance with a standard treatment course. The patient should be questioned about recent sexual relations, since treatment failure in an adolescent girl often occurs because of reexposure to an untreated contact. It should be remembered that several infections may coexist; a patient may be adequately treated for one infection and still have a second or third infection. For example, an adolescent may have *C. trachomatis* cervicitis, *Trichomonas* vaginitis, and vulvar condyloma. In addition, the use of oral broad-spectrum antibiotics for the treatment of the vaginitis may be followed by a second infection with *Candida.*

An adolescent may have symptoms for weeks or months before seeking medical help because of anxiety about a pelvic examination or because of guilt or trauma from a previous episode of rape, intercourse, or sexual abuse. Therefore, it is important to explain carefully to her both the details of the pelvic examination and the possible causes of vaginal discharge.

The microbiologic flora of the adolescent vagina and cervix are shown in Fig. 1 (1). Assessment usually includes a speculum examination to obtain specimens of the vaginal discharge for wet preparations, pH, and in sexually active patients endocervical tests for *N. gonorrhoeae* and *C. trachomatis* (see Chapters 1 and 12). A speculum examination is usually omitted in the virginal adolescent 12 to 13 years old who has a whitish mucoid discharge, since samples for wet preparations obtained with a saline-moistened, cotton-tipped applicator or Calgiswab gently inserted through the hymenal opening are sufficient to confirm the diagnosis of leukorrhea and exclude candida. Recent studies have focused on whether vaginal complaints can be diagnosed on the basis of urine testing for gonorrhea and *Chlamydia* and provider- or patient-obtained vaginal swabs for wet preps, pH, and *Trichomonas* culture. Other studies have found that adult women can be successful at obtaining introital samples (a dacron swab placed 1 inch into the distal vagina for 10 seconds) that have a high sensitivity and specificity for detection of

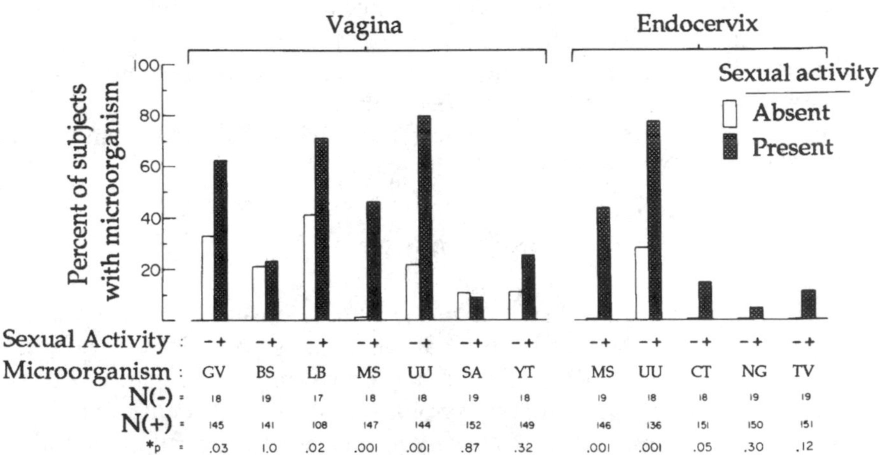

FIG. 1. Microbiologic isolations from vagina and endocervix in adolescent girls by presence or absence of sexual activity. BS, group B streptococcus; CT, *Chlamydia trachomatis*; GV, *Gardnerella vaginalis*; LB, lactobacillus; MS, *Mycoplasma* species; NG, *Neisseria gonorrhoeae*; SA, *Staphylococcus aureus*; TV, *Trichomonas vaginalis*; UU, *Ureaplasma urealyticum*; YT, yeast. *Chi-square statistic except for CT, NG, and TV Fischer exact test. (From Shafer MA, Sweet RL, Ohm-Smith MJ. Microbiology of the lower genital tract in postmenarcheal adolescent girls: Differences by sexual activity, contraception, and presence of nonspecific vaginitis. *J Pediatr* 1985;107:974; with permission.)

gonorrhea, *Chlamydia,* and *Trichomonas* (2). Although there may be some advantages to this approach, adolescents may provide less adequate vaginal pool self-sampling, the vulva is not visualized (the patient may have a dermatoses, condyloma accuminata, or genital herpes as an etiology for symptoms), and lesions of the cervix and vagina would be missed. Thus careful selection of patients with vaginitis who might be appropriate for this methodology is important.

Inspection of the vulva is often helpful in the differential diagnosis of vulvovaginitis. A small magnifying glass can be of immense help. A red, edematous vulva with satellite red papules is characteristic of acute *Candida* vulvovaginitis. Fissures and excoriations are seen with subacute or chronic *Candida* infections. Vulvar dermatoses may present with red, scaly, cutaneous plaques (Table 1). Small vesicles or ulcers are typical of herpetic vulvitis. Symptomatic gonococcal cervicitis and pelvic inflammatory disease (PID) may be accompanied by a greenish yellow discharge from the vagina and urethra.

The appearance of the vaginal secretions often gives a clue to the diagnosis. A thick, curdy discharge is typical of *Candida*; a yellow or white, bubbly, frothy discharge can be typical of *Trichomonas vaginalis*. In patients with *Trichomonas* infections and those with cervicitis, the cervix may be friable and may bleed during collection of the samples. A cervical ectropion is present in many adolescents; large ectropions may be responsible for persistent vaginal discharge in adolescents, even in the absence of infection. Cervical ectopy has been associated with younger age, *C. trachomatis*, and OC use (3). Mucopurulent cervicitis (MPC) is variably defined by the presence of mucopurulent discharge, quantitation of leukocytes in cervical exudate, easily induced cervical bleeding, and histologic examination of the cervix. The Centers for Disease Control and Prevention (CDC) definition of MPC is the presence of mucopurulent secretion visible in the endocervical canal or on an endocervical swab. Mucopus is evident if a yellow color is noted on a white cotton-tipped applicator inserted into the endocervical canal and twirled; the yellow color is associated with *C. trachomatis* cervicitis in clinics that treat sexually transmitted diseases (STDs). *N. gonorrhoeae* may also cause MPC, but often other infectious agents, not yet well defined, cause persistent mucopus.

Microscopic examination of the wet preparations usually provides the diagnosis (see Chapter 1, and Figs. 2 and 3). On the saline preparation slide, trichomonads are seen as motile flagellated organisms. Sheets of epithelial cells are characteristic of leukorrhea. So-called clue cells (epithelial cells coated with large numbers of refractile bacteria that obscure the cell borders) are seen in bacterial vaginosis. The potassium hydroxide (KOH) preparation is used to demonstrate the pseudohyphae of *Candida*. If the discharge is itchy or cheesy and yet no pseudohyphae are seen on the KOH preparation, a culture for *Candida* on Biggy agar is helpful.

Large numbers of leukocytes may be seen in the presence of *Trichomonas*, to a lesser extent with *Candida* vaginitis, and with cervicitis. The presence of leukocytes in the absence of a diagnosis suggests that further tests and a followup visit in 2 weeks may be necessary. For example, the wet preparation may miss the diagnosis of *Trichomonas* because of a sensitivity of only 50% to 75%.

TABLE 1. *Differential diagnosis of the vulvar dermatoses*

Condition	Clinical appearance	Diagnostic test	Therapy
Psoriasis	Red plaques with silvery scale; also on knees, elbows, scalp; nail pitting	Clinical appearance; cutaneous biopsy;	Topical steroids (triamcinolone 0.1%); systemic antimetabolite Rx if severe
Seborrheic dermatitis	Scaling/erythema; also on eyebrows; nasolabial folds, hairline, occasional axillae	Clinical appearance; KOH preparation of scale negative	Dandruff shampoos, hydrocortisone 1% cream
Dermatophyte (tinea cruris)	Annular plaque with central clearing and peripheral scale	KOH preparation of of scale positive	Topical imidazole creams bid until clear for 1 week
Chronic dermatitis (contact or irritant)	Often eczematous and oozing; may involve congruent areas; eyelids; may generalize	Careful history and patch testing if indicated	Cool compresses, Crisco or hydrocortisone 2.5% ointment, no allergens
Lichen simplex chronicus	Thick, furrowed vulva; other common sites are ankle, arm, or nape of neck	Cutaneous biopsy	Triamcinolone 0.1% ointment for 4–6 weeks; rule out vaginal *Candida*
Lichen planus	"Purple polygonal papules and plaques," lacy white pattern or erosions on oral and vulvar mucosa, wrists, shins common	Cutaneous biopsy	Topical steroids: cream or suppositories (clobetasol × 1–2 weeks, taper to hydrocortisone 1%)
Lichen sclerosus	White, wrinkly; usually only vulva, anus ("keyhole" pattern); dermis thick, epidermis atrophic; occasional patchy on trunk	Clinical appearance, cutaneous biopsy	Topical steroids (clobetasol x 2 weeks, then taper, 1% hydrocortisone ointment or cream); emollients, hygiene

(Adapted from McKay M. Vulvitis and vulvovaginitis: cutaneous considerations. *Am J Obstet Gynecol* 1991;165:1176; with permission.)

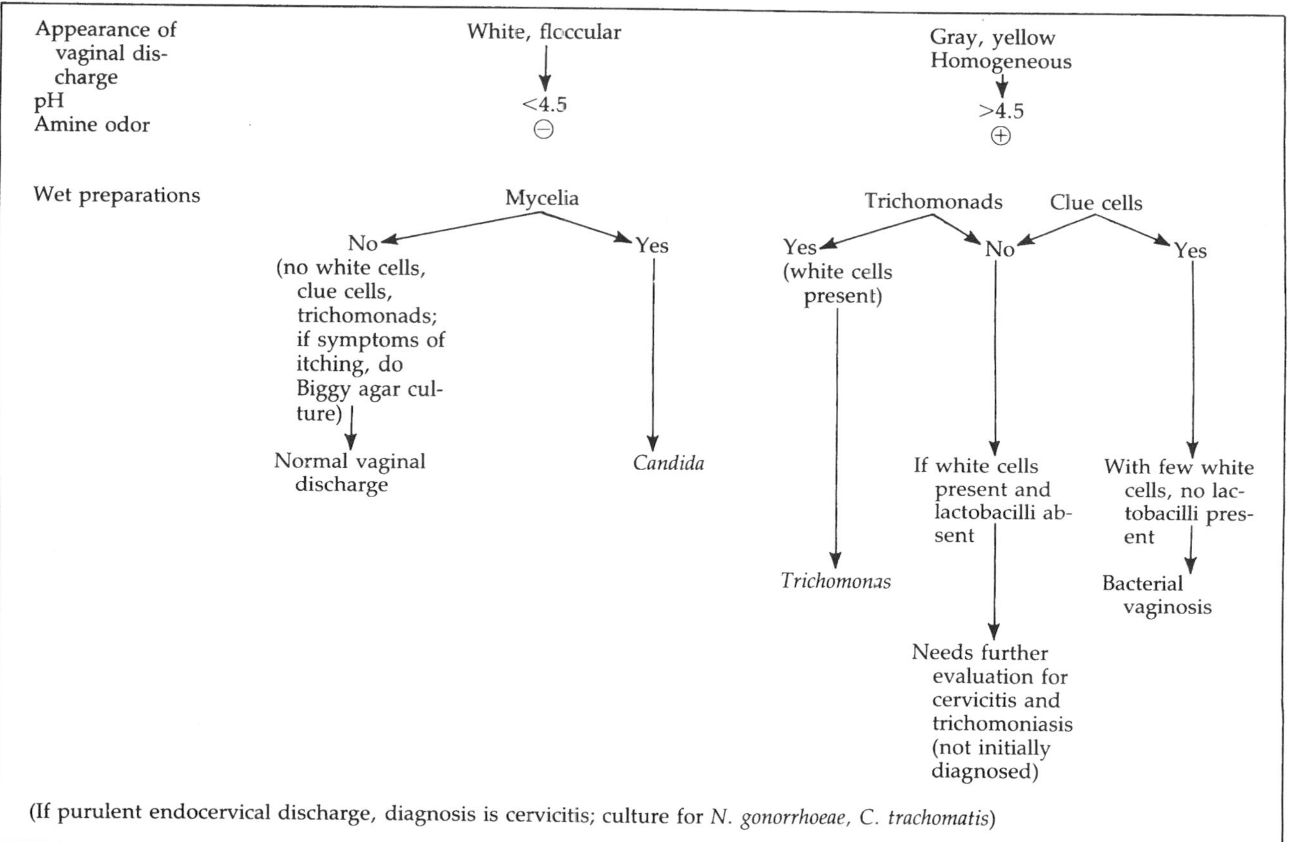

FIG. 2. Differential diagnosis of vaginitis.

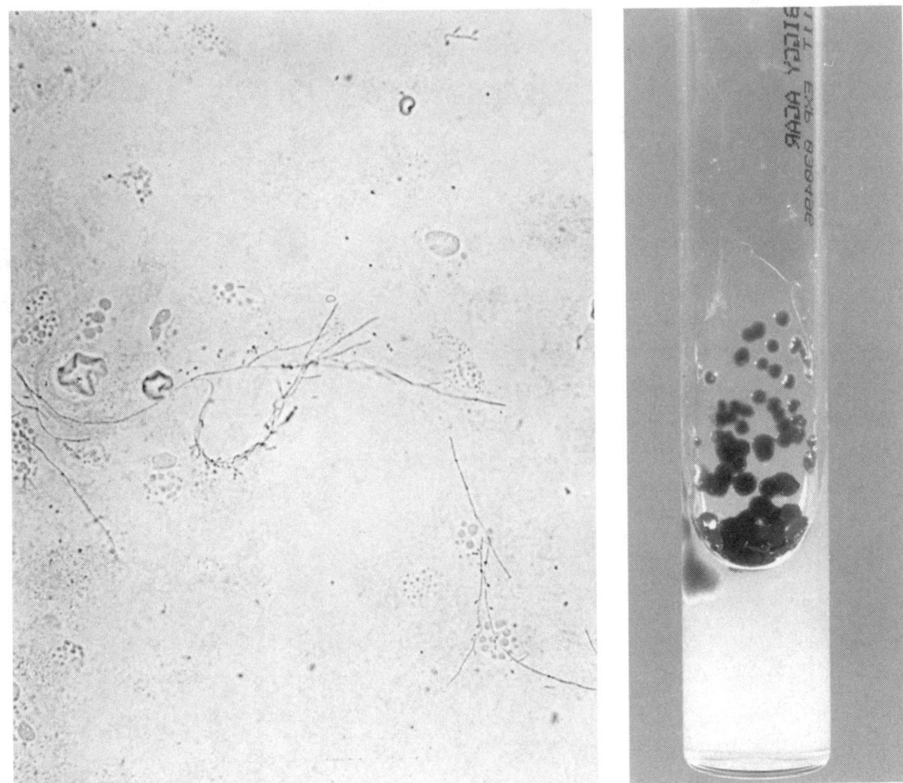

FIG. 3. *Candida* vaginitis. **(A)** Potassium hydroxide preparation showing pseudohyphae. (From Syntex slide collection, Palo Alto, CA; with permission.) **(B)** Biggy agar culture with multiple brown colonies.

An amine fishy odor when a drop of discharge is mixed with 10% KOH is a positive "whiff" test result; it occurs most commonly with bacterial vaginosis but may sometimes occur with *Trichomonas* as well. The pH of the vaginal secretions is helpful in the differential diagnosis. A normal pH of <4.5 is found in patients with normal leukorrhea and *Candida* vaginitis, whereas the pH is elevated above 4.5 (4.7 in some studies) in patients with *Trichomonas* vaginitis and bacterial vaginosis. Gram stain of the vaginal discharge can be used to identify lactobacilli, typical of normal discharge, and to detect alterations in the flora seen in bacterial vaginosis in which gram-variable coccobacilli and curved gram-negative rods are observed. Gram stain of the endocervical mucopus can be examined for increased numbers of polymorphonuclear leukocytes and the presence of gram-negative intracellular diplococci (see Chapter 12). Cultures or tests should be done to detect *N. gonorrhoeae* and *C. trachomatis* in sexually active adolescents.

The Papanicolaou (Pap) smear can also be helpful in the diagnosis. Herpes simplex is associated with intranuclear inclusions and multinucleate giant cells, and HPV with koilocytosis, squamous atypia, and squamous intraepithelial lesions. *Chlamydia* has been associated with inflammation, cytoplasmic inclusions, and transformed lymphocytes or increased histiocytes. *Trichomonas* may be seen on Pap smear, but false-positive smears are not infrequent and should be confirmed with a wet preparation or culture in the asymptomatic patient. The Pap smear has been noted to have a sensitivity of 17% to 58% for the detection of *C. trachomatis,* 3% to 49% for *Candida,* 25% for bacterial vaginosis, 33% to 79% for *Trichomonas,* and 25% to 66% for herpes simplex (4). In a study of STD patients, Paavonen and colleagues (5) found on colposcopic evaluation that endocervical mucopus was associated with *N. gonorrhoeae*, *C. trachomatis*, and herpes simplex; ulcers, necrotic areas, and increased surface vascularity with herpes simplex; strawberry cervix (uniformly arranged red spots or stippling of a few millimeters in size, located on the squamous epithelium covering the ectocervix) with *Trichomonas*; hypertrophic cervicitis with *C. trachomatis*; and immature metaplasia with *C. trachomatis* and cytomegalovirus.

Therapy is aimed at the specific cause. Patients should avoid douches, because douching has been associated with an increased risk of PID. When one STD has been detected, the clinician should test the patient for others, including serology for syphilis. Counseling about prevention, abstinence, safer sex, and the use of condoms is essential.

In most situations, therapy should include the following:

1. Warm baths once or twice a day (baking soda may be added if the vulva is irritated). Only bland soaps should be used.
2. Careful drying after the bath and application of a small amount of baby powder (no talc) to the vulva.
3. Frequent changes of white cotton underpants or panty shields to absorb the discharge.
4. Good perineal hygiene (including wiping from front to back after bowel movements).
5. Avoidance of bubble bath or other chemical irritants.

Leukorrhea

Agent: A normal estrogen effect.

Symptoms: A whitish mucoid discharge that usually starts before menarche and may continue for several years. With the establishment of more regular cycles, the adolescent may notice a cyclic variation in vaginal secretions: copious watery secretions at midcycle and then a stickier, scantier discharge in the second half of the cycle associated with rising progesterone levels.

Diagnosis: The wet preparation reveals epithelial cells without evidence of inflammation.

Treatment: Most health classes that discuss puberty and menarche do not include an explanation of the change in vaginal secretions. The clinician can reassure the patient by explaining vaginal physiology and can suggest measures to help if she is bothered by the discharge—baths, cotton underpants, and, as needed, some form of panty shield that she can change frequently. If an older adolescent is troubled by excessive discharge, especially during jogging or athletics, evaluation of the cervix and vagina may be indicated. The use of a conventional tampon (not a superabsorbent tampon) during athletics for a few hours at midcycle can help the adolescent cope with the heavy discharge. It is extremely important that she not be overtreated with vaginal creams and given the impression that the leukorrhea represents an infection. It is also important to discourage the daily use of tampons because of the possibility of vaginal ulcers.

Trichomonal Vaginitis

Agent: Trichomonas vaginalis, a small, motile, flagellated parasite.

Symptoms: Frothy, malodorous, yellow or white discharge that may cause itching, dysuria, postcoital bleeding, dyspareunia, or any combination of these symptoms. May be asymptomatic and found on culture, Pap smear, or wet preparation (6,7).

Source: Usually sexually acquired. Males are usually asymptomatic but may reinfect the female after she is treated. Since *Trichomonas* may survive for several hours in urine and wet towels, the possibility of transmission by sharing washcloths has been suggested but not proved; it is unlikely to occur frequently, given the association of this infection with other sexually transmitted diseases. The incubation time has been estimated to be between 4 and 20 days with an average of 7 days. The incidence of *Trichomonas* has decreased over the past two decades (8).

Diagnosis: The vulva may be erythematous or excoriated, with a visible discharge evident on inspection. The classic yellow-green discharge is seen in 20% to 35% of patients; more often the discharge is gray or white. A frothy discharge is seen in about 10% of women and may also occur with bacterial vaginosis. Grossly visible punctate hemorrhages and swollen papillae (strawberry cervix) are seen in only about 2% of patients (15% of a STD population evaluated by colposcopy). By colposcopy, this special finding had a 45% sensitivity and a 99% specificity for *Trichomonas* (5).

The wet preparation may show flagellated organisms dancing under the coverslip along with an increase in the number of leukocytes, which can be visualized using both low and high power of the microscope (6–13). The vaginal wet mount is far from a perfect tool; it detects 64% of infections in asymptomatically infected women, 75% of those with clinical vaginitis, and 80% of those with characteristic symptoms. Philip and coworkers (14) found that the wet mount gave a positive result only in patients whose cultures had $>10^5$ colony forming units/ml. The use of Feinberg-Whittington or Diamond culture has a sensitivity of 86% to 97%. Pap smears have a detection rate of only 50% to 86%, and false-positive results can occur. If asymptomatic women are treated only on the basis of a positive Pap smear, 20% to 30% may be treated unnecessarily (12). Monoclonal antibody staining has been reported to detect 86% of positive specimens, including 92% of those with positive wet mounts and 77% of those missed on wet mount (9). The InPouch TV system also has a better sensitivity than the wet mount. Bacterial vaginosis and *Trichomonas* vaginitis may occur simultaneously, and *Trichomonas* facilitates the growth of anaerobic bacteria (15).

Treatment: Metronidazole, 2.0 g orally all in one dose, is effective in 86% to 95% of patients (16,17). It is important that the sexual partner be treated with the same dose at the same time. The side effects of metronidazole include nausea, vomiting, headache, metallic aftertaste, and rarely blood dyscrasias. The patient should be instructed to avoid alcohol and intercourse until both partners have been treated. If the clinician does not wish to provide treatment for the partner, the partner can be referred to his own clinician (although trichomonads are difficult to document in the male).

If the organisms persist in the vagina after two courses of single-dose metronidazole, and if reinfection is not the cause, a longer course of metronidazole can be tried: 500 mg orally twice daily for 7 days. Recurrent infection necessitates retreating the partner and making sure the relationship is monogamous; otherwise, the patient should understand the futility of repeated treatment.

Rarely, a patient will have a *Trichomonas* infection that has relative resistance to metronidazole and is refractory to treatment (9,18,19). The patient can be treated with 2 g/day of metronidazole orally for 3 to 5 days. Patients not responding to the regimen should be managed in consultation with an expert, and the susceptibility of the *Trichomonas* to metronidazole should be determined. Lossick and colleagues (18) reported the need for an average oral dose of 2.6 g/day of metronidazole for a mean period of 9 days to cure refractory *Trichomonas*. Neurologic side effects are common if >3 g is taken orally in a day. A complete blood count should be done before prolonged therapy is undertaken.

Pregnancy: No birth defects have been associated with the drug (20). Patients with symptoms may be treated with a single 2-g dose of metronidazole.

Candida Vaginitis

Agent: Candida albicans accounts for 60% to 80% of vaginal fungal infections; other *Candida* species, including *Candida glabrata* (20%) and *Candida tropicalis* (6% to 23%), also cause similar symptoms (8,21,22). Non-*albicans* species may be more difficult to eradicate with current therapies.

Symptoms: Thick, white, cheesy, pruritic discharge. The vulva may be red and edematous. Itching may occur before and after menses and, in some patients, seems to remit at midcycle. Patients may experience dyspareunia with an increase in symptoms after intercourse. Many patients have external irritation and dysuria.

Source: The predisposing factors to *Candida* vaginitis include diabetes mellitus, pregnancy, antibiotics, corticosteroids, obesity, and tight-fitting undergarments. The frequency of positive cultures rises from 2.2% to 16% by the end of pregnancy. The increase in clinical infections appears to be associated with the rise in pH that occurs in late pregnancy as well as premenstrually (23). Infections are more common in the summer. *Candida* may occur as part of the normal flora in 10% to 20% of women; eradication of *Candida* as determined by culture, however, appears to be important in patients with frequent recurrences. Recurrent *Candida* vaginitis may be the first presenting symptom of HIV disease in women.

Candida is not seen more commonly in STD clinics than in other settings, and sexual transmission rarely plays a role (24,25). Males may have symptomatic balanitis or penile dermatitis.

Diagnosis: The vulva is usually red and may be edematous, with small satellite red papules or fissures at the posterior forchette. The KOH preparation shows filamentous forms in 80% to 90% of symptomatic patients (Fig. 3A). In patients with suggestive signs or symptoms and especially in patients previously labeled as having recurrent *Candida* infections, it is important to obtain specimens for culture from the vagina before more aggressive therapy is undertaken. The easiest office culture medium is Biggy agar, which can be read for the presence of brown colonies after 3 to 7 days of incubation (Fig. 3B). Sabouraud agar can also be used. Most patients with symptomatic infections have a large number of colonies; however, even a few colonies may be significant in the woman with frequent infections who has recently finished a treatment course. In cases difficult to diagnose, the patient may be shown how to inoculate a culture at home with a cotton-tipped applicator when her symptoms increase.

Treatment: The options for therapy include intravaginal preparations and oral agents. The azoles are the mainstay of intravaginal treatment. Courses of therapy range from a single dose to 3 to 7 days of therapy with creams or suppositories for uncomplicated infections (mild to moderate, sporadic, normal host, susceptible *Candida albicans*). Complicated infections (severe local or recurrent infections in an abnormal host or less susceptible pathogen such as *Candida glabrata*) require 10–14 days of topical or oral azoles. The suppositories are less messy but may not treat vulvar infection as well. The symptomatic male partner can use the cream as well. Some packaging contains both suppositories and cream (e.g., Monistat Dual-Pak, Gynelotrimen Combination Pack). The efficacy of treatment, as judged by symptomatic improvement and negative cultures after any of the available treatment courses with azoles, is approximately 85% to 90% at the end of therapy and 70% to 80% 3 weeks later. Allergic symptoms to the azoles are often manifested by increased burning and itching after several days of therapy. Nystatin is probably less effective because it requires the patient to comply with 2 weeks of therapy; however, it is useful in women who develop allergic symptoms to the azoles. A small study found topical boric acid (600 mg powder in a gelatin capsule administered intravaginally once daily for 14 days) to yield a moderate success rate in women with *T. glabrata*, which has been more difficult to treat with some antifungal creams (26). The intravaginal treatment doses are as follows (27–31):

Clotrimazole, 100-mg vaginal tablet for 7 nights*
Clotrimazole, 200-mg vaginal tablets for 3 nights*
Clotrimazole, 1% cream, one applicatorful (5 g) for 7 nights*
Clotrimazole, 500-mg vaginal tablet for 1 night
Miconazole, 200-mg vaginal suppository for 3 nights*
Miconazole, 100-mg vaginal suppository for 7 nights*
Miconazole, 2% cream, one applicatorful (5 g) for 7 nights*
Butaconazole, 2% cream, one applicatorful (5 g) for 3 nights*
Tioconazole, 6.5% ointment, one applicatorful (4.6 g) for 1 night*
Terconazole, 0.4% cream, 1 applicatorful (5 g) for 7 nights
Terconazole, 0.8% cream, 1 applicatorful (5 g) for 3 nights
Terconazole, 80-mg vaginal suppository for 3 nights
Nystatin, 100,000-unit vaginal tablet for 14 nights

The base of some of these suppositories and creams may interact with latex products, including diaphragms and condoms, and thus the patient should be informed of this possibility.

Oral therapy with fluconazole 150 mg given as a single dose has the same efficacy as 3- and 7-day courses of the azole antifungal topical agents (32–35). The reported adverse effects of oral therapy have included headache (13%), nausea (7%), and abdominal pain (6%); rare cases of angioedema, anaphylaxis, and hepatotoxicity have been reported. The important drug interactions include those with terfenadine, rifampin, astemizole, phenytoin, cyclosporin A, coumarin-like agents, oral hypoglycemic agents, and possibly OCs (34,36). In contrast, the primary side effects of topical agents are local burning and dysuria. Patients may prefer the ease of a single oral dose but should be counseled about the risks and benefits. For complicated infections, fluconazole can be given on days 1, 4, and 7.

Only topical agents should be used during pregnancy (for significant symptoms); treatments that have been studied for use in the second and third trimesters include clotrimazole, miconazole, butoconazole, and terconazole. Absorption is negligible with tioconazole and clotrimazole and does not occur with nystatin (37). Pregnant patients should be treated for 7 days.

Recurrent vulvovaginal candidiasis, defined as four or more symptomatic episodes annually, can be very difficult to treat. The most important issue is to make sure that the diagnosis is in fact *Candida*. Patients may have inflammation of the minor vestibular glands, HPV infection, or allergies to soaps, spermicides, or rarely semen. Once the diagnosis of *Candida* has been confirmed, the clini-

*Available over the counter.

cian should check for predisposing factors such as diabetes. Looser-fitting clothing and nondeodorized panty shields can be recommended. Any douching equipment should be cultured or discarded. The potential for a gastrointestinal reservoir in the patient or partner should be considered. In addition, the patient may not have purchased the medication because of cost or may not have finished the previously prescribed dosage. In adolescents with recurrent *Candida* infections and risk factors, HIV infection should be considered.

Many patients who have experienced frequent recurrences of *Candida* vulvovaginitis in the past can be maintained symptom free with *one* of the following treatments: vaginal clotrimazole (100 mg) 6 days a month *or* vaginal clotrimazole (500 mg) once a month *or* an antifungal vaginal cream for 2 to 3 days before and after each menses *or* a vaginal cream "always on Sunday" *or* a vaginal cream for 1 to 3 days at the first sign of itching or other symptoms. While prophylactic monthly clotrimazole treatment results in fewer episodes over a 6-month period, empiric self-treatment for symptoms is less expensive and is preferred by many (38).

Ketoconazole, itraconazole, and fluconazole have been studied as agents for chronic or recurrent candidiasis in women with a decrease in symptomatic recurrences. The doses given have included 400 mg of ketoconazole for 5 days at the onset of each menses for six cycles, 100 mg of ketoconazole daily for 6 months (39), 200 mg of intraconazole once monthly for 6 months (40), and fluconazole once weekly or once monthly (37). Relapse after treatment is common even with long-term oral therapy, and the risks of using these and other oral agents needs to be carefully considered because of their potential for hepatotoxicity. Sexual partners are treated if they have symptomatic balanitis or penile dermatitis.

Bacterial Vaginosis

Agent: Bacterial vaginosis (BV) results from the complex alteration of microbial flora of the vagina. Although *Gardnerella vaginalis* is found in most patients with this diagnosis, it is also found in many asymptomatic patients, including nonsexually experienced young women. Bacterial vaginosis results from an increased concentration of *G. vaginalis,* anaerobic organisms (especially *Bacteroides* and *Mobiluncus* species) and *Mycoplasma hominis* with an absence of normal hydrogen peroxide–producing lactobacilli (13,41–46). The overgrowth results in an elevated vaginal pH and the production of amines, putrescine and cadaverine, which cause the typical fishy malodor that patients experience. Gas-liquid chromatographic studies show an increase in acetate, proprionate, isobutyrate, butyrate, and isovalerate, with an increase in the succinate/lactate ratio of 0.4. Bacterial vaginosis occurs in 4% to 15% of college students, 10% to 25% of pregnant women, and 30% to 37% of women attending an STD clinic. The presence of BV has been associated with postpartum endometritis, premature labor and premature rupture of membranes, preterm delivery of low-birthweight infants, irregular menstrual bleeding, and PID (especially following invasive procedures) (46–48). The treatment of bacterial vaginosis with metronidazole or a combination of metronidazole and erythromycin appears to be effective in reducing preterm births in patients with a history of prematurity in the previous pregnancy (49,50)

Symptoms: Malodorous discharge; associated symptoms may be abdominal pain and irregular or prolonged menses.

Source: Usually occurs in sexually active patients. Risk factors have included the presence of an intrauterine device, prior STD, smoking, low socioeconomic status, and an uncircumcised partner. The anaerobes associated with bacterial vaginosis are commonly found in the rectum of women with this diagnosis (51). Although the urethra of males can be colonized with similar anaerobic organisms, the use of a condom for 2 weeks eliminates the organisms in most men (51).

Diagnosis: The pelvic examination reveals a homogeneous, malodorous, yellow, white, or gray discharge adherent to the vaginal walls, in contrast to the normal clumped or floccular discharge. Three of four criteria should be met to make the clinical diagnosis: (a) homogeneous white noninflammatory discharge adherent to the vaginal walls, (b) pH ≥4.5 [in one study, pH ≥4.7 (42)]; (c) positive "whiff" test result (a fishy or amine odor noted before or after addition of 1 drop of 10% KOH to a sample of the vaginal discharge); and (d) the presence of clue cells, making up at least 20% of the cells (Fig. 4).

Gram stain of the vaginal discharge can also be useful (44,45,52). A positive determination is made if four or fewer lactobacilli are seen per oil immersion field and if *Gardnerella* morphologic types plus one or more other bacterial morphologic types (gram-positive cocci, small gram-negative rods, curved gram-variable rod, or fusiforms) are detected. Making a diagnosis only on the basis of Gram stain findings or a Pap smear may result in overdiagnosis of bacterial vaginosis (8). In a high-prevalence STD clinic population, the Gram stain had a 97% sensitivity, 79% specificity, and 69% positive predictive value for bacterial vaginosis (42). Homogeneous discharge was found in 69%, pH ≥4.7 in 97%, positive "whiff" test result in 43%, and clue cells (≥20% of epithelial cells) in 78% of patients with bacterial vaginosis. The "whiff" test was the least sensitive test, and the pH was the least specific test, since 47% of patients without bacterial vaginosis had elevated pH. A pH of ≤4.4 and a predominance of lactobacilli on wet mount or Gram stain are useful in excluding the diagnosis of bacterial vaginosis. The finding of clue cells on Pap smears can be moderately sensitive and specific for BV, and most clinicians treat the adolescent who has symptoms, atypia, or other abnormalities on the Pap smear. Cultures for *G. vaginalis* are not helpful and should not be obtained in diagnosing this condition.

Treatment: Treatment is usually prescribed only to symptomatic women. However, because of the link between BV and PID and invasive procedures, as well as the evidence that metronidazole reduces postabortion PID, the treatment of symptomatic and asymptomatic BV may be considered before surgical abor-

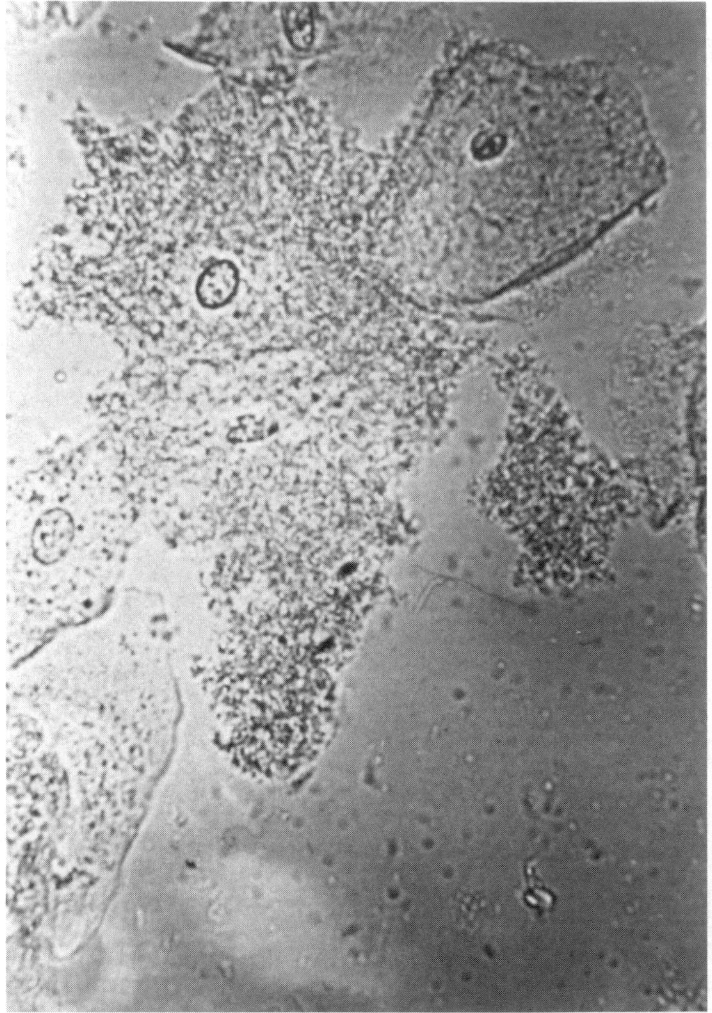

FIG. 4. Clue cells in bacterial vaginosis. (From Syntex slide collection, Palo Alto, CA; with permission.)

tion procedures are performed (37,47). The standard therapies for nonpregnant patients are oral metronidazole, 500 mg twice a day for 7 days, which results in cure rates of 95% (53,54); clindamycin cream 2%, one applicatorful (5 g) intravaginally at bedtime for 7 days; or metronidazole gel 0.75%, one applicatorful (5 g) intravaginally once or twice a day for 5 days (55). Alternatives are clindamycin 300 mg, orally twice a day for 7 days (56) or single-dose metronidazole (2 g), which is less effective (84%, with a range of 67% to 90%), especially if followup is done at 3 weeks instead of just 1 week after the completion of therapy (54,57–59). Treatment of the partner with metronidazole has not diminished recurrences in the woman and is not recommended (60–62). Condoms should be recommended for several weeks, with the hope of altering flora. Recurrences are common in the year following treatment, and to date no method for recolonizing the vagina with lactobacilli has been proved effective.

Low-risk pregnant women with symptomatic BV should be treated with metronidazole 250 mg 3 times a day for 7 days (alternatives: metronidazole 2 g single dose; clindamycin 300 mg twice a day; or metronidazole gel). Clindamycin gel is not recommended during pregnancy, and data on metronidazole gel are limited. Asymptomatic high-risk pregnant women (with previous preterm birth) may be screened in the second trimester and treated (36).

Vaginitis Secondary to a Foreign Body

Agent: In adolescents, usually a retained tampon.

Symptoms: Foul-smelling, often bloody discharge.

Diagnosis: Examination.

Treatment: Removal of the foreign body and irrigation of the vagina with warm water.

Gonorrhea

Agent: Neisseria gonorrhoeae.

Symptoms: Often asymptomatic. In symptomatic patients, *N. gonorrhoeae* may cause a purulent vaginal discharge from cervicitis, urethritis, PID, proctitis, pharyngitis, or arthritis (see Chapter 12).

Source: Sexual contact.

Diagnosis: Culture on Thayer-Martin-Jembec medium, DNA probe test, or other test. Gram stain of the discharge may reveal gram-negative, intracellular diplococci (suggestive but not conclusive evidence of infection in women).

Treatment: See Chapter 12.

Chlamydial Infection

Agent: *Chlamydia trachomatis* serotypes D through K.

Symptoms: The serotypes D through K of *C. trachomatis* have been associated with nongonococcal urethritis in men, and mucopurulent cervicitis, salpingitis, perihepatitis, and the urethral syndrome in women.

Source: Sexually transmitted.

Diagnosis: Culture on McCoy cells; direct immunofluorescent smear (MicroTrak), enzyme immunoassays, DNA probes, ligase chain reaction (LCR), polymerase chain reaction (PCR), and transcription-mediated amplification (TMA) tests (see Chapters 1 and 12).

Treatment: See Chapter 12.

Genital Herpes

Agent: Usually herpes simplex virus type 2 (HSV-2), but 5% to 15% of first episodes are caused by type 1 (HSV-1). Herpes infections can be divided into primary first episodes, in which the patient has no antibody to HSV-1 or HSV-2; nonprimary first episodes, in which the patient does have antibody to one type (usually a type 2 infection with antibodies to type 1); and recurrences. Primary first episodes are responsible for approximately 60% of first episodes and nonprimary infections for the other 40% of first episodes. Three percent of nonprimary first episodes and 2% of recurrences are caused by HSV-1 (63,64).

When Lafferty and associates (65) examined patients with simultaneous oral and genital HSV infections, their results showed that oral labial recurrences occurred in 5 of 12 patients with HSV-1 and 1 of 27 with HSV-2, whereas genital recurrences occurred in 2 of 27 with HSV-1 and 24 of 27 with HSV-2. Mean monthly recurrences were 0.33/month for genital HSV-2, 0.12/month for oral HSV-1, 0.02/month for genital HSV-1, and 0.001/month for oral HSV-2. Over the course of a year after the first episode, 14% of patients with HSV-1 and 60% of those with HSV-2 will have a recurrence. The recurrence rate may decrease after the first year (64–68).

Asymptomatic genital shedding of HSV has been reported in 1.6% to 8.0% of women seen in STD clinics and 0.25 to 1.5% of women seen in private gynecology practices. Although symptomatic patients are most infectious, asymptomatic patients may spread HSV to their sexual partners (69,70). Seroepidemiologic studies in adults have suggested that the prevalence of HSV-2 is greater than was previously thought (<1% in under-15-year-olds to 20% in 30- to 40-year-olds) (71). Twenty-two percent of women attending a family planning clinic (72), 46% of women attending a STD clinic, and 8.8% of university students (73) had serologic evidence of HSV-2 infection. Among the HSV-2–seropositive women in the STD clinic, only 22% had symptoms, 4% had viral shedding without symptoms, 16% had formerly had symptomatic episodes, and 58% had neither shedding nor a history of clinical episodes (74). The characteristic external genital ulcers were present in only 66% of patients with positive HSV cultures. Atypical lesions included fissures, furuncles, excoriations, and nonspecific vulvar erythema. Also, HSV was noted to cause 29 of 33 cervical ulcers; anorectal infections (both symptomatic and asymptomatic) were common. Herpes simplex may occur in 5% of women with dysuria and frequency.

Symptoms: In primary infections, vesicles appear on the labia, vestibule, vagina, and/or cervix; they rupture in 1 to 3 days and produce small painful ulcers. The patient experiences local burning and irritation, dysuria, and inguinal adenopathy. Systemic symptoms are often present, including headache, fever, myalgia, and malaise. Patients may also have neurologic symptoms such as aseptic meningitis, sacral anesthesia, urinary retention, and constipation that may last for 4 to 8 weeks. Anorectal symptoms in primary infections include discharge, pain, and tenesmus. Large numbers of virus are shed from the lesions and, usu-

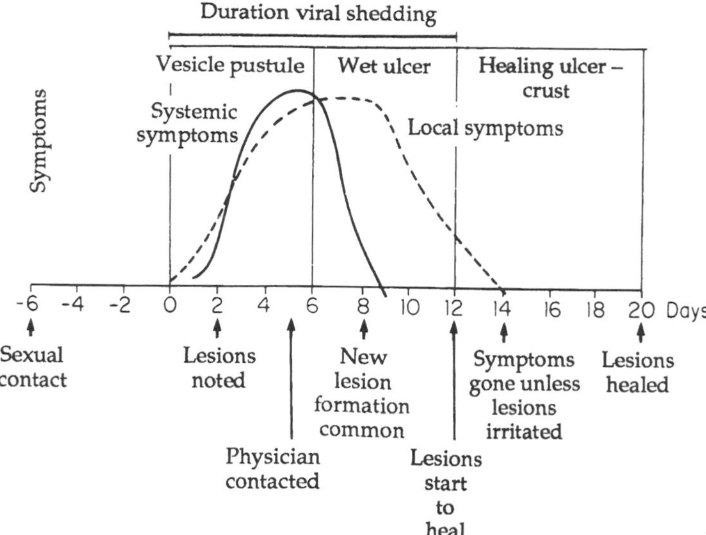

FIG. 5. The clinical course of primary genital herpes. (From Corey L, Adams HG, Brow ZA, et al. Genital herpes simplex virus infections: clinical manifestation, course, and complications. *Ann Intern Med* 1983;98:958; with permission.)

ally, from the cervix. Positive cultures persist for 8 to 10 days and sometimes for as long as 2 weeks. Symptoms improve in 10 days to 3 weeks (Fig. 5).

The symptoms associated with recurrences are less marked and shorter in duration (3 to 5 days) than those of primary infections. The number of lesions is also less, and the lesions are generally external rather than vaginal or cervical and may be atypical (fissures as well as ulcers). The mean healing time was 8.0 ± 2.8 days in a study by Guinan and coworkers (75) of college students. Many patients experience a prodrome of neuralgia in the buttocks, groin, or legs and itching or burning 24 hours before the herpetic lesions recur. Virus is shed in lesser amounts for 4 to 5 days and is usually markedly diminished by the 6th to 7th day.

Nonprimary first-episode infections with HSV have a time course for symptoms and viral shedding that is intermediate between those for primary herpes and recurrent herpes (Fig. 6).

Extragenital sites may occur on the buttocks, groin, thighs, pharynx, fingers, and conjunctiva. HIV-infected patients and other immunocompromised young women may have severe persistent herpes infection and often require prolonged therapy with antiviral agents.

Source: Sexually acquired. The incubation period is 2 to 10 days but may be 1 to 28 days or longer (76). The partner who transmits the genital herpes may be asymptomatic.

Diagnosis: Inspection and cultures. A tender, painful vesicle, pustule, or yellowish ulcer should make the clinician think of HSV. A scraping from the base

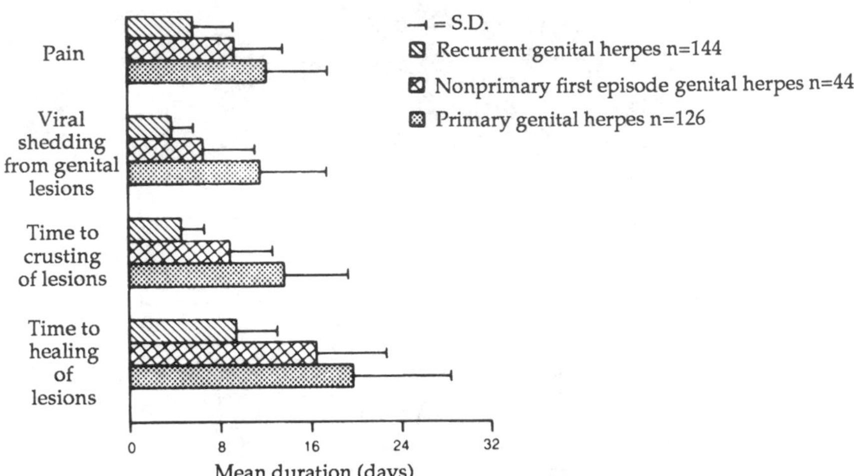

FIG. 6. Comparison of the mean duration of symptoms and signs in female patients with first episode, nonprimary first episode, and recurrent genital herpes. SD, standard deviation. (From Corey L, Adams HG, Brow ZA, et al. Genital herpes simplex virus infections: clinical manifestation, course, and complications. *Ann Intern Med* 1983;98:958; with permission.)

of a lesion, which is stained with Wright's stain (a Tzanck preparation), may reveal multinucleate giant cells and inclusions but the sensitivity is low (30% to 50%). The Pap smear may show characteristic changes of intranuclear inclusions and multinucleated cells (40% to 50% sensitive). Colposcopy of the cervix may reveal ulcers and necrotic areas and increased surface vascularity (68% sensitive and 98.5% specific for the diagnosis of cervical HSV) (5).

The best diagnostic technique is viral culture. The virus grows rapidly, and within several days a definitive diagnosis of HSV-1 or HSV-2 can usually be made (laboratories generally hold the culture for 2 weeks before reporting a negative). The rate of positivity of the culture depends on the timing and the type of infection. For example, HSV can be cultured from 94% of vesicles, 70% of ulcers (82% first episode, 42% recurrent), and 27% of crusted lesions. Culture of the cervix will yield HSV in 80% to 88% of primary first episodes, 65% of nonprimary first episodes, and 12% of recurrent episodes (67,68). In culturing a genital lesion, the vesicle should be unroofed and a sterile swab rubbed vigorously over the base. An ulcer can be similarly swabbed. The swab should then be placed immediately into viral transport media and processed as soon as possible. It is cost effective to swab several lesions and place the separate swabs into the same viral media (74).

Immunofluorescent techniques using fluorescein-labeled anti-HSV are 50% to 60% sensitive, depending in part on the site of sampling; vulvar lesions are more likely to be positive than cervical swabs. The sensitivity of the commercial enzyme immunoassay, Herp Chek direct Herpes Simplex Virus Antigen test, is similar to that of the culture of early vesiculopustular lesions but better than that of the culture of later-stage, crusted lesions (58% Herp Chek positive, 26% culture positive) (77). The test is rapid (5 hours), but it is expensive when single patient samples are run and the test cannot differentiate between HSV-1 and HSV-2. PCR tests are likely to become the preferred method.

Documenting a conversion from negative titer (no antibodies detected) to a positive titer in a previously uninfected patient (no HSV-1 or HSV-2) can be useful in some clinical situations in which cultures are negative and primary infection is suspected. The absence of antibody on two occasions 2 to 3 weeks apart can help eliminate the diagnosis. A rise of IgM antibody followed by IgG antibody is most convincing of recent infection. A fourfold rise in titer is more difficult to interpret because it may indicate a new infection with a different type or a significant recurrence. In addition, the antibody tests done by many commercial laboratories have cross-reactivity between HSV-1 and HSV-2. Assays vary in sensitivity, and thus interpretation can be problematic. Titers with type-specific assays are useful in research settings and for retrospective diagnosis.

Treatment: Antiviral therapy with acyclovir and other similar drugs can shorten the duration of symptoms and viral shedding, prevent the formation of new lesions, and reduce systemic symptoms, but it is not curative and initial therapy does not prevent later recurrences (78–81). Oral acyclovir 200 mg five times a day, or 400 mg three times a day (37), for 7 to 10 days (or until clinical resolution) is recommended for symptomatic primary genital herpes. Acyclovir 400 mg five times a day, or 800 mg three times a day, for 10 days (or until clinical resolution) is recommended for herpes proctitis. Higher doses of acyclovir for genital herpes does not decrease the symptoms or modify the time to first recurrence (82). Valacyclovir 1 g oral twice daily for 10 days and famciclovir 250 mg three times a day for 10 days are effective for first-episode genital herpes. Adjunctive measures include sitz baths in tepid water or Burow's solution, dry heat (low or cool setting on a hair dryer), and/or lidocaine jelly 2% applied to the genital area. Patients may need to void in the shower or into a sitz bath if the lesions cause urinary retention. Analgesics may be necessary, but narcotics have the potential to worsen urinary retention. Occasionally, patients with severe genital lesions and systemic symptoms require hospitalization and treatment with oral or intravenous acyclovir, urinary catheterization, and bed rest. The side effects of intravenous acyclovir include phlebitis and transient reversible elevation of serum creatinine. Care must be taken to ensure adequate hydration. Nausea, vomiting, diarrhea, and headache may occur with intravenous or oral acyclovir. Except in the rare patient who cannot tolerate oral acyclovir, topical acyclovir should not be used. *Candida* vaginitis often accompanies or follows genital HSV.

Recurrences can usually be treated symptomatically with local measures in immunocompetent patients. However, if recurrences are severe and treatment can be started during the prodrome, acyclovir 400 mg three times a day for 5 days, or 800 mg twice a day for 5 days, or 200 mg five times a day for 5 days, valacyclovir 500 mg twice daily for 5 days can be prescribed or famciclovir 125 mg twice a day for 5 days (36,83). Frequent recurrences (at least six times per year) can be suppressed with acyclovir, 400 mg twice a day for 1 year; however, such a course does not change the natural history of HSV, and recurrences usually begin anew after the treatment has ended (80,84). Other options are famciclovir 250 mg twice a day and valacyclovir 250 mg twice a day or 1 g once a day. Toxicity of acyclovir does not appear to be a problem even when treatment lasts as long as 3 years, but treatment should be stopped once a year so that the clinical course can be reassessed. Acyclovir-resistant strains can be recovered from healthy immunocompetent patients but have not been a treatment problem (85). Resistant strains among immunosuppressed and HIV-positive patients require alternative therapy. Acyclovir should not be used for recurrent herpes in pregnancy.

Cultures from pregnant women with a previous history of HSV have not been found to be cost effective in preventing neonatal HSV. Women at high risk of transmitting infection to their newborns are those with a primary infection during the third trimester and those with active genital lesions at the time of vaginal delivery. Unfortunately, many mothers who give birth to babies with severe HSV are asymptomatic. In identifying HSV-2–seropositive patients, a detailed history of genital symptoms has not been found to be superior to a simple question asking the woman whether she has ever had genital herpes (86). The current guidelines of the American College of Obstetrics and Gynecology and the Infectious Disease Society for Obstetrics and Gynecology should be followed.

Patients with genital lesions from HSV should not have intercourse until the lesions heal. Although condoms can prevent the transmission of virus, the location of the lesions makes protection with barrier methods difficult. Patients should be educated about the risk of recurrence, the possibility of transmission (especially with the onset of prodromal symptoms but also during asymptomatic shedding), and the avoidance of self-inoculation to the mouth and fingers. Cultures and tests should be done for other sexually transmitted diseases.

Pediculosis Pubis (Crabs)

Agent: Phthirius pubis (crab lice).

Symptom: Pruritus.

Source: Close physical contact, infested blankets and clothing.

Diagnosis: On inspection, small, moving adult lice or minute, firmly attached flakes (1- to 2-mm nits, eggs) are visible on the pubic hair, often near the base of the hair follicle.

Treatment: 1% permethrin creme rinse (Nix) is applied for 10 minutes and washed off, or 1% lindane shampoo is lathered into the pubic hair, left on for 4 minutes, and then thoroughly washed off (not recommended for pregnant or lactating women or for children <4 years old). Alternatively, pyrethrins (RID, A-200 Pyrinate, Lice) may be applied for 10 minutes and washed off. After rinsing, the hair should be cleaned with a fine-tooth comb. If symptoms persist, the patient should be reevaluated in 1 week to check for lice or nits at the hair–skin junction; if lice or nits are found, the patient is retreated. Sex partners within the last month should be treated. Clothing and blankets should be laundered and machine-dried using the heat cycle or dry cleaned, or set aside for 1 week.

Pinworms

Agent: Enterobius vermicularis (pinworm).

Symptoms: Pruritus, mostly around the anus.

Source: Oral–anal spread; more common in young children.

Diagnosis: The parent or patient may have observed the actual pinworms, especially in the middle of the night. The diagnosis by observation of the characteristic ova can be made using a piece of Scotch tape or a commercial pinworm tape blotted around the anus as soon as the patient awakens in the morning. The tape is affixed to a glass slide and examined for the ova. Rarely, an adult pinworm may be seen in the vagina during an examination.

Treatment: Mebendazole, 100 mg orally once, repeated in 2 weeks.

VULVAR DISORDERS

The differential diagnosis of vulvar dermatosis is shown in Table 1. Psoriasis, allergic and irritant reactions, lichen sclerosus, seborrheic dermatitis, and vesiculobullous disease can cause symptoms in the adolescent. Lichen simplex chronicus and lichen planus also can occur. Vesiculobullous conditions include erythema multiforme, pemphigus, benign familial pemphigus, bullous and cicatricial pemphigoid, linear IgA disease, and dermatitis herpetiformis (87,88). The definitive diagnosis of most vulvar disorders is made by biopsy.

The most common causes of vulvitis among adolescents are specific vaginal infections (e.g., *Candida*), genital herpes, and irritative vulvitis. Nonspecific vulvar irritation may be caused by hot weather, nylon underpants, tight bluejeans, obesity, poor hygiene, or sitting on sand. The patient may also experience pruritus, pain, and dysuria. The vulva appears erythematous. The diagnosis is made by exclusion of a specific vaginitis, allergy, or HPV of the vulva (see Chapter 13). The application of hydrocortisone cream 1% applied three times daily to the vulva for several days to weeks, the use of white cotton underpants, and the avoidance of precipitating factors is usually effective.

An entity that can be troubling to the adolescent is vulvodynia, characterized by vulvar discomfort and burning, stinging, and irritation. No one causative factor can be identified. The International Society for the Study of Vulvar Disease (ISSVD) has defined certain subsets. Vulvar vestibulitis is a chronic and persistent condition characterized by severe pain when the vestibule is touched or vaginal entry is attempted, tenderness to pressure localized within the vulvar vestibule, and physical findings confined to vestibular erythema of various degrees (89). Some cases have been attributed to local inflammation, irritation, and/or infection with bacteria, *Candida*, or HPV. The therapeutic options reviewed by the ISSVD found favorable results with vestibular resection and interferon therapy and less favorable results with laser therapy or local excision of sensitive lesions. There are no series dealing only with adolescent patients, but first-line therapy is twice daily plain water rinsing; the avoidance of soaps, pads, and irritants; sparing use of topical lidocaine ointment or low potency corticosteroids; the use of emollients, and the application of vaginal lubricants for intercourse.

Vestibular papillomatosis is a descriptive term for the presence of multiple papillae that may cover the entire mucosal surface of the labia minora. Although it can be a sign of HPV infection, it can also be a nonspecific finding.

Essential vulvodynia refers to a condition in which patients lack physical findings and complain of constant burning. These patients are more likely to be postmenopausal, and tricyclic antidepressants have been helpful for some patients. Idiopathic vulvodynia is characterized by dull, continuous pain; therapies have not been established (87,89).

VULVAR ULCERS AND NEVI

The diagnosis of vulvar ulcers is sometimes difficult; some helpful features are outlined in Table 2. The most common cause of ulcers in adolescents is genital herpes; other much less common causes are chancroid, found in fewer than 1 in 1000 patients in the University of Washington STD clinic (74), and syphilis. All three have been associated with an increased risk of HIV infection. Syphilis is characterized by a nonpainful hard ulcer (see Chapter 12). Genital herpes is characterized by painful, usually multiple, and shallow ulcers (see above). Epstein-Barr virus infection (mononucleosis) can be associated with painful genital ulcers (90). Patients with myelocytic leukemia receiving chemotherapy may develop genital ulcers (91). Varicella zoster rarely causes ulcers.

Chancroid typically appears as multiple purulent ulcers, often with ragged edges, and tender unilateral or bilateral inguinal adenopathy. Suppurative inguinal adenopathy is almost pathognomonic. The diagnosis is made by excluding the diagnosis of genital herpes or syphilis, although these diseases may occur simultaneously. If the diagnosis is unclear, or if the patient resides in a community with a high prevalence or outbreak of chancroid (92), treatment for both syphilis and chancroid may be indicated, as well as followup serology tests for syphilis. Culture of *Haemophilus ducreyi* is the only sure means of diagnosis, but special media and conditions are necessary. Detection from the direct smears of the base of the genital lesion is a method used by clinicians, although the sensitivity and specificity are lower than those of cultures. The specimen is obtained from the ulcer base, which may involve peeling off the crust or wiping away excess pus (but not extensive cleaning). The cotton swab is used to touch first

TABLE 2. *Clinical features of genital ulcers*

	Syphilis	Herpes	Chancroid	Lymphogranuloma venereum	Donovanosis
Incubation period	2–4 weeks (1–12 weeks)	2–7 days	1–14 days	3 days–6 weeks	1–4 weeks (up to 6 months)
Primary lesion	Papule	Vesicle	Papule or pustule	Papule, pustule, or vesicle	Papule
Number of lesions	Usually one	Multiple, may coalesce	Usually multiple, may coalesce	Usually one	Variable
Diameter (mm)	5–15	1–2	2–20	2–10	Variable
Edges	Sharply demarcated, elevated, round or oval	Erythematous	Undermined, ragged, irregular	Elevated, round or oval	Elevated, irregular
Depth	Superficial or deep	Superficial	Excavated	Superficial or deep	Elevated
Base	Smooth, nonpurulent	Serous, erythematous	Purulent	Variable	Red and rough ("beefy")
Induration	Firm	None	Soft	Occasionally firm	Firm
Pain	Unusual	Common	Usually very tender	Variable	Uncommon
Lymphadenopathy	Firm, nontender, bilateral	Firm, tender, often bilateral	Tender, may suppurate, usually unilateral	Tender, may suppurate, loculated, usually unilateral	Pseudoadenopathy

(From Piol P, Plummer FA. Genital ulcer adenopathy syndrome. In: KK Holmes, P Mardh, Sparling PF, et al eds. *Sexually transmitted diseases*, 2nd ed. New York: McGraw-Hill, 1990:711; with permission.)

the base and then the edges of the ulcer. The swab is then rolled onto a slide in a circle about the size of a dime, and the slide is allowed to air dry and is gram stained. An indirect immunofluorescence of ulcer smears using a monoclonal antibody directed against *H. ducreyi*, a dot-immunobinding serologic test, and new PCR tests are promising techniques. Thus, patients with ulcers without a history of blisters who do not have herpes or syphilis (no evidence of *Treponema pallidum* on darkfield examination or by serologic test at least 7 days after the onset of ulcers, and no evidence of herpes by clinical presentation or HSV tests) and who have have significant painful inguinal adenopathy should be treated for chancroid with azithromycin 1 g orally in one dose, or ceftriaxone 250 mg IM in a single dose, erythromycin base, 500 mg orally four times a day for 7 days (36,93), or ciprofloxacin 500 mg twice a day for 3 days (only in nonpregnant patients over 17 years old). A clinical response should be evident within several days; patients should be seen in 7 days to make sure that ulcer healing is occurring and that adenopathy is less painful. Nodes may become fluctuant in spite of adequate medical therapy and require needle aspiration (94). If a response to therapy has not occurred by day 7, the diagnosis may be different (e.g., herpes), the patient may be noncompliant with medication, the organisms may be resistant to the antibiotic chosen, or the patient may be infected with HIV. Sexual contacts within the 10 days preceding the onset of symptoms should be examined and treated. Serologic testing for syphilis and HIV should be performed 3 months after therapy.

Lymphogranuloma venereum is caused by three serotypes (L-1, L-2, and L-3) of *C. trachomatis*. The ulcer is usually transient, and the patient is usually seen by the clinician for the late sequelae: enlarged inguinal nodes and rectal strictures. Diagnosis is made by isolation of the organism, immunofluorescence of inclusion bodies in leukocytes of a node aspirate, or most commonly serologic test. Treatment is doxycycline 100 mg twice a day for 21 days.

The diagnosis of carcinoma, pemphigus, or granuloma inguinale generally requires a biopsy specimen. Granuloma inguinale, a rare disease, causes painful ulcerations with red granulation tissue or keloid-like depigmented scars, elephantoid enlargement of the external genitalia, and fistulas. Ulcers can also occur with chronic fistulas or Crohn's disease; the local application of zinc oxide paste may help alleviate symptoms. A course of oral metronidazole or other antibiotics in addition to medications to suppress the Crohn's disease has proved beneficial in some patients with chronic ulcers and fistulas.

Hidradenitis suppurativa is a disorder involving apocrine glands. This condition develops after puberty, and usually involves the breasts, axillae, and the anogenital region. The etiology is unclear. The earliest lesions present as subepithelial swellings that may be firm or appear fluctuant, but if incised they are usually fleshy and do not drain purulent material. Initial therapy should include local care with warm baths and nonirritating clothing. Oral antibiotics and topical antiseptics may be helpful; oral contraceptives and antiandrogens may also improve the condition. For severe cases, surgery is the best treatment with incision and healing secondarily. Local excision of affected areas can also be performed with primary closure of the surrounding nonaffected tissue.

The mouth should always be examined in patients with vulvar ulcers. Behçet's disease is a multisystem disorder characterized by recurrent oral and genital ulcers, often associated with uveitis (70% to 80%) and, less commonly, arthritis, phlebitis, and rashes. Although the disease usually does not appear until the third decade of life, rare cases in young children and adolescents have been reported (95,96). Therapy is often unsatisfactory and has included oral contraceptives, corticosteroids, colchicine, and immunosuppressive agents.

Although most darkly pigmented lesions on the vulva of adolescent girls represent lentigo (a benign freckle-like increase in the concentration of melanocytes in the basal layer of the epithelium) or a compound, junctional, or intradermal nevus, the rare occurrence of melanoma or other forms of carcinoma makes it important to perform an excisional biopsy to establish a diagnosis.

An atlas of vulvar pathology can be very helpful to the clinician who sees adolescents with gynecologic problems.

TOXIC SHOCK SYNDROME

Toxic shock syndrome (TSS) received much publicity in the early 1980s as a disease that was occurring in young women primarily in association with one brand of tampon (Rely). Since that time, there has been recognition of milder cases than the original CDC definition as well as newer information on toxin production and risk factors.

Although the original description of TSS by Todd and associates (97) suggested that it was a disease of boys and girls, the increased awareness of TSS in the early 1980s stemmed from the recognition that it occurred in young menstruating women who used tampons. Subsequently, both menstrual and nonmenstrual cases were recognized. Almost all cases in men and nonmenstruating women have been associated with a focal infection such as an infected wound, abscess, augmentation mammoplasty, or pneumonia (especially associated with influenza); similar presentations have also been linked to toxin-producing strains of *Streptococcus pyogenes*. The disease in menstruating young women is associated with the elaboration of an exotoxin, toxic-shock syndrome toxin (TSST-1), and an enterotoxin A (SEA) by *Staphylococcus aureus* (98–101). *S. aureus* has been cultured from the vagina of 98% of women with TSS versus 7% of controls. TSS has a peak occurrence on the fourth day of the menses and has been associated with continuous tampon use.

In a study of time intervals based on the change in tampon types, Pettiti and Reingold (102) reported the incidence of TSS per 100,000 women to be 0.4 from 1972 to 1977 (tampon absorbency low), 1.5 from 1977 to 1979 (superabsorbent tampons, not Rely), 2.4 from 1979 to 1980 (Rely and other superabsorbent tampons), and 2.2 from 1980 to 1985 (Rely off the market). The incidence from April 1985 to December 1987 was 1.5 in 100,000 women (95% CI: 0.8, 2.6) in the interval after the removal of polyacrylate rayon products from the market and reductions in absorbency (103); further decreases occurred through 1990 (104). Factors that appear to promote TSS are the neutral pH of the vagina during menstruation and the introduction of oxygen into the vagina when tampons are inserted. Cases of TSS do, however, occur during menses in women not using tampons. Contraceptive sponges and, to a lesser extent, diaphragms have been associated with rare cases of TSS.

The toxin TSST-1 has been isolated in 84% to 100% of menstrual cases of TSS, whereas this toxin has been reported in only 50% to 62% of nonmenstrual cases, which suggests that other toxins are involved in the pathogenesis of nonmenstrual TSS. Most individuals develop antibody to TSST-1 by the age of 20 years. Toxic shock syndrome occurs predominantly in the population that lacks antibody, because of either a genetic factor or lack of exposure. Young patients, especially adolescents, can be expected to be at increased risk for TSS. Almost half of the 30 patients studied by Bergdoll and associates (105) had no antibody to this toxin during convalescence. This toxin appears to block B-lymphocytes from making antibody. Women who have not made antibody to TSST-1 by the time of followup are at a high risk of recurrence with future menses and tampon use.

Milder cases of TSS have also been described; physicians and patients need to be aware of the more minor symptoms occurring with tampon (or diaphragm) use in order to intervene effectively. The criteria set up by the CDC to study the epidemiology of TSS is for the more severe manifestation of the syndrome. Toxic shock is probable when four of five major criteria are fulfilled. These criteria are as follows:

1. Fever of ≥38.9°C.
2. Rash: diffuse macular erythroderma (looks like sunburn).
3. Desquamation 1 to 2 weeks after the onset of the illness, particularly of palms and soles.
4. Hypotension (systolic blood pressure ≤90 mm Hg for adults, or below the fifth percentile by age for children under 16 years, or orthostatic decrease ≥15 mm Hg in diastolic blood pressure, or orthostatic syncope or orthostatic dizziness).
5. Involvement of three or more of the following organ systems:
   a. Gastrointestinal (vomiting or diarrhea).
   b. Muscular (severe myalgia or creatinine phosphokinase level at least two times the upper limits of normal).
   c. Mucous membranes (vaginal, oropharyngeal, or conjunctival hyperemia).
   d. Renal (blood urea nitrogen or creatinine at least two times the upper limit of normal or >5 leukocytes/high power field in the absence of urinary tract infection).
   e. Hepatic (total bilirubin, AST, ALT at least two times the upper limit of normal).
   f. Hematologic (platelet count <100,000/mm^3).
   g. Central nervous system (disorientation or alterations in consciousness when fever and hypotension are absent).

In addition, if cultures from blood and cerebrospinal fluid are obtained, they must be negative (except for *S. aureus*). Serologic tests for Rocky Mountain spotted fever, leptospirosis, or measles also must be negative. Adolescents with any of these symptoms or with vomiting, diarrhea, and a rash during menstruation should be instructed to remove the tampon and go to the emergency room. Toxic shock syndrome should be managed in the same way as other forms of shock; the administration of fluid is most important. Laboratory tests include hematology and chemistry profiles, along with coagulation parameters. Hypocalcemia and hypomagnesemia and elevated creatine phosphokinase are common findings. A vaginal examination should be done, and the tampon should be removed if it is still in place. Gram stain of the vaginal pool should be done. Cultures from the blood, rectum, vagina, oropharynx, anterior nares, and urine should be obtained. Penicillinase-resistant antistaphylococcal antibiotics should be administered for 2 weeks (IV, p.o.). Although evidence is lacking, many clinicians favor irrigating the vagina with saline, povidone–iodine solution, or vancomycin or gentamicin solution. In patients with deep abscesses in which the toxin-producing staphylococci are unlikely to be eradicated rapidly, or in particularly severe cases of TSS, therapy with immunoglobulin (which has high levels of antibody to TSST-1) and possibly steroids may improve the outcome. Further studies are needed.

Because there is an approximately 30% risk of recurrence, patients should be warned to avoid tampons for at least 6 months. The presence of high levels of antibody to TSST-1 at followup in a patient with no antibody at presentation is reassuring. Serial cultures of the vagina may be difficult to interpret, since other strains of *S. aureus* may be present. Testing for TSST-1–producing strains requires a specialized laboratory. Sources of antibody testing to TSST-1 at baseline and followup can be arranged through some academic centers or the CDC. Tampon use can be resumed when seroconversion occurs.

There is insufficient knowledge on which to base absolute guidelines to patients, but we suggest that patients (a) avoid superabsorbent tampons, (b) use tampons intermittently and use pads at night, (c) change tampons every 4 to 6 hours, and especially (d) remove tampons and call a physician if vomiting, diarrhea, rash, or fever occur. The recommendation about the frequency of changing tampons has not been subjected to critical study.

DYSURIA

Dysuria is common in adolescent girls and is discussed in this section because vaginitis and vulvar lesions may produce symptoms usually associated with a urinary tract infection (UTI) (Table 3). The clinician needs to do a careful gynecologic assessment of adolescents with dysuria (106–108). In one study, only one-half of adult women with dysuria had bacteriuria with more than 10^5 organisms/ml (108). Vaginitis, vulvitis, genital herpes, *N. gonorrhoeae*, *C. trachomatis*, and bacteriuria with fewer than 10^5 organisms per milliliter are responsible

TABLE 3. *Differential diagnosis of dysuria in adolescent girls*

Bacterial urinary tract infection
Vulvovaginitis/cervicitis/urethritis
Candida
Trichomonas
Bacterial vaginosis
N. gonorrhoeae
C. trachomatis
Herpes simplex
Vulvar dermatoses
Skene's gland abscess
Traumatic urethritis
Urethral syndrome of unclear etiology

for most of the remaining group. Pyuria on urinalysis can occur with a UTI, *Trichomonas* vaginitis, and gonococcal or chlamydial infections. Stamm and associates (108,109) have suggested that women with dysuria and pyuria who do not have bacteriuria of $>10^4$ organisms per milliliter, gonorrhea, or vaginitis have either low counts of bacteriuria (coliforms or *Staphylococcus saprophyticus*) or infection with *C. trachomatis*. In contrast, of the undiagnosed group of women with dysuria but no pyuria, few had demonstrable infection. In women with dysuria and frequency (in whom the usual causes were excluded), doxycycline 100 mg orally twice a day for 10 days led to improvement only in those with pyuria (8 or more leukocytes/mm^3 of urine on hemocytometer chamber) (110).

In assessing dysuria in an adolescent, the clinician should take a history about the onset of symptoms, sexual activity (recent and past), symptoms of urethritis in the male partner(s), previous UTIs, and internal dysuria (pain felt inside the body) versus external dysuria (pain felt as urine passes over the inflamed labia) (Fig. 7). If the patient reports a clear-cut history of external dysuria and discharge, her symptoms are likely due to vaginitis or a vulvar cause. Although adult women who have internal dysuria and frequency usually have a UTI, many adolescent girls have vaginitis, gonorrhea, or *Chlamydia* infection alone or in combination with a UTI. In contrast to older women, adolescents may be less able to differentiate internal versus external dysuria. Pain occurring only at the end of urination and/or hematuria suggests a UTI.

The laboratory evaluation of dysuria in an adolescent should include urinalysis, urine culture (if UTI is suspected), wet preparations of the vaginal secretions, and, in sexually active patients, endocervical or urine tests for gonorrhea and *C. trachomatis*. A 1+ or 2+ leukocyte esterase result and a positive nitrite result on the urine dipstick favor a diagnosis of UTI, as does a positive Gram stain (1 organism per high-power field) of unspun urine. However, many adolescents with a UTI do not have a positive urine nitrite test. Inspection of the genitalia should be done to exclude urethral or vulvar pathology such as genital herpes. Samples for wet preparations should be obtained as noted earlier. A cul-

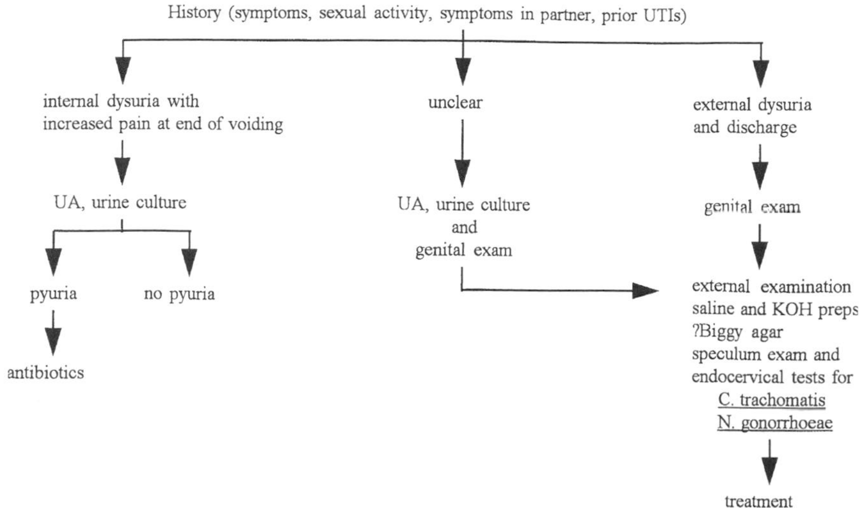

FIG. 7. Evaluation of dysuria in the adolescent girl. UTI, urinary tract infection; UA, urinalysis; KOH, potassium hydroxide.

ture for *Candida* should be done in patients with itching, vulvar erythema, or external dysuria in whom the KOH preparation does not reveal *Candida*.

The adolescent with dysuria usually has a UTI or a specific gynecologic infection (106). In patients with undiagnosed dysuria and persistent pyuria on urinalysis, a course of antibiotics effective against both low-count UTIs and *C. trachomatis* is recommended. Patients without pyuria or a diagnosis fall into the small category of urethral syndrome of unclear etiology, and antibiotics are not beneficial.

Adolescents with uncomplicated cystitis are treated with single-dose antibiotics or preferably a 3- to 7-day course (111–113). Single-dose regimens include trimethoprim/sulfamethoxazole (320 mg/1600 mg), ofloxacin 400 mg, and amoxicillin 3 g (112). In a comparative trial of single-dose versus 10 days of trimethoprim/sulfamethoxazole, Fihn and coworkers (112) found that a 10-day course yielded higher rates of cure at 2 weeks from the start of therapy, but at 6 weeks the difference was not significant. The 10-day course increases the cost and the possibility of allergic symptoms, diarrhea, and *Candida* vaginitis. The quinolones (ciprofloxacin, norfloxacin, ofloxacin) are effective in a 3- to 7-day course for nonpregnant young women over the age of 17. Other oral antibiotics include cephalexin, cefuroxime axetil, cefprozil (107), and cefixime. Hooten and colleagues (113) reported that a 3-day regimen of trimethoprim/sulfamethaxazole (160 mg/800 mg twice a day) was more effective and less costly than 3-day courses of macrocrystalline nitrofurantoin, cefadroxil, or amoxicillin for therapy of uncomplicated cystitis. Although some clinicians have suggested that single-dose antibiotics without testing is a cost-effective strategy in treating young women with dysuria, the adolescent may be less precise in describing her symptoms, less likely to return for followup diagnosis, and more likely to have *Chlamydia* infection. Thus, we recommend that a diagnosis be made in adolescents at the same time a 3- to 7- day treatment is begun. The exception is the young women with recurrent UTIs who can clearly recognize the onset of symptoms.

Ultrasonography of the kidneys should be performed in adolescents with complicated UTIs, pyelonephritis, inadequate response to antibiotics, and recurrent cystitis. In contrast to the recommendations for children, in which ultrasonography of the kidneys and voiding cystourethrogram (VCUG) or radionucleotide cystogram is usually performed with the *first* UTI, VCUG or a radionucleotide cystogram is generally ordered in adolescents who have an abnormal ultrasound, a family history of vesicoureteral reflux (VUR), or clinical pyelonephritis. In centers where the finding of VUR would change management (i.e., be considered an indication for surgery), radionucleotide studies are recommended for all patients with clinical pyelonephritis. Radionucleotide scans involve less radiation than standard VCUGs. A ^{99m}Tc-dimercaptosuccinic acid (DMSA) scan is useful for detecting renal cortical defects due to pyelonephritis or renal scars and is indicated to clarify the clinical management of a lower-tract UTI and an uncertain diagnosis of pyelonephritis (114).

Patients often have recurrent UTIs in relation to coitus. Diaphragm use or condom use with spermicides are also risk factors; spermicides change vaginal flora (see Chapter 17) (115). Other diaphragm designs or other methods of contraception may need to be considered. Coitus-related UTI can be treated with voiding every 2 hours during the day; voiding after intercourse (although no effect was noted in one study [115]), and suppressive antibiotics. Antibiotic regimens include trimethoprim/sulfamethoxazole, 40/200 mg (one-half of a 80/400-mg tablet) a day or one-half tablet three times per week, postcoital antibiotics (116–118), or single-dose therapy with each infection (119–120). Administration of 40 mg/200 mg of trimethoprim/sulfamethoxazole within 2 hours of intercourse (only one tablet every 24 hours) has been highly effective in reducing the number of UTIs (118). The use of prophylactic antibiotics is considered cost-effective when women experience more than two infections per year. Self-administration of antibiotics at the time of the UTI appears to be most useful in women who are accurate at self-diagnosis and have only one to two infections per year. Patients can be taught how to perform their own culture tests at home for diagnosis and to follow up symptoms. One drawback to self-therapy is the failure to reduce the proportion of patients with enterobacterial colonization of the urethra and vagina (120).

REFERENCES

1. Shafer MA, Sweet RL, Ohm-Smith MS, et al. Microbiology of the lower genital tract in postmenarchal adolescent girls: differences by sexual activity, contraception, and presence of nonspecific vaginitis. *J Pediatr* 1985;107:974.
2. Wiesenfeld HC, Heine RP, Rideout A, et al. The vaginal introitus: a novel site for *Chlamydia trachomatis* testing in women. *Am J Obstet Gynecol* 1996;174:1542.

3. Critchlow CW, Wolner-Hanssen PW, Eschenbach DA, et al. Determinants of cervical ectopia and of cervicitis: age, oral contraception, specific cervical infection, smoking, and douching. *Am J Obstet Gynecol* 1995;173:534.
4. Roongpisuthipong A, Grimes DA, Hadgu A. Is the Papanicolaou smear useful for diagnosing sexually transmitted diseases? *Obstet Gynecol* 1987;69:820.
5. Paavonen J, Stevens CD, Wohler-Hanssen P, et al. Colposcopic manifestations of cervical and vaginal infections. *Obstet Gynecol Survey* 1988;43:373.
6. Wolner-Hanssen P, Krieger JN, Stevens CE, et al. Clinical manifestations of vaginal trichomoniasis. *JAMA* 1989;261:571.
7. Lossick JG. The diagnosis of vaginal trichomonias. *JAMA* 1988;259:1230.
8. Kent HL. Epidemiology of vaginitis. *Am J Obstet Gynecol* 1991;165:1168.
9. Krieger JN, Tam MR, Stevens CE, et al. Diagnosis of trichomoniasis: Comparison of conventional wet-mount examination with cytologic studies, cultures, and monoclonal antibody staining of direct specimens. *JAMA* 1988;259:1223.
10. Fouts AC, Kraus SJ. *Trichomonas vaginalis:* reevaluation of its clinical presentation and laboratory diagnosis. *J Infect Dis* 1980;141:137.
11. Rein MF, Muller M. *Trichomonas vaginalis* and trichomoniasis. In: Holmes KK, Mardh P, Sparling PF, et al, eds. *Sexually transmitted diseases*, 2nd ed. New York: McGraw-Hill, 1990.
12. Weinberger MW, Harger JH. Accuracy of the Papanicolaou smear in the diagnosis of asymptomatic infection with trichomonas vaginalis. *Obstet Gynecol* 1993;82:425.
13. Wathne B, Holst E, Hovelius B, et al. Vaginal discharge—comparison of clinical, laboratory and microbiological findings. *Acta Obstet Gynecol Scand* 1994;73:802.
14. Philip A, Carter-Scott P, Rogers C. An agar culture technique to quantitative *Trichomonas vaginalis* in women. *J Infect Dis* 1987;55:304.
15. James JA, Thomason JL, Gelbart SM, et al. Is trichomoniasis often associated with bacterial vaginosis in pregnant adolescents? *Am J Obstet Gynecol* 1992;166:859.
16. Hager WD, Brown ST, Kraus SJ, et al. Metronidazole for vaginal trichomoniasis: seven day vs. single dose regimen. *JAMA* 1980;244:1219.
17. Dykers J. Single dose metronidazole for *Trichomonas:* patient and consort. *N Engl J Med* 1975;293:23.
18. Lossick JG, Muller M, Garrell TE. In vitro drug susceptibility and doses of metronidazole required for cure in cases of refractory vaginal trichomoniasis. *J Infect Dis* 1986;153:948.
19. Grossman JH, Galask RP. Persistent vaginitis caused by metronidazole-resistant trichomonas. *Obstet Gynecol* 1990;76:521.
20. Piper JM, Mitchel EF, Ray WA. Prenatal use of metronidazole and birth defects: no association. *Obstet Gynecol* 1993;82:348.
21. Horowitz BJ, Edelstein SW, Lippman L. *Candida tropicalis* vulvovaginitis. *Obstet Gynecol* 1985;66: 229.
22. Robertson WH. Mycology of vulvovaginitis. *Am J Obstet Gynecol* 1988;158:989.
23. Galask RP. Vaginal colonization by bacteria and yeast. *Am J Obstet Gynecol* 1988;158:993.
24. Horowitz BJ, Edelstein SW, Lippman L. Sexual transmission of *Candida. Obstet Gynecol* 1987;69: 883.
25. Bisschop MP, Merkus JM, Scheygrand H, et al. Cotreatment of the male partner in vaginal candidiasis: a double blind randomized control study. *Br J Obstet Gynaecol* 1986;93:79.
26. Sobel JD, Chaim W. Treatment of *Torulopis glabrata* vaginitis: retrospective review of boric acid therapy. *Clin Infect Dis* 1997;24:649.
27. Leonderslot EW, Goormans E, Wiesenhaan PE, et al. Efficacy and tolerability of single-dose versus six-day treatment of candidal vulvovaginitis with vaginal tablets of clotrimazole. *Am J Obstet Gynecol* 1985;152:953.
28. Adamson GD. Three-day treatment of vulvovaginal candidiasis. *Am J Obstet Gynecol* 1988;158:1002.
29. Corson SL, Kapikian RR, Nehring R. Terconazole and miconazole cream for treating vulvovaginal candidiasis, a comparison. *J Reprod Med* 1991;36:561.
30. Horowitz BJ. Antifungal therapy in the management of chronic candidiasis. *Am J Obstet Gynecol* 1988;158:996.
31. Topical drugs for vaginal candidiasis. *Med Lett* 1991;33:81.
32. Stein GE, Christensen S, Mummaw N. Comparative study of fluconazole and clotrimazole in the treatment of vulvaginal candidiasis. *DICP Ann Pharmacother* 1991;25:582.
33. Oral fluconazole for vaginal candidiasis. *Med Lett* 1994;36:81.
34. *Physicians' Desk Reference*, 1996. Fluconazole (Diflucan).
35. Sobel JD, Brooker D, Stein GE, et al. Single oral dose fluconazole compared with conventional clotrimazole topical therapy of Candida vaginitis. *Am J Obstet Gynecol* 1995;172:1263.

36. CDC 1998 Sexually Transmitted Disease Treatment Guidelines. *MMWR* 1998;47(RR-1):1.
37. Drugs for sexually transmitted diseases. *Med Lett* 1995;37:117.
38. Fong IW. The value of prophylactic (monthly) clotrimazole versus empiric self-treatment in recurrent vaginal candidiasis. *Genitourin Med* 1994;70:124.
39. Sobel JD. Recurrent vulvovaginal candidiasis: a prospective study of the efficacy of maintenance ketoconazole therapy. *N Engl J Med* 1986;315:1455.
40. Creatsas GC, Charalambidis VM, Zagotzidou EH, et al. Chronic or recurrent vaginal candidiasis: short-term treatment and prophylaxis with itraconazole. *Clin Ther* 1993; 15:662.
41. Speigel CA, Amsel R, Eschenbach D, et al. Anaerobic bacteria in nonspecific vaginitis. *N Engl J Med* 1980;303:601.
42. Eschenbach DA, Hillier S, Critchlow C, et al. Diagnosis and clinical manifestations of bacterial vaginosis. *Am J Obstet Gynecol* 1988;158:819.
43. Larsson PB, Bergman BB. Is there a causal connection between motile curved rods, *Mobiluncus* species, and bleeding complications? *Am J Obstet Gynecol* 1986;154:107.
44. Speigel CA, Amsel R, Holmes KK. Diagnosis of bacterial vaginosis by direct gram stain of vaginal fluid. *J Clin Microbiol* 1983;18:170.
45. Hay PE, Taylor-Robinson D, Lamont RF. Diagnosis of bacterial vaginosis in a gynaecology clinic. *Br J Obstet Gynaecol* 1992;99:63.
46. Briselden AM, Moncla BJ, Stevens CE, Hillier SL. Sialidases (neuraminidases) in bacterial vaginosis and bacterial vaginosis-associated microflora. *J Clin Microbiol* 1992;30:663.
47. Gravett MG, Nelson HP, DeRouen T, et al. Independent associations of bacterial vaginosis and *Chlamydia trachomatis* infection with adverse pregnancy outcome. *JAMA* 1986;256:1899.
48. Hillier SL, Nugent RP, Eschenback DA, et al. Association between bacterial vaginosis and preterm delivery of a low birth weight infant. *N Engl J Med* 1995;333:1737.
49. Morales WJ, Schorr S, Albritton J. Effect of metronidazole in patients with preterm birth in precedintg pregnancy and bacterial vaginosis: a placebo-controlled, double-blind study. *Am J Obstet Gynecol* 1994;171:345.
50. Hauth JC, Goldenberg RL, Andrews WW, et al. Reduced incidence of preterm delivery with metronidazole and erythromycin in women with bacterial vaginosis. *N Engl J Med* 1995;333:1732.
51. Holst E. Reservoir of four organisms associated with bacterial vaginosis suggests lack of sexual transmission. *J Clin Microbiol* 1990;28:2035.
52. Nugent RP, Krohn MA, Hillier SL. Reliability of diagnosing bacterial vaginosis is improved by a standardized method of Gram stain interpretation. *J Clin Microbiol* 1991;29:297.
53. Pheifer T, Forsyth P, Durfee M, et al. Non-specific vaginitis: role of *Haemophilus vaginalis* and treatment with metronidazole. *N Engl J Med* 1978;298:1429.
54. Swedberg J, Steiner JF, Deiss F, et al. Comparison of single-dose vs. one week course of metronidazole for symptomatic bacterial vaginosis. *JAMA* 1985;254:1046.
55. Hillier SL, Lipinski C, Briselden AM, Eschenbach DA. Efficacy of intravaginal 0.75% metronidazole gel for the treatment of bacterial vaginosis. *Obstet Gynecol* 1993;81:963.
56. Greaves WL, Chungafung J, Morris B, et al. Clindamycin versus metronidazole in the treatment of bacterial vaginosis. *Obstet Gynecol* 1988;72:799.
57. Purdon A, Hanna JH, Morse PL, et al. An evaluation of single-dose metronidazole treatment for *Gardnerella vaginalis* vaginitis. *Obstet Gynecol* 1984;64:271.
58. Jerve F, Berdal TB, Bohman P, et al. Metronidazole in the treatment of non-specific vaginitis (NSV). *Br J Vener Dis* 1984;60:171.
59. Lugo-Miro VI, Green M, Mazur L. Comparison of different metronidazole therapeutic regimens for bacterial vaginosis. *JAMA* 1992;268:92.
60. Vejtorp M, Bollerup L, Vejtorp E, et al. Bacterial vaginosis: a double-bind randomized trial of the effect of treatment of the sexual partner. *Br J Obstet Gynaecol* 1988;95:920.
61. Moi H, Erkkola R, Jerve F, et al. Should male consorts of women with bacterial vaginosis be treated? *Genitourin Med* 1989;65:263.
62. Vutyavanich T, Pongsuthirak P, Vannareumol P, et al. A randomized double-blind trial of tinidazole treatment of the sexual partners of females with bacterial vaginosis. *Obstet Gynecol* 1993;82:550.
63. Reeves WC, Corey L, Adams HG, et al. Risk of recurrence after first episodes of genital herpes. *N Engl J Med* 1981;305:315.
64. Corey L. First episode, recurrent, and asymptomatic herpes simplex infections. *J Am Acad Dermatol* 1988;18:169.
65. Lafferty WE, Coombs RW, Benedetti J, et al. Recurrences after oral and genital herpes simplex virus infection: influence of site of infection and viral type. *N Engl J Med* 1987;316:1444.

66. Piot P, Plummer FA. Genital ulcer adenopathy syndrome. In: Holmes KK, Mardh P, Sparling PF, et al, eds. *Sexually transmitted diseases*, 2nd ed. New York: McGraw-Hill, 1990:711.
67. Corey L, Adams HG, Brown ZA, et al. Genital herpes simplex virus infections: clinical manifestations, course and complications. *Ann Intern Med* 1983;98:958.
68. Corey L, Holmes KK. Genital herpes simplex virus infections: current concepts in diagnosis, therapy, and prevention. *Ann Intern Med* 1983;98:973.
69. Wald A, Zeh J, Selke S, et al. Virologic characteristics of subclinical and symptomatic genital herpes infections. *N Engl J Med* 1995;333:770.
70. Rooney JF, Felser JM, Ostrove JM, et al. Acquisition of genital herpes from an asymptomatic sexual partner. *N Engl J Med* 1986;314:1561.
71. Johnson RE, Nahmias AJ, Magdar LS, et al. A seroepidemiologic survey of the prevalence of herpes simplex virus type 2 infection in the United States. *N Engl J Med* 1989;321:7.
72. Breinig MK, Kingsley LA, Armstron JA, et al. Epidemiology of genital herpes in Pittsburgh: serologic, sexual, and racial correlates of apparent and inapparent herpes simplex infections. *J Infect Dis* 1990;152:299.
73. Koutsky LA, Ashley RL, Holmes KK, et al. The frequency of unrecognized type 2 herpes simplex virus infection among women, implications for the control of genital herpes. *Sex Trans Dis* 1990;17:90.
74. Koutsky LA, Stevens CE, Holmes KK, et al. Underdiagnosis of genital herpes by current clinical and viral-isolation procedures. *N Engl J Med* 1992;326:1533.
75. Guinan ME, MacCalman J, Kern ER. The course of untreated recurrent genital herpes simplex infection in 27 women. *N Engl J Med* 1981;304:759.
76. Thin RN. Does first episode genital herpes have an incubation period? A clinical study. *Int J STD AIDS* 1991:2:285.
77. Cone RW, Swenson PD, Hobson AC, et al. Herpes simplex virus detection from genital lesions: a comparative study using antigen detection (HerpChek) and culture. *J Clin Microbiol* 1993; 31:1774.
78. Bryson YJ, Dillon M, Lovett M, et al. Treatment of first episodes of genital herpes simplex virus infection with oral acyclovir. *N Engl J Med* 1983;308:916.
79. Mertz GJ, Jones CC, Mills J, et al. Long-term acyclovir suppression of frequently recurring genital herpes simplex virus infection: a multicenter double-blind trial. *JAMA* 1988;260:201.
80. Straus SE, Takiff HE, Seidlin M, et al. Suppression of frequently recurring genital herpes: a placebo-controlled double-blind trial of oral acyclovir. *N Engl J Med* 1984;310:1545.
81. Crumpacker CS. Molecular target of antiviral therapy (Seminars in Medicine). *N Engl J Med* 1989;321:163.
82. Wald A, Benedetti J, Davis G, et al. A randomized, double-blind, comparative trial comparing high- and standard-dose oral acyclovir for first-episode genital herpes infections. *Antimicrob Agents Chemother* 1994;38:174.
83. Sacks SL, Aoki FY, Diaz-Mitoma F, et al. Patient-initiated twice-daily oral famcyclovir for early recurrent genital herpes. *JAMA* 1996;276:44.
84. Douglas JM, Critchlow C, Benedetti J, et al. A double-blind study of oral acyclovir for suppression of recurrences of genital herpes simplex virus infection. *N Engl J Med* 1984;310:1551.
85. Lehrman SN, Douglas JM, Corey L, et al. Recurrent genital herpes and suppressive oral acyclovir therapy: relation between clinical outcome and in-vitro drug sensitivity. *Ann Intern Med* 1986; 104:786.
86. Brown ZA, Benedetti JK, Watts DH, et al. A comparison between detailed and simple histories in the diagnosis of genital herpes complicating pregnancy. *Am J Obstet Gynecol* 1995:172:1299.
87. McKay M. Vulvitis and vulvovaginitis: cutaneous consideration. *Am J Obstet Gynecol* 1991;165:1176.
88. Marren P, Wojnarowska F, Venning V, et al. Vulvar involvement in autoimmune bullous diseases. *J Reprod Med* 1993;38:101.
89. McKay M, Frankman O, Horowitz BJ, et al. Vulvar vestibulitis and vestibular papillomatosis report of the ISSVD committee on vulvodynia. *J Reprod Med* 1991;36:413.
90. Portnoy J, Ahronheim GA, Ghibu F, et al. Recovery of Epstein-Barr virus from genital ulcers. *N Engl J Med* 1984;311:966.
91. Muram D, Gold SS. Vulvar ulcerations in girls with myelocytic leukemia. *South Med J* 1993;86:293.
92. Flood JM, Sarafian SK, Bolan GA, et al. Multistrain outbreak of chancroid in San Francisco, 1989–1991. *J Infect Dis* 1993;176:1106.
93. Schmid GP, Sanders L Jr, Blount JH, et al. Chancroid in the United States: reestablishment of an old disease. *JAMA* 1987;258:3265.

94. Schmid GP. The treatment of chancroid. *JAMA* 1986;255:1757.
95. Silber TJ, Olsen J. Recurrent genital ulcer in an adolescent as a manifestation of Behçet's disease. *J Adolesc Health Care* 1988;9:231.
96. Ammann AJ, Johnson A, Fyfe G, et al. Behçet syndrome. *J Pediatr* 1985;107:41.
97. Todd J, Fishaut M, Kapral F, et al. Toxic shock syndrome associated with phage group-1 staphylococci. *Lancet* 1978;2:1116.
98. Mills JT, Parsonnet J, Tsai Y, et al. Control of production of toxic-shock syndrome toxin-1 (TSST-1) by magnesium IM. *J Infect Dis* 1985;151:1158.
99. Kain KC, Schulzer M, Chow AW. Clinical spectrum of nonmenstrual toxic shock syndrome (TSS): Comparison with menstrual TSS by multivariate discriminant analyses. *Clin Infect Dis* 1993;16:100.
100. Marples RR, Wieneke AA. Enterotoxins and toxic-shock syndrome toxin-1 in non-enteric staphylococcal disease. *Epidemiol Infect* 1993;110:477.
101. Berkley SF, Hightower AW, Broome CV, et al. The relationship of tampon characteristics to menstrual toxic shock syndrome. *JAMA* 1987;258:917.
102. Petitti DB, Reingold A. Tampon characteristics and menstrual toxic shock syndrome. *JAMA* 1988; 259:686.
103. Petitti DB, Reingold AL. Recent trends in the incidence of toxic shock syndrome in Northern California. *Am J Public Health* 1991:81:1209.
104. CDC. Reduced incidence of menstrual toxic-shock syndrome—United States, 1980–1990. *MMWR* 1990;39:421.
105. Bergdoll MS, Reiser RF, Crass BA, et al. A new staphylococcal enterotoxin F, associated with toxic-shock-syndrome *Staphylococcus aureus* isolates. *Lancet* 1981;1:1017.
106. Demetriou E, Emans SJ, Masland RP. Dysuria in adolescent girls. *Pediatrics* 1982;80:299.
107. Komaroff AL, Pass TM, McCue JD, et al. Management strategies for urinary and vaginal infections. *Arch Intern Med* 1978;138:1069.
108. Stamm WE, Wagner KF, Amsel R, et al. Causes of the acute urethral syndrome in women. *N Engl J Med* 1980;303:409.
109. Stamm WE, Counts GW, Running KR, et al. Diagnosis of coliform infection in acutely dysuric women. *N Engl J Med* 1982;307:463.
110. Stamm WE, Running K, McKevitt M, et al. Treatment of acute urethral syndrome. *N Engl J Med* 1981;304:956.
111. Komaroff AL. Acute dysuria in women. *N Engl J Med* 1984;310:368.
112. Fihn SD, et al. Trimethoprim-sulfamethoxazole for acute dysuria in women: a single-dose or ten-day course: a double-blind, randomized trial. *JAMA* 1988;260:627.
113. Hooten TM, Winter C, Tiu F, Stamm WE. Randomized comparative trial and cost analysis of a 3-day antimicrobial regimens for treatment of acute cystitis in women. *JAMA* 1995;273:41.
114. Jakobsson B, Soderlundh S, Berg U. Diagnostic significance of ^{99m}Tc-dimercaptosuccinic acid (DMSA) scintigraphy in urinary tract infection. *Arch Dis Child* 1992; 67:1338.
115. Hooten TM, Scholes D, Hughes JP, et al. A prospective study of risk factors for symptomatic urinary tract infection in young women. *N Engl J Med* 1996;335:468.
116. Plau A, Sachs T, Englestein D. Recurrent urinary tract infection in premenopausal women. Prophylaxis based on an understanding of the pathogenesis. *J Urol* 1983;129;1152.
117. Vosti KL. Recurrent urinary tract infection prevention by prophylactic antibiotics after sexual intercourse. *JAMA* 1975;1231:934.
118. Stapleton A, Latham RH, Johnson C, Stamm WE. Postcoital antimicrobial prophylaxis for recurrent urinary tract infection: a randomized, double-blind, placebo-controlled trial. *JAMA* 1990;264:703.
119. Stamm WE. Prevention of urinary tract infections. *Am J Med* 1984;76.
120. Wong ES, McKevitt M, Running K, et al. Management of recurrent urinary tract infections with patient-administered single-dose therapy. *Ann Intern Med* 1985;102:302.

FURTHER READING

Kaufman RH, Friedrich EG, Gardner HL. *Benign diseases of the vulva and vagina.* Chicago: Yearbook, 1989.

Wilkinson EJ, Stone IK. *Atlas of vulvar disease*. Baltimore: Williams & Wilkins, 1995.

12

Sexually Transmitted Diseases: Gonorrhea, *Chlamydia trachomatis*, Pelvic Inflammatory Disease, and Syphilis

Sexually transmitted diseases (STDs) are a major threat to the health of adolescents in the 1990s. An estimated 3 million teenagers—roughly 1 of 8 persons aged 13 to 19 years—acquire an STD every year (1). The high prevalence of STDs in teens is the result of many factors, including earlier onset of sexual activity, low rates of consistent condom use, increased health facilities for teenagers allowing better diagnosis and reporting, and the recognition of asymptomatic infections in males and females (2). Adolescents infected with *Neisseria gonorrhoeae* and *Chlamydia trachomatis* are at particular risk of upper genital tract infections including pelvic inflammatory disease (PID) and the possible sequelae of infertility, ectopic pregnancy, and chronic pain. Although the highest number of gonococcal and chlamydial infections occur in young women between 15 and 24 years of age, very young teenagers who are sexually active have an especially high risk of acquiring these pathogens. The recent Institute of Medicine report calls for bold national leadership to address STDs in the United States and notes that the health consequences and costs associated with the high prevalence of STDs remain largely hidden (11).

More widespread screening to detect asymptomatic infections of *N. gonorrhoeae* and *C. trachomatis* and improved recognition of the symptoms of upper urinary tract infections are needed to enhance the health care of teenage women. The finding of one STD should lead to the diagnostic suspicion of other potential STDs, including syphilis and human immunodeficiency virus (HIV). Given the risk of transmitting and acquiring hepatitis B infection during the adolescent years, all adolescents deserve appropriate immunization to prevent this infection. Family planning clinics should provide adequate screening and treatment for STDs, and STD clinics should counsel their clients about appropriate methods of contraception if pregnancy is not desired. Potential effects of contraceptives on STDs are considered in Chapter 17.

GONOCOCCAL INFECTIONS

An estimated 1 million new infections of *N. gonorrhoeae* occur in the United States each year, costing $288 million annually (1,3). Adolescents aged 15 to 19 years have higher rates of gonorrhea than sexually active men and women in any 5-year age group between 20 and 44 years (1). Approximately 24% to 30% of the reported morbidity from gonorrhea is in adolescent age groups. From 1981 to 1991, gonorrhea rates among adolescents increased or remained unchanged while rates among older groups decreased (4). Overall rates of gonococcal infections continue to decrease in the 1990s.

Gonococcal infections may be symptomatic or asymptomatic. Screening endocervical cultures indicates that the asymptomatic rate of gonorrhea ranges from 0.2% to 13% in adolescent women, depending on the clinical setting. Adolescents seen in private practices in the suburbs and college health centers have significantly lower rates than adolescents seen in large outpatient hospital clinics serving an inner city population (5–8) or in juvenile detention centers (18%) (5) (Table 1). A history of prior sexual abuse is particularly associated with the detection of gonorrhea in incarcerated teens (5). Risk markers for gonorrhea are *sexual behaviors* such as early onset of sexual intercourse, large numbers of casual partners, selection of partners with a high risk of gonorrhea, as well as "survival sex" and *health behaviors* such as failure to recognize symptoms, delay in seeking treatment, delay in notifying partners, nonuse of barrier contraception, and noncompliance with therapy (7). Screening sexually active adolescents at low risk once a year or less and teens with high-risk behaviors at least every 6 months appears to be a prudent policy. A young woman who has recently changed sexual partners or has symptoms should also be tested.

Although it has been estimated that 75% to 90% of all gonococcal infections in women, and 10% to 40% of infections in men are asymptomatic, many of these patients on careful questioning do, in fact, have symptoms. Although urine tests for gonorrhea are becoming increasingly sensitive, specific, and available, culturing the endocervix is the best screening test for detecting infection in adolescent girls. Routinely culturing the rectum and pharynx is not cost effective in asymptomatic adolescent populations (9,10). Pharyngeal gonorrhea was reported in 2.2% of an adolescent clinic population in 1982 but a followup of the same clinic 8 years later showed that 0 of 319 had pharyngeal gonorrhea (the earlier study may have included some *Neisseria* species that were misidentified) (10). Treatment regimens currently used generally take into account the eradication of *N. gonorrhoeae* at all sites.

Isolating *N. gonorrhoeae*, a fastidious gram-negative diplococcus, requires special techniques. Culture swabs should always be plated directly onto the

TABLE 1. *Prevalence of* Chlamydia trachomatis *in the cervix*[a]

Reference	No.	Age (yrs)	Characteristics	% Chlamydia	% GC
Shafer et al (50)	363	13–20	50% black 32% white 11% Hispanic Symptoms in 24%	14	7
Bump et al (51)	68	14–17	72.5% black 27.5% white Asymptomatic	19	6
Chacko (52)	70	13–18	Pregnant—black, urban, low SES	27	
	190	13–18	Nonpregnant	23	
Fraser et al (53)	125	14–20	52% black—urban clinic	8	12
Bell et al (54)	100		Adolescents in a juvenile detention center	20	18
Fisher et al (55)	150	14–21	Suburban clinic	14.5	
McCormack et al (56)	439		College students (1974–75)	4.9	0.4
Ismail et al (57)	201	13–19	Pregnant, low SES	21.3	
Khurana et al (58)	49	15–19	Pregnant, low SES	18.4	
Harrison et al (59)	162		53% undergraduate college health center 86% white 10% Hispanic	8	1.2
Johnson (60)	2271	17–40 (mean 20.8)	Student health center	9	
Biro (63)	479	12–22	Asymptomatic Symptomatic	11 21	
Hsuih et al (84)	189	13–25	Symptomatic and Asymptomatic	9.8	1.3

[a]GC, *N. Gonorrhoeae*; SES, socioeconomic status.

appropriate medium (see Chapter 1). It is critical that *N. gonorrhoeae* be properly identified, since cultures of vaginal discharge in prepubertal girls may yield other *Neisseria* species such as *N. cinerea* that may initially be diagnosed as *N. gonorrhoeae*. In prepubertal children with presumptive *N. gonorrhoeae*, accurate confirmatory testing is essential.

DNA probes for screening genital sites for gonorrhea such as the Gen-Probe PACE system (direct chemiluminescent DNA probe test) have sensitivities of 90% to 97% (12,13). In a study of 1750 specimens in the Netherlands with an overall positive rate of 8.7%, sensitivity was 97.1%, specificity 99.1%, positive predictive value 90.1%, and negative predictive value 99.8% (13). The Gen-Probe PACE-2 is a reliable test of cure as early as 6 days after treatment (14). The only drawback for DNA probes is the inability to test the organisms for antibiotic resistance, but all recommended treatment regimens are effective against penicillin-resistant organisms. The advantage of the DNA probes is the ability to test simultaneously with the same swab for *C. trachomatis*. Polymerase chain reaction (PCR) tests are especially promising when utilized in fluids with low rates of detection; PCR has been reported to have a sensitivity of 79% and specificity of 96% for synovial fluid for *N. gonorrhoeae* (15). The development of ligase chain reaction tests (LCR) has allowed the use of sensitive screening tests for *N. gonorrhoeae* on endocervical samples (97.3% sensitivity and 99.6% specificity) (16) and on first-void urine specimens (94.6% sensitivity and 100% specificity) among women attending an STD clinic (17). The use of urine for screening may particularly enhance STD screening.

Gram stain of genital secretions is another method for detecting gonorrhea. The Gram stain is considered positive if gram-negative intracellular diplococci are seen within polymorphonuclear leukocytes. Although the specificity of this finding is 95% for the diagnosis of *N. gonorrhoeae*, the sensitivity is variable, close to 100% in men with symptomatic urethritis but <60% for cervical and rectal infections (18).

Gonococcal Cervicitis and Urethritis

The presenting complaints of patients with gonococcal cervicitis include vaginal discharge, dysuria, urinary frequency, and dyspareunia. On examination, the cervix may be tender to palpation; Gram stain of the purulent discharge may be positive, but the diagnosis of gonorrhea in women must be confirmed by culture DNA probe or other test. However, treatment can be instituted on the basis of symptoms and a positive smear.

Gonococcal urethral and cervical infections often coexist in the woman. The urethral infection may be asymptomatic, or the patient may present with urinary frequency, dysuria, suprapubic pain, and/or purulent discharge from the urethra or Skene's glands. Urinalysis may show pyuria, and Gram stain of the purulent discharge may be positive for gram-negative intracellular diplococci. The urethral discharge should be tested for *N. gonorrhoeae*. As noted in Chapter 11, the differential diagnosis of dysuria includes (low count) urinary tract infections, chlamydial urethritis, and vulvovaginal infections.

Labial pain and swelling may be present if the young woman has a Bartholin's gland infection (which may be associated with infections caused by *N. gonorrhoeae*, *Chlamydia*, or other organisms) (Fig. 1). Depending on assessment, the abscess is usually treated with incision and drainage using a Word catheter, cultures are taken, and the patient is given a course of antibiotics. Marsupialization is necessary for recurrent infections.

Treatment of Asymptomatic Infections, Contacts, Urethritis, and Cervicitis

Treatment of *N. gonorrhoeae* must take into account the sites infected, the prevalence of antibiotic resistance, the high rate of coexisting *C. trachomatis* infections in adolescents, allergies, pregnancy, and the likelihood of compliance.

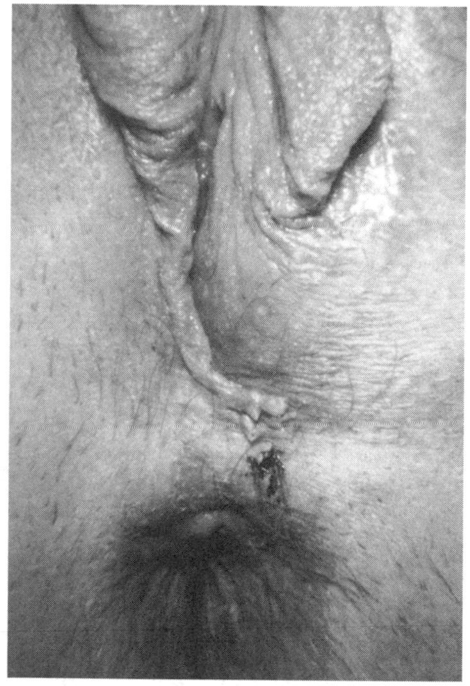

FIG 1. Bartholin's gland abscess.

Antibiotic resistance can be plasmid-mediated, chromosomally mediated, or both. Important variations currently identified in the United States are plasmid-mediated penicillin resistance (β-lactamase–producing *N. gonorrhoeae*), plasmid-mediated tetracycline resistance, and chromosomally mediated resistance to penicillin or tetracycline (3,19–22). Resistance to quinolones has also become a recent problem in some communities.

Because of the 15% to 40% prevalence of coexisting *C. trachomatis* infections in heterosexual patients with gonorrhea, the single-dose therapy should be followed with medication effective against this organism.

The recommendation of the 1998 Sexually Transmitted Diseases Treatment Guidelines (3) for gonorrhea is as follows:

Ceftriaxone, 125 mg IM in a single dose
or
Cefixime, 400 mg orally in a single dose
or
Ciprofloxacin, 500 mg orally in a single dose
or
Ofloxacin, 400 mg orally in a single dose
PLUS
a regimen effective against possible coinfection with *C. trachomatis*:

Azithromycin, 1 g in a single dose
or
Doxycycline, 100 mg orally two times a day for 7 days
Alternative therapy for *C. trachomatis*:
Ofloxacin, 300 mg twice daily for 7 days
or
Erythromycin base, 500 mg orally four times a day for 7 days
or
Erythromycin ethylsuccinate, 800 mg orally four times a day for 7 days.

Some patients (especially those who are pregnant) cannot tolerate the 500-mg dose of erythromycin because of nausea and vomiting; in these cases the erythromycin base can be given 250 mg orally four times a day for 14 days.

Ceftriaxone can be mixed with 1% lidocaine (without epinephrine) to reduce patient discomfort with the injection (23). The 250-mg dose and the 125-mg dose appear equally effective, although the vial currently supplied provides a 250-mg dose. Ceftriaxone combined with a 7-day course of doxycycline is considered effective against incubating syphilis. A history of allergy to penicillin and cephalosporins should be obtained before initiating treatment. Fortunately, the cross-reactivity between third-generation cephalosporins and penicillin is rare; the type of penicillin allergy should be determined before treatment is initiated.

Many clinics prefer the ease of administering oral cefixime directly to the patient to avoid the intramuscular injection. In a multicenter study, the cure rate of 400 mg of cefixime was 96% compared to 98% with 250 mg of ceftriaxone (24); two other studies have found 97% and 98% success rates with cefixime (25,26). Minimal gastrointestinal side effects were observed with both treatments. The two regimens were both effective against the small number of patients with pharyngeal and rectal gonorrhea although ceftriaxone and ciprofloxacin are recommended for known pharyngeal infection (3).

The quinolones (ciprofloxacin and ofloxacin) are effective for the treatment of gonorrhea and are less expensive than ceftriaxone. The quinolone ciprofloxacin is effective against pharyngeal gonorrhea, and in a small study of ofloxacin 88% of pharyngeal infections were cured. Quinolones are not active against incubating syphilis. Resistance of the gonococcus to the quinolones may become an increasing problem in the 1990s with reports of decreased susceptibility in several states (27,28). The quinolones should not be prescribed to pregnant or nursing women or to patients under 18 years old.

Spectinomycin, 2.0 g IM, is useful in patients who cannot tolerate cephalosporins or quinolones; it is not effective against *Treponema pallidum* or pharyngeal gonococcal infections.

Other alternatives for the treatment of gonorrhea for which there are fewer data include norfloxacin, 800 mg orally once; ceftizoxime, 500 mg IM once; cefotaxime, 500 mg IM once; cefotetan 1 g IM, cefoxitin 2 g IM, and trovafloxacin 100 mg orally once (3). All of the regimens above are followed by a regimen effective

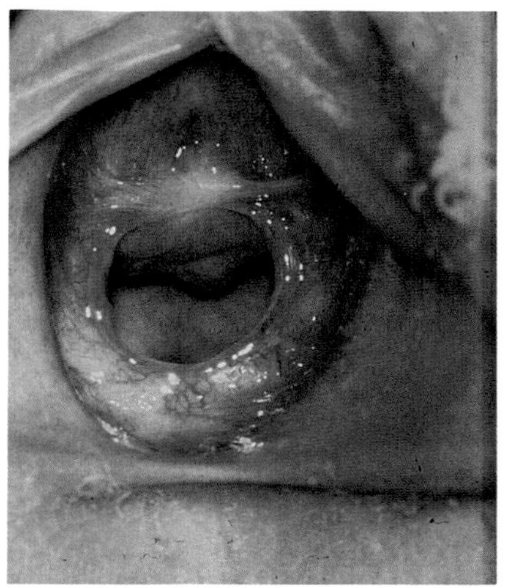

Plate 1. Normal hymen in prepubertal girl.

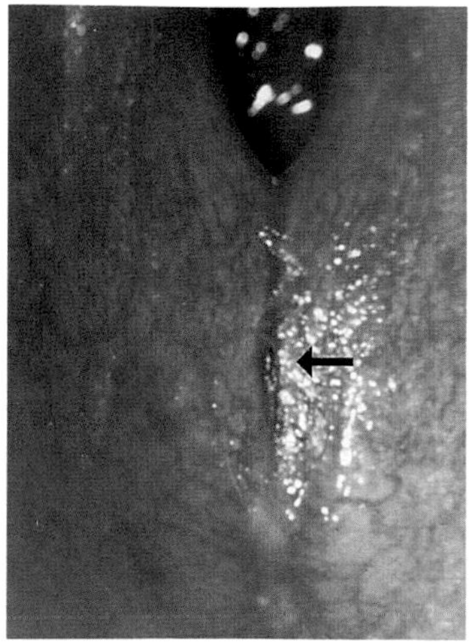

Plate 2. Labial/vulvar adhesion.

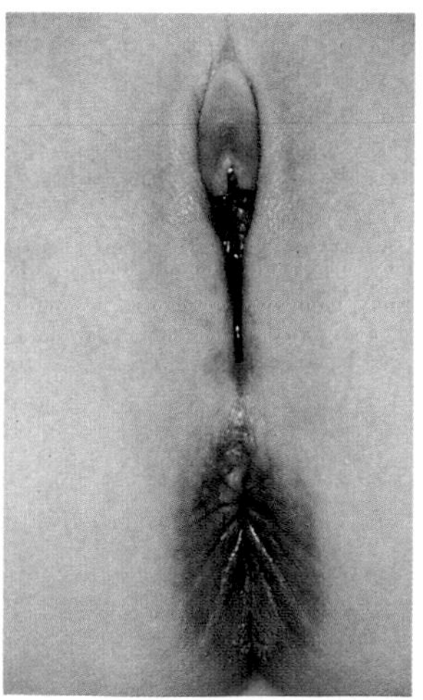

Plate 3. Lichen sclerosus in a prepubertal child.

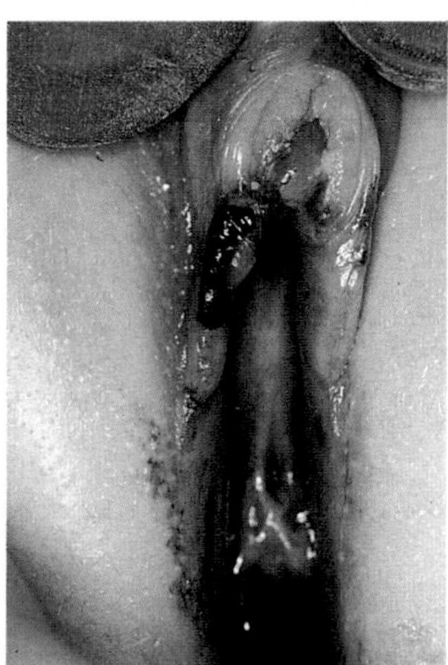

Plate 4. Close up of lichen sclerosus from Plate 3.

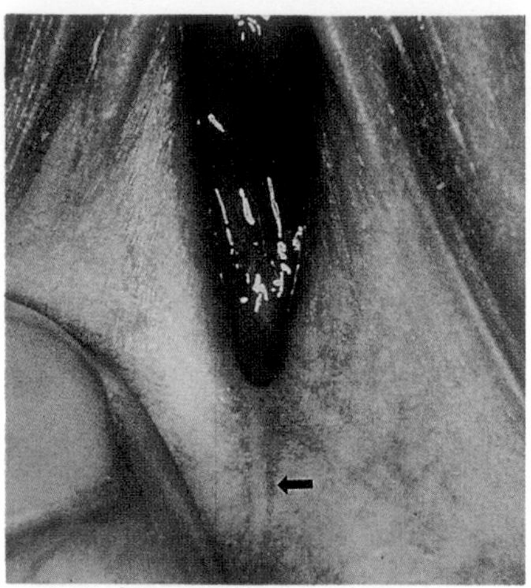

Plate 5. Linea vestibularis (midline sparing, midline avascular area) in a prepubertal girl. (From Heger A, Emans SJ, et al. *Evaluation of the sexually abused child.* New York: Oxford University Press 1992;92; with permission.)

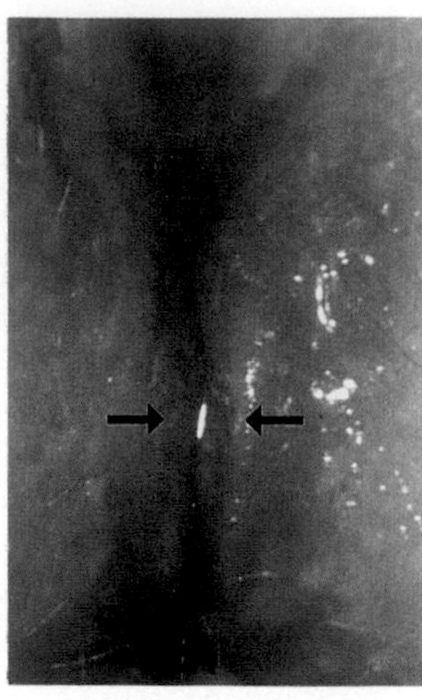

Plate 6. Failure of midline fusion (*arrows*) between the posterior fourchette (P) and the anus (A).

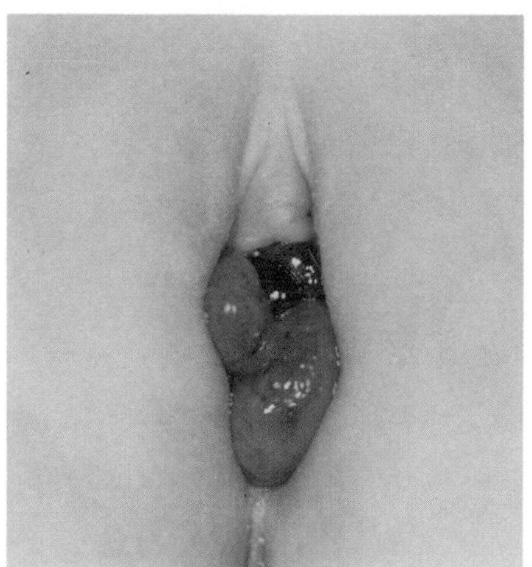

Plate 7. Rhabdomyosarcoma of the vagina (sarcoma botryoides).

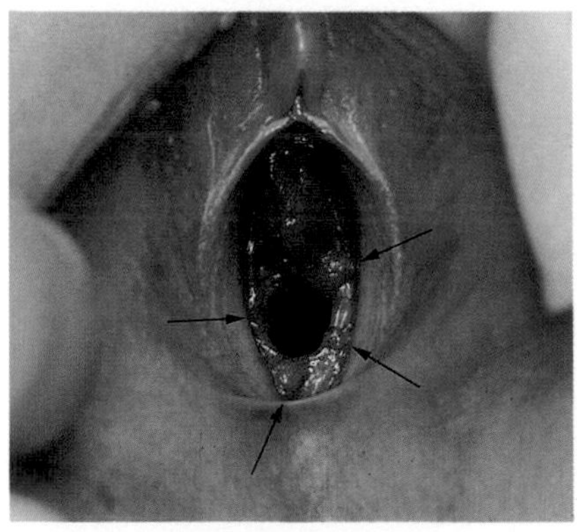

Plate 8. Condyloma acuminata (at arrows) on the hymen of a prepubertal girl.

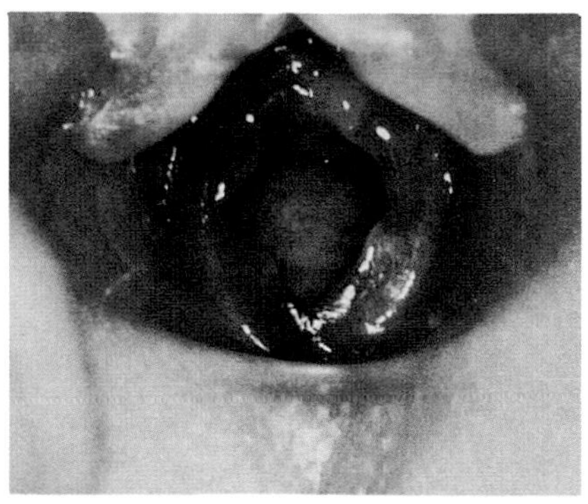

Plate 9. Three-year-old girl with submucosal hemorrhage at 6 o'clock and from 8 to 10 o'clock. Traumatic shallow transection at 9 o'clock from acute sexual abuse. (From Heger A, Emans SJ, et al. *Evaluation of the sexually abused child.* New York: Oxford University Press 1992:119; with permission.)

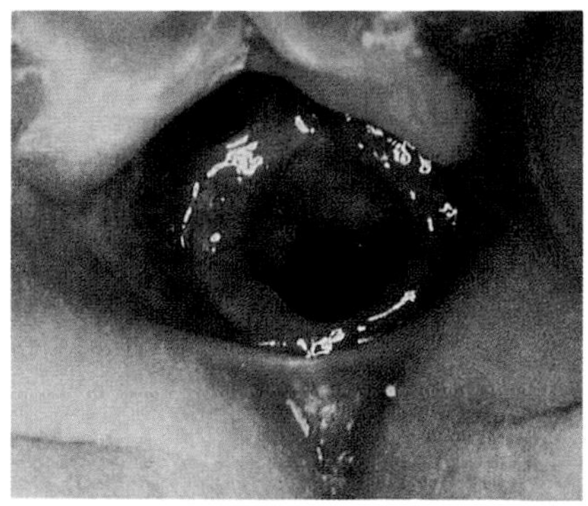

Plate 10. Same patient as Plate 9 with followup 10 days later showing a well healed hymen without any clear indication of previous trauma. (From Heger A, Emans SJ, et al. *Evaluation of the sexually abused child.* New York: Oxford University Press 1992; 119; with permission.)

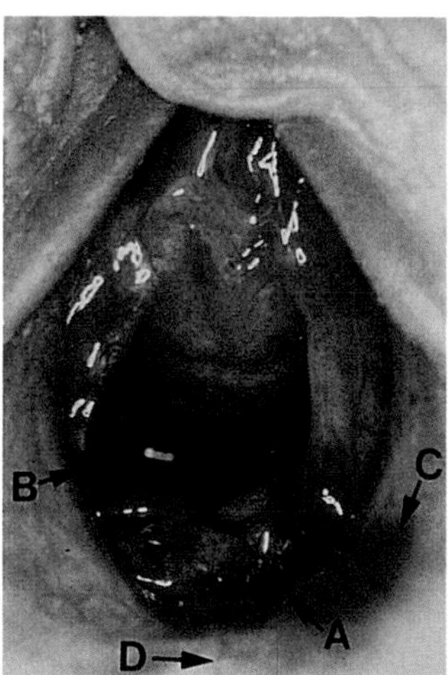

Plate 11. Three days post sexual assault of a 9-year-old girl. Supine traction with jagged edges at 5 o'clock (A). A second transection at 9 o'clock is obscured by edematous tissue (B). Contusion of the vestibular wall (C) and small midline posterior fourchette adhesion (D). (From McCann J, Voris J, Simon M. Genital injuries resulting from sexual abuse: a longitudinal study. *Pediatrics* 1992;89:307; with permission.)

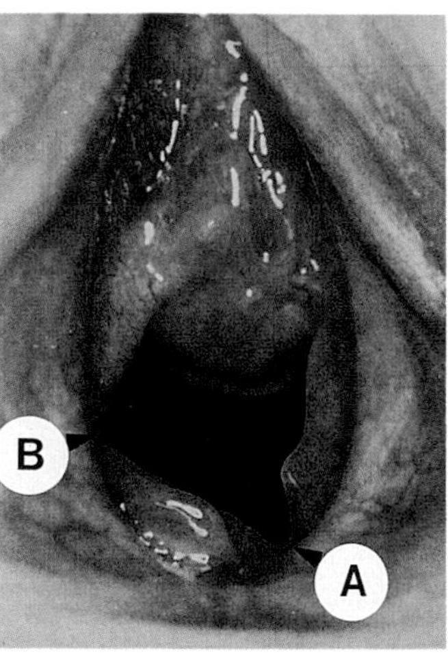

Plate 12. Eleven days post assault in the patient described in Plate 11. Transections (complete clefts) of the hymen at 5 and 9 o'clock. (From McCann J, Voris J, Simon M. Genital injuries resulting from sexual abuse: a longitudinal study. *Pediatrics* 1992; 89:307; with permission.)

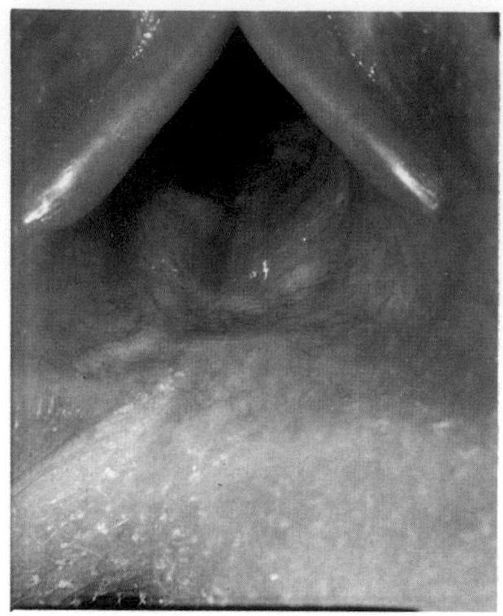

Plate 13. Dilated hymenal orifice and transection of hymen at 6 o'clock in a 9-month-old sexually and physically abused infant.

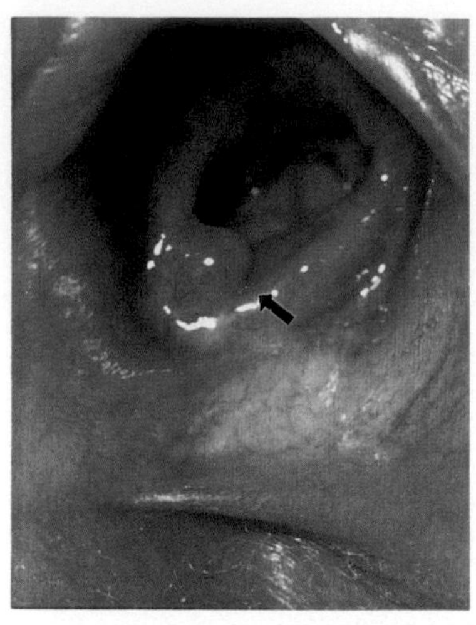

Plate 14. Incomplete transection of the hymen at 6 o'clock (*arrow*) with an adjacent bump in a 3-year-old with a history of sexual abuse and insertion of a magic marker 4 days before the examination. (From Emans SJ, Woods ER, Flagg NT, et al. Genital findings in sexually abused, symptomatic and asymptomatic girls. *Pediatrics* 1987:79:778; with permission.)

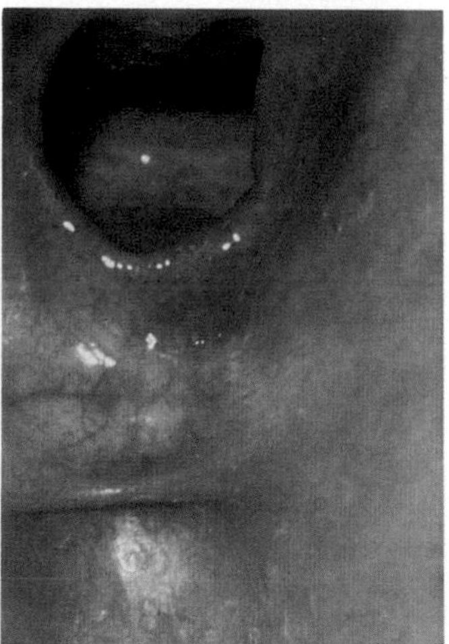

Plate 15. Scarring and rounding of the lower half of the hymen with an adhesion between the hymen and the vagina at 5 o'clock in a 9-year-old girl with a two-year history of chronic sexual abuse. (From Emans SJ, Woods ER, Flagg NT, et al. Genital findings in sexually abused, symptomatic and asymptomatic girls. *Pediatrics* 1987:79:778; with permission.)

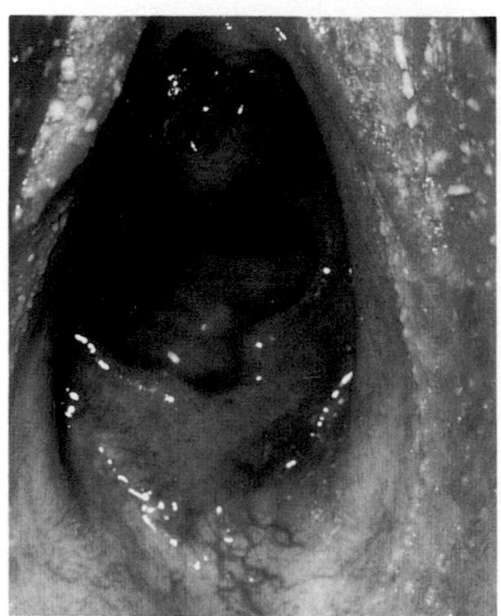

Plate 16. Rounded and distorted lower hymenal border with an indentation at 6 o'clock with two adjacent bumps in an 11-year-old girl with a long history of sexual abuse.

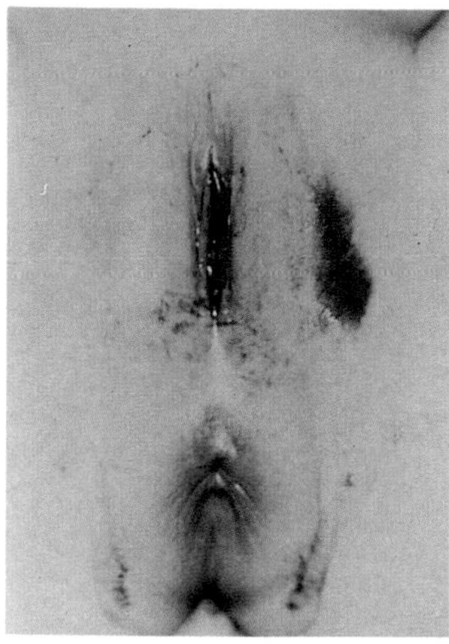

Plate 17. Ecchymoses and bleeding in a child following a straddle injury to the perineum.

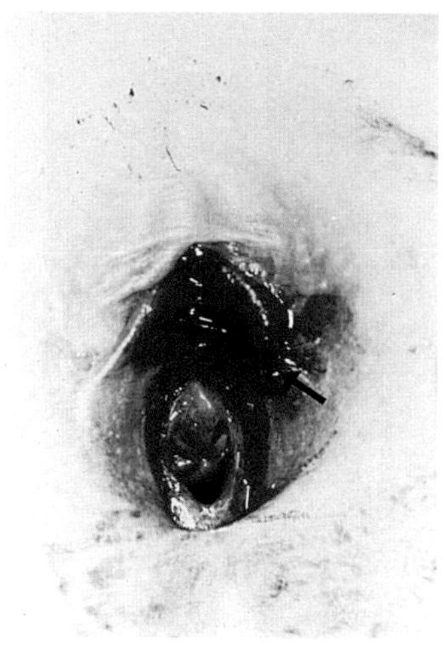

Plate 18. Same child as Plate 17. Close-up of the vulva with laceration by the labia minora and periurethral tissues *(arrow)*. (Note the normal hymen.)

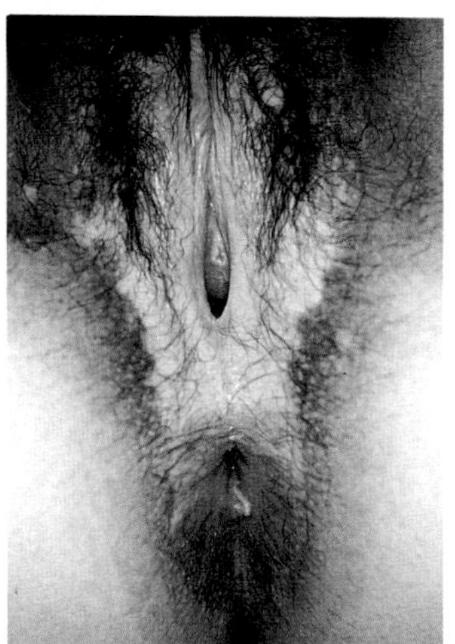

Plate 19. Postpubertal girl with lichen sclerosus.

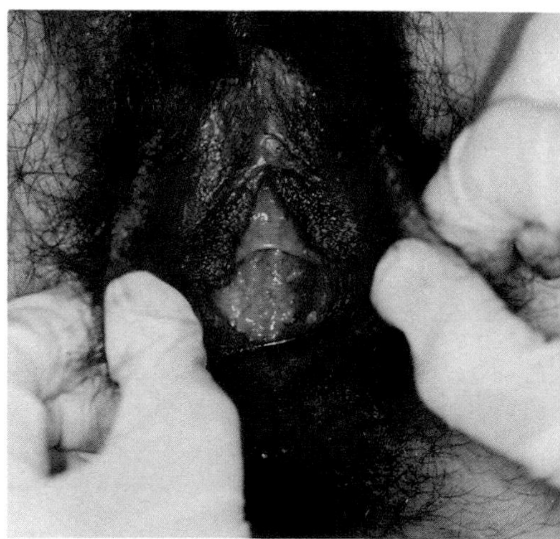

Plate 20. Vaginal agenesis.

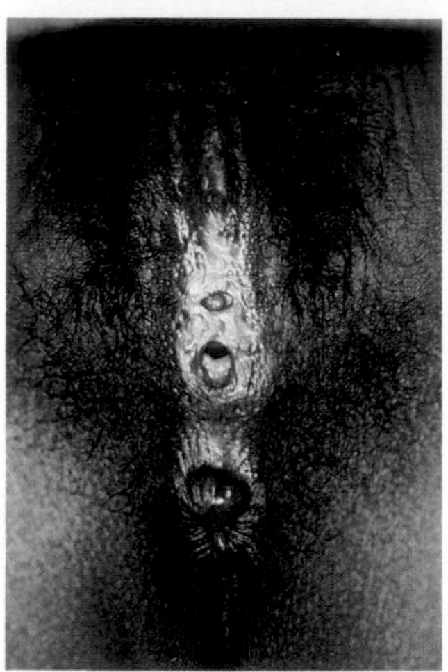

Plate 21. Status post ritual genital mutilation of a young woman from Somalia.

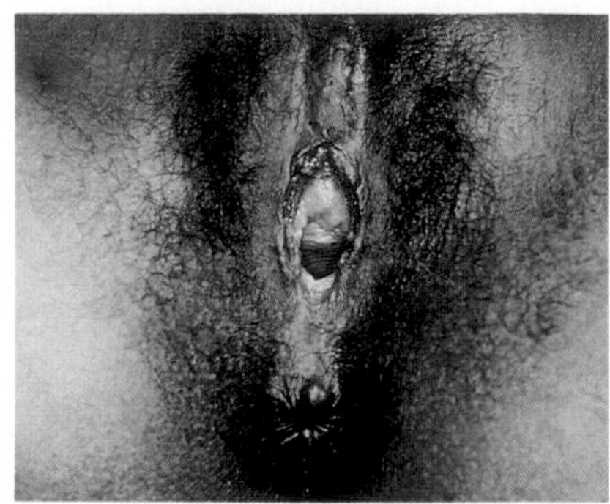

Plate 22. Re-creation of the introitus of the young woman's vulva from Plate 21, performed at the request and specification of the young woman.

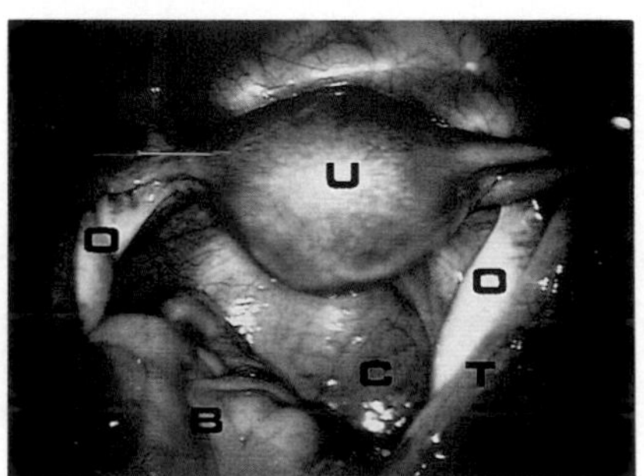

Plate 23. Laparoscopic view of normal pelvis (U, uterus; C, cul-de-sac; O, ovary; T, fallopian tube; B, bowel).

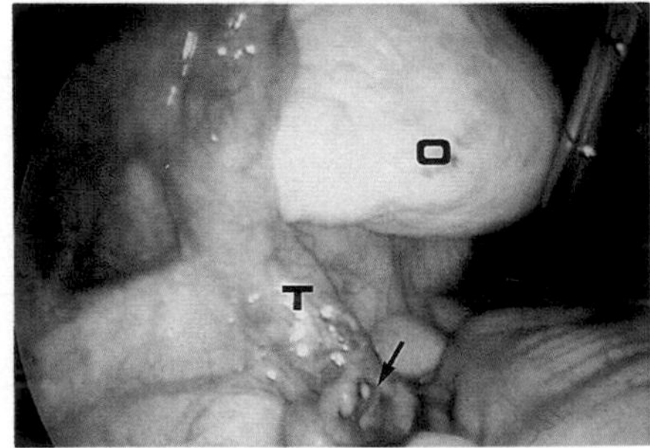

Plate 24. Laparoscopic view of normal ovary (O) and fallopian tube (T). Chromopertubation shows free spill of blue dye from fimbriae *(arrow).* Note that the distal end of the fallopian tube is not directly attached to the ovary.

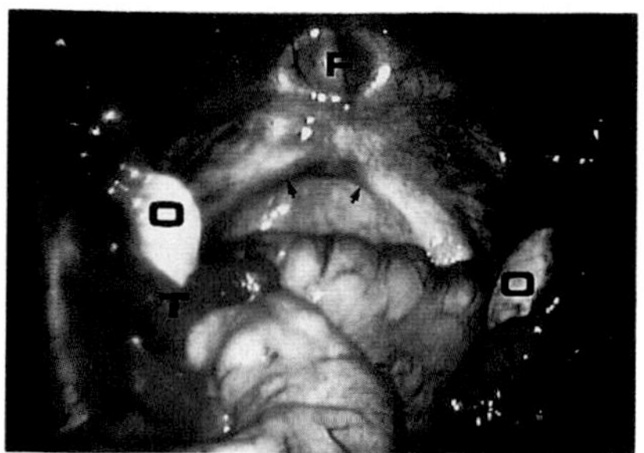

Plate 25. Seventeen-year-old girl with vaginal agenesis and bilateral rudimentary uterine horns. (F, Foley catheter balloon; O, ovary; T, fallopian tube; small arrows demonstrate uterosacral ligaments, large arrows demonstrate rudimentary uterine horns).

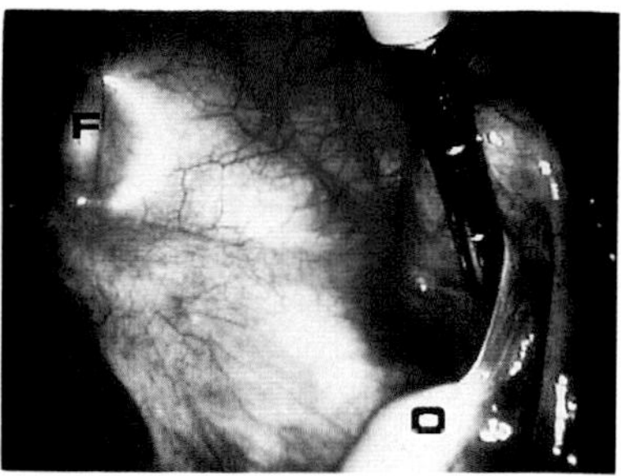

Plate 26. Close-up of rudimentary uterine horn (hemiuterus) shown in Plate 25 (O, ovary; F, Foley catheter balloon).

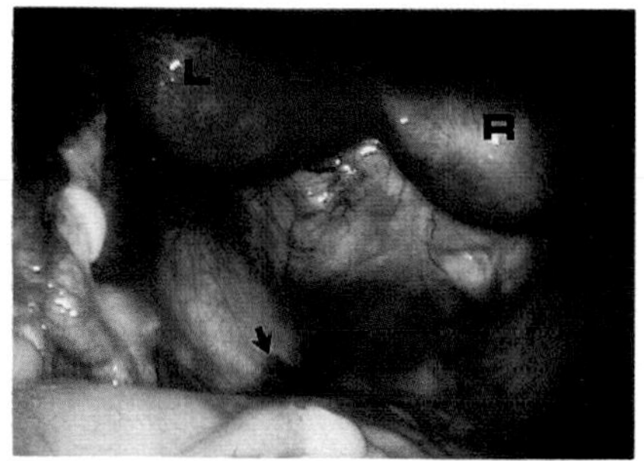

Plate 27. Laparoscopic view of left hemiuterus (L) communicating with single cervix as demonstrated by flow of blue dye injected through the cervix freely spilling from left fallopian tube *(arrow).* Right hemiuterus (R) does not communicate with the cervix and was removed laparoscopically as shown in Figs. 70 to 72 in Chapter 8.

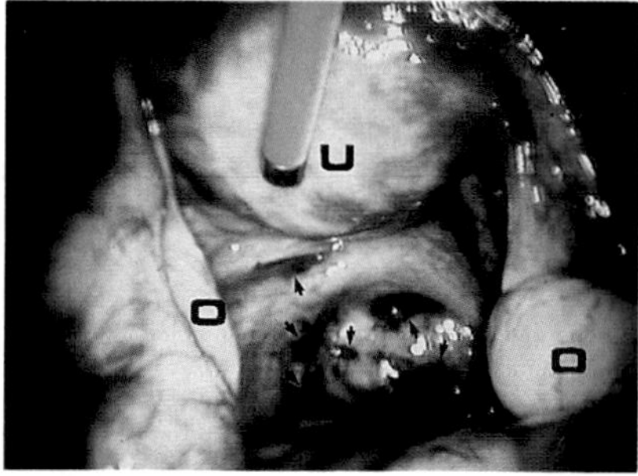

Plate 28. Atypical endometriosis with flame lesions (*arrows*) (U, uterus; O, ovary).

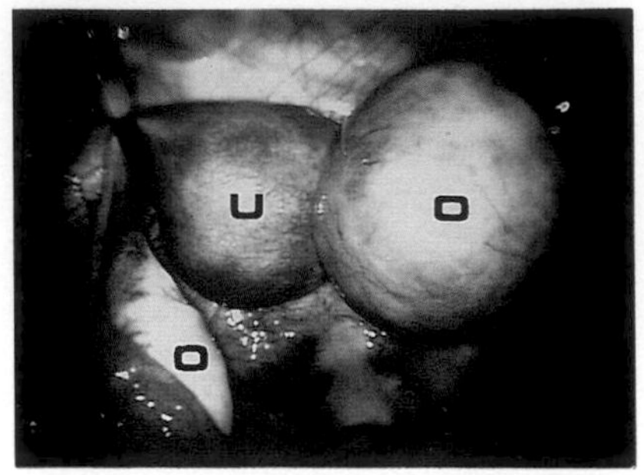

Plate 29. Right simple symptomatic ovarian cyst (U, uterus; O, ovary). (Of note, the photograph post laparoscopic ovarian cystectomy is shown in Fig. 3 in Chapter 15.)

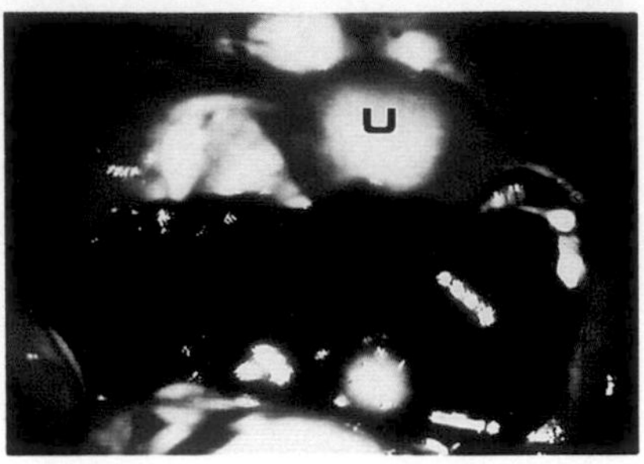

Plate 30. Laparoscopic view of blood and clot filling the pelvis from a ruptured corpus luteal cyst.

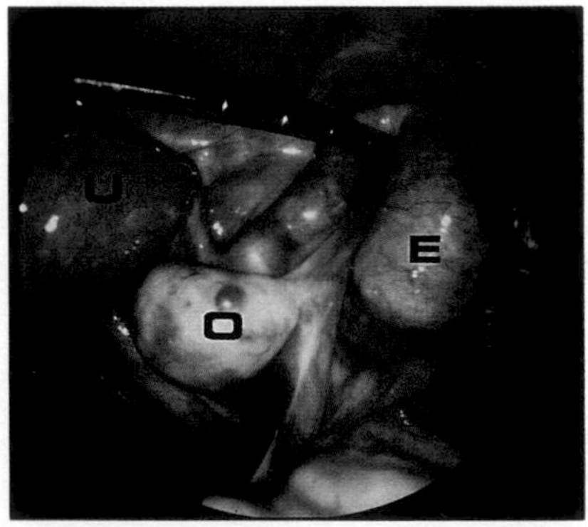

Plate 31. Laparoscopic view of right ectopic pregnancy (U, uterus; O, ovary; E, ectopic pregnancy in right fallopian tube). (Courtesy of Robert B. Hunt, M.D., Department of Obstetrics, Gynecology, and Reproductive Biology, Harvard Medical School, Boston, MA.)

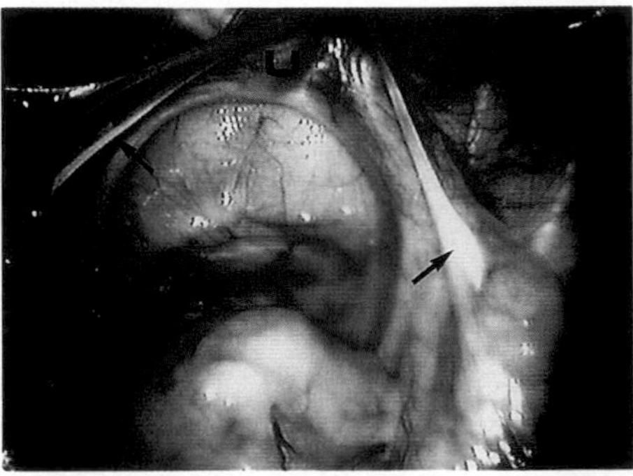

Plate 32. Streak gonads *(small arrows)* and prepubertal uterus (U) in 15-year-old diagnosed with gonadal dysgenesis.

against coexisting *C. trachomatis* (29). A single dose of azithromycin has been reported to cure 93% of patients (101 of 118 male) with *N. gonorrhoeae* (30), and a 2-g dose has been recently approved by the Food and Drug Administration (FDA). Further studies are needed of cost and side effects. Oral medications may be preferred for rape victims who may be further traumatized by an intramuscular injection.

A serologic test for syphilis should be sent at the time of therapy. If the initial test result is negative, a followup blood test 1 month later is necessary only if the patient was treated with spectinomycin or a quinolone. HIV counseling and availability of testing as well as individual counseling about risk reduction and "safer sex" are important parts of care. Patients are instructed to abstain from sexual relations for 7 days. Since treatment failure is rare with the recommended regimens, a rescreening test for gonorrhea done 1 to 2 months after treatment allows the opportunity to test for reinfection. Adolescents who have had one gonococcal infections are likely to acquire a second one. Among teens with an *N. gonorrhoeae* infection in our clinics, 23% developed one or more additional infections with *N. gonorrhoeae* and 19% developed another chlamydial infection in the ensuing 8 to 14 months of followup (31). Persistent symptoms also call for retesting.

Every patient should be interviewed to find contacts within 60 days before symptoms or diagnosis. Regardless of symptoms, all contacts should be tested and treated at the same visit.

Gonococcal Pharyngitis

Gonococcal pharyngeal infection is usually asymptomatic, but may occur as patchy erythema (virus-like throat) or less commonly with a red, edematous uvula with vesiculopustular lesions on the soft palate and tonsillar pillars (strep-like) (32,33). This infection spontaneously clears in 10 to 12 weeks; however, patients are at risk for disseminated disease during this time. Diagnosis is by culture on selective media. Recommended treatment is ceftriaxone, 125 mg IM once, or ciprofloxacin, 500 mg orally as a single dose, or ofloxacin 400 mg orally as a single dose plus treatment for Chlamydia.

Gonococcal Proctitis

Gonococcal infection of the rectum may occur asymptomatically, or the patient may have an anal discharge of blood and pus (acute proctitis) or a low-grade proctitis with pain on defecation. In suspected cases, a cotton-tipped applicator should be inserted into the rectum to obtain a sample of the pus for culture; the specimen should be obtained by direct visualization if possible (34). Proctitis can be more difficult to treat than urethritis, but the treatment courses for women are the same as noted for cervicitis.

Disseminated Gonococcal Infection

Disseminated gonococcal infection (DGI) results from gonococcal bacteremia and the patient may present with skin lesions, migratory arthralgias, tenosynovitis, arthritis, and rarely hepatitis, meningitis, or endocarditis.

The diagnosis of gonococcal arthritis depends largely on clinical suspicion because the source of the gonococcus in adolescent girls is usually an asymptomatic or low-grade cervicitis or pharyngeal infection (33,35). Two forms of gonococcal arthritis have been described by Holmes and others (36,37), although many patients do not fit this classic description. In young women, the early form begins at the onset or just following a menstrual period and is characterized by migratory polyarthralgias, tenosynovitis, fever, chills, and skin lesions (pinpoint erythematous papules that may progress to purpuric vesiculopustular lesions) (Fig. 2). There are usually <20 skin lesions, chiefly in a peripheral distribution. Gram stain and culture from these lesions are positive in about 10% of patients (35), but direct fluorescent antibody staining of biopsies detects *N. gonorrhoeae* in more than half of these patients. Blood cultures may be positive if taken within 2 days of the onset of symptoms. Joint fluid, usually scanty, is often negative by culture for the gonococcus.

The late form of gonococcal arthritis is characterized by a monarticular effusion, most often involving the knee, followed by elbows, ankles, wrists, small joints of the hands and feet, and shoulders. A positive synovial fluid culture occurs in 20% to 50% of cases. Cultures of synovial fluid containing <20,000 leukocytes/mm^3 are usually negative, whereas fluids containing >80,000/mm^3 are usually positive. PCR is a more sensitive detection technique (15). Blood cultures are negative and systemic symptoms are usually absent in the late form.

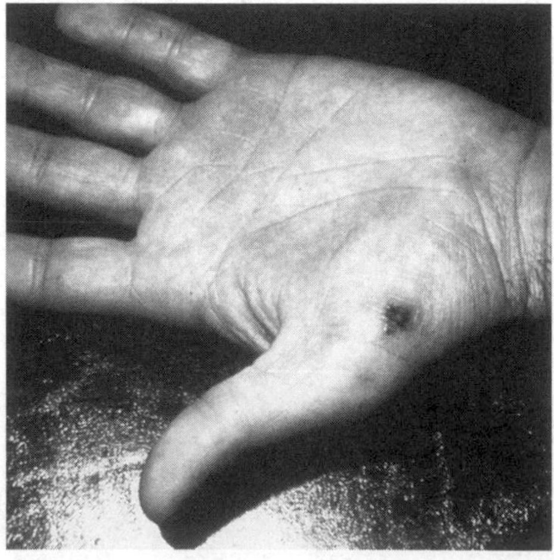

FIG. 2. Skin lesion of gonococemia.

In a recent study of 41 cases of gonococcal arthritis from 1985 to 1991, Wise and colleagues (21) reported positive cultures from 86% of urogenital samples, 14 (44%) synovial fluid samples, 7 rectal samples (39%), 4 blood samples (12%), and 2 throat samples (7%). Clinical features included migratory arthralgias in 27, urogenital symptoms or signs in 26, fever in 21, and skin lesions in 16.

Hospitalization is recommended for initial therapy and is essential in those who are unreliable for followup, have purulent joint effusions, an uncertain diagnosis, or evidence of meningitis or endocarditis.

Treatment of DGI includes *one* of the following: ceftriaxone 1 g IV or IM daily, or cefotaxime, 1 g IV, every 8 hours, or ceftizoxime, 1 g IV, every 8 hours, or for patients allergic to β-lactam drugs ciprofloxacin, 500 mg IV every 12 hours, or spectinomycin, 2 g IM every 12 hours. All regimens are continued for 7 to 10 days or at least 1 to 2 days intravenously or until improvement and then followed by cefixime 400 mg orally twice a day or ciprofloxacin 500 mg orally twice a day (not in pregnant or lactating women or adolescents under 18 years) to complete 7 days' total therapy (3,38). Immobilization of the joint is helpful. Although open drainage of joints other than the hip is not indicated, repeated aspiration may be necessary (3).

Gonococcal endocarditis and meningitis should be treated with ceftriaxone 1 to 2 g intravenously every 12 hours for 10 to 14 days (meningitis) or for 4 weeks (endocarditis). The possibility of a complement deficiency should be investigated in patients with serious DGI (39).

Reiter's Syndrome

Reiter's syndrome is characterized by the triad of arthritis, urethritis, and ocular abnormalities, frequently following a disease such as *N. gonorrhoeae* or *C. trachomatis* urethritis, or enteric infections such as *Shigella*, *Salmonella*, or *Yersinia*. Evidence of *Chlamydia* infections has been found in 42% to 69% of patients with Reiter's syndrome (40). Reiter's syndrome is associated with HLA-B27 and -B7 determinants. The joints affected are primarily knees, ankles, feet, and wrists in an oligo- or monarticular pattern; sacroilitis and spondyloarthropathies can also occur. Ocular problems include iritis and conjunctivitis. Dermatologic findings include keratoblennorrhagica, mucocutaneous lesions, balanitis circinate, nail changes, and oral ulcers. Treatment should aim at the detection and antimicrobial therapy of the genital infection and the use of nonsteroidal antiinflammatory agents for the reactive arthritis. The eyes should be carefully monitored by an ophthalmologist and treated with topical and systemic agents as indicated (41,42).

Gonococcal Eye Infections

Although gonococcal ophthalmia in the newborn is well known to pediatricians, adolescents can develop purulent discharge from gonococcal conjunctivitis. Periorbital edema and pain, gaze restriction, keratitis, and preauricular adenopathy can occur. Ceftriaxone, 25 to 50 mg/kg (maximum 1 g) IM should be administered, and evaluation and followup by an ophthalmologist are essential. The possibility of concurrent chlamydial eye infection or genital infections with *N. gonorrhoeae* or other STDs should be evaluated.

Gonococcal Infections in the Prepubertal Child

Gonococcal infection in the prepubertal child is typically manifested as a purulent vulvovaginitis rather than a cervicitis. The infection may rarely be asymptomatic or be evident as a thin mucoid discharge (see Chapters 3 and 20). Although the Gram stain is helpful, *Neisseria meningitides* and other *Neisseria* species can be associated with vaginal discharge. Other nonculture tests such as DNA probes should not be used for diagnosis in children. Cultures should be confirmed with two tests using different principles (biochemical, enzyme substrate, or serologic). Isolates should be preserved to permit additional testing if needed.

Rectal infections occur in about half of girls with gonococcal vaginitis and may be asymptomatic or cause perianal itching, burning, purulent discharge, and tenesmus. Oropharyngeal infections have been rarely reported alone (43). Conjunctivitis may occur alone or in association with vulvovaginitis. Once a diagnosis is made, the child should be interviewed by an experienced social worker, psychologist, nurse practitioner, or pediatrician to try to elicit a history of sexual abuse (see Chapter 20). Culturing all family members and caretakers of the child can be helpful in determining the source of the infection, frequently an older male relative or step-parent. Although it is potentially possible that *N. gonorrhoeae* can be transmitted by sexual play between siblings and peers, the clinician should assume that sexual abuse is involved in all cases of prepubertal gonorrhea. Since sexual abuse often involves vulvar coitus or oral sex rather than vaginal penetration, a physical examination in many abused girls shows a normal hymen. Cases of gonorrhea must be reported to the mandated state agency.

Prior to treatment, rectal and pharyngeal cultures for *N. gonorrhoeae* should be obtained from the child with vaginal gonorrhea since anorectal and pharyngeal infections are frequently asymptomatic. A vaginal culture for *C. trachomatis* and a serology for syphilis should also be obtained. HIV counseling and testing should be considered initially and at followup.

For children over 100 pounds (≥45 kg), adult regimens for treating cervicitis and urethritis are used. For children under 100 pounds (<45 kg), the recommended regimen is ceftriaxone, 125 mg IM once. Children allergic to cephalosporins are treated with spectinomycin, 40 mg/kg (maximum 2 g) IM once. Patients under 45 kg with bacteremia or arthritis are treated with ceftriaxone, 50 mg/kg (maximum 1 g) once daily for 7 days (3). Coinfection with *C. trachomatis* should be treated with erythromycin, 50 mg/kg/day in 4 divided doses (<45 kg, ≤8 years), and with azithromycin 1 g single dose, or with doxycycline in children older than 8 years (see also Chapter 3). Children ≥45 kg and <8 years may be treated with azithromycin 1 g.

Followup cultures of the throat, rectum, and vagina should be taken 7 to 14 days after treatment. Reinfection is likely if the source is not identified and treated. Persistent vaginal discharge in a girl who has been adequately treated and had negative cultures for gonorrhea may result from a coinfection with *C. trachomatis* that was not adequately treated.

Only a few cases of salpingitis secondary to *N. gonorrhoeae* have been reported in prepubertal girls, and thus no data exist on the best form of treatment (43–45). Antibiotics with similar spectrum as used in adolescent and adult PID are appropriate. Disseminated gonococcal disease has also been rarely reported.

CHLAMYDIA TRACHOMATIS INFECTIONS

The past two decades have delineated the importance of the epidemic of *C. trachomatis* infections among sexually active patients, especially adolescents. There are an estimated 4 million new cases of *Chlamydia* infection each year in the United States with treatment and sequelae costing over $2 billion annually (3,46,47). In 1995, a total of 477,638 cases of *Chlamydia* were reported to the Centers for Disease Control and Prevention (CDC) with the highest rates in the western and midwestern states. The annual rate of *Chlamydia* test positivity has generally declined from 1988 to 1995, with the highest rates occurring among teens who are at high risk of acquiring this infection.

The serotypes D through K have been associated with nongonococcal urethritis and epididymitis in men and mucopurulent cervicitis, salpingitis, urethritis (see pyuria-dysuria syndrome in Chapter 11), postabortal and postpartum endometritis, and perihepatitis in women. Cervical infection with *C. trachomatis* has been associated with premature rupture of membranes, preterm labor, and low birth weight (48). Chlamydial DNA is found more commonly in the cervix of infertility patients, especially those with tubal factors as the cause of infertility (49). Both men and women may have conjunctivitis, Reiter's syndrome, and rectal infections. Infants born to mothers with chlamydial genital infections may have conjunctivitis and pneumonia.

C. trachomatis is a common infection, occurring in 5% to 15% of asymptomatic sexually active adolescent and young adult patients, 20% to 30% of patients seen in STD clinics, 40% to 50% of symptomatic patients, and 15% to 50% of patients with *N. gonorrhoeae*. Adolescents have an increased number of partners, are inconsistent users of condoms, and often have a significant cervical ectropion. The columnar cells on the cervical ectropion are exposed to the vaginal environment and are thus more easily colonized with *Chlamydia*. If the patient has an ectropion, the presence of infecting *Chlamydia* is also more easily detected. Oral contraceptives have been reported in some studies, but not others, to be associated with *Chlamydia* infections. Oral contraceptives may also affect the prevalence by contributing to the persistence of the ectropion. Adolescents also may be at increased risk of developing a chlamydial infection because of their "immunologic immaturity" and lower levels of antichlamydial antibodies. It is estimated that sexually active women less than 20 years old have chlamydial infection rates two- to threefold higher than adult women. Prevalence figures vary depending on the population studied, with rates from 4.9% in a college population in the mid-1970s to 27% in inner-city pregnant teens (50–67). Among 16-to 24-year-old female entrants into the U.S. Job Corps, positivity results have ranged from 4.2% to 17.1% (71). Most clinics can expect that 6% to 15% of sexually active adolescents screened will have *C. trachomatis* endocervical infections (Table 1).

Several studies of risk profiles for women with chlamydial infections have been done (60–73). In a study of 1059 women attending family planning clinics with a 9.3% prevalence of *C. trachomatis* infection, Handsfield and coworkers (64) reported that the presence of two or more of the following risk factors identified 90% of infections: age under 25 years, intercourse with a new partner within 2 months, examination showing purulent or mucopurulent cervical exudate, bleeding induced by swabbing the endocervical mucosa, and use of no contraception or a nonbarrier method. In a study of eight high-risk family planning and STD clinics (prevalence 17.6%) in New York and two low-risk college and private clinics (prevalence 5.7%), Han and colleagues (65) identified the following demographics as risk factors for *Chlamydia* infection among women (mean age of 24.5 years): age under 20 years [odds ratio (OR) 1.6], use of oral contraceptives (OR 2.0), a history of more than one sexual partner in 6 months (OR 1.7), and inflammation on Papanicolaou (Pap) smear (OR 2.1). A study of four family planning clinics in San Francisco (prevalence 9.2%) revealed five factors associated with infection: age under 25 years, cervical friability, single marital status, a new sexual partner within the past 3 months, and lack of barrier contraception (66). In a university student health center with a *Chlamydia* infection prevalence of 9%, Johnson and colleagues (60) identified a new sexual partner within 2 months, more than one partner within 6 months, cervical ectopy, cervical friability, at least 20 polymorphonuclear leukocytes per high power field in cervical secretions, and leukocytes in vaginal secretions as important contributors to their model. In a primary care clinic at Group Health Cooperative of Puget Sound (prevalence 3.7% overall, and 13% for those under 20 years), Stergachis and colleagues (61) reported seven characteristics independently predictive of *Chlamydia* infection: being unmarried, examination showing ectopy, black race, douching, nulliparity, age 24 years or under, and intercourse with two or more partners in the preceding year.

In STD clinics, the presence of mucopurulent cervical discharge, a positive yellow swab test (a white cotton-tipped applicator is twirled in the endocervical canal and the color compared to a white background), and the presence of leukocytes on a Gram stain of the endocervical discharge have all been associated with *C. trachomatis* infection. Brunham and associates (68) in a study of 100 women in an STD clinic found that of those with *C. trachomatis* isolated, 89% had 10 or more polymorphonuclear leukocytes per oil immersion field; in contrast, only 17% of those without *C. trachomatis* had 10 or more leukocytes. However, examining this test in an adolescent clinic, Moscicki et al (69) found the positive predictive value of finding more than 5 leukocytes per oil immersion field (1000×) to be only 36%. Although in STD clinics patients may have signs and symptoms of chlamydial infections, in lower risk settings such as college health centers most patients are asymptomatic and detected only by screening tests.

Given the difficulty in identifying risk factors for individual sexually active teenagers, the best policy is to screen adolescents once or twice a year, after a change in sexual partners, and with any suggestive symptoms (70). In the presence of a positive endocervical culture, Jones and coworkers (72) found that 40% of women have positive cultures from the endometrium and evidence of silent upper tract infection. More adolescents with endocervical infection with *C. trachomatis* go on to develop salpingitis than do adult women, so screening becomes particularly important.

Recurrent *Chlamydia* infections are particularly problematic because of the increased incidence of resulting tubal damage and subsequent infertility. In a retrospective study of women in Wisconsin, young age at first infection was the strongest predictor of recurrent *C. trachomatis* (69). In 54% of those under 15 years old at initial infection and 30% of those 15 to 19 years old, recurrence developed in the following 1 to 6 years.

Diagnosis

A number of detection methods for diagnosing *C. trachomatis* are now available, and improved methods are likely to be expanded in clinical use soon (74–84) (Table 2). Female endocervical samples can be screened using cultures, direct immunofluorescent smears (MicroTrak), enzyme immunoassays (Chlamydiazyme, Abbott; IDEIA, Dako), DNA probes (Pace 2, Gen-Probe), ligase chain reaction (LCR, Abbott), polymerase chain reaction (PCR, Amplicor, Roche), and transcription-mediated amplification (TMA, Gen-Probe Amplified) (85). Urine screening is possible with many of the new LCR, PCR, and TMA technologies, which are likely to revolutionize the screening of teens at intervals between their annual gynecologic evaluation. In prepubertal children, in whom the diagnosis of sexual abuse must be considered, culture is essential because of the possibility of

TABLE 2. *Sensitivity and specificity of test for* Chlamydia trachomatis

	Sensitivity (%)	Specificity (%)
Cell culture	80–90	100
Direct fluorescent antibody test (DFA)	61–93	82–97
Enzyme immunoassay (EIA)	74–89	93–98
Enzyme-amplified monoclonal immunoassay (IDEIA)	93–97	97–99
Nucleic acid hybridization (DNA probe)	71–95	97–100
Polymerase chain reaction (PCR)	93–97	99–100
Ligase chain reaction (LCR)	87–94	99–100
Transcription-mediated amplification (TMA)	98–100	98–100

false-positive indirect tests. In adolescents, if the data are being collected for medical-legal reasons, appropriate cultures are important. It is critical that in choosing tests for screening adolescents the package insert of the test be read carefully to determine what sites have been approved for use of the tests. For example, rectal flora can give false-positive results for enzyme immunoassay (EIA) tests. Thus culture is currently indicated for nasopharyngeal specimens in infants, rectal specimens in all patients (regardless of age), and vaginal specimens in prepubertal girls (47). Studies are gradually evolving on the utility of PCR, LCR, and TMA testing on specimens related to sexual abuse and sexual assault and new gold standards may evolve over the next few years (see Chapter 20).

In adolescents, culture using McCoy cells and subsequent identification using fluorescent antibody stain 2 to 3 days later has been considered the gold standard against which other methods are judged. Culture will not detect nonviable organisms of the lower genital tract while viable organisms may coexist in the upper genital tract. Care must be taken when cultures are obtained to make sure that a Dacron swab is used and that the endocervix is scraped to obtain cells, since *C. trachomatis* is an intracellular organism. Although the specificity is 100%, it is estimated that the sensitivity of the culture is only 80% to 90%. The use of a special cervical cytobrush may improve detection of the organism.

The SYVA MicroTrak system includes urethral and cervical swabs and a cytobrush for making a direct smear. After applying a fluorescein-conjugated monoclonal antibody, the microscopist looks for the presence of yellow-green elementary bodies. The value of this test depends on the prevalence of *C. trachomatis* in the population studied, whether single- or double-pass cultures are used as the standard, and whether 1, 5, or 10 elementary bodies are considered a positive test result. The sensitivity of this test has ranged from a low of 61% in an adolescent clinic (50) to 93% in an STD clinic (76). The positive predictive value of this test ranges from 80% in populations with a 10% prevalence of infection to a predictive value of 95% in populations with a prevalence of 30%.

Enzyme immunoassays include chlamydiazyme and IDEIA. Chlamydiazyme is an enzyme-linked immunoabsorbent assay and requires a spectrophotometer. This test also has had a range of sensitivities and specificities depending on the study; Amortegui and Meyer (77) found a sensitivity of 82% in a population with a prevalence of 8.8%, compared to a study by Baselski and coworkers (78) that found a sensitivity of 96% in a pregnant group with a prevalence of 21.1%. Positive predictive values have ranged from 32% to 87% depending on the population studied. Lebar and associates (83) reported a 97% sensitivity in a population with a 16% prevalence of infection using another immunoassay (Boots CellTech IDEIA III).

The DNA probes can provide testing for both gonorrhea and *Chlamydia* infection with a single swab. Sensitivities have been reported for chlamydial DNA tests to be 65% to 92% with specificities of 95% to 99% (63,79,80,84). In a study of adolescents, Biro and colleagues (63) reported that the Gen-Probe PACE 2 system had a sensitivity of 72%, specificity of 96%, positive predictive value of 67%, and negative predictive value of 96% in asymptomatic girls (prevalence 11%) and sensitivity of 65%, specificity of 96%, positive predictive value of 81%, and negative predictive value of 91% in symptomatic girls (prevalence 20.7%). Office-based tests such as Kodak Surecell have a reported sensitivity of 67% to 84% (81). Similar technologies offer promise because of the ability to test and treat at the same visit. LCR and PCR techniques provide marked amplification of specific DNA sequences and TMA an amplified RNA assay; all three have yielded a new standard for chlamydial detection. Several of these tests are also approved for screening of urine in adolescents and thus noninvasive screening for *Chlamydia* is possible. In addition, some methods allow for detection of *Chlamydia* and gonorrhea simultaneously. Loeffelholz et al (82) reported a rapid and sensitive PCR assay (Amplicor) with a sensitivity of 97% and specificity of 99.7%, compared to culture sensitivity of 85.7% and specificity 100%. Hsuih et al (84) reported a sensitivity of 82.4% and specificity of 93.3% for Amplicor PCR in comparison with a sensitivity of 99.4% and specificity of 98.3% for GenProbe PACE II. LCR, an *in vitro* nucleic acid amplification technique that exponentially amplifies selected DNA sequences, has proved sensitive and specific in the detection of *Chlamydia* in the cervix and urine of women. In a study of 2132 endocervical specimens at five sites with 10.9% confirmed as having *Chlamydia*, the sensitivity for LCR (Abbott LCx) was 94% and cell culture 65%; specificity of both was >99.9% (86). TMA has a sensitivity and specificity of 98% to 100%.

Given the limitations of all the tests for *Chlamydia*, symptomatic patients with mucopurulent cervical infection and their partners should be treated even if these detection methods yield negative results. However, young women with cervical ectopy may have persistent or recurrent mucopus in spite of the eradication of *N. gonorrhoeae* and *C. trachomatis*, and thus additional research is needed to elucidate other infectious agents responsible for this condition.

In choosing a test for office practice, clinicians need to look at the comparison of the test with culture, the expense, the time to obtain results, and the sensitivity and predictive value in the population of patients for whom they will be providing care (88–91). Cultures are of greatest value in screening populations with a low risk of chlamydial infection. Trachtenburg and colleagues (87) have estimated that with a prevalence of >2%, screening would pay for itself. Analyzing costs of various strategies, Phillips and coworkers (89) found that using a rapid test to detect *C. trachomatis* would reduce overall health costs if the prevalence was ≥7% and that routine cultures would be cost effective with a prevalence >14%. Screening also markedly reduces the risk of PID (90). Doing urethral cultures in addition to endocervical screening detects a small number of additional patients—4.5% in one study (91)—who are infected with *C. trachomatis* but adds to cost and is uncomfortable to the patient.

Results were initially conflicting on testing first catch urine with several methods in women to detect chlamydial infections without the need for endocervical swabs (62,91–93); more recent studies of new methodology have shown considerable success. In a Swedish study, Svensson et al (92) reported that among 619 asymptomatic teens in a family planning clinic, 7.8% had positive results on endocervical screening and 6% on first catch urine (IDEIA media). At the same time 751 asymptomatic high school students were screened by first catch urine with a positive rate of 2.1%. In contrast, Sellors et al (91) found that only 37.3% of all *Chlamydia*-positive women had a positive first catch urine test result using an enzyme immunoassay, Chlamydiazyme. The new Abbott LCR test, recently approved by the FDA, detected 30% more *Chlamydia* infections in the first void urine samples (first 15 to 20 ml) than endocervical swabs (93). The TMA (Gen-Probe Amplified) also provides urine testing for *Chlamydia*.

In Pap smears from women seen in STD clinics, increased numbers of histiocytes and polymorphonuclear leukocytes and the presence of transformed leukocytes have been associated with *C. trachomatis* infection with sensitivities of 17% to 95%, specificities of 61% to 100%, and positive predictive values of 40% to 100% (94,95). Since it is likely that an adolescent would already have been screened for *C. trachomatis*, reports of the Pap smear are difficult to use in selective screening but certainly should encourage followup evaluation if findings suggestive of *Chlamydia* are noted. Colposcopic evaluation has suggested an association between *C. trachomatis* infection and endocervical mucopus, hypertrophic cervicitis, and immature metaplasia (96).

Serologies for IgG and IgM to *C. trachomatis* are primarily a research tool. A conversion from lack of antibody to the presence of a titer 3 weeks after PID, the presence of IgM, and a fourfold rise in antibody titer have been used to confirm the role of *C. trachomatis* retrospectively in clinical cases of salpingitis and some sexual abuse cases. Antibodies to *C. trachomatis* are more common in women with PID, tubal infertility, and ectopic pregnancy than in control women without these disorders. In children, infections with so-called TWAR agents may give cross-reacting rises in antibody titers to *C. trachomatis*.

In addition to genital tract infections, *C. trachomatis* has been recognized increasingly as an etiologic agent in perihepatitis or Fitz-Hugh-Curtis syndrome (97). Salpingitis may or may not be present. The patient typically presents with right upper quadrant pain, often pleuritic, and laboratory evaluation reveals an increased sedimentation rate and a positive endocervical culture for *C. trachomatis*. Ultrasonography may be necessary to exclude biliary tract disease in patients with this type of pain. Liver function tests are usually normal in chlamydial perihepatitis, in contrast to the abnormal liver function tests that may accompany gonococcal perihepatitis.

Although *C. trachomatis* has been cultured from the pharynx in 3.7% of men and 3.2% of women in an STD clinic (98), a positive culture was not associated with symptoms. This organism is rarely cultured from patients with symptomatic pharyngitis and thus does not appear to be an important etiologic agent for this disease. Similarly, *C. trachomatis* has been cultured from the rectum of 5.2% of women attending an STD clinic. A positive rectal culture in women tends to correlate with concurrent genital infection, not rectal symptoms (100), although mild proctitis has been associated with nonlymphogranuloma venereum immunotypes in homosexual men (99).

Treatment

Treatment of *C. trachomatis* cervical and urethral infections in women is *one* of the following (3,47,100):

Azithromycin 1.0 g orally once
or
Doxycycline, 100 mg orally two times a day for 7 days

Alternate regimens:
Ofloxacin 300 mg two times a day for 7 days
or
Erythromycin base, 500 mg four times a day for 7 days
or
Erythromycin ethylsuccinate, 800 mg four times a day for 7 days

Doxycycline and azithromycin are similar in efficacy and side effects (100). In one study, 17% of patients treated with azithromycin and 20% of those treated with doxycycline had side effects, mainly gastrointestinal (100). Azithromycin, an azalide antibiotic, has the advantage of a long half-life and single dosing, which can be administered by a health professional, but the medication is also more costly. Ofloxacin and trovafloxacin have similar efficacy to doxycycline and can also be used to treat *N. gonorrhoeae* (101) but quinolones cannot be used in pregnancy, lactation, or adolescents under 18 years of age. Trimethoprim/sulfamethazole (160 mg/800 mg), twice a day for 10 days, has a higher failure rate of 8% to 10%. Clindamycin is effective against *Chlamydia* in vitro and results in clinical and bacteriologic cure in patients given clindamycin and gentamicin for PID. In a small study of 56 women with *C. trachomatis* treated with clindamycin 450 mg four times daily for 10 days, 86% completed the course and had microbiologic and clinical cures (102).

Pregnant patients are generally treated with erythromycin 500 mg four times a day for 7 days or amoxicillin 500 mg three times daily for 7 days (103,104). For those who cannot tolerate the high doses, a lower dose of 250 mg of erythromycin base or 400 mg of erythromycin ethylsuccinate can be given four times daily for 14 days. Erythromycin estolate has been associated with hepatotoxicity and should not be used in pregnant women. Azithromycin is a category B drug; a small randomized trial involving 30 pregnant women comparing azithromycin and erythromycin showed similar efficacy (100% for azithromycin and 93% for erythromycin) (105) and it is an alternative regimen (3). Azithromycin is secreted in breast milk (106).

Patients should be examined for other STDs, and partners should receive adequate diagnosis and treatment at the same visit. It is important to remember that *C. trachomatis* can remain asymptomatic in the cervix for months and probably years (56), and pinpointing the source can be problematic in some adolescents. Thus the usual recommendation is to evaluate and treat partners within 60 days of the onset of symptoms or identification in the asymptomatic patient. If the last intercourse was >60 days previously, the last sexual partner should be assessed and treated. Patients and partners should abstain from intercourse until the treatment course is completed and they are without symptoms. As with all STDs, patients should be thoroughly counseled about the need to have monogamous relationships and the use of barrier contraception or abstinence.

Because of the high risk of reexposure to an untreated partner, the possibility of noncompliance, and the morbidity associated with the infection in young women, clinicians should rescreen adolescents in 1 to 2 months and continue to advise ongoing screening. Cerin and colleagues (107) have reported that cell culture, a direct immunofluorescence test (MicroTrak), and an EIA test (IDEIA, CellTech) all gave negative results by day 6 of treatment with doxycycline; other tests may give false positives up to 3 weeks.

PELVIC INFLAMMATORY DISEASE

The term *pelvic inflammatory disease* refers to infection in the upper genital tract that involves the fallopian tubes. PID may occur as a sexually acquired acute salpingitis, a postpartum or postabortal infection, or the chronic sequela to a previous acute or silent salpingitis.

It has been estimated that 1 million women in the United States are treated for acute salpingitis each year, with 16% to 20% of cases occurring in adolescents. About 250,000 to 300,000 women are hospitalized each year. In the 1988 National Center for Health Statistics report, almost 11% of women reported prior treatment for clinical PID (108). Risk factors included age, race, vaginal douching, age at first intercourse, STD history, and number of lifetime partners. Determinants of risk of PID include the size of inoculum, the number of infecting pathogens, the virulence of infecting organisms, host susceptibility, and environmental factors. Several authors have begun to differentiate between *risk markers* and *risk factors*. For example, most demographic and social indicators (socioeconomic status, residence, substance abuse) appear to be *risk markers* whereas contraceptive practices, sexual behaviors, health care behaviors, smoking, and douching are *risk factors* (110). Young age may be seen as both a risk marker and a risk factor. Thus adolescents represent an especially high-risk group because they often have multiple sexual partners, have a high prevalence of *N. gonorrhoeae* and *C. trachomatis* infections, and have less access to screening and diagnosis of both STDs and PID. Women with multiple partners have a 4.6-fold increased risk of PID. The use of nonbarrier methods of contraception makes adolescents more likely to acquire endocervical infections, and the immaturity of their immune systems with low levels of protective antibody appears to increase their susceptibility to ascending infection. It has been estimated that adolescents with a gonococcal or chlamydial endocervical infection have a 30% chance of developing PID, as opposed to a 10% risk in the older woman. Sexually active 10- to 15-year-old women appear to be seven to ten times more likely to contract PID than sexually active women 20 to 29 years old.

The cost of acute PID has been estimated at over $4.2 billion (for medical services and lost work) in 1990 with an estimated increase to $9 billion by 2000 (111). Asymptomatic pelvic infection and minimally symptomatic PID can also lead to adhesions, infertility, and ectopic pregnancy and thus have additional costs. Of women with infertility due to obstructed fallopian tubes, up to 70% have serum antibodies to *Chlamydia* (112) and many have no history of PID.

Barrier contraceptives such as condoms and spermicides lower the risk of acquiring STDs and PID. The role of oral contraceptives is less clear. As noted in the section on *Chlamydia*, oral contraceptives may contribute to the ease of detection of *Chlamydia* by contributing to the persistence of the ectopy or to altered attachment of organisms to endocervical cells in the presence of estrogen. However, the use of the oral contraceptives appears to lessen the risk of hospitalization for PID, postulated to occur because of changes in cervical mucus, lighter menstrual flow, diminished uterine contractions, less retrograde menstruation, less canal dilatation, and modification of immune response (110,113–118). Initial studies demonstrated protection by oral contraceptives primarily against gonococcal PID; however, a second study suggested that the protection was primarily for symptomatic PID in women infected with *Chlamydia* (117). A study from Sweden (118) in adult women has also suggested that chlamydial PID rates are lower in oral contraceptive users. However, another study found that women with unrecognized endometritis were four times more likely to be using oral contraceptives than were women with overt endometritis (109). Thus protection against asymptomatic chlamydial upper tract disease needs further study. There appears to be no change in the risk of tubal infertility (110).

A history of previous PID is a risk factor for PID and up to one-third of women will have a second episode of PID. The sequelae of infertility, ectopic pregnancy, and pelvic pain are also related to the number of episodes of PID.

PID is usually divided into gonococcal, chlamydial, and nongonococcal-nonchlamydial PID on the basis of the presence or absence of *N. gonorrhoeae* and *C. trachomatis* on endocervical tests. Patients with gonorrhea or chlamydial infection can also have other pathogens present. A positive cervical culture for gonorrhea is found in 20% to 80% of patients with PID, with most estimates around 25% to 40%. Holmes and colleagues (119) found gonorrhea in 49% of initial episodes of PID versus 34% with recurrent attacks. It is uncommon to isolate gonococci after three or more episodes of PID. In patients with positive gonococcal cultures from the endocervix, the fallopian tube culture is most likely to be positive during the first 2 days of symptoms. Eschenbach and associates (120) found *N. gonorrhoeae* in the peritoneal exudate from 8 out of 21 patients with, and in none of the 33 patients without, cervical gonococcal infections, and Sweet and coworkers (121) isolated *N. gonorrhoeae* from the cul-de-sac in 32% of 26 patients and from the fallopian tube in 19%.

Chlamydial infection is found in 25% to 40% of patients with PID. In patients with acute PID, Mårdh and collaborators (122) isolated *C. trachomatis* from 19 of 53 cervical cultures and from 6 of 20 specimens of the fallopian tube. The course of chlamydial PID can be subacute and indolent, and adolescents frequently delay seeking medical attention.

Mixed aerobic and anaerobic infections account for 25% to 60% of cases of PID and may have different risk factors (123). The polymicrobial flora include coliforms, *Gardnerella vaginalis*, *Hemophilus influenzae*, group B streptococci, *Bacteroides* species (e.g., *Bacteroides fragilis*, *disiens,* and *bivius*), *Peptostreptococcus*, *Peptococcus*, and *Mycoplasma hominis* (116,118–126). *M. hominis* appears to be associated with PID although the organism is frequently cultured from the cervix of both women with PID and those without PID (127,128). The aerobic and anaerobic flora of PID is strikingly similar to that occurring in bacterial vaginosis (BV) (129), suggesting to some that BV may be a risk factor for PID (130). Although it has been suggested that the gonococcus paves the way for other invaders from the lower genital tract, anaerobic organisms are frequently found within the first 24 hours of symptoms.

Both gonococcal and chlamydial PID have been reported to be temporally related to menses. Sweet and coworkers (131) found that 81% of women with PID occurring within 7 days of the onset of menses had an infection with either gonorrhea or *Chlamydia*. In contrast, of the occurrences of PID seen >14 days after the onset of menses, 66% were nongonococcal nonchlamydial infections. Overall, 55% of gonococcal PID and 57% of chlamydial PID occurred in the first 7 days of the cycle. Oginski and colleagues (132) found that 83% of patients with gonococcal PID had the onset of symptoms within the first week compared to 32% with *Chlamydia* and 30% with neither. Slap and colleagues (133) found that adolescent patients with tubo-ovarian abscess (TOA) tended to present later in their menstrual cycle (>18 days from the last menstrual period) than those without TOA. The increased risk of ascending infection during the menses may occur because of loss of the cervical mucus plug; shedding of the endometrium, which may have offered protection from infection; the presence of menstrual blood, which is an excellent culture medium; and the reflux of blood into the fallopian tubes. It appears that once the gonococci reach the tubal epithelium, they penetrate the cells and cause cell destruction with production of a purulent exudate. The gonococcus produces extracellular products that may damage host cells. The infection then reaches the fimbriated ends of the tubes and causes pelvic peritonitis. If the tubes are blocked, a pyosalpinx may develop; if the ovaries are involved, a tubo-ovarian abscess may occur. About one-fourth of hospitalized PID patients have palpable adnexal swelling, and 3% to 17% develop an abscess. It is likely that chlamydial infection spreads in a similar fashion to gonococcal infection by direct canalicular spread along the endometrial surface to the tubes. It appears that *C. trachomatis* has an acute phase with influx of polymorphonuclear leukocytes and a chronic or persistent phase that involves the presence of mononuclear cells (delayed hypersensitivity) (115). Thus the long-term damage may occur because of recurrent infection, which stimulates host responses. Simultaneous infection with gonorrhea appears to facilitate replication of *Chlamydia* in cervical epithelium. Other postulated modes of spread for bacteria include transport via attachment to sperm or *Trichomonas*, transfer with retrograde menstruation, or perhaps lymphatic spread (which may occur with mycoplasma). Sexual intercourse during menses was associated with an OR of 5.2 (95% CI: 1.9, 14.4) for the development of PID (134). Douching more than three times per month has been associated with PID (135) but the pathogenesis of the proposed increased risk has not been elucidated.

Diagnosis

The classic picture of acute salpingitis includes lower abdominal pain, vaginal discharge, and fever, usually following the onset of menses in a sexually active young woman. Symptoms may be much less specific and include menstrual irregularities, dyspareunia, nausea, vomiting, diarrhea, constipation, dysuria, and urinary frequency. Historical symptoms are usually not statistically significant indicators of PID and when they are, they have low sensitivity and specificity (136). Signs found to be different between a group of PID patients and a group of women with a visually normal pelvis have included longer duration of pain and irregular bleeding (137). A history of urethritis or an STD in the patient's sexual partner helps the clinician to make the appropriate diagnosis.

The physical findings associated with PID are lower abdominal tenderness, adnexal tenderness, and cervical motion tenderness. The frequency of other findings such as fever, elevated leukocyte count, increased C-reactive protein, signs of genital infection, or abnormal vaginal discharge varies considerably. The abdominal tenderness and adnexal tenderness are typically bilateral, although Falk (138) reported an 8% incidence of unilateral salpingitis confirmed by laparoscopy. Pain on cervical motion is usually present but is nonspecific and may also occur with other pathologic conditions such as appendicitis, gastroenteritis, urinary tract infection, pyelonephritis, and an ovarian cyst. Rebound tenderness may not be present early in the disease if peritonitis is not present. Liver tenderness caused by perihepatitis (Fitz-Hugh-Curtis) may occur in both gonococcal and chlamydial infections (97,139); the patient may complain of pleuritic right upper quadrant pain with radiation to the right shoulder and back. A palpable adnexal mass has a 24% to 49% sensitivity and a 74% to 79% specificity for PID (138). Fever is present only in 33% of patients with PID (temperature over 38°C has a sensitivity of 24% to 39% and a specificity of 79% to 91%) (136).

The laboratory tests should include a complete blood count (CBC), erythrocyte sedimentation rate (ESR), serologic test for syphilis, Gram stain of the endocervical discharge, cultures or other tests for *N. gonorrhoeae* and *C. trachomatis*, urinalysis, urine culture (if any symptoms suggest pyelonephritis or cystitis), and a sensitive pregnancy test (such as the urine or serum ICON). The CBC may show a normal or elevated leukocyte count. In a study of adolescents with PID, Oginski and colleagues (140) found that depending on the cause of the PID 33% to 71% of patients had normal leukocyte counts. The ESR is >15 mm/h in 75% to 80% of patients. In a study by Wolner-Hanssen and associates (118) in women subjected to laparoscopy because of signs and symptoms of acute salpingitis, 75% of those with PID compared to 31% of those with a visually normal pelvis had an elevated ESR. Kahn and colleagues (136) found that C-reactive protein had a sensitivity of 74% to 93% (with specificity 50% to 90%) and ESR >15 and >20, a sensitivity of 71% to 81% and 64% to 81% and specificity of 35% to 57% and 43% to 69%, respectively. Vaginal discharge (purulent or unspecified) was reported to be a significant indicator in three of four studies with sensitivities of 26% to 81% and specificity of 42% to 83%. Cervical discharge was studied only once and was not found to be discriminating (136); the Gram stain of a purulent cervical discharge reveals gram-negative intracellular diplococci in only about half of patients with gonococcal PID. The absence of any leukocytes in the cervical secretions and vaginal discharge suggests a different diagnosis from PID. It is important to remember that the "classic" picture of pelvic pain, purulent cervical discharge, adnexal tenderness, fever, leukocytosis, and increased ESR is seen in only about 20% of laparoscopically verified PID cases.

Several groups have tried to examine whether clinical or historical indicators can help differentiate types of PID before the culture or other endocervical tests for gonorrhea and *Chlamydia* return. Patients with chlamydial PID have been observed to be less likely to be febrile and more likely to have long-standing milder symptoms and breakthrough bleeding on oral contraceptives than those with gonococcal or mixed aerobic–anaerobic PID. The markedly elevated sedimentation rate may contrast with the mild symptoms of chlamydial PID. Golden and colleagues (125) found that adolescent patients with *Chlamydia*-associated PID in contrast to girls with gonococcus-associated PID had a longer duration of symptoms (6.2 vs. 3.1 days), lower temperature (37.8°C vs. 38.5°C), and lower leukocyte count (11,055 vs. 14,648/mm^3). Such associations have not been found in all studies (140).

A pregnancy test should always be obtained and the possibility of an ectopic pregnancy considered in the adolescent with acute abdominal pain; it is important to remember that an adolescent may have more than one diagnosis, such as chlamydial PID and ectopic pregnancy (see Case 19 in Chapter 6). Despite the past view that pregnancy and PID are rarely coincident, Acquavella and colleagues (141) reported a series of adolescents with both diagnoses in the first trimester.

Ultrasonography (especially transvaginal) can be extremely useful in ruling out other diagnoses and defining adnexal masses. Mean adnexal volume appears to be greater in adolescents with PID versus controls, even in those PID patients without tubo-ovarian abscesses (142). Tubo-ovarian abscesses are also monitored serially with ultrasound. Radionucleotide studies using labeled leukocytes have been proposed for the diagnosis of PID (143).

The diagnosis of PID is sometimes problematic. Laparoscopic studies of patients with a presumptive diagnosis of acute salpingitis have concluded that the clinical diagnosis is confirmed by visual inspection in only 60% to 70% of cases (144–148). An additional 5% of patients with negative examinations by laparoscopy do have gonococci present in the cervical culture. Jacobson (144,145) found that 12% of patients with "clinical PID" had in fact a different diagnosis—acute appendicitis, ectopic pregnancy, ruptured corpus luteum, ovarian abscess, or endometriosis. In a significant number of patients, no pathologic condition of the pelvis was found. Westrom (146) found that the diagnosis of PID was much more likely if it was based not only on finding signs of genital infection, lower abdominal pain, and pelvic tenderness, but also included one or more of the following: (a) ESR >15 mm/h, (b) a rectal temperature greater than 38°C, or (c) palpable adnexal masses. If all these criteria were present, the diagnosis of PID was confirmed in 96% of patients. A clinical diagnosis plus a positive culture or rapid diagnostic test for *N. gonorrhoeae* or *C. trachomatis* allows correct diagnosis in 90% of patients. Clearly, a clinician cannot expect all the criteria to be present to initiate therapy; otherwise many adolescents would be undertreated and would be likely to develop sequelae.

TABLE 3. *Criteria for diagnosis of pelvic inflammatory disease*

Minimum criteria

Empiric treatment of pelvic inflammatory disease (PID) should be based on the presence of all three of the following minimum clinical criteria for pelvic inflammation and the absence of an established cause other than PID:

- Lower abdominal tenderness
- Adnexal tenderness
- Cervical motion tenderness

Additional criteria

For women with severe clinical signs, more elaborate diagnostic evaluation is warranted because incorrect diagnosis and management may cause unnecessary morbidity. These additional criteria may be used to increase the specificity of the diagnosis.

Routine criteria

- Oral temperature >38.3°C
- Abnormal cervical or vaginal discharge
- Elevated erythrocyte sedimentation rate
- Elevated C-reactive protein
- Laboratory documentation of cervical infection with *N. gonorrhoeae* or *C. trachomatis*

Definitive criteria

- Histopathologic evidence of endometritis on endometrial biopsy
- Tubo-ovarian abscess or thickened fluid-filled tubes on sonography or other radiologic tests
- Laparoscopic abnormalities consistent with PID

Although initial treatment decisions can be made before bacteriologic diagnosis of *C. trachomatis* or *N. gonorrhoeae* infection, such a diagnosis emphasizes the need to treat sexual partners.

(From CDC 1998 Sexually Transmitted Diseases Guidelines. *MMWR* 1998;47(RR-1):1; with permission.)

UNCOMPLICATED PELVIC INFLAMMATORY DISEASE CLINICAL PRACTICE GUIDELINE INCLUSION CHECKLIST

Patient MUST meet <u>all</u> of the following criteria, in the absence of another established cause:

- ☐ lower abdominal pain
- ☐ cervical motion tenderness
- ☐ adnexal tenderness

Patient MUST meet *at least one* of the following criteria:

- ☐ oral temp. > 38.3 C
- ☐ WBC ≥ 13,000 K/mm^3
- ☐ abnormal cervical or vaginal discharge
- ☐ ESR >20 mm/hr
- ☐ laboratory documentation of cervical infection with *N. gonorrheae* or *C. trachomatis*

All patients should have the following as part of the initial evaluation:

- ☐ pelvic exam
- ☐ endocervical culture for *gonorrheae*
- ☐ endocervical EIA or culture for chlamydia
- ☐ CBC with differential
- ☐ ESR or C reactive protein
- ☐ RPR
- ☐ urine *B*hCG
- ☐ urine dipstick
- ☐ urine culture

The following should be considered:

- ☐ serum *B*hCG if urine *B*hCG is negative and suspect ectopic
- ☐ U/S if mass or difficult exam
- ☐ GYN consult immediately if pregnant or if needs U/S
- ☐ surgical consult if suspect appendicitis or other surgical problem

DIFFERENTIAL DIAGNOSIS (partial list):
GI - appendicitis, constipation, diverticulitis, gastroenteritis, IBD, irritable bowel syndrome

GYN - rupture or torsion of ovarian cyst, endometriosis, dysmenorrhea, ectopic pregnancy, mittelschmerz, ruptured follicle, septic or threatened abortion, tubo-ovarian abscess

Urinary tract - cystitis, pyelonephritis, urethritis, nephrolithiasis

A ☐ *Check box if patient was placed on the PID clinical practice guideline.*

FIG. 3. [Forms used at Children's Hospital, Boston, in the treatment of pelvic inflammatory disease (PID) (Principal authors: L Shrier, Chair; M Laufer, SJ Emans, E Woods, D Goldman, S Moszczenski, M Harper, R Lindemann).] **(A)** Uncomplicated PID inclusion checklist for placing a patient on the Clinical Pathway Guideline for PID.

Laparoscopy has proved invaluable in clarifying the etiologic agents and the clinical accuracy of diagnosis in PID. Laparoscopy is indicated if the diagnosis is in doubt, especially in patients recurrently labeled with PID but never meeting satisfactory criteria and not responding to antibiotic therapy. It should also be used in research settings, especially when clinical trials of antibiotics are undertaken. Care should be taken in making sure that cultures taken at laparoscopy are processed so that fastidious organisms will not be missed. Laparoscopy, however, does not detect endometritis and may miss incipient inflammation of the fallopian tubes (3).

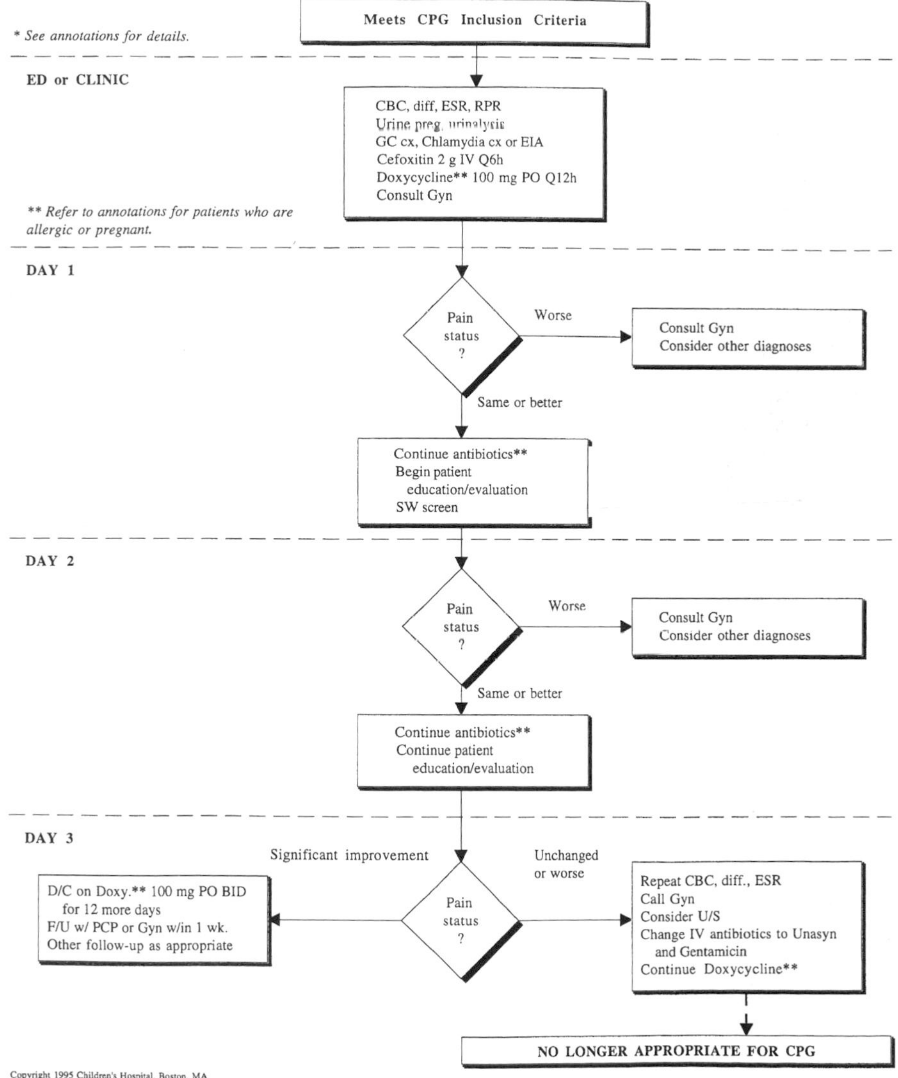

FIG. 3. (B) Algorithm for patients meeting the inclusion critera.

Uncomplicated PID
Clinical Practice Guideline
PATIENT EDUCATION/EVALUATION

SW screen completed ☐
Full SW evaluation? ☐ No ☐ Yes
Complete below

Please initial under appropriate column as activities are completed:	MD	RN	SW
Explain diagnosis and encourage questions **Explain transmission and encourage questions** **Assess parental knowledge of disease/diagnosis (if appropriate)**			
Assess use of contraception **Explain need for contraception/condoms/spermicide** **Patients understands need for use of contraception/condoms/spermicide** **Patient states plans for obtaining and using birth control**			
Assess risk behaviors - smoking, ETOH/drug use, previous STDs, pregnancy **Explain how ETOH/drugs may lessen use of barrier contraceptives** **HIV/STD education for risk reduction & information on testing and counseling given** **Educational material given on HIV/STD** **Patient understands risks and how to reduce them**			
Assess use of primary care **Explain importance of primary care for prevention, early diagnosis, treatment**			
Assess living situation, child care arrangements (if applicable)			
Explain need to notify sexual partner(s) for treatment **Patient asked to identify sexual partner(s)** **Patient verifies that contact(s) agree(s) to be evaluated/treated** **If not, name given to State** **Give letter detailing treatment to each partner's provider**			
Explain how to identify pain/discomfort using the pain scale 1-10			
Explain need to abstain from intercourse & use of tampons for 1 week after tx completed **Explain that patient should not douche**			
Assess insurance/prescription **Patient is able to fill prescription**			
Patient understands: **•how to take prescription** **•STD/HIV prevention** **•importance of antibiotic therapy and follow-up** **•symptoms of recurrence and when to notify doctor** **•use of condoms and abstinence**			
Discharge: **•patient has adequate family supports/living situation to which to be discharged** **•patient understands she has f/u within one week of diagnosis (Gyn or PCP)** **•appointment with primary care on _________ date** **•primary care provider notified** **•patient able to fill prescription**			

Initials: ______ Signature: ____________ Initials: ______ Signature: ____________

a:\edueval.wpd

C

FIG. 3. (C) Clinical Practice Guideline Tracking sheet for PID for diagnostic tests and results.

Children's Hospital Uncomplicated Pelvic Inflammatory Disease Clinical Practice Guideline (PID CPG) **CPG DATA TRACKING SHEET**	*Use addressograph*

	DIAGNOSTIC TESTS	RESULTS			
INITIAL TESTS	Pelvic Exam	☐CMT	☐AT	☐Abnormal discharge	
	Endocervical culture for gonorrhea	☐ Negative (-)	☐ Positive (+)	☐ Not done	Reason: ______
	Endocervical EIA/culture for chlamydia	☐ Negative (-)	☐ Positive (+)	☐ Not done	Reason: ______
	CBC with Differential	WBC ______	Diff. ______		
	ESR	______			
	RPR	☐ Reactive	☐ Non-reactive		
	Urine βhCG	☐ Negative (-)	☐ Positive (+)		
	Urine dipstick	☐ Negative (-)	☐1+ ☐2+ ☐3+		
	GYN consult for surgical assessment	☐ PID	☐ Non-PID		
	Urine culture	☐ Negative (-)	☐ Positive (+) : ______		
CONDITIONAL TESTS	Serum βhCG **IF** urine βhCG is negative and suspect ectopic	☐ Negative (-)	☐ Positive (+)		
	U/S **IF** mass or difficult exam	☐ Negative (-)	☐ Positive (+) : ______		
	Surgical consult **IF** suspect appendicitis or other surgical problem:				
ADDITIONAL TESTS	**If abdominal pain not improving by Day 3:** CBC with Differential	WBC ______	Diff. ______		
	ESR	______			
	U/S	☐ Negative (-)	☐ Positive (+) :		
	Reconsult GYN:				

D **DISCHARGE DIAGNOSIS:** ______________________

FIG. 3. (D) Clinical Practice Guideline Tracking Sheet for patient education and evaluation. CMT, cervical motion tenderness; AT, adnexal tenderness.

Endometrial biopsy also improves the accuracy of the diagnosis of PID, but is not used in the routine clinical diagnosis. Histologic diagnosis of endometritis based on the presence of plasma cells had a sensitivity of 89% and specificity of 67% in detecting laparoscopically confirmed PID (149).

Kahn et al. (136) have suggested that the criteria for PID should be modified given the current studies on sensitivity and specificity of history, clinical signs, and laboratory tests for PID. They would include the following indicators in their model: abnormal vaginal discharge on examination, elevated C-reactive protein, elevated ESR, endometritis by biopsy and laparoscopic evidence of PID. Suggestive evidence would include evidence of gonococcal or chlamydial infection, elevated temperature, and palpable mass. They suggest that if both adnexal and cervical motion tenderness are present, PID can be diagnosed in women with a mild presentation, especially if one indicator is present. In women with more severe presentations, more indicators would need to be present. See Table 3 for CDC criteria.

In order to improve care for adolescents at our hospital, we have a Clinical Pathway Guideline, which continues to evolve (150,151) (Fig. 3). Given the frequency of noncompliance with medical therapy during adolescence and the risk of future reproductive problems, we admit all adolescents to the hospital.

Inpatient (Parenteral) Therapy for Acute Pelvic Inflammatory Disease

Antibiotic therapy must be directed at the known pathogens for PID, but education and skill building for future risk reduction, assessment of other risk behaviors, planning for followup medical, contraceptive, and STD screening care, and treatment of partners are equally important in the hospitalization of the adolescent.

Broad-spectrum antibiotics result in the resolution of symptoms in most patients; however, the long-term results of treatment are still far from satisfactory. All patients who have questionable diagnosis, suspected pelvic abscess, upper quadrant pain, peritoneal signs, temperature higher than 38°C, vomiting, or are prepubertal, pregnant, possibly noncompliant to outpatient treatment (including medication and followup appointments), immunodeficient, or fail to respond to outpatient treatment within 48 hours require inpatient therapy. Some experts believe that all women with PID should be hospitalized if future fertility is desired (124).

Effectiveness of therapy for PID is improved with prompt institution of antibiotic therapy. Viberg (152) found that none of the patients treated within 2 days of the onset of symptoms were involuntarily infertile, and all had patent fallopian tubes. In contrast, if treatment was instituted after the sixth day, only 70% had tubal patency.

In selecting antibiotics for treatment of PID, the clinician needs to take into account the polymicrobial cause of the disease, regardless of whether *N. gonor-*

rhoeae or *C. trachomatis* is cultured. It is especially important to make sure that the antibiotics are known to be effective against *Chlamydia,* since clinical improvement may occur in spite of persistence of positive endometrial cultures for *Chlamydia.* For example, in a study of women treated with parenteral second- and third-generation cephalosporins, 94% showed prompt clinical improvement and yet *C. trachomatis* was recovered from 87% of the posttreatment endometrial aspirates (153). In contrast, patients treated with clindamycin plus tobramycin had negative posttreatment cultures for *Chlamydia.* In patients with severe disease or abscess formation, parenteral antibiotics effective against anaerobes must be included.

Several drug regimens have been used in the past for the treatment of uncomplicated PID and ongoing trials of new drug combinations are in progress (3,124,154–159). The CDC Guidelines have recommended *one* of two regimens:

1. Cefoxitin, 2 g IV every 6 hours, or cefotetan, 2 g IV every 12 hours, plus doxycycline, 100 mg orally or IV every 12 hours. The doxycycline can be given orally if gastrointestinal function is normal. The above regimen is continued for at least 24 hours after the patient improves clinically. After discharge from the hospital, the patient is continued on doxycycline 100 mg orally twice daily for a total of 14 days. (Alternative cephalosporins such as ceftizoxime, cefotaxime, and ceftriaxone, which give adequate coverage of gonococci, facultative gram-negative aerobes, and anaerobes, have been utilized [3] although the regimens above remain the standard preferred therapy.)
2. Clindamycin, 900 mg IV every 8 hours plus gentamicin, 2.0 mg/kg loading dose IM or IV followed by a maintenance dose of 1.5 mg/kg every 8 hours (in patients with normal renal function). The regimen is continued for at least 24 hours after the patient improves clinically. After discharge from the hospital the patient is continued on doxycycline, 100 mg orally twice daily for a total of 14 days. Clindamycin, 450 mg orally four times a day can be used as an alternative to complete 14 days of therapy. Doxycycline remains the regimen of choice for out-patient therapy for chlamydial PID.

Despite concerns about whether the second regimen would cover gonococci and *Chlamydia*, patients treated with these drugs do experience comparable clinical and bacteriologic cure rates of PID. Even though clindamycin provides better anaerobic coverage than doxycycline and *in vitro* and some *in vivo* data suggest efficacy against chlamydial infection, doxycycline is the preferred therapy when *Chlamydia* is known or highly suspected to be present (124). There is synergism between gentamicin and clindamycin, but the magnitude does not appear to be sufficient to explain the beneficial clinical effect against gonococci. Some clinicians prefer the second regimen with clindamycin for treatment of an abscess; however, Reed and colleagues (161) found that the two regimens had equal efficacy for tubo-ovarian abscess with a 75% success rate. The three current alternative therapies for PID include ofloxacin and metronidazole;

ampicillin/sulbactam and doxycycline; and ciprofloxacin, doxycycline, and metronidazole. The quinolones alone have limited *in vitro* efficacy against anaerobes and should be used with other drugs. In a study of three antibiotic regimens (159), ciprofloxacin failed to eradicate anaerobic bacteria (especially *Bacteroides bivius* and *Peptococcus asaccharolyticus*) from the endometrial cavity as effectively as cefoxitin/doxycycline or clindamycin/gentamicin in spite of initial clinical improvement.

Most patients with PID respond well clinically to broad-spectrum antibiotics. However, patients with tubo-ovarian abscesses can be difficult to manage. Ultrasonography, and in some cases computed tomography (CT) and magnetic resonance imaging (for patients in whom sonography does not provide adequate information), can be used along with clinical assessment to make the diagnosis and document improvement (Fig. 4). Anaerobic organisms, in particular *Bacteroides fragilis,* are strongly associated with abscess formation. A study of 232 abscesses by Landers and Sweet (160) found that 68% of patients treated with a regimen that included clindamycin responded to medical management, measured by improved symptoms, decreased fever and tenderness, lowered leukocyte count, and shrinkage of adnexal masses. The combination of tobramycin and clindamycin covers most organisms cultured from abscesses, and clindamycin has excellent penetration into abscess cavities. Other antibiotics with good activity against the anaerobes and good penetration of abscesses include cefoxitin and metronidazole. Although a trial of metronidazole plus tobramycin gave equivalent results in the treatment of a variety of pelvic infections as did clindamycin and tobramycin, metronidazole in combination with an aminoglycoside does not provide adequate coverage against aerobic streptococci, *N. gonorrhoeae*, or microaerophilous streptococci (160). Some centers prefer to use triple antibiotics in patients with tubo-ovarian abscesses, such as gentamicin and ampicillin plus either metronidazole or clindamycin.

Thirty to forty percent of women with TOA fail to respond within 48 to 72 hours as defined by persistent fever, increasing size of the abscess, persistent leukocytosis, increasing sedimentation rate, or suspicion of rupture (158,163). It should be noted that the sedimentation rate may lag several days behind clinical improvement and may even rise initially. Bilateral abscesses and those >8 cm in diameter are less likely to respond to medical management alone; >50% of patients with TOAs ≥10 cm required surgical therapy. With the advent of better anaerobic drug combinations in the last 5 years, it is likely that fewer patients will fail to respond to medical management. Surgical intervention may include percutaneous drainage (anterior abdomen, posterior transgluteal, transvaginal) guided by CT or real-time ultrasound (162–164) (the majority that have been drained have been unilocular abscesses), transabdominal laparotomy with drainage or extirpation of the abscess, with or without unilateral adnexectomy, or total abdominal hysterectomy and bilateral salpingo-oophorectomy. Although long-term data are not available on fertility outcomes and are criti-

A

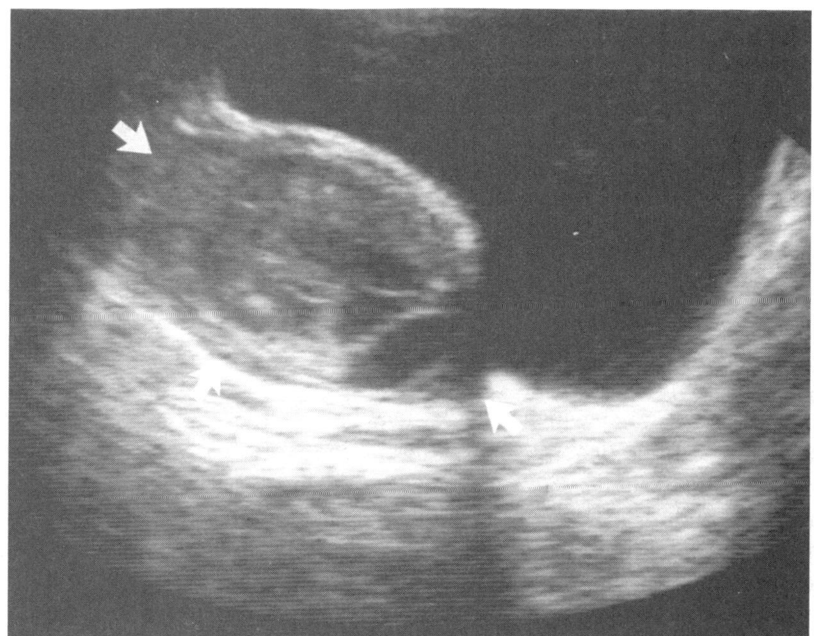

B

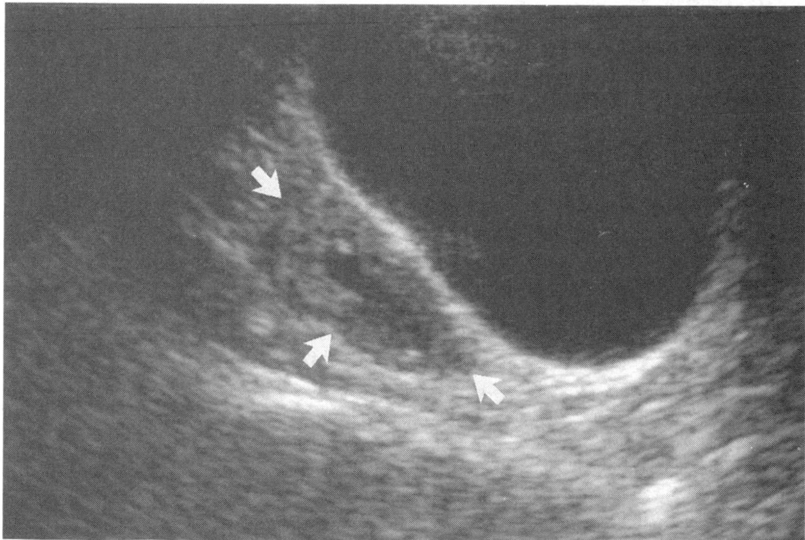

FIG. 4. Pelvic ultrasonograms of an adolescent referred to Children's Hospital, Boston, after 1 month of pelvic pain, negative pregnancy test result, elevated sedimentation rate, a positive cervical culture for *C. trachomatis,* and noncompliance with outpatient antibiotics. **(A)** Longitudinal sonogram of the right adnexa, showing a complex mass behind the bladder (*arrows*). A right ovary separate from this structure could not be identified. These findings can be seen with several disorders, including tubo-ovarian abscess, hemorrhagic ovarian cyst, ectopic pregnancy, or inflammation of nongynecologic origin, such as appendicitis. The patient was treated with cefoxitin and doxycycline for 10 days as an inpatient and then took an additional 14-day course of oral metronidazole and doxycycline as an outpatient. **(B)** Resolution of the tubo-ovarian abscess 4 weeks after therapy. The right ovary is now well visualized and is normal, except for a small amount of residual fluid within it (*arrows*). (Readings of scans courtesy of Jane Share, M.D., Children's Hospital, Boston.)

cally needed to evaluate new approaches, some centers have advocated a more aggressive early surgical approach to large tubo-ovarian abscesses with aspiration of the abscess, gentle washing of the abscess cavity, instillation of antibiotics, and closed drainage to gravity. Other centers (including ours) have taken a more conservative surgical approach and feel that preservation of fertility is more likely if the patient is treated medically with appropriate antibiotics with performance of surgery only if the patient does not improve with medical therapy. Fertility after treatment of tubo-ovarian abscesses may be 20% to 50% with conservative medical and surgical approaches.

After inpatient parenteral therapy, oral antibiotics are continued to complete a 14-day course. Patients with severe disease including tubo-ovarian abscesses are usually treated for a longer course with oral clindamycin or a two-drug regimen such as oral doxycycline plus metronidazole.

In most studies, HIV-infected patients appear to be at increased risk for acquiring PID and may also have serious infections. Irwin and colleagues (165) have questioned whether bias has confounded studies on the recognition of PID incidence, clinical presentation and course, and microbiology of PID in HIV-infected women. HIV-positive patients should be hospitalized for parenteral antibiotics.

Pregnant adolescents require aggressive inpatient management (parenteral therapy for 7 to 14 days is often recommended). Gonococcal infection during pregnancy is associated with septic abortion, preterm delivery, postpartum infection, and transmission to the newborn. Both chlamydial and gonococcal infection increase the risk for postabortal infection.

With discharge from the hospital, the patient should be seen weekly, and sexual contacts should be identified and treated with regimens effective against both *C. trachomatis* and *N. gonorrhoeae* to prevent reinfection. Rescreening for *Chlamydia* and *N. gonorrhoeae* at 4 to 6 weeks is essential because of the possibility of reinfection in these young women. STD counseling is important to minimize the chance of reinfection and to protect against other infections such as human papillomavirus (HPV) and HIV.

Outpatient (Oral) Therapy for Acute Pelvic Inflammatory Disease

Although most, if not all, adolescents with PID should be treated as inpatients, outpatient regimens for the reliable adult patient with *mild* signs and symptoms, a temperature under 38°C, and no vomiting are single-dose ceftriaxone, 250 mg IM (or cefoxitin, 2 g IM plus probenecid, 1 g orally, or equivalent cephalosporin), followed by doxycycline, 100 mg orally twice daily for 14 days (166). Wolner-Hanssen and colleagues (166) reported a clinical cure rate of 92%. An alternative therapy is ofloxacin 400 mg orally twice a day for 14 days plus metronidazole 500 mg twice a day for 14 days. Changing gonococcal sensitivities to the quinolones may alter this treatment course.

It is essential that the clinician feel comfortable that the patient has the resources to purchase the antibiotics and will return in 48 to 72 hours to assess whether the treatment is effective. A lack of response, vomiting of the antibiotics, or noncompliance should prompt hospitalization since timely therapy is felt to be critical to fertility outcome. The patient is advised to abstain from intercourse for 3 to 4 weeks and her sexual partner(s) should be seen for appropriate cultures and treatment.

Consequences of Acute Pelvic Inflammatory Disease

Infertility, ectopic pregnancies, and chronic abdominal pain are the principal sequelae of acute PID. Thus, the aim of the clinician must be to treat adequately and promptly and to prevent recurrences. Women with a first episode of PID have a two- to threefold increased risk of a second episode of PID compared to women who have never had PID. During the treatment of the infection, it should be explained to the patient how the disease is sexually transmitted and how to prevent recurrences. The importance of monogamous relationships, consistent use of the condom, and treatment of both partners should be stressed. A single episode of gonococcal salpingitis appropriately treated carries a low risk of later infertility, and patients can generally be reassured of this.

Tubal occlusion may be more common in nongonococcal infections, although newer data have questioned this. Longer duration of abdominopelvic pain before admission and younger age at first intercourse have been associated with infertility and subsequent PID (167). Hillis and colleagues (168) also found delayed care a risk factor for infertility. The clinician needs to be skillful at counseling adolescents about the risks of infertility. If the issue of possible infertility is overemphasized, the teen may discontinue effective contraception and take risks to prove her own fertility. In a study of laparoscopically proven PID, tubal occlusion was verified after one infection in 12.8% of patients, after two infections in 35.5%, and after three or more infections in 75% (168). In another study (112), Westrom and colleagues reported tubal occlusion in 8% after one episode, 19.5% after two, and 40% after three or more. Other studies have suggested an infertility risk of 10% to 12% with the first infection, 23% to 25% with the second, and 50% with the third (169–171). In general, the more severe the PID, the higher the risk of future infertility.

In addition to infertility, previous salpingitis is a major cause of ectopic pregnancy. Studies have found a six- to ten-fold increase in ectopic pregnancy in PID patients (113). Adolescents who have had PID should be counseled about this risk, and ectopic pregnancy should always be considered in the differential diagnosis of the adolescent with acute abdominal pain (see Chapter 18). The clinician should maintain a high index of suspicion in monitoring the pregnancy of an adolescent with a history of PID.

PID may also result in chronic pain. Safrin et al (167) found that 24% of patients with PID had pelvic pain for 6 months or more post hospitalization. Physical examination may reveal adnexal tenderness or masses. The sedimentation rate may be normal or elevated. Laparoscopy is necessary to establish the diagnosis and to evaluate the extent of the disease. Adolescents with endometriosis (see Chapter 9) can be incorrectly diagnosed as having PID, and they may receive multiple courses of antibiotics before the correct diagnosis is made by laparoscopy.

Therapy for chronic PID must be individualized. Treatment may include an extended course of oral antibiotics such as doxycycline, clindamycin, amoxicillin/clavulanate, or metronidazole; and nonsteroidal antiinflammatory drugs for pain. The patient should be cultured and treated with appropriate antimicrobial agents for subsequent episodes of PID and the sexual partner also examined and treated.

Prevention of PID is key and must include prevention of exposure to *Chlamydia* and *N. gonorrhoeae* (e.g., delaying the age of intercourse), prevention of acquisition of chlamydial and gonorrheal infections (e.g., condoms, investigations of methods of transmission), prevention of PID (e.g., screening, antibiotic regimens), and prevention of PID sequelae (172). Adolescents at risk of PID need education to be able to assess symptoms, to access health care services for screening and evaluation of symptoms, to receive therapy that is effective and takes into account compliance issues, and to be able to refer sexual partners for treatment in a timely manner.

SYPHILIS

In 1990, 50,223 cases of primary and secondary syphilis were reported, a 9% increase from 1989 (173). After a steady decline in primary and secondary syphilis and congenital syphilis in the early 1980s, a dramatic increase in disease occurred beginning in 1987. Reported cases increased 23% in the first 3 months of 1987 as compared to the first 3 months of 1986 (174). The areas reporting large increases were California, Florida, New York City, Texas, and other parts of the southeastern United States with the disease showing a striking increase among blacks and Hispanics (175).

From 1981 to 1991, 10% to 12% of the reported morbidity from primary and secondary syphilis affected the adolescent age group (4). Primary and secondary syphilis rates were much higher for adolescent girls 15 to 19 years in 1991 than 1981. Rates among females increased 112% from 1984 to 1991 (4). Fortunately, the 1990s have witnessed an overall decline in syphilis rates from the high levels of the late 1980s.

Guidelines have not been developed for the routine screening of adolescent patients for syphilis; however, clinical criteria have been used for both symptomatic and asymptomatic teens. Sexually active adolescents should be screened for syphilis when they present with any suspicious oral or genital lesions, unexplained skin rash or lymphadenopathy, other STDs (such as gonorrhea, chlamydial infection, PID, HPV, HIV), or pregnancy. Asymptomatic adolescents with multiple partners, nonuse of barrier methods, involvement in prostitution, drug abuse, or juvenile delinquency, and/or a history of STDs should be considered for annual syphilis screening since adolescents frequently do not present at the time of symptoms (176). For example, in a detention center in New York City serving juveniles 9 to 18 years of age, the prevalence rate for syphilis was 0.6% for boys and 2.5% for girls (177).

The presence of genital ulcers increases the risk of acquiring HIV infection, and adolescents at risk for HIV acquisition are also at risk for syphilis exposure. In a blinded study of sera from a comprehensive adolescent health center and two school-based clinics in an area of New York with a high seroprevalence of HIV, McCabe and associates (178) reported that of the 59 specimens positive for syphilis, 15% were HIV seropositive; 84% of the patients with positive syphilis serology (positive rapid plasma reagin [RPR] and fluorescent treponemal antibody absorbed [FTA-ABS] or just positive FTA-ABS) were female and 80% of these young women had had a prior STD, most commonly chlamydial infection (35%).

Screening serum for syphilis involves the use of nontreponemal tests that can be accurately quantitated: the Venereal Disease Research laboratory [VDRL] and RPR tests. Only the VDRL is used for cerebrospinal fluid (CSF) determinations. A rising titer is indicative of recently acquired infection, a reinfection, or a relapse. A decline in titer is generally indicative of adequate treatment of the early stage of syphilis. Patients with primary syphilis will often have a nonreactive RPR within 1 year; patients with secondary syphilis can become nonreactive within 2 years; those in the macular and maculopapular stage of the rash at diagnosis and treatment return to seronegativity more rapidly than patients with papular and/or pustular rashes (179). Patients who are reinfected with syphilis also take longer to revert to a nonreactive RPR test. Patients who have early latent syphilis for <1 year generally revert to a negative test result within 4 years, whereas only 20% to 45% of late latent patients become nonreactive within 5 years. Many in the latter group remain serofast (180–182). Brown and coworkers (183) analyzed data from the Early Syphilis Study and generated curves describing the VDRL decline with time. The curves describe an approximately fourfold decline in titer at 3 months and an eightfold decline in 6 months in patients with primary and secondary syphilis. Retreatment rates for the less effective regimens of erythromycin and spectinomycin exceeded 10%. Romanowski and coworkers (184) and others have found the rate of decline was slower than previously noted. Successful treatment of primary and secondary syphilis results in a fourfold decrease in serum RPR by 6 to 12 months. The FTA-ABS result became negative in 24% of patients treated for primary syphilis and the microhemagglutination assay for antibody to *T. pallidum* (MHA-TP) negative in 13% of these patients. The same laboratory and the same test (either VDRL or RPR) should be used to monitor a patient after therapy.

Darkfield examination and direct fluorescent antibody test for *T. pallidum* (DFA-TP) of the lesion exudate or tissue are definitive methods for diagnosing early syphilis. Serologic tests, the RPR and VDRL, are the most frequently used tests for diagnosing syphilis, and if the results are positive, they should be reported quantitatively with titers. The RPR is an extremely sensitive test and gives positive results by the seventh day of the chancre, at the time many patients actually seek medical help. However, different states use different nontreponemal tests that have varying sensitivities, some of which may not show positive results for 2 to 3 weeks after the chancre has appeared. Thus, clinicians seeing adolescents should gather information from the state-run STD clinics periodically to keep abreast of current information on testing available in their centers. In <2% of patients with secondary syphilis, the RPR test may appear to give a false-negative result because of a prozone reaction. Most laboratories do not do titers unless the undiluted specimen gives a positive result. Thus, if syphilis is suspected and the reagin test appears nonreactive or weakly reactive, a second serum specimen should be sent with instructions to dilute the serum.

False-positive reagin tests occur in 1 out of 3000 to 5000 healthy patients; in some populations it may be 1% to 2% (74). Conditions such as mononucleosis, hepatitis, malaria, vaccinia, measles, chickenpox, pneumococcal pneumonia, scarlet fever, rickettsial disease, tuberculosis, pregnancy, drug abuse, immunizations, and connective tissue diseases may result in false-positive RPR tests (188). The specific or treponemal tests are useful to make the diagnosis in situations in which false-positive reactions might occur and in the diagnosis of late syphilis. The most commonly used treponemal tests are the FTA-ABS and the MHA-TP. False-positive results for FTA-ABS and MHA-TP are infrequent but have been reported in patients with elevated globulins, Lyme disease, leprosy, malaria, infectious mononucleosis, relapsing fever, leptospirosis, and systemic lupus erythematosus (185). The FTA-ABS and MHA-TP tests are not recommended for routine screening of low-risk populations because the test results remain positive for life in most individuals whether the syphilis has been treated or not. Special tests, which include DNA and Reiter absorptions for the FTA test, eliminate most of the false-positive results and can be performed by the STD Laboratory Program of the CDC on request (which may sometimes be indicated in the diagnosis and treatment of the pregnant woman). If a patient has a reactive nontreponemal test (e.g., RPR) and a nonreactive treponemal test (e.g., MHA-TP) and no clinical or epidemiologic evidence of syphilis, no treatment is necessary but both tests should be repeated in 4 weeks.

In caring for seropositive women, the clinician should always attempt to document previous titers and forms of treatment. A fourfold change in titer, equivalent to 2 dilutions (1:16 to 1:4 or 1:8 to 1:32) is necessary to demonstrate a change in status (3). Patients should be retreated if there is clinical (darkfield-positive lesions) or serologic evidence of a sustained fourfold increase in quantitative nontreponemal test or a history of recent sexual exposure to an infectious person. Treponemal tests (FTA-ABS or MHA-TP) should not be used to monitor disease activity. In general, high-risk seropositive women should be considered infected and treated unless the clinician is certain about recent therapy. The diagnosis and treatment of syphilis during pregnancy is particularly urgent to prevent congenital syphilis.

No single test can be used to determine if neurosyphilis is present. The diagnosis is made on the basis of reactive VDRL-CSF, CSF leukocyte count >5 leukocytes/mm^3, and elevated CSF protein. The sensitivity of the CSF-VDRL is 30% to 70%, but it is very specific, and thus a positive test result is sufficient to diagnose neurosyphilis but a negative test is not sufficient to exclude the diagnosis. FTA-ABS on CSF is more sensitive but less specific (more false positives), but a negative test result appears to exclude the diagnosis (3,200). Lukehart and colleagues (186) reported that 41% of 39 patients with untreated primary and secondary syphilis had pleocytosis and 24% of 33 patients with secondary syphilis (none of 7 primary syphilis patients) had reactive CSF VDRL tests.

It is essential that patients with syphilis have appropriate counseling and testing for HIV infection because of the difficulty with potential failed treatment and persistent neurosyphilis.

Stages of Syphilis

The stages of syphilis are as follows:

1. Primary syphilis. Ten to 90 days (average 3 weeks) after oral or genital exposure to an infected partner, the young woman may develop a hard, painless chancre on her vulva, vagina, cervix, anal area, or mouth, accompanied by nontender lymphadenopathy. The lesions are often asymptomatic and may be missed. The serologic test for syphilis gives a positive result 4 to 6 weeks after exposure; thus, a negative test result at the time a lesion is first noted does not rule out the diagnosis. The RPR test result, however, is positive if the chancre has been present for 7 days. If the result of the initial VDRL or RPR is negative but the lesion arouses suspicion, repeat tests are indicated at 1 week, 1 month, and 3 months to exclude syphilis. If possible, a darkfield examination of the clear fluid expressed from the chancre or a DFA-TP of the lesion should be done by an experienced clinician. The darkfield examination can be repeated for 3 consecutive days, and the serologic test repeated. Even without therapy, the lesion(s) will heal spontaneously in 2 to 4 weeks, leaving a small scar.

2. Secondary syphilis. If the chancre is untreated, the patient may experience, 6 weeks to several months later, the symptoms of secondary syphilis, including a generalized rash (often present on the palms and soles), fever, malaise, alopecia, weight loss, lymphadenopathy, condyloma lata, or mucous membrane lesions. The rash generally progresses from macular to maculopapular, to papular, and lastly, to pustular lesions. The serum RPR test result at this time is positive.

3. Latent syphilis. By definition, this is the state of syphilis in which the patient has no symptoms and the spirochete is "hidden." However, the patient may be infectious and may later develop symptoms of tertiary syphilis. This stage is divided by history and serology into early latent (under 1 year), late latent of more than 1 year's duration, and latent syphilis of unknown duration. Patients can be documented to have acquired syphilis within the preceding year on the basis on seroconversion, a fourfold or greater increase in titer on a RPR or VDRL test, history or symptoms of primary or secondary syphilis, or a sex partner with primary, secondary, or latent syphilis (documented as duration <1 year) (3). All others are considered to have late latent syphilis.

4. Late syphilis. Except for gummas, which are probably a hypersensitivity phenomenon, the late manifestations of syphilis (neurologic and cardiovascular problems) are the result of a vasculitis. Late syphilis usually occurs in patients beyond the adolescent age group, although very rarely neurosyphilis or cardiovascular lesions can develop in adolescents as a sequela of untreated congenital syphilis.

Treatment

Primary or Secondary Syphilis or Contact History

Benzathine penicillin G, 2.4 million units IM at a single session is the treatment of choice. (Massachusetts uses benzathine penicillin, 2.4 million units once weekly for 2 weeks: a total dose of 4.8 million units.)

Parenteral penicillin is the drug of choice for all stages of syphilis, and alternative therapy should be selected only for nonpregnant patients in whom there is documented penicillin allergy and for whom compliance is not a problem. Some patients will experience the Jarisch-Herxheimer reaction to the penicillin therapy—an acute febrile reaction with headache and myalgia that may occur within the first 24 hours of therapy for syphilis (antipyretics can be recommended) (3).

Nonpregnant penicillin-allergic patients should be treated with doxycycline, 100 mg orally twice a day for 2 weeks or tetracycline, 500 mg orally 4 times a day for 2 weeks. Compliance with this regimen is extremely important, as is serologic followup. Patients who cannot tolerate doxycycline or tetracycline should have their penicillin allergy confirmed; choices are erythromycin, 500 mg orally 4 times a day for 2 weeks with close serologic followup, or penicillin desensitization so that benzathine penicillin can be used. Preliminary data suggest that ceftriaxone, 250 mg IM for 10 days should be effective, but close followup of serologies is mandatory.

Patients should be reexamined and serologic tests checked at 3 and 6 months. Patients who have persistent signs or symptoms or who have a sustained fourfold increase in nontreponemal test titer compared with baseline or subsequent result can be considered to have failed therapy or be reinfected. They should be tested for HIV infection and retreated. Unless reinfection is likely, the CSF should be evaluated. If nontreponemal antibody titers have not declined fourfold by 6 to 12 months, the patient should be considered at risk for failure (see 1997 STD Guidelines).

Latent Syphilis

Early latent syphilis of <1 year's duration can be treated with a single dose of penicillin (in Massachusetts a total of 4.8 million units), as above for primary syphilis.

Syphilis of more than 1 year's duration or unknown duration, except neurosyphilis, should be treated with 2.4 million units of benzathine penicillin G, IM once a week for 3 consecutive weeks. Ideally all patients with syphilis of >1 year's duration should have a CSF examination. A CSF examination is indicated in patients with neurologic or ophthalmic signs and symptoms, treatment failure, other evidence of active syphilis (aortitis, gumma, iritis), or a positive HIV antibody test result (with late latent syphilis or syphilis of unknown duration). If neurosyphilis is found, then patients should be treated with the regimen below.

The efficacy of alternative drugs to penicillin in the treatment of syphilis of >1 year's duration is less well established. Penicillin-allergic (nonpregnant) patients who have had neurosyphilis excluded may be treated with doxycycline, 100 mg orally twice a day for 4 weeks or tetracycline, 500 mg orally four times a day for 4 weeks. The duration of therapy is 2 weeks for infections known to be <1 year (3). In patients who cannot tolerate tetracycline, penicillin allergy should be confirmed by history and testing, and penicillin desensitization should be considered.

Neurosyphilis

A dose of aqueous penicillin G, 18 to 24 million units is administered as 3 to 4 million units every 4 hours IV for 10 to 14 days. If outpatient compliance can be ensured, an alternative treatment is procaine penicillin, 2.4 million units IM daily plus probenecid, 500 mg orally 4 times a day, both for 10 to 14 days. Many then give benzathine penicillin G, 2.4 million units IM weekly for 1 to 3 doses.

If pleocytosis was initially present in the CSF, CSF examination should be repeated every 6 months until the cell count is normal. If no decrease occurs by 6 months or if the cell count is not normal by 2 years, retreatment should be strongly considered.

Syphilis and HIV Infection

Published case reports and series have suggested that HIV-infected patients have an increased risk of treatment failures and neurosyphilis (3,185–187). More data are needed on the optimal therapy in these patients. Although unusual serologic responses may occur in HIV-infected patients, both treponemal and nontreponemal tests are usually accurate for most patients. Current recommendations call for the usual treatment schedule for early syphilis (although some treat with two to three injections) with careful quantitative nontreponemal tests done at 1, 2, and 3 months and then at 6, 9, 12, and 24 months. If the titer does not decrease appropriately, the patient should be reevaluated and the CSF examined. Consultation with an infectious disease expert, state laboratory, or the CDC is recommended.

Syphilis in Pregnancy

Pregnant patients should be screened in the first trimester and, depending on the state and risk, also at term for syphilis. High-risk patients should also be screened early in the third trimester. Pregnant patients with syphilis should be treated as soon as the diagnosis is made to prevent fetal death and congenital syphilis. Patients who are not allergic to penicillin should be treated with the same dosage schedules recommended for nonpregnant patients. Penicillin should be given to pregnant women even if they have a history of penicillin allergy if their skin test results to minor and major determinants are negative or their skin test results are positive and they have been desensitized. Ziaya and colleagues (188) have described an intravenous method of penicillin desensitization, and the CDC has provided a recommended management strategy for patients (3). These methods of desensitization should be used only in consultation with an expert and in a facility with emergency procedures available. Tetracycline is not recommended during pregnancy because of adverse effects on the fetus, and erythromycin is not optimal because of the possibility of inadequate treatment of the mother and fetus. Following treatment, pregnant women should have monthly quantitative nontreponemal serologic tests for the remainder of the pregnancy. Women should be retreated if they show a fourfold rise in titer or do not show a fourfold decrease in titer in 3 months.

Followup

Adolescent patients should have careful tracing of contacts performed by the state health department. Contacts should be evaluated clinically and with serologic tests. Patients exposed within the preceding 90 days may have negative test results in spite of infection and should be presumptively treated. Patients exposed more than 90 days previously can await the results of serologic tests if followup is certain; otherwise they too should be treated. The time periods for determining at-risk sex partners are 3 months plus duration of symptoms for primary syphilis, 6 months plus duration of symptoms for secondary syphilis, and 1 year for early latent syphilis (3). Serologic screening in locations where crack cocaine is used has been another strategy for case finding in the syphilis epidemic (189).

Serologic tests should be carefully monitored in the patient diagnosed with syphilis. State and CDC health care professionals can be extremely helpful in the interpretation of titers. Compliance with testing is especially important in individuals treated with nonpenicillin regimens. Counseling about risk reduction is crucial in adolescents who have had syphilis since the same risk factors associated with the acquisition of syphilis place the patient at risk of acquiring HIV.

REFERENCES

1. Sexually Transmitted Diseaseas (STDs) in the United States. *Facts in brief.* New York: The Alan Guttmacher Institute, 1993.
2. Committee on Adolescence. Sexually transmitted diseases. *Pediatrics* 1994;94:568.
3. CDC. 1998 Sexually Transmitted Diseases Treatment Guidelines. *MMWR* 1998;47(RR-1):1.
4. Webster LA, Berman SM, Greenspan JR. Surveillance for gonorrhea and primary and secondary syphilis among adolescents, United States—1981–1991. *MMWR* 1993;41:1.
5. Vermund SH, Alexander-Rodriquez T, MacLeod S, Kelley KF. History of sexual abuse in incarcerated adolescents with gonorrhea or syphilis. *J Adolesc Health Care* 1990;11:449.
6. Saltz GR, Linnemann CC, Brookman RR, et al. *Chlamydia trachomatis* cervical infections in female adolescents. *J Pediatr* 1981;98:981.
7. Rice RJ, Roberts PL, Handsfield HH, Holmes KK. Sociodemographic distribution of gonorrhea incidence: implications for prevention and behavioral research. *Am J Public Health* 1991;81:1252.
8. McCormack WM, Eveard JR, Laughlin CF, et al. Sexually transmitted conditions among women college students. *Am J Obstet Gynecol* 1981;139:130.
9. Keith L, Mass W, Berger G, et al. Gonorrhea detection in a family planning clinic: a cost-benefit analysis of 2000 triplicate cultures. *Am J Obstet Gynecol* 1975;121:399.
10. Roochvarg LB, Lovchik JC. Screening for pharyngeal gonorrhea in adolescents. *J Adolesc Health* 1991;12:269.
11. Eng TR, Butler WT, eds. *The hidden epidemic: confronting sexually transmitted diseases.* Washington, DC: Institute of Medicine, 1996.
12. Granato PA, Roefaro FM. Evaluation of a prototype DNA probe test for noncultural diagnosis of gonorrhea. *J Clin Microbiol* 1989;27:632.
13. Vlaspolder F, Mutsaers JAEM, Blog F, Notowicz A. Value of a DNA probe assay (Gen-probe) compared with that of culture for diagnosis of gonococcal infection. *J Clin Microbiol* 1993;31:107.
14. Hanks JW, Scott CT, Butler CE, Wells DW. Evaluation of a DNA probe assay (Gen-probe Pace 2) as the test of cure for *Neisseria gonorrhoeae* genital infections. *J Pediatr* 1994;125:161.

15. Liebling MR, Arkfeld DG, Michelini GA, et al. Identification of *Neisseria gonorrhoeae* in synovial fluid using the polymerase chain reaction. *Arthritis Rheum* 1994;37:702.
16. Ching S, Lee H, Hook EW, et al. Ligase chain reaction for detection of *Neisseria gonorrhoeae* in urogenital swabs. *J Clin Microbiol* 1995:33:3111.
17. Smith KR, Ching S, Lee H. Evaluation of ligase chain reaction for use with urine for identification of *Neisseria gonorrhoeae* in females attending a sexually transmitted disease clinic. *J Clin Microbiol* 1995;33:455.
18. Hook EW, Holmes KK. Gonococcal infections. *Ann Intern Med* 1985;102:229.
19. Handsfield HH, Sandstrom EG, Knapp JS, et al. Epidemiology of penicillinase-producing *Neisseria gonorrhoeae* infections: analysis by auxotyping and serogrouping. *N Engl J Med* 1982;306:950.
20. CDC. Penicillinase-producing *Neisseria gonorrhoeae*—United States, 1986. *MMWR* 1987;36:107.
21. Wise CM, Morris CR, Wasilauskas BL, Salzer WL. Gonococcal arthritis in an era of increasing penicillin resistance. *Arch Intern Med* 1994;154:2690.
22. Schwarcz SK, Zenilman JM, Schnell D, et al. National surveilllance of antimicrobial resistance in *Neisseria gonorrhoeae*. *JAMA* 1990;264:1413.
23. Schichor A, Bernstein B, Weinerman H, et al. Lidocaine as a diluent for ceftriaxone in the treatment of gonorrhea. *Arch Pediatr Adolesc Med* 1994;148:72.
24. Handsfield HH, McCormack WM, Hook EW III, et al. A comparison of single-dose cefixime with ceftriaxone as treatment for uncomplicated gonorrhea. *N Engl J Med* 1991;325:1337.
25. Portilla I, Lutz B, Montalvo M, Mogabgab WJ. Oral cefixime versus intramuscular ceftriaxone in patients with uncomplicated gonococcal infections. *Sex Transm Dis* 1992;19:94.
26. Plourde PJ, Tyndall M, Agoki E, et al. Single-dose cefixime versus single-dose ceftriaxone in the treatment of antimicrobial-resistant *Neisseria gonorrhoeae* infection. *J Infect Dis* 1992;166:919.
27. CDC. Decreased susceptibility of *Neisseria gonorrhoeae* to fluoroquinolones—Ohio and Hawaii, 1992–1994. *MMWR* 1994;43:325.
28. CDC. Fluoroquinolone resistance in *Neisseria gonorrhoeae*—Colorado and Washington, 1995. *MMWR* 1995;44:761.
29. Stamm WE, Guinan ME, Johnson C, et al. Effect of treatment regimens for *Neisseria gonorrhoeae* on simultaneous infection with *Chlamydia trachomatis*. *N Engl J Med* 1984;310:545.
30. Waugh MA. Open study of the safety and efficacy of a single oral dose of azithromycin for the treatment of uncomplicated gonorrhoea in men and women. *J Antimicrob Chemother* 1993;31:193.
31. Laras L, Craighill M, Woods ER, Emans SJ. Epidemiologic observations of adolescents with *Neisseria gonorrhoeae* genital infections treated at a children's hospital. *Adolesc Pediatr Gynecol* 1994;7:9.
32. Wiesner PJ, Tronca E, Bonin P, et al. Clinical spectrum of pharyngeal gonococcal infection. *N Engl J Med* 1973;288:181.
33. Cramolino GM, Litt IF. The pharynx as the only positive culture site in an adolescent with disseminated gonorrhea. *J Pediatr* 1982;100:644.
34. Felman YV, Nikitas JA. Anorectal gonococcal infection. *NY State J Med* 1980;80:1631.
35. Al-Suleiman SA, Grimes EM, Jonas HS. Disseminated gonococcal infections. *Obstet Gynecol* 1983; 61:48.
36. Holmes KK, Counts GW, Beaty HW, et al. Disseminated gonococcal infection. *Ann Intern Med* 1971; 74:979.
37. Keiser H, Rubin FL, Wolinsky E, et al. Clinical forms of gonococcal arthritis. *N Engl J Med* 1968; 279:234.
38. Drugs for sexually transmitted diseases. *Med Lett* 1995;37:117.
39. O'Brien JP, Goldenberg DL, Rice PA. Disseminated gonococcal infection: a prospective analysis of 49 patients and a review of pathophysiology and immune mechanisms. *Medicine* (*Baltimore*) 1983; 62:395.
40. Rahman MU, Cheema MA, Schumacher HR, Hudson AP. Molecular evidence for the presence of chlamydia in the synovium of patients with Reiter's syndrome. *Arthritis Rheum* 1992;35:521.
41. Keat A. Reiter's syndrome and reactive arthritis in perspective. *N Engl J Med* 1983;309:1606.
42. Jay MS, Seymore C, Jay WM, et al. Reiter's syndrome in an adolescent female with systemic sequelae. *J Adolesc Health Care* 1987;8:280.
43. Ingram DL. *Neisseria gonorrhoeae* in children. *Pediatr Ann* 1994;23:345.
44. Burry VF. Gonococcal vulvovaginitis and possible peritonitis in prepubertal girls. *Am J Dis Child* 1971;121:536.
45. Kulhanjian JA, Hilton NS. Gonococcal salpingitis in a premenarchal female following sexual assault. *Clin Pediatr* 1991;30:5355.

46. Washington AE, Johnson RE, Sanders LL. *Chlamydia trachomatis* infections in the United States. *JAMA* 1987;257:2072.
47. CDC Recommendations for the prevention and management of *Chlamydia trachomatis* infections, 1993. *MMWR* 1993;42(RR-12):1.
48. Gravett MG, Nelson HP, DeRouen T, et al. Independent association of bacterial vaginosis and *Chlamydia trachomatis* with adverse pregnancy outcome. *JAMA* 1986;256:1899.
49. Soong YK, Kao SM, Lee CJ, et al. Endocervical chlamydial deoryribonucleic acid in infertile women. *Fertil Steril* 1990;54:815.
50. Shafer MA, Vaughan E, Lipkin ES, et al. Evaluation of fluorescein conjugated monoclonal antibody test to detect *Chlamydia trachomatis* endocervical infection in adolescent girls. *Pediatrics* 1986;108: 779.
51. Bump RC, Sachs LA, Buesching WJ, et al. Sexually transmissible infectious agents in sexually active and virginal asymptomatic adolescent girls. *Pediatrics* 1986;77:488.
52. Chacko MR. *Chlamydia trachomatis* infection in sexually active adolescents: prevalence and risk factors. *Pediatrics* 1984;73:836.
53. Fraser GJ, Rettig PJ, Kaplan DW. Prevalence of cervical *Chlamydia trachomatis* and *Neisseria gonorrhoeae* in female adolescents. *Pediatrics* 1983;71:333.
54. Bell TA, Farrow JA, Stamm WE, et al. Sexually transmitted diseases in females in a juvenile detention center. *Sex Transm Dis* 1985;12:140.
55. Fisher M, Swenson PO, Risucci D, et al. *Chlamydia trachomatis* in suburban adolescents. *J Pediatr* 1987;111:617.
56. McCormack WM, Alpert S, McComb DE, et al. Fifteen-month follow-up study of women infected with *Chlamydia trachomatis*. *N Engl J Med* 1979;300:123.
57. Ismail MA, Chandler AE, Beem MO, et al. Chlamydial colonization of the cervix in pregnant adolescents. *J Reprod Med* 1985;30:549.
58. Khurana CM, Deddish PA, delMundo F. Prevalence of *C. trachomatis* in the pregnant cervix. *Obstet Gynecol* 1985;66:241.
59. Harrison HR, Costin M, Meder JB. Cervical *Chlamydia trachomatis* infection in university women: relationship to history, contraception, ectopy and cervicitis. *Am J Obstet Gynecol* 1985;153: 244.
60. Johnson BA, Poses RM, Fortner CA, Meier FA, Dalton HP. Derivation and validation of a clinical diagnostic model for chlamydial cervical infection in university women. *JAMA* 1990;264:316.
61. Stergachis A, Scholes D, Heidrich FE, Sherer DM, Holmes KK, Stamm WE. Selective screening for *Chlamydia trachomatis* infection in a primary care population of women. *Am J Epidemiol* 1993;138: 143.
62. Svensson LOL, Mares I, Mardh PA, Olsson SE. Screening voided urine for *Chlamydia trachomatis* in asymptomatic adolescent females. *Acta Obstet Gynecol Scand* 1994;73:63.
63. Biro FM, Reising SF, Doughman JA, Kollar LM, Rosenthal SL. A comparison of diagnostic methods in adolescent girls with and without symptoms of chlamydia urogenital infection. *Pediatrics* 1994;93:476.
64. Handsfield HH, Hasman LL, Roberts PL, et al. Criteria for selective screening for *Chlamydia trachomatis* infection in women attending family planning clinics. *JAMA* 1986;255:1730.
65. Han Y, Morse DL, Lawrence CE, et al. Risk profile for chlamydia infection in women from public health clinics in New York State. *J Commun Health* 1993;18:1.
66. Weinstock HS, Bolan GA, Kohn R, et al. *Chlamydia trachomatis* infection in women: a need for universal screening in high prevalence populations? *Am J Epidemiol* 1992;135:41.
67. Ramstedt K, Forssman L, Giesecke J, Granath F. Risk factors for *Chlamydia trachomatic* infection in 6810 young women attending family planning clinics. *Int J STD AIDS* 1992;3:117.
68. Brunham RC, Paavonen J, Stevens CE, et al. Mucopurulent cervicitis—the ignored counterpart in women of urethritis in men. *N Engl J Med* 1984;311:1.
69. Moscicki B, Shafer MA, Millstein SG, et al. The use and limitations of endocervical gram stain and mucopurulent cervicitis as predictors for *Chlamydia trachomatis* in female adolescents. *Am J Obstet Gynecol* 1987;157:65.
70. Mosure DJ, Berman S, Fine D, et al. Genital chlamydia infection in sexually active female adolescents: do we really need to screen everyone? *J Adolesc Health* 1997;20:6.
71. CDC. Chlamydia trachomatis genital infections–US 1995. *MMWR* 1997;46(9):193.
72. Jones RB, Mammel JB, Shepard MK, et al. Recovery of *Chlamydia trachomatis* from the endometrium of women at risk for chlamydial infection. *Am J Obstet Gynecol* 1986;155:35.

73. Hillis SD, Nakashima A, Marchbanks PA, Addiss DG, Davis JP. Risk factors for recurrent *Chlamydia trachomatis* infections in women. *Am J Obstet Gynecol* 1994;170:801.
74. Judson FN, Ehret J. Laboratory diagnosis of sexually transmitted infections. *Pediatr Ann* 1994;23: 361.
75. Schubiner HH, Lebar W, Jemal C, Hershman B. Comparison of three new non-culture tests in the diagnosis of *Chlamydia* genital infections. *J Adolesc Health* 1990;11:505.
76. Tam MR, Stamm WE, Handsfield HH, et al. Culture-independent diagnosis of *C. trachomatis* using monoclonal antibodies. *N Engl J Med* 1984;310:1146.
77. Amortegui AJ, Meyer MP. Enzyme immunoassay for detection of *C. trachomatis* from the cervix. *Obstet Gynecol* 1985;65:523.
78. Baselski VS, McNeeley SG, Ryan G, et al. A comparison of non–culture-dependent methods for detection of *C. trachomatis* infections in pregnant women. *Obstet Gynecol* 1987;70:47.
79. Pao CC, Lin SS, Yang TE, et al. Deoxyribonucleic acid hybridization analysis for the detection of urogenital *Chlamydia trachomatis* infections in women. *Am J Obstet Gynecol* 1987;156:195.
80. Clarke LM, Sierra MF, Daidone BJ, et al. Comparison of the Syva microtrak enzyme immunoassay and Gen-probe pace 2 with cell culture for diagnosis of cervical *Chlamydia trachomatis* infection in a high-prevalence female population. *J Clin Microbiol* 1993;31:968.
81. Hook EW III, Quinn TC, Spitters C. Sensitivity of rapid antigen detection tests for *Chlamydia trachomatis* screening [In Reply]. *JAMA* 1995;273:918.
82. Loeffelholz MJ, Lewinski CA, Silver SR, et al. Detection of *Chlamydia trachomatis* in endocervical specimens by polymerase chain reaction. *J Clin Microbiol* 1992;30:2847.
83. Lebar W, Herschman B, Jemal C, Pierzchala J. Comparison of DNA probe, monoclonal enzyme immunoassay, and cell culture for the detection of *Chlamydia trachomatis*. *J Clin Microbiol* 1989; 27:1918.
84. Hsuih TCH, Guichon A, Diaz A, et al. Chlamydial infection in a high-risk population: comparison of Amplicor PCR and Gen-probe II for diagnosis. *Adolesc Pediatr Gynecol* 1995;8:71.
85. Black CM. Current methods of laboratory diagnosis of *Chlamydia trachomatis* infections. *Clin Microbiol Rev* 1997;10:160.
86. Schachter J, Stamm WE, Quinn TC, et al. Ligase chain reaction to detect *Chlamydia trachomatis* infection of the cervix. *J Clin Microbiol* 1994;32:2540.
87. Trachtenberg AI, Washington E, Halldorson S. A cost-based decision analysis for *Chlamydia* screening in California family planning clinics. *Obstet Gynecol* 1988;81:101.
88. Sanders LL, Harrison HR, Washington AE. Treatment of sexually transmitted chlamydial infections. *JAMA* 1986;255:1750.
89. Phillips RS, Aronson MD, Taylor WC, et al. Should tests for *Chlamydia trachomatis* cervical infection be done during routine gynecologic visits? *Ann Intern Med* 1987;107:188.
90. Scholes D, Stergachis A, Heidrich FE, et al. Prevention of pelvic inflammatory disease by screening for cervical chlamydial infection. *N Engl J Med* 1996;334:1362.
91. Sellors JW, Mahony JB, Jang D, et al. Comparison of cervical, urethral, and urine specimens for the detection of *Chlamydia trachomatis* in women. *J Infect Dis* 1991;164:205.
92. Svensson LO, Mares I, Olsson SE. Detection of *Chlamydia trachomatis* in urinary samples from women. *Genitourin Med* 1991;67:117.
93. Lee HH, Chernersky MA, Schacter J, et al. Diagnosis of *Chlamydia trachomatis* genitourinary infection in women by ligase chain reaction assay of urine. *Lancet* 1995;345:213.
94. Kiviat NB, Paavonen J, Brockway J, et al. Cytologic manifestations of cervical and vaginal infections: 1. Epithelial and inflammatory cellular changes. *JAMA* 1985;253:989.
95. Roongpisuthipong A, Grimes DA, Hadgu A. Is the Papanicolaou smear useful for diagnosing sexually transmitted diseases? *Obstet Gynecol* 1987;69:820.
96. Paavonen J, Stevens CE, Wolner-Hanssen P, et al. Colposcopic manifestation of cervical and vaginal infections. *Obstet Gynecol* 1988;47:373.
97. Katzman DK, Friedman IM, McDonald CA, et al. *Chlamydia trachomatis* Fitz-Hugh-Curtis syndrome without salpingitis in female adolescent. *Am J Dis Child* 1988;142:996.
98. Jones RB, Rabinovitch RA, Katz BP. *C. trachomatis* in the pharynx and rectum of heterosexual patients at risk for genital infections. *Ann Intern Med* 1985;102:757.
99. Quinn TC, Goodell SE, Mkrtichian E, et al. *Chlamydia trachomatis* proctitis. *N Engl J Med* 1981; 305:195.
100. Martin DH, Mroczkowski TF, Dalu ZA, et al. A controlled trial of a single dose of azithromycin for the treatment of chlamydial urethritis and cervicitis. *N Engl J Med* 1992;327:921.

101. Faro S, Martens MG, Maccato M, et al. Effectiveness of ofloxacin in the treatment of *Chlamydia trachomatis* and *Neisseria gonorrhoeae* cervical infection. *Am J Obstet Gynecol* 1991;164:1380.
102. Campbell WF, Dodson MG. Clindamycin therapy for *Chlamydia trachomatis* in women. Am J Obstet Gynecol 1990;162:343.
103. Crombleholme WR, Schachter J, Grossman M, et al. Amoxicillin therapy for *Chlamydia trachomatis* in pregnancy. *Obstet Gynecol* 1990;75:752.
104. Magat AH, Alger LS, Nagey DA, et al. Double-blind randomized study comparing amoxicillin and erythromycin for the treatment of *Chlamydia trachomatis* in pregnancy. *Obstet Gynecol* 1993;81:745.
105. Bush MR, Rosa C. Azithromycin and erythromycin in the treatment of cervical chlamydial infection during pregnancy. *Obstet Gynecol* 1994;84:61.
106. Kelsey JJ, Moser LR, Jennings JC, Munger MA. Presence of azithromycin breast milk concentrations: a case report. *Am J Obstet Gynecol* 1994;170:1375.
107. Cerin A, Grillner L, Persson E. Chlamydia test monitoring during therapy. *Int J STD AIDS* 1991;2:176.
108. Aral SO, Mosher WD, Cates W Jr. Self-reported pelvic inflammatory disease in the United States, 1988. *JAMA* 1991;266:2570.
109. Ness RB et al. Oral contraception and the recognition of endometritis. *Am J Obstet Gynecol* 1997;176:580.
110. Washington AE, Aral SO, Wolner-Hanssen P, et al. Assessing risk for pelvic inflammatory disease and its sequelae. *JAMA* 1991;266:2581.
111. Washington AE, Katz P. Cost of and payment source for pelvic inflammatory disease: trends and projections, 1983 through 2000. *JAMA* 1991;266:2565.
112. Westrom L, Joesoef R, Reynolds G, et al. Pelvic inflammatory disease and fertility: a cohort study of 1,844 women with laparoscopically verified disease and 657 control women with normal laparoscopic results. *Sex Transm Dis* 1992;19:185.
113. Washington AE, Sweet RL, Shafer MB. Pelvic inflammatory disease and its sequelae in adolescents. *J Adolesc Health Care* 1985;6:298.
114. Washington AE, Gove S, Schachter J, et al. Oral contraceptives, *Chlamydia trachomatis* infection, and pelvic inflammatory disease. *JAMA* 1985;253:2246.
115. Rice PA, Schachter J. Pathogenesis of pelvic inflammatory disease. What are the questions? *JAMA* 1991;266:2587.
116. McCormack WM. Pelvic inflammatory disease. *N Engl J Med* 1994;330:115.
117. Wolner-Hanssen P, Eschenbach OA, Paavonen J, et al. Decreased symptomatic chlamydial pelvic inflammatory disease associated with oral contraceptive use. *JAMA* 1990;263:54.
118. Wolner-Hanssen P, Svensson L, Mårdh PA, et al. Laparoscopic findings and contraceptive use in women with signs and symptoms suggestive of acute salpingitis. *Obstet Gynecol* 1985;66:233.
119. Holmes KK, Eschenbach DA, Knapp JS. Salpingitis, an overview of etiology. *Am J Obstet Gynecol* 1980;138:893.
120. Eschenbach D, Buchanan TM, Pollack HM, et al. Polymicrobial etiology of acute pelvic inflammatory disease. *N Engl J Med* 1975;293:166.
121. Sweet RL, Mills J, Hadley KW, et al. Use of laparoscopy to determine the microbiologic etiology of acute salpingitis. *Am J Obstet Gynecol* 1979;134:68.
122. Mårdh PA, Ripa T, Svensson L, et al. *Chlamydia trachomatis* infection in patients with acute salpingitis. *N Engl J Med* 1977;296:1377.
123. Jossens MOR, Schachter J, Sweet RL. Risk factors associated with pelvic inflammatory disease of differing microbial etiologies. *Obstet Gynecol* 1994;83:989.
124. Peterson HB, Walker CK, Kahn JG, et al. Pelvic inflammatory disease. Key treatment issues and options. *JAMA* 1991;266:2605.
125. Golden N, Neuhoff S, Cohen H. Pelvic inflammatory disease in adolescents. *J Pediatr* 1989;114:138.
126. Paavonen J. *Chlamydia trachomatis* in acute salpingitis. *Am J Obstet Gynecol* 1980;138:957.
127. Cassell GH, Cole BC. Mycoplasmas as agents of human disease. *N Engl J Med* 1981;304:80.
128. Taylor-Robinson D, McCormack WM. The genital mycoplasmas. *N Engl J Med* 1980;302:1003.
129. Soper DE, Brockwell NJ, Dalton HP, Johnson D. Observations concerning the microbial etiology of acute salpingitis. *Am J Obstet Gynecol* 1994;170:1008.
130. Faro S, Martens M, Maccato M. Vaginal flora and pelvic inflammatory disease. *Am J Obstet Gynecol* 1993;169:470.
131. Sweet RL, Blankfort-Doyle M. Robbie MO, et al. The occurrence of chlamydial and gonococcal salpingitis during the menstrual cycle. *JAMA* 1986;255:2062.

132. Oginski WF, Rosenfeld WD, Bijur PE. Acute pelvic inflammatory disease in adolescents. *Adolesc Pediatr Gynecol* 1992;5:243.
133. Slap GB, Forke CM, Cnaan A, et al. Recognition of tubo-ovarian abscess in adolescent with pelvic inflammatory disease. *J Adolesc Health* 1996;18:397.
134. Jossens MO, Eskenazi B, Schachter J, et al. Risk factors for pelvic inflammatory disease. A case control study. *Sex Transm Dis* 1996;23:239.
135. Wolner-Hanssen P, Eschenbach DA, Paavonen J. Association between vaginal douching and acute pelvic inflammatory disease. *JAMA* 1990;263:1936.
136. Kahn JG, Walker CK, Washington AE. Diagnosing pelvic inflammatory disease. A comprehensive analysis and considerations for developing a new model. *JAMA* 1991;266:2594.
137. Wolner-Hanssen P, Mardh PA, Svensson L, et al. Laparoscopy in women with chlamydial infection and pelvic pain: a comparison of patients with and without salpingitis. *Obstet Gynecol* 1983;61:299.
138. Falk V. Treatment of acute non-tuberculous salpingitis with antibiotics alone and in combination with glucocorticoids. *Acta Obstet Gynecol Scand* 1965;44(Suppl 16):65.
139. Kornfeld SJ, and Worthington MG. Culture-proved Fitz-Hugh-Curtis syndrome. *Am J Obstet Gynecol* 1981;139:106.
140. Oginski WF, Rosenfeld WD, Bijar PE. Acute pelvic inflammatory disease in adolescents. *Adolesc Pediatr Gynecol* 1992;5:243.
141. Acquavella AP, Rubin A, D'Angelo J. The co-incident diagnosis of pelvic inflammatory disease and pregnancy: are they compatible? *J Pediatr Adolesc Gynecol* 1996;9:129.
142. Golden N, Cohen H, Gennari G, et al. The use of pelvic ultrasonography in the evaluation of adolescents with pelvic inflammatory disease. *Am J Dis Child* 1987;141:1234.
143. Mozas J, Castilla JA, Alarcon JL, et al. Diagnosis of pelvic inflammatory disease with 99mtechnetium-hexamethylpropylenamine-oxime-labeled autologous leukocytes and pelvic radionuclide scintigraphy. *Obstet Gynecol* 1993;81:797.
144. Jacobson L. Laparoscopy in the diagnosis of acute salpingitis. *Acta Obstet Gynecol Scand* 1964;43:160.
145. Jacobson L, Westrom L. Objectivized diagnosis of acute pelvic inflammatory disease. *Am J Obstet Gynecol* 1969;105:1088.
146. Westrom L. Incidence, prevalence and trends of acute PID and its consequences in industrialized countries. *Am J Obstet Gynecol* 1980;138:1006.
147. Jacobson L. Differential diagnosis of acute PID. *Am J Obstet Gynecol* 1980;138:1006.
148. Hager WD, Eschenbach DA, Spence MR, et al. Criteria for diagnosis and grading of salpingitis. *Obstet Gynecol* 1983;61:113.
149. Paavonen J, Aine R, Teisala K, et al. Comparison of endometrial biopsy and peritoneal fluid cytologic testing with laparoscopy in the diagnosis of acute pelvic inflammatory disease. *Am J Obstet Gynecol* 1985;151:645.
150. Rome ES. Pelvic inflammatory disease in the adolescent. *Curr Opin Pediatr* 1994;6:383.
151. Rome ES, Moszczenski SA, Craighill M, et al. A clinical pathway for pelvic inflammatory disease for use on an inpatient service. *Clin Perform Quality Health Care* 1995;3:185.
152. Viberg L. Acute inflammatory conditions of the uterine adnexa. *Acta Obstet Gynecol Scand* 1964;43:5.
153. Sweet RL, Schachter J, Robbie MO. Failure of β-lactam antibiotics to eradicate *Chlamydia trachomatis* in the endometrium despite apparent clinical cure of acute salpingitis. *JAMA* 1983;250:2641.
154. Sweet RL, Schachter J, Landers DV, et al. Treatment of hospitalized patients with acute pelvic inflammatory disease: comparison of cefotetan plus doxycycline and cefoxitin plus doxycycline. *Am J Obstet Gynecol* 1988;158:737.
155. Wasserheit JN, Bell TA, Kiviat NB, et al. Microbial causes of proven pelvic inflammatory disease and efficacy of clindamycin and tobramycin. *Ann Intern Med* 1986;104:187.
156. Hemsell DL, Wendel GD Jr, Hemsell PG, et al. Inpatient treatment for uncomplicated and complicated acute pelvic inflammatory disease: ampicillin/sulbactam vs. cefoxitin. *Infect Dis Obstet Gynecol* 1993;1:123.
157. McGregor JA, Crombleholme WR, Newton E, et al. Randomized comparison of ampicillin-sulbactam to cefoxitin and doxycycline or clindamycin and gentamicin in the treatment of pelvic inflammatory disease or endometritis. *Obstet Gynecol* 1994;83:998.
158. Dodson MG, Faro S, Gentry LO. Treatment of acute pelvic inflammatory disease with aztreonam, a new monocyclic β-lactam antibiotic and clindamycin. *Obstet Gynecol* 1986;67:657.
159. Ohm-Smith M, Crombleholme WR, Sweet RL. In vitro activity of ciprofloxacin against anaerobic

bacteria recovered from patients with acute PID (Abstract #28). Presented at Interscience Conference on Antimicrobial Agents and Chemotherapy, 1988.
160. Landers DV, Sweet RL. Current trends in the diagnosis and treatment of tuboovarian abscess. *Am J Obstet Gynecol* 1985;151:1098.
161. Reed SD, Landers DV, Sweet RL. Antibiotic treatment of tuboovarian abscess: comparison of broad-spectrum lactam agents versus clindamycin-containing regimens. *Am J Obstet Gynecol* 1991;164: 1556.
162. Casola G, vanSonnenberg E, D'Agostino HB, et al. Percutaneous drainage of tubo-ovarian abscesses. *Radiology* 1992;182:399.
163. vanSonnenberg E, D'Agostino HB, Casola G, et al. US-guided transvaginal drainage of pelvic abscesses and fluid collections. *Radiology* 1991;181:53.
164. Teisala K, Heinonen PK, Punnonen R. Transvaginal ultrasound in the diagnosis and treatment of tubo-ovarian abscess. *Br J Obstet Gynaecol* 1990;97:178.
165. Irwin KL, Rice RJ, Sperling RS, et al. Potential for bias in studies of the influence of human immunodeficiency virus infection on the recognition, incidence, clinical course, and microbiology of pelvic inflammatory disease. *Obstet Gynecol* 1994;84:463.
166. Wolner-Hanssen P, Paavonen J, Kiviat N, et al. Outpatient treatment of pelvic inflammatory disease with cefoxitin and doxycycline. *Obstet Gynecol* 1988;81:595.
167. Safrin S, Schachter J, Dahrouge D, Sweet RL. Long-term sequelae of acute pelvic inflammatory disease. A retrospective cohort study. *Am J Obstet Gynecol* 1992;166:1300.
168. Hillis SD, Joesoef R, Marchbanks PA, et al. Delayed care of pelvic inflammatory disease as a risk factor for impaired fertility. *Am J Obstet Gynecol* 1993;168:1503.
169. Westrom L. Effect of acute pelvic inflammatory disease on fertility. *Am J Obstet Gynecol* 1975; 121:707.
170. Svenson L, Mårdh PA, Westrom L. Infertility after acute salpingitis with special reference to *Chlamydia trachomatis*. *Fertil Steril* 1983;40:322.
171. Westrom L. Influence of sexually transmitted diseases on sterility and ectopic pregnancy. *Acta Eur Fertil* 1985;16:21.
172. Washington AE, Cates W Jr, Wasserheit JN. Preventing pelvic inflammatory disease. *JAMA* 1991; 266:2574.
173. CDC. Primary and secondary syphilis—United States, 1981–1990. *MMWR* 1991;40:314.
174. CDC. Increases in primary and secondary syphilis—United States. *MMWR* 1987;36:393.
175. Rolfs RT, Nakashima AK. Epidemiology of primary and secondary syphilis in the United States, 1981 through 1989. *JAMA* 1990;264:1432.
176. Silber TJ, Niland NF. The clinical spectrum of syphilis in adolescence. *J Adolesc Health Care* 1984;5:112.
177. Alexander-Rodriguez T, Vermund SH. Gonorrhea and syphilis in incarcerated urban adolescents: prevalence and physical signs. *Pediatrics* 1987;80:561.
178. McCabe E, Jaffe LR, Diaz A. Human immunodeficiency virus seropositivity in adolescents with syphilis. *Pediatrics* 1993;92:695.
179. Fiumara NJ. Treatment of primary and secondary syphilis. *JAMA* 1980;243:2500.
180. Fiumara NJ. Treatment of early latent syphilis of less than a year's duration. *Sex Transm Dis* 1978; 5:85.
181. Fiumara NJ. Serologic responses to treatment of 128 patients with late latent syphilis. *Sex Transm Dis* 1979;6:243.
182. Felman YM, Nikitas JA. Syphilis serology today. *Arch Dermatol 1980;*116:84.
183. Brown ST, Zaidi A, Larsen SA, et al. Serological response to syphilis treatment: a new analysis of old data. *JAMA* 1985;253:1296.
184. Romanowski B, Sutherland R, Fick GH, et al. Serologic response to treatment of infectious syphilis. *Ann Intern Med* 1991;114:1005.
185. Hook EW III, Marra CM. Acquired syphilis in adults. *N Engl J Med* 1992;326:1060.
186. Lukehart SA, Hook EW III, Baker-Zander SA, et al. Invasion of the central nervous system by *Treponema pallidum*: implications for diagnosis and treatment. *Ann Intern Med* 1988;109:855.
187. Gordon SM, Eaton ME, George R, et al. The response of symptomatic neurosyphilis to high-dose intravenous penicillin G in patients with human immunodeficiency virus infection. *N Engl J Med* 1994;331:1469.
188. Ziaya PR, Hankins GD, Gilstrap LC, et al. Intravenous penicillin desensitization and treatment during pregnancy. *JAMA* 1986;256:2561.

189. CDC. Alternative case-finding methods in a crack-related syphilis epidemic—Philadephia. *MMWR* 1991;40:77.

FURTHER READING

Holmes KK, Mårdh P, Sparling PF, et al., eds. *Sexually transmitted diseases*, 2nd ed. New York: McGraw-Hill, 1990.

13

Human Papillomavirus in Children and Adolescents, with Evaluation of Pap Smears in Adolescents

The importance of human papillomavirus (HPV) as a sexually transmitted disease became evident during and after the Korean War. The wives of servicemen who returned from the war with penile warts were noted to develop similar lesions after a 4–6-week incubation period (1). With the advent of recombinant DNA techniques in the 1970s, it became clear that the genital warts caused by certain types of HPV are very different from common skin warts. Even with an increased understanding of HPV biology and epidemiology, there are still many unanswered questions, particularly in pediatric and adolescent populations.

VIRAL CHARACTERISTICS

Human papillomaviruses are DNA viruses that are mucosotropic and cutaneotropic. They most commonly involve the skin, lower genital tract, larynx, oral cavity, urethra, bladder, and anal/perianal epithelium. HPV replicates in the nucleus of epidermal cells. The virus attacks cells in the basal layer of the epidermis or mucosa, where a viral reservoir is established. Active expression of the viral genome occurs as the cells differentiate during their migration toward the epithelial surface. Certain types of HPV, particularly those that cause malignant transformation of the cell, become integrated in the host DNA. Expression of HPV genes, unlike that of other viruses, is tied to the cellular events of squamous differentiation and keratinization. Because genital epithelium has a limited ability to keratinize, the viral replicative cycle does not always proceed to lysis of the cell. This may result in an abortive infection in which the human cell is not destroyed but instead becomes malignant (2). These papillomaviruses generally infect mammals and are resistant to freezing, desiccation, or inactivation (3). Serologic typing is confounded by antisera cross-reacting between HPV types. To date, the most reliable method of identification of specific HPV types is DNA hybridization.

A new HPV type is identified if there is <50% hybridization with other known types. However, despite this established criterion, the actual DNA sequence homology may be 90% among the distinct types. There are currently over 65 types known by this convention. When the virus would otherwise be considered a known HPV type but has a distinct restrictive endonuclease pattern, then a subtype is designated by adding a letter (e.g., HPV-6b) (4). Among the first 55 types, the common skin types are 1, 2, 4, 7, 26, 27, 28, and 29, with 1, 2, and 4 being the most frequent. HPV type 2 is specific for common skin warts, and types 1 and 4 are seen with deep plantar and palmar warts. The genital warts are represented by types 6, 11, 16, 18, 30, 31, 32, 33, 34, 35, 39, 42, 43, 44, 48, 51, 52, 53, 54, and 55; types 6, 11, 16, and 18 are the predominant types in clinical genital findings (4). Types 6 and 11 are most often associated with exophytic "cauliflower" genital warts. These types often involve the posterior fourchette and labia minora (Fig. 1) and have also been associated with laryngeal papillomas and conjunctival lesions (5). Types 16, 18, 31, 33, and 35 cause flat condylomata and are associated with cervical dysplasia and anogenital cancers, as well as squamous cell cancers of the respiratory tract and other cutaneous sites (Table 1).

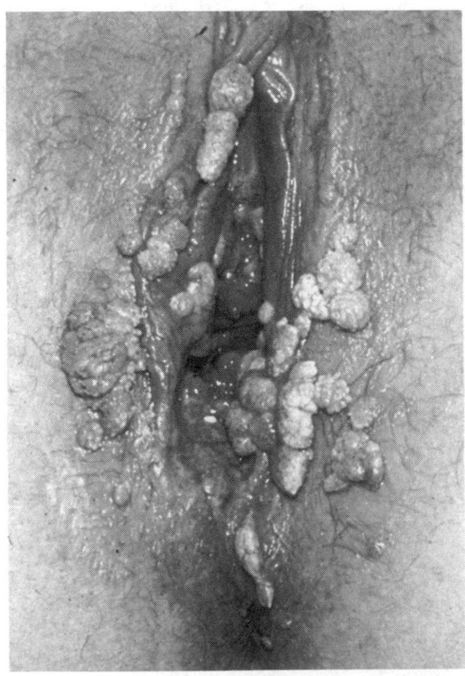

FIG. 1. Vulvar condyloma acuminatum.

TABLE 1. *Classification of HPV types by risk of neoplasia and cancer*

	Low risk	Intermediate risk	High risk
HPV type	6	30[a]	16
	11	31	18
	42	33	45
	43	35	56
	44	39	
	53	51	
	54	52	
	55	58	
		66	

[a]It is not clear whether HPV-30 is of intermediate or high risk.

(Adapted from Lorincz AT, Reid R, Jenson AB, et al. Human papillomavirus infection of the cervix: relative risk associations of 15 common anogenital types. *Obstet Gynecol* 1992; 79:328–337; with permission from The American College of Obstetricians and Gynecologists.)

EPIDEMIOLOGY

The population prevalence of genital HPV infection is unclear at this date. The use of a DNA method of detection yields a prevalence of HPV infection that is much higher than would be observed by clinical evaluations alone. In a survey of female students attending a university health service for routine annual gynecologic examinations, 46% were infected with HPV when a cervical swab was analyzed by the polymerase chain reaction (PCR) technique (6). PCR amplifies the DNA before detection and makes the assay more sensitive. In the same study, a dot blot hybridization technique (ViraPap) showed a prevalence of 11%. Only 1% had vulvar, anal, or vaginal warts detected by gross visual examination, and 9% had a history of genital warts. Whether the detection of the DNA alone is an indicator of the disease is controversial.

The human immune system, particularly the cell-mediated T-cell responses, plays a role in clinically manifested HPV disease (4). Healthy subjects can have spontaneous regression of disease, especially if the lesions have been present for <1 year and if specific immunoglobulins have developed (4,7). Immunosuppression from a variety of disease states has been associated with a greater incidence of HPV, including patients with renal transplants (8,9), neoplastic syndromes, and human immunodeficiency virus (HIV) infection (10,11). Genital warts may first appear or may grow markedly during pregnancy because of hormonal upregulation and amplification of the viral DNA and/or suppression of the immune system (12).

Since the advent of DNA detection, the HPV genome has been identified as a predominant factor associated with invasive cervical cancer (2,13). Similar disease associations have been noted in dysplasias of the vulva, vagina, penis, and anus. Rare squamous cell carcinoma of the lung and head and neck cancers have also been reported to be associated with genital types of HPV (14). Despite this evidence, HPV has been established as a necessary but not the sole factor in oncogenesis (15). Other cofactors may be cigarette smoking (16,17), immunosuppression (9,18), and other vaginal infections, including allergic responses to *Candida* organisms (19) and genital herpes simplex, as well as extension of the squamocolumnar junction into the vagina as occurs with *in utero* exposure to diethylstilbestrol (20).

DIAGNOSIS

Detection of genital HPV infections involves visual inspection and a variety of cytologic, histologic, and molecular techniques. Infection with HPV may be apparent clinically with or without the aid of magnification. Special stains with 3% to 5% acetic acid, Schiller's iodine, or toluidine blue with or without the magnification of the colposcope may help in the diagnosis. The infection is more often subclinical and thus apparent only at the time of the evaluation of an abnormal Papanicolaou (Pap) smear or with the biopsy of clinically unusual-appearing tissues (21,22). Single or multiple viral types may be involved (23).

Several techniques have been developed for the detection of subclinical HPV. *In situ* hybridization uses a labeled RNA or DNA probe to detect HPV in a specimen, and it will detect as few as 20 copies of HPV DNA/RNA per cell (5). Southern blot hybridization with restriction-endonuclease pattern analysis is sensitive and specific for HPV and detects 0.1 copies of HPV DNA per cell. The Southern blot technique is time consuming and expensive but was the primary research tool in the initial studies on genital HPV (12). Commercially available kits, such as ViraPap and ViraType (Life Technologies, Bethesda Research Labs, Gaithersburg, MD), use dot blot techniques and can identify seven HPV types. Newer tests, including the HPV Profile and the Hybrid Capture Microtiter DNA test (Digene, Beltsville, MD), can identify up to 14 types and are being further refined in Pap smears and cervical biopsies (24–27). PCR techniques can detect as little as one genome of HPV DNA per 100,000 cells; whether this amount is sufficient to cause infection is not known (5). All of these techniques can be performed on fresh tissue; however, *in situ* hybridization and PCR can also be used on fixed, paraffin-embedded tissue.

HPV IN CHILDREN

Transmission

Condyloma acuminata (venereal warts) represents the most common clinical manifestation of HPV in infants and young children. These warts may have the typical verrucous appearance around the vulva and anus (Fig. 2) also seen in adolescents or may have an atypical appearance resembling a fleshy tumor at the introitus (Fig. 3 and Color Plate 8). HPV can be transmitted to an infant at the time of delivery from an infected symptomatic or asymptomatic mother. The

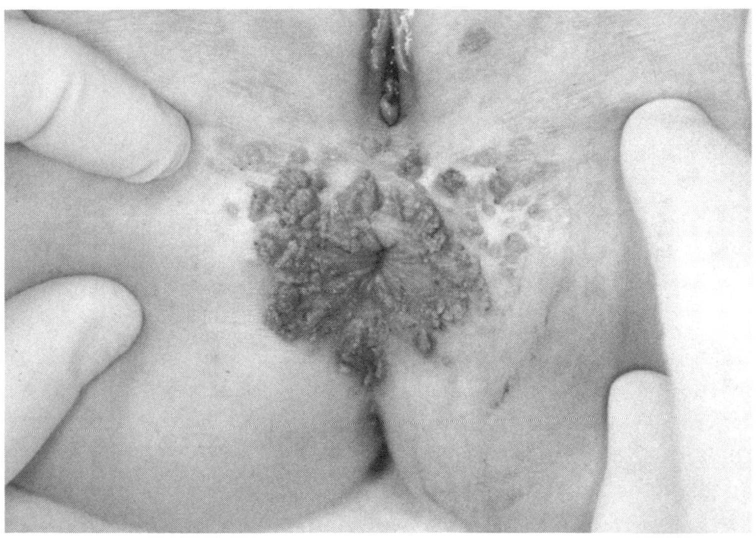

FIG. 2. Perianal condyloma in prepubertal child.

chance of perinatal transmission has been variably reported. Pakarian and colleagues (28) reported that of 31 women who had a past history of cervical intraepithelial neoplasia (CIN) and/or genital warts, 20 (65%) were positive for HPV DNA prior to delivery by PCR on cervical swab. Twelve of the 32 infants (38%; one set of twins) were positive for HPV DNA on either buccal or genital swabs at 24 hours. At 6-week followup, eight infants were positive for HPV DNA. The recent finding of HPV in the oral cavity of normal children has suggested that the virus is more prevalent than previously known (29). Sedlacek and colleagues (30) found HPV using Southern blot hybridization in the nasopharyngeal swabs of 11 of 23 (48%) neonates delivered vaginally from mothers who had detectable levels of HPV DNA in cervical cells. The exact mode of perinatal transmission is still unclear, with evidence for hematologic, transamniotic, and cervicovaginal transmission (30-32). Since the incubation period from exposure to clinical expression may be many months, a child with warts in the first 24 months of life may have been infected at birth. Whether longer intervals of latency to clinical expression occur is still unknown.

When condyloma are noted in a child, the possibility of sexual abuse needs to be explored regardless of age. The data reported from several studies in dermatology centers have been conflicting and showed a greater prevalence of nongenital wart types than that observed in gynecologic and sexual abuse clinics (33–37). The great majority of warts found in the genital area of prepubertal girls seen in our clinic are caused by HPV types 6 and 11 (38). Even when a hand wart virus is found, a nonsexual-contact explanation may not be the only mode of spread. It is possible, although yet unproved, that caregivers can transmit the

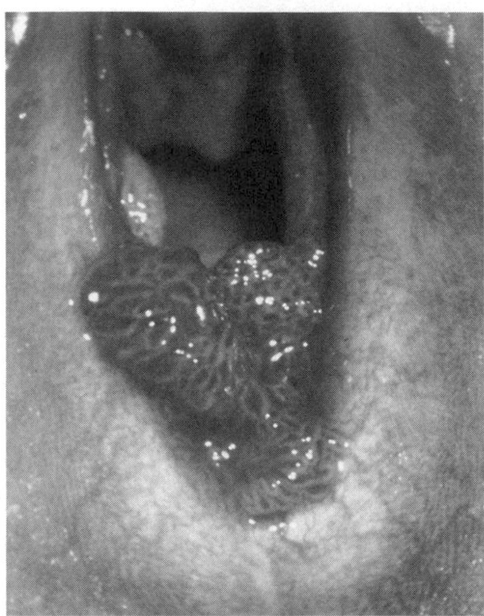

FIG. 3. Hymeneal condyloma in prepubertal girl.

genital wart virus during shared bathing. The issues of transmission were highlighted in a 5-year-old evaluated in our clinic with a single wart on her inner thigh that appeared shortly after birth; 5 years later she developed extensive hymeneal and vulvar warts (35). Psychological evaluation revealed that she had been involved in coercive sexual play with a peer. The warts on the inner thigh and the vulva were identical genital types.

In a study of 1538 children aged 1 to 12 years being evaluated for possible abuse, Ingram and colleagues (39) concluded that a history of sexual contact could be established in 43% of the 28 children with condyloma acuminata. In children comprehending questions regarding sexual contact (i.e., were verbal), 63% with condyloma had a history of sexual contact. In a study of vaginal-wash samples, 5 of 15 girls with a history of sexual abuse (3 had visible warts) and none of 17 controls were positive for HPV types 6, 11, or 16 (40). Prepubertal girls with external genital warts may have atypia or dysplasia on cervicovaginal wash specimens or on Pap smears (41).

Given the uncertainties regarding the mode of HPV transmission in individual patients, the clinician needs to pursue a careful history of abuse, even if the source seems apparent. Because of the long latency, identifying a perpetrator or determining whether the virus was acquired at birth is often not possible, but the child should continue to be followed to try to ensure her safety in her environment. The careful multidisciplinary approach to possible sexual abuse evaluation should take place when the clinician is faced with a patient with condyloma. Gutman and coworkers (42) proposed using four criteria in the evaluation:

1. Behavioral indications of abuse,
2. Medical examination to identify physical indications of abuse,
3. Microbiologic assessment for other sexually transmitted diseases, and
4. Age-appropriate interviews of the child and caretakers by skilled personnel.

Cultures for other sexually transmitted infections (*Neisseria gonorrhoeae* and *Chlamydia trachomatis)* and serology for syphilis (*Treponema pallidum)* and hepatitis B (if not immunized) should be obtained. In children with other risk factors or extensive HPV infections, immunosuppression from HIV should be considered. It should be kept in mind, when embarking on this often difficult but necessary work-up of the child with an HPV infection (see Chapter 20), that the patient's protection and welfare are the greatest issues.

Diagnosis

The diagnosis of condyloma acuminata can be made definitively by a single biopsy, which can then be split for routine histologic examination and for HPV-DNA typing (4). In pediatric patients, DNA typing has the utility of firmly establishing that an infection has been caused by a genital type of HPV and not by a common skin type, which cannot be differentiated using histology alone (4). However, even if the DNA typing reflects a genital source, it cannot be used to identify or exclude a specific perpetrator of sexual abuse because genital HPV types are quite prevalent and a single person can carry multiple types of virus. Even if a mother has the same type as her child, her partner will also be exposed to the same types, and so the mode of transmission cannot be validated. On the other hand, a negative DNA typing does not exclude the diagnosis of a genital HPV type. Problems in processing a specimen, such as delay in transport, or infection with one of the numerous genital types that are not included in the commercial kits will produce a false-negative test result (4).

There are several conditions that mimic the appearance of condyloma, including molluscum contagiosum, skin tags, urethral prolapse, and sarcoma botryoides (see Chapter 3 and Color Plate 7).

Laryngeal papillomatosis can also occur in children secondary to perinatal transmission of HPV. This troubling infection, usually from HPV type 11, often presents with hoarseness in the first 5 years of life and may require multiple interventions. Most children with juvenile laryngeal papillomas are born to mothers with a history of genital HPV infection (43). However, the exact risk of laryngeal disease for a child born to a mother with HPV is unknown but may be between 1:200 and 1:1500 (44). HPV laryngeal disease has also occurred among infants delivered by cesarean section. Hence, delivery by cesarean section is generally determined by maternal indications (e.g., if the outlet is obstructed or vaginal delivery would result in excessive bleeding) (45).

Treatment

Treatment of anogenital condyloma in children is controversial. Although some prefer to treat a few warts, particularly in the anal area, with trichloroacetic acid using EMLA (a eutectic mixture of local anesthetics, lidocaine 2.5%, and prilocaine 2.5%) in advance, others feel that genital typing is important for future followup and assessment. Hence, operative treatment under anesthesia provides the opportunity to obtain biopsies before destructive therapies are undertaken. We generally use carbon dioxide laser under general anesthesia to treat these lesions. The laser should be attached to the colposcope or an operating microscope with a micromanipulator to best define the dermatologic planes. Using the superpulse mode at a low wattage leaves minimal adjuvant tissue damage. This technique allows the depth of destruction to be confined to the epidermis and superficial papillary dermis. During the laser procedure, the vaporized debris is frequently wiped away with 5% acetic acid–soaked gauze so that the classic appearance of the white papillations can be observed. At the end of the procedure, infiltrating with 0.25% bupivacaine HCl will assist with postoperative analgesia. Immediate postoperative application of ice reduces local swelling.

The child with only a few lesions can be treated in an ambulatory setting. For more extensive lesions, admission to the hospital the night after the procedure may be indicated if the child has difficulty voiding and needs bladder catheterization. Sitz baths and/or a squeeze bottle of warm water to irrigate the area can help relieve pain. Voiding into a bathtub of warm water and using stool softeners may lessen discomfort of bowel and bladder function (4). A thin application of silver sulfadiazine cream is used topically four times a day, and oral analgesics are given as needed. Long-term followup is important because of the potential for recurrences.

Systemic use of retinoic acid as possible therapy for recalcitrant HPV infection has been proposed (46,47). In a study using human keratinocytes, retinoic acid was shown to suppress the infectivity and proliferation of HPV. Its use in a very small number of immunosuppressed patients was associated with complete resolution of their warts (46,47).

The long-term risk of neoplasia, especially of the vulva, is unknown but remains a significant worry. An unresolved issue for clinicians in this field is the frequency and methodology of followup of children with an HPV infection. This is particularly difficult to answer in those children who have HPV-16/18 identified from their lesions. We and others (41) have several young children with atypical cells or dysplasia on their Pap smears. A case of vulvar malignancy has been reported in a 14-year-old who had been diagnosed with condyloma acuminatum in infancy (48). At present, we are obtaining yearly "blind" Pap smears in prepubertal girls with a previously documented abnormal Pap smear. It is unclear when to recommend standard Pap smear screening after puberty in girls with known HPV-16/18 with or without a previously documented abnormal cytology.

HPV INFECTIONS IN ADOLESCENTS

Transmission

Epidemiologic studies have found a high prevalence of HPV infection in sexually active adolescents and young adults. The prevalence of HPV detected by DNA techniques far exceeds the clinical expression of this virus. This is particularly significant since both sexual intercourse at an early age and the occurrence of HPV are associated with an increased risk of cervical cancer (49). Risk factors notable in the adolescent population for acquisition of this virus include multiple sexual partners, lack of condom use, previous sexually transmitted diseases, and sexual relations with an infected partner. HPV is found widely in both urban low-socioeconomic-status adolescents and suburban adolescents (50–54). In an inner city adolescent clinic, cervicovaginal washings for HPV DNA were positive in 32% of sexually active patients (50). Fisher and colleagues (51) reported that HPV was found by cervicovaginal lavage in 32% of 106 sexually active middle-class adolescents; 18% had evidence of HPV infection with either type 16 or type 18. Risk factors associated with HPV in this study were more than two sexual partners, sexual activity for >2 years, menarche before age 12 years, and a history of a sexually transmitted disease. Logistic regression found that age of menarche and number of sexual partners were independent risk factors for HPV. In a study of 661 sexually active teenagers attending family planning clinics, Moscicki and colleagues (52) found that 15% were positive by RNA-DNA dot blot hybridization and >60% of HPV-infected individuals had types 16, 18, 31, 33, or 35. The high prevalences of HPV-16 and -18 in the adolescent age group is particularly worrisome (55,56) (Table 1). In a study of 25 adolescent patients aged 15 to 20 years with CIN 3 or high-grade dysplasia, 21 (84%) had detectable HPV-16 and/or HPV-18 (55). Shew and colleagues (53) have suggested that the high prevalence of HPV among adolescents may be related to early sexual activity and exposure to HPV during early adolescence, close to the time of menarche. The immature cervix of adolescents, with a large transformation zone and squamous metaplasia, is more likely to become infected with exposure to HPV (53,54). Although Bergeron and colleagues (57) have reported that swabs taken from the underwear of 74 patients were positive for genital HPV using filter hybridization techniques, no studies in adolescents have documented this as a mode of transmission.

Over time, the type of HPV may not remain stable because of latency, new infection, or other unknown factors. Rosenfeld and colleagues (58) in a study of 51 sexually active 13- to 21-year-old patients found that 39% were infected with HPV at the first screening and 25.5% at a followup visit 6–36 months later. Although 57% (29 of 51) had HPV at some time, only 4 had HPV at both visits, with only 1 subject showing the same HPV type over time. Thus, diagnosis based on screening for HPV with DNA probes does not appear to be a cost-effective strategy at this time (59).

Male partners of women infected with HPV have been studied, particularly in the last decade (60–64). Barrasso and coworkers (60) found that 64.4% of male sexual partners of women with cervical flat condyloma or CIN had evidence of HPV infection; in 42.5%, the lesions were detected only after the application of acetic acid. Many men are not aware of the existence of lesions, and some may have penile intraepithelial neoplasia at the time of evaluation. Although colposcopy has been useful in the detection of condyloma in men, there is no practical screening test for subclinical infection with HPV. Krebs and Helmskamp (64) found no difference between treatment failure rates of women in whom the male partner was examined and treated versus those with no treatment. Thus, most recurrences of HPV disease in women are probably from reactivation rather than reinfection. Male partners should be treated for obvious exophytic warts and as in all persons with HPV should be counseled about their ability to transmit the virus to uninfected partners. It is still not known whether those with subclinical HPV infection are as contagious as those with exophytic warts (45). Although condom use is efficacious in preventing some HPV spread, mainly in primary infections, the contact of vulva and scrotum may further spread the infection, and thus the female condom may be more effective.

Diagnosis

The most common clinical manifestation of HPV disease in the sexually active adolescent is the appearance of warty condyloma on the vulva or anus 4–6 weeks after an exposure to HPV (1). Urethral condyloma (Fig. 4) may also occur. However, because of the long latency, the lesions may appear months to years after sexual contact due to the presence of virus in the previously normal-appearing tissues (65). Condyloma acuminata are associated primarily with types 6 and 11; however, types 16 and 18 and other subtypes may be present. Perianal warts occur commonly in homosexual males and in females engaging in anal intercourse but also occur in girls denying anal intercourse. Cigarette smoking appears to increase the risk of progression from asymptomatic HPV infection to genital warts in both HIV-positive and HIV-negative women (66).

In addition to gross warts, HPV can be detected by the application of 3% to 5% acetic acid to the vulva, vagina, and cervix; however, the test is not a specific test for HPV infection and can yield false-positive results. The procedure causes slight burning or a cold sensation and is time consuming but can be used to identify probable subclinical HPV. The aceto-white lesions may be seen with the naked eye but are particularly visible with the use of magnification of a colposcope. Lesions on the vulva are often referred to as microcondyloma of the labia and should not be confused with the normal, usually symmetric, vestibular papillae that usually do not stain aceto-white. HPV lesions may cause vestibular pruritus, burning, and dyspareunia. When the presence of HPV is questioned, punch biopsy for pathologic evaluation should be obtained.

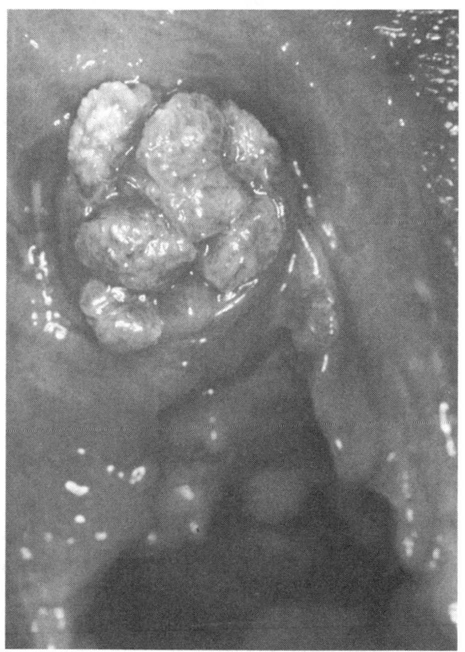

FIG. 4. Urethral condyloma. (Courtesy of Ann Davis, M.D., Beth Israel Deaconess Hospital, Boston, MA)

Treatment

Because HPV infection is often multicentric and normal-appearing skin is often infected with latent HPV, treatment is directed at clinical disease, such as warts, cervical squamous intraepithelial lesions (SILs), vulvar intraepithelial neoplasia, and vaginal intraepithelial neoplasia.

Most genital warts are benign growths and cause only local, if any, symptoms. Treatment of external exophytic warts probably does not influence the development of cervical or penile disease and is 22% to 94% effective in eradicating visible disease (usually 25% at 3 months) (45). The goal is local destruction of the lesions with the hope that the patient's own host responses will augment the treatment for a complete resolution. Any treatment must be compared against the possibility of spontaneous resolution; exophytic warts usually regress over 3–5 years (45). In placebo-controlled studies, genital warts cleared within 3 months without treatment in 20% to 30% of patients. Treatment is more successful if genital warts are small and have been present for <1 year.

Destructive therapies include podophyllin, trichloroacetic acid (TCA), liquid nitrogen, cryotherapy, and laser and should take into account the extent of lesions and patient preference. Application of 25% podophyllin in tincture of benzoin has problems with use. This compound needs to be washed off after 4 to 6 hours (1 to 4 hours with first application) and must be applied frequently.

Podophyllin is contraindicated in pregnancy and in well-vascularized perianal and vaginal tissue because of absorption and the possibility of toxic reactions. Efficacy is 32% to 79%, with recurrences among 27% to 65% of patients (45).

Podofilox 0.5% solution is a self-administered agent for external genital warts only (67). The solution is applied with a cotton swab to the warts twice daily for 3 days, followed by 4 days of no therapy. This cycle may be repeated as necessary for a total of four cycles. The total wart area should not exceed 10 cm^2, and total volume of podofilox used should not exceed 0.5 ml/day. A self-administered medication should be prescribed only for the mature adolescent capable of complying with the procedure. The initial application should optimally be done in the office with the use of a mirror. The compound does not have to be washed off. Local adverse effects include pain, burning, inflammation, and erosion in half of patients treated. Efficacy is 45% to 88%, with recurrence among 33% to 60% of patients (45). This compound is also contraindicated during pregnancy.

Many clinicians prefer to use another chemical compound, TCA, in strengths of 80% to 90%. TCA must be applied carefully to prevent chemical burns of normal adjacent tissue and must be applied only to the abnormal lesion. Immediately afterward, baking soda, aloe vera gel, or normal saline can be used to ease the burning sensation. Unlike podophyllin, TCA does not need to be washed off and is reapplied weekly. Few data are available on efficacy; one trial in men found a 81% efficacy with 36% recurrence rate (45).

The newest therapy, imiquimod 5% cream, is applied by the patient three times a week to external genital and perianal warts for up to 16 weeks. The area is washed 6 to 10 hours later. Side effects include moderate erythema, peeling, and swelling. Sexual contact should be avoided while the cream is on the skin; the cream may weaken diaphragms and condoms. Success rates are 50% to 70%. There are no published data in patients <18 years or in pregnancy (45).

If the lesions fail to respond or progress between treatments over 6 weeks, laser or cryocautery can be discussed with the patient. Cryotherapy is relatively inexpensive and does not require anesthesia. Most patients experience moderate pain. Efficacy is 63% to 88%, with recurrences among 21% to 39% of patients (45). Electrodesiccation has been used in some centers; it is contraindicated in patients with pacemakers and for lesions proximal to the anal verge (54).

The advantages of treatment with the carbon dioxide laser are that cure rates are high and vulvar, vaginal, cervical, and perianal lesions can be treated concurrently. The disadvantages of laser treatment are that general anesthesia is generally required, costs are high, and postoperative pain can be significant. After laser therapy, the patient needs to be instructed in using sitz baths, voiding into the water if dysuria causes urinary retention, drying the vulva with a hair dryer, rinsing with a squirt bottle after a bowel movement or urination, application of silver sulfadiazine cream in a thin layer every 4 to 12 hours for 10 to 30 days, use of narcotics/analgesics for pain, avoidance of sex for at least 1 month and thereafter use of a condom, and use of a stool softener (68). Problems include postoperative pain, bleeding, and scarring (vulvar coaptations, vaginal strictures, and cervical stenosis). It is important to remember that the laser cannot effectively eliminate all multicentric subclinical HPV infection of the lower genital tract, even with the use of extensive therapy (69). Although controversial, incorporating surrounding tissue into the field of destruction may reduce the chance of recurrence for vulvar epithelial neoplasia and vulvar and/or anal/perianal condyloma (68,70). Physicians using laser technology for treatment of HPV infections need to avoid contact with the laser vapor, which contains intact HPV DNA and may result in nasal or vocal cord HPV infections (71).

Treatment of vaginal warts have included cryotherapy using liquid nitrogen, 80% to 90% TCA (powdered with baking soda to remove unreacted acid), or podophyllin (10% to 25%). The Centers for Disease Control and Prevention (CDC) caution against the use of a cryoprobe in the vagina because of the risk of vaginal perforation and/or fistula formation. Urethral meatus warts have been treated with cryotherapy and podophyllin, and anal warts with cryotherapy, TCA, and surgical resection. Oral warts are treated with cryotherapy with liquid nitrogen, electrodesiccation, or surgical removal (45).

5-Fluorouracil (5-FU) cream, although not approved by the U.S. Food and Drug Administration (FDA) for the therapy of HPV infection, has been used successfully in some centers for the treatment of vaginal and urethral condyloma (72,73). Controlled studies are lacking, however. Protocols modeled on those of Krebs have proved useful in the care of a very few, carefully selected patients at our hospital (24,72,73). 5-FU has been used as prophylaxis for HPV recurrence following laser therapy, especially for immunosuppressed patients who have a high risk of relapse. For prophylaxis, the patient applies 4 to 5 ml (applicator size of 5 mL or 10 mL must be determined by pharmacy availability) of 5% 5-FU *deeply* into the vagina once every 2 weeks just prior to bedtime, with subsequent insertion of a tampon after the application to prevent seepage of the medication onto the vulva. A small amount of petroleum jelly can be placed at the introitus, although the efficacy of treating coexisting vulvar disease may be lessened. The tampon should be removed the next morning, and the patient should bathe. A very thin film of 5-FU is applied over the vulva at night once every 2 weeks, with care taken to apply it in the areas previously involved with HPV. The first application of 5-FU is started as soon as sufficient healing has occurred following laser therapy but not later than 4 weeks. At a followup of 9 to 22 months after complete ablation of clinical HPV, 13% of patients treated with prophylactic 5-FU and 38% of those without additional treatment had recurrent lesions (73).

When employed for the treatment of vaginal condyloma, 5-FU in a 3-ml dose can also be used on a weekly basis for 10 weeks; care must be taken, as noted above, to prevent seepage from the introitus by inserting a tampon. Krebs (72) reported that 85% of women treated with 10 weekly applications of 5% 5-FU (approximately 1.5 g per vaginal treatment) had no evidence of disease at 3-month followup. Alternatively, 2 ml of 5-FU can be applied every third night for 2 weeks (24). 5-FU has also been used for urethral condyloma and can be applied every third night, and the patient is then instructed to void 4 hours later and bathe. However, the clinician needs to be aware of the potential for *serious* side effects. This involves close monitoring of patients, with immediate discontinuance for any sign of redness externally on the vulva or internally on the vaginal mucosa. 5-FU is contraindicated in pregnancy, and adolescents must be using a reliable form of contraception consistently and must understand the risks of noncompliance. Counseling should be documented in the medical record. In addition, the adolescent must be able to follow directions, since erosive vulvitis will occur if 5-FU is improperly used; hands must be washed thoroughly after every application. Bone marrow suppression and gastrointestinal side effects have not been a problem with gynecologic uses of 5-FU because of the small amount of the total dose absorbed. However, the amount of absorption may increase when applied to eroded epithelium, and this may lead to side effects.

Interferon has been used in some centers with variable results but is not recommended by the CDC due to cost and its association with a high frequency of side effects (45,74,75). Friedman-Kien and colleagues (75) found that therapy eliminated warts in 62% of patients treated with intralesional interferon alfa twice weekly for up to 8 weeks, compared with only 21% treated with placebo. However, two randomized trials did not find it more effective than placebo (45). Side effects included fever, flu-like symptoms, myalgia, and malaise and usually disappeared by the end of the third week of therapy. Gall and colleagues (76) in a small randomized study showed that previously reported intramuscular injections are inferior to intralesional injections. Safety has not been established in patients <18 years of age. Effective contraception must be used since it is currently unknown whether this drug is harmful to the fetus or a woman's reproductive capacity.

EVALUATION AND MANAGEMENT OF PAP SMEARS

A Pap smear screening is recommended for any adolescent who has ever been sexually active or exposed to HPV or is ≥18 years old (77). Cervical dysplasia and rarely carcinoma *in situ* can occur during adolescence, especially in adolescents who become sexually active with multiple partners shortly after menarche or who have been exposed to HPV, especially types 16 and 18 (9,15–19,53,78–82). The techniques for obtaining a Pap smear are described in Chapter 1. For accurate cytologic diagnosis, the collection of the sample must be representative of normal and abnormal cell populations and must include the squamocolumnar junction and the endocervix. The laboratory should be provided with essential history such as last menstrual period, use of oral contraceptives, presence of an intrauterine device, and prior abnormal Pap smear or treatment for dysplasia. It should be remembered that Pap smears may have a false-negative rate of 20% to 60%, depending on quality control in individual laboratories (83). An abnormal growth on the cervix regardless of Pap smear results should be assessed with colposcopy and biopsy.

TABLE 2. *The Bethesda System II (TBS II) for reporting cervicovaginal cytologic diagnoses*[a]

Statement on specimen adequacy

Satisfactory for evaluation
Satisfactory for evaluation but limited by ... (reason)
Unsatisfactory for evaluation

General categorization (optional)

Within normal limits
Benign cellular changes (see Descriptive diagnoses)
Epithelial cell abnormality (see Descriptive diagnoses)

Descriptive diagnoses

- Benign cellular changes
  - Infection
    - *Trichomonas vaginalis*
    - Fungal organisms morphologically consistent with *Candida* spp.
    - Predominance of coccobacilli consistent with shift in vaginal flora
    - Bacteria morphologically consistent with *Actinomyces* spp.
    - Cellular changes associated with herpes simplex virus
  - Other
- Reactive changes
  - Reactive cellular changes associated with:
    - Inflammation (including typical repair)
    - Atrophy with inflammation (atrophic vaginitis)
    - Radiation
    - Intrauterine contraceptive device
    - Other
- Epithelial cell abnormalities
  - Squamous cell
    - Atypical squamous cells of undetermined significance (ASCUS): qualify premalignant/malignant or reactive process favored
    - Squamous intraepithelial lesion
      - Low grade
        - Cellular changes with HPV
        - Mild dysplasia/CIN 1
      - High grade
        - Moderate dysplasia/CIN 2
        - Severe dysplasia/CIN 3
        - Carcinoma *in situ*/CIN 3
      - Squamous cell carcinoma
  - Glandular cell
    - Endometrial cells, cytologically benign, in a postmenopausal woman
    - Atypical glandular cells of undetermined significance: qualify premalignant/malignant or reactive process favored
    - Adenocarcinoma
      - Endocervical
      - Endometrial
      - Extrauterine
      - Unspecified
  - Other malignant neoplasms: specify
  - Hormonal evaluation (applies to vaginal smears only)

[a]CIN, cervical intraepithelial neoplasia; HPV, human papillomavirus.

TABLE 3. *Comparison of the Bethesda System II (TBS II) with previous Pap smear classification systems*[a]

Expected histology	Unknown	Normal	Squamous metaplasia	Atypical squamous metaplasia	Mild dysplasia	Moderate dysplasia	Severe dysplasia	Carcinoma *in situ*	Invasive cancer
National Cancer Institute (TBS II)	Unsatisfactory	Within normal limits	Infection	Atypia	Low-grade SIL	High-grade SIL			Squamous cancer
Richart classification	Class 0	Class I		Class II	CIN 1	CIN 2	CIN 3		
World Health Organization	Unsatisfactory	Normal			Mild dysplasia	Moderate dysplasia	Severe dysplasia	Epidermoid carcinoma *in situ*	Invasive epidermoid carcinoma
Papanicolaou classification	Class 0	Class I		Class II	Class II or III	Class III	Class IV		Class V
Cytologic description	Few cells, WBCs/RBCs, dried, distorted cells, broken slide	Normal differentiated cells, metaplasia, mild inflammation		Significant inflammation, nuclear enlargement	<10% basal or undifferentiated cells	10%–20% basal or undifferentiated cells	>30% basal or undifferentiated cells on slide		Malignant cells

[a]CIN, cervical intraepithelial neoplasia; SIL, squamous intraepithelial lesions (this category includes cytologic changes of koilocytosis/HPV); WBCs/RBCs, ratio of white blood cells to red blood cells.

In response to the variable systems of cytologic nomenclature, a new system of terminology, known as the Bethesda system (TBS) (84), was published and subsequently modified (TBS II) at a 1991 National Cancer Institute workshop. TBS II, now being used by >80% of the cytology laboratories in the United States (85,86), is abbreviated in Table 2. A correlative Table 3 compares TBS II with previous reporting systems.

The Pap smear in the HPV-infected adolescent may reveal koilocytes (squamous cells with dense, sometimes granular, "raisinoid" nuclei and a perinuclear halo, also termed *balloon* cells), dyskeratosis, and/or evidence of a squamous intraepithelial lesion. Narrative summaries of Pap cytologic findings are important, and careful consultation between the clinician and the cytology laboratory is essential to ensure that the terminology used (including koilocytosis, koilocytotic atypia) is being interpreted similarly. Although Pap smears are not perfect, they remain a useful screening technique for cervical dysplasia and cancer (15,87,89). Studies in teenagers have shown varying rates of abnormal cervical cytology, from 3% to 17% depending on the inclusion criteria (SIL, atypical squamous cells of undetermined significance [ASCUS]) and the population studied (87,88,90–94). In 1984, Sadeghi and coworkers (90) reported CIN 1, 2, or 3 in 3651 (1.9%) of 194,069 adolescents 15 to 19 years old. Schydlower and colleagues (91) found that 3% of adolescents (age 13 to 21 years) receiving medical care at a military medical center had SIL, and Russo and Jones (93) reported that among 1207 women aged 16 to 19 years seen in a public health department

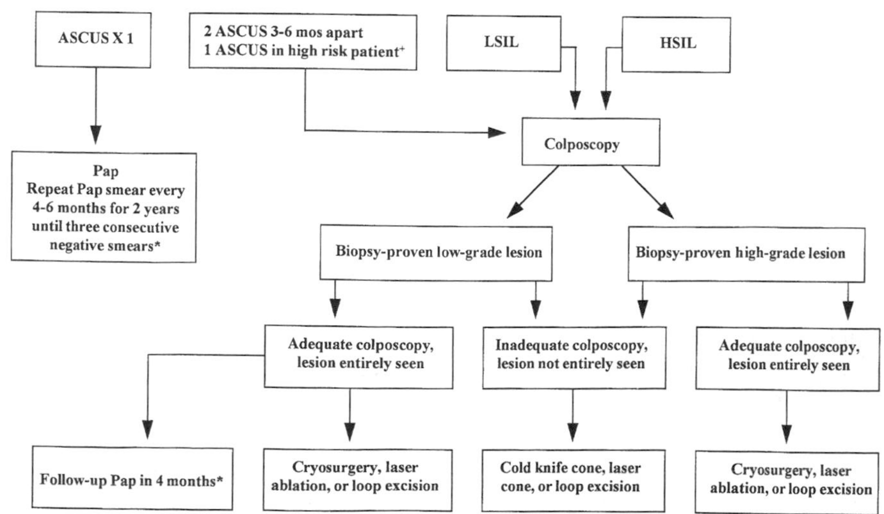

FIG. 5. Management strategies for abnormal Papanicolaou (Pap) smears.

family planning clinic, 8.5% had atypia and 2.5% dysplasia. In our adolescent medicine clinic in 1994 to 1995, 10.9% of patients 11 to 23 years old had ASCUS and 2.5% SIL (94). Thus, screening and close followup are essential in the adolescent population.

Abnormal Pap smears in the adolescent population are treated using the paradigm in Fig. 5. For those Pap smears reported as benign cellular change, if a specific infective agent is identified, we evaluate the patient and treat if confirmed. For the ASCUS Pap smear that is unqualified or reactive, followup Pap smears are done every 4 to 6 months for 2 years or until the person has three consecutive negative Pap smears in a row.

Intervention in the case of an ASCUS Pap smear that favors a premalignant process remains controversial. The standard has been to repeat the Pap smear in 3 to 6 months and, if persistent, to refer for colposcopy. The problem exists that at least 20% of ASCUS Pap smears in adults and teens are actually some degree of SIL (94–96). Hence, some authors have tried using viral DNA-typing methods to distinguish high-risk ASCUS and even low-grade SIL (LSIL) Pap smears. If the HPV typing shows a high-risk type, the patient with one ASCUS is referred for immediate colposcopy. Cox and associates (97) determined that CIN (low and high grade) was present in 21% of ASCUS ViraPap-negative and 66% of ASCUS ViraPap-positive patients. However, the current ViraPap test detects only seven HPV types. With the advent of a new generation of more sensitive HPV-typing tests, clinical usefulness may improve. An ASCUS/LSIL Triage Study has been initiated by the National Cancer Institute and will enroll 7000 women who will receive care every 6 months for 3 years with the aim of addressing HPV testing (the Hybrid Capture microliter DNA test) and other forms of clinical management and diagnostic procedures including computer-assisted Pap smears.

All patients with Pap smears that show persistent atypia, any degree of SIL, or carcinoma require further evaluation and treatment. Most centers have noted an increase in abnormal Pap smears in the past decade in adolescent and young adult women, and many special cervical clinics have been established or expanded (63,70,71). Colposcopy (visualization of the cervix with a 15×-power binocular microscope) and use of 3% to 5% acetic acid allow appropriate biopsies. Schiller's iodine stain can also assist in visualizing abnormal areas. The glycogen-producing squamous cervical and vaginal epithelial cells take up the stain, producing a brown color, whereas the columnar epithelium of the endocervix and nonglycogenated abnormal areas do not take up the stain. Adolescents tolerate cervical biopsies better if they are given a dose of a nonsteroidal antiinflammatory medication prior to the procedure (unless there is a contraindication). Compliance with referrals to colposcopy can remain problematic in adolescents and barriers may include lack of insurance, confidentiality, lack of knowledge, transportation, and fear, although definitive studies have not been done.

Technical advances such as cervicograms and computer-imaging digital colposcopy for evaluating the cervix are under investigation. Cervicography, a magnified photographic analytic process for evaluation of the transformation zone, was developed by Stafl in the late 1970s (98). Of Stafl's 700 patients who had cervicography, 296 (42%) who had abnormal cytology were referred for colposcopic evaluation. Directed biopsies in these 296 patients revealed that 136 (46%) had dysplasia or carcinoma. Among patients with biopsy-proven neoplasia, 91% had both colposcopic and cervicographic findings that were suspicious. In 1988, Tawa and colleagues (99) reported their experience with simultaneous cervical cytology and cervicography in screening a group of 3271 patients enrolled in a managed care health plan. There were 373 suspicious cervicograms and 39 positive Pap smears. In the same group, dysplasia was detected in 72 patients by cervicograms and in 14 by cytology. A recent study comparing digital computerized colposcopy with traditional methods in 188 patients found diagnosis was in agreement with histology in 85.1% of the cases utilizing the computer versus 66% by the traditional means (100).

Another technique, called speculoscopy, was recently approved by the FDA. The special activated blue-white Speculite chemoluminescent light (Trylon Corporation, Torrance, CA) is attached to the inner aspect of the upper dilator blade of the speculum. With the lights in the room dimmed, the cervix and vaginal vault are inspected through magnifying loupes. Any speculoscopic examination demonstrating aceto-white areas is considered positive, and the patient is referred for colposcopy (101). Use of speculoscopy has been reported to increase the detection of cervical dysplasia in high-risk women from 9 of 29 (31%) by Pap smear alone to 24 of 29 (83%) with chemoluminescent exam. Patients in whom the results of both tests were negative were extremely unlikely to harbor significant pathology (<1% of the 243 women studied) (102).

In addition, the recent release of new types of Pap smear preparations, including the thin prep system and PAPNET system (an automated interactive instrument for analysis of Pap smears), may also increase the sensitivity of this screening test and reduce the false-negative rate of Pap smears. Further studies are under way (103,104).

HPV infection and SIL represent a continuum, *not* a stepwise change (105). HPV DNA is present in cervical cells from 90% of patients with SIL versus 10% of controls (106). Although rates of both koilocytes and HPV antigen decrease in both high-grade SIL and invasive cancer, HPV DNA can still be recovered from cellular DNA. HPV types 16 and 18 are present in 70% of SIL and cancer, with small percentages for types 10, 11, 31, 33, and 35; type 6 is rarely present in cervical cancer. Reid and colleagues (107) found that only 1 of 80 cervical biopsy specimens that were positive for type 6 or type 11 had a diagnosis of CIN greater than grade 2. In contrast, 42 of 48 (88%) of cervical biopsies that showed CIN 3 or invasive cancer were positive for types 16, 18, or 31. However, 10% of condyloma and CIN 1 were associated with types 16, 18, or 31. Only 31% of patients with HPV type 6 or type 11 presented with abnormal Pap smears in contrast to 93% of those with types 16, 18, or 31. Evidence of seroconversion with the detection of HPV type 16 antibodies has also been associated with SIL (108).

The rate of progression from HPV cervical disease to dysplasia is variably reported, with higher degrees of dysplasia more likely to progress to carcinoma (109–111). Nash and colleagues (109) found that about one-third of patients with histologically confirmed HPV cervical infection progressed to CIN within 1 year. Nasiell and coworkers (110) calculated that a woman with mild dysplasia had a yearly risk for the development of severe dysplasia/carcinoma *in situ* 560 times greater than a woman without dysplasia. Lesions with aneuploidy are much more likely to progress to invasive disease than polyploid lesions. These percentages of progression may be lower than those that occur in natural history studies because the biopsy itself may be helpful in stimulating the patient's immune system to work against HPV. Spontaneous regression of HPV-16 lesions is low. Colposcopy alone without the use of biopsy cannot be used to predict the outcome or progression of HPV lesions.

Many patients with vulvar HPV disease have coexisting cervical disease. Although numbers vary in studies, Spitzer and associates (112) reported that 78% of patients with overt vulvar condyloma had HPV cervical disease by colposcopy and biopsy. Patients with genital warts should be evaluated with more frequent Pap smears than the annual examination recommended for sexually active teenagers. For example, we typically obtain Pap smears every 6 months during active disease and then, after resolution of the warts, every 6 months for at least 2 to 3 years. In addition, invasive vulvar cancers can be associated with types 6, 11, and 16 (107,113). Vulvar carcinoma is most often found in older women and not associated with HPV, but younger women who have vulvar carcinoma are more likely to have a coexisting HPV infection (56).

Treatment of cervical HPV infections depends on the results of colposcopy and cervical biopsy (22,114). If the biopsy confirms HPV without dysplasia and there are exophytic warts, options include observation or ablative therapy. Observation may be difficult to rationalize in an adolescent population in which followup may be unreliable and infected partners may not be treated. On the other hand, ablative therapy for mild disease that may not progress and may even regress can hardly be justified in persons just beginning their reproductive years. Ablative therapies include TCA, laser therapy, and cryotherapy. In our program, we have embarked on a more conservative treatment regimen and have chosen to observe these patients with Pap smears every 6 months.

However, if the biopsy of the HPV lesion shows a SIL, appropriate therapy includes cryotherapy, laser therapy, loop electrosurgical excision procedure (LEEP), or cone biopsy, depending on the grade of abnormality. Cryotherapy had been the most common form of treatment and has a failure rate of approximately 12% with one treatment. It has been replaced by LEEP because of less long-term compromise to the cervix and better long-term eradication of the disease (115). Although LEEP is performed as an outpatient procedure in the adult population, it may not be well tolerated by adolescents in this setting, and use of the operating room and anesthesia personnel may be indicated.

LSIL has been shown to progress in 15% of cases to high-grade lesions, and in these cases ablation or excision is reasonable treatment (116). Spontaneous regression has been shown to occur in 60% of low-grade lesions. Observation may be indicated in those patients with low-grade lesions who appear reliable and have had extensive patient education concerning their diagnosis. Pap smears should be repeated every 4 months. If the lesion persists, treatment is indicated (116).

High-grade lesions are now more frequently encountered in adolescents. After the extent of the lesion has been determined and a negative endocervical curettage has been obtained, careful but thorough ablative and/or excisional therapy should be completed. This can be accomplished by laser conization or ablation, LEEP, or cold-knife conization if indicated. In many centers such as ours, cold-knife conization in the adolescent population is being reserved for cases in which invasion is suspected.

Careful followup at 3 to 4 months after treatment for preinvasive lesions of the cervix is important. Falcone and Ferenczy (117) have recommended combined cytologic testing and colposcopy and, if appropriate, histologic examination at 3 months, followed by cytologic followup (Pap smears) at subsequent visits (116). In our program, we have chosen to follow the Pap smears at 4-month intervals after treatment for preinvasive lesions of the cervix for 2 years, and if consecutively negative, then at 6-month intervals for 2 years, with colposcopic exams at yearly intervals.

Immunocompromised Patients

HPV lesions in immunocompromised patients are particularly difficult to treat. The risk of vulvar and anal carcinoma in renal transplant patients is significantly higher than in normal patients; the risk of CIN has been estimated to be 16-fold higher than in the general population (9). Since these lesions often recur, treatment should be conservative with topical agents, local measures, and observation, unless there are pathologic diagnoses of abnormal cells. When there are pathologic abnormalities, our treatment has tended to use multiple modalities: LEEP for cervical SIL and laser therapy for vaginal, vulvar, or anal lesions, occasionally followed by long-term prophylaxis with 5-FU to prevent recurrences.

HIV in adolescence is increasingly more common than in the past (see Chapter 14). HIV effects on the immune system often accelerate HPV infection in the host. In a study of HIV-positive women, 33 of whom were symptomatic and 18 asymptomatic, 23 (70%) of the symptomatic women were positive for HPV compared with only 4 (22%) of the asymptomatic (119).

The strategy for detection of cervical disease in the HIV-infected person is controversial (45,118,119). The CDC recommend annual Pap smear testing if the specimen is adequate and remains normal (45). The American College of Obstetrics and Gynecology recommends semiannual testing (118). The question still remains whether there is a need to increase Pap smear testing in seropositive women when the T-cell count diminishes. Although confirmatory data are still needed, a unpublished study was done in 32 HIV-infected women to determine the accuracy of routine Pap smear screening in determining cervical disease. Initially, three women (9%) had abnormal Pap smears; after colposcopy and biopsies were done, 27 (84%) were found to have abnormal histology and 13 (41%) of the patients had CIN (119). Given the risk-taking behavior of many adolescents, including those with HIV infection, increased and more intense surveillance may be indicated (118,120). CD4 lymphocyte counts and HIV RNA levels may be helpful in guiding assessment of cervical disease. At present, our center continues to screen HIV-positive adolescents every 6 months for all sexually transmitted diseases, including obtaining a Pap smear. If the patient can be observed closely, subclinical cervical HPV infections and low-grade cervical and other genital dysplasias are followed with Pap smears every 4 months and yearly colposcopy rather than frequent ablative treatments.

CONCLUSIONS

Prevention of HPV infection in the adolescent population is imperative. Many of the barrier methods discussed in Chapters 14, 17, and 22 (HIV prevention, contraception, sexuality education) are applicable to the prevention of HPV. Abstinence and, for the sexually active, condoms and other barrier methods (vaginal condoms) are the only methods known to decrease HPV infections. Increasing evidence has shown that cigarette smoking in the presence of HPV acts as a cofactor to decrease the transit time to carcinoma. Because immunocompromised adolescents are at special risk from this virus, they require adequate counseling prior to becoming sexually active. They need to know about the importance of using condoms and avoiding infected partners.

When dealing with the adolescent who receives the diagnosis of HPV infection or a parent whose child has HPV, the health care provider needs to continue to provide education and support. It is essential to explore the individual's feelings and beliefs surrounding this infection because tremendous psychosocial trauma often goes along with a diagnosis of HPV infection. Compliance with care will be significantly improved if the provider assists with acceptance and understanding of this diagnosis.

REFERENCES

1. Barrett TJ, Silber JD, McGinley JP. Genital warts—a venereal disease. *JAMA* 1954;154:333.
2. Zazove P, Caruthers, BS, Reed, BD. Genital human papillomavirus infection. *Am Fam Physician* 1991;43:1279.
3. Cobb MW. Human papillomavirus infection. *J Am Acad Dermatol* 1990;22:547.
4. Craighill M. Human papillomavirus infection in children and adolescents. *Semin Pediatr Infect Dis* 1993;4:85.
5. Frasier LD. Human papillomavirus infections in children. *Pediatr Ann* 1994;23:354.

6. Bauer HM, Ting Y, Greer CE, et al. Genital human papillomavirus infection in female university students as determined by a PCR-based method. *JAMA* 1991;265:472.
7. Pyrhonen S, Penttinen K. Wart virus antibodies and the prognosis of wart disease. *Lancet* 1972;2:1330.
8. Barr BB, Benton EC, McLaren K, et al. Human papillomavirus infection and skin cancer in renal allograft recipients. *Lancet* 1989;1:124.
9. Halpert R, Fruchter RG, Sedlis A, et al. Human papillomavirus and lower genital neoplasia in renal transplant patients. *Obstet Gynecol* 1986;68:251.
10. Johnson JC, Burnett AF, Willett GD, et al. High frequency of latent and clinical human papillomavirus cervical infections in immunocompromised human immunodeficiency women. *Obstet Gynecol* 1992;79:321.
11. Vermund SH, Kelley KF, Klein RS, et al. High risk of human papillomavirus infection and cervical squamous intraepithelial lesions among women with symptomatic human immunodeficiency virus infection. *Am J Obstet Gynecol* 1991;165:392.
12. Zur Hausen H. Human papillomaviruses in the pathogenesis of anogenital cancer. *Virology* 1991;184:9.
13. Kadish AS, Burk RD, Kress Y, et al. Human papillomaviruses of different types in precancerous lesions of the uterine cervix. *Hum Pathol* 1986;17:384.
14. Byrne JC, Tsao MS, Fraser RS, et al. Human papillomavirus-11 DNA in a patient with chronic laryngotracheo-bronchial papillomatosis and metastatic squamous-cell carcinoma of the lung. *N Engl J Med* 1987;317:873.
15. Pfister H. Relationship of papillomaviruses to anogenital cancer. *Obstet Gynecol Clin North Am* 1987;14:349.
16. Hellberg D, Nilsson S, Haley NJ, et al. Smoking and cervical intraepithelial neoplasia: nicotine and cotinine in serum and cervical mucus in smokers and nonsmokers. *Am J Obstet Gynecol* 1988;158:910.
17. Slattery ML, Robison LM, Schuman KL, et al. Cigarette smoking and exposure to passive smoke are risk factors for cervical cancer. *JAMA* 1989;261:1593.
18. Sillman FH, Sedlis A. Anogenital papillomavirus infection and neoplasia in immunodeficient women. *Obstet Gynecol Clin North Am* 1987;14:437.
19. Witkin SS, Roth DM, Ledger WJ. Papillomavirus infection and an allergic response to *Candida* in women with recurrent vaginitis (letter to the editor). *JAMA* 1989;261:1584.
20. Bornstein J, Kaufman RH, Adam E, et al. Human papillomavirus associated with vaginal intraepithelial neoplasia in women exposed to diethylstilbestrol in utero. *Obstet Gynecol* 1987;70:75.
21. Reid R, ed. Human papillomavirus. *Obstet Gynecol Clin North Am* 1987;14:329.
22. Davis A, Emans SJ. Human papilloma virus infection in the pediatric and adolescent patient. *J Pediatr* 1989;115:1.
23. Bergeron C, Ferenczy A, Shah KV, et al. Multicentric human papillomavirus infections of the female genital tract: correlation of viral types with abnormal mitotic figures, colposcopic presentation, and location. *Obstet Gynecol* 1987;69:736.
24. Burmer GC, Parker JD, Bates J, et al. Comparative analysis of human papillomavirus detection by polymerase chain reaction and Virapap/Viratype kits. *Am J Clin Pathol* 1990;94:554.
25. Richart RM. HPV DNA testing comes of age. *Contemp Obstet Gynecol* 1995;79.
26. Cox JT, Lorincz AT, Schiffman MH, et al. Human papillomavirus testing by hybrid capture appears to be useful in triaging women with a cytologic diagnosis of atypical squamous cells of undetermined significance. *Am J Obstet Gynecol* 1995;172:946.
27. Sun XW, Ferenxzy A, Johnson D, et al. Evaluation of the hybrid capture human papillomavirus deoxyribonucleic acid detection test. *Am J Obstet Gynecol* 1995;173:1432.
28. Pakarian F, Kaye J, Cason J, et al. Cancer-associated human papillomaviruses: perinatal transmission and persistence. *Br J Obstet Gynaecol* 1994;101:514.
29. Jenison SA, Xu XP, Valentine JM. Evidence of prevalent genital-type human papillomavirus infections in adults and children. *J Infect Dis* 1990;62:60.
30. Sedlacek TV, Lindheim S, Eder C, et al. Mechanism for human papillomavirus transmission at birth. *Am J Obstet Gynecol* 1989;161:55.
31. Pao CC, Lin SS, Lin CY, et al. Identification of human papillomavirus DNA sequences in peripheral blood mononuclear cells. *Am J Clin Pathol* 1991;95:540.
32. Tseng CJ, Lin CY, Wang RL, et al. Possible transplacental transmission of human papillomaviruses. *Am J Obstet Gynecol* 1992;166:35.

33. Obalek S, Misiewicz J, Jablonska S, et al. Childhood condyloma acuminatum: association with genital and cutaneous human papillomaviruses. *Pediatr Dermatol* 1993;10:101.
34. Goerzen JL, Robertson DI, Inoue M, Trevenen, CL. Detection of HPV DNA in genital condyloma acuminata in female prepubertal children. *Adolesc Pediatr Gynecol* 1989;2:224.
35. Davis AJ, Emans SJ, Craighill MC, et al. HPV autoinoculation: a case report. *Adolesc Pediatr Gynecol* 1989;2:165.
36. Vallejos H, Del Mistro A, Kleinhaus S, et al. Characterization of human papilloma virus types in condyloma acuminata in children by in situ hybridization. *Lab Invest* 1987;56:611.
37. Hanson RM, Glasson M, McCrossin I, Rogers M. Anogenital warts in childhood. *Child Abuse Negl* 1989;13:225.
38. Craighill M, O'Connell, B, McLachlin C, et al. HPV PCR analysis of prepubertal lesions. Presented at the North American Society of Pediatric Gynecology annual meeting, April, 1993.
39. Ingram DL, Everett D, Lyna PR, et al. Epidemiology of adult sexually transmitted disease agents in children being evaluated for sexual abuse. *Pediatr Infect Dis J* 1992;11:945.
40. Gutman LT, St. Claire K, Herman-Giddens ME, et al. Evaluation of sexually abused and nonabused young girls for intravaginal human papillomavirus infection. *Am J Dis Child* 1992;146:694.
41. Gutman LT, St. Claire KK, Everett VD, et al. Cervical-vaginal and intra-anal human papillomavirus infection of young girls with external genital warts. *J Infect Dis* 1994;170:339.
42. Gutman LT. Sexual abuse and human papillomavirus infection (letter to the editor). *J Pedriatr* 1990;3:495.
43. Bennett RS, Powell KR. Human papillomaviruses: association between laryngeal papillomas and genital warts. *Pediatr Infect Dis J* 1987;6:229.
44. Kashima HK, Shah K. Recurrent respiratory papillomatosis: clinical overview and management principles. *Obstet Gynecol Clin North Am* 1987;14:581.
45. Centers for Disease Control. 1998 sexually transmitted disease guidelines. *MMWR* 1998;47:88.
46. Khan MA, Jenkins GR, Tolleson WH, et al. Retinoic acid inhibition of human papillomavirus type 16-mediated transformation of human keratinocytes. *Cancer Res* 1993;53:905.
47. Shimomaye S. Recent developments in the treatment of human papillomavirus. *Dermatology* 1994;160:365.
48. Boutselis JG. Intraepithelial carcinoma of the vulva. *Am J Obstet Gynecol* 1972;113:733.
49. Crowther ME. Is the nature of cervical carcinoma changing in young women? *Obstet Gynecol Surv* 1995;50:71.
50. Rosenfeld W, Vermund S, Wentz S, et al. High prevalence rate of human papillomavirus infection and association with abnormal Papanicolaou smears in sexually active adolescents. *Am J Dis Child* 1989;143:1443.
51. Fisher M, Rosenfeld WD, Burk RD. Cervicovaginal human papillomavirus infection in suburban adolescents and young adults. *J Pediatr* 1991;119:821.
52. Moscicki AB, Palefsky J, Gonzales J, et al. Human papillomavirus infection in sexually active adolescent females: prevalence and risk factors. *Pediatr Res* 1990;28:507.
53. Shew ML, Fortenberry JD, Miles P, et al. Interval between menarche and first sexual intercourse, related to risk of human papillomavirus infection. *J Pediatr* 1994;125:661.
54. Moscicki AB, Winkler B, Irwin CE, et al. Differences in biologic maturation, sexual behavior, and sexually transmitted disease between adolescents with and without cervical intraepithelial neoplasia. *J Pediatr* 1989;115:487.
55. Johnson TL, Joseph CLM, Caison-Sorey TJ, et al. Prevalence of HPV 16 and 18 DNA sequences in CIN III lesions of adults and adolescents. *Diagn Cytopathol* 1994;10:276.
56. Messing MJ, Gallup DG. Carcinoma of the vulva in young women. *Obstet Gynecol* 1995;86:51.
57. Bergeron C, Ferenczy A, Richart R. Underwear: contamination by human papillomaviruses. *Am J Obstet Gynecol* 1990;162:25.
58. Rosenfeld WD, Rose E, Vermund SH, et al. Follow-up evaluation of cervicovaginal human papillomavirus infection in adolescents. *J Pediatr* 1992;121:307.
59. Sheets EE, Crum CP. Current status and future clinical potential of human papillomavirus infection and intraepithelial neoplasia. *Curr Opin Obstet Gynecol* 1993;5:63.
60. Barrasso R, DeBrux J, Croissant O, et al. High prevalence of papillomavirus-associated penile intraepithelial neoplasia in sexual partners of women with cervical intraepithelial neoplasia. *N Engl J Med* 1987;317:916.
61. Sand PK, Bower LW, Blischke SO, et al. Evaluation of male consorts of women with genital human papillomavirus infection. *Obstet Gynecol* 1986;68:679.

62. Maymon R, Shulman A, Maymon B, et al. Penile condyloma: a gynecological epidemic disease: a review of the current approach and management aspects. *Obstet Gynecol Surv* 1994;49:790.
63. Rosenberg SK, Greenberg MD, Reid R. Sexually transmitted papillomaviral infections in men. *Obstet Gynecol Clin North Am* 1987;14:495.
64. Krebs HB, Helmskamp F. Treatment failure of genital condyloma acuminata in women: role of the male sexual partner. *Am J Obstet Gynecol* 1991;165:337.
65. Hillman RJ, Ryait BK, Botcherby M, Taylor-Robinson D. Changes in HPV infection in patients with anogenital warts and their partners. *Genitourin Med* 1993;69:450.
66. Feldman J, Chirgwin K, Dehovitz JA, et al. The association of smoking and risk of condyloma acuminatum in women. *Obstet Gynecol* 1997;89:346.
67. Beutner KR, Friedman-Kien AE, Artman NA, et al. Patient-applied podofilox for treatment of genital warts. *Lancet* 1989;1:831.
68. Ferenczy A. Laser treatment of patients with condyloma and squamous carcinoma precursors of the lower female genital tract. *CA Cancer J Clin* 1987;37:334.
69. Riva JM, Sedlacek TV, Cunnane MF, et al. Extended carbon dioxide laser vaporization in the treatment of subclinical papillomavirus infection of the lower genital tract. *Obstet Gynecol* 1989;73:25.
70. Ferenczy A, Mitao M, Nagai N, et al. Latent papillomavirus and recurring genital warts. *N Engl J Med* 1985;313:784.
71. Garden JM, O'Banion MK, Shelnitz LS, et al. Papillomavirus in the vapor of carbon dioxide laser-treated verrucae. *JAMA* 1988;259:1199.
72. Krebs HB. Treatment of vaginal condyloma acuminata by weekly topical application of 5-fluorouracil. *Obstet Gynecol* 1987;70:68.
73. Krebs HB. Prophylactic topical 5-fluorouracil following treatment of human papillomavirus-associated lesions of vulva and vagina. *Obstet Gynecol* 1986;68:837.
74. Trofatter KF. Interferon. *Obstet Gynecol Clin North Am* 1987;14:569.
75. Friedman-Kien AE, Eron LJ, Conant M, et al. Natural interferon alfa for treatment of condyloma acuminata. *JAMA* 1988;259:533.
76. Gall SA, Hughes CE, Mounts P, et al. Efficacy of human lymphoblastoid interferon in the therapy of resistant condyloma acuminatum. *Obstet Gynecol* 1986;67:643.
77. Cannistra S, Niloff JM. Cancer of the uterine cervix. *N Engl J Med* 1996;334:1030.
78. Kurman RJ, Shiffman MH, Lancaster WD, et al. Analysis of individual human papillomavirus types in cervical neoplasia: a possible role for type 18 in rapid progression. *Am J Obstet Gynecol* 1988;159:293.
79. Crum CP, Ikenberg H, Richart RM, et al. Human papillomavirus type 16 and early cervical neoplasia. *N Engl J Med* 1984;310:880.
80. Lancaster WD, Castellano C, Santos C, et al. Human papillomavirus deoxyribonucleic acid in cervical carcinoma from primary and metastatic sites. *Am J Obstet Gynecol* 1986;154:115.
81. Reeves WC, Brinton LA, Garcia M, et al. Human papillomavirus infection and cervical cancer in Latin America. *N Engl J Med* 1989;320:1437.
82. Lister UM, Ahinla O. Carcinoma of the vulva in childhood. *J Obstet Gynaecol Br Commonw* 1972;79:470.
83. Peters RK, Thomas D, Skultin G, et al. Invasive squamous cell carcinoma of the cervix after recent negative cytology test results—a distinct subgroup. *Am J Obstet Gynecol* 1988;158:926.
84. National Cancer Institute Workshop. The 1988 Bethesda system for reporting cervical/vaginal cytologic diagnoses. *JAMA* 1989;262:931.
85. Richart RM, Jones H, Nolle K, et al. Managing patients with low-grade pap smears. *Contemp Obstet Gynecol* 1993;38:82.
86. Isacson C, Kurman RJ. The Bethesda system: a new classification for managing pap smears. *Contemp Obstet Gynecol* 1995;40:67.
87. Delke IM, Veridiano NP, Russell SH, et al. Abnormal cervical cytology in adolescents. *J Pediatr* 1981;98:985.
88. Hein K, Schreiber K, Cohen MI, et al. Cervical cytology: the need for routine screening in the sexually active adolescent. *J Pediatr* 1977;91:123.
89. Koss LG. The Papanicolaou test for cervical cancer detection: a triumph and a tragedy. *JAMA* 1989;261:737.
90. Sadeghi SB, Hsieh EW, Gunn SW. Prevalence of cervical intraepithelial neoplasia in sexually active adolescents. *Am J Obstet Gynecol* 1981;148:726.
91. Schydlower M, Greenberg J, Patterson PH. Adolescent with abnormal cervical cytology. *Clin Pediatr* 1981;20:723.

92. McQuiston C. The relationship of risk factors for cervical cancer and in HPV college women. *Nurse Pract* 1989;14:18.
93. Russo JF, Jones DDE. Abnormal cervical cytology in sexually active adolescents. *J Adolesc Health Care* 1984;5:269.
94. Lavin C, Goodman E, Perlman S, Emans SJ. Follow-up of abnormal Pap smears in a hospital-based adolescent clinic *J Pediatr Adolesc Gynecol* (in press).
95. Jones DE, Creasman WT, Dombroske RA, et al. The evaluation of the atypical smear. *Am J Obstet Gynecol* 1987;157:544.
96. Wright TC, Sun XW, Koulos J. Comparison of management algorithms for the evaluation of women with low-grade cytologic abnormalities. *Obstet Gynecol* 1995;85:202.
97. Cox JT, Schiffman MH, Winzelberg AJ, Patterson JM. An evaluation of human papillomavirus testing as part of referral to colposcopy clinics. *Obstet Gynecol* 1992;80:389.
98. Stafl A. Cervicography: a new method for cervical cancer detection. *Am J Obstet Gynecol* 1981;139:815.
99. Tawa K, Forsythe A, Cove JK, et al. A comparison of the Papanicolaou smear and the cervigram: sensitivity, specificity, and cost analysis. *Obstet Gynecol* 1988;71:229.
100. Cristoforoni PM, Gerbaldo D, Perino A, et al. Computerized colposcopy: results of a pilot study and analysis of its clinical relevance. *Obstet Gynecol* 1995;85:1011.
101. Massad LS, Lonky NM, Mutch DG, et al. Use of speculoscopy in the evaluation of women with atypical Papanicolaou smears. *J Reprod Med* 1993;38:163.
102. Mann W, Lonky N, Massad S, et al. Papanicolaou smear screening augmented by a magnified chemiluminescent exam. *Int J Gynaecol Obstet* 1993;43:289.
103. Koss LG, Schreiber K, Elgert P, et al. Evaluation of the PAPNET cytologic screening system for quality control of cervical smears. *Am J Clin Pathol* 1994;101:220.
104. Halford JA, Wright RG, Sitchman EJ. Quality assurance in cervical cytology screening. Comparison of rapid rescreening and the PAPNET testing system. *Acta Cytol* 1997;41:79.
105. Noumoff JS. Atypia in cervical cytology as a risk factor for intraepithelial neoplasia. *Am J Obstet Gynecol* 1987;156:628.
106. Lorincz AT, Temple GF, Kuram RJ, et al. Oncogenic association of specific human papillomavirus types with cervical neoplasia. *J Natl Cancer Inst* 1987;79:671.
107. Reid R, Greenberg M, Jenson AB, et al. Sexually transmitted papillomaviral infections. I. The anatomic distribution and pathologic grade of neoplastic lesions associated with different viral types. *Am J Obstet Gynecol* 1987;156:212.
108. Carter JJ, Koutsky LA, Wipf GO, et al. The natural history of human papillomavirus type 16 capsid antibodies among a cohort of university women. *J Infect Dis* 1996;174:927.
109. Nash JD, Burke TW, Hoskins WJ. Biologic course of cervical human papillomavirus infection. *Obstet Gynecol* 1987;69:160.
110. Nasiell K, Roger V, Nasiell M. Behavior of mild cervical dysplasia during long-term follow-up. *Obstet Gynecol* 1986;67:665.
111. Reid R. Physical and surgical principles governing expertise with the carbon dioxide laser. *Obstet Gynecol Clin North Am* 1987;14:515.
112. Spitzer M, Krumholz BA, Seltzer VL. The multicentric nature of disease related to human papillomavirus infection of the female lower genital tract. *Obstet Gynecol* 1989;73:303.
113. Sutton GP, Stehman FB, Ehrlich CE, et al. Human papillomavirus deoxyribonucleic acid in lesions of the female genital tract: evidence for type 6/11 in squamous carcinoma of the vulva. *Obstet Gynecol* 1987;70:564.
114. Reid R. Human papillomaviral infection: the key to rational triage of cervical neoplasia. *Obstet Gynecol Clin North Am* 1987;14:407.
115. Wright TC, Richart RM, Loop excision of the uterine cervix. *Curr Opin Obstet Gynecol* 1995;7:30–34.
116. *Cervical cytology:* evaluation and management of abnormalities. ACOG Technical Bulletin 183. American College of Obstetrics and Gynecology, 1993:1.
117. Falcone T, Ferenczy A. Cervical intraepithelial neoplasia and condyloma: an analysis of diagnostic accuracy of posttreatment follow-up methods. *Am J Obstet Gynecol* 1986;154:260.
118. *Human immunodeficiency virus infection.* ACOG Technical Bulletin 169. American College of Obstetrics and Gynecology, 1992:1.
119. Minkoff H, Dehovitz JA. HIV infection in women. *AIDS Clin Care* 1991;3:33.
120. Stratton P, Gupta P, Kalish L, et al. Immune status, STDs and cervical dysplasia on Pap smear in HIV positive pregnant and non-pregnant women in the women and infants transmission study (WITS). 3rd Con Retro and Opportun Infect 1996;1:133.

14

Human Immunodeficiency Virus in Young Women

As of December 30, 1996, 581,102 cases of acquired immunodeficiency syndrome (AIDS) have been reported in the United States, and 362,004 people have died (1). In most of the world outside North America and Europe, the human immunodeficiency virus (HIV) is spread primarily as a sexually transmitted disease within heterosexual relationships, with essentially a 1:1 ratio between male and female cases (2). The pandemic has progressed to the point that any clinician caring for young women will need to consider HIV as part of the differential diagnosis for many signs and symptoms, to offer HIV counseling and testing and risk reduction advice to young women, and to be prepared to inform and provide care for young women who test positive for HIV infection. The clinician may also be caring for girls and adolescents born with HIV and presenting with reproductive health concerns, and/or managing the routine or specialized health care of adolescents and young adults with HIV infection acquired during or after puberty. This chapter updates current epidemiologic information describing both risk factors for and prevalence of AIDS and HIV infection in young women. It also describes the gynecologic symptoms and signs associated with HIV infection and discusses the clinician's role in case finding, prevention, diagnosis, and management, as well as reviewing the impact of HIV on reproductive health.

EPIDEMIOLOGY

Description of the HIV epidemic in adolescents in the United States relies on information from several sources: AIDS case reports, seroprevalence studies, surveys of risk behavior and of indicator diseases, mortality data, and voluntary testing data. True population-based prevalence and incidence data are not currently available, although back calculation, serosurveillance, and household surveys have been used to estimate the number of people living with HIV infection in the United States (3).

AIDS Case Reports

Table 1 describes persons reported with AIDS during the periods 1981 to 1987, 1988 to 1992, and 1993 to October, 1995 (4). Important trends are seen in the increase in the proportions of persons with AIDS who are female, persons of color, injection drug users, and alive at the time of the report. There are also decreases in the proportions of cases in whites, men who have sex with men, and blood or blood-product recipients. The largest proportionate increases of reported cases among adolescents and young adults (ages 13 to 29 years) occurred in the South. In the South and Midwest, higher proportions of cases occurred in small cities (<500,000 population) and rural areas. The proportion of adolescent and young adult cases resulting from heterosexual transmission also differed by region (South, 32%; Midwest, 22%; West, 18%; Northeast, 7%) (4). Of the more than 30,000 people <25 years of age diagnosed with AIDS in the United States, 31% have been female (49% of <13-year-olds, 37% of 13–19-year-olds, and 25% of 20–24-year-olds) (3) (Table 2). Since the time from infection with HIV to the development of AIDS-defining conditions or criteria averages 5–10 years, most 20–24-year-olds with AIDS acquired their infection during adolescence. The epidemiology of HIV infection in newly diagnosed youth in the United States resembles the distribution of much of the developing world. Using Centers for Disease Control and Prevention (CDC) exposure categories, most girls (90%) <13 years of age were infected through their mothers, and most young women (53%) aged 13 to 24 years were infected through heterosexual transmission (see Table 2). The unknown/other risk category also includes young women whose only risk was sexual contact with a partner of unknown risk (5) and young women whose risk factor is still undetermined. A small number (2%) of 13 to 19-year-old women with AIDS are youths with perinatal HIV who have survived into adolescence. To date, 79% of girls and young women with AIDS have been black or Hispanic. The 1993 change in case definition caused a greater proportional increase in AIDS cases in women than in men (128% for women, 113% for men), and the yearly case rate has been increasing at 9.8% for women and 2.5% for men (6). Since 1992, AIDS has become the fourth leading cause of death for 25- to 44-year-old women and the sixth for 15- to 24-year-old women. It is the leading cause of death for black women, the third leading cause among Hispanic women, and the leading cause of death for all 25- to 44-year-old women in at least nine cities in the United States (7,8).

HIV Seroprevalence

Table 3 summarizes several studies of HIV-antibody prevalence in selected populations, using unlinked, blinded samples of blood obtained for other reasons or results of routine linked testing in special populations such as the military and Job Corps (9–17). Among Job Corps entrants aged 16 to 21 years, seropreva-

TABLE 1. *Number and percentage of persons with AIDS by selected characteristics and period of report—United States, 1981–October 1995*[a]

Characteristic	1981–1987 No. (%)	1988–1992 No. (%)	1993–October 1995 No. (%)	Cumulative No. (%)
Sex				
Male	46,317 (92.0)	177,807 (87.5)	204,356 (82.5)	423,480 (85.5)
Female	4,035 (8.0)	25,410 (12.5)	43,383 (17.5)	72,828 (14.5)
Age group (yr)				
0–4	653 (1.3)	2,766 (1.4)	2,013 (0.3)	5,432 (1.1)
5–12	100 (0.2)	669 (0.3)	616 (0.2)	1,385 (0.3)
13–19	199 (0.4)	758 (0.4)	1,343 (0.5)	2,300 (0.5)
20–29	10,531 (20.9)	38,662 (19.0)	41,861 (16.9)	91,054 (18.2)
30–39	23,269 (46.2)	92,493 (45.5)	111,992 (45.3)	227,754 (45.4)
40–49	10,491 (20.8)	47,088 (23.1)	64,990 (26.2)	122,569 (24.4)
50–59	3,690 (7.3)	14,537 (7.2)	18,413 (7.5)	36,640 (7.3)
≥60	1,419 (2.3)	6,244 (3.1)	6,513 (2.6)	14,176 (2.8)
Race/ethnicity				
White, non-Hispanic	30,104 (59.8)	102,551 (50.5)	105,516 (42.6)	238,171 (47.5)
Black, non-Hispanic	12,794 (25.4)	63,319 (31.2)	94,158 (38.0)	170,271 (34.0)
Hispanic[b]	7,039 (14.0)	35,213 (17.3)	45,135 (18.2)	87,33 (17.4)
Asian, Pacific Islands	309 (0.5)	1,339 (0.7)	1,800 (0.7)	3,457 (0.7)
American Indian, Alaskan Native	67 (0.1)	438 (0.6)	183 (0.3)	1,283 (0.3)
HIV-exposure category				
Men who have sex with men	32,246 (64.0)	110,934 (54.6)	111,257 (44.9)	254,437 (50.8)
Injecting drug use	8,539 (17.2)	49,093 (24.2)	67,708 (27.3)	125,440 (25.0)
Men who have sex with men and inject drugs	4,193 (8.3)	14,257 (7.0)	13,984 (5.6)	32,429 (6.5)
Hemophilia	505 (1.0)	1,744 (0.9)	2,009 (0.8)	4,258 (0.8)
Heterosexual contact	1,248 (2.5)	12,335 (6.1)	24,958 (10.1)	38,541 (7.7)
Transfusion recipients	1,285 (2.6)	3,894 (1.9)	2,521 (1.0)	7,700 (1.6)
Perinatal transmission	608 (1.2)	3,084 (1.5)	2,439 (1.0)	6,124 (1.2)
No risk reported	1,628 (3.2)	7,881 (3.9)	22,872 (9.2)	32,331 (6.4)
Region[c]				
Northeast	19,544 (38.8)	62,282 (30.6)	74,769 (30.2)	156,595 (31.2)
Midwest	3,770 (7.5)	20,352 (10.0)	24,914 (10.1)	49,036 (9.8)
South	12,960 (25.7)	65,926 (32.4)	86,462 (34.9)	165,348 (33.0)
West	13,550 (26.9)	46,675 (23.0)	53,729 (21.7)	113,954 (22.7)
U.S. territories	516 (1.0)	7,889 (3.9)	7,566 (3.1)	15,971 (3.2)
Vital status				
Living	2,779 (5.5)	32,144 (15.8)	155,006 (62.6)	189,929 (37.9)
Deceased	47,573 (94.5)	171,073 (84.2)	92,735 (37.4)	311,381 (62.1)
Total[d]	50,352 (100.0)	203,217 (100.0)	247,741 (100.0)	501,310 (100.0)

[a]AIDS, acquired immunodeficiency syndrome; HIV, human immunodeficiency virus.

[b]Persons of Hispanic origin may be of any race.

[c]Northeast: Connecticut, Maine, Massachusetts, New Hampshire, New Jersey, New York, Pennsylvania, Rhode Island, and Vermont; Midwest: Illinois, Indiana, Iowa, Kansas, Michigan, Minnesota, Missouri, Nebraska, North Dakota, Ohio, South Dakota, and Wisconsin; South: Alabama, Arkansas, Delaware, District of Columbia, Florida, Georgia, Kentucky, Louisiana, Maryland, Mississippi, North Carolina, Oklahoma, South Carolina, Tennessee, Texas, Virginia, and West Virginia; West: Alaska, Arizona, California, Colorado, Hawaii, Idaho, Montana, Nevada, New Mexico, Oregon, Utah, Washington, and Wyoming.

[d]Includes persons for whom sex, race ethnicity, or region are missing.

(Data from CDC. First 500,000 AIDS cases–United States, 1995. *MMWR* 1995;44:849.)

TABLE 2. *AIDS cases in girls and young women, United States, through December, 1996*[a]

	Age (yr)		
	<13	13–19	20–24
Proportion of cases female			
Females (n)	3708	1010	5539
Female (%)	49	37	26
Female race/ethnicity category (%)			
White/non-Hispanic	16	18	23
Black/non-Hispanic	60	65	55
Hispanic	23	16	21
Asian/Pacific Islander	0.5	1	0.5
American Indian/Alaskan Native	0.4	0.1	0.4
Other/unknown	0.3	0.1	3
HIV exposure category (%) (n = 7629)[b]			
Perinatal	90	2	
Injection drug use		15	30
Hemophilia	3	1	0.2
Blood transfusion	5	7	2
Heterosexual		54	53
Other/unknown[c]	2	22	15

[a]AIDS, acquired immunodeficiency syndrome; HIV, human immunodeficiency virus.
[b]Includes boys and girls in HIV exposure category <13 years.
[c]Risk not reported or identified. Includes women who had heterosexual contacts not known to be infected or at risk.
[Adapted from Centers for Disease Control and Prevention (1).]

TABLE 3. *Selected HIV seroprevalence in adolescent and young adult populations*[a]

Group (no. of sites)	Dates	Age and sex	Population	% HIV Positive
Military recruits[b]	10/85–3/89	<20	1,141,164	0.03
		<18 F	112,604	0.03
		<18 M	763,872	0.02
Active duty military[b]	1/87–4/88	17–19	322,506	0.01
		20–24	568,920	0.12
Job corps entrants[b]	1988	16–21 M		0.36
		16–21 F		0.21
	1992	16–21 M		0.22
		16–21 F		0.42
Adolescent clinics (22 F, 15 M)[c]	1990–92	<20 F	8,491	0.2 (0–2.5)
		<20 M	3,205	0.0 (0–1.2)
Correctional facilities (31 M, 8 F)[c]	1990–92	<20 F	1,601	1.2 (0–2.1)
		<20 M	14,571	0.2 (0–6.3)
Homeless youth centers (5)[c]	1990–92	<20 F	2,178	0.9 (0–1.7)
		<20 M	1,658	3.6 (0–6.6)
STD clinics (Baltimore)[b]	2/87–4/87	15–19 F	434	2.5
		15–19 M	509	2
STD clinics (70)[c]	1990–92	<20 F	22,230	0.5 (0–5.0)
		<20 M	25,447	0.5 (0–3.6)
Mothers of newborns, New York[b]	11/87–11/88	<20 upstate NY	12,344	0.13
		<20 NYC	12,871	0.72

[a]HIV, human immunodeficiency virus; STD, sexually transmitted disease.
[b]Source: OTA: Adolescent Health-Vol. II (14), with permission.
[c]Source: Sweeney et al. (17), with permission. (Figures in parentheses represent the number of sites serving youth of each gender.)

lence in young women increased between 1988 and 1992, and rates were highest in urban northeast and rural southern women and nonwhite women (15,18). Using cord blood of newborn infants screened for HIV in 1992, 1.7 of 1000 women were seropositive at delivery nationally, while in New York City 7.2 of 1000 women <20 years of age and 13 of 1000 women aged 20 to 29 were seropositive in 1987 to 1989 (12,16). Studies of homeless youth have shown seroprevalence rates ranging from 0.41% to 7.4% (14,17,19,20). In Baltimore sexually transmitted disease (STD) clinics, HIV seroprevalence studies from 1979 to 1989 showed an increase in seroprevalence in both men and women, with a dramatic drop in the male/female ratio to 1:1. The greatest age-specific increases in seroprevalence in STD clinic users were among teenagers (from 0.18% in 1979 to 1983 to 2.1% in 1987 to 1989) (21). Few studies have documented the rate of HIV infection in healthy adolescents, but one study in Washington, DC, showed the highest seroprevalence rate (0.47%) in females attending an adolescent clinic (22). Our own blinded seroprevalence study in 1993 showed that 0.4% of 1028 healthy adolescent clinic patients receiving a routine blood test were seropositive (0.73% when only sexually active teenagers were included in the denominator) (23). Overall, recent CDC seroprevalence studies showed higher seroprevalence rates and ranges among girls than among boys <20 years old in adolescent clinics, correctional facilities, and STD clinics between 1990 and 1992, with heterosexual sex with a partner of unknown risk as the only risk factor for most young women (17,21,22,24). HIV seroprevalence increases proportionately with age during adolescence (from 1.3% of 15-year-old to 8.6% of 20-year-old homeless youths in New York City, for example), but few have looked at seroincidence or seroconversion (18,20). In a study of 5164 patients in Miami STD clinics with at least two HIV test results documented between December 1987 and December 1990, 4% seroconverted. The highest seroconversion rates were among patients having primary or secondary syphilis, as well as among black teenagers and black women (25).

Description of Girls and Young Women with HIV

In addition to AIDS case reports, mortality rates, and seroprevalence data, a few descriptions of young women with HIV have now been published (26–28). A New York study comparing hospitalized and outpatient HIV-positive (n = 72) and HIV-negative (n = 1142) youths aged 13 to 21 years showed that the 26 seropositive females were more likely than seronegative females to have the following risk factors: sexual abuse (33% vs. 28%), survival sex (27% vs. 2%), sex while under influence (69% vs. 27%), STD history (73% vs. 38%), cigarette use (73% vs. 30%), injection drug use (IDU) (8% vs. 0%), incarceration (42% vs. 7%), psychiatric care (27% vs. 12%), out of school (46% vs. 22%), and out of home (77% vs. 16%) (27). IDU was rare, but crack cocaine use was common in HIV-infected youths in New York City. Most young women had heterosexual contact as their only transmission risk but were rarely aware of their partner's risk at the time of contact (28).

A final picture of girls and young women with HIV can be obtained from examining data from those states that mandate reporting of HIV infection. By December 30, 1996, 82,284 cases had been reported. For the 16,971 0- to 24-year-olds with reported HIV infection, the male/female ratio is 1.8:1 (1.1:1 for 0- to 12-year-olds, 1:1 for 13- to 19-year-olds, and 2.4:1 for 20- to 24-year-olds). For 13- to 24-year-old females with reported HIV infection, 12% had IDU as their primary mode of transmission, 43% were heterosexual contacts of a known infected or high-risk partner, and 44% were other (most presumably heterosexual contacts of partners whose risk or HIV status was unknown) (1). Back calculation using age-specific AIDS incidence suggests that the age of onset for HIV infection is declining and that 25% of new infections are in persons <22 years of age (29). Recent projections of HIV prevalence suggest that the female proportion of United States residents living with HIV infection increased steadily between 1984 and 1992 and that male/female ratios are lower in black and Hispanic populations (3).

CLINICAL CHARACTERISTICS

To date, little information is available on the clinical manifestations and natural history of AIDS and HIV infection in women, and even less information on adolescents and long-term pediatric survivors.

Susceptibility

Young and adolescent girls have increased susceptibility to sexually transmitted infections due in part to cervical ectopy, to low estrogen effect on the prepubertal vagina, and perhaps to normal fluctuations in cell-mediated immunity during puberty. Although studies of HIV serotypes prevalent in Asia and sub-Saharan Africa report equivalent male/female and female/male transmission, in Europe and the United States studies of couples discordant for HIV status have repeatedly shown that women are two to ten times more susceptible to seroconversion due to vaginal sex than men, though consistent use of condoms dramatically lowers that risk (5,19,29–31). The likelihood of a woman's seroconverting in a discordant couple or in an area of high seroprevalence is increased by factors such as sexual trauma, current or prior genital ulcer disease (syphilis, chancroid, herpes), atrophic vaginitis, chlamydial infection, trichomonal infection, oral contraceptive use, vaginal sex during menses, and receptive anal sex (31–34). Host factors of the transmitting partner included viral load, severity of HIV disease, presence of genital ulcer disease, and in some studies lack of circumcision. Women with multiple partners or with a history of prostitution or survival sex were more likely to be infected, but women who were married or had had lifetime sexual experience with only one partner were not protected from infection.

Clinical Manifestations of HIV Infection and AIDS

Clinical manifestations discussed here include those that are AIDS defining, specific to girls and women, or likely to be seen as presenting conditions. The list of AIDS-defining diagnoses for adults and adolescents has been expanded twice, in 1987 and 1993 (6). The 1993 change included one gender-specific diagnosis, invasive cervical cancer, which added 489 female cases by December 1996. Women were more likely to be reported retroactively after the 1993 change for immunosuppression (T-lymphocyte CD4 count <200 cells/mm^3, or <14%) as an AIDS-defining condition. *Pneumocystis carinii* pneumonia (PCP) has been the most common AIDS-defining condition in both men and women (52% and 53% of 1988 to 1991 cases). Candidal esophagitis, chronic herpes simplex infection, and wasting syndrome have been more common among women than men, and Kaposi's sarcoma much less common.

Several common gynecologic conditions are more aggressive, severe, persistent, or likely to recur in women with HIV infection. Some young women present with these symptoms early in the disease, often with the initial drop in immune function (measured by CD4 counts) that occurs during seroconversion but also years later as cell-mediated immunity is gradually lost. For both girls and young women, vulvovaginal candidiasis that is recurrent or resistant to treatment is extremely common; we have also found bacterial vaginosis and trichomoniasis more likely to be recurrent or persistent. Cervical dysplasia is more common in young women with HIV infection, perhaps because of increased likelihood of exposure to sexually transmitted human papillomavirus (HPV) infection and decreased ability to respond to the HPV infection (see Chapter 13). Women with cervical cancer and severe dysplasia have higher HIV seroprevalence, and several studies have concluded that there is an increased risk and rate of progression in women with HIV that is related to loss of immune function and viral interaction (35–37). In a review analyzing 21 controlled studies on this association, Mandelblatt and colleagues (38) reported a summary odds ratio that HIV-infected women were 4.9 (95% confidence interval [CI]: 3, 8.2) times more likely to have cervical neoplasia than uninfected women. Vulvovaginal and anal condyloma acuminata are also more common in HIV-infected girls and women and more difficult to treat. Anal neoplasia is reported more often in those who have had anal sex, and we have also seen vulvar intraepithelial neoplasia in HIV-infected adolescents. Pelvic inflammatory disease is reported more frequently in HIV-infected women and is also more likely to recur or cause chronic symptoms or complications such as tubo-ovarian abscess (see Chapter 12). Genital ulcer diseases such as syphilis, chancroid, and herpes simplex are more common and extensive in women with HIV infection and may have atypical presentations. Vulvar molluscum contagiosum and herpes zoster may also occur. The features of these diseases may be exacerbated by declining immune function (39).

Menstrual disorders are common in girls and young women with HIV. Girls infected since birth or infancy may be referred for delayed puberty or menarche or growth failure, but many do progress normally through puberty. Dysfunctional uterine bleeding may occur, especially in women with thrombocytopenia as a result of HIV disease or therapy, and severe bleeding may need hormonal therapy (see Chapter 6). Young women with wasting syndrome may present with oligomenorrhea or menorrhagia.

Other clinical manifestations of early HIV infection include those associated with acute seroconversion and those that occur as immune function begins to deteriorate. Seroconversion syndromes may range from a nonspecific febrile flu-like viral syndrome with lymphadenopathy and malaise to a striking systemic illness with fever, diarrhea, desquamating skin rash, lymphadenopathy, stomatitis, *Candida* vaginitis, or thrush. Standard HIV-antibody tests are negative during and for several weeks after an acute retroviral illness, though viral cultures and HIV-antigen tests such as qualitative polymerase chain reaction (PCR) may be positive. Symptoms and recurring illnesses seen months to years later, but usually when CD4 lymphocyte counts fall to <500 cells/mm^3, may include lymphadenopathy, increased acne and other dermatitis or skin infection (seborrhea, zoster, molluscum, warts), parotitis, malaise, persistent diarrhea, cholelithiasis, weight loss (or failure to thrive in children), and recurrent bacterial infections such as sinusitis, pneumonia, and pyelonephritis. Many young women will have no unusual symptoms or illness during the first few years of their infection or may have constitutional signs and laboratory analyses (e.g., a high erythrocyte sedimentation rate) suggesting collagen vascular disease or other chronic illness. The complete blood cell count and differential usually reflect a viral process.

IDENTIFYING HIV BY COUNSELING AND TESTING

As the prevalence of HIV grows and available therapies improve, it has become clear that counseling and testing only people who are symptomatic or members of previously defined risk groups is inadequate for both prevention and access to care and support, especially for adolescent and young adult females. Specific HIV prevention counseling and offering of testing are essential components of reproductive health care. However, HIV testing should not be done without informed consent and assessment of sexual behavior, substance use and abuse, and psychosocial issues, as well as attention to the skills needed for risk reduction and personal protection. Guidelines and recommendations have been developed to address these issues in adolescents (40–43).

Indications for Testing

In July 1995, the CDC issued new guidelines recommending routine HIV counseling and voluntary testing for all pregnant women (44). In addition, counseling and testing should be available to any young woman who requests them, and they are recommended for all young women with risk behaviors (including

TABLE 4. *Indications for recommending or offering HIV counseling and testing*[a]

Medical or gynecologic conditions consistent with HIV-related illness or immune dysfunction
History of injection drug use (IDU) or IDU in sexual partner
Men who have had sex with other men
History of other substance abuse associated with unprotected sex (especially crack or cocaine)
History of survival sex or prostitution
Partner known or suspected to be HIV infected or at high risk
History of exposure to blood products between 1978 and 1985 or in a country with relatively unsafe blood supply
Victim of rape or sexual abuse (baseline and 3–9 months later)
Sexually transmitted disease diagnosis or history (especially genital ulcer disease)
Pelvic inflammatory disease diagnosis or history
Cervical dysplasia
Pregnant or seeking pregnancy (male and female)
History of unprotected sex with multiple partners, strangers, older men, or any partner in or from an area where HIV is very prevalent
Child born to an HIV-infected mother
Prior to mandatory testing to enter military or job corps
Occupational exposure
Confirmation of results of home testing or anonymous testing
Patient desires testing

[a]HIV, human immunodeficiency virus.

unprotected vaginal or anal sex), indicator conditions, life circumstances suggestive of increased risk for HIV, or increased desire to modify behavior and/or seek care (Table 4). Young women are more likely to seek HIV testing if encouraged by their clinician (45). When new sexually transmitted infections or relationships prompt testing, it is important to assess the timing of potential risk exposure and to recommend avoidance of risk behavior, as well as repeat testing 3 to 8 months after the last exposure if an initial test is negative. The care provider discussing HIV infection with clients must be aware of applicable state laws regarding HIV testing, consent, confidentiality, release of information, and reporting, as well as available sources of anonymous and/or free testing. (In 25 states, all HIV infections are reportable, and in 4 only pediatric infections are reportable, while AIDS diagnosis is reportable in all states and United States territories.) Some states have specific laws or policies allowing adolescents to access testing without parental consent, while in others the right to testing is assumed to be part of a youth's right to confidential STD diagnosis and treatment. Testing of children and preadolescents usually requires parental or guardian consent (with assent of preadolescents usually recommended also), and most states have policies for decision making for children in state custody.

Pre- and Posttest Counseling

The counseling accompanying HIV testing should be done by a compassionate and nonjudgmental care provider who allows time for questions and feedback. The counseling should be tailored to the cognitive skills, knowledge, and emotional status of the adolescent. Young adolescents testing without parental support or involvement should be asked to involve another trusted adult or support person in the process, if possible. Pretest counseling may require more than one visit for some adolescents, especially those whose life circumstances are unstable (Table 5). Youths with cognitive delay, learning disabilities, depression, history of psychiatric hospitalizations, and active substance abuse require special care, and permission to discuss testing with ongoing therapists or counselors may be helpful. Safety plans may need to be developed for young women in domestic violence situations prior to testing. In addition to seeing some patients more than once for pretest counseling, we also often schedule one or more visits during the time spent waiting for a test result. At these visits, we assess the emotional impact of the testing decision, offer support, answer questions, and review the plan. Results should never be given until the result of the confirmatory test (usually a Western blot) is known if the enzyme-linked immunosorbent assay for antibody is positive; therefore, it is advisable to schedule the results visit far enough in advance to ensure that both screening and confirmatory results will be ready. Posttest counseling is reviewed in Table 6. Although testing positive often precipitates an emotional crisis, even negative HIV-test results may have a serious impact and require counseling time. Information and support may need to be provided over several visits. Many HIV-positive youths go through a period of denial in which they are unable or unwilling to seek care.

TABLE 5. *Components of pretest HIV counseling for youths (1–3 visits)*[a]

Education about AIDS
Education about HIV infection (course, lack of cure, availability of treatment, asymptomatic infection, routes of transmission, window period)
Assessment of current and past sexual and substance-using behavior'
Assessment of psychosocial history and supports
Screen for domestic violence
Risks and benefits of testing
Previous HIV testing dates and results, including home testing
Meaning of positive, negative, and indeterminate test results
Availability of confidential or anonymous testing
Applicable protection of HIV-related information in record
Reporting requirements
Review of safe sex and other risk-reduction practices
Development of a personal plan for risk reduction and for protecting others
Discuss plans for disclosure and support during the testing process
Discuss and assess impact of a positive test
Discuss implications of a positive test for pregnant women, strategies to reduce perinatal transmission
Describe care available
Assess and discuss need for testing of any living children if the mother is positive
Obtain informed, noncoerced consent
Draw blood
Discuss need for retesting if recent possible exposure or unsafe behavior in future
Schedule followup visit(s) for more pretest counseling and support, if indicated
Schedule results visit (far enough in advance to allow confirmation of a positive test)

[a]HIV, human immunodeficiency virus; AIDS, acquired immunodeficiency syndrome.

TABLE 6. *Components of posttest HIV counseling (always done in person, not by phone or letter)*[a]

Negative result
Explain result is ready
Give result, allow person to express feelings
Meaning of a negative result, review window period
Review personal protection plan and plans for notifying support person or partner
Reassess risk, including risky behavior since the test was done (if any)
Plan and schedule for retesting after window interval, if indicated
Discuss documentation of test result and release of test information
Stress a negative test does not confer immunity or protection
Positive result
Review psychosocial needs with care team prior to visit, have crisis intervention plan in place
When patient arrives, explain result is ready
Give result, allow person to express feelings, give comfort and listen
Reassess emotional state and need for support, offer to involve family or support person, if patient chooses
Reassure that treatment, care, support are available, that HIV infection is a chronic disease
Discuss importance of followup and education, and schedule followup appointment as soon as possible, assuming patient will retain little of what you discuss today
Stress hope, optimism, availability of support (hotlines, support groups)
Review how to avoid transmission, reinfection
Review self-care plan to monitor immune function and stay healthy (lifestyle, nutrition, substance use)
If pregnant, rediscuss options, including treatment options to reduce transmission, impact of HIV on prenatal care
Reassess reproductive health care plans (contraception, plans for children, etc.)
Begin or schedule baseline assessment
Indeterminate result
Give result, allow person to react
Review meaning of an indeterminate result (may be caused by other conditions, seroconversion)
Stress need to continue risk-reduction plan
Schedule followup test in 3–6 months
Evaluate clinically for evidence of recent infection, other conditions
If pregnant, repeat test immediately, consider viral culture or polymerase chain reaction test, consult with HIV infectious disease expert

[a]HIV, human immunodeficiency virus.

Newly licensed home testing kits for HIV may result in broader knowledge of serostatus but also in confusion for some youths. Confirmatory tests will be indicated for young women utilizing this anonymous method. We do not recommend this method for young or immature adolescents because of the great advantage of an individual client-centered approach to both testing and education of future risk.

A new oral mucosal transudate (OMT) antibody testing system was recently licensed, not for home testing but for use by a clinician or trained HIV counselor. The OMT samples are used for both an enzyme immunoassay screening test and a confirmatory Western blot test on the same sample. OMT testing is accurate, has sensitivity (99.9%) and specificity (>99.9%) comparable to serum testing,

and may be a useful technique for youths with needle phobia or in nonclinical settings offering testing (46).

Reproductive Health Issues, Pregnancy, Parenting

The new CDC guidelines recommending testing of all pregnant women for HIV infection were developed in response to the 1994 results of Protocol 076 of the AIDS Clinical Trials Group (44,47). In this trial, a regimen of treatment of asymptomatic pregnant women with zidovudine beginning in the second trimester, as well as intrapartum intravenous administration and 6-week treatment of the newborn child with oral drug, resulted in a highly significant drop in transmission rates to the infants (from 25.5% to 8.3%) of the treated mothers (47,48). The fact that breast-feeding increases the risk of transmission to the infant and therefore is *not* recommended for HIV-positive mothers (or those uncertain of their or their partners' HIV status) also supports prenatal testing. Obstetric care can also be modified to reduce maternal–fetal transmission risk and risk of obstetric complications if HIV status is known. The current recommendations for diagnosis and care of infants born to HIV-infected mothers include the use of PCR and other antigen testing and viral culture beginning at birth (which results in identification of the vast majority of infected infants by 6 months of age). All infants born to HIV-infected women should receive prophylaxis against PCP from the age of 1 month until proved HIV negative (or until age 1 year if infected), regardless of their immune function. HIV education and pre- and posttest counseling of young women who are pregnant or seeking pregnancy (or not using effective contraception) and their partners should incorporate this information. A negative HIV test early in pregnancy does not entirely eliminate the possibility of recent or future antenatal infection, so repeat testing and/or continued condom use is recommended if the partner's serostatus is positive or unknown, and is also advisable if the partner's serostatus is unknown or he is at increased risk.

Issues of HIV and sexual assault are discussed in Chapter 20.

HIV CARE AND SUPPORT

Caregivers providing medical and reproductive health care to young women and girls with HIV infection should be familiar with current developments in HIV care or have the consultative support of providers with HIV primary care and infectious disease experience. Providers of gynecologic, family planning, and prenatal care services may be seeing patients whose primary HIV care provider is elsewhere, necessitating close communication and care coordination. Many young women with HIV do not learn their status until they or their child become seriously ill with AIDS. For patients entering care in the absence of life-threatening illness, a methodical baseline evaluation assists in establishing the current state of the patient's general health and immune function, identifying the timing of seroconversion, determining symptoms attributable to HIV, identifying coexisting infections and/or neoplastic disorders, assessing protection against vaccine-preventable diseases, making recommendations for antiretroviral treatment, and identifying and preventing opportunistic infections. Better understanding of the pathogenesis of HIV has demonstrated persistent viral replication during all stages of HIV infection and a correlation between viral load (numbers of copies per milliliter of plasma) and prognosis. A quantitative HIV-RNA PCR test was recently licensed for commercial use, and two other viral-load measures are proceeding to licensing. Viral load should be assessed as part of the initial baseline evaluation and results incorporated into patient education and treatment recommendations (49). Viral load may be increased and T-lymphocytes decreased during acute illnesses or shortly after immunizations, so timing of assessments is important.

Many adolescents with HIV infection will be asymptomatic or have mild non-specific symptoms when initially diagnosed, though they may have high viral load or detectable alterations of immune function indicating need for antiretroviral treatment. The initial evaluation and subsequent monitoring should focus on detecting and treating illnesses that may hasten the progression of HIV, screening for latent infections that may reactivate as immune function fails, and assessing immune function, viral load, and immunization and nutrition status (7,28,50–52) (Table 7). The infection is staged as:

Primary, during which there is rapid viral replication after new onset of HIV infection, characterized by high viral loads, decreased CD4 lymphocyte counts, and in some cases symptoms characteristic of seroconversion illness
Asymptomatic with normal immune function
Asymptomatic with abnormal immune function
Symptomatic with non-AIDS–defining symptoms or infections
Symptomatic with opportunistic infections, cancers, a CD4 count of <200 cells/mm^3, or syndromes meeting criteria for AIDS diagnosis.

This staging, along with careful assessment of immune function and viral load, is essential to advising the patient and family about likely disease progression over time, to recommending appropriate treatment and prophylaxis, and to improving the patient's quality of life.

History and Review of Systems

Care providers should pay particular attention to past medical history (hospitalizations, transfusions, surgery, lymphadenopathy) that may determine the timing of acquisition of infection, history of STDs and other infectious and parasitic diseases, immunizations, drug allergies, growth and development, menstrual history, sexual and reproductive history (with special attention to contacts and prac-

TABLE 7. *Baseline evaluation and monitoring of asymptomatic or mildly symptomatic HIV-infected young women*

Evaluation or screening test	Frequency/interval
Medical and social history	Annual
Review of systems	3 mo[a]
Sexual and substance-use behavior	Every visit
Complete physical examination	Annual
Targeted physical, symptom screen	3 mo[a]
Pap smear	6 mo[a]
STD screen (three sites)	6 mo[a]
Tuberculin skin test (PPD) and controls	Annual
Chest X-ray	Baseline; annual if anergic[a]
Ophthalmologic examination	Baseline; annual
CMV+/toxo+	6–12 mo[a]
CD4[a] <100 mm^3	3–6 mo
Dental maintenance	3–6 mo
Hepatitis B screen	Baseline
CBC and differential, platelets, reticulocytes, ESR	6 mo[a,b]; 3 mo if CD4 <500
T-lymphocyte profile or subsets (number, percent, CD4/CD8 ratio)	6 mo if CD4 >600; 3 mo[a,c] if CD4 <500
Urinalysis	Annual[a]
Chemistries	Annual[a,b]
Viral serologies (CMV, toxo, VZV, ?EBV, ?HepC)	Annual until positive
RPR/VDRL	6 mo[a]
HIV viral load	Baseline; every 3–6 mo[a,c,d]

CBC, complete blood cell count; CMV, cytomegalovirus; EBV, Epstein-Barr virus; ESR, erythrocyte sedimentation rate; HIV, human immunodeficiency virus; PPD, purified protein derivative; RPR, rapid plasma reagin test; STD, sexually transmitted disease; toxo, toxoplasmosis; VDRL, venereal Disease Research Laboratory test; VZV, varicella-zoster virus.

[a]More frequently if clinically warranted or unstable.

[b]Certain therapies require more frequent monitoring.

[c]Acute illness or recent immunizations may temporarily lower CD4 count and increase viral load. Avoid testing in these circumstances, or repeat when resolved.

[d]Repeat 3–5 weeks after initiation or change in antiretroviral therapy.

tices and children conceived or born) before and after estimated time of infection, date and result of last Papanicolaou smear, contraceptive history and use of barrier methods, use of licit and illicit drugs, needle exposure, medications, family history, and psychosocial history (including substance use, previous psychiatric hospitalization or suicidal ideation or attempts, housing, custody status, family structure, sources of income, health insurance, education and work status, and peer supports). Much of this information can be gathered during pretest counseling. Review of systems should ask about the presence or absence of malaise, fatigue, weight loss, fever, chills, night sweats, swollen lymph or salivary glands, skin rashes (discolorations, alopecia, scaling, eruptions, nodules, infections, and purpura), oral lesions and thrush, dysphagia, vision problems, headache, persistent cough, dyspnea, easy bruising, diarrhea, anorexia, nausea, vomiting, anal pain, abdominal pain, genital sores or dysuria or discharge, limb pains and weakness, problems in memory and concentration, or loss of coordination and sensation. Exposure to pets and foreign travel should also be assessed, as should diet and food preparation and storage methods.

Physical Examination

The examination should include assessment of vital signs, growth and Tanner staging, and nutritional status, as well as a careful description of skin, hair, and nails. Lymphadenopathy location and size should be documented. The examination should include visual acuity, funduscopic examination, oral and dental examination, and palpation of salivary glands, as well as screening for otitis, sinus infection, and pharyngitis. Lung examination should look for signs of pneumonia or bronchospasm, and any organomegaly or abdominal tenderness should be documented. Genital examination should elicit the presence of lesions or discharge, as well as anal lesions, and include STD testing. Neurologic and mental status examination should especially look for signs of peripheral neuropathy, intracranial lesions, dementia, and mental illness, as well as signs of current drug or alcohol use or withdrawal.

Baseline and Periodic Assessments

Some experts recommend early combination antiretroviral therapy for young women with early primary infection with a goal of maintaining nondectable viral load. Clinicians should consult HIV experts in their community for available clinical trials or current recommendations. The asymptomatic adolescent who has a negative baseline evaluation and a CD4 lymphocyte count >500 to 600 cells/mm^3 (or 20%) and a low viral load (<5000 to 10,000 copies/ml) has little likelihood of rapid progression of disease over the next few months (53). She or he should be offered immunization against childhood diseases (substituting inactivated poliovaccine for oral poliovaccine), if not already immunized. Other immunizations that should be given include *Hemophilus influenzae* type B conjugate vaccine and pneumococcal vaccine. Hepatitis B vaccine should be offered if there is no evidence of prior infection, and annual influenza virus vaccine is often recommended for the patient and for household contacts. Varicella vaccine has not been tested in HIV-infected adolescents, and HIV is currently a contraindication to its use, though nonimmune family members should receive it. Infectious disease consultation is recommended when immunizations in patients with low CD4 counts (<100 cells/mm^3) are being considered. Follow-up examination frequency is dependent on the patient's psychological and health status, CD4 count, illnesses present, and treatment being monitored. Many youths are lost to followup for months to a year or more after being tested for HIV, and many already have CD4 counts <500 cells/mm^3 at the time of diagnosis (54). Each time the adolescent is seen, behavior and lifestyle should be assessed and healthy practices reinforced. Systems review and examination should screen for manifestations of HIV-related diseases, and education and support should be routinely offered. Few peer support groups address the particular needs of youth, but when available they may be important local resources for young women and their families. Introduction to another adult or peer living with HIV infection may be more acceptable than a group approach.

Care and Support

Other components of care include assessment of cognitive function, mental status, and language and literacy, as well as reviews of biologic and practical family relationships and social supports (including disclosure—who does and does not know about the HIV diagnosis), continuing risk reduction, partner notification needs and plans, substance use and abuse and treatment history, criminal justice involvement, legal guardianship, practical needs (housing, food, income, health insurance), and education and school status (including disclosure preferences). Patient (and sometimes family or support person) education to promote self-care should cover HIV natural history, signs and symptoms of progression, currently available treatment alternatives and standards of care, frequency of visits, nutrition, exercise, importance of regular dental care and ophthalmologic examinations, sources of information about HIV and treatment, assistance with disclosure, reproductive options, hygiene and blood precautions, support services available, assistance with disclosure, dating, and safe sex and harm reduction, as well as education and counseling specific to the patient's problems. Given the rapid changes in HIV treatments, clinicians should regularly update clients on changing standards of care and new developments in research.

Reproductive Health Issues

As recommendations for prenatal screening are implemented, more young women will be diagnosed during pregnancy. Transmission may be intrauterine, intrapartum, or postpartum, and its likelihood is increased in women with low CD4 lymphocyte counts, traumatic deliveries, high viral load, and previous infected infants, as well as with breast-feeding. Antenatal and infant treatment with zidovudine (ZDV) lessens the likelihood of infection in the offspring (46). Pregnant seropositive youths and their partners should be counseled on available options, risks, treatments to decrease transmission (e.g., zidovudine for mothers and babies), and prognoses. For those who decide to continue a pregnancy, collaboration with the obstetrician and the pediatrician who will care for and monitor the baby is essential. If a young woman is already on antiretroviral therapy prior to pregnancy or clinically needs antiretroviral treatment, treatments should be based on maternal health and clinicians should seek consultation on the latest treatment recommendations and availability of local perinatal clinical trials.

Currently ZDV monotherapy is recommended for asymptomatic women with CD4 count >500 cells/mm^3 not already on antiretroviral drugs, but combination therapies are also being used and studied in women whose own health warrants more aggressive treatment.

A seropositive patient who is or might become sexually active should be counseled about the risks of pregnancy and childbearing, and exposure to STDs and new HIV strains posed by intercourse, and should be offered both barrier and hormonal methods of contraception. Seropositive women considering pregnancy may be offered alternatives (e.g., artificial insemination) to unprotected intercourse for conception. Intrauterine devices are not recommended for HIV-positive women because of the risk of pelvic infection. Oral contraceptives may have interactions with some of the medications used for treating HIV or opportunistic infections or may cause increased side effects, but they are generally effective, as are other methods such as depot medroxyprogesterone injections and levonorgestrel subdermal implants. Finally, seropositive pregnant and parenting adolescents should be given support for planning for the future care of their children in the event of their incapacitation or death.

Gynecologic Management

Frequent monitoring for cervical dysplasia, sexually transmitted diseases, and reproductive tract infections is needed. In general, HIV-infected patients require more prolonged and aggressive therapy for cervical dysplasia and genitourinary infections, with hospitalization usually indicated for pelvic inflammatory disease and primary herpes infection. Recurrent vulvovaginal candidiasis (see Chapter 11) may be treated by monthly short courses of topical medication or oral fluconazole treatment or prophylaxis. In addition to cervical cancer and neoplasia (see Chapter 13), young women with HIV may be more susceptible to other reproductive malignancies (e.g., ovarian cancer) and lymphoma.

Treatment and Prophylaxis

The standard of care for management of HIV infection is constantly changing, with several new drugs recently approved for antiretroviral therapy that were previously available only to research protocol patients. The goal of antiretroviral therapy is reduction in viral replication and viral load, and prolongation of the slope of decline in immune function with resultant improvements in survival and quality of life (53,54). Management of sick adolescents and adolescents on antiretroviral treatment should be done in conjunction with infectious disease or other specialists knowledgeable about HIV management and new developments. Several new guidelines for antiretroviral treatment were issued in June, 1997 (55,56,57). Initiation of antiretroviral therapy is recommended for youths with AIDS or symptomatic HIV disease. Therapy is also recommended for the asymptomatic patient with decreased or rapidly declining cellular immunity (indicated by a CD4 lymphocyte count <500 cells/mm^3, or 20%, on two occasions) or a high viral load ($>10{,}000$ copies/ml) if the youth is willing and able to adhere to treatment regimens. Aggressive treatment of documented new primary infections or seroconversion syndromes is recommended by some experts, and clinical trials are in progress to determine the optimal agents and duration for such therapy.

ZDV monotherapy is no longer recommended, and no monotherapy is the best choice for antiretroviral treatment. Though ACTG Protocol 152 showed both didanosine (ddI) monotherapy and ZDV/ddI combination to be superior to ZDV alone in children, a more recent trial (PACTG 300) was stopped in June, 1997, because both ZDV/3TC and ZDV/ddI were superior to ddI alone in young children. Viral load is a better indicator of treatment efficacy than CD4 cell count, and both should be monitored when antiretroviral therapy is initiated or changed. Currently available antiretroviral agents include nucleoside analog reverse transcriptase inhibitors (RTIs): zidovudine, zalcitabine (ddC), ddI, stavudine, lamivudine and abacavir; protease inhibitors: saquinavir, indinavir, ritonavir and nelfinavir; and nonnucleoside RTIs (NNRTI): nevaripine and delavirdine and effavirenz. In addition, new drugs in each category are nearing approval. In most cases, adolescent treatment doses are empirically the same as those for adults for youths who are Tanner stage 4 or greater, and pediatric doses are used for Tanner stages 1 to 2 youths. The first line of therapy should probably now be two RTIs plus a protease inhibitor, to maximize impact on viral replication, and diminish development of resistance, but these complex regimens demand excellent adherence. Youths unwilling to begin or adhere to such an extensive regimen may benefit from less intensive regimens, such as two RTIs plus an NNRTI, two RTIs alone, or ddI monotherapy. In our experience, such twice a day regimens are more feasible for adherence by youths, but may diminish later therapeutic choices or increase the likelihood of resistance. A therapeutic regimen that does not affect a decreased viral load or improved immunologic and clinical status after 4–6 weeks should probably be changed to another combination regimen with at least two new drugs, which may produce a dramatic response. Early combination therapy with the goal of obtaining a nondetectable viral load is now the standard of care for most experts and prolongs both survival and time before progression to AIDS if successful (58). Protease inhibitors can induce rapid development of resistance when used intermittently, and some have a high incidence of side effects and serious interactions with medications and street drugs, so their use in young women requires a level of motivation and compliance rare in our experience. In addition, the impact of a complex medication regimen on a patient's mental health and quality of life must also be considered. Management of HIV infection requires constant patient education and input, as well as knowledge of the doses, side effects, drug interactions, and monitoring needed for each regimen, together with constant efforts to monitor changes in treatment guidelines and standards of care. Successful treatment of youths with HIV infection should include the young women as partners, with the clinicians explaining strategies and offering hope, as well as options and choices, with attention to lifestyle issues that affect compliance and tolerance. Antiretroviral treatment guidelines are revised annually and are widely available on the Internet (59).

As immune function declines with CD4 counts <200 cells/mm^3, patients become vulnerable to a cascade of life-threatening opportunistic infections. Guidelines for primary and secondary prevention of opportunistic infections in pregnant and nonpregnant persons living with HIV infection were summarized in a 1995 supplement of *Clinical Infectious Diseases* (60), which was updated in June, 1997 (61). One opportunistic infection indicating poor prognosis and decreased life expectancy is PCP. Prophylaxis designed to prevent PCP is recommended for all seropositive individuals who have a CD4 count <200 cells/mm^3, or 14%, an AIDS diagnosis, or a history of PCP disease. Prophylaxis with oral trimethoprim/sulfamethoxazole or alternatively with oral dapsone and pyrimethamine or aerosolized pentamidine is currently recommended. The first two regimens also prevent toxoplasmosis. Prophylaxis against *Mycobacterium avium-intracellulare* (MAI) infection is often recommended for youths with a CD4 count of <100 cells/mm^3. MAI infection prophylaxis options are daily clarithromycin, weekly azithromycin, rifabutin plus azithromycin, or daily rifabutin, with rifabutin alone the least effective option (62). Vigorous preventive treatment of tuberculin-positive individuals with HIV infection is also recommended, with 12 months of isoniazid as the standard treatment. Other primary and secondary prophylactic regimens are being studied for PCP, toxoplasmosis, cytomegalovirus, and fungal infections. Lifestyle alterations can also help patients avoid exposure to opportunistic pathogens. As new potent antiretroviral combinations produce dramatic CD4 cell count increases, further study will be needed to determine whether prophylaxis against opportunistic infections needs to be continued. A conservative approach assumes that cell lines immune to certain agents may *not* be regained and therefore that continued prophylaxis is warranted.

PREVENTION, CARE COORDINATION, AND ADVOCACY

All health care professionals should be knowledgeable about HIV infection and comfortable doing individual risk assessments and providing counseling and access to testing and care. Every family planning, gynecology, prenatal, health maintenance, or medical visit is an opportunity to engage in active prevention and case finding. Familiarity with community resources available for children, youths, and families infected with HIV is essential. Consultation with infectious disease experts experienced in HIV management improves awareness of current therapeutic and prophylactic guidelines, assists in the diagnosis and management of opportunistic infections, and helps to assess eligibility for clinical research.

DiClemente (63) has recently reviewed adolescent HIV risk, prevention research, and policy and legal issues. Children and women have traditionally been considered more difficult research subjects, and trials of therapeutic modalities in adolescents, children, and women have generally lagged behind those for adults and men. In the early years of HIV research, adolescents were systematically excluded from treatment protocols. Since 1989, some protocol eligibility ages have been lowered or raised to allow enrollment of adolescents, but many barriers still exist to youths' access to care. Some youths are under too much psychosocial stress and in such unstable living situations that participation in clinical protocols is unrealistic without first addressing survival needs. Many HIV-positive youths are still involved in risky behavior such as drug or alcohol use or unprotected sex, and many may not have a supportive adult guardian. Although most legal experts feel adolescents are entitled to diagnosis and treatment of HIV as an STD, minors living on their own and minors in custody of the state cannot generally consent alone to research, unless they meet the legal definition of emancipated.

More data are needed on the seroprevalence, seroincidence, and natural history of HIV. Studies are needed both in those who enter puberty while infected and in those who acquire infection during adolescence to determine the effects, if any, of changes in hormonal levels, body composition, and acquisition of other illnesses on disease progression and course. Twelve sites recently federally funded as members of the Adolescent Medicine HIV/AIDS Research Network are beginning collaboration on this effort. Research is also needed to define the impact of HIV infection on the social, cognitive, and behavioral functioning of youths, to determine which therapeutic, support, and educational services help, to develop and assess effective prevention programs and to pilot and implement effective models for case finding, primary care, treatment, and case management. Funding from the CDC and the Health Resources and Services Administration's Ryan White program (Title IV: Pediatric and Adolescent Care Projects and Title V: Special Projects of National Significance) is assisting these efforts.

Health care providers have an essential role as advocates and spokespersons on behalf of youth, who are often undervalued and disenfranchised. They often have unique opportunities to impact community policies, advocate for adolescent access to services, and become involved in prevention, education, and intervention at the community level through schools and community-based programs (see Chapter 22). Care providers can use their experience with the health care needs of at-risk and HIV-infected youths to advocate with local, state, and national policy makers for increased funding of research and early intervention efforts targeting adolescents and joint efforts to unify adolescent data collection efforts, clarify definitions, and include adolescents as a target group in federally funded programs. Like other youths with chronic diseases, young women living with HIV infection need the support and assistance of health professionals sensitive to their needs, knowledgeable about their disease, and willing to engage as active partners in sustaining health and optimizing quality of life.

REFERENCES

1. Centers for Disease Control and Prevention. HIV/AIDS surveillance report. *U.S. HIV and AIDS cases reported through December 1996.* 1997;8.
2. AIDS Bureau, MA Department of Public Health. AIDS: The Global Picture. 1995;1:1.
3. Karon J, et al. Prevalence of HIV infection in the United States, 1984-1992. *JAMA* 1996;276:126.
4. Centers for Disease Control and Prevention. First 500,000 AIDS cases—United States, 1995. *MMWR* 1995;44:849.
5. Greenspan A, Castro KG. Heterosexual transmission of HIV infection. *SIECUS Report* 1990;19:1.
6. Centers for Disease Control and Prevention. 1993 Revised classification system for HIV infection and expanded surveillance case definition for AIDS among adolescents and adults. *MMWR* 1992; 44(RR-17).

7. El Sadr W, Oleske JM, Agins BD, et al. *Clinical practice guideline: evaluation and management of early HIV infection.* Agency for Health Care Policy and Research publication 94-0572. US Public Health Service, 1994.
8. National Center for Health Statistics. Annual summary of births, marriages, divorces, and deaths: United States, 1993. *Mon Vital Stat Rep* 1994;43(13).
9. Quinn TC, Glasser D, Cannon RO, et al. Human immunodeficiency virus infection among patients attending clinics for sexually transmitted diseases. *N Engl J Med* 1987;318:197.
10. Kelen GD, Frutz S, Quaqish B, et al. Unrecognized human immunodeficiency virus infection in emergency department patients. *N Engl J Med* 1987;318:1645.
11. Hoff R, Berardi VP, Weiblen BJ, et al. Seroprevalence of human immunodeficiency virus among childbearing women. *N Engl J Med* 1988;318:525.
12. Novick LF, Berns D, Stricof R, et al. HIV seroprevalence in newborns in New York state. *JAMA* 1989;261:1745.
13. Hahn RA, Ontario IM, Jones S, et al. Prevalence of HIV infection among intravenous drug users in the United States. *JAMA* 1989;261:2677.
14. *Adolescent health, volume II: background and the effectiveness of selected prevention and treatment services.* Office of Technology Assessment.
15. Conway GA, Epstein MR, Hayman CR, et al. Trends in HIV prevalence among disadvantaged youth: survey results from a national job training program, 1988-1992. *JAMA* 1993;269:2887.
16. *National HIV seroprevalence summary: results through 1992.* Centers for Disease Control and Prevention, 1994.
17. Sweeney P, Lindegren ML, Buehler JW, et al. Teenagers at risk of human immunodeficiency virus type 1 infection: results from seroprevalence surveys in the United States. *Arch Pediatr Adolesc Med* 1995;149:521.
18. St Louis ME, Conway GA, Hayman CR, et al. Human immunodeficiency virus infection in disadvantaged adolescents: findings from the US Job Corps. *JAMA* 1991;266:2387.
19. Chaisson MA. Heterosexually acquired HIV infection in New York City. *AIDS Reader* 1995;5:88.
20. Stricof RL, Kennedy JT, Nattell TC, et al. HIV seroprevalence in a facility for runaway and homeless adolescents. *Am J Public Health* 1991;81(suppl):50.
21. Quinn TC, Groseclose SL, Spence M, et al. Evolution of the human immunodeficiency virus epidemic among patients attending sexually transmitted disease clinics: a decade of experience. *J Infect Dis* 1992;165:541.
22. D Angelo LJ, Getson PR, Luban NL, et al. Human immunodeficiency virus infection in urban adolescents: can we predict who is at risk? *Pediatrics* 1991;88:982.
23. Melchiono M, Samples C, Mann R, et al. Adolescent and young adult seroprevalence survey. North American Society for Pediatric and Adolescent Gynecology (Abstract), 1993.
24. Young RA, Feldman S, Brackin BT, et al. Seroprevalence of human immunodeficiency virus among adolescent attendees of Mississippi sexually transmitted disease clinics: a rural epidemic. *South Med J* 1992;85:460.
25. Otten MW Jr, Zaidi A, Peterman TA, et al. High rate of HIV seroconversion among patients attending urban sexually transmitted disease clinics. *AIDS* 1994;8:549.
26. Ilegbodu AE, Frank ML, Poindexter AN, Johnson D. Characteristics of teens tested for HIV in a metropolitan area. *J Adolesc Health* 1994;15:479.
27. Hein K, Dell R, Futterman D, et al. Comparison of HIV+ and HIV- adolescents: risk factors and psychosocial determinants. *Pediatrics* 1995;95:96.
28. Futterman D, Hein K. Medical management of adolescents with HIV infection. In: Pizzo P, Wilfert R, eds. *Pediatric AIDS.* Baltimore: Williams & Wilkins, 1993.
29. Rosenberg PS, Biggar RJ, Goedert JJ. Declining age at HIV infection in the United States. *N Engl J Med* 1993;330:789.
30. Padian NS, Shiboski SC, Jewell NP. Female to male transmission of human immunodeficiency virus. *JAMA* 1991;266:1664.
31. Johnson AM. Condoms and HIV transmission. *N Engl J Med* 1994;331:391.
32. Meulen J, Mgaya HN, Chang-Claude J, et al. Risk factors for HIV infection in gynaecological inpatients in Dar es Salaam, Tanzania, 1988-1990. *East Afr Med J* 1992;69:688.
33. Plourde PJ, Plummer FA, Pepin J, et al. Human immunodeficiency virus type 1 infection in women attending a sexually transmitted diseases clinic in Kenya. *J Infect Dis* 1992;166:86.
34. Plummer PA, Simonsen JN, Cameron DW, et al. Cofactors in male-female sexual transmission of human immunodeficiency virus type 1. *J Infect Dis* 1991;163:233.

35. Maiman M. Cervical neoplasia in women with HIV infection. *Oncology* 1994;8:83.
36. Stratton P, Ciacco KH. Cervical neoplasia in the patient with HIV infection. *Curr Opin Obstet Gynecol* 1994;6:86.
37. Northfelt DW. Cervical and anal neoplasia and HPV infection in persons with HIV infection. *Oncology* 1994;8:33.
38. Mandelblatt JS, Fahs M, Garibaldi K, et al. Association between HIV infection and cervical neoplasia: implications for clinical care of women at risk for both conditions. *AIDS* 1992;6:173.
39. Shah PN, Kell PD, Barton SE. Gynaecological disorders and human immunodeficiency virus infection. *Int J STD AIDS* 1994;5:383.
40. Recommendations of the Work Group. AIDS testing and epidemiology for youth. *J Adolesc Health Care* 1989;10(3s):52s.
41. Friedman LS, Goodman E. Adolescents at risk for HIV infection. *Prim Care* 1992;19:171.
42. *Adolescent HIV counseling and testing policy: recommended guidelines*. Massachusetts Department of Public Health, 1990.
43. *HIV blood test counseling: physician guidelines,* 2nd ed. Chicago: American Medical Association, 1993.
44. US Public Health Service. Recommendations for human immunodeficiency virus counseling and voluntary testing for pregnant women. *MMWR* 1995;44(RR-7).
45. Goodman E, Tipton AC, Hecht L, et al. Perseverance pays off: health care providers impact on HIV testing decisions by adolescent females. *Pediatrics* 1994;6:878.
46. Gallo D, Georg JR, Fitchen JH, et al. Evaluation of a system using oral mucosal transudate for HIV-1 antibody screening and confirmatory testing. Orasure HIV Clinical Trials Group. *JAMA* 1997; 277:254.
47. Zidovudine for the prevention of HIV transmission from mother to infant. *MMWR* 1994;43:285.
48. Recommendations of the USPHS task force on the use of zidovudine to reduce perinatal transmission of human immunodeficiency virus. *MMWR* 1994;43(RR-11).
49. HIV viral load markers in clinical practice (commentary and review). *Nature Med* 1996;2:625.
50. Jewett JF, Hecht FM. Preventive health care for adults with HIV infection. *JAMA* 1993;269:1144.
51. Futterman D, Hein K. Medical care of HIV-infected adolescents. *AIDS Clin Care* 1992;4:95.
52. Kunins H, Hein K, Futterman D, et al. Guide to adolescent HIV/AIDS program development. *J Adolesc Health* 1993;14(suppl 5).
53. Carpenter CJ. Antiretroviral therapy for HIV infection: recommendations of an international panel. *JAMA* 1996;276:146.
54. Futterman D, Hein K, Reuben N, et al. Human immunodeficiency virus-infected adolescents: the first 50 patients in a New York City program. *Pediatrics* 1993;91:730.
55. Draft report of the NIH panel to define principles of therapy HIV infection, available at http://www.cdcnac.org, June, 1997. Final publication in *MMWR* anticipated summer, 1997.
56. Panel for clinical practices for treatment of HIV infection convened by the Department of Health and Human Services and the Henry J. Kaiser Family Foundation. Draft guidelines for the use of antiretroviral agents in HIV-infected adults and adolescents, available at http://www.cdcnac.org. Final publication in *MMWR* anticipated summer, 1997.
57. Carpenter C, Fischi M, Hammer S, Hirsch M, et al. Antiretroviral therapy for HIV infection in 1997: updated recommendations of the International AIDS Society-USA Panel. *JAMA* 1997;277:1962.
58. Englund JA, Baker CJ, Raskino C, et al. Zidovudine, didanosine, or both as the initial treatment for symptomatic HIV-infected children. *N Engl J Med* 1997;336:1704.
59. Centers for Disease Control and Prevention. Guidelines for the use of antiretroviral agents in HIV-infected adults and adolescents. *MMWR* 1998;47(suppl):RR-5.
60. Kaplan JE, et al. USPHS/IDSA guidelines for prevention of opportunistic infections in persons infected with human immunodeficiency virus. *Clin Infect Dis* 1995;21(suppl 1).
61. Centers for Disease Control and Prevention. 1997 USPHS/IDSA Guidelines for the prevention of opportunistic infections in persons infected with human immunodeficiency virus. *MMWR* 1997;46 (suppl)(RR-12).
62. Pierce M Crampton S, Henry D, et al. A randomized trial of clarithromycin as prophylaxis against disseminated MAI complex infection in patients with AIDS. *N Engl J Med* 1996;335:384.
63. DiClemente RJ, ed. *Adolescents and AIDS: a generation in jeopardy.* Sage Publications, 1992.

15

Benign and Malignant Ovarian Masses

Ovarian masses in infants, children, and adolescents may result from functional cysts or benign or malignant neoplasms. Ovarian tumors are the most common genital neoplasms that occur during childhood, accounting for about 1% of all malignant neoplasms found in the age range of 0 to 17 years (1,2). Historically, it was widely believed that all ovaries containing masses discovered in infants, children, and adolescents should be removed surgically, but with the identification of serum tumor markers and advances in radiologic imaging, a more rational and conservative approach to thc management of these ovarian masses has been developed. The purpose of this chapter is to review the incidence, presentation, physical findings, evaluation, and management of various types of ovarian masses that are encountered in neonates, children, and adolescents.

CLASSICATION OF OVARIAN MASSES

Ovarian masses may result from functional (nonneoplastic) cysts or benign or malignant neoplasms. In 1973, the World Health Organization classified ovarian neoplasms into nine major categories and 26 subtypes, based on histologic cell type and benign versus malignant state (3). An abbreviated and modified version is shown in Table 1 (3,4). In contrast to the adult experience, in which epithelial tumors account for the significant proportion of neoplasms, the majority of tumors in the younger population are of germ cell origin (Table 2) (5). Although the majority of lesions in childhood are benign, it is important for the clinician to make the diagnosis early to lessen the possibility of ovarian torsion and loss of an adnexa and to improve the prognosis for malignant lesions.

FUNCTIONAL OVARIAN CYSTS

Functional cysts (20% to 50% of ovarian tumors) are not true neoplasms but rather should be considered a variation of a normal physiologic process (see

TABLE 1. *Modified World Health Organization's international histologic classification of ovarian tumors*

Common "epithelial" tumors
Serous
Mucinous
Endometrioid
Clear cell
Brenner
Transitional
Small cell
Malignant mixed mesodermal
Unclassified
Sex cord–stromal tumors
Granulosa stromal cell
Granulosa cell
Thecoma-fibroma
Sertoli stromal cell
Sertoli cell tumors
Sertoli-Leydig cell tumors
Well differentiated
Intermediately differentiated
Poorly differentiated
With heterologous element
Sex cord tumor with annular tubules
Leydig (hilus) cell tumors
Lipid (lipoid) cell tumors
Gynandroblastoma
Germ cell tumors
Dysgerminoma
Endodermal sinus tumor
Embryonal carcinoma
Polyembryoma
Choriocarcinoma
Teratomas
Immature
Mature (dermoid cyst)
Monodermal (struma ovarii, carcinoid)
Mixed forms
Gonadoblastoma
Metastatic
Other

(Adapted from Serov SF, Scully RE, Sobin LH. *International histological classification of tumours. No. 9. Histologic typing of ovarian tumours.* Geneva: World Health Organization, 1973; and Rice LW, Barbieri RL. The ovary. In: Ryan RJ, Berkowitz RS, Barbieri RL, eds. *Kistner's gynecology,* 6th ed. Boston: Mosby-Year Book, 1995;187; with permission.)

Chapters 4, 6, and 9). Functional cysts include follicular, corpus luteum, and theca-lutein types, all of which are benign and usually self-limited. The incidence of cysts and nonmalignant tumors in the community is probably even higher than indicated in most series, as percentages are based on referred cases and it is not possible to determine the underlying incidence of nonidentified or asymptomatic cysts or masses (5,6).

TABLE 2. *Primary ovarian tumors treated at the Children's Hospital, Boston (1928–1982)*

Tumor type	No.	%
Mature (benign) teratomas	78	47
Cystic (76)		
Solid (2)		
Common "epithelial" tumors	27	16
Mucinous (12)		
Serous (14)		
Mixed (1)		
Sex cord–stromal tumors	21	13
Granulosa cell (10)		
Thecoma (2)		
Fibroma (1)		
Sertoli-Leydig (7)		
Unclassified (1)		
Immature teratomas	17	10
Endodermal sinus tumor	14	8
Dysgerminoma	8	5
Choriocarcinoma[a]	1	<1

[a]Mixed malignant germ cell tumor with predominant element being choriocarcinoma.
(From Lack EE, Goldstein DP. Primary ovarian tumors in childhood and adolescence. *Curr Probl Obstet Gynecol* 1984;8:1;with permission.)

Fetal Ovarian Cysts

Ovarian cysts in fetuses range in frequency from 30% to 70%, depending on the gestational age; the true incidence is unknown (7). These cysts are commonly detected prenatally on routine obstetric ultrasound (8–10). The etiology of fetal ovarian cysts is unclear, but most likely they result from a combination of ovarian stimulation by maternal and fetal gonadotropins (see Fig. 4-4) (11,12). The differential diagnosis of fetal cystic intraabdominal masses is shown in Table 3 (13). An increased incidence of fetal and neonatal follicular cysts has been reported in association with preeclampsia, diabetes mellitus, polyhydramnios, and isoimmunization disease (7,11,14,15).

The majority of antenatal ovarian cysts are unilateral, although both ovaries may be involved (14). Spontaneous regression occurs in both simple and complex fetal cysts both antenatally and postpartum, and thus the management of the patient with antenatally diagnosed ovarian cysts is observation (8–10,16,17). The risks to the fetus of an ovarian cyst may include intracystic hemorrhage, rupture of the cyst with possible hemorrhage, gastrointestinal and urinary tract obstruction, ovarian torsion and necrosis, incarceration into a congenital inguinal hernia, difficulty with delivery due to abdominal dystocia, and respiratory distress at birth due to the mass effect (18). In some fetuses with large cysts (>6 cm), elective cesarean section may be the preferred route to prevent rupture. The rate of malignancy is so low that it need not be considered in making therapeutic decisions. Antenatal cyst aspiration has been advocated to reduce the potential

TABLE 3. *Differential diagnosis of fetal/neonatal intraabdominal cystic masses*

Differential diagnosis
Genitourinary tract disorders
Ovarian cyst
Hydrometrocolpos
Cloacal anomaly
Urinary tract obstruction
Renal cyst
Megaloureter or megalocystis
Urachal cyst
Adrenal cyst
Gastrointestinal tract disorders
Mesenteric cyst
Enteric duplication cyst
Meconium cyst
Duodenal atresia
Volvulus
Miscellaneous disorders
Choledochal cyst
Pancreatic cyst
Splenic cyst
Presacral cystic teratoma
Anterior meningocele
Neuroblastoma
Lymphangioma

(From Lack EE, Goldstein DP. Primary ovarian tumors in childhood and adolescence. *Curr Probl Obstet Gynecol* 1984;8:1;with permission.)

complications of fetal ovarian cysts (19); however, the role of antenatal cyst aspiration is questionable because of potential misdiagnosis and complications of the aspiration procedure.

Neonatal Ovarian Cysts

If *in utero* torsion occurs, the ovary may undergo necrosis and develop into a calcified persistent mass or resorb. The most common genitourinary cystic mass not related to the kidney is an ovarian cyst (20). The differential diagnosis of a neonate with a cystic intraperitoneal mass is extensive and includes a number of congenital cystic masses of other intraperitoneal organs, as well as congenital anomalies (see Table 3) (13,21). As noted above, the etiology of fetal and neonatal ovarian cysts is unknown. As neonates have a shallow pelvis, the cysts are often displaced to the mid- or upper abdomen, at which time they are palpable abdominally. On abdominal examination, the ovary containing the cyst is generally freely mobile. Ultrasound reveals a cystic mass (Fig. 1) that may have a simple (clear, fluid-filled) or complex (fluid, debris, septa, solid components, echogenic wall) sonographic pattern. The complex appearance on ultrasound may make a precise diagnosis more difficult (13).

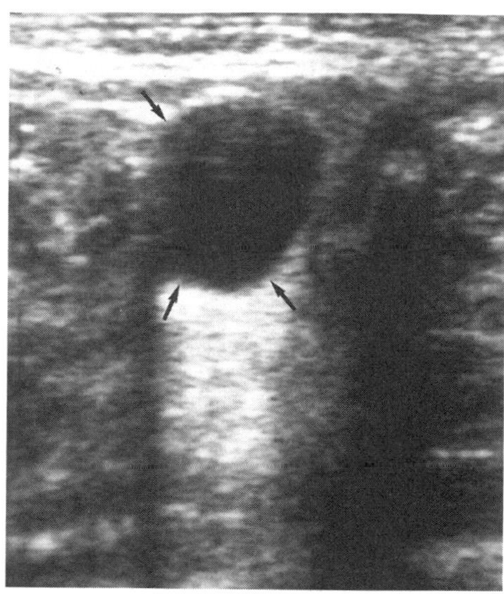

FIG. 1. Ultrasound shows a simple cyst *(arrows)* in a neonate. (Courtesy of Carol Barnewolt, M.D., Children's Hospital, Boston, MA.)

Spontaneous regression occurs in these cysts postpartum usually by 4 months of age. They should be followed with serial ultrasound examinations to ensure regression. The greatest concern in the neonate with an ovarian cyst is the possibility of torsion with subsequent ovarian loss. If the cyst does not resolve, then either neoplasia is present (unlikely) or torsion with hemorrhage and/or necrosis (see Fig. 1 in Chapter 9) has occurred (10,22). Torsion can occur with a cyst of any size, just as it does with normal adnexa, particularly when long pedicles are present (23,24). When known cysts are followed conservatively, parents or other caregivers should be made aware of the signs and symptoms of torsion (see Chapter 9) and urged to contact the child's physician without delay.

Postpartum cyst aspiration has been advocated to reduce the likelihood of torsion (19). In contrast to antenatal cyst aspiration, the use of neonatal cyst aspiration has been clearly established, because the diagnosis is more certain and the risk of complications is low (24). Aspiration of persistent large cysts (>5 to 6 cm) is recommended. If the cysts recur, surgical removal is indicated.

The traditional management of neonatal cysts increasing in size or persisting for >4 months is surgery. Although every attempt should be made to salvage the ovary in cases of persistent ovarian cysts, in many instances, especially in cases of torsion with ovarian necrosis, oophorectomy is necessary (10,22). It should be noted that infants and children may also have torsion of normal ovaries (see Chapter 9) (25–27). Depending on the condition of the torsed ovary, it may be possible to untwist the vascular pedicle in an attempt to salvage the ovary (28).

Ovarian Cysts During Childhood

Childhood ovarian cysts develop as a result of gonadotropin stimulation of the ovary, and thus the incidence of ovarian cysts decreases in early childhood and then increases as puberty is approached (29,30). Most simple ovarian cysts in children result from failure of the normal mature follicle to involute. Some functional cysts will be hormonally active and result in precocious pseudopuberty, with the patient presenting with an episode of vaginal bleeding or premature breast development (31–34). Hormone-secreting cysts may cause sexual precocity, as is seen in association with the McCune-Albright syndrome (35). Cysts may also occur in patients with idiopathic central precocious puberty and would be expected to resolve with the institution of gonadotropin-releasing hormone analog therapy (36) (see Chapter 5). When prepubertal ovaries are found to be enlarged and multicystic, an evaluation for thyroid disease is indicated (see Chapter 5). If a child has a cystic mass without precocity, the cyst may well be a parovarian (see Fig. 7 in Chapter 8) or mesothelial cyst and, if symptomatic, requires excision (see Figs. 8 to 10 in Chapter 8). In young children, an ovarian cyst is often discovered by a parent or clinician as an asymptomatic abdominal mass or as increasing abdominal girth. The embryologic ovary migrates from the level of T-10 (in early life it is characteristically abdominal in location) and during maturation descends to the true pelvis by puberty. Thus, ovarian tumors are felt to present as abdominal masses in the young child (1). Chronic abdominal aching pain, either periumbilical or located in one lower quadrant, may be present. Acute severe pain simulating appendicitis or peritonitis may develop secondary to torsion, perforation, infarction, or hemorrhage from or into a tumor or cyst (see Chapter 9). Patients may experience intermittent pain, presumably because of partial torsion, that subsequently resolves without therapy. This may also be the warning sign of impending torsion and the need for emergency surgery. Nonspecific symptoms including nausea, vomiting, a sense of abdominal fullness or bloating, and urinary frequency or retention may signal the presence of a tumor.

The management of an ovarian cyst in the prepubertal age group depends on the appearance of the cyst on ultrasound and the presence of significant symptomatology. A patient with acute rupture of an ovarian cyst with hemorrhage needs to be assessed to determine whether the bleeding appears to be self-limited (in which case the patient can be observed with serial hematocrit readings and examinations) or whether it is resulting in a significant decrease in hematocrit or changes in vital signs. If it is determined that the patient needs surgery, then she is stabilized and laparoscopy or laparotomy undertaken (37). Free blood and clots (see Color Plate 30) can be aspirated and hemostasis ensured by fulguration of areas of bleeding via laparoscopy. A hemoperitoneum is not a contraindication to laparoscopy. If the surgeon is not comfortable with laparoscopy for children or if the patient is hypotensive, then a laparotomy is undertaken. In cases of ovarian torsion, surgery is indicated at the time of the diagnosis. As noted in Chapter 9, ultrasound may be helpful in determining the

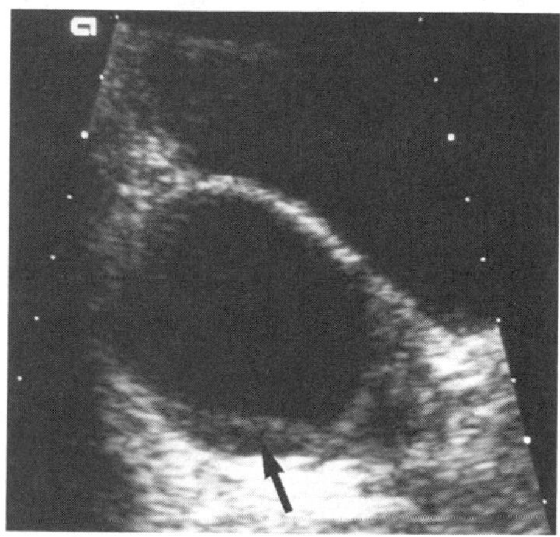

FIG. 2. Ultrasound shows an ovarian cyst containing debris *(arrow)*. (Courtesy of Carol Barnewolt, M.D., Children's Hospital, Boston, MA.)

presence of ovarian torsion. Torsed ovaries can be "detorsed" laparoscopically with salvage of the ovary (28,38–40). Whether pexis of the contralateral ovary can be helpful in preventing a second episode of ovarian torsion of a normal ovary needs evaluation. If oophoropexy is elected, it can be safely accomplished by operative laparoscopy (41).

If, on the other hand, the ovarian mass is purely cystic or has few internal echoes/debris suggestive of hemorrhage and no other complex features such as septation or calcification (Fig. 2), it is almost certainly benign and can be managed by observation (34,37). A followup ultrasound scan in 4 to 8 weeks should reveal a decrease in size. If the cyst has not resolved and the ultrasonic characteristics are still reassuring, then continued observation is still appropriate. Warner and associates (42) reported on the conservative management of 51 children with both simple and complex cysts, all >5 cm in diameter. Of these cysts, 90% spontaneously resolved, largely within 2 weeks. Of the 23 children treated surgically either because of initial ultrasonic appearance or for persistence, 10 were found to have neoplasms (six teratomas, two cystadenomas, one granulosa cell tumor, one Sertoli-Leydig cell tumor) (42). Thind and colleagues (43) found that in 64 children with simple cysts <5.5 cm in diameter, all of the cysts resolved. These girls, however, tended to have persistent symptoms for a few months followed by spontaneous resolution. The cysts sometimes recurred, although new ovarian cysts also occurred on the contralateral side (43).

Ovarian Cysts During Adolescence

The development of simple cysts is quite common in adolescents. Most simple cysts result from the failure of the maturing follicle to ovulate and involute. Adolescent ovaries may contain multiple follicles in different stages of development (see Fig. 9-4). Cysts in the postmenarchal adolescent may be asymptomatic

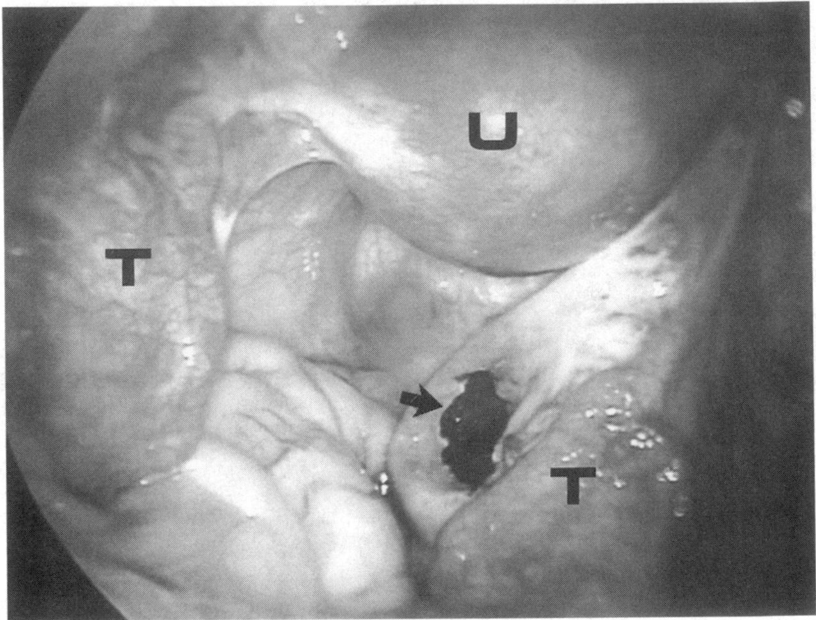

FIG. 3. Postlaparoscopic ovarian cystectomy (*arrow* at site) of right simple symptomatic ovarian cyst shown in Color Plate 29. T, fallopian tubes; U, uterus.

or cause menstrual irregularities, pelvic pain, or, if large, urinary frequency, constipation, or pelvic heaviness. Cysts can rupture, causing intraabdominal hemorrhage (see Color Plate 30). Torsion of a cyst causes acute pain, nausea, vomiting, and pallor, often followed by less severe localized pain. The white blood cell count may be elevated with a shift to the left. Examination reveals induration of the pelvic floor and a tender mass.

In most cases, follicular cysts found on routine examination resolve spontaneously in 1 to 2 months. If a cyst <6 cm is palpated in an asymptomatic patient and ultrasound or pelvic examination confirms a simple, fluid-filled cyst, the patient may be observed with or without the addition of an oral contraceptive prescribed to suppress the hypothalamic–ovarian axis. The oral contraceptive pill does not "shrink" the existing cyst, but with suppression of the hypothalamic–ovarian axis another ovarian cyst will not develop and confuse the clinician as to whether the first cyst resolved and a new one formed or whether the original cyst has persisted. The patient should be examined monthly or followup ultrasound performed. Patients incidentally found to have small follicular cysts at the time of surgery (e.g., appendectomy) should not undergo cyst aspiration or cystectomy, as these cysts will resolve spontaneously and ovarian or paratubal adhesions may form from ovarian surgery and result in infertility and/or pelvic pain (see Chapter 9) (44,45). If a fluid-filled cyst increases in size, is >6 cm, or causes symptoms, then a laparoscopic cyst aspiration (with the cyst fluid sent for cytology) or cystectomy (with the cyst wall sent for pathologic evaluation) can be performed (see Color Plate 29 and Fig. 3) (46). If surgery is undertaken, ovarian cystectomy is preferred to cyst aspiration due to the high rate of recurrence after aspiration (47). It should be noted that asymptomatic simple cysts of 6 to 10 cm may also spontaneously resolve and can be safely observed in some patients. If the cyst recurs or operative intervention is needed, the procedure should be conservative and preserve as much ovarian tissue as possible.

Corpus luteum cysts occur often and can reach 5 to 10 cm in diameter. These cysts are the result of the normal formation of a corpus luteum after ovulation (see Chapter 4). Ultrasound is useful to suggest the appearance of a corpus luteum cyst, which contains increased echoes (Fig. 4). There may be bleeding into the cyst or rupture with intraperitoneal hemorrhage. Color Plate 30 shows a laparoscopic view of blood and clot filling the pelvis after rupture of a corpus luteum cyst. Although such cysts are often asymptomatic, they may cause pain. In the absence of pain or intraperitoneal bleeding, therapy with an oral contraceptive pill (to suppress a new cyst from forming) and observation for 3 months are indicated. If hemorrhage or severe pain occurs or the cyst is large (>6 cm) on initial examination, laparoscopy or laparotomy may be necessary. Due to increased ovarian size and weight, corpus luteum cysts may increase the risk of ovarian torsion.

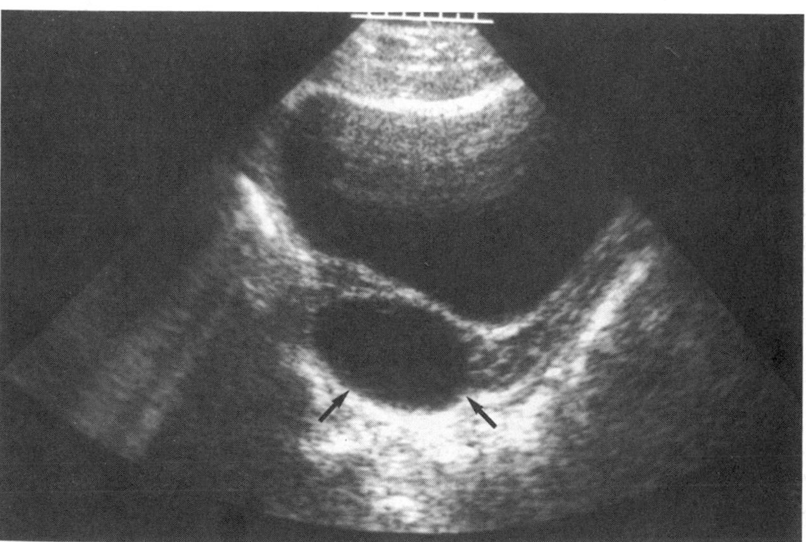

FIG. 4. Ultrasound shows a corpus luteum cyst *(arrows)* in a young woman reporting dull pain. (Courtesy of Carol Barnewolt, M.D., Children's Hospital, Boston, MA.)

OVARIAN TUMORS/NEOPLASMS

Presentation and Examination

Patients with an ovarian tumor may present with abdominal pain or complaints of increasing abdominal girth, nausea, and vomiting, or they may be totally asymptomatic, with the mass being found on routine examination. The wide variety of symptoms caused by ovarian tumors suggests that abdominal palpation and rectal examination in the lithotomy position is important in any girl with nonspecific abdominal or pelvic complaints (5,44). A large, thin-walled cyst may be confused with ascites. The size of the tumor is not indicative of its malignant potential. Exquisite tenderness suggests torsion or hemorrhage of the cyst but may also occur with appendicitis and rupture.

Imaging

Ultrasound is extremely helpful in the evaluation of an ovarian mass (20,37,43,48–50). Although ultrasound has revolutionized the management of patients with ovarian masses, not all tumors that are palpated will be visualized on ultrasound, and not all "masses" will turn out to be of significance. Ultrasound is routinely used to to determine overall size and identify whether a mass is simple, complex, solid, bilateral, or associated with free fluid. This information is helpful in forming a differential diagnosis and correlating with age, presentation, and tumor markers to determine the appropriate therapy. Much has been reported on the use of the ultrasound/color flow Doppler imaging appearance of an ovarian mass in predicting malignancy in older women (51–53). A solid ovarian mass in childhood is always viewed as malignant until proven otherwise by surgical removal. The differential diagnosis of solid tumors includes dysgerminoma, neuroblastoma, Wilms' tumor, rhabdomyosarcoma, lymphoma, leukemia, or other nongenital tumors. For large tumors or those suspected of being malignant, additional information can be obtained with the use of computed tomography (CT) or magnetic resonance (MR) imaging to evaluate the tumor and identify liver or lung metastases (37,54,55).

Tumor Markers

Some ovarian neoplasms secrete protein tumor markers that can be assayed from peripheral blood samples (Table 4). These tumor markers are helpful in making a diagnosis of an ovarian tumor and in following clinical response and possible recurrences (56). α-Fetoprotein (AFP) is an oncofetal antigen that is a glycoprotein. It is produced by endodermal sinus tumors, mixed germ cell tumors, and immature teratomas (57,58). Lactate dehydrogenase (LDH) is found

TABLE 4. *Serum tumor markers*

Marker	Associated tumor
CA 125	Epithelial tumors (especially serous) Immature teratoma (rare)
α-Fetoprotein	Endodermal sinus tumors Embryonal carcinomas Mixed germ cell tumors Immature teratoma (rare) Polyembryoma (rare)
Human chorionic gonadotropin	Choriocarcinoma Embryonal carcinomas Mixed germ cell tumors Polyembryoma Dysgerminoma (rare)
Carcinoembryonic antigen	Serous tumors Mucinous tumors
Lactate dehydrogenase	Dysgerminoma Mixed germ cell tumors
Estradiol	Thecomas Adult granulosa cell tumors
Testosterone	Sertoli cell tumors Leydig (hilus) cell tumors
F9 embryoglycan	Embryonal carcinoma Yolk sac tumor Choriocarcinoma Immature teratoma
Inhibin	Granulosa-theca cell tumor
Müllerian inhibiting substance	Granulosa-theca cell tumor

to be elevated in cases of dysgerminoma (59). CA 125, a marker for epithelial ovarian cancer (60), is highly sensitive but not very specific; it will be elevated with many intraperitoneal processes, such as endometriosis, pelvic inflammatory disease, pregnancy, Crohn's disease, and other abdominal malignancies (61). Human chorionic gonadotropin (hCG) is produced by trophoblastic cells and thus will be elevated with pregnancy, hydatidiform moles, placental site tumors, choriocarcinoma, and embryonal ovarian carcinomas. Carcinoembryonic antigen (CEA) can be produced by epithelial and germ cell tumors. A human antibody against an embryoglycan present on the mouse teratocarcinoma cell line F9 (F9 embryoglycan) has been identified in the sera of patients with embryonal carcinoma, yolk sac tumor, choriocarcinoma, and immature teratoma, but it has not been identified in patients with dysgerminoma or mature teratoma (62). Levels of inhibin and müllerian inhibiting substance have been shown to be elevated in children with granulosa-theca cell tumors (63,64).

TABLE 5. *International Federation of Gynecology and Obstetrics (FIGO) staging of carcinoma of the ovary*

Staging of ovarian carcinoma is based on findings at clinical examination and by surgical exploration. The histologic findings are to be considered in the staging, as are the cytologic findings as far as effusions are concerned. It is desirable that a biopsy be taken from suspicious areas outside of the pelvis.

Stage I	Growth limited to the ovaries
Stage IA	Growth limited to one ovary; no ascites present containing malignant cells. No tumor on the external surface; capsule intact
Stage IB	Growth limited to both ovaries; no ascites present containing malignant cells. No tumor on the external surfaces; capsules intact
Stage IC[a]	Tumor classified as either stage IA or IB but with tumor on the surface of one or both ovaries; or with ruptured capsule(s); or with ascites containing malignant cells present; or with positive peritoneal washings
Stage II	Growth involving one or both ovaries, with pelvic extension
Stage IIA	Extension and/or metastases to the uterus and/or tubes
Stage IIB	Extension to other pelvic tissues
Stage IIC[a]	Tumor either stage IIA or IIB but with tumor on the surface of one or both ovaries; or with capsule(s) ruptured; or with ascites containing malignant cells present; or with positive peritoneal washings
Stage III	Tumor involving one or both ovaries with peritoneal implants outside the pelvis and/or positive retroperitoneal or inguinal nodes. Superficial liver metastasis equals stage III. Tumor is limited to the true pelvis but with histologically proven malignant extension to small bowel or omentum
Stage IIIA	Tumor grossly limited to the true pelvis with negative nodes but with histologically confirmed microscopic seeding of abdominal peritoneal surfaces
Stage IIIB	Tumor of one or both ovaries with histologically confirmed implants of abdominal peritoneal surfaces, none >2 cm in diameter; nodes are negative
Stage IIIC	Abdominal implants >2 cm in diameter and/or positive retroperitoneal or inguinal nodes
Stage IV	Growth involving one or both ovaries, with distant metastases. If pleural effusion is present, there must be positive cytologic findings to allot a case to stage IV. Parenchymal liver metastasis equals stage IV.

[a]To evaluate the impact on prognosis of the different criteria for allotting cases to stage IC or IIC, it would be of value to know whether the rupture of the capsule was spontaneous or caused by the surgeon and if the source of malignant cells detected was peritoneal washings or ascites.

(Adapted from International Federation of Gynecology and Obstetrics (FIGO) Cancer Committee. Staging announcement. *Gynecol Oncol* 1986;25:303; FIGO. Changes in definitions of clinical staging for carcinoma of the cervix and ovary. *Am J Obstet Gynecol* 1987;156:263–264; Creasman WT. Changes in FIGO staging. *Obstet Gynecol* 1987;70:138; FIGO. Annual report on the results of treatment in gynecological cancer. *Int J Gynaecol Obstet* 1989;28:189–190; Creasman WT. New gynecologic cancer staging. *Obstet Gynecol* 1990;75:287–288; and FIGO. Changes in gynecologic cancer staging by the International Federation of Gynecology and Obstetrics. *Am J Obstet Gynecol* 1990;162:610; with permission.)

Staging

The staging of malignant ovarian tumors has been defined by the International Federation of Gynecology and Obstetrics (FIGO) (Tables 5 and 6) (65–70). This staging system standardizes nomenclature of ovarian malignancies for defining appropriate surgery and cytotoxic therapy and comparing outcome on the basis of clinical staging. The modified FIGO staging for germ cell tumors results in a significantly different grouping of patients, most notably that stage IC patients in the initial FIGO staging are now classified as stage III by the modified classification.

Surgery

Surgical intervention should aim, whenever possible, at preservation of reproductive potential. Unless a malignancy is diagnosed on frozen section at the time of the procedure, conservative surgery should be undertaken with excision of the lesion and ovarian reconstruction or unilateral salpingo-oophorectomy. It is preferable to subject the patient to a second procedure after the final pathology specimens are reviewed rather than perform unnecessary ablative procedures. If, however, malignancy is found or suspected, adequate staging, including abdominal and pelvic exploration, peritoneal washings, biopsies of suspicious areas, and periaortic and pelvic lymph node sampling, is crucial. Pathologic consultation may be invaluable in determining the exact diagnosis, so that appropriate therapy can be undertaken postoperatively, especially since advances in effective adjuvant chemotherapy for many ovarian tumors have improved the prognosis of many patients.

TABLE 6. *Modified FIGO staging classification for germ cell tumors*

Stage	Extent of disease
I	Limited to ovary, peritoneal washings negative for malignant cells; no clinical, radiographic, or histologic evidence of disease beyond the ovaries. The presence of gliomatosis peritonei does not result in changing stage I disease to a higher stage. Tumor markers normal after appropriate half-life decline
II	Microscopic residual or positive lymph nodes <2 cm; peritoneal washings negative for malignant cells. The presence of gliomatosis peritonei does not result in changing stage II disease to a higher stage; tumor markers positive or negative
III	Lymph node involvement (metastatic nodule) >2 cm; gross residual or biopsy only; contiguous visceral involvement (omentum, intestine, bladder); peritoneal washings positive for malignant cells; tumor markers positive or negative
IV	Distant metastases, including liver

(Adapted from International Federation of Gynecology and Obstetrics (FIGO) Cancer Committee. Staging announcement. *Gynecol Oncol* 1986;25:303; FIGO. Changes in definitions of clinical staging for carcinoma of the cervix and ovary. *Am J Obstet Gynecol* 1987;156:263–264; Creasman WT. Changes in FIGO staging. *Obstet Gynecol* 1987;70:138; FIGO. Annual report on the results of treatment in gynecological cancer. *Int J Gynaecol Obstet* 1989;28:189–190; Creasman WT. New gynecologic cancer staging. *Obstet Gynecol* 1990;75:287–288; and FIGO. Changes in gynecologic cancer staging by the International Federation of Gynecology and Obstetrics. *Am J Obstet Gynecol* 1990;162:610; with permission.)

SPECIFIC BENIGN AND MALIGNANT OVARIAN TUMORS/NEOPLASMS

Endometriosis

Endometriosis is discussed in detail in Chapter 9, where it is noted that in the ovary large endometrial cysts may develop, so-called endometriomas or "chocolate cysts." Since endometrial tissue is dependent on hormones for growth, the ovary is an optimal site and is in fact the most common single site of endometriosis in adults (71). Endometriosis within the ovary is much less common in adolescents and may represent disease progression. Ultrasound may be helpful in identifying an ovarian endometrioma (72). As noted in Chapter 9, endometriomas do not adequately respond to hormonal therapy and thus require surgical intervention. The use of laparotomy to treat endometriosis is decreasing as laparoscopic surgeons become more experienced. Endometriomas encountered in adolescent patients can safely be removed through the laparoscope (Fig. 5A). Adequate endometrioma surgery requires excision, including resection of the endometrioma's cyst wall (Fig. 5B and C)

Germ Cell Tumors

Germ cell tumors are the most common ovarian tumor in childhood and adolescence. This diverse group of tumors is derived from germ cells (Fig. 6) (73)

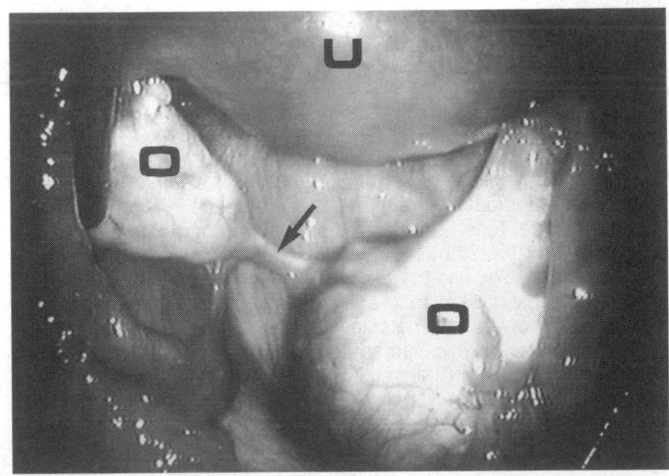

FIG. 5. (A) Laparoscopic view of the pelvis of a young woman with pelvic pain in whom a non-resolving, 4-cm right ovarian endometrioma was identified on ultrasound. Note the abnormal dense adhesion between the right and left ovaries *(arrow)*. This woman had previous surgery for a left ovarian dermoid cyst.

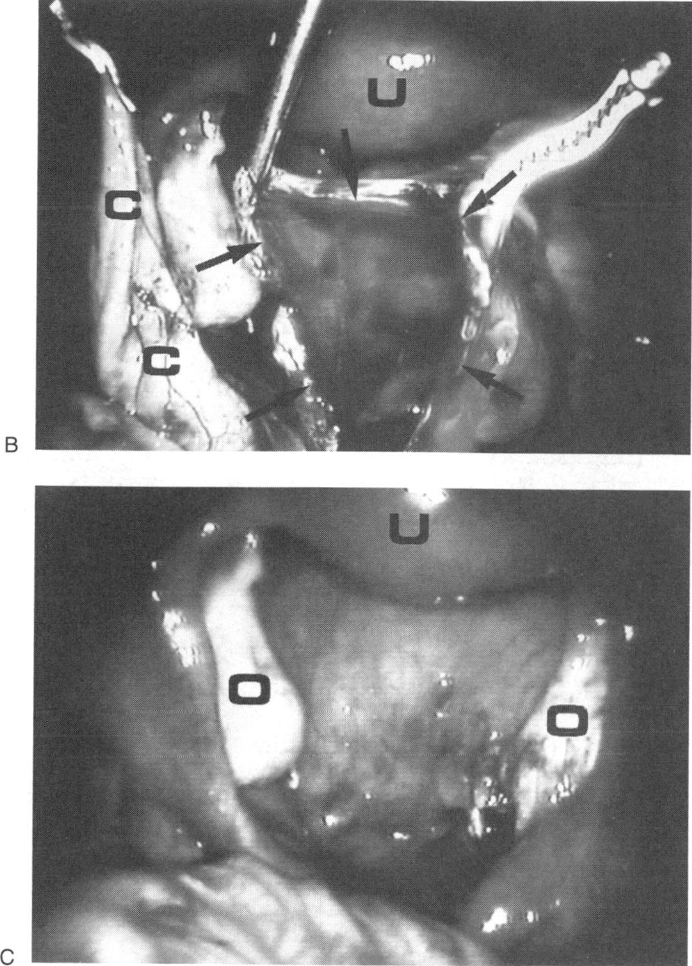

FIG. 5. *Continued* **(B)** After lysis of the adhesion, a right ovarian cystectomy of a 4-cm endometrioma has been performed. *Arrows* identify the edges of normal ovarian cortex remaining after the ovarian cystectomy. The endometrioma cyst wall has been removed from within the ovary and is now ready for removal from the intraperitoneal cavity. **(C)** View of patient after lysis of adhesions and ovarian cystectomy. C, cyst wall; O, ovary; U, uterus.

and includes both embryonic and extraembryonic tumors. The benign germ cell tumors include gonadoblastoma and teratoma; the malignant germ cell tumors include dysgerminoma, mixed germ cell tumor, endodermal sinus tumor, immature teratoma, embryonal tumor, choriocarcinoma, and polyembryoma.

Gonadoblastoma is a rare tumor composed of germ cells mixed with sex cord derivatives (74). Scully (75) regarded them as a type of *in situ* cancer from

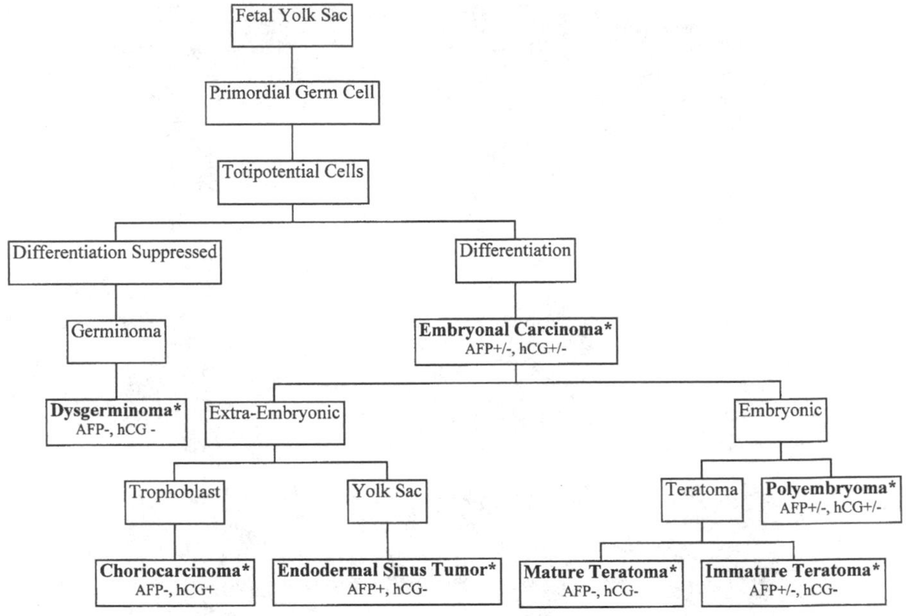

FIG. 6. Germ cell tumor derivation. AFP, α-fetoprotein; hCG, human chorionic gonadotropin. (Adapted from Teilum G. Classification of endodermal sinus tumour (mesoblastoma vitellinum) and so-called embryonal carcinoma of the ovary. *Acta Pathol Microbiol Scand* 1965;64:407; with permission.)

which a malignant germ cell tumor such as dysgerminoma can develop. Although this tumor is benign, it is associated with a malignant germ cell tumor (dysgerminoma) in approximately 25% to 50% of cases (76). Gonadoblastoma is almost always found in patients with gonadal dysgenesis associated with a Y chromosome or a Y-chromosomal fragment. Thus, if a Y chromosome or antigen is identified, the risk that patients who have this tumor will develop a malignancy is sufficiently high to require prophylactic bilateral gonadectomy. The exception to the need for immediate gonadectomy is the androgen insensitivity syndrome (AIS) (testicular feminization), in which the gonads should remain *in situ* until after puberty to allow normal secondary sexual development; the risk of a malignancy developing from a gonadoblastoma in this case is low prior to the completion of the development of secondary sexual characteristics. Thus, in the case of AIS, the gonads are removed once breast development is complete. In cases of gonadal dysgenesis, the gonads appear as streaks as shown in Color Plate 32. Bilateral gonadectomy can be accomplished by either conventional laparotomy or laparoscopy (77–79); the best approach (laparoscopy vs. laparotomy) is controversial and not yet determined. It is known that germ cells can be present in the upper area of the infundibulopelvic ligament, and thus if a laparoscopic procedure is performed, there is a risk of persistence of gonadal tissue. In either approach, we recommend that frozen sections should be performed to determine whether residual gonadal tissue is present at the upper border of resection. At this time, we are currently recommending the more conservative laparotomy approach.

The most common germ cell tumor is the *benign cystic teratoma,* more commonly known as a *dermoid cyst.* Dermoid cysts are mature cystic teratomas and are benign by definition; the malignant potential of teratomas (immature teratomas) is related to the histologic differentiation of the cells. Dermoid cysts are bilateral in 10% to 25% of cases in adults and 0% to 9% of those reported in children (7% of those in a series at Children's Hospital, Boston [5]). Patients may present with abdominal pain or nausea or may be asymptomatic. Due to the weight of the dermoid contents, the ovary is at increased risk of torsion, and thus the patient may present with symptoms of torsion (see Chapter 9). An adnexal mass is often palpated on physical examination. Plain X-ray studies of the pelvis and abdomen may reveal a calcification in the pelvis. Ultrasonography can identify an ovarian mass as consistent with a dermoid cyst (Fig. 7A) due to the presence of thick sebaceous fluid, hair, and calcium (80,81). The contralateral ovary should also be examined carefully by ultrasound to exclude bilateral disease (82). As dermoid cysts are germ cell tumors, they will not resolve spontaneously and thus require surgical intervention. Optimal treatment should preserve reproductive function, and thus there is much controversy of professional opinion as to the appropriate surgical approach (laparoscopy vs. laparotomy) (83). The endoscopic approach may be ideal with many of these tumors to shorten hospital length of stay, improve cosmetic results (smaller incisions), and decrease overall cost; however, the risk of spillage of the cyst fluid may result in a chemical peritonitis with resulting adhesion formation and possible infertility (83). On the other hand, laparoscopic surgery itself may have a decreased risk of adhesion formation as compared to laparotomy (84,85). Due to the risk of spillage of cyst contents and the possible adverse effect on reproductive function, some surgeons recommend a minilaparotomy approach to these lesions. In addition, there is the possibility that what was thought to be a benign lesion is in fact a malignancy and that the tumor cells are spread intraperitoneally with spillage of the cyst contents (86,87). It is our practice to present the risks and benefits of each surgical approach to each patient and her parents in order to make an appropriate individual surgical plan. With either surgical approach, the dermoid cyst is excised and the remaining normal ovary salvaged (Fig. 7B and C). Historically, it was recommended to bivalve the contralateral ovary in order to identify possible bilateral disease, but now with the

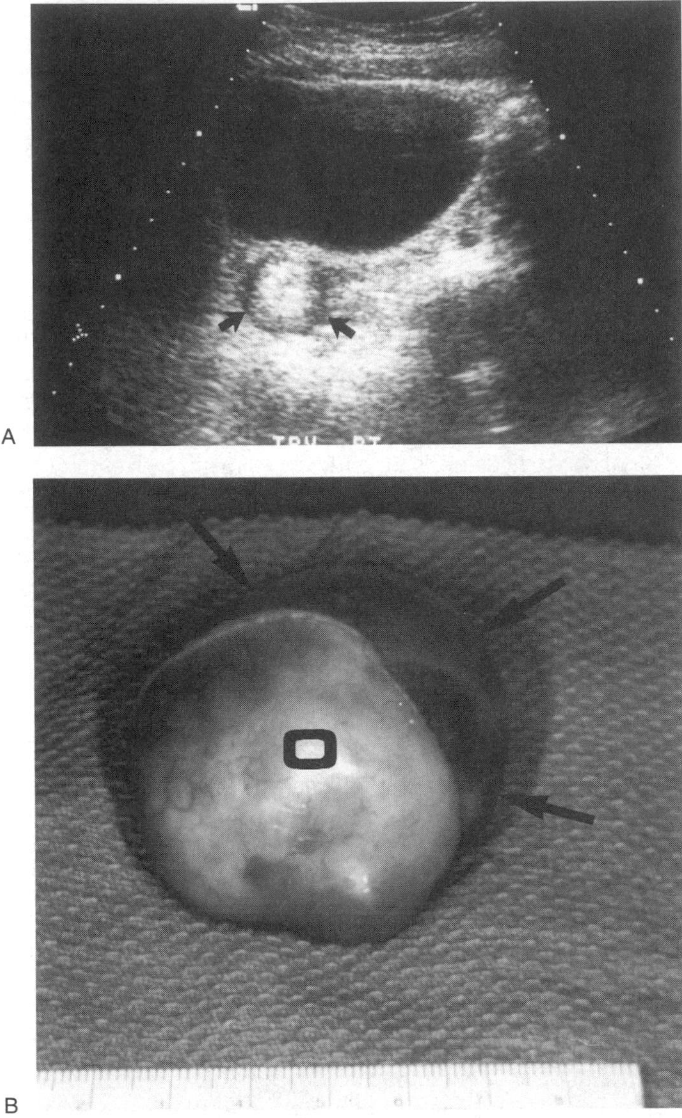

FIG. 7. (A) Ultrasound shows a dermoid cyst in a young woman with pelvic pain and a palpable ovarian mass; *arrows* mark the edges of the cyst. (Courtesy of Carol Barnewolt, M.D., Children's Hospital, Boston, MA.) **(B)** The cyst is removed intact through a minilaparotomy incision. *Arrows* indicate the edges of the cyst; note the thin layer of ovarian cortex that remains on its surface.

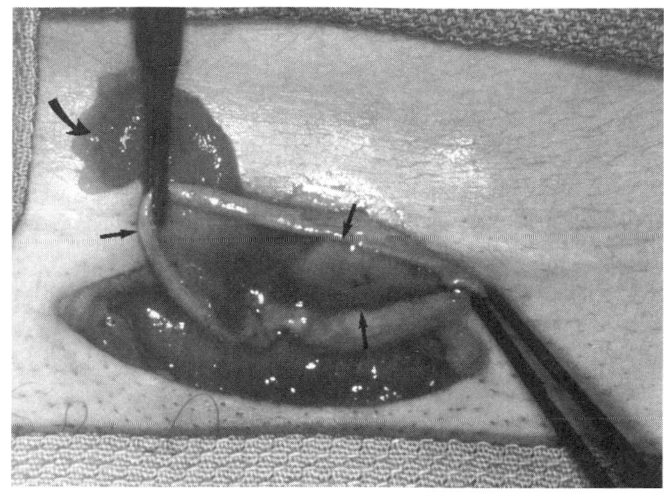

C

FIG. 7. *Continued* **(C)** After ovarian cystectomy, note the thin normal ovarian cortex that remains *(small arrows)* and the fimbriated end of the fallopian tube *(larger curved arrow).*

use of preoperative ultrasound and careful inspection of the ovary intraoperatively, routine bivalving of the opposite ovary is no longer necessary.

Functional teratomas are those that are hormonally active. When thyroid tissue is present, the term *struma ovarii* is applied. This condition is extremely rare, but when it does occur, thyrotoxicosis may develop. Carcinoid tumors can also occur in functional teratomas.

The younger the patient is, the more likely it is that the teratoma will be of the immature germ cell type, so-called *immature teratoma* (5). Patients present with abdominal pain, complaint of an abdominal mass, or nausea/vomiting. A mass may be palpable on abdominal (Fig. 8) or pelvic examination. Abdominal symptoms may occur acutely due to torsion or rupture of the tumor. MR imaging (Fig. 9) or CT may be helpful in further evaluation of the tumor and assessment for liver or lung metastases. Although levels of tumor markers such as AFP and hCG are usually negative or slightly elevated, they should be measured preoperatively (see Table 4) (57,58).

Management in our institution involves preoperative imaging, testing for serum tumor markers, and a consultation with a pediatric oncologist. The surgical approach is a vertical midline skin incision, with standard staging procedure for ovarian cancer. After the pelvic washings, a unilateral salpingo-oophorectomy, distal omentectomy, and Papanicolaou smear of the diaphragm, pelvic, and periaortic lymph node sampling is performed by the gynecologist or a pediatric surgeon (Fig. 10). The malignancy is staged according to the modified FIGO

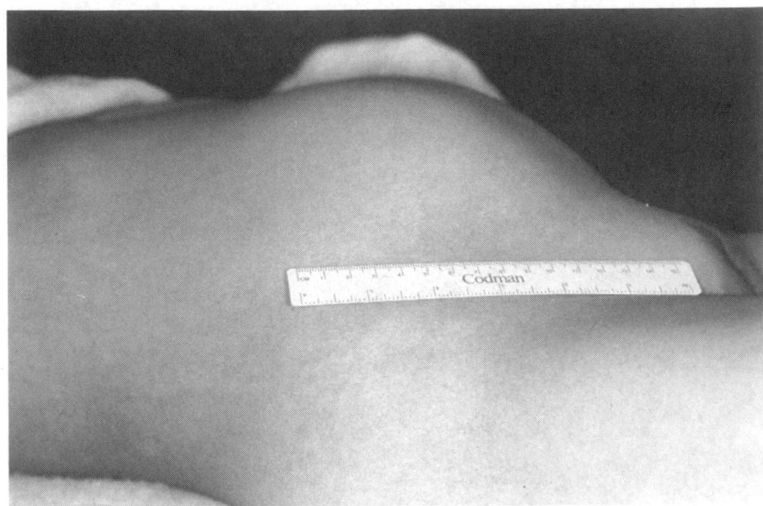

FIG. 8. A 12-year-old presented with vomiting, increasing abdominal girth, and a palpable abdominal mass. It was notable that the upper edge of the mass was not palpable as it extended under the rib cage.

staging classification for germ cell tumors (Table 6). Immature teratomas are graded based on a histology grading system (Table 7) (88), with grade 1 being the most differentiated (with the least risk of malignancy) and grade 3 being the least differentiated (with the greatest malignant potential). The immature component considered most important for grading is the neural component. Peritoneal implantation of mature glial tissue (gliomatosis peritonei) is thought to be

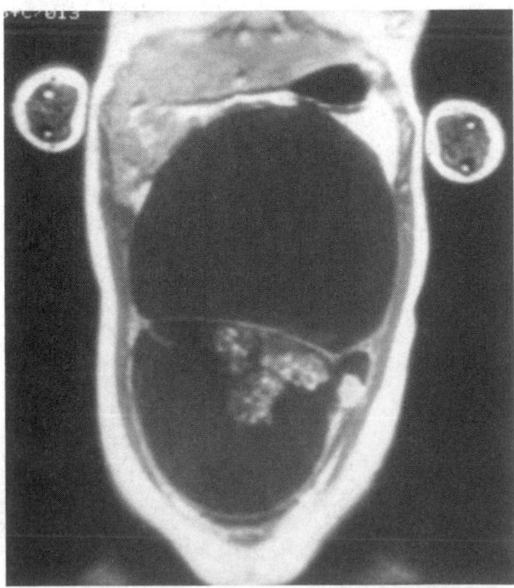

FIG. 9. MR image of the patient shown in Fig. 8. (Courtesy of Carol Barnewolt, M.D., Children's Hospital, Boston, MA.)

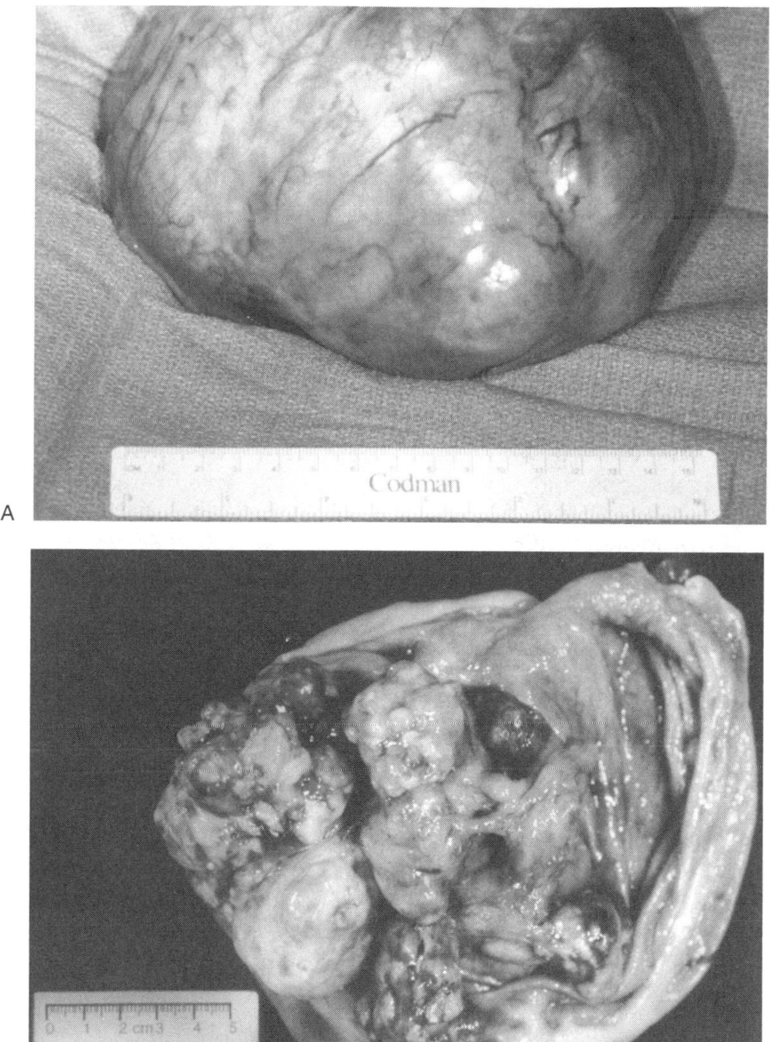

FIG. 10. (A, B) Gross pathology of a large ovarian mass (immature teratoma) removed from a 9-year-old girl with increasing abdominal girth and a palpable abdominal mass.

a separate and distinct entity, does not represent malignant spread, and, if present, does not change the stage of the tumor (89,90). The grade and stage of the disease are determined by the final pathologic evaluation. Tumor size, stage, and histologic grade are factors in predicting survival (88,91–93). In the Air Force study of 1972 (94), all patients with tumors <10 cm at greatest dimension survived regardless of stage or grade. The survival rate fell to 67% for tumors 10 to 19.9 cm and to 54% for tumors >20 cm. With pure immature teratomas, it has

TABLE 7. *Grading of immature ovarian teratomas*

Grade 0	All tissues mature; no mitotic activity
Grade 1	Some immaturity but with neuroepithelium absent or limited to one low-magnification field; no more than one focus in a slide
Grade 2	Immaturity present; neuroepithelium common but no more than three low-power microscopic fields in one slide
Grade 3	Immaturity and neuroectoderm prominent; no more than four low-power fields per section

[From Norris HJ, Zirkin HJ, Benson WL. Immature (malignant) teratoma of the ovary: a clinical and pathologic study of 58 cases. *Cancer* 1976;37:2359–2372; with permission.]

been observed that 5-year survival is based on stage (74% survival for all grades of stage I and 38% survival for stages II and III) and histologic grade (grade I, 81%; grade II, 60%; grade III, 30%) (88,92). Chromosomal analysis of the tumor suggests that immature ovarian teratomas of premeiotic origin show a greater malignant potential (95) and deviations in karyotype suggest a worse prognosis (96,97).

The current recommended therapy for immature teratomas is evolving. If a serum tumor marker is positive, it can be followed pre- and postoperatively to detect treatment response and early recurrence. In numerous reports, unilateral salpingo-oophorectomy appeared adequate for treatment of stage I grade 1 or 2 tumors (98–101). The prognosis for patients with higher stages has improved significantly in the last 15 years with the use of adjuvant chemotherapy (5,44, 102,103). Most trials utilizing chemotherapy use a multiagent approach (Table 8) (90,91,98–101,104,105). For those patients treated only with surgery who have a recurrence, the response to chemotherapy is excellent (90). In a report of 10 years' experience of 32 prospectively treated patients with pure immature teratoma, 30 patients had fertility-sparing surgery and were treated with chemotherapy only if they had stage I or II grade 3 or stage III disease; 10 patients who were initially treated with surgery alone relapsed and were treated

TABLE 8. *Examples of multiagent combination chemotherapy regimens (given in cycles intravenously every 3–4 weeks)*[a]

VAC	Vincristine Actinomycin Cyclophosphamide
PVB	Cisplatin Vinblastine Bleomycin
BEP	Cisplatin Etoposide Bleomycin
EP	Etoposide Cisplatin

[a]These regimens are provided as informational background; specific chemotherapy and dosages for individual patients should be determined by a medical or gynecologic oncologist.

with chemotherapy (90). At the time of the report, all patients were alive. Long-term followup studies of patients with malignant germ cell tumors report that the majority have normal menstrual function and a reasonable probability of having normal reproductive outcomes (106,107).

Dysgerminoma

Dysgerminoma is a malignant tumor derived from the primordial, sexually undifferentiated germ cells (see Fig. 6). In the Children's Hospital series, the average age of patients was 14 years (range, 6.5 to 21 years) (5). Dysgerminoma has the same histology as seminoma in males. As mentioned above, it can occur in phenotypic females with abnormal karyotypes (46,XY) and abnormal gonads containing gonadoblastomas (76). Several cases of dysgerminoma have also been reported in girls with Turner's syndrome, one of whom had male-specific sequences of the Y chromosome detected by DNA probes (108). The symptoms and signs associated with the tumor are similar to those discussed for other germ cell tumors. Rarely (2%), a pure dysgerminoma will contain syncytiotrophoblastic cells and produce low levels of hCG (109). In many instances, tumor cells are mixed with other cell types that may also produce hCG. LDH is elevated in some patients with dysgerminoma, and the levels and the isoenzyme pattern (LDH-1 and LDH-2) may be useful in suggesting the diagnosis preoperatively, but data are needed on whether this enzyme has any useful role as a marker in postoperative followup (44,59,110). Other tumor markers such as AFP and CEA should be measured, although they are usually negative.

At surgery, the tumor appears grossly as a lobulated, solid, yellow-white mass. Most patients with dysgerminoma have stage I disease, and thus surgery alone is adequate for cure. The mass should be removed intact, and an adequate staging procedure performed. A conservative surgical approach with unilateral salpingo-oophorectomy is usually undertaken in young women with stage IA tumors (<10 cm, removed unruptured, without evidence of metastatic spread) (44). Approximately 8% to 15% of dysgerminomas are bilateral, and thus the contralateral ovary is closely inspected, and any suspicious areas are biopsied (111). If there is bilateral ovarian involvement, then the uterus can be left *in situ* for reproduction options with donor oocytes and assisted reproductive technologies. Since the spread of this tumor is usually lymphatic with early involvement of pelvic and paraaortic lymph nodes followed by mediastinal and supraclavicular nodes, ipsilateral pelvic and paraaortic lymph nodes should be sampled to adequately stage the patient. Staging is critical for determining therapy and prognosis. In addition, some studies have shown a benefit with chromosomal analysis of the tumor in that deviations in karyotype suggest a worse prognosis (97).

All patients with greater than stage I disease should undergo cytoreductive surgery with removal of all operable tumor, and require additional therapy (112).

The 10-year survival rates for patients with dysgerminoma confined to one ovary and treated with surgery alone was shown to be 92%; however, there was a 17% recurrence rate and a 6% mortality (111). The 5-year survival rate for patients with dysgerminoma confined to one or both ovaries is excellent (80% to 96%), and two-thirds of those with recurrences can be successfully treated later with radiation (5,44). Dysgerminoma is extremely radiosensitive; however, radiation therapy has adverse effects on reproductive endocrine function (see Chapter 19) and is reserved for cases of metastatic disease or recurrence (44,113). Because these tumors occur in young women and reproductive preservation is of great importance, multiagent chemotherapy (see Table 8) has replaced radiation therapy as the treatment of choice of advanced disease and appears promising in preserving reproductive potential (101,104,106,114,115). The 5-year survival of patients with dysgerminoma with extraovarian spread drops to 63%. Patients with advanced or bilateral disease should have abdominal hysterectomy, bilateral salpingo-oophorectomy, nodal biopsies, omental biopsy, and tumor debulking (44). A dysgerminoma with mixed elements of endodermal sinus tumor has an increased malignant potential and poorer prognosis.

Endodermal Sinus Tumor

Endodermal sinus tumor, also termed yolk sac tumor, is of extraembryonic germ cell origin (see Fig. 6). It is rare but in our series ranked second in frequency among germ cells tumors (5). The average age of our patients was 10 years (range, 18 months to 16 years), while other series have shown the average age at presentation to be 19 years (116,117). Endodermal sinus tumor is usually very aggressive, and patients usually seek medical attention rapidly due to abdominal pain (5). The serum tumor marker AFP can be useful during preoperative evaluation, as most of these tumors have a positive result, and can be used to follow the course of therapy. An unusual case of ataxia-telangiectasia and endodermal sinus tumor has been reported, emphasizing the association of both conditions with abnormal production of AFP (118). Yolk sac tumors are usually unilateral stage I (116,117), and thus appropriate surgery is a staging exploratory laparotomy with unilateral salpingo-oophorectomy. Intraperitoneal and hematogenous spread is common, while lymph node metastasis is unusual. The histology reveals Schiller-Duval bodies (a central capillary surrounded by simple papillary projections). Unlike dysgerminoma, these tumors are not radiosensitive (116,117), and prior to the use of multiagent chemotherapy they were usually fatal. Long-term outcomes have improved for patients with stage I tumor treated with unilateral salpingo-oophorectomy followed by aggressive chemotherapy (101,104–106,114,115,119–121). Based on the current results, it appears that conservative surgery for early-stage endodermal sinus tumor or conservative surgery with cytoreduction followed by multiagent chemotherapy is the best means to achieve complete remission and preserve reproductive function in young women.

Embryonal Carcinoma

Embryonal cell carcinoma (see Fig. 6) is a highly malignant and very rare germ cell tumor (122). In 60% of cases, the tumor is hormonally active and may produce precocious puberty in the child and menstrual irregularity or hirsutism in the adolescent (122). The markers AFP and hCG may be secreted by this tumor. It is rarely bilateral and tends to spread intraperitoneally. Standard staging laparotomy with unilateral salpingo-oophorectomy should be performed. Postoperative chemotherapy has been shown to be useful in reducing the likelihood of recurrence (119,121).

Polyembryoma

This is a very rare tumor of germ cell origin (see Fig. 6) that usually presents in premenarchal patients. Elevated levels of both AFP and hCG have been documented (123). Prognosis is poor, as chemotherapy has only rarely induced remission.

Choriocarcinoma

Pure ovarian choriocarcinoma may develop without an association with a gestation. Although rare, this is a very aggressive tumor. As with gestational choriocarcinoma, hCG is an accurate tumor marker (124). Multiagent chemotherapy (see Table 8) is used in the treatment after surgical resection and staging (1,2,44,101,104).

Mixed Germ Cell Tumors

A mixed germ cell tumor consists of two or more germ cell tumors and usually has a prognosis based on the "worst" cell element. These tumors usually present as stage I disease, and the mean age at presentation is 16 years (125). Tumor markers should be measured, since hCG, AFP, and sometimes LDH are elevated. Appropriate surgical therapy includes a staging laparotomy with unilateral salpingo-oophorectomy. Postoperative multiagent chemotherapy (see Table 8) is selected based on the pathologic elements identified (104,125,126).

Sex Cord–Stromal Tumors

Thecoma-fibroma is rare in the pediatric age group. Thecoma is uncommon before age 30. Fibromas account for <2% of all ovarian tumors of children and young women (127). Thecoma-fibroma is benign. Fibromas with ascites and pleural effusions (Meigs' syndrome) have been seen in children. Gorlin's syn-

TABLE 9. *Comparison of adult granulosa cell tumors (GCT) and juvenile GCT*

Adult GCT	Juvenile GCT
<1% prepubertal	50% prepubertal
Usual after age 30 years	Rare after age 30 years
Follicles usually regular, without mucin	Follicles often irregular, contain mucin
Call-Exner bodies common	Call-Exner bodies rare
Nuclei pale, commonly grooved	Nuclei dark, rarely grooved
Luteinization infrequent	Luteinization frequent
Recurrence rarely early, often very late	Recurrence typically early

(From Young RH, Dickersin GR, Scully RE. Juvenile granulosa cell tumor of the ovary: a clinicopathologic analysis of 125 cases. *Am J Surg Pathol* 1984;8:575–596; with permission.)

drome is an autosomal-dominant disorder consisting of ovarian fibroma, basal cell nevi, dental cysts, and skeletal abnormalities. A thecoma can be hormonally active and produce estrogen, although there is a report of a testosterone-producing thecoma (128). It is highly unusual for this tumor to be malignant.

Tumors of sex cord–stromal cell origin make up 10% to 20% of childhood ovarian tumors. Approximately one-half are hormonally active. Granulosa cell tumors are divided into adult and juvenile subtypes (Table 9) (129). Juvenile granulosa cell tumors secrete estrogen and in the young child may therefore produce pseudoprecocious puberty with breast enlargement and vaginal bleeding (130). In 2 of 10 patients in our series, pubic hair and clitoral enlargement were also noted (130). In the adolescent, these tumors may cause menstrual irregularities, including hypermenorrhea. Juvenile granulosa cell tumors have a more favorable prognosis than the typical adult tumor (5,44,129,130–133). Since <5% of tumors are bilateral, unilateral salpingo-oophorectomy with appropriate staging is usually adequate, since almost all children have stage IA tumors (5, 133,134). Call-Exner bodies are pathognomonic of the adult granulosa cell tumor but are rare in the juvenile type (129). Bilateral oophorectomy, chemotherapy, and/or radiation therapy have not been shown to improve outcome in patients with stage I disease (130). Postoperatively, estrogen levels and vaginal maturation index should return to normal prepubertal levels in young girls. Serum inhibin levels appear promising as a marker to reflect the size of the tumor and the presence of recurrent disease in adult women. Prognosis is excellent, with 84% to 92% survival. More advanced disease may be treated with chemotherapy (133).

Sertoli-Leydig Cell Tumors

Sertoli-Leydig cell tumor was previously termed androblastoma or arrhenoblastoma. In our pediatric series, the average age at diagnosis was 13 years (range, 5 to 17 years) (5). This tumor may secrete androgens and thus produce heterosexual precocity in young children and hirsutism or virilization in adolescents (135). Two adolescents have been reported to have elevated levels of serum AFP, which initially suggested endodermal sinus tumor but AFP returned to undetectable levels after surgery for Sertoli-Leydig cell tumor (136). Prognosis is dependent on the stage and degree of differentiation of the tumor; in most cases, it is a low-grade malignant tumor. Unilateral salpingo-oophorectomy and staging are important; prognosis is usually good.

Gynandroblastoma is a rare ovarian tumor consisting of both male and female sex cord cells. It may cause premature breast development in girls and either hyperestrogenism or hyperandrogenism in adolescents (137–139).

Sex cord tumors with annular tubules have been associated with Peutz-Jeghers syndrome (gastrointestinal polyposis and oral cutaneous pigmentation), a condition also associated with adenocarcinoma of the cervix (137) (see Chapter 19).

Common "Epithelial" (Coelomic) Tumors

Cystadenoma, an epithelial tumor filled with pseudomucinous (pseudomucinous cystadenoma) or cystic fluid (serous cystadenoma), accounts for 10% to 20% of ovarian tumors. In most cases, it is diagnosed after menarche, and the youngest patient in our series was 11.5 years old (5). Cystadenoma is usually benign, with about 7% being borderline and 4% malignant (140–143). Conservative surgery with unilateral salpingo-oophorectomy is appropriate for stage IA borderline tumors involving only one ovary (140–144). Biopsy of the contralateral ovary (with serous cystadenoma and if the ovary appears suspicious in mucinous cystadenoma) and staging are important. Careful and prolonged followup is essential since recurrences may appear many years later. Tumors of borderline malignancy have a more favorable prognosis than higher-grade carcinomas (140–144).

In the rare invasive tumor, patients with other than stage IA should be managed, in similar fashion to adult women, with a staging laparotomy, cytoreductive surgery, and multiagent chemotherapy (145).

Families have been identified with increased rates of epithelial ovarian and breast cancers; affected individuals have been found to have a deletion of chromosome 17 in the q21-q23 region suggestive of a tumor suppressor gene (146–148) (see Chapter 16). This finding of genetic abnormalities initially related to an increased risk of breast cancer has been named breast cancer gene-1 (BRCA-1). It has been suggested that this gene may be mutated in 1 in 800 American women. An estimated 5% of ovarian cancer before age 70 years is associated with mutations in BRCA-1 (150). Of those carrying the BRCA-1 mutation, the ovarian cancer risk has been estimated to be 26% to 85% by age 70 years (149,151), although a more recent analysis found a lower risk of 16% (152). The BRCA-1 frameshift gene mutation (185delAG) in Ashkenazic Jewish women is believed to occur at a carrier frequency of 1% and to account for approximately 39% of ovarian cancer cases occurring prior to age 50 years (153). Ovarian cancer developed in 20% of women of Ashkenazic descent with the 185delAG mutation, as compared with none of the Jewish women without the mutation (154). Provisional recommendations for women with BRCA-1 mutations, published in 1997, included annual or semiannual screening using transvaginal ultrasonography (ideally with color flow Doppler and a morphologic index) and serum CA 125 levels beginning at age 25 to 35 years. These recommendations have been based on expert opinion and thus the efficacy has not been proved (151).

Familial ovarian cancer centers currently exist in many locations throughout the world and provide families with genetic counseling and screening for both ovarian and breast cancer. Clinicians caring for adolescents will need to be involved in decision making with their patients to make the best use of the emerging genetic technology without increasing anxiety in these young women and their families.

Other Tumors

Lipid (lipoid) cell tumor is rare (155,156). Wentz and coworkers (157) reported a 17-year-old adolescent with hirsutism and oligomenorrhea in association with a lipid cell tumor.

Fibrosarcomas and undifferentiated sarcomas are rare and rapidly fatal.

Lymphoma may occur as a primary ovarian tumor (158), and other tumors may be metastatic to the ovary. Rarely, leukemia will relapse with ovarian enlargement simulating an ovarian tumor (94,159).

REFERENCES

1. Breen JL, Maxson WS. Ovarian tumors in children and adolescents. *Clin Obstet Gynecol* 1977;20:607.
2. Breen JL, Bonamo JF, Maxson WS. Genital tract tumors in children. *Pediatr Clin North Am* 1981; 28:355.
3. Serov SF, Scully RE, Sobin LH. *International histological classification of tumours. No. 9. Histologic typing of ovarian tumours.* Geneva: World Health Organization, 1973.
4. Rice LW, Barbieri RL. The ovary. In: Ryan RJ, Berkowitz RS, Barbieri RL, eds. *Kistner's gynecology,* 6th ed. Boston: Mosby-Year Book, 1995;187.
5. Lack EE, Goldstein DP. Primary ovarian tumors in childhood and adolescence. *Curr Probl Obstet Gynecol* 1984;8:1.
6. Diamond M, Baxter J, Peerman C, et al. Occurrence of ovarian malignancy in childhood and adolescence: a community-wide evaluation. *Obstet Gynecol* 1988;17:858.
7. DeSa DJ. Follicular ovarian cysts in stillborns and neonates. *Arch Dis Child* 1975;50:45.
8. Nussbaum AR, Sanders RC, Hartman DS, et al. Neonatal ovarian cysts: sonographic-pathologic correlation. *Radiology* 1988;168:817–821.
9. Lindeque BG, du Toit J, Muller LM, et al. Ultrasonographic criteria for the conservative management of antenatally diagnosed fetal ovarian cysts. *J Reprod Med* 1988;33:196.
10. Brandt ML, Luks FI, Filiatrault D, et al. Surgical indications in antenatally diagnosed ovarian cysts. *J Pediatr Surg* 1991;26:276.
11. Kirkinen P, Jouppila P. Perinatal aspects of pregnancy complicated by fetal ovarian cyst. *J Perinat Med* 1985;13:245.

12. Speroff L, Glass RH, Kase NG. *Clinical gynecologic endocrinology and infertility*, 5th ed. Philadelphia: Williams & Wilkins, 1994.
13. Case records of the Massachusetts General Hospital. *N Engl J Med* 1995;332:522.
14. Bower R, Dehner LP, Ternberg JL. Bilateral ovarian cysts in the newborn: a triad of neonatal abdominal masses, polyhydramnios, and maternal diabetes mellitus. *Am J Dis Child* 1974;128:731.
15. Nguyen KT, Reid RL, Sauerbrei E. Antenatal sonographic detection of a fetal theca lutein cyst: a clue to maternal diabetes mellitus. *J Ultrasound Med* 1986;5:665.
16. Spence JEH, Domingo M, Pike C. The resolution of fetal and neonatal ovarian cysts. *Adolesc Pediatr Gynecol* 1992;5:27
17. Murray S, London S. Management of ovarian cysts in neonates, children, and adolescents. *Adolesc Pediatr Gynecol* 1995;8:64.
18. Siegel M. Pediatric gynecologic sonography. *Radiology* 1991;179:593.
19. Landrum B, Ogburn PL, Feinberg S, et al. Intrauterine aspiration of a large fetal ovarian cyst. *Obstet Gynecol* 1986;68(suppl):11S.
20. Meizner I, Levy A, Katz M, et al. Fetal ovarian cysts: prenatal ultrasonographic detection and postnatal evaluation and treatment. *Am J Obstet Gynecol* 1991;164:874.
21. Teele RL, Share JC. The abdominal mass in the neonate. *Semin Roetgenol* 1988;23:175.
22. Croitoru DP, Aaton LE, Laberge JM, et al. Management of complex ovarian cysts presenting in the first year of life. *J Pediatr Surg* 1991;26:1366.
23. Mordehai A, Mares Y, Bakri R, et al. Torsion of uterine adnexa in neonates and children: a report of 20 cases. *J Pediatr Surg* 1991;26:1195.
24. Salkala E, Leon Z, Rouse G. Management of antenatally diagnosed fetal ovarian cysts. *Obstet Gynecol Surv* 1991;46:407.
25. Schultz R, Newton WA, Clatworthy HW. Torsion of previously normal tube and ovary in children. *N Engl J Med* 1963;268:343–346.
26. Worthington-Kirsch R, Raptopoulos V, Cohen I. Sequential bilateral torsion of normal ovaries in a child. *J Ultrasound Med* 1986;5:663.
27. Davis AJ, Feins NR. Subsequent asynchronous torsion of normal adnexa in children. *J Pediatr Surg* 1990;25:687.
28. Shalev E, Mann S, Romano S, et al. Laparoscopic detorsion of adnexa in childhood: a case report. *J Pediatr Surg* 1991;26:1193.
29. Cohen HL, Eisenberg P, Mandel F, et al. Ovarian cysts are common in premenarchal girls: a sonographic study of 101 children 2–12 years old. *AJR* 1992;159:89.
30. Cohen HL, Shapiro MA, Mandel FS, et al. Normal ovaries in neonates and infants: a sonographic study of 77 patients 1 day to 24 months. *AJR* 1993;160:583.
31. Kosloske AM, Goldthorn JF, Kaufman E, et al. Treatment of precocious pseudopuberty associated with follicular cysts of the ovary. *Am J Dis Child* 1984;138:147.
32. Chasalow FI, Granoff AB, Tse TF, et al. Adrenal steroid secretion in girls with pseudoprecocious puberty due to autonomous ovarian cysts. *J Clin Endocrinol Metab* 1986;63:828.
33. Freedman SM, Kreitzer PM, Elkowitz SS, et al. Ovarian microcysts in girls with isolated premature thelarche. *J Pediatr* 1993;122:246.
34. Millar DM, Blake JM, Stringer DA, et al. Prepubertal ovarian cyst formation: 5 years' experience. *Obstet Gynecol* 1993;81:434.
35. Frisch LS, Copeland KC, Boepple PA. Recurrent ovarian cysts in childhood: diagnosis of McCune-Albright syndrome by bone scan. *Pediatrics* 1992;90:102.
36. Arisaka O, Shimura N, Nakayama Y, et al. Ovarian cysts in precocious puberty. *Clin Pediatr* 1989; 28:44.
37. Van Winter JT, Simmons PS, Podratz KC. Surgically treated adnexal masses in infancy, childhood, and adolescence. *Am J Obstet Gynecol* 1994;170:1780.
38. Gordon JD, Hopkins KL, Jeffrey RB, Giudice LC. Adnexal torsion: color Doppler diagnosis and laparoscopic treatment. *Fertil Steril* 1994;61:383.
39. Mage G, Canis M, Manhes H, et al. Laparoscopic management of adnexal torsion: a review of 35 cases. *J Reprod Med* 1989;34:520.
40. Shalev E, Peleg D. Laparoscopic treatment of adnexal torsion. *Surg Gynecol Obstet* 1993;176:448.
41. Laufer MR, Billett A, Diller L et al. A new technique for laparoscopic prophylactic oophoropexy prior to craniospinal irradiation in children with medulloblastoma. *Adolesc Pediatr Gynecol* 1995;8:77.
42. Warner B, Kuhn J, Barr L. Conservative management of large ovarian cysts in children: the value of serial pelvic ultrasonography. *Surgery* 1992;112:749.

43. Thind CR, Carty HM, Pilling D. The role of ultrasound in the management of ovarian masses in children. *Clin Radiol* 1989;40:180.
44. Kennedy AW. Ovarian neoplasms in childhood and adolescence. *Semin Reprod Endocrinol* 1988; 6:79.
45. Goldstein DP, deCholnoky C, Emans SJ, et al. Laparoscopy in the diagnosis and management of pelvic pain in adolescents. *J Reprod Med* 1980;24:251.
46. Mettler L, Irani S, Semm K. Ovarian surgery via pelviscopy. *J Reprod Med* 1993;38:130.
47. Lipitz S, Seidman DS, Menczer J, et al. Recurrence rates after fluid aspiration from sonographically benign-appearing ovarian cysts. *J Reprod Med* 1992;37:845.
48. Wilson DA. Ultrasound screening for abdominal masses in the neonatal period. *Am J Dis Child* 1982;136:147.
49. Wu A, Siegel MJ. Sonography of pelvic masses in children: diagnostic predictability. *AJR* 1987; 148:1199.
50. Fleischer AC. Transabdominal and transvaginal sonography of ovarian masses. *Clin Obstet Gynecol* 1991;34:433.
51. Kawai M, Kano T, Kikkawa F, et al. Transvaginal Doppler ultrasound with color flow imaging in the diagnosis of ovarian cancer. *Obstet Gynecol* 1992;79:163.
52. Weiner Z, Thaler I, Beck D, et al. Differentiating malignant from benign ovarian tumors with transvaginal color flow imaging. *Obstet Gynecol* 1992;79:159.
53. Timor-Tritsch IE, Lerner JP, Monteagudo A, et al. Transvaginal ultrasonographic characterization of ovarian masses by means of color flow-directed Doppler measurements and a morphologic scoring system. *Am J Obstet Gynecol* 1993;168:909.
54. Fedele L, Dorta M, Brioschi D, et al. Magnetic resonance evaluation of gynecologic masses in adolescents. *Adolesc Pediatr Gynecol* 1990;3:83.
55. Scoutt LM, McCarthy SM. Imaging of ovarian masses: magnetic resonance imaging. *Clin Obstet Gynecol* 1991;34:443.
56. Schwartz PE. Ovarian masses: serologic markers. *Clin Obstet Gynecol* 1991;34:423.
57. Perrone T, Steeper T, Dehner L. Alpha-fetoprotein localization in pure ovarian teratoma: an immunohistochemical study of 12 cases. *Am J Clin Pathol* 1987;88:713.
58. Kawai M, Furuhashi Y, Kano T, et al. Alpha-fetoprotein in malignant germ cell tumors of the ovary. *Gynecol Oncol* 1990;39:160.
59. Schwartz PE, Morris JMcL. Serum lactic dehydrogenase: a tumor marker for dysgerminoma. *Obstet Gynecol* 1989;32:191.
60. Bast RC, Klug TL, St. John E, et al. A radioimmunoassay using a monoclonal antibody to monitor the course of epithelial ovarian cancer. *N Engl J Med* 1983;309:883.
61. Rubal A, Encabo G, et al. CA-125 serum levels in non-malignant pathologies. *Bull Cancer (Paris)* 1988;71:751.
62. Kawata M, Sekiya S, Tamkamizawa H, et al. Molecular properties of F9 embryoglycan recognized by a unique antibody in sera from patients with germ cell tumors. *Cancer Res* 1987;47:2288.
63. Gustafson ML, Lee MM, Scully RE, et al. Müllerian inhibitory substance as a marker for ovarian sex cord tumor. *N Engl J Med* 1992;326:466.
64. Lappohn RE, Burger HG, Bouma J, et al. Inhibin as a marker for granulosa cell tumor. *Acta Obstet Gynecol Scand Suppl* 1992;155:61.
65. International Federation of Gynecology and Obstetrics (FIGO) Cancer Committee. Staging announcement. *Gynecol Oncol* 1986;25:303.
66. International Federation of Gynecology and Obstetrics (FIGO). Changes in definitions of clinical staging for carcinoma of the cervix and ovary. *Am J Obstet Gynecol* 1987;156:263.
67. Creasman WT. Changes in FIGO staging. *Obstet Gynecol* 1987;70:138.
68. International Federation of Gynecology and Obstetrics (FIGO). Annual report on the results of treatment in gynecological cancer. *Int J Gynaecol Obstet* 1989;28:189.
69. Creasman WT. New gynecologic cancer staging. *Obstet Gynecol* 1990;75:287.
70. International Federation of Gynecology and Obstetrics (FIGO). Changes in gynecologic cancer staging by the International Federation of Gynecology and Obstetrics. *Am J Obstet Gynecol* 1990; 162:610.
71. Jenkins S, Olive DL, Haney AF. Endometriosis: pathogenetic implications of the anatomic distribution. *Obstet Gynecol* 1986;67:335.
72. Mais V, Guerriero S, Ajossa S, et al. The efficiency of transvaginal ultrasonography in the diagnosis of endometrioma. *Fertil Steril* 1993;60:776.

73. Teilum G. Classification of endodermal sinus tumour (mesoblastoma vitellinum) and so-called embryonal carcinoma of the ovary. *Acta Pathol Microbiol Scand* 1965;64:407.
74. Scully RE. Gonadoblastoma: gonadal tumor related to dysgerminoma (seminoma) and capable of sex hormone production. *Cancer* 1953;6:455.
75. Scully RE. Gonadoblastoma: a review of 74 cases. *Cancer* 1970;25:1340.
76. Trochir V, Hernandez E. Neoplasia arising in dysgenetic gonads. *Obstet Gynecol Surv* 1988;41:74.
77. Droesch K, Droesch J, Chumas J, et al. Laparoscopic gonadectomy for gonadal dysgenesis. *Fertil Steril* 1990;53:360.
78. Shalev E, Zabari A, Romano S, et al. Laparoscopic gonadectomy in 46,XY female patient. *Fertil Steril* 1992;57:459.
79. Arici A, Kutteh WH, Chantilis SJ, et al. Laparoscopic removal of gonads in women with abnormal karyotypes. *J Reprod Med* 1993;38:521.
80. Sisler CL, Siegel MJ. Ovarian teratomas: a comparison of the sonographic appearance in prepubertal and postpubertal girls. *AJR* 1990;154:139.
81. Mais V, Guerriero S, Ajossa S, et al. Transvaginal ultrasonography in the diagnosis of cystic teratoma. *Obstet Gynecol* 1995;85:48.
82. Ayhan A, Aksu T, Develioglu O, et al. Complications and bilaterality of mature ovarian teratomas (clinicopathological evaluation of 286 cases). *Aust N Z J Obstet Gynaecol* 1991;31:83.
83. Howard FM. Surgical management of benign cystic teratoma: laparoscopy vs. laparotomy. *J Reprod Med* 1995;40:495.
84. Nezhat CR, Nezhat FR, Metzger DA, et al. Adhesion reformation after reproductive surgery by videolaseroscopy. *Fertil Steril* 1990;53:1008.
85. Operative Laparoscopy Study Group. Postoperative adhesion development after operative laparoscopy: evaluation at early second-look procedures. *Fertil Steril* 1991;55:700.
86. Maiman M, Seltzer V, Boyce J. Laparoscopic excision of ovarian neoplasms subsequently found to be malignant. *Obstet Gynecol* 1991;77:563.
87. Nezhat F, Nezhat C, et al. Four ovarian cancers diagnosed during laparoscopic management of 1011 women with adnexal masses. *Am J Obstet Gynecol* 1992;167:790.
88. Norris HJ, Zirkin HJ, Benson WL. Immature (malignant) teratoma of the ovary: a clinical and pathologic study of 58 cases. *Cancer* 1976;37:2359.
89. Nielsen SNJ, Scheithauer BW, Gaffey TA. Gliomatosis peritonei. *Cancer* 1985;56:2499.
90. Bonazzi C, Peccatori F, Colombo N, et al. Pure ovarian immature teratoma, a unique and curable disease: 10 years' experience of 32 prospectively treated patients. *Obstet Gynecol* 1994;84:598.
91. Ayhan A, Aksu T, Selcuk Tuncer Z, et al. Immature teratoma of the ovary. *Eur J Gynaecol Oncol* 1993;14:205.
92. O'Connor DM, Norris HJ. The influence of grade on the outcome of stage I ovarian immature (malignant) teratomas and the reproducibility of grading. *Int J Gynecol Pathol* 1994;13:283.
93. Ayhan A, Tuncer ZS, Yanik F, et al. Malignant germ cell tumors of the ovary: Hacettepe hospital experience. *Acta Obstet Gynecol Scand* 1995;74:384.
94. Norris HJ, Jensen RD. Relative frequency of ovarian neoplasms in children and adolescents. *Cancer* 1972;30:713.
95. King ME, DiGiovanni LM, Yung JF, et al. Immature teratoma of the ovary grade 3, with karyotype analysis. *Int J Gynecol Pathol* 1990;9:178.
96. Ihara T, Ohama K, Satoh H, et al. Histologic grade and karyotype of immature teratoma of the ovary. *Cancer* 1984;54:2988.
97. Palmquist MB, Webb MJ, Lieber MM, et al. DNA ploidy of ovarian dysgerminomas: correlation with clinical outcome. *Gynecol Oncol* 1992;44:13.
98. Nielsen SNJ, Gaffey TA, Malkasian GD. Immature ovarian teratoma: a review of 14 cases. *Mayo Clin Proc* 1986;61:110.
99. Gershenson DM, DelJunco G, Silva EG, et al. Immature teratoma of the ovary. *Obstet Gynecol* 1986;68:624.
100. Kouolos JP, Hoffman JS, Steinhoff MM. Immature teratoma of the ovary. *Gynecol Oncol* 1989;34:46.
101. Schwartz PE, Chambers SK, Chambers JT, et al. Ovarian germ cell malignancies: the Yale University experience. *Gynecol Oncol* 1992;45:26.
102. Pippitt CH Jr, Cain JM, Hakes TB, et al. Primary chemotherapy and the role of second-look laparotomy in non-dysgerminomatous germ cell malignancies of the ovary. *Gynecol Oncol* 1988;31:268.
103. Ablin AR, Krailo MD, Ramsay NK, et al. Results of treatment of malignant germ cell tumors in 93 children: a report from the Children's Cancer Study Group. *J Clin Oncol* 1991;9:1782.

104. Schwartz PE. Combination chemotherapy in the management of ovarian germ cell malignancies. *Obstet Gynecol* 1984;64:564.
105. Wong LC, Ngan HYS, Ma HK. Primary treatment with vincristine, dactinomycin, and cyclophosphamide in nondysgerminomatous germ cell tumor of the ovary. *Gynecol Oncol* 1989;34:155.
106. Gershenson DM. Menstrual and reproductive function after treatment with combination chemotherapy for malignant ovarian germ cell tumors. *J Clin Oncol* 1988;6:270.
107. Wu PC, Huang RL, Lang JH, et al. Treatment of malignant ovarian germ cell tumors with preservation of fertility: a report of 28 cases. *Gynecol Oncol* 1991;40:2.
108. Shah KD, Kaffe S, Gilbert F, et al. Unilateral microscopic gonadoblastoma in a prepubertal Turnaer mosaic with Y chromosome material identified by restriction fragment analysis. *Am J Clin Pathol* 1988;90:622.
109. Kapp DS, Kohorn EI, Merino MJ, et al. Pure dysgerminoma of the ovary with elevated serum human chorionic gonadotropin: diagnostic and therapeutic considerations. *Gynecol Oncol* 1985;20:234.
110. Pressley RH, Muntz HG, Falkenberry S, et al. Serum lactic dehydrogenase as a tumor marker in dysgerminoma. *Gynecol Oncol* 1992;44:281.
111. Gordon A, Lipton D, Woodruff JD. Dysgerminoma: a review of 158 cases from the Emil Novak ovarian tumor registry. *Obstet Gynecol* 1981;58:497.
112. Thomas GM, Dembo AJ, Hacker NF, et al. Current therapy for dysgerminoma of the ovary. *Obstet Gynecol* 1987;70:268.
113. Bjorkholm E, Lundell M, Gyftodimos A, et al. Dysgerminoma: the Radiumhemmet series 1927-1984. *Cancer* 1990;65:38.
114. Gershenson DM, Morris M, Cangir A, et al. Treatment of malignant germ cell tumors of the ovary with bleomycin etoposide, and cisplatin. *J Clin Oncol* 1990;8:715.
115. Gershenson DM. Update on malignant ovarian germ cell tumors. *Cancer* 1993;71:1581.
116. Kurman RJ, Norris HJ. Endodermal sinus tumor of the ovary: a clinical and pathologic analysis of 71 cases. *Cancer* 1976;38:2404.
117. Gershenson DM, DelJunco G, Herson J, et al. Endodermal sinus tumor of the ovary: the M.D. Anderson experience. *Obstet Gynecol* 1983;61:194.
118. Pecorelli S, Sartori E, Favalli G, et al. Ataxia-telangiectasia and endodermal sinus tumor of the ovary: report of a case. *Gynecol Oncol* 1988;29:240.
119. Williams SD, Birch R, Einhorn LH, et al. Treatment of disseminated germ-cell tumors with cisplatin, bleomycin, and either vinblastine or etoposide. *N Engl J Med* 1987;316:1435.
120. Athanikar N, Saikia TK, Ramkrishnan G, et al. Aggressive chemotherapy in endodermal sinus tumor. *J Surg Oncol* 1989;40:17.
121. Kawai M, Kano T, Furuhashi Y, et al. Prognostic factors in yolk sac tumors of the ovary: a clinicopathologic analysis of 29 cases. *Cancer* 1991;67:184.
122. Kurman RJ, Norris HJ. Embryonal carcinoma of the ovary: a clinicopathologic entity distinct from endodermal sinus tumor resembling embryonal carcinoma of the adult testis. *Cancer* 1976;38:2420.
123. Takeda A, Ishizuka T, Goto S, et al. Polyembryoma of ovary producing alpha-fetoprotein and hCG: immunoperoxidase and electron microscopic study. *Cancer* 1982;49:1878.
124. Axe SR, Klein VR, Woodruff JD. Choriocarcinoma of the ovary. *Obstet Gynecol* 1985;66:111.
125. Gershenson DM, DelJunco G, Copeland LJ, et al. Mixed germ cell tumors of the ovary. *Obstet Gynecol* 1984;64:200.
126. Carlson RW, Sikic BI, Turbow MM, et al. Cisplatin, vinblastine and bleomycin (PVB) therapy for ovarian germ cell tumors. *J Clin Oncol* 1983;1:645.
127. Bosch-Banyeras JM, Lucaya X, Bernet M, et al. Calcified ovarian fibroma in prepubertal girls. *Eur J Pediatr* 1989;148:749.
128. Givens JR, Andersen RN, Wiser WL, et al. A testosterone-secreting gonadotropin-responsive pure thecoma and polycystic ovarian disease. *J Clin Endocrinol Metab* 1975;41:845.
129. Young RH, Dickersin GR, Scully RE. Juvenile granulosa cell tumor of the ovary: a clinicopathologic analysis of 125 cases. *Am J Surg Pathol* 1984;8:575.
130. Lack EE, Perez-Atayde AR, Murthy ASK, et al. Granulosa theca cell tumors in premenarchal girls: a clinical and pathologic study of ten cases. *Cancer* 1981;48:1846.
131. Bjorkholm E, Silfversward C. Prognostic factors in granulosa-cell tumors. *Gynecol Oncol* 1981; 11:261.
132. Biscotti CV, Kennedy AW. Ovarian juvenile granulosa cell tumors. *Adolesc Pediatr Gynecol* 1990;3:15.
133. Powell JL, Johnson NA, Bailey CL, et al. Management of advanced juvenile granulosa cell tumor of the ovary. *Gynecol Oncol* 1993;48:119.

134. Zaloudek C, Norris HJ. Granulosa tumors of the ovary in children: a clinical and pathologic study of 32 cases. *Am J Surg Pathol* 1982;6:503.
135. Young RH, Scully RE. Ovarian Sertoli-Leydig cell tumors: a clinicopathological analysis of 207 cases. *Am J Surg Pathol* 1985;9:543.
136. Mann WJ, Chumas J, Rosenwaks Z, et al. Elevated serum α-fetoprotein associated with Sertoli-Leydig cell tumors of the ovary. *Obstet Gynecol* 1986;67:141.
137. Simmons PS, Backes RJ, Kaufman GH, et al. Gynandroblastoma of the ovary in a young child. *Adolesc Pediatr Gynecol* 1988;1:57.
138. Scully RE. Sex cord tumor with annular tubules: a distinctive ovarian tumor of the Peutz-Jeghers syndrome. *Cancer* 1970;25:1107.
139. Young RH, Welch WR, Dickersin GR, et al. Ovarian sex cord tumor with annular tubules: review of 74 cases including 27 with Peutz-Jeghers syndrome and four with adenoma malignum of the cervix. *Cancer* 1982;50:1384.
140. Deprest J, Moerman P, Corneillie P, et al. Ovarian borderline mucinous tumor in a premenarchal girl: review on ovarian epithelial cancer in young girls. *Gynecol Oncol* 1992;45:219.
141. Leake JF, Currie JL, Rosenshein NB, et al. Long-term follow-up of serous ovarian tumors of low malignant potential. *Gynecol Oncol* 1992;47:150.
142. Elchalal U, Dgani R, Piura B, et al. Current concepts in management of epithelial ovarian tumors of low malignant potential. *Obstet Gynecol Surv* 1995;50:62.
143. Barakat RR. Borderline tumors of the ovary. *Obstet Gynecol Clin North Am* 1994;21:93.
144. Casey AC, Bell DA, Lage JM, et al. Epithelial ovarian tumors of borderline malignancy: long-term follow-up. *Gynecol Oncol* 1993;50:316.
145. Cannistra SA. Cancer of the ovary. *N Engl J Med* 1993;329:1550.
146. Hall JM, Lee MK, Newman B, et al. Linkage of early-onset familial breast cancer to chromosome 17q21. *Science* 1990;250:1684–1689.
147. Narod SA, Feunteun J, Lynch HT, et al. Familial breast-ovarian cancer locus on chromosome 17q21-q23. *Lancet* 1991;338:82.
148. Easton DF, Ford D, Bishop DT. Breast and ovarian cancer incidence in BRCA1-mutation carriers. *Am J Hum Genet* 1995;56:265.
149. Ford D, Easton DF, Bishop DT, et al. Risks of cancer in BRCA1-mutation carriers. *Lancet* 1994; 343:692.
150. Stratton JF, Gayther SA, Russell P, et al. Contribution of BRCA1 mutations to ovarian cancer. *N Engl J Med* 1997;336:1125.
151. Burke W, Daly M, Garber J, et al. Recommendations for follow-up care of individuals with an inherited predisposition to cancer. *JAMA* 1997;277:997.
152. Struewing JP, Hartge P, Wacholder S, et al. The risk of cancer associated with specific mutations of BRCA1 and BRCA2 among Ashkenazi Jews. *N Engl J Med* 1997;336:1401.
153. Struewing JP, Abeliovich D, Peretz T, et al. The carrier frequency of the BRCA1 185delAG mutation is approximately one percent of Ashkenazi Jewish individuals. *Nat Genet* 1995;11:198.
154. Muto MG, Cramer DW, Tangir J, et al. Frequency of the BRCA1 185delAG mutation among Jewish women with ovarian cancer and matched population controls. *Cancer Res* 1996;56:1250.
155. Hayes MC, Scully RE. Ovarian steroid cell tumors (not otherwise specified): a clinicopathological analysis of 63 cases. *Am J Surg Pathol* 1987;11:835.
156. Padilla SL. Androgen-producing tumors in children and adolescents. *Adolesc Pediatr Gynecol* 1989;2:135.
157. Wentz AC, Gutai JP, Jones GS, et al. Ovarian hyperthecosis in the adolescent patient. *J Pediatr* 1976; 88:488.
158. Fox H, Langley FA, Govan AD, et al. Malignant lymphoma presenting as an ovarian tumour: a clinicopathological analysis of 34 cases. *Br J Obstet Gynaecol* 1988;95:386.
159. Heaton DC, Duff GB. Ovarian relapse in a young woman with acute lymphoblastic leukemia. *Am J Hematol* 1989;30:42.

16

The Breast: Examination and Lesions

Breast development in the majority of girls begins between the ages of 8 and 13 years. As breast development is often regarded as a sign of feminine sexuality, young women and their families may worry about minor asymmetry or "inadequate" development. It is often difficult for the teenager to acknowledge smaller breasts as "normal." On the other hand, reassurance is in order only if the remainder of the examination and history excludes an endocrine or developmental disorder.

Increasing publicity about the frequency of breast cancer among women in the United States and the occurrence of breast cancer among relatives and mothers of adolescent patients has made many adolescents exceptionally nervous about breast masses, even though malignancy in this age group is rare (1,2). This concern may be used constructively to encourage young women to seek routine preventive health assessments and information about normal breast development and the techniques of breast self-examination.

BREAST EXAMINATION

All pediatric and adolescent patients should have a breast examination at the time of their annual physical examination regardless of whether specific complaints are mentioned. Examination of breasts is initiated during the newborn examination when breast tissue is usually evident secondary to stimulation from maternal hormones. In addition, neonates may have bilateral "white" nipple discharge ("witches' milk"), which is also due to maternal hormonal stimulation. Neonates and infants may have breast problems such as accessory nipples, infection, hemangioma, lipoma, and lymphangioma. For the prepubertal child, the assessment includes inspection and palpation of the chest wall for masses, pain, nipple discharge, or signs of premature thelarche or precocious development (see Chapter 5).

For the adolescent examination, the patient is asked to lie supine with one arm under her head. Breast development is recorded as Sexual Maturity Ratings, also called Tanner stages B1 to B5 (see Fig. 9 in Chapter 4). If asymmetry or disorders of development are a concern, then exact measurements of the areola, glandular breast tissue, and overall breast size should be included at each examination (Fig. 1). For example, one might record the following:

	Areola (cm)	Breast gland (cm)	Overall (cm)
Right	2.5	5 × 6	9
Left	2.4	4 × 5	8.5

The first number in the breast gland figure is the upper-to-lower measurement; the second number is the right-to-left measurement. The overall size is the right-to-left measurement of the border of the fatty tissue of the breast mound.

There are several techniques for the orderly examination of the breast of the adolescent. In the first method, the examiner palpates the breast tissue in a pattern similar to spokes of a wheel, that is, in a straight line from the margin of the breast inward and clockwise around the breast starting with the tail of the breast in the axilla (Fig. 2). In a second method, the breast is palpated by the examiner using a circular clockwise pattern with either concentric circles or a spiral pattern inward. In a third method, the vertical or horizontal strip method, the breast

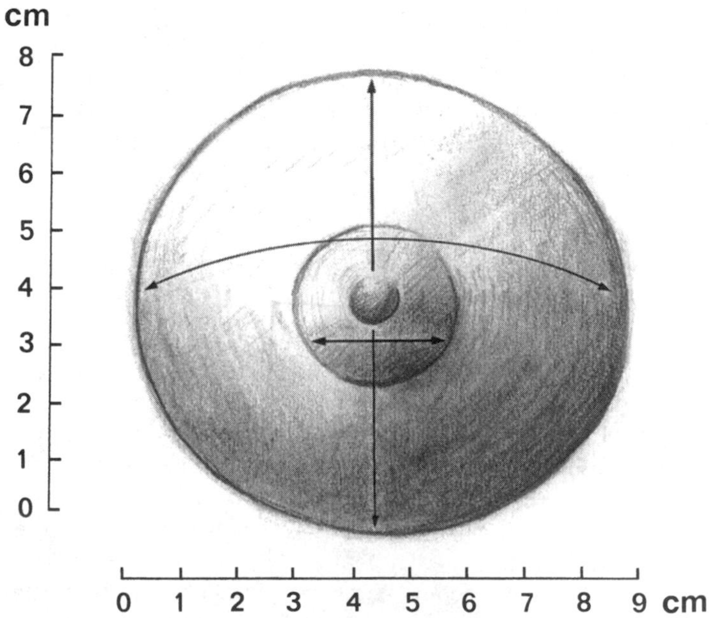

FIG. 1. Measurement of the developing breast (see text).

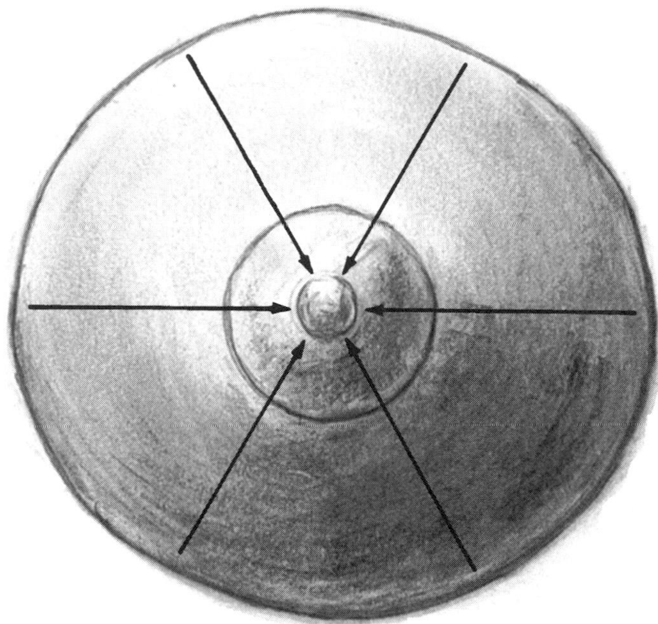

FIG. 2. Palpation of the breast. The fingers are moved in a straight line inward going clockwise around the breast.

is palpated in a linear systematic approach to cover all of the breast tissue. This last method appears to be particularly effective for self-examination (3). In all the methods, the flat finger pads should be moved in a slightly rotatory fashion (about the size of a dime) to feel for abnormalities. Normal glandular tissue has an irregular, granular surface (like tapioca pudding); a fibroadenoma feels firm, rubbery, or smooth. The areola should be compressed to assess for the existence of nipple discharge. As part of the overall health assessment, supraclavicular, infraclavicular, and axillary lymph nodes are palpated.

During the examination, the teenager can be educated as to what the examiner is doing; in addition, breast self-examination skills can be discussed and demonstrated. Educating an adolescent about the techniques of self-examination at the time of the breast examination may increase understanding of the ongoing examination and make her feel more at ease (4,5). Breast self-examination is often taught in schools as part of health education classes and thus provides a link to examinations in the office. Although adolescents can become quite proficient in learning the necessary techniques, adolescents appear to practice self-examination only sporadically and often not at the end of menses (6). Studies on the value of self-examination during adolescence toward promoting lifelong health habits or early detection of breast cancer have not been done (7). The rationale for teaching breast self-examination is to contribute to an adolescent's understanding and acceptance of her body, enhance her level of comfort with the clinical examination, and provide an opportunity for discussion about women's health issues (8). However, a number of authors have questioned whether early teaching of breast examination promotes anxiety, extra visits to health care facilities, and surgery in adolescents; these authors have also queried whether time in the office visit is better spent with other risk-reduction strategies, given the extraordinary rarity of breast cancer in the adolescent age group (8–10). Although techniques may be discussed with adolescents, adolescents should not be made to feel guilty for not adhering to a self-examination schedule. Teaching self-examination techniques is most appropriate for older adolescent and young adult women who are usually more interested in learning these techniques and want to participate in this aspect of their health care. There is some evidence that breast self-examination is the primary mode by which adolescent breast masses are detected; Hein and colleagues (4) found that 81% of a group of 95 teenagers with breast masses found them by self-detection. Nevertheless, adolescents should be reassured that cancer is extraordinarily unlikely in their age group but that a new breast mass that does not disappear after a menstrual period or is associated with pain, fever, or erythema should be evaluated in an expedient fashion.

With increasing knowledge about predisposing risk factors for breast cancer such as genetic markers, family history, and previous radiation and cancer, clinicians will be better able to target those with increased risks of developing breast cancer with appropriate in-office instruction and take-home educational materials. Adolescent women with previous radiation of the chest, who have an increased risk of second tumors including cancers of the breast (11–14), and those with malignancies that may metastasize to the breast should have early teaching of breast self-examination during adolescence.

Breast self-examination should be performed at the end of each menstrual period. Instructions include having the adolescent:

1. Look in the mirror for asymmetry while undressing for a shower,
2. Examine the breasts while standing in the shower (soap on the hands facilitates the examination), and
3. Reexamine the breasts that night supine (before going to sleep) with one hand behind the head and a small pillow under the shoulder.

She should be shown how to press gently with the middle three finger pads in one of the systematic approaches described above. Patient information pamphlets, videos, or posters (such as those published by the American Cancer Society) should be available in the health care provider's office. It is particularly helpful for the patient to begin self-examination the night after a normal examination at the office visit so that she can be assured that she has a normal baseline for comparison. She can then continue to perform a breast self-examination after each annual check-up in addition to her monthly examinations to reinforce normal breast findings.

MASTALGIA

Mild breast tenderness often occurs premenstrually in association with fibrocystic changes or exercise or as a sign of early pregnancy. Severe breast tenderness is not a major complaint of healthy adolescents. Thus, the clinician providing office care to adolescents must be prepared to do a breast assessment and a pregnancy test in young women complaining of mastalgia. In spite of much anecdotal evidence that elimination of caffeine from the diet may benefit individual adolescents with fibrocystic changes and mastalgia, the majority of case-control studies have not demonstrated an association between benign breast disease and caffeine and methylxanthines (15,16) or benefit from elimination diets (15,17,18). We usually suggest that teenagers with cyclic or noncyclic breast discomfort wear a comfortable supporting bra, use ibuprofen as needed, and undertake a 3-month trial of elimination of substances such as coffee, tea, cola, and chocolate. Depending on the patient's self-assessment of how she is doing, she can continue to avoid caffeine as she wishes. A number of sexually active adolescents also notice improvement of symptoms from taking low-dose progestin-dominant oral contraceptives, although some adolescents report new symptoms from oral contraceptives. Evening primrose oil (1000 mg three times a day for 3 months) has been reported to have a response rate of 44% improvement in mastalgia (19,20); the mode of action is thought to be related to the high fatty acid content and its resulting action on the prostaglandin pathway, but more data are needed.

With the active participation of many young women in sports, the brassiere industry has responded with the design of many new styles with smooth cups and support that are particularly helpful to those with large breasts involved in activities such as jogging, basketball, and weightlifting (21).

PROBLEMS OF BREAST DEVELOPMENT

Asymmetry

Asymmetry of the breasts is a common complaint, especially from girls in the early stages of breast development. Since the breast bud may initially appear on one side as a tender, granular lump, parents are often concerned about the possibility of a malignancy. In all individuals with breast asymmetry, a careful examination should be performed to rule out a breast mass, cyst, or abscess. Giant fibroadenomas may blend into normal breast tissue and may be missed initially during palpation.

The clinician can play an important role in counseling the patient with true asymmetric breast development. The young adolescent needs to hear that many other adolescents and adult women have breast asymmetry; it should be pointed out that she may be unaware of the degree of asymmetry in other girls because her observations are based on seeing them fully clothed.

It is helpful to let the 13- or 14-year-old girl know that most 18- or 19-year-olds are coping well with the amount of breast asymmetry they have and that most elect not to have surgical intervention. The clinician should acknowledge that many younger adolescents (14 or 15 years old) are most anxious to have their body image equalized and "made normal" as quickly as possible without regard for the possible risks and long-term complications involved in augmentation or reduction mammoplasty. The young teenager can benefit from being told that the clinician understands that the asymmetry may cause worries for her and that an annual examination is important to determine the degree of asymmetry and to help her decide at the end of full growth (no further change in measurements) whether any consideration of intervention is warranted.

Since bathing suit fittings can be particularly difficult for girls with asymmetry, girls should be encouraged to try on a large number of styles that offer breast support, before coming to a final decision about the need for surgical intervention. For many youngsters, the use of slightly padded bras or simple bra pads also makes the asymmetry much less of a problem. A major difference in breast size can be treated with a foam insert (available in department stores for mastectomy patients).

If asymmetry is still marked at age 15 to 18 years and serial measurements show no further increase in size of either breast, patients may wish to explore the option of augmentation or reduction mammoplasty. A plastic surgeon can delineate the risks and benefits. Potential long-term sequelae of implants have been an increasing concern, and newer materials are needed. Referral to a plastic surgeon willing to discuss the options without pushing the patient inordinately in the direction of surgery is essential. Success can be quite dramatic, as illustrated in Fig. 3.

Hypertrophy

Some adolescents develop very large breasts that are associated with back pain, postural kyphosis, breast discomfort, shoulder soreness from bra straps, intertrigo, and psychological distress. Surgical reduction of large breasts at the end of breast growth can yield rewarding benefits to many young women. However, as is the case with augmentation mammoplasty, adolescents need to understand the results and risks of surgery, including infection, scars, and potential difficulty with breast-feeding.

True virginal hypertrophy occurs rarely in adolescents and causes the breasts to continue to enlarge in size beyond normal; unilateral or segmental enlargement may occur. The differential diagnosis includes juvenile fibroadenomas and cystosarcoma phyllodes. For cases of true virginal hypertrophy, surgical reduction should be delayed, if possible, until growth has ceased (Fig. 4).

Tuberous Breasts

Tuberous breasts are a variant of breast development in which the base of the breast is limited in size and the nipple–areola complex is overdeveloped, giving the appearance of a tuberous plant root. The glandular tissue may be totally

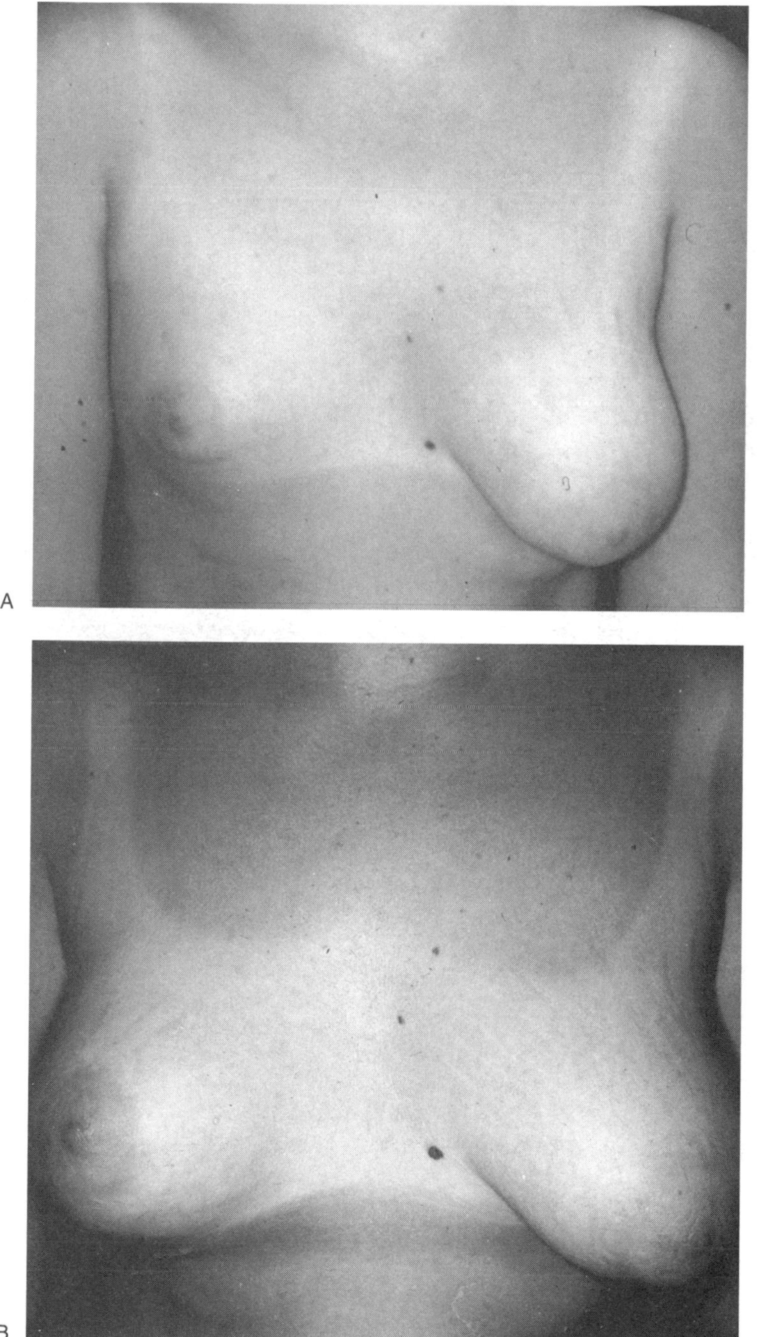

FIG. 3. (A) Preoperative view of a 16-year-old girl with hypoplasia of the right breast. **(B)** Appearance after augmentation mammoplasty with a Cronin prosthesis. (Courtesy of George E. Gifford, M.D., Children's Hospital, Boston, MA.)

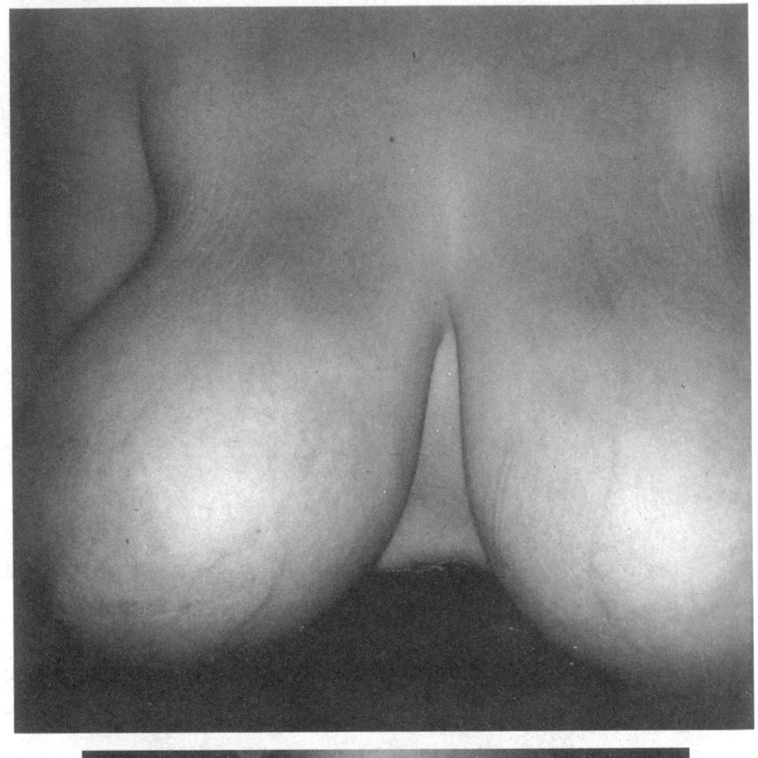

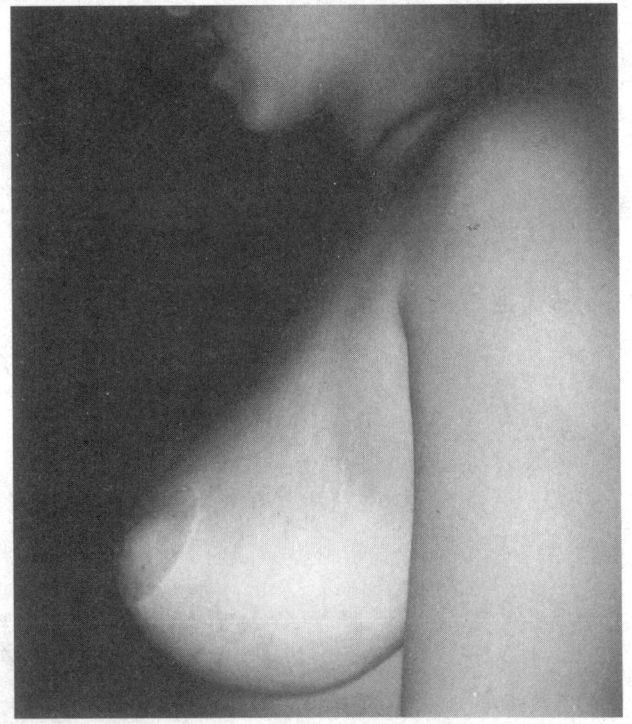

FIG. 4. (A) Preoperative view of a 19-year-old woman with virginal hypertrophy of both breasts, resulting in back pain and kyphosis. **(B)** Appearance after reduction mammoplasty. (Courtesy of George E. Gifford, M.D., Children's Hospital, Boston, MA.)

within the distended, enlarged areolae. Plastic surgery may be undertaken for cosmetic reasons. This condition is sometimes associated with breasts that develop with the induction of secondary sexual characteristics from exogenous hormones prescribed for treatment of premature ovarian failure, abnormalities of gonadotropin-releasing hormone secretion, or gonadal dysgenesis.

Lack of Breast Development

Lack of breast development may be secondary to congenital absence of glandular tissue (amastia), a systemic disorder (e.g., malnutrition, Crohn's disease), radiation therapy, congenital adrenal hyperplasia (CAH), gonadal dysgenesis, hypogonadotropic hypogonadism, or rarely an intersex disorder or 17α-hydroxylase deficiency. Amastia is extremely rare and usually unilateral; it also may be associated with Poland's syndrome (aplasia of pectoralis muscles, rib deformities, webbed fingers, radial nerve aplasia). The congenital absence of one or both nipples (athelia) is very rare and may not be associated with absent breast tissue.

The evaluation of adolescents with amastia depends on the history and physical findings (see Chapter 6). Any evidence of androgen excess, such as mild enlargement of the clitoris, hirsutism, or severe acne, should suggest a disorder

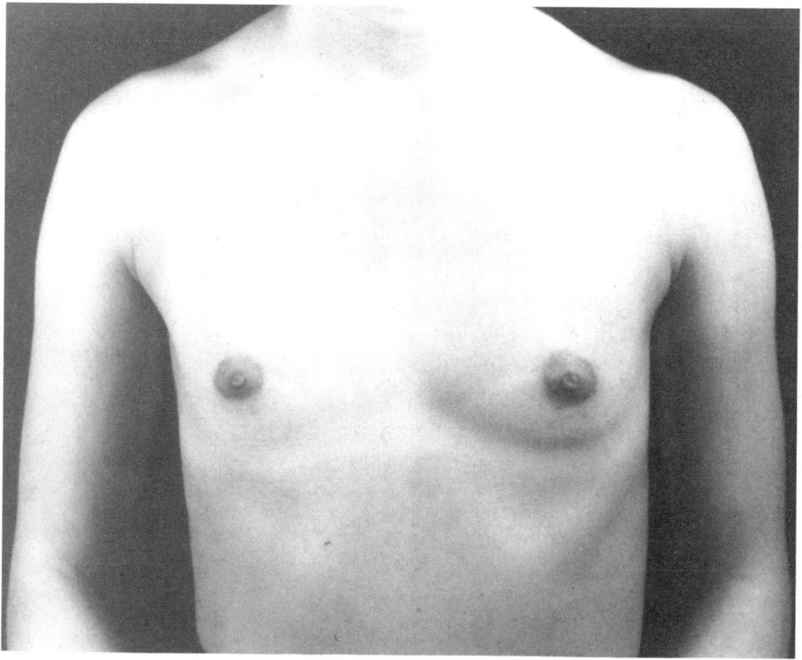

FIG. 5. A 19-year-old patient presented with irregular periods and lack of glandular tissue; late-onset 21-hydroxylase deficiency (CAH) was diagnosed.

such as CAH, an intersex disorder, polycystic ovary syndrome, or possibly an adrenal or ovarian tumor (see Chapter 7). Figure 5 shows a 19-year-old patient who had irregular menses, lack of glandular breast development, normal pubic and axillary hair, mild clitoromegaly, and mild hirsutism. Adrenocorticotropic hormone testing was consistent with late-onset 21-hydroxylase deficiency (CAH) (see Chapter 7). Suppression of adrenal androgens with corticosteroids resulted in regular menses and normal breast development.

Despite the need to consider endocrinologic problems, the clinician should be aware that the great majority of adolescents with small breasts, normal sexual hair, and regular menses are healthy young women and deserve reassurance. Sports bras, which tend to compress the breast further, can be avoided. The oversized sweater and sweatshirt look can be reassuring to young teenagers who are often self-conscious in tank tops. Augmentation mammoplasty may be considered by some young women in their late teens and early 20s, and an understanding of the risks and benefits is essential. Athletes with small breasts are generally counseled to avoid augmentation mammoplasty until their careers are completed, since the change could potentially alter performance (21).

Premature Thelarche and Precocious Puberty

A discussion of premature thelarche and precocious puberty can be found in Chapter 5.

Accessory Nipples or Breasts

Accessory nipples (polythelia) or breasts (polymastia) occur in 1% to 2% of healthy patients. In some cases, all three components of the breast—glandular tissue, areola, and nipple—are present. More commonly, only a small areola and nipple are found, usually along the embryologic milk line between the axillae and groin. The most common sites are medial and just inferior to the normal breast tissue and in the axilla. These abnormalities are usually asymptomatic. No therapy is usually undertaken, unless at a later date the patient wishes to have the tissue removed for cosmetic reasons. Although studies have been conflicting on the association of supernumerary nipples and renal anomalies (22,23) and further studies are needed, a reasonable approach is to perform renal ultrasonography in an infant with multiple congenital anomalies and supernumerary nipples.

Engorgement of accessory breasts is common during pregnancy and lactation. If no outlet is present, the breast tissue spontaneously involutes within several days to weeks after delivery.

NIPPLE DISCHARGE

Nipple discharge is unusual during the teen years. The discharge may be milky, purulent, watery, serous, serosanguineous, or bloody. Most discharges, even bloody ones, do not signify cancer. A milky discharge is characteristic of galactorrhea, which occurs in adolescents following a pregnancy (full-term or after an abortion) or is associated with drug use (prescription and illicit), hypothyroidism, or prolactin-secreting tumors. The evaluation of galactorrhea and hyperprolactinemia is discussed in Chapter 6.

A purulent discharge is suggestive of infection. A sticky green or serosanguineous discharge or a multicolored discharge may be associated with duct ectasia. A serosanguineous discharge may occur with intraductal papilloma, fibrocystic changes, or rarely cancer. A small amount of yellow, clear serous material can be expressed in early adolescence or in the later teen years, associated with fibrocystic changes.

Occasionally, a periareolar gland of Montgomery (Morgagni's tubercles) will drain a small amount of clear to brownish fluid through an ectopic opening on the areola for several weeks. A small subareolar lump may be palpable. Usually no treatment is necessary, and the discharge and lump resolve spontaneously over several weeks to months (20,24). If the cyst persists, however, excision is advisable.

Intraductal papillomas arise from abnormal proliferation of mammary duct epithelium projecting into a dilated lumen. Slight local trauma may rupture the vascular stalk and cause a bloody discharge. The mass may enlarge sufficiently to make it palpable. In adolescents, these masses may be subareolar or located in ducts in the periphery of the breast (25). In an extensive review of breast masses, Neinstein (20) found that intraductal papillomas accounted for only 1.2% of lesions biopsied in adolescents. Intraductal papillomas should be surgically excised.

Hyperprolactinemia has also been associated with mammary duct ectasia, a clinical syndrome of nipple discharge, nipple inversion, breast mass, and/or periareolar sepsis (nonpuerperal mastitis). In a study of 108 patients, Peters and Schuth (26) found that 27% of the patients had transiently elevated prolactin (42 ± 22 μg/L) during the period of inflammation with return to normal within 4 weeks and that 20% of the patients had more severe hyperprolactinemia (78 ± 56 μg/L), often associated with a previously undiagnosed prolactinoma. The authors suggested that the former group may have neurogenic hyperprolactinemia in response to the inflammation, whereas the latter group may be predisposed to the infection because nipple secretion might facilitate bacterial invasion. Of the patients in this study, 19 (18%) were between 12 and 20 years of age.

Apocrine chromhidrosis, the secretion of colored sweat by the apocrine glands of the areola, may sometimes be confused with bloody nipple discharge. Characteristically, the discharge occurs when the patient exercises or manually exerts pressure around the areola. Both cytologic examination and cultures are negative. No treatment is indicated for this condition (27).

PERIAREOLAR HAIR

Periareolar hair is not uncommon in the healthy adolescent. Cosmetic treatment (usually unnecessary) can be accomplished by cutting the hairs. Plucking or shaving may be uncomfortable and can lead to mastitis/cellulitis.

OTHER PROBLEMS

Joggers may experience sore or scaling nipples in response to friction. Lubrication of the nipple, a soft cotton bra without a seam in the cup, or Band-Aids over the nipples in the girl with small breasts not using a bra are often curative (21). Bicyclists may have difficulty with cold, painful nipples after several days of riding in the colder climates; a wind-breaking jacket and increased insulation over the chest should be advised.

Overweight girls with large pendulous breasts may have local infections on the undersurface of the breast with agents such as *Candida*, which results in a bright red rash. Topical antifungal drugs are usually sufficient, although florid cases with axillary involvement have responded better to oral antifungal agents.

BREAST MASSES

Breast masses in adolescents, found either at the time of routine examination or during self-examination, provoke much anxiety for both the individuals and their families. The evaluation should include a history of previous breast disease, previous or intercurrent malignancy, chest radiation, menstrual history, pregnancy, constitutional symptoms, duration, size, symptoms associated with the breast mass, nipple discharge, and family history of breast disease and breast cancer. The work-up includes a complete physical examination (checking for hepatosplenomegaly and lymphadenopathy) and assessment of the mass including evaluation of consistency, size, mobility, tenderness, warmth, overlying skin changes, and associated discharge.

Importantly, the majority of adolescents who present to clinicians with the complaint of a "breast lump" have normal physiologic breast tissue or fibrocystic changes (28). Adolescents typically have very dense breast tissue. Fibrocystic changes are characterized by diffuse cord-like thickening and lumps that may become tender and enlarged prior to menses each month. Physical findings tend to change each month, so that suspected cysts can often be followed clinically. Love and colleagues (29) have questioned whether these findings should be characterized as a disease since the process occurs in 50% of women clinically and 90% histologically. The etiology of fibrocystic changes is unknown and, as noted earlier, does not appear to be related to methylxanthine consumption (30). One possible etiology is an imbalance of estrogen/progesterone (17,20).

In a survey of English-language articles published since 1960 on breast lesions evaluated by biopsy, Neinstein (20) determined that 18.5% showed fibrocystic changes. The long-term risk of cancer in women with fibrocystic changes relates to the histology of the lesions found. In a study of 10,366 consecutive breast biopsies followed up for a median duration of 17 years, DuPont and Page (31) reported that women having proliferative disease without atypical hyperplasia had a risk of cancer that was 1.9 (95% confidence interval [CI]: 1.2, 2.9) times the risk of women with nonproliferative lesions; the risk in women with atypical hyperplasia (atypia) was 5.5 (95% CI: 3.1, 8.8) times that in women with nonproliferative lesions. The risk in women with atypia and a family history of breast cancer was 11-fold that of women with no atypia and a negative family history. Seventy percent of the women undergoing breast biopsy for benign disease did not have risk factors detected and were not at increased risk of later breast cancer.

Although most breast "lumps" seen in the office setting in adolescents are normal nodularity or fibrocystic changes, most breast masses that are surgically excised in this age group are fibroadenomas (1,5,10,32). Surgical series (10,20) have provided a demonstration of the types of breast masses surgically removed in adolescents; Table 1 shows the data from these two reviews that included 21 studies (1,5,10,15,32–48). In a review of 51 patients, aged 8 to 20 years, who underwent excision of breast masses at Children's Hospital, Boston, 81.4% of the masses were fibroadenomas (5). The pathology report on the remainder of the biopsy specimens showed fibrocystic disease, simple cysts, capillary hemangiomas, fat necrosis, adenomatous hyperplasia, and (in one patient) normal breast tissue. This is similar to the spectrum of breast disease reported by Daniel and Mathews (32), who found that fibroadenomas accounted for 94% of breast tumors in the 12- to 21-year age group. Neinstein's (20) review of 15 series in the literature demonstrated that fibroadenomas represented 68.3% of the lesions in 1797 cases involving patients <22 years old. In clinical series of adolescents in office settings, the percentage of breast masses attributed to fibroadenomas is only 15% (28).

Fibroadenomas are typically firm or rubbery and mobile, and usually have a clearly defined edge. Pathologically, they have stromal proliferation surrounding aggregates of compressed or uncompressed, elongated and distorted ducts (39). They tend to be eccentric in position and occur more frequently in the lateral breast quadrants than the medial quadrants. The breast mass may remain unchanged or increase in size with subsequent menstrual cycles. The average duration of symptoms is 5 months (38), and the average size is 2 to 3 cm with a range of <1 cm to >10 cm. Recurrent or multiple fibroadenomas have been reported in 10% to 25% of cases (28). Giant fibroadenomas grow more rapidly to >5 cm and have a greater degree of stromal cellularity; they may replace and compress most of the normal breast tissue. Because of the soft consistency, these lesions may be mistaken initially for normal tissue. They accounted for 1.1% of lesions in Neinstein's review (20).

A question that has frequently been raised is whether patients with a history of fibroadenoma are at increased risk of breast cancer. In a retrospective cohort study of 1835 patients with fibroadenoma diagnosed between 1950 and 1968, Dupont et al (49) compared these patients with two control groups (Connecticut Tumor Registry) and women chosen from among patients' sisters-in-law. They reported that the risk of invasive breast cancer among patients with fibroadenoma was 2.15 (95% CI: 1.5, 3.2) times that of controls. The risk for complex fibroadenoma (cysts, sclerosing adenosis, epithelial calcifications, or papillary apocrine changes) was 3.1-fold (95% CI: 1.9, 5.1). Patients with benign prolifer-

TABLE 1. *Summary of studies involving breast disease in young women*[a]

Reference	No.	Age (yr)	Normal	Cyst	Fibroadenoma	FC/prolif	CP	Hypertrophy	IP	Other benign lesion/tumor	Infection	Malignancy
32	63	10–20	0	0	40	9	2	0	0	4	5	3
33	429	<21	0	0	338	76	0	0	2	2	10	1
34	118	10–20	0	0	0	118	0	0	0	0	0	0
35	59	8–20	2	2	41	4	0	0	1	3	0	0
36	237	10–20	0	8	169	25	0	0	13	5	2	3
37	111	<16	2	1	84	2	0	4	1	7	9	1
38	42	12–18	—	—	30	—	—	—	—	—	8	0
39	134	0–16	—	—	102	4	—	—	—	—	9	1
40	145	<21	0	0	104	26	2	0	4	4	4	1
1	143	11–20	—	—	103	9	—	—	—	—	4	1
41	63	10–20	—	—	42	9	—	—	—	—	5	3
42	40	12–22	0	0	19	11	1	5	0	2	0	2
43	249	11–30	—	—	167	37	—	—	—	—	—	5
44	151	<21	0	0	119	7	0	0	0	5	20	0
45	5	10–16	0	0	5	0	0	0	0	0	0	0
5	51	8–20	0	3	48	3	0	0	0	4	1	0
46	95	12–21	0	0	90	0	0	0	1	2	2	0
47	30	<21	0	0	18	9	0	1	0	1	1	0
15	34	12–18	0	1	29	1	0	0	0	0	1	1
48	95	12–21	0	9	71	0	2	0	0	2	11	0
10	185	<18	0	0	100	44	0	24	0	11	2	4
Totals	2479	—	4	24	1719	394	7	34	22	52	94	26
%	100	—	0.16	0.97	69.34	15.89	0.28	1.37	0.89	2.10	3.79	1.05

[a]CP, Cytosarcoma phyllodes; FC/prolif, Fibrocystic/proliferative; IP, Intraductal papillomas.

ative disease in the parenchyma adjacent to the fibroadenoma had a risk of 3.88 (95% CI: 2.1, 7.3). In their series, two-thirds of the patients had noncomplex fibroadenomas, no family history of breast cancer, and no increased risk. However, among patients with a family history of breast cancer and either a complex fibroadenoma or proliferative disease, the incidence of breast cancer during the first 25 years after diagnosis of the fibroadenoma was 20%.

Cystosarcoma phyllodes is a rare primary tumor that is usually benign but is sometimes malignant (50). This tumor accounted for 0.4% of cases in the Neinstein series (20). The lesions are usually large and circumscribed; Briggs and coworkers (51) found an average size of 6 cm (range, 2 to 13 cm) in nine adolescents. Overlying skin may be taut and shiny with distended veins apparent; skin retraction, necrosis, nipple discharge, and retraction may occur. Classification of the lesion as benign or malignant is based on stromal findings (20).

Cancer of the breast is extremely rare in children and adolescents (32,33, 52–55). In a series of 237 patients 10 to 20 years of age with breast lesions, Farrow and Ashikari (56) reported only one patient with primary breast carcinoma and two patients with sarcomas metastatic to breast tissue. In a retrospective review of surgically treated breast disease in 185 adolescents (11 to 17 years old) at the Mayo Clinic, four patients had malignant neoplasms (primary rhabdomyosarcoma, metastatic rhabdomyosarcoma, metastatic neuroblastoma, and non-Hodgkin's lymphoma) (10). Primary lymphoma may present as a breast mass in adolescents (57). In Neinstein's series (20), 0.9% of lesions were cancer (range, 0% to 2% in various series) with 5/16 adenocarcinoma. Up to 30% of teenagers with breast cancer have a family history. The size of tumors has varied from 1 cm to 2.5 cm. Patients with previous radiation therapy to the chest have an increased risk of developing cancer of the breast at a young age and therefore require careful ongoing surveillance including breast self-examination, clinical examination, and mammography (11–14).

It has been recognized that breast cancers cluster in families. There is an increased risk of breast cancer in women whose relatives have been found to have breast cancer. The risk is highest if there are multiple affected relatives and if the relatives are closer (mothers or sisters). It is thought that the risk of genetic transmission is greater from the maternal side than from the paternal side (58). Several genetic syndromes have been associated with an increased risk for breast cancer. The Li-Fraumeni syndrome includes brain, breast, and lung malignancies, lymphomas, and sarcomas that develop at an early age; this syndrome has been found to result from a germline mutation of the p53 tumor suppressor gene (59). Families have been identified with increased rates of breast and ovarian cancers; these individuals have been found to have a deletion of chromosome 17 in the q21-q23 region suggestive of a tumor suppressor gene (60,61). This finding of genetic abnormalities related to an increased risk of breast cancer has been named breast cancer gene-1 (BRCA-1) (62). A second mutation, BRCA-2, has also been identified and other genetic patterns are likely to be delineated. An estimated 5% to 10% of breast cancers have been thought to be due to the BRCA-1 and BRCA-2 mutations although more recent evidence suggests that the number is probably lower. Risks for carriers of these mutations were originally derived from high-risk families enrolled in protocols and required cautious interpretation. The cumulative risk for breast cancer for women with BRCA-1 mutations was originally estimated to be 3.2% by age 30, 19.1% by age 40 years, and 85% by age 70 years (63). Ovarian cancer risk with this mutation was estimated to be 26% to 85% by age 70. The risk of breast cancer for those with the BRCA-2 mutations appears to be less than the risk for women with the BRCA-1 mutation, and the ovarian cancer risk is <10% by age 70 years. A more recent analysis of Jewish women in the Washington area with a specific BRCA-1 or a BRCA-2 mutation found lower estimates of breast cancer (56%) and ovarian cancer (16%) by age 70 years (64). Provisional recommendations for women with these mutations were published in 1997 and have included breast self-examination beginning at age 18 to 21 years, annual or semiannual clinical breast examination beginning at age 25 to 35, and mammography screening beginning at age 25 to 35 years. These recommendations have been based on expert opinion and thus the efficacy has not been proved (63). Clinicians caring for these adolescents will need to be involved in decision making with them to make the best use of emerging technology without increasing their anxiety.

Juvenile papillomatosis is a rare breast tumor of young women, first described in 1980. The findings in 180 patients from the Juvenile Papillomatosis Registry

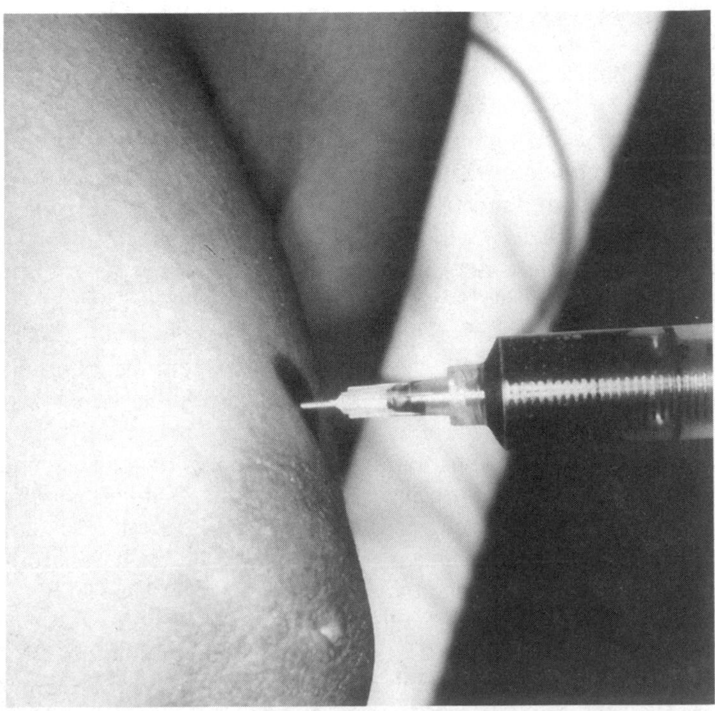

FIG. 6. Needle aspiration of simple cyst of the breast.

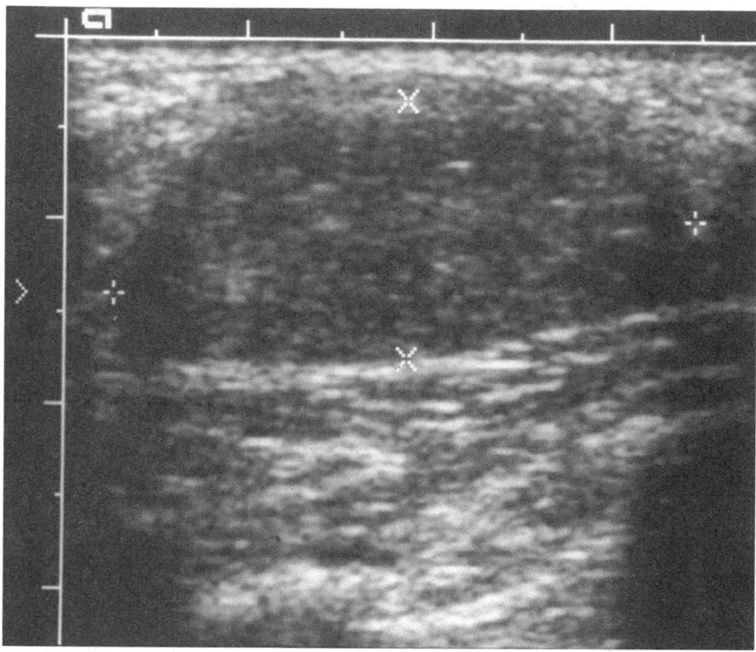

FIG. 7. Ultrasound of a fibroadenoma. (Courtesy of Carol Barnewolt, M.D., Children's Hospital, Boston, MA.)

were reported in 1985 (65). The tumor features atypical papillary duct hyperplasia and multiple cysts. The mean age at presentation was 23 years (range, 12 to 48 years). The localized tumor was often initially mistaken for a fibroadenoma. In 28% of cases, patients had a relative with breast cancer, and 7% had a first-degree relative with breast cancer. A small number of patients had breast cancer diagnosed concurrently with the juvenile papillomatosis, and several patients developed cancer at followup. Bilateral juvenile papillomatosis may especially increase the risk of later developing cancer, and thus careful surveillance is indicated in patients with this diagnosis based on excisional biopsy. Papillary hyperplasia without the cystic component of juvenile papillomatosis appears to be a more benign condition in young patients (66).

If the adolescent presents with the complaint of a breast mass, palpation may make the diagnosis evident with findings such as the thickening of fibrocystic disease or the tenderness and erythema consistent with a breast infection or abscess. Trauma may cause a breast mass, but examination immediately following a contusion may locate a preexisting lesion. If the differential diagnosis is a cyst or fibroadenoma, the lesion can be measured and the patient instructed to return after her next menstrual period. If the lesion has disappeared, then a cyst was probably present. If the lesion is still present and the patient is cooperative, needle aspiration of the mass can be performed in the office using a 23-gauge

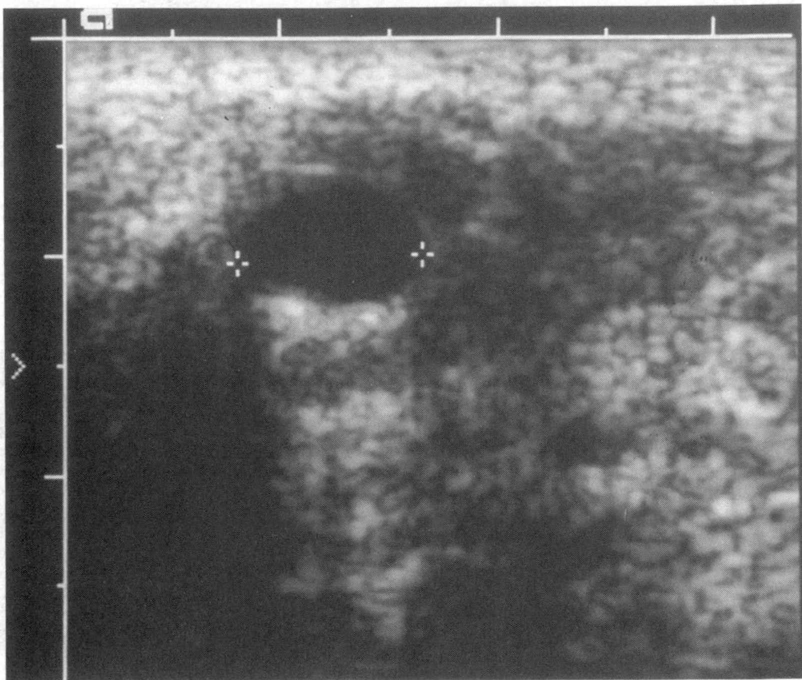

FIG. 8. Ultrasound of a simple cyst of the breast. (Courtesy of Carol Barnewolt, M.D., Children's Hospital, Boston, MA.)

needle on a 3-ml syringe (Fig. 6). A small amount of lidocaine can be used to infiltrate the skin with a 25-gauge needle (67). A cyst can be aspirated, whereas a fibroadenoma gives a characteristic gritty, solid sensation. Material obtained (even if just on the tip of the needle) may be smeared on a ground glass frosted slide, fixed, and sent for cytology examination. If the mass collapses after aspiration, it is assumed to be a cyst and is reevaluated in 3 months. Ultrasound of the breast tissue can also be helpful in delineating a fibroadenoma (Fig. 7) from a simple cyst (Fig. 8) or a galactocele (Fig. 9), as well as in localizing the extent of an abscess (52). Mammography is rarely used to evaluate breast masses in the adolescent age group, since the breast tissue is very dense, the risk of the patient's having carcinoma is negligible, and radiographic features have not influenced clinical management (68).

Ductal ectasia can be associated with a nipple discharge and/or breast mass usually occurring in the subareolar region. Ultrasound can be helpful in determining the diagnosis. The abnormal duct should be surgically excised if the patient is symptomatic.

When aspiration of a persistent, discrete mass is not feasible or is nonproductive or when masses are nonmobile and hard, enlarging, tender, or a source of considerable anxiety, the patient should have a surgical excision of the mass (Fig. 10). Unless there are underlying medical conditions, such as cardiac or pulmonary disease, an excisional biopsy can be done in an ambulatory setting under

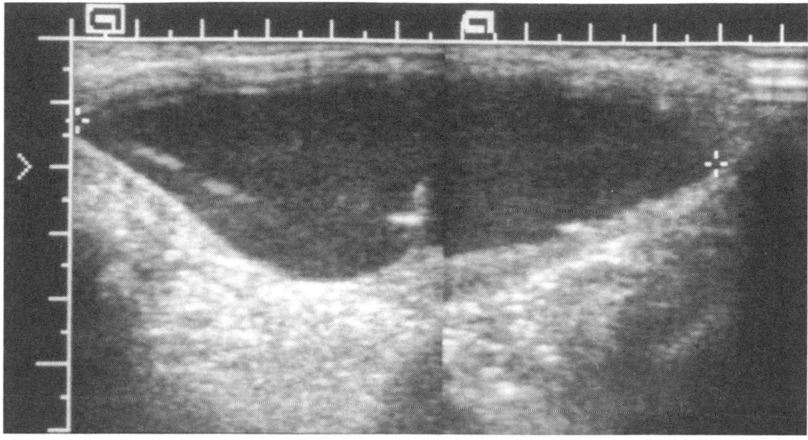

FIG. 9. Ultrasound of a galactocele. (Courtesy of Carol Barnewolt, M.D., Children's Hospital, Boston, MA.)

general or local anesthesia, depending on technical considerations and the patient's preference and ability to cooperate. Since breast scars can be cosmetically deforming, the optimal incision of the breast is circumareolar (Fig. 11). Tissue adjacent to the fibroadenoma should be obtained to examine for atypical proliferative changes (see above) (49). Curvilinear or semilunar incisions are superior to radial incisions in terms of wound healing and cosmetic results. Periareolar ectopic lobules, which often have clear or dark discharge from the areola (not the nipple), can be excised with a circumareolar incision. Fine needle aspi-

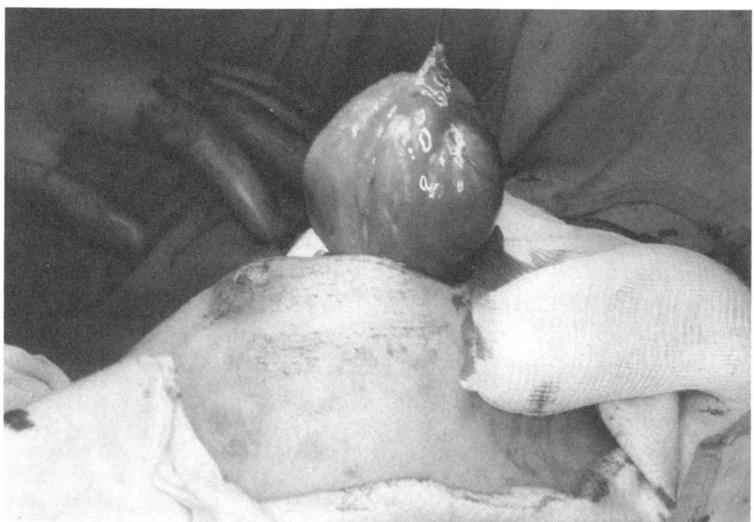

FIG. 10. Resection of a giant fibroadenoma.

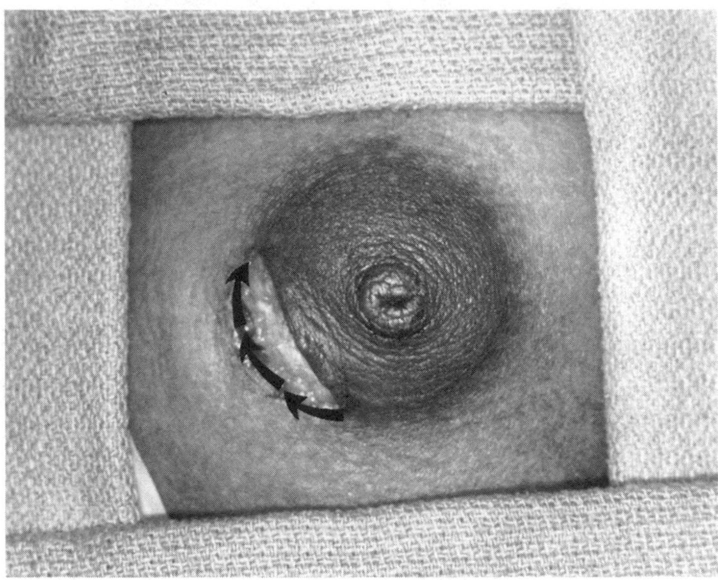

FIG. 11. Circumareolar incision for resection of breast mass.

ration has not been extensively studied in adolescents (69); however, it might allow prolonged observation in adolescents with fibroadenomas or altered therapy in an adolescent diagnosed with a primary carcinoma and suspected of having metastatic disease to the breast. Followup is particularly important after excision because new cysts and fibroadenomas can occur.

Contusion

A contusion to the breast may result in a poorly defined, tender mass that resolves over several weeks. Trauma may result from sports or other accidental injuries or from physical or sexual abuse. A hematoma resulting from trauma should be managed with pain medications, ice packs, and binding of the breast with a sports bra or elastic wrap. A mass from severe trauma may take several months to resolve, and occasionally scar tissue remains palpable indefinitely. Fat necrosis may also result from trauma, although the patient may not notice the growing lesion until several months later. Biopsy is frequently indicated in such circumstances. It should be remembered that the examination immediately following trauma to the breast may locate a preexisting lesion. A sharply delineated, nontender mass is probably unrelated to the recent injury.

Infection

Infection of the breast is seen chiefly in newborns and lactating women. In a review of neonatal mastitis at Children's Hospital, Boston, Walsh and McIntosh

(70) found that infections occurred in full-term infants 1 to 5 weeks of age with a female/male sex ratio of 2:1. All but a few cases were caused by *Staphylococcus aureus,* and most infants (10 of 17) treated after 1971 responded to appropriate β-lactamase-resistant antibiotics without the need for incision and drainage. Recurrent infections or persistence of a mass after treatment for an infection may signal an underlying lesion such as a hemangioma, lymphangioma, or cystic hygroma.

Breast infections in adolescents are most common during lactation. Bacteria such as staphylococci and streptococci enter through cracks in the nipples; cellulitis is often associated with streptococci and abscesses with staphylococci. Nonlactating adolescents may also develop breast infections, usually beneath the areola or at the margin between the areola and the normal skin. The etiology of these infections is unclear, but they may occur because of duct ectasia or metaplasia of the duct epithelium. In addition, the adolescent may give a history of having recently shaved around the areola or having plucked a periareolar hair. Sexual play may also cause breast trauma. Subareolar inflammatory masses may occur secondary to rupture of an areolar gland. The patient may present with a tender mass or, in the early stages of infection, with erythema and warmth of the skin adjacent to the areola. In agreement with our experience, Beach (30) found that infections may be more extensive and deeper than initial superficial findings suggest. As in the neonate, staphylococci are the most common pathogens. Aspiration of the mass (with or without the aid of ultrasound) can help make the clinical and bacteriologic diagnosis. Mastitis associated with duct ectasia usually has a visible discharge, which can be Gram-stained and cultured. If diagnosed early when the predominant feature is cellulitis, most cases will respond to oral antibi-

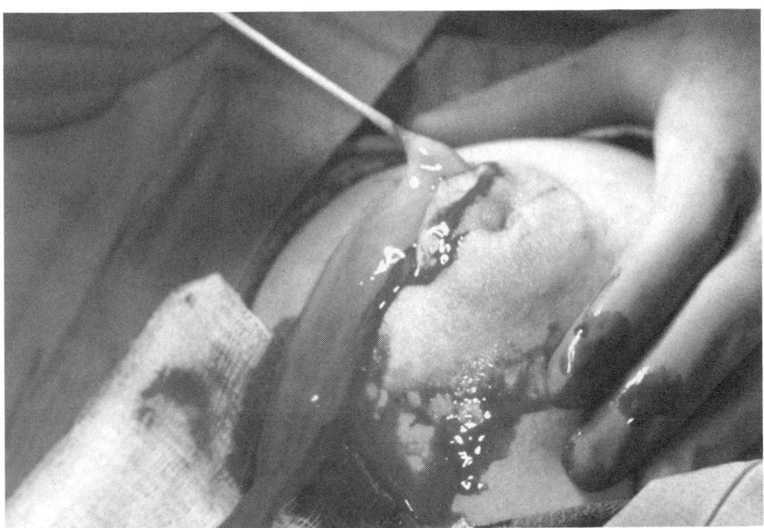

FIG. 12. Incision and drainage of a breast abscess.

otics such as dicloxacillin or a cephalosporin given for 3 to 4 weeks. If the mass becomes fluctuant or if symptoms progress or fail to resolve, incision, drainage (Fig. 12), and packing are performed on an inpatient basis or in the ambulatory operating room setting. Antibiotics should be continued postoperatively. Subareolar abscesses may become recurrent and require elective excision of the dilated milk ducts and associated inflammatory tissue (30,53,71,72).

REFERENCES

1. Stone AM, Shanker IR, McCarthy K. Adolescent breast masses. *Am J Surg* 1977;134:275.
2. West KW, Resoorla FJ, Schere LR III, et al. Diagnosis and treatment of symptomatic breast masses in the pediatric population. *J Pediatr Surg* 1995;30:182.
3. Atkins JE, Solomon LJ, Worden JK, et al. Relative effectiveness of methods of breast self-examination. *J Behav Med* 1991;14:357.
4. Hein K, Dell R, Cohen MI. Self-detection of a breast mass in adolescent females. *J Adolesc Health Care* 1982;3:15.
5. Goldstein DP, Miler V. Breast masses in adolescent females. *Clin Pediatr* 1982;21:17.
6. Cromer BA, Frankel ME, Keder LM. Compliance with breast self-examination instruction in healthy adolescents. *J Adolesc Health Care* 1989;10:105.
7. O'Malley MS, Fletcher SW. Screening for breast cancer with breast self-examination: a critical review. *JAMA* 1987;257:2196.
8. Simmons PS. Diagnostic considerations in breast disorders of children and adolescents. *Obstet Gynecol Clin North Am* 1992;19:91.
9. Goldbloom R. Self-examination by adolescents. *Pediatrics* 1985;76:126.
10. Simmons PS, Wold LE. Surgically treated breast disease in adolescent females: a retrospective review of 185 cases. *Adolesc Pediatr Gynecol* 1989;2:95.
11. Bhatia S, Robinson LL, Oberlin O, et al. Breast cancer and other second neoplasms after childhood Hodgkin's disease. *N Engl J Med* 1996;334:745.
12. Ivins JC, Taylor WF, Wold LE. Elective whole-lung irradiation in osteosarcoma treatment: appearance of bilateral breast cancer in two long-term survivors. *Skeletal Radiol* 1987;16:133.
13. Tucker MA, Coleman CN, Cox RS, et al. Risk of second cancers after treatment for Hodgkin's disease. *N Engl J Med* 1988;318:76.
14. Squire R, Bianchi A, Jakate SM. Radiation-induced sarcoma of the breast in a female adolescent. *Cancer* 1988;61:2444.
15. Lubin F, Ron E, Wax Y, et al. A case-control study of caffeine and methylxanthines in benign breast disease. *JAMA* 1985;253:2388.
16. Shairer C, Brinton LA, Hoover RN. Methylxanthines and benign breast disease. *Am J Epidemiol* 1986;124:603.
17. Vorherr H. Fibrocystic breast disease: pathophysiology, pathomorphology, clinical picture, and management. *Am J Obstet Gynecol* 1986;154:161.
18. Heyden S, Fopdor JG. Coffee consumption and fibrocystic breasts: an unlikely association. *Can J Surg* 1986;29:208.
19. Pye JK, Mansel RE, Hughes LE. Clinical experience of drug treatments for mastalgia. *Lancet* 1985; 2:373.
20. Neinstein LS. Review of breast masses in adolescents. *Adolesc Pediatr Gynecol* 1994;7:119.
21. Haycock CE. How I manage breast problems in athletes. *Phys Sports Med* 1987;15:89.
22. Kenney RD, Flippo JL, Black EB. Supernumerary nipples and renal anomalies in neonates. *Am J Dis Child* 1987;141:987.
23. Hersh JH, Bloom AS, Cromer AO, et al. Does a supernumerary nipple/renal field defect exist? *Am J Dis Child* 1987;141:989.
24. Watkins F, Giacomantonio M, Salisbury S. Nipple discharge and breast lump related to Montgomery's tubercles in adolescent females. *J Pediatr Surg* 1988;23:718.
25. Organ CH Jr, Organ BC. Fibroadenoma of the female breast: a critical clinical assessment. *J Natl Med Assoc* 1983;75:701.
26. Peters F, Schuth W. Hyperprolactinemia and nonpuerperal mastitis (duct ectasia). *JAMA* 1989;261: 1618.

27. Saff D. Apocrine chromhidrosis. *Pediatr Dermatol* 1995;12:48.
28. Diehl T, Kaplan DW. Breast masses in adolescent females. *J Adolesc Health Care* 1985;6:353.
29. Love SM, Gelman RS, Silen W. Fibrocystic "disease" of the breast—a nondisease? *N Engl J Med* 1982;307:1010.
30. Beach RK. Routine breast exams: a chance to reassure, guide, and protect. *Contemp Pediatr* 1987; 70:100.
31. Dupont WD, Page DL. Risk factors for breast cancer in women with proliferative breast disease. *N Engl J Med* 1985;312:146.
32. Daniel W, Mathews M. Tumors of the breast in adolescent females. *Pediatrics* 1968;41:743.
33. Simpson L, Barson A. Breast tumors in infants and children: a 40-year review of cases at a children's hospital. *Can Med Assoc J* 1969;101:100.
34. Oberman HA, Stephens PJ. Carcinoma of the breast in childhood. *Cancer* 1971;30:470.
35. Nichini FM, Goldman L. Inflammatory carcinoma of breast in a 12-year-old girl. *Arch Surg* 1972; 105:505.
36. Kern WH, Clark RW. Retrogression of fibroadenomas of the breast. *Am J Surg* 1973;126:59.
37. Seashore JH. Breast enlargements in infants and children. *Pediatr Ann* 1975;4:542.
38. Turbey WJ, Buntain WL, Dudgeon DL. The surgical management of pediatric breast masses. *Pediatrics* 1975;56:736.
39. Bower R, Bell MJ, Ternberg JL. Management of breast lesions in children and adolescents. *J Pediatr Surg* 1976;11:337.
40. Ashikari R, Jun MY, Farrow JH. Breast carcinoma in children and adolescents. *Clin Bull* 1977;7:55.
41. Gogas J, Sechas M, Skalkeas GR. Surgical management of disease of the adolescent female breast. *Am J Surg* 1979;137:634.
42. Oberman HA. Breast lesions in the adolescent female. *Pathol Ann* 1979;1:175.
43. Ligon R, Stevenson D, Diner W, et al. Breast masses in young women. *Am J Surg* 1980;140:799.
44. Seltzer MH, Skiles MS. Diseases of the breast in young women. *Surg Gynecol Obstet* 1980;150:360.
45. Hammar B. Childhood breast carcinoma: report of a case. *J Pediatr Surg* 1981;16:77.
46. Ernster VL, Goodson WH, Hunt T, et al. Vitamin E and benign breast "disease": a double-blind, randomized, clinical trial. *Surgery* 1985;4:490.
47. London RS, Sundaram GS, Murphy L, et al. The effect of vitamin E on mammary dysplasia: a double-blind study. *Obstet Gynecol* 1985;65:104.
48. Raju CG. Breast masses in adolescent patients in Trinidad. *Am J Surg* 1985;149:219.
49. Dupont WD, Page DL, Parl FF, et al. Long-term risk of breast cancer in women with fibroadenoma. *N Engl J Med* 1994;331:10.
50. Hart J, Layfield LJ, Trumbull WE, et al. Practical aspects in the diagnosis and management of cystosarcoma phyllodes. *Arch Surg* 1988;123:1079.
51. Briggs RM, Walters M, Rosenthal D. Cystosarcoma phyllodes in adolescent female patients. *Am J Surg* 1983;146:712.
52. McNicholas NM, Mercer PM, Miller JC, et al. Color Doppler sonography in the evaluation of palpable breast masses. *AJR* 1993;161:765.
53. Ekland D, Zeigler M. Abscess in the nonlactating breast. *Arch Surg* 1971;107:398.
54. Oberman H, Stephens P. Carcinoma of the breast in childhood. *Cancer* 1972;30:470.
55. Karl SR, Ballantine TV, Zaino R. Juvenile secretory carcinoma of the breast. *Br J Surg* 1987;74:214.
56. Farrow J, Ashikari H. Breast lesions in young girls. *Surg Clin North Am* 1969;49:261.
57. Dixon JM, Lumsden AB, Krajewski A, et al. Primary lymphoma of the breast. *Br J Surg* 1987;74:214.
58. Smith BL. The breast. *Curr Probl Obstet Gynecol Fertil* 1996;19:1.
59. Levine AJ. The p53 tumor-suppressor gene. *N Engl J Med* 1992;326:1350.
60. Hall JM, Lee MK, Newman B, et al. Linkage of early-onset familial breast cancer to chromosome 17q21. *Science* 1990;250:1684.
61. Narod SA, Feunteun J, Lynch HT, et al. Familial breast-ovarian cancer locus on chromosome 17q21-q23. *Lancet* 1991;338:82.
62. Ford D, Easton DF, Bishop DT, et al. Risks of cancer in BRCA1-mutation carriers. *Lancet* 1994; 343:692.
63. Burke W, Daly M, Garber J, et al. Recommendations for follow-up care of individuals with an inherited predisposition to cancer. *JAMA* 1997;277:997.
64. Struewing JP, Hartge P, Wacholder S, et al. The risk of cancer associated with specific mutations of BRCA1 and BRCA2 among Ashkenazi Jews. *N Engl J Med* 1997;336:1401.
65. Rosen PP, Holmes G, Lesser ML, et al. Juvenile papillomatosis and breast carcinoma. *Cancer* 1985; 55:1345.

66. Rosen PP. Papillary duct hyperplasia of the breast in children and young adults. *Cancer* 1985; 56:1611.
67. Hindle WH, Payne PA, Ran EY. The use of fine needle aspiration in the evaluation of persistent palpable dominant masses. *Am J Obstet Gynecol* 1993;168:1814.
68. William SM, Kaplan PA, Peterson JC, et al. Mammography in women under age 30: is there clinical benefit? *Radiology* 1986;161:49.
69. Markovic-Glamoçak M, Suçiç M, Boban D. Fine-needle aspiration and nipple discharge cytology in the diagnosis of breast lesions in adolescent and young women: cytologic findings as compared with those obtained in older women. *Adolesc Pediatr Gynecol* 1994;7:205.
70. Walsh M, McIntosh K. Neonatal mastitis. *Clin Pediatr* 1986;25:395.
71. Osuch JR. Benign lesions of the breast other than fibrocystic change. *Obstet Gynecol Clin North Am* 1987;14:703.
72. Greydanus DE, Parks DS, Farrell EG. Breast disorders in children and adolescents. *Pediatr Clin North Am* 1989;36:601.

17

Contraception

Contraceptive counseling of adolescents requires knowledge of adolescent development and the available forms of contraception. The clinician needs to develop an ongoing therapeutic alliance with the adolescent. The adolescent needs to be in partnership with the health care professional to make healthy choices, including postponement of sexual relationships and use of effective contraceptive "safer sex" methods. Correct and effective use of contraception by adolescent girls and young women is dependent on a number of factors including the personal characteristics of the user (age, educational level, socioeconomic status, parity, and social context), the characteristics of the method (dosage, side effects, ease of use, and cost), and the service system providing the method (access, counseling, educational methods, and choices offered, including backup emergency contraception) (1). Too often, clinicians think only of the user without reflecting on the other two important areas that have a major impact on compliance.

Although clinicians providing health care to adolescents may promote postponement of sexual activity, many teenagers are engaging in intercourse at early ages and often without any form of contraception. In the 1990s, 56% of women and 73% of men reported having had intercourse before age 18 years, compared to 35% of women and 55% men in the early 1970s (2). The 1997 Youth Risk Behavior Survey found that there was a decline in the number of adolescents reporting sexual intercourse between 1990 and 1997 (3,4). In 1997, 48% of high school students (9th to 12th grade) reported ever having had sexual intercourse; 48.9% of males were sexually experienced versus 47.7% of girls. Among 9th graders, 34.0% of girls report ever having been sexually active, compared to 60.1% of 12th grade girls. These percentages are higher for out-of-school youths (5). The 1995 Survey of Family Growth found that 21.4% of 15-year-old girls, 38% of 16-year-old, 49.6% of 17-year-old, 62.7% of 18-year-old, and 72.4% of 19-year-old never married women reported ever being sexually active, with an overall rate for 15- to 19-year-old never married women of 48.1% (6). Use of any contraceptive method at first intercourse rose from 51.4% for those under 16 years to 60% for 19-year-olds. Among 15- to 19-year-old women, 61.6% had used a coitus-dependent method "every time" in the three months prior to the interview (6). The percentage of adolescents using contraception increased from 48% to 65% during the 1980s, almost entirely because of the increase in condom use from 23% to 48% (2). Black and Hispanic teenagers are somewhat less likely (77% and 65%, respectively) to use contraception than white teens (81%) (2), but the differences may be linked to cultural differences, poverty, family structure, and acceptability of early pregnancy and parenting.

Earlier onset of sexual behavior is associated with more lifetime partners and a higher number of recent partners (7). Among sexually active 15- to 17-year-old women, 55% have had two or more partners, and 13% have had at least six (8). Adolescents who become sexually active in their early teens are often involved in other risk-taking activities such as substance abuse and smoking and are especially likely to have an unplanned pregnancy or acquire a sexually transmitted disease (STD) (7,8). Eighty-two percent of pregnancies in adolescents are unintended. Other age groups of women, however, also have unintended pregnancies; for example, 77% of pregnancies in women aged 40 to 44 years are unintended (9).

The increasing awareness of STDs, especially the acquired immunodeficiency syndrome (AIDS), has allowed more open discussion of adolescent sexuality. Sex education in schools and at home, peer counseling, access to contraceptive services, and efforts to help adolescents understand the sexual messages in magazines, billboards, television, books, and movies are essential to address the problems associated with early sexual intercourse. The adolescent patient should be asked about menses and sexual history at each visit to her health care provider. A 14- or 15-year-old teenager will rarely make a specific request for a contraceptive from her primary care clinician unless she knows that the topic can be discussed confidentially. A college student aged 18 or 19 years is much more likely to seek gynecologic care on her own and deal with the issue of contraception. Setting up barriers for access to contraceptive services or mandating parental involvement will increase the number of unwanted pregnancies rather than decrease the number of sexually active adolescents.

Who should prescribe a contraceptive for an adolescent? This depends on whether the physician or nurse practitioner is familiar with routine pelvic examinations and knowledgeable about the indications and contraindications for using the various contraceptive methods. Above all, it is important that clinicians be supportive and empathetic listeners to adolescents and that they not be prejudiced against certain birth control methods. Primary care clinicians need to be familiar with the efficacy and side effects of the various methods, even if the patient is referred to a gynecologist or family planning clinic.

For sexually active 15- to 24-year-old women, friends and family members remain the major source of referral to clinics and private physicians, respectively (10). The age at first visit, ethnicity, and income level of the young woman may impact on her access to services and influence her choice of provider. Black, low-income, and younger women are more likely to select clinics. Adolescents often prefer clinics because of confidentiality, anonymity, low cost, and proximity to home (11). In a study of family planning clinics, teenagers reported that they chose clinics because "it doesn't tell my parents," "the people there care about teens," "it is the closest," "my friends come to it," "it is the only one I know of" (12). Too often, the first visit to a family planning clinic results from a pregnancy scare.

The interval between first intercourse and clinic visit varies from 2 weeks to several years, with mean intervals of 9 to 23 months in different studies (10–16). In our study (16), the interval between first intercourse and a clinic visit to initiate oral contraceptive (OC) use was not different among patients seen in an urban adolescent clinic (10.7 months), a family planning clinic (8.5 months), and a suburban private practice of adolescent medicine (10.9 months). However, the suburban adolescents were much more likely to have used some type of contraceptive method (usually condoms) before making an appointment; 57% of urban adolescents compared to 14% of suburban adolescents had *never* used a method before coming to the clinic.

Since pregnancy frequently occurs in the first 6 months of sexual activity, a major health care challenge is to reach adolescent patients earlier. Potential solutions include offering community education programs for teenagers, enlisting the support of religious organizations, developing relationships with youth groups, opening clinics during evening and weekend hours, and accepting teenagers as walk-in patients, as well as school-based clinics or school-linked services (see Chapters 18 and 22). Adolescents who have had sex education courses are less likely to become sexually active and more likely to use condoms (17).

Since effective contraception involves the ability to think abstractly, plan ahead, and take action including visiting a clinic or doctor, young adolescents may not have reached the developmental stage in which they can organize a plan. Risk taking and a sense of invulnerability are often a part of adolescence. In addition, the risks of contraception, especially OCs, are often significantly overrated in the adolescent mind (18), and in fact by the general public as well. Strategies are needed to delay the onset of sexual activity, make barrier contraceptives more available and acceptable to adolescents, improve access to services, tailor patient education, and develop better long-acting contraception. It becomes particularly critical to combine the resources of family planning clinics and STD clinics so that teenagers accessing family planning services can be screened for STDs and those accessing STD clinics can discuss family planning needs. In addition, overall changes are needed in the psychosocial environment of youth, especially those who are disadvantaged and/or live in poverty. Males need to be involved early and included in family planning educational programs and services. More holistic approaches to teenage pregnancy prevention are expensive but have long-term benefits to individuals and society (see Chapter 18).

In providing medical care to the sexually active adolescent, the clinician should obtain a complete medical history and determine whether there are any specific indications or contraindications to the use of a particular form of contraception. If the patient has already practiced contraception, she may be more apt to comply with the method chosen. The degree to which one or both partners can take responsibility for avoiding an unwanted pregnancy should be assessed. Multiple partners, low self-evaluation, and feelings of hopelessness have been associated with noncompliance with OC regimens (19). The future plans of the adolescent should be assessed, since those bound for college are more likely to be successful using birth control methods (16,20,21). In contrast, the 15-year-old adolescent who has dropped out of school and has no future plans may have ambivalent feelings about a pregnancy (see Chapter 18).

Rates of successful use of contraceptives can vary with the population of adolescents served. In a study of adolescents prescribed OCs, only 48% of those seen in the urban clinic returned for their 3-month followup visit and continued to take the pill, compared to 65% of patients seen in a family planning clinic and 84% of patients seen in a suburban private practice (16). At long-term followup (13.5 ± 3.7 months), 34% of urban and 55% of suburban teens continued to take the pill; factors associated with contraceptive compliance included health care in a private practice, suburban residence, white race, college-bound, higher level of father's education, satisfaction with the OC, and absence of side effects. Ten pregnancies occurred among noncompliant urban patients. A second study done in our clinic demonstrated that the compliance was similar for monophasic and triphasic OCs at 1-year followup (22). Furstenberg and associates (13) made similar observations in a study of compliance among family planning patients, in which continuing use of contraception was associated with older age, white race, adolescents who had working parents with higher levels of education, being college-bound, above-average grades, a steady sexual relationship, and satisfaction with the method chosen. A study of San Francisco teens found that intention to use contraception was related to actual use of contraception 1 year later (23,24). Several models to explain contraceptive compliance have been suggested (25,26).

In rethinking appropriate counseling, Oakley (27) has suggested that since demographic factors related to contraceptive compliance are difficult to change, counseling of women should focus on use behaviors and assessment of abilities and intentions to carry out those behaviors. The woman who is particularly in need of new counseling approaches is one without prior experience to draw on (no successful analogous behavior from which to generalize), no future plans, no support for avoiding unplanned pregnancy, previous unplanned pregnancies, short-term sexual relationships, cognitive impairment, having a visit not initiated by her, and the acceptance of a pregnancy in the next 6 to 12 months. The emphasis of the counseling has to be on future orientation, reviewing the complex behaviors necessary for effective use, assessing intentions, interpreting problems with contraception correctly, and mobilizing self-planning so that effective actions can be taken to resolve problems. Discontinuation and misuse of OCs are frequent causes of unintended pregnancy in adolescents and adult women (28). It is important for health care providers to realize that young women may underreport missed OCs (29).

Before prescribing contraceptives, the health care provider should discuss the risks of being sexually active, including the emotional consequences, STDs, and pregnancy. Behavioral change is often slow. Some teenagers have not even thought that they could get pregnant with sexual intercourse and have not contemplated the use of contraception. Others have already thought about contraceptive options and made a choice. The adolescent may later forget about her commitment and no longer be using condoms or other protection because of sporadic relationships. Clinicians are challenged by assisting young people through the stages of change by education, personalizing the risk, and skills building (see Chapter 1).

The possibility of parental involvement should be assessed with the adolescent, particularly because some adolescents can share the information with a parent, particularly the mother. Payment for the visit and laboratory tests and issues of confidentiality should be discussed early in the provision of contraceptive services. Involvement of the male partner is ideal but often not achieved in clinical practice. For the teen who has been successfully using condoms and now wishes to use hormonal contraception, discussion about the need for continuing protection against STDs is paramount. Although in one study two-thirds of patients stated that they planned to continue to use condoms after initiating hormonal contraception, Loeb and colleagues (30) found that only 28% were using condoms at last intercourse at the 3-month followup visit. An adolescent girl needs to discuss with the health care provider whether to tell her partner about her decision to initiate hormonal contraception. She may be concerned that his knowledge of her method will negatively affect his condom use.

Some states have passed laws that specifically allow minors to give their own informed consent for birth control. Adolescents who are emancipated minors or "mature minors" can consent to their own contraception (see Chapter 21). This highly charged issue is best dealt with at the first visit. If the clinician is providing continuity of care from childhood to adolescence, a comprehensive preventive services visit when the girl is 11 or 12 years old is an ideal time to explain the need for privacy and confidentiality in the adolescent years. The parents can understand that a new phase of health care is beginning and that the physician will share as much as possible, but that certain information about school, friends, drugs, and sexuality needs to remain confidential. The parents should be encouraged to call with any of their concerns. Most families welcome knowing that physicians and nurse practitioners are concerned about psychosocial and health issues. The clinician can explicitly state the confidentiality policy before contraceptive issues arise, letting families know that their input is valued and that issues will be shared as needed (or if clearly life threatening). In some situations, prescribing an OC for dysmenorrhea or irregular menses may be better accepted by parents and preserve confidentiality for the patient.

The teen who does not share the information about birth control with her parents should at least think through with the clinician what she would do if her parents found the contraceptive pills or device. In volatile situations, the clinician

TABLE 1. *Lowest expected and typical percentages of accidental pregnancy in the United States during the first year of use of a method*

Method	Lowest expected[a]	Typical[b]
Chance[c]	85	85
Spermicides[d]	3	21
Periodic abstinence		20
Calendar	9	
Ovulation method	3	
Symptothermal[e]	2	
Postovulation	1	
Withdrawal	4	18
Cap[f]	6	18
Sponge		
Parous women	9	28
Nulliparous women	6	18
Diaghragm[f]	6	18
Condom[g]	2	12
Intrauterine device		
Progesterone-impregnated T (Progestasert)	2	3
Copper T 380A (ParaGard)	0.8	
Pill		3
Combined	0.1	
Progestogen only	0.5	
Injectable progestogen		
DMPA	0.3	0.3
NET	0.4	0.4
Implants		
Norplant (6 capsules)	0.04	0.04
Norplant-2 (2 rods)	0.03	0.03
Female sterilization	0.2	0.4
Male sterilization	0.1	0.15

DMPA, medroxyprogesterone acetate; NET, norethindrone enanthate.

[a]Among couples who initiate use of a method (not necessarily for the first time) and who use it perfectly (both consistently and correctly), these percentages represent the authors' best guesses regarding those who can expect to experience an accidental pregnancy during the first year if they do not stop use of the method for any other reason.

[b]Among typical couples who initiate use of a method (not necessarily for the first time), these are the percentages that will experience an accidental pregnancy during the first year if they do not stop use for any other reason.

[c]The lowest expected and typical percentages are based on data from populations in which contraception is not used and from women who cease using contraception in order to become pregnant. These represent the authors' best guess of the percentage who would conceive among women now relying on reversible methods of contraception if they abandoned contraception altogether. The lowest reported percent is based on U.S. women who use no contraception, even though they do not wish to become pregnant. This group is selected for low fecundity or low coital frequency, and some fraction may use an unreported variant of periodic abstinence.

[d]Foams and vaginal suppositories.

[e]Cervical mucus (ovulation) method is supplemented by calendar in the preovulatory phase and by basal body temperature in the postovulatory phase.

[f]With spermicidal cream or jelly.

[g]Without spermicides.

(Adapted from Trussell J, Hatcher R, Cates W, et al. Contraceptive failure in the United States: an update. *Stud Fam Plann* 1990;21:(1), Table 1; with permission of the Population Council.)

should offer to be the mediator to help both sides come to a solution around responsible sexuality. The clinician can facilitate communication by asking both the parent(s) and the daughter to come in for counseling at the end of the office day. Each health care provider has his or her own style of communication, but it is helpful to empathize with the parents' concerns for their daughter and to acknowledge the change in sexual mores. At the same time, the parent(s) should be congratulated on raising a daughter who is being responsible about contraception instead of becoming pregnant, as with so many of her peers. Acknowledging to parents how difficult it is to raise adolescents and listening to their issues can facilitate solutions.

The pregnancy rates of 100 women using different contraceptive devices for 1 year (100 woman-years of use) are listed in Table 1 (31–34). Trussell and colleagues (33,34) have written eloquently about the problems of developing these numbers, including the varying definitions and measurements of efficacy from study to study, the lack of randomized clinical trials, selection bias, concepts of use and exposure, assessment of failures (pregnancies, lost-to-followup rates), recent OC use, and conflict of interest of investigators. Estimates for use failure rates for a first year of contraception in fact may be 30% higher because of underreporting of abortions. For some teenagers, the pregnancy rate with the combined OC may climb to 9 to 12 pregnancies per 100 woman-years or even higher because of missed pills and misunderstanding the directions (Table 2). It is critical for teens to know how to use backup methods and how to obtain emergency contraception. The teenager must feel that she has actively participated in the decision about the best method of contraception for her lifestyle; the dialogue between clinician and patient is of supreme importance (35,36). For example, a patient will sometimes discontinue a form of contraception because she perceives that the health care provider is unhelpful, the time in the waiting room too long, or the pelvic examination distressing. Regardless of what the patient initially states as her preferred form of contraception, it is important for the clinician to discuss all available forms of birth control, because method switching is common. Writing the methods of contraception (including abstinence), the preg-

TABLE 2. *Contraceptive failure (%) during the first 12 months of use by method, race, and age (yr) for unmarried women*

	White		Nonwhite	
Method	<20	20–24	<20	20–24
Pill	9.3	5.9	18.1	11.7
Condom	13.3	22.5	22.3	36.3
Diaphragm	12.4	22.5	35.5	57.0
Spermicide	35.0	38.7	34.0	37.6

(From Jones EF, Forrest JD. Contraceptive failure in the United States: revised estimates from the 1982 National Survey of Family Growth. *Fam Plann Perspect* 1989;21:103, with permission.)

nancy rates, and the risks and benefits on a sheet of paper can help the patient make a good choice.

Coitus interruptus (withdrawal) is still practiced by a large number of adolescents who believe it to be an effective form of contraception. More effective forms of contraception should be strongly encouraged. The clinician should also discuss abstinence and help patients learn to say "No" when they are not ready for intercourse or wish to reinstitute abstinence. Many excellent pamphlets are available and can allow patients to read factual information and contemplate their decision away from the medical clinic (see Appendix 1).

Since few women use the same form of contraception throughout their reproductive lives, it is important to emphasize to the young teenager that even if she chooses an OC initially, she may well make other choices in the future depending on her need for contraception, the frequency with which she is having intercourse, her age, parity, and her partner's preferences.

The mortality in young, sexually active women is shown in Table 3. The risk of combined OCs is substantially less than that of carrying a pregnancy to term. However, hormonal contraception, such as OCs, medroxyprogesterone contraceptive injections, and levonorgestrel subdermal implants, offers no protection from acquiring a STD, and thus the use of condoms needs to be emphasized.

Health care providers also need to address the sexuality issues of adolescents with chronic diseases, disabilities, and developmental delay (see Chapter 19). Adolescents with chronic diseases, especially those with delayed development and undernutrition, are frequently assumed to be too sick to be sexually active or may be infantilized by parents and health care providers. A discussion of sexuality and contraceptive methods is important for all adolescents. Many ill patients take chances because they falsely assume their disease has made them infertile. Patients who are immunosuppressed must be educated about their increased risks of persistent human papillomavirus (HPV) infection (see Chapter 13) and should be encouraged to use condoms with every sexual relationship. Permanent sterilization can be considered by young women with conditions such as severe heart disease or cystic fibrosis, depending on the wishes of the patient.

TABLE 3. *Annual number of birth- or method-related deaths associated with control of fertility per 100,000 nonsterile women by fertility control method according to age (yr)*

Method of control and outcome	15–19	20–24	25–29	30–34	35–39	40–44
No fertility control methods[a]	7.0	7.4	9.1	14.8	25.7	28.2
Oral contraceptives, nonsmoker[b]	0.3	0.5	0.9	1.9	13.8	31.6
Oral contraceptives, smoker[b]	2.2	3.4	6.6	13.5	51.1	117.2
Intrauterine device[b]	0.8	0.8	1.0	1.0	1.4	1.4
Condom[a]	1.1	1.6	0.7	0.2	0.3	0.4
Diaphragm/spermicide[a]	1.9	1.2	1.2	1.3	2.2	2.8
Periodic abstinence[a]	2.5	1.6	1.6	1.7	2.9	3.6

[a]Deaths are birth related.
[b]Deaths are method related.
(From *Physicians' desk reference,* Montvale, NJ: Medical Economics Data, 1996.)

Patients with disabilities need sensitive counseling to help them through a pelvic examination, reassurance about their normal anatomy, and provision of contraception that meets their needs. Female barrier methods may not be possible for some teens. Patients with myelodysplasia have an increased incidence of latex allergy and thus often require the use of nonlatex gloves for pelvic examinations and may need to avoid latex condoms. In all young women with medical and psychiatric disorders, the clinician needs to carefully weigh the risk of pregnancy, the probability that the patients will use the method, the effectiveness of the method chosen, and the risk of the method associated with the disorder (37). Too often, only issues related to the risk of the method in a particular disease are considered in the equation, and often those data are extrapolated from anecdotal evidence, case reports, or suppositions based on studies in healthy women.

Parents often bring in adolescent girls with developmental delay to discuss contraception. These patients, especially those with mild retardation, appear to be at increased risk of sexual assault or abuse. Thus, depending on the social environment and available supervision, risk, and age of the adolescent, thoughtful discussion is needed about the choices: observation, prophylactic hormonal contraception (an OC, injectable progestins, or implants), or sterilization (depending on the needs of the patient and the legal issues involved). These adolescents can also benefit from education about hygiene, reproduction, contraception, and responsible sexuality.

PATIENT EVALUATION

The indications and contraindications of each method are discussed below. Adolescents deserve information on all methods, including emergency contraception. Clinicians should take a complete medical history including baseline information on problems such as weight gain, headaches, acne, breast tenderness, dysmenorrhea, irregular menses, and nausea/vomiting, so that issues that arise at future visits can be better assessed. It is also important to perform a general physical examination, including a blood pressure reading and breast and pelvic examination. Fear of the first pelvic examination can be a barrier to teens wishing to obtain contraceptives (18). Thus, delaying the first pelvic examination for 3 to 6 months in adolescents who might otherwise postpone use of effective contraception has been helpful in building trust (38). For most adolescents, the pelvic examination can be done at the initial visit. In fact, sometimes adolescents fear returning for the examination when it could have been easily accomplished at the initial visit. Thus, decisions about the timing of the examination need to be individualized. Delay may also prevent the early identification and treatment of asymptomatic STDs although this is less a problem with newer urine testing techniques.

Questions that are appropriate to ask the teen are shown in Table 4. Whichever method is chosen should be demonstrated for the teen. Younger adolescents are concrete thinkers and need to have the OC package opened and the exact method

TABLE 4. *Questions to pose to teens choosing a contraceptive method*

What methods have you used before?
What are your worries about this method?
Do you have friends who have used this method?
What were their experiences? Did they have problems?
Do you think you can use this method effectively?
Have you ever had problems with your weight? Have you ever dieted?
Is your partner in favor or opposed to this method?
How will you be able to handle unexpected bleeding? or extra bleeding?
Do you have questions I haven't answered?

of taking the pill demonstrated. Similarly, the use of condoms or spermicides requires a hands-on demonstration. Any handouts that will be given should be read with the teen and open-ended questions asked. The factors related to compliance should be taken into account as the clinician helps the patient form appropriate plans for the future.

Initial laboratory studies for adolescents typically include hemoglobin level, Papanicolaou (Pap) smear, tests for *Neisseria gonorrhoeae* and *Chlamydia trachomatis*, and urinalysis (or dipstick urine test). The prevalence of gonococcal and chlamydial infections in sexually active adolescents in general and in a given adolescent population should be considered in developing guidelines for screening. All sexually active adolescents should be screened for *C. trachomatis* at least annually and more often if the patient is symptomatic or there is a change in partners. Screening for *N. gonorrhoeae* is particularly cost effective in urban teens, those with multiple partners and early age of coitus, pregnant adolescents, symptomatic patients, and those with other STDs. The incidence of *N. gonorrhoeae* infection is very low in college students and suburban adolescents in monogamous relationships, and thus gonorrhea screening may be selective and less frequent in some populations. The availability of a single screening test swab for both gonorrhea and chlamydia obviates such choices and allows simplified testing. A blood test for syphilis is indicated in high-risk patients (those with multiple partners, a sexual partner at risk, sex in exchange for drugs or money, homelessness, residence in an area with high prevalence) and in those with other STDs. Adolescents should be offered counseling and testing for human immunodeficiency virus (HIV) infection; all adolescents should receive counseling on disease prevention and risk reduction, especially with regard to HPV and HIV. Adolescents should be immunized against hepatitis B.

Although guidelines vary because of the difficulty of obtaining accurate family histories, we recommend obtaining serum total cholesterol and high-density lipoprotein cholesterol levels once during adolescence (preferably before the initiation of hormonal contraception). At minimum, lipid screening should be done in patients who have a family history of early arteriosclerotic heart disease or hypercholesterolemia and in those age 19 years or older.

Other risk-taking behaviors (substance use, nonuse of seat belts, violence) should also be assessed and addressed as part of preventive health services to teens. Providing effective counseling on tobacco avoidance and smoking cessation is particularly important in the context of adolescent health care.

COMBINED ORAL CONTRACEPTIVES

Many teenagers choose an OC because of the low failure rate, the relief from dysmenorrhea, and the ease of use of a method that is not directly related to the episode of intercourse. Common pills and their hormone content are listed in Table 5. The majority of OCs are combination pills containing an estrogen and a progestin. The so-called minipill is a progestin-only pill.

TABLE 5. *Oral contraceptives available in the United States*

Proprietary name	Estrogen	μg	Progestin	mg
Demulen 1/50	Ethinyl estradiol	50	Ethynodiol diacetate	1
Ovral	Ethinyl estradiol	50	Norgestrel	0.5
Ovcon 50	Ethinyl estradiol	50	Norethindrone	1
Norinyl 1 + 50	Mestranol	50	Norethindrone	1
Ortho-Novum 1/50	Mestranol	50	Norethindrone	1
Demulen 1/35	Ethinyl estradiol	35	Ethynodiol diacetate	1
Norinyl 1 + 35[a]	Ethinyl estradiol	35	Norethindrone	1
Ortho-Novum 1/35[a]	Ethinyl estradiol	35	Norethindrone	1
Ortho-Cyclen	Ethinyl estradiol	35	Norgestimate	0.25
OrthoTri-Cyclen	Ethinyl estradiol	35	Norgestimate	0.180 × 7 d 0.215 × 7 d 0.250 × 7 d
Brevicon[a], Modicon[a]	Ethinyl estradiol	35	Norethindrone	0.5
Ovcon 35	Ethinyl estradiol	35	Norethindrone	0.4
Lo/Ovral	Ethinyl estradiol	30	Norgestrel	0.3
Loestrin 1.5/30	Ethinyl estradiol	30	Norethindrone acetate	1.5
Levlen, Nordette	Ethinyl estradiol	30	Levonorgestrel	0.15
Desogen, Ortho-Cept	Ethinyl estradiol	30	Desogestrel	0.15
Jenest-28	Ethinyl estradiol	35	Norethindrone	0.5 × 7 d 1.0 × 14 d
Ortho-Novum 7/7/7	Ethinyl estradiol	35	Norethindrone	0.5 × 7 d 0.75 × 7 d 1.0 × 7 d
Tri-Norinyl	Ethinyl estradiol	35	Norethindrone	0.5 × 7 d 1.0 × 9 d 0.5 × 5 d
Tri-Levlen, Triphasil	Estradiol	30	Levonorgestrel	0.05 × 6 d 0.075 × 5 d 0.125 × 10 d
Estrostep	Ethinyl estradiol Ethinyl estradiol Ethinyl estradiol	20 × 5 d 30 × 7 d 35 × 9 d	Norethindrone acetate	1
Loestrin 1/20	Ethinyl estradiol	20	Norethindrone acetate	1
Alesse, Levlite	Ethinyl estradiol	20	Levonorgestrel	0.1
Mircette	Ethinyl estradiol	10 × 5 d 20 × 21 d	Desogestrel	0.15 × 21 d
Ovrette			Norgestrel	0.075
Micronor, Nor-QD			Norethindrone	0.35

[a]Generics are available for some of the pills.

The estrogen contained in the combination pills is either *mestranol* or *ethinyl estradiol* and varies in dose from 20 to 50 μg. Ethinyl estradiol (31) is rapidly absorbed, with peak levels in 60 to 120 minutes. Mestranol is converted in the liver to ethinyl estradiol; therefore, peak serum levels of ethinyl estradiol are lower and occur later after ingestion of mestranol than after ingestion of the same dose of ethinyl estradiol. Some patients may have incomplete conversion of mestranol to ethinyl estradiol. All of the low-dose OCs have ≤35 μg ethinyl estradiol. OCs with 50 μg estrogen have either mestranol or ethinyl estradiol. It is difficult to assess the exact potency of these two compounds in relation to each other because the progestin may potentiate or lessen the effects of a particular dose of the estrogen. However, many authors consider that 50 μg of mestranol is equivalent to 35 μg of ethinyl estradiol (39). The plasma levels of ethinyl estradiol seen with an OC containing 50 μg mestranol and 1 mg norethindrone were the same as those with a pill containing 35 μg ethinyl estradiol and 1 mg norethindrone (40).

The progestins used in OCs, termed 19-nortestosterone derivatives, are related to 19-carbon androgens and include norethindrone, norethindrone acetate, norethynodrel, ethynodiol diacetate, norgestrel, levonorgestrel, desogestrel, norgestimate, and gestodene. These progestins have varying qualities of being estrogenic, antiestrogenic, progestational (anabolic), and androgenic. Potencies are extremely controversial because of the varying tests used, including animal models, delay of menses, and ability to induce glycogen vacuoles in human endometrium (41–44). Generally, the estranes—norethindrone, norethindrone acetate, and ethynodiol diacetate—are considered fairly equipotent; norgestrel is estimated to be 5 to 10 times more potent, and levonorgestrel is 10 to 20 times more potent. Gestodene is considered less androgenic and more progestational than levonorgestrel. Norgestimate is estimated to be three times the potency of norethindrone on the test of percentage of rabbits ovulating (levonorgestrel is seven to eight times more potent than norethindrone on this test). Norgestimate has four to five times less binding affinity for rabbit uterine receptors than levonorgestrel and much less affinity for androgen receptors and sex hormone–binding globulin than levonorgestrel. Desogestrel is more progestational than levonorgestrel but less androgenic; this compound also binds to corticoid receptors (1,39). Half-lives have been estimated to be about 7 to 8 hours (range, 4 to 11 hours) for norethindrone, 10 to 12 hours for gestodene, 16 hours (range, 8 to 30 hours) for levonorgestrel, 45 to 71 hours for norgestimate, and 20 hours (range, 11 to 24 hours) for desogestrel. There are variations in elimination half-lives between subjects and within the same subject, as well as evidence of differences when the progestin is given alone, when it is given for multiple doses, and when it is administered with estrogen (41). Some progestins, such as norethindrone, have a loss of drug with the first pass through the liver after absorption, and others, such as levonorgestrel, do not. Long half-lives and other aspects of binding and metabolism of certain progestins likely contribute to the lowered incidence of breakthrough bleeding. Newer progestins, such as drospirenone, a progestin related to the 21-carbon antimineralocorticoid 17α-spironolactone, are being tested and are notable for weight loss and mild decline in blood pressure.

The combination OCs prevent pregnancy by suppressing the ovarian–hypothalamic axis and thus inhibiting ovulation. In addition, they alter the endometrium to make implantation unlikely, increase the viscosity of the endocervical mucus, and may have a direct effect on corpus luteum steroidogenesis. Fortunately, even with missed pills, ovulation usually remains suppressed (45). Women taking an OC with 35 μg ethinyl estradiol with monophasic 1 mg norethindrone appear to have less follicular development than those taking the same dose of estrogen with 0.5 mg norethindrone or a triphasic norethindrone dose (Ortho-Novum 7/7/7) (46).

Selection of a particular combined OC depends on the patient's needs and response, the availability of samples and supplies to family planning clinics and physician offices, and cost (typically $12 to $30 per cycle). Typical starter combination OCs containing 30 to 35 μg ethinyl estradiol include pills such as norethindrone 1 mg/ethinyl estradiol 35 μg, Ortho-Novum 7/7/7, or Tri-Norinyl, levonorgestrel triphasic pills (Triphasil, Tri-Levlen), and norgestimate pills (Ortho-Cyclen, OrthoTri-Cyclen). OCs with less estrogen (Alesse, Estrostep, Mircette) have recently been introduced and are also good first start OCs. Some pills are more estrogen dominant and others more progestin dominant. An OC with low androgenicity would be a good choice for adolescents with acne, hirsutism, or polycystic ovary syndrome. An OC with more progestin is helpful in patients with dysmenorrhea, hypermenorrhea, previous breakthrough bleeding, or dysfunctional uterine bleeding. A patient with previous nausea or vomiting on OCs may benefit from using a very low-dose estrogen pill with 20 μg ethinyl estradiol (47). The triphasic pills have the theoretical advantage of delivering less total milligrams of contraceptive steroids per cycle than some monophasic pills and often provide improved cycle control. However, a pill with 0.5 mg norethindrone still has less progestin than the triphasic Ortho-Novum 7/7/7. Although some adolescents may find the particular packaging or the presence of many different colored tablets confusing, most do well if the package is demonstrated at the time of the visit (22).

Breakthrough bleeding rates appear to be lower with some of the newer OCs and the levonorgestrel OCs, although studies are often difficult to compare because of varying definition of bleeding and spotting (49). For example, the triphasic levonorgestrel pill has a low rate of breakthrough bleeding (6.9% of first cycle and 3.2% of total cycles) and amenorrhea (0.6% of cycles) (23), with less breakthrough bleeding in the first four cycles than norethindrone triphasics (50). Desogestrel- and norgestimate-containing pills also have extremely low rates of breakthrough bleeding and amenorrhea (51–54). In a comparative study, Corson (52) reported that 11.3% of women taking a norgestimate/ethinyl estradiol pill and 10.6% of women taking a norgestrel/ethinyl estradiol pill experienced breakthrough bleeding in the first 6 months and 1.1% and 1.8%, respectively, experienced amenorrhea in the same interval. Studies of OCs containing 0.15 mg desogestrel and 30 μg ethinyl estradiol have shown similar low levels of problems with cycle control (53). Absence of side effects can be important for adolescents to enhance continued use of OCs. All of the combined OCs are remarkably effective, with 0.28 to 0.33 pregnancies per 100 woman-years of use.

The side effects and contraindications of OCs must be carefully understood before the pill is prescribed. Clinicians are encouraged to read in detail the package insert to have a good understanding of the risks, precautions, and potential problems and to become aware of the information that the patient will be reading prior to starting the pill. Absolute contraindications include thromboembolic disease, cerebrovascular or coronary artery disease, breast cancer, estrogen-dependent neoplasia, undiagnosed genital bleeding (applicable primarily to adult women), pregnancy, and liver tumors.

Counseling about risks and benefits should be documented in the medical record; some clinics use a standard informed-consent form outlining any increased risks that the individual may have (see Appendix 2). Although physicians are usually concerned about the serious but highly unlikely side effects of OCs, patients often have very different worries related to pill use, and their intention to use and actual use of OC may be influenced by concerns about health and physical appearance (55). In our Boston study (16), urban teens were concerned about weight gain (32%), blood clots (22%), birth defects (11%), and future fertility (10%), whereas suburban teens were almost exclusively worried about the possibility of weight gain (86%). Although birth defects and future fertility are not related to OC use, failure to address patients' worries may lead to noncompliance. The statements such as "Some adolescents I see are worried about gaining weight" or "Some adolescents are worried about not being able to have children" help initiate the dialogue between the adolescent and the health care provider. Our studies as well as others have found no significant mean weight gain associated with the use of low-dose OCs (1,16,56). Carpenter and Neinstein (56) reported no significant difference between an OC group and a control group in initial weight and weight after 1 year of use. However, because weight gain is such an issue for teens and there are some teens who appear to be particularly prone to gain weight with the use of hormonal methods, it is important to weigh the patient at each visit and provide appropriate dietary assessment and counseling. Avoiding all fast foods and decreasing TV viewing time for the first 3 months of use of hormonal contraception can be an important preventive strategy. Encouraging the sedentary teen to increase her exercise level is also important.

A handout should be given to patients, and this can serve as an important point of discussion. To avoid confusion, the clinic handout should either be the new Food and Drug Administration (FDA) patient package insert or reflect its content. Instructions for missed pills should be uniform. Although written instructions can save phone calls, they are not a substitute for careful counseling in the office because many patients misplace these sheets soon after the visit (16). The possible occurrence of breakthrough bleeding for the first few cycles should be explained in detail, with patients being shown the actual pill package and where breakthrough bleeding might occur (usually the second week). Patients should be encouraged to call if any problems are worrying them and counseled not to stop taking the pill without calling. Documenting in the chart the baseline occurrence of headaches, weight issues, nausea, and other complaints is essential so that these problems can be assessed at followup. Patients are instructed in possible side effects using the acronym ACHES: A—abdominal pain (severe); C—chest pain (severe), cough, shortness of breath; H—headache (severe), dizziness, weakness, numbness, speech problems; E—eye problems (vision loss or blurring); S—severe leg pain (calf or thigh) (31).

The benefits of the pill should be stressed. These include less iron-deficiency anemia, less dysmenorrhea, a lowered incidence of benign breast disease and uterine and ovarian cancers, less pelvic inflammatory disease (PID), less acne, and probably increased bone density (57). For example, among teens seen in an urban family planning clinic, those girls with severe dysmenorrhea who experienced a reduction of their symptoms on OCs were eight times more likely to be consistent users (58).

Patients should then be given a prescription or a 3-month supply of pills and asked to return to the clinic in 1 to 3 months to check weight, blood pressure, and side effects. The patient who is older and who sought medical care specifically to obtain a contraceptive may be seen in 3 months and encouraged to call if any special problems arise. It is helpful if each office has one professional designated to take patients' phone calls at the time they are initiated, as adolescents may be calling from school or another location where the call may be difficult to return. Younger teenagers, those who have been having intercourse for months to years without adequate contraception, and those with multiple partners, school failure, or other high-risk behaviors, or the sibling of a parenting teen should be encouraged to return in 6 weeks or even sooner to continue the dialogue on contraceptive choices and address other risky behaviors if present.

Most pills are available in 21- and 28-day packages; the latter have seven tablets that are placebos (except Loestrin and Estrostep, which contain iron, and Mircette, which has 5 days of estrogen). The majority of teenagers do best using a 28-day pill, since it is easier to remember to take a pill every day rather than for 21 days of hormones followed by a 7-day rest. In our experience, 21-day pills frequently result in confusion. To start the first package of pills, patients may start on the Sunday following the first day of menses (unless menses starts on a Sunday, in which case the pills are started that day); on the first day of menses (some OCs are packaged only for Sunday starts; others have stickers or mechanisms that allow any day start); or on day 5 of menses (if necessary because of the timing of arrival of patients in the office). Patients who are amenorrheic and need to start an OC can be asked to refrain from intercourse for 2 weeks, a sensitive pregnancy test can be performed, and medroxyprogesterone (10 mg for 5 days) prescribed to initiate withdrawal flow before starting an OC.

Patients are instructed to take one pill daily at about the same time each day, preferably after dinner or at bedtime. It is essential that adolescents cue pill taking to a daily activity such as a meal or tooth brushing. Adolescents frequently miss pills and thus should receive careful instructions on methods of dealing with this problem (the specific instructions are in the handout in Appendix 3). The importance of a backup method and emergency contraception should be stressed. Patients will likely experience breakthrough bleeding with missed pills.

The followup visit includes a blood pressure and weight check. Teens should be questioned about consistent use, concerns, and side effects of the method, and the benefits should be reviewed. Not infrequently, the nausea and breakthrough bleeding that patients experience during the first cycle of pills have disappeared by the third cycle. Adjustments in pill dosage can be made as suggested in the section below on side effects. Adolescent patients' ability to obtain or pay for refills should be reviewed.

Young adolescents are then seen at least every 6 months for renewal of the pill prescription, blood pressure and weight check, and counseling. Screening for *C. trachomatis* and *N. gonorrhoeae* every 6 months in high-risk teens or with a change in sexual partner and every 12 months in lower-risk teens is appropriate. Older adolescents who are consistent contraceptive users can be seen annually for STD and Pap screening. Teens at high risk for other problem behaviors need much more frequent visits to deal not only with contraceptive use but with the many other behavioral and social issues in their lives.

Side Effects, Contraindications, and Precautions

Weight Change

Weight gain is uncommonly caused by the low-dose OCs (see previous section); however, weight should be checked at each visit. Fluid retention can sometimes occur secondary to the estrogen or progestin. Progestins can have an anabolic effect and increase appetite. Teens may lose weight because of self-imposed dieting, nausea, or depression.

Often an adolescent believes she has gained 5 to 10 lbs, when in fact the gain is a perception and not an actual change. Thus, if teens call about significant weight gain, it is important to have them come to the office for a weight measurement. If weight gain occurs, a lower-calorie, lower-salt diet, an increase in exercise, a decrease in TV time, and, if needed, a change to a pill low in both estrogen and progestin usually solve the problem.

Nausea

Nausea is generally considered an estrogenic side effect. Many patients will experience mild nausea for the first few days of taking OCs and sometimes for the first day of the subsequent one or two cycles. Generally, this mild nausea disappears without treatment over the first three cycles, and most patients tolerate the low-dose OCs that contain 30 to 35 µg ethinyl estradiol quite well. If patients take the pill ½ hour after dinner or with a snack at bedtime rather than in the morning, nausea is less likely to be a problem. However, if the nausea is persistent or bothersome, it is wise to reduce the amount of estrogen (e.g., from 35 to 30, or to 20 µg). Changing to Loestrin 1/20, Alesse, or Mircette can be particularly helpful, although the tradeoff may be more irregular cycles.

Nausea and vomiting can obviously have many other etiologies, including pregnancy, viral syndromes, and gastrointestinal diseases, and thus may need further evaluation. Patients who have vomiting or gastroenteritis may risk pill failure and should use a backup method. If vomiting occurs within 1 hour of taking the pill, taking an extra pill from a different pill pack is recommended.

Breakthrough Bleeding

Breakthrough bleeding is the occurrence of endometrial bleeding per vagina while the patient is taking hormone tablets. It occurs most frequently in the first one or two cycles, generally during the second week of the cycle; it usually diminishes with subsequent cycles on the same pill. The patient should be told in advance about the possibility of breakthrough bleeding so that she will not stop taking the pill because of excessive concern about this common side effect. Most patients with breakthrough bleeding for several days in the first few cycles can be reassured that the bleeding will disappear with subsequent cycles. In adolescents who develop breakthrough bleeding after several months to years of use, missed pills are a common cause, but chlamydial infection should always be kept in mind, as this is another frequent etiology of breakthrough bleeding. Thus, when patients call concerned about irregular bleeding, the clinician should assess the pill dose, duration of use, and possibility of missed pills ("Some patients find it hard to remember all their pills. Have you missed any?"), as well as previous gynecologic problems, pelvic pain, new sexual partners, other medications, gastrointestinal problems, and symptoms of pregnancy. Usually, there is a benign explanation such as missed pills or the early months of pill use. In fact, among 15- to 17-year-old OC users, 28% had missed two or more pills in the previous 3 months. Among university women, self-report of missed pills was much lower than observed on the basis of electronic data (59). If there are worrisome factors in the history, an evaluation should be undertaken to exclude pregnancy (including ectopic), chlamydial or gonococcal infection (60), pelvic inflammatory disease, neoplasia, and other gynecologic pathology.

For breakthrough bleeding in the early months of pill taking, patients can usually be reassured and observed over several months. They need to know that the use of lower-dose pills has resulted in breakthrough bleeding for some women. Patients who have skipped or missed pills should make them up, as indicated in Appendix 3. If patients desire treatment or the bleeding is heavy for >2 or 3 days or present for >5 days, there are several approaches that patients can take. One approach is to take one pill in the morning and another in the evening for several days until the breakthrough bleeding stops, with additional pills drawn from a separate package of pills. Another is to add 20 µg ethinyl estradiol or conjugated estrogens (0.625 mg) 12 hours after the OC for 7 days at the first sign of breakthrough bleeding or even throughout one to three cycles (31). However, for teens, obtaining a second prescription for estrogen is likely to be difficult. If the breakthrough bleeding is a persistent problem after the first three cycles or lasts an entire cycle, a change to a more progestin-dominant pill should be tried; for example, changing *from* a pill with 0.5 mg norethindrone (e.g., Modicon) or a triphasic norethindrone pill (Ortho-Novum 7/7/7 [61]) *to* a pill containing 1 mg norethindrone (e.g., Ortho-Novum 1/35 or Norinyl 1 + 35), or *from* a pill with 1 mg norethindrone *to* a triphasic levonorgestrel pill (e.g., Triphasil or Tri-Levlen), a norgestrel pill (e.g., Lo/Ovral), or one of the new progestins such as norgestimate (Ortho-Cyclen). Occasionally, a 50-µg ethinyl estradiol pill (e.g., Ovral) is necessary for 1 to 2 cycles to regain cycle control, after which patients can resume a 35-µg pill or a triphasic pill. Breakthrough bleeding may be a sign of decreased efficacy, especially if patients are taking other medications, and a backup method of contraception is advisable.

Headaches

Headaches occur in 10% to 30% of healthy adolescents on a weekly basis. Thus, it is important for the clinician to obtain a history of headache type, frequency, and severity before prescribing an OC. Some patients, especially those with an increase in headaches in the premenstrual phase, may actually find that headaches are ameliorated with the use of monophasic pills. Some patients with migraine or other headaches experience an increase in headaches. Other patients have new onset of headaches associated with OC use. Whenever patients call with an increase in or new onset of headaches, a history of associated factors, prior headaches, caffeine and alcohol use, fatigue and stress at school, psychosocial issues, sinus infections, and the presence of neurologic symptoms should be obtained. A blood pressure reading should be obtained and a neurologic and physical examination performed, if indicated. If the findings of these examinations are normal but headaches are significant and appear to be related to OC use, the pill can be discontinued for a month or two and an alternative method of contraception used. Alternatively, a lower-dose OC or progestin-only pill can be prescribed.

It is unclear whether there is any increased risk of stroke with migraine headaches with or without the use of OCs (62). Most physicians prescribe OCs to patients with a history of tension headaches and common migraine headaches and monitor frequency of symptoms, changing dose or prescribing a progestin-only method as needed. In patients with a history of classic migraine (with aura) and focal neurologic symptoms (e.g., loss of speech, hemiparesis, field cuts) during the headache, the potential but unknown risk should be discussed, and alternative contraception such as use of a progestin-only or a barrier method should be selected. However, in patients with infrequent symptoms or at high risk of pregnancy, the risks and benefits of using OCs should be discussed. Further evaluation is needed if patients experience new sudden, severe, or persistent headaches, headaches in which neurologic symptoms persist after the headaches resolve, or headaches waking them from sleep.

Hypertension

A combination OC is not recommended for patients with untreated hypertension. At most 1% to 2% of normotensive individuals have been observed to develop hypertension (a blood pressure >140/90 mm Hg) within weeks to several months of starting an OC, with the risk of hypertension increasing with age, parity, and obesity.

The mechanism of development of the hypertension is still a matter of considerable controversy and may be related to both the estrogen and the progestin (1). OCs increase plasma renin substrate, renin activity, angiotensin, and aldosterone. OC users in whom hypertension develops may have a predisposition to a hypertensive response to mineralocorticoids, a failure in feedback response, or inadequate inactivation of angiotensin.

In the rare adolescents in whom new-onset hypertension develops while taking OCs, the elevated blood pressure usually returns to normal within 2 to 12 weeks after the pill is discontinued. Preferably, nonhormonal contraception should be used until the blood pressure returns to normal, but in some patients effective contraception with a progestin-only method is indicated, given the evidence that this method does not alter blood pressure (1). For example, if mild hypertension develops in a patient taking a 35-μg ethinyl estradiol pill and subsequently resolves, a pill lower in estrogen and progestin (e.g., Loestrin 1/20) or a progestin-only pill may be prescribed, with monitoring of the blood pressure. If hypertension recurs, the patient should use another form of contraception. Sustained hypertension requires an evaluation. Most clinicians will prescribe OCs if the patient (especially a nonsmoker) has well-controlled hypertension (diastolic pressure <90 mm Hg).

Vascular Thrombosis

The estimated risk of deep vein thrombosis and pulmonary embolism has varied among studies, and several studies have questioned whether there is an increased risk in nonsmoking women (63–71). The large Puget Sound Study involving 37,807 woman-years of OC use found three cases of venous thrombosis with a relative risk (RR) of 2.8 (64). The Walnut Creek Study found no increase in thromboembolism (65), and the comparison of intrauterine device users and OC users in Finland found an RR of 1.2 (95% confidence interval [CI]: 0.37, 3.62) for deaths from pulmonary embolism (66). In a study of 230,000 women, 15 to 44 years old, receiving Michigan Medicaid, the RR of OCs with <50 μg estrogen was 1 (67,68). Some of the older studies on thrombosis risk have been questioned because of the difficulty of making a clinical diagnosis of thrombophlebitis, case ascertainment, and lack of controlling for factors such as smoking (69–71). The rate of false-positive clinical diagnosis varies from 25% to 83%. Other factors influencing incidence rates are family history, low antithrombin III, hypercoagulability states (e.g., polycythemia, protein C and protein S deficiency, factor V Leiden mutation), postpartum, lupus erythematosus, obesity, chronic disease such as diabetes, and immobility (72).

Lower-dose estrogen pills also may pose a lowered risk because of the lesser impact on clotting factors (73–75). For some OCs, slightly increased levels of coagulation factors II, VII, VIII, and X, unchanged or reduced antithrombin III activity and protein S levels, and mildly increased fibrinolytic activity are observed. Even when changes do occur, the levels of factors are usually still within the normal range and the decrease in antithrombin III noted is not in the range noted in familial disorders associated with thrombophlebitis (70). Studies on pills with the newer progestins have shown little or no impact on clotting factors (49); however, several epidemiologic studies have suggested that certain progestins, including desogestrel and gestodene, are associated with a higher risk (1.5 to 2.0) of thromboembolism than norethindrone- and levonorgestrel-containing OCs (76–79). The annual risk for nonfatal venous thrombosis has been estimated to be 4/100,000 for healthy women, 10 to 15/100,000 for women taking norethindrone- and levonorgestrel-containing pills, 20 to 30/100,000 for women taking desogestrel- or gestodene-containing pills, and 60/100,000 for pregnant women (76–79). The risk of thromboembolism is higher in patients with the recently recognized and moderately prevalent factor V Leiden mutation. The carrier frequency of factor V Leiden [a mutation of factor V that renders activated factor V relatively resistant to degradation by activated protein C (APC)] is 5.3% among Caucasian Americans, 2.2% among Hispanic Americans, 1.2% among African Americans, and 0.45% among Asian Americans (80). Risks and benefits of prescribing oral contraceptives need to be weighed since the presence of factor V Leiden is common and unintended pregnancy will also increase the risk of venous thromboembolism. However, use of newer progestins by those with this mutation appears to particularly enhance risk of thromboembolism. Some researchers have argued that bias is a significant problem in this observational research, as new starters on OCs are more likely to experience thrombosis because those with preexisting clotting disorders may be detected during the first 3 months of OC use, that is, each time a new contraceptive is introduced, the risk is enhanced due to new use among susceptibles (81). In addition, clinicians may have used the new progestins in patients particularly at risk for problems (such as obesity and smoking). In contrast, the newer progestins were associated with a lowered rate of myocardial infarction compared to older progestins (82). Current tests do not allow the prediction of which of the rare patients on OCs will develop thrombosis. However, young women who have a strong family history of thrombosis or who develop thrombosis on OCs should be evaluated for familial disorders (73).

Since prior thrombophlebitis is a contraindication to OC use, rigorous medical criteria should be used to determine whether a patient has thrombophlebitis. Adolescents who have significant pleuritic chest pain, hemoptysis, shortness of breath, or other symptoms suggestive of pulmonary embolism should have appropriate medical evaluation, including chest X-ray film, electrocardiogram, arterial blood gas measurement, ventilation–perfusion lung scan, and in suspected cases angiography or magnetic resonance angiography, to confirm the diagnosis (83). Two studies have found an increased risk of postoperative thromboembolism in women using OCs prior to major (especially abdominal) surgery (72,84), and thus some clinicians favor discontinuing OC use 4 weeks before major elective surgery. The possibility of an unplanned pregnancy, however, is a significant risk for adolescents, and thus temporary discontinuation is usually suggested only if the procedure involves prolonged bed rest and immobilization in plaster casts and alternative contraceptive methods can be reliably used.

OCs are generally considered contraindicated in patients with cyanotic heart disease or pulmonary artery hypertension. The risk of taking OCs by patients with mitral valve prolapse (especially symptomatic) is controversial, although smoking likely contributes substantially to the morbidity that has been reported (85). The presence of varicose veins is not a contraindication to OC use. Although in the past many clinicians avoided OCs in patients with sickle cell disease, many centers now use them because of the lack of data showing any difference between users and nonusers in side effects (1,85–87). Even in the few centers reporting thrombosis in those with sickle cell disease, it is unclear that the pill was a contributing factor, and higher-dose pills were prescribed. More studies are needed to define the potential risks contrasted with needed benefits. Progestin-only methods may have a beneficial effect of decreasing sickle cell crises.

An association between OC use and stroke (including subarachnoid hemorrhage) was reported by some earlier studies, but not by most current studies. The Puget Sound Study (64) and the updated Oxford Study (88) found no increase in RR for cerebral vascular accident. The Nurses' Health Study (89) found no change in the risk of mortality from stroke in ever-users of OCs (RR: 1.05; 95% CI: 0.75, 1.45; multivariate RR: 1.03); there was a slight increase in RR in current users in 1976, but the numbers were small and the CIs large and included 1.0 (RR: 1.45; 95% CI: 0.72, 2.95 for current users, and RR: 0.99; 95% CI: 0.68, 1.42 for past users). A case–control study at Kaiser Health Plan (92) found that for current users of OCs, the RR for ischemic stroke was 1.18 (95% CI: 0.54, 2.59) and for hemorrhagic stroke 1.14 (95% CI: 0.60, 2.16). For hemorrhagic stroke, there was an increased RR for OCs and smoking of 3.64 (95% CI: 0.95, 13.87). Past users had a decreased risk of stroke. An increase in ischemic stroke in smokers and those with hypertension was also noted in the World Health Organization (WHO) international study but no increase in hemorrhagic stroke in women <35 years (90,91). Factors that appear to contribute to the reduction of risk include a reduction of hormone doses, better screening of users, and better epidemiologic studies that control for confounding factors (1,93).

The data initially suggesting an association between myocardial infarction and OC use have been extensively reevaluated and new studies carried out (64–66,89,94–96). The Walnut Creek Study (65) found an increased incidence of acute myocardial infarction with OCs only in smokers >40 years old. The Puget Sound Study (64) found no cases of myocardial infarction among 36,807 woman-years of use. A study of 119,061 women in the Nurses' Health Study found that past use of OCs did not increase the risk of subsequent cardiovascular disease (95). In a 12-year followup study of 166,755 nurses, Colditz (89) reported that ever-use of OCs was associated with a RR of mortality from coronary heart disease of 0.82 (95% CI: 0.66, 1.02), and current use with a RR of 0.70 (95% CI: 0.33, 1.51). Smoking is a major contributing factor to elevated risk in older women. The increased risk of myocardial infarction is felt to be primarily related to thrombosis, not atherosclerosis, since the risk is not related to past use or duration of OC use. The current or past use of OCs alone in young women has no effect on the incidence of myocardial infarction (31,96). Rare case reports of mesenteric artery thrombosis and retinal artery thrombosis have been reported (1,97).

Diabetes and Carbohydrate Metabolism

Early studies using older, higher-dose OC pills suggested that these compounds impaired glucose tolerance. Ethynodiol diacetate and norethindrone given alone in moderate doses cause significant increases in blood glucose and insulin levels, but the most pronounced effect seems to occur with norgestrel (98,91). More recent studies using the lower-dose formulations now available appear to show minimal, if any, impact (99–103). Contraceptives with 35 μg ethinyl estradiol and 0.4 or 0.5 mg norethindrone, the triphasic preparations, and those containing the progestins desogestrel and norgestimate appear to have no clinically significant impact on glucose tolerance (49,104).

Patients who are >30% overweight for height or who have a sibling or parent with diabetes have an increased risk for glucose intolerance. Although the benefits of screening have not been assessed, some clinicians favor obtaining a fasting blood glucose or 2-hour postprandial glucose in these adults before prescribing OCs. The OCs low in progestin can be provided to adolescents with gestational diabetes, glucose intolerance, or insulin-dependent diabetes, with monitoring and discussion of the risks and benefits (105,106). Insulin requirements rarely change on low-dose pills. Because of concern about the potential for greater effect of some of the higher dose norgestrel-containing pills, many clinicians prefer to start adolescents with diabetes mellitus on pills that contain low doses of other progestins although there are no comparative studies. Although barrier forms of contraception may seem preferable because of the association of premature atherosclerosis and diabetes and the potential increased risk of thrombotic events, recent studies of small numbers of diabetic patients on OCs have been reassuring (107).

Lipid Metabolism

There has been tremendous interest and concern about the role of OCs in altering plasma lipids (71,108–112). The interpretation has been difficult because of lack of knowledge as to whether changes observed have any relationship to long-term morbidity and mortality. Conclusions about the association of high-density lipoprotein (HDL) cholesterol on the lower incidence of myocardial infarction are drawn from epidemiologic studies in men in their midlife, not from young women taking OCs. In addition, the benefit of altering HDL cholesterol in a supposedly beneficial direction has not been demonstrated. Because factors other than triglycerides, total cholesterol, and HDL and low-density lipoprotein (LDL) cholesterol play roles in atherosclerosis, interest has emerged in studying subfractions of HDL cholesterol, apolipoproteins, and other factors. An elevated level of apolipoprotein (apo) B or depressed level of apo A-1 (or a high ratio of apo B to apo A-1) has been associated with coronary heart disease.

Oral estrogens in high doses can increase liver synthesis and release of very low-density lipoproteins (VLDL), triglycerides, HDL cholesterol, and total cholesterol. Progestins are associated with a decline in HDL cholesterol and in the most antiatherogenic subfraction, HDL_2. The balance of estrogen to progestin, the amount of contraceptive steroid, and the response of the individual patient determine the changes in lipid levels. Because of widely different protocols, including numbers and characteristics of subjects, duration of OCs, and nature of the lipoproteins studied, results must be interpreted with caution. Speroff and DeCherney (49) have pointed out that most studies are short term (a steady state may not be reached in 6 months), a number of factors are often not controlled (phase of menstrual cycle, postpartum state), and untreated controls are not included in the design. In general, the HDL/total cholesterol and HDL/LDL cholesterol ratios do not appear to change significantly with OCs containing <1 mg norethindrone and 35 μg ethinyl estradiol or with most of the newer estrogen/progestin combinations. Speroff and DeCherney (49) reviewed 23 reports of desogestrel-containing pills and found changes (some small or variable) in total cholesterol (+3%), HDL cholesterol (+13%), LDL cholesterol (+2%), triglycerides (+29%), apo B (+10%), and apo A-1 (+11%). Monophasic norgestimate pills showed changes in triglycerides (+4%), total cholesterol (+5%), LDL cholesterol (+3%), and HDL cholesterol (+7%). It is important to note that, contrary to assumptions that have been made on an epidemiologic basis in humans, studies in nonhuman primates have suggested that even a progestin-dominant combination pill that lowered HDL cholesterol reduced the amount of arteriosclerosis because the estrogen component appears to have a protective effect (112).

Given the problems of epidemiology, controlled studies, and extrapolation of risks to women, the most prudent course for practitioners is to select a balanced contraceptive with a low dose of progestin and estrogen. Instruction in low-cholesterol, low-saturated fat, high-fiber diets, avoidance of smoking, and exercise are useful adjuncts in the care of young women.

Combination OCs should not be offered to patients with known hypertriglyceridemia because of the risk of pancreatitis (113). Progestin-only pills have a negligible effect on lipids and thus appear preferable in the presence of hypertriglyceridemia (108).

Changes in Laboratory Values

Several laboratory tests are potentially altered by the ingestion of OCs (1,31,114). Of particular importance to clinicians is the change observed in some thyroid function tests. Although there is no change in the free thyroxine (free T_4) level or the clinical status of patients, the increase in thyroid-binding globulin (TBG) leads to an increase in measured total T_4 and a decrease in resin triiodothyronine (resin T_3) levels and in the TBG index. In some studies but not others, the serum folate concentration has been reported to be decreased (115,116). This could be potentially significant in adolescents with inadequate diets and in women who become pregnant shortly after discontinuing OC use.

Of interest to clinicians treating adolescents with polycystic ovary syndrome and androgen excess is the increase in sex hormone–binding globulin (SHBG) secondary to the estrogen component of the pill; the increase is greater in pills containing low doses of norethindrone (0.4 or 0.5 mg) and the newer progestins (desogestrel and norgestimate) than those containing norgestrel (51,53). For example, the mean SHBG level more than doubled in users of a norgestimate/ethinyl estradiol pill, compared to only a 10% increase in users of a norgestrel/ethinyl estradiol pill (117). However, *all* OCs markedly reduce free testosterone levels. Levels of SHBG continue to rise at 6 months after initiating OCs, and free testosterone levels continue to fall (118). OCs not only decrease free testosterone but also frequently decrease dehydroepiandrosterone sulfate (an adrenal androgen often elevated in polycystic ovary syndrome) (119).

Gastrointestinal Diseases

A recent review found a odds ratio of 1.36 for OC use and gallbladder disease (95% CI: 1.15, 1.62) (120); the recent Oxford Family Planning Study found no association, with a RR of 1.1 (95% CI: 0.9, 1.3) (121). Grodstein and colleagues (122) found no increase for ever-users in symptomatic gallstones but did find a slight increase in long-term users (RR: 1.5, 95% CI: 1.0, 2.2 for 10 to 14 years of use). Increased body mass index was the strongest predictor of risk. Others have suggested that rather than increasing the lifetime risk, OCs might accelerate gallbladder disease in women with susceptibility to this problem (1).

Studies of the risk of OC use and inflammatory bowel disease have been conflicting. In two recent data sets (123,124), the RRs of Crohn's disease and ulcerative colitis were higher in current users, but the results were not statistically significant (1). A Puget Sound Study found that women who had used OCs within 6 months of disease onset had a RR of 2.0 (95% CI: 1.2, 3.3) for ulcerative colitis and a RR of 2.6 (95% CI: 1.2, 5.5) for Crohn's disease, compared to never-users. Use for >6 years was associated with a RR of 5.1 for Crohn's disease but no increased risk for ulcerative colitis (125). Duration of use of >6 years and an estrogen dose >35 μg also appear to increase the RRs (1). Use of OCs reduced the risk of colorectal cancer in one study (126).

Women who have reduced hepatic reserve because of an inherited or acquired defect may become jaundiced while taking OCs. Women with a history of recurrent cholestatic jaundice of pregnancy should not be given OCs. OCs are generally contraindicated in patients with active hepatitis, but a negative impact on the course or outcome has not been proved (127). Patients with mononucleosis and hepatitis A have frequently completely recovered before the issue of use is raised or therapy altered. Some clinicians feel that liver function tests should be checked prior to reinstituting OCs. The potential risks and benefits need to be balanced in adolescents with chronic hepatitis, cystic fibrosis, or other conditions associated with changes in liver function tests.

Contraceptive steroids are generally contraindicated in patients with porphyria because of the chance of triggering an attack (127).

Collagen Vascular Disease

Women with systemic lupus erythematosus (SLE) have an increased risk of thrombosis that may be enhanced in those with antiphospholipid antibodies and also in those taking OCs (85,128–131). Most studies are case reports or involve a small series of adults with SLE. Julkunen and colleagues (129,130) estimated a RR of 2.3 for thrombosis, but with a wide CI (0.5, 10.3). For that reason, progestin-only agents are often suggested, especially for those with a history of thrombosis, antiphospholipid antibodies, or active nephritis. Julkunen and associates did, however, report that 25 (78%) of 32 women who used a progestin-only method discontinued use because of side effects (mostly gynecologic but one case of thrombosis was noted). Thus, low-dose OCs have been prescribed for adolescents with SLE when the risks and likelihood of a pregnancy outweigh the potential increased risks of OCs and the patients are appropriately counseled (1,128).

Most patients with rheumatoid arthritis will tolerate an OC well; however, occasionally, increased symptoms of the disease appear to be related to OC therapy. Conflicting studies have shown either no effect or a protective effect of OCs on the development of rheumatoid arthritis (131–134).

Epilepsy

Several studies have demonstrated no increase in seizures with current formulations (62,135–137). In fact, patients with a history of an increase in seizures in the premenstrual and/or menstrual phase of the cycle may benefit from OC use.

The major problem with the use of OCs in adolescents with seizure disorders is the potential for lowered efficacy of the OC and decreased anticonvulsant levels. Anticonvulsants such as phenobarbital, phenytoin, carbamazepine, primidone, and oxcarbazepine increase the metabolism of synthetic steroids by increasing conjugation in the gut and enzyme induction in the liver. In addition, these drugs increase the production of sex hormone–binding globulin to which the progestin is bound (137). The pregnancy rate for women taking enzyme-inducing anticonvulsants and OCs has been estimated at 3.1/100 woman-years of use (129). Use of progestin-only pills or levonorgestrel subdermal implants does not provide sufficient efficacy for patients on enzyme-inducing anticonvulsants. Sodium valproate has not been associated with OC failure but has been associated with polycystic ovary syndrome (see Chapter 7). Most of the new antiepileptic agents such as gabapentin, lamotrigine, and felbamate do not interfere with OCs.

A pill with 35 to 50 μg ethinyl estradiol is generally prescribed, although some clinicians suggest pills with 50 to 100 μg daily (139). The patient should be counseled about the potential increased risk of pregnancy and a backup method such as condoms strongly suggested. Although not proved, the persistence of breakthrough bleeding in patients on anticonvulsant therapy may imply lowered efficacy and the need to change to a pill with more estrogen (50 μg) and a more potent progestin. A barrier method should be used in cycles with breakthrough bleeding. Some clinicians reduce the pill-free interval from 7 days to 4 to 5 days with the hope of lowering the pregnancy risk; others advise prescribing only 50-μg OC pills; still others recommend four packs of 21-day hormone pills followed by a tablet-free interval of 5 to 6 days (140,141).

Drug Interactions

Drugs may interact with OCs by changing absorption, altering serum protein binding, and increasing hepatic metabolism with the induction of cytochrome P-450 enzymes (140,141). Some women are rapid metabolizers of steroids, and some women may have liver enzyme systems that are particularly likely to induction (1). As noted, anticonvulsants and OCs have important drug interactions. In addition, the use of rifampin also diminishes the efficacy of OCs (140–143). Whether other antibiotics such as ampicillin or tetracycline alter efficacy is debatable. Most studies show no effect of these antibiotics on steroid hormone levels (144,145). Although antibiotic usage has been associated with 23% and 34% of the failures reported in series of pill users (146,147), studies of clinical pharmacology have been unable to demonstrate altered kinetics in a small number of women (1,144). It is possible that some women are particularly susceptible or that there are changes in bowel flora or bioavailability of estrogen that account for the rare reported failures. It is probably best to advise the use of a barrier method, especially if breakthrough bleeding occurs. Griseofulvin may affect OC efficacy although studies are conflicting; a backup method or higher-dose pill should be prescribed if breakthrough bleeding occurs.

The clearance of benzodiazepines (such as chlordiazepoxide and diazepam), theophylline, prednisolone, caffeine, metoprolol, and cyclosporine is reduced in OC users (140,141). Thus, toxicity, drug levels, and clinical effectiveness need to be followed. Levels of tricyclic antidepressants may be altered by OC use, and thus levels should be monitored to avoid toxicity. Decreased concentrations of acetylsalicylic acid, clofibric acid, morphine, paracetamol, and temazepam have been observed in OC users (140,141). Although mineral oil and OC pills should not be taken at the same time, absorbents such as antacids and kaolin have not been shown to have any effect on OCs. Vitamin C does not appear to alter OC kinetics (148).

Oligomenorrhea or Amenorrhea

Scanty or absent withdrawal flow, most commonly associated with progestin-dominant and low-estrogen pills, may develop months or even several years after continuous use. If a patient becomes amenorrheic, she should continue taking her pills, and the possibility of pregnancy should be evaluated promptly. Menses may return spontaneously, or amenorrhea may persist. The patient should be reassured that the lack of menses is in no way harmful and is not associated with postpill amenorrhea. The options are to continue pregnancy tests every 1 to 2 months (it may be best to err of the side of more frequent tests in questionably compliant patients), to have the patient check basal body temperatures during the placebo week each month, or to change to an OC more likely to result in menstrual flow.

For patients who can take their temperatures easily and understand the instructions (usually college students), the procedure involves checking basal body (oral) temperature for 3 days during the 7-day hormone-free interval (on placebos). If no pills have been missed and the temperature is <98°F, pill amenorrhea is likely and the pills can be continued. Temperatures >98°F may imply a viral infection or incorrectly measured temperature, but a sensitive pregnancy test should be done.

If patients desire a change of pill, selecting one with less progestin is often helpful, for example, switching to a pill containing 0.4 mg (Ovcon 35) or 0.5 mg (e.g., Modicon) norethindrone from one containing 1 mg, or from Lo/Ovral (0.3 mg norgestrel) to a triphasic levonorgestrel pill (Triphasil, Tri-Levlen), or from any pill to a norgestimate pill. Some clinicians also add a small amount of supplemental estrogen (ethinyl estradiol 20 μg or conjugated estrogens 0.625 mg) for 21 days for one to three cycles, although it is clearly best to try to find a pill with 30 to 35 μg of estrogen for long-term use. Patients on OC therapy should be reassured that a 1- to 3-day light withdrawal flow is perfectly normal.

After discontinuation of the pill, 1% to 2% of patients have postpill amenorrhea, similar to the incidence of amenorrhea in control populations (149). Approximately 95% of these patients revert to regular periods within 12 to 18 months. Most patient with postpill amenorrhea have irregular cycles before initiating OC use, and thus the cause of oligomenorrhea should be investigated before an OC is prescribed. For example, a patient with polycystic ovary syndrome and hirsutism may appropriately be treated with an OC, but she will likely experience oligomenorrhea again after it is discontinued. Patients who lose weight or engage in endurance sports while taking OCs appear to be more susceptible to postpill amenorrhea just as they would be if they were not taking OCs.

Patients with amenorrhea for >6 months after the cessation of OCs or with galactorrhea or headaches should have an appropriate evaluation (see Chapter 6). In adolescents, pregnancy must be an important consideration regardless of the number of weeks or months of amenorrhea.

Depression

Subjective symptoms such as depression, nervousness, or emotional lability have been associated with OC use in some studies, but not in others (1,93). Most adolescents do well on OCs without any impact on psychological well-being, but some—perhaps because of a predisposition (family history or personal history) or intervening life stresses—do feel symptoms of irritability or depression that appear to coincide with the initiation of OC use. Depressive symptoms are common during adolescence, and thus the clinician is often faced with trying to assess whether the OC is part of the problem and to determine the severity of the depression or other mood changes and the need for psychiatric intervention. It is crucial to have a baseline history of previous psychiatric symptoms as the adolescent begins OC use, since patients with a family or personal history of depression or significant symptoms of premenstrual syndrome may be more likely to experience psychological problems while using OCs. Expectations about OC use may also play a role. After other causes for the depression or emotional lability are explored, the clinician can suggest a change to a different hormone preparation with less progestin or discontinuing the pill to see if the subjective effects are improved. Although some clinicians recommend supplementation with 20 mg vitamin B_6 daily, patients should be counseled about the potential for side effects with excessive doses.

Pregnancy Outcome

There is no increase in the incidence of congenital anomalies over the background rate of 2% to 3% in patients who have previously taken OCs or in those who have inadvertently taken OCs during early pregnancy (150). Dating of pregnancies is improved if patients wait a cycle or two after discontinuing OCs to attempt conception.

Neoplasms

Most studies to date, including the Centers for Disease Control and Prevention data on >4700 women, have found no increase in breast cancer (lifetime RR: 1.0) associated with the use of OCs, although this issue is a source of controversy and ongoing reassessments (1,151–155). A number of studies have examined subgroups of women to determine whether younger women, those using OCs before a first pregnancy, or long-term users face special risks. Part of the difficulty with the epidemiologic studies is the issue of recall of use, the decreasing number of women who are never-users, the change in estrogen dose over the past 20 years, and the change in users to adolescents of younger age. Coker and associates (156) assigned a RR of 1.2 to women aged 15 to 49 years and 1.0 for women ≥50 years; Petitti and Porterfield (157) suggested a RR of 1.7 for ages 15 to 44 years and 1.0 for age ≥45 years. The Cancer and Steroid Hormone (CASH) study (151) found a slightly increased RR for women 20 to 34 years old at diagnosis, no association for those aged 35 to 44 years, and a slightly decreased risk for women aged 45 to 54 years. A subgroup of women who used OCs >4 years and who used previous higher-dose formulations may have a RR of 1.5. In an analysis of 54 epidemiologic studies of over 53,000 women with breast cancer and over 100,000 women without breast cancer, the Collaborative Group on Hormonal Factors in Breast Cancer concluded that there was a small relative risk of having breast cancer diagnosed in current users of 1.24 (95% CI: 1.15, 1.33), which decreased to 1.16 (95% CI: 1.08, 1.23),1 to 4 years after stopping OCs, and to 1.01 (95% CI: 0.96, 1.05) by 10 years after use (158,159). The cancers diagnosed in OC users were less advanced compared to never-users and more likely to be localized to the breast. It may be that women receiving OC prescriptions are more likely to have breast cancer diagnosed early. There was no effect on duration of use, age at first use, type of formulation, parity, reproductive or family history, or a number of other factors. The consensus of the FDA, the U.S. Institute of Medicine, and the WHO is that the overall risk is approximately 1.0 and that no change in prescribing patterns is indicated (1). Genetic markers for breast cancer may also begin to help elucidate risk factors (160) (see Chapter 16). OCs appear to offer some protection against benign breast disease, at least the older formulations; the newer, lower-dose pills may not have the same effect (1,155).

Although an increased incidence of cervical dysplasia and progression to carcinoma *in situ* has been reported in some studies of OC users, these women have higher rates of sexual activity, an increased number of partners, and an earlier age of beginning coitus, as well as more substance use (including cigarettes) (1,149,156,161–165). The nonuse of a barrier method by OC users increases the likelihood of infection with HPV (see Chapter 13), and the immature cervix of the adolescent is likely more susceptible to the effect of HPV exposure. OC users are also under increased surveillance with Pap smears because of the need for a prescription, and thus detection bias in studies is also a problem. Most studies, but not all, have reported that long-term use is associated with a small increased risk of cervical cancer. A WHO study (165) found that ever-users of OCs had a RR of 1.75 for carcinoma *in situ* with an even greater risk for long-term (>5 years) users. Coker and colleagues (156,164) suggested that the most reasonable RR for cervical cancer for ages 15 to 49 years was 1.2, with a RR of 1.0 after age 49. However, they did not find any relationship between OCs and preinvasive cervical cancer. In a case–control study, cases were slightly less likely to be ever-users of OCs (0.7; 95% CI: 0.3, 1.6) when investigators controlled for age, socioeconomic status, barrier method use, smoking history, age at first sexual intercourse, number of sexual partners, current marital status, and number of Pap smears (164).

Ever or current use of combination OCs reduces the incidence of endometrial cancer, with age-adjusted RRs of 0.2 to 0.7 (1,166–170). The CASH study (159) found a RR of 0.6 for ever-use, with the protective effect lasting ≥15 years. The protective effect increases with duration of use. For a duration of use ≥2 years, there appears to be a 38% reduction in risk, compared to estimated risk reduction of 51% with 4 years of use, 64% with 8 years, and 70% with 12 years (162).

Benign ovarian cysts are less common in all OC users. OCs with higher doses of estrogen, however, are more suppressive if the prime indication is suppression of ovarian cysts. OCs have a strong protective effect against ovarian cancer (1,171–177), with the RR of 0.64 (95% CI: 0.57, 0.73) for ever-use of OCs in a recent metaanalysis (174). Using data from several sources, Gross and Schlesselman (175) have estimated that 5 years of OC use by nulliparous women can reduce their ovarian cancer risk to the level observed in parous women and that 10 years of use by women with a positive family history can reduce their risk below that of a never-user with a negative family history. The protective effect occurred with as little as 3 to 6 months of use and continued for 15 years after use ended.

In modeling the hypothetical incidence of all reproductive cancers ascribed to OC use, Coker and colleagues (156) suggested that if ≥5 years of use was associated with a 20% increase in breast cancer before age 50 years, a 20% increase in cervical cancer risk, and a 50% reduction in ovarian and endometrial cancer, then for every 100,000 pill users there would be 44 fewer reproductive cancers.

Studies on the RR of liver cancer have yielded variable results in different populations. In low-risk populations in Western countries, the RR, based on small numbers of cases, has been estimated at 2.6 for ever-use and 9.6 for long-term use

(>5 or 8 years of use) (176), yielding an estimate of one death in 100,000 long-term users per year among women <35 years old and two deaths in women aged 35 to 44 years (1,177). In the Nurses Health Study (89), ever-use of OCs was not related to an increased risk for liver cancer mortality (RR: 0.43; 95% CI: 0.08, 2.42). Interestingly, in high-risk populations, studies have found no elevated risk (1,127,178), and thus the impact, if present, is quite small. Although the data have been interpreted in different ways, the development of benign liver adenomas may be increased by OCs, and the risk appears to increase with duration of use and higher doses (1). The risk of hepatocellular adenoma has been estimated at 1 to 2/100,000 OC users (179). However, in British studies that included over a quarter million woman-years of use, no liver tumors were found. A study at the Armed Forces Institute of Pathology suggested that one type of hepatic tumor (fibrolamellar) occurs in the same age group that would be taking OCs, and thus an age-related bias may have occurred in establishing an association (180). Patients with hepatocellular adenoma may have an abdominal mass, vague upper abdominal pain, or acute pain with circulatory collapse following hemorrhage. No prospective studies of OCs have identified any hepatomas (127).

Skin

The majority of OC users note an improvement in acne and hirsutism. Essentially all OCs lower free and total testosterone, although there are minor differences in the extent of these changes and the magnitude of the increase in SHBG (181). For patients with preexisting acne, OCs should be selected that have a particularly beneficial effect on acne; formulations recommended by many clinicians include pills with 0.4 or 0.5 mg norethindrone (e.g., Ovcon 35, Modicon), with 1 mg ethynodiol diacetate (Demulen 1/35), and with the new progestins (e.g., OrthoTri-Cyclen). Patients taking pills with higher doses of progestins may occasionally have a mild exacerbation of acne and may need a change to a different or lower-dose progestin. Familiarity with acne therapy is also important for clinicians providing care to teenagers.

Chloasma (the darkening of the upper lip and forehead and under the eyes) has been noted in a small number of OC users; it usually fades slowly after discontinuing OCs but may be permanent. It is more common in dark-skinned patients who are exposed to sunlight and taking higher-dose OCs.

There is no association of OCs and melanoma (1), but all patients should be advised to use sunscreens.

Hair loss may be due to many stresses; therefore, it is difficult to establish the OC as a definite cause in most cases. Most reports stem from the use of higher-dose pills, not current formulations (182).

Ocular Problems

Much of the literature on the occurrence of eye problems is related to case reports and experiences with higher-dose OCs (1), in which concern was raised about the possibility of dry eyes or corneal edema from combined OCs. In a review, Petursson and coworkers (183) found only seven cases of difficulty in wearing contact lenses; several studies have found no statistical differences in the rates of eye pathology or the ability to wear contact lenses (1). Optic nerve or retinal disease is a contraindication to OC therapy. The pill should be discontinued immediately if visual symptoms, especially transient loss of vision, occur, since retinal thrombosis, optic neuritis, and migraine with focal ophthalmic symptoms may occasionally be associated with OC use.

Bone Density

Although there are a number of studies on the relationship of OCs to bone density, the results are conflicting. Most show a beneficial effect, but some have found no effect (1,184–187). In a prospective longitudinal study of up to 5 years in 156 college-aged women, Recker and associates (186) reported that OC use contributed a further, independent positive effect beyond physical activity and dietary calcium. If a beneficial effect is present, premenopausal OC users may enter menopause with 2% to 3% more bone density (185). The adolescents most likely to benefit would be those at risk of low bone density, including those with hypoestrogenic amenorrhea, eating disorders, and late menarche.

Infections

Although OCs were earlier thought to be associated with an increased possibility of candidal vaginitis, more recent data on low-dose pills have not confirmed this association (131).

OC use lessens the risk of being hospitalized with PID (188), but adolescent OC users are at an increased risk of having *C. trachomatis* isolated from the cervix (see Chapter 12). The increased risk in adolescent pill users may be secondary to factors such as the nonuse of barrier methods and the presence of a prominent and persistent cervical ectropion, which increases replication and detection of this organism.

Studies are conflicting on the risk of acquiring HIV infection in OC users. Postulated causes have included persistence of the cervical ectropion, higher rates of chlamydial cervicitis, and immunologic changes (1).

PROGESTIN-ONLY PILL

Progestin-only oral contraceptive pills (POPs) are a choice for teenagers who cannot tolerate the estrogen in the combined OC pill or have a medical contraindication to the use of the combined pill (1,189). The available options include a low-dose (0.35 mg) norethindrone pill (Micronor, Nor-QD) and a 0.075-mg norgestrel pill (Ovrette). Because norethindrone is inactivated as it passes through the liver, it is roughly 60% bioavailable, whereas the norgestrel pill is 100% bioavailable. These two POPs are considered approximately equivalent in terms of progestin dose and effect on metabolism. POPs have several modes of action. Foremost, they alter the cervical mucus, inhibiting sperm penetration. They also alter the endometrium in most women, slow movement of the ovum in the fallopian tube, and prevent ovulation in about 50% of women.

POPs must be taken daily at approximately the same time to be effective in the prevention of pregnancy because serum progestin levels peak about 2 hours after oral administration and then rapidly decline because of rapid distribution and elimination (1) (Fig. 1). For increased effectiveness in the evening, it is thus preferable for a woman to take the pill in the late afternoon or what has been termed "tea time." If a woman is 3 hours late taking the pill, she should be instructed to use a backup method (e.g., condom) for 48 hours. The failure rate in typical use probably approaches 3% to 5%, but this rate is lower in older

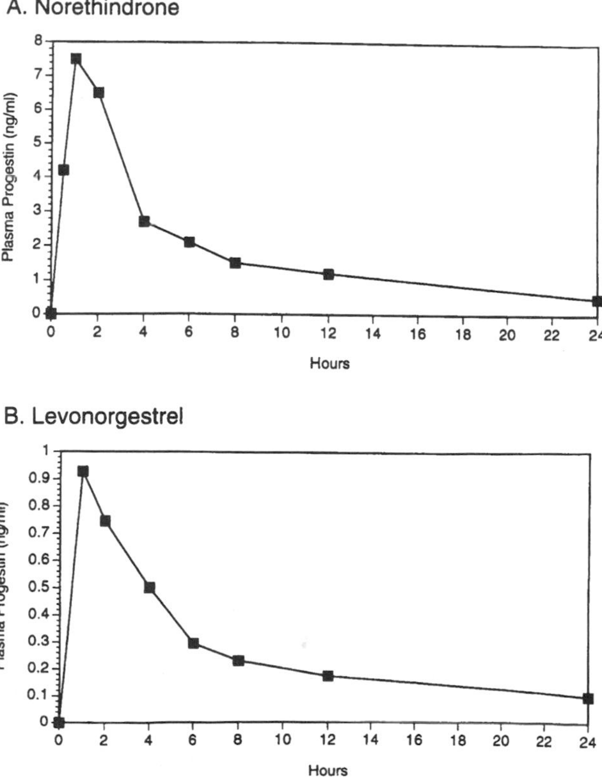

FIG. 1. Mean plasma levels during first 24 hours after oral intake. **(A)** Norethindrone 0.35 mg (n = 16). **(B)** Levonorgestrel 0.03 mg (n = 5). (From McCann MF, Potter LS. Progestin-only oral contraception: comprehensive review. *Contraception* 1994;50(suppl 1):S23; with permission.)

women (who are subfertile) and in women <112 lbs, who are more likely to have short cycles with ovulation inhibited (1). Since ovulation is not inhibited in many patients, pregnancy should be considered in patients with irregular bleeding or amenorrhea. If pregnancy does occur, ectopic pregnancy should be considered since the risk appears to be about 10% among POP failures. Ovarian cysts are also more likely to occur in POP users than combined OC pill users. Irregular menses are the usual reason that women decide to discontinue this method, and careful counseling in advance about menstrual changes is important for users. Often, the menses are most irregular in the first 3 to 4 months, after which the cyclicity improves.

The risk of thrombophlebitis has not been established but appears to be minimal. The coagulation changes associated with combination pills are not evident with POPs in short-term studies. Hypertension is usually not a problem. Carbohydrate and lipid metabolism is probably not affected in most patients. Liver disease is not considered a contraindication to the use of POPs (1).

POPs are acceptable choices for women with diabetes mellitus, SLE, sickle cell disease, hypertension, cyanotic and other cardiac disease, migraine headaches exacerbated by combined OCs, and lipid problems, as well as during lactation. Teenage mothers who are on supplements or not breast-feeding at all should start a POP at 3 weeks postpartum (some start immediately postpartum); breast-feeding teens should begin POPs by 3 months postpartum (earlier if a first menses occurs). POPs are not a good choice for patients taking anticonvulsants that enhance liver metabolism of contraceptive steroids, rifampin, or griseofulvin. In addition, patients with polycystic ovary syndrome are not good candidates because the estrogen of the combined OC is necessary to increase sex hormone–binding globulin production and lower free testosterone.

If teenagers are switching from a POP to a combined OC, they should be instructed to start on the first day of menses; if they are switching from an OC to a POP, the first POP should be taken at the end of the 21 active hormone tablets (discarding the placebos) (1).

MEDROXYPROGESTERONE ACETATE (DEPO-PROVERA) AND OTHER INJECTABLE HORMONES

Medroxyprogesterone acetate (Depo-Provera) is a synthetic progestin derived from progesterone. A 150-mg dose of this aqueous micronized suspension is injected IM every 3 months. Depot medroxyprogesterone suppresses the hypothalamic–ovarian axis and prevents the midcycle luteinizing hormone surge. In addition, it produces thinning and sometimes profound atrophy of the endometrium and increases the viscosity of the cervical mucus. The pregnancy rate of women given Depo-Provera is 0 to 0.4/100 woman-years (190–193).

The 100-mg/ml formulation of Depo-Provera should be used to ensure greater drug availability. The first injection should be given within the first 5 days of the menstrual cycle (after a sensitive pregnancy test). Postpartum women should be given the injection within 5 days of delivery if not breast-feeding or at the 6th week postpartum if breast-feeding. A reminder system that encourages patients to return at 12 weeks after the previous injection can be very helpful so that 1 week of "grace" period is provided. However, there are no clear protocols for adolescents, who may return for appointments at variable times; the benefits of excellent pregnancy protection with this method have to be weighed against the small risk of giving an injection to a patient who may have a very early pregnancy (but the test is not yet positive). Generally, if it is 14 weeks or less (91 to 98 days) since the adolescent's last Depo-Provera injection, a sensitive pregnancy test is done and the next injection given. If it is more than 14 weeks, then a sensitive pregnancy test is obtained; if she has not had intercourse in the previous 2 weeks or has used condoms 100% of the time, the risks and benefits are explained and the injection is given. If, however, she has been sexually active without protection in the previous 2 weeks, she is asked to return in 2 weeks for another sensitive pregnancy test after abstaining from intercourse and then given the injection.

The most important side effect of depot medroxyprogesterone is menstrual irregularity; patients often experience irregular spotting and, occasionally, very heavy menses during the first few months of therapy. Weight gain can be another important side effect; it has been estimated that women gain about 5 lbs each year for the first 3 years (although control groups have not been included in these studies). The package insert reports an average gain of 13.8 lbs for 4 years of use and 16.5 lbs for 6 years of use. Other side effects include depression, nervousness, breast tenderness, headaches, nausea, vomiting, decreased glucose tolerance, and lowered HDL cholesterol (1,194). The risk of thromboembolic disease is probably not increased (1). Liver cancer is not increased in humans, and medroxyprogesterone has a protective effect from endometrial cancer (1,193). A recent analysis of a pooled data set of the WHO and New Zealand studies reported a RR of 1.1 (95% CI: 0.97, 1.4) for breast cancer in women who had ever used medroxyprogesterone, with no increase in risk with increasing duration of use (195). However, recent or current use within the past 5 years was associated with a RR of 2.0 (95% CI: 1.5, 2.8), raising the possibility that enhanced detection of tumors or acceleration of the growth of preexisting tumors may be occurring.

Another concern with special importance for teenagers is the potential impact of medroxyprogesterone on bone density. A cross-sectional study in adult women suggested that bone density was lower in women given medroxyprogesterone than in premenopausal control women, but no relationship to duration of use was observed (196). Based on small numbers, the researchers did find that bone density measurements increased after discontinuation. Although estradiol levels are in the low follicular range (193), they are lower than those that occur during use of subdermal levonorgestrel implants. Since women gain a major portion of their ultimate bone density during their adolescent years, especially between 11 and 15 years, it is critical to know whether the use of medroxyprogesterone enhances, diminishes, or leaves unchanged the normal gains in bone density. In a longitudinal study of adolescents receiving Depo-Provera, Norplant, OCs, or no hormonal therapy, Cromer and colleagues (197) reported that lumbar vertebral bone density decreased slightly in the Depo-Provera users and increased in the other groups; however, the numbers were small in this preliminary study and larger numbers of adolescents are needed to confirm this observation. Thus the unknown risks contrasted with the benefits of pregnancy prevention with the use of Depo-Provera in the first 2 years after menarche have to be weighed by the clinician and the adolescent.

Depo-Provera is a good choice for teens who have difficulty remembering to take a daily pill and do not desire the long-term effectiveness, potential side effects, or cost of levonorgestrel implants (198). Injectable contraceptives may be particularly culturally acceptable to teens who have experience with the popularity of injectables in their native countries. Of importance, medroxyprogesterone appears to lessen the risk of sickle cell crises in users (199), and there are no drug interactions with anticonvulsants in young women with epilepsy.

The indications for medroxyprogesterone contraceptive injection include postpartum and lactating women and women with hypertension, hemoglobinopathies (SS disease), seizure disorders, and mental retardation (to help with menstrual hygiene problems). Women using teratogenic medications and those experiencing side effects with estrogen are also good candidates. Very little is known about continuation rates in adolescents; in a study of 50 teens, Smith and colleagues (200) reported that 72% continued to use Depo-Provera at 1 year, 56% at 2 years, and 18% at 3 years.

Patients planning to use Depo-Provera need to be counseled in advance about irregular menses. Most patients will have amenorrhea after three shots, but some have problems with frequent or heavy menses. By 12 months of use, 57% of women have amenorrhea, and by 24 months 68% have amenorrhea; most patients are happy about the amenorrhea. Adolescents are often concerned about irregular or heavy bleeding. This bleeding usually responds to counseling or 21 days of estrogen therapy (20 μg ethinyl estradiol) or one or two packages of OCs. For patients with mental retardation in whom the clinician wishes to ensure that the progestin is likely to be tolerated without significant mood change and the patient does not need immediate contraception, a 2- to 3-week course of oral medroxyprogesterone, 10 mg daily, can be helpful to assess side effects.

After a 150-mg injection of Depo-Provera, the mean interval before the return of ovulation is 4.5 months. In long-term users, the return of fertility is delayed, with a median time to conception of 10 months (range, 4 to 31 months). Of former Depo-Provera users, 70% conceive within 12 months (compared to 94% for OCs) and >90% by 24 months (190).

Another injectable contraceptive (not yet available in the United States) is norethindrone enanthate (Noristerat), with pregnancy rates <2/100 woman-years of use (two studies have found a rate of 0.4/100 and 0.6/100). Because a large

WHO study showed a failure rate of 3.6 at 12 months, with pregnancies occurring 10 to 12 weeks following the last dose, the dosage was altered to 200 mg every 2 months for the first 6 months and then 200 mg every 2 to 3 months thereafter. Side effects are similar to those of medroxyprogesterone, although bleeding tends to be more regular (191,201). Mean time to return of ovulation was 2.6 months.

Two other monthly injectable contraceptives of estrogen and progestin have been noted to be highly effective, with improved bleeding patterns over medroxyprogesterone alone (202). These include medroxyprogesterone acetate 25 mg/estradiol cypionate 5 mg (Cyclo Provera) and norethindrone enanthate 50 mg/estradiol valerate 5 mg (Mesigyna).

SUBDERMAL IMPLANTS

Levonorgestrel subdermal implants (Norplant System) were approved in the United States in 1990 and have been used in many other countries (31,203–207). The first Norplant System involves six nonbiodegradable Silastic rods that are implanted through a small incision in the upper or lower arm and slowly release levonorgestrel; they are effective for 5 years. Initially, 85 μg/day levonorgestrel are released with a decline to 50 μg/day by 9 months, 35 μg/day by 18 months and 30 μg/day thereafter. The pregnancy rate is 0.03 to 0.4/100 woman-years of use. Women who have regular cycles on Norplant (presumably those who ovulate) are at higher risk of failure than women with irregular cycles (182). Insertion should be performed in the immediate postabortion or postpartum period or within the first 7 days of the cycle. A sensitive pregnancy test should be obtained before insertion.

Insertion, which takes about 10 to 15 minutes, needs to be done carefully so that capsules can later be removed (182,207–210). Much of the current controversy concerning this method of contraception stems from the difficulty of removal, which could be lessened by proper insertion techniques, careful preinsertion counseling, and knowledge of several different removal techniques including the Population Council method, the Emory method (208) (video available), the pop-out method (209) (video available), and the "U" technique (210). Removal usually takes 15 to 30 minutes. Potential complications with insertion include infection, expulsion, hematoma/bleeding, increased pigmentation over the implant area, and scarring. Similar complications occur with removal and include breakage of the implants, scarring, and the need for a second incision or procedure.

The main reason for discontinuation of the Norplant System is menstrual problems, chiefly frequent irregular bleeding. Thus, counseling before insertion is critical, because patients must be prepared for irregular bleeding and must have plans made about how they and their partners will react to the extra bleeding. The menstrual abnormalities can include amenorrhea, prolonged bleeding, spotting, and an increase in spotting/bleeding days. Although the total number of days of bleeding increases, the overall blood loss is often less, and thus the pattern rarely results in anemia. Other side effects include headache, mood change, acne, hirsutism, scalp hair loss, and weight gain. No unfavorable changes in carbohydrate metabolism, liver function, blood pressure, ectopic pregnancy rate, or total menstrual blood loss have been reported. It appears that the total cholesterol/HDL cholesterol ratio is unchanged or only minimally decreased (211). Norplant users do have more functional ovarian cysts than do normally cycling women (1). Initial continuation rates in adults were reported at 85% to 90% at 1 year (204). After removal of the implants, women experience a prompt return of fertility; by 1 month, 25% are pregnant, by 3 months 49%, and by 12 months 86% (212).

Several studies of Norplant use in adolescents have found that they have similar reasons for use and side effects as adult women. Ease of use and high effectiveness are important benefits for teenagers and adult women (30,204, 213–222), and teens are often influenced by their mothers to consider use (220). Nonparenting adolescents, however, may have more objections to the visibility of the device than adult women. Teenage Norplant users appear to return for annual examinations at a rate similar to that of adolescents not using the system (229). Continuation rates are also similar to those of adults. In a study of teenage mothers who selected OCs or Norplant, Polaneczky and colleagues (217) found that at 15 months 95% of 48 teens were using Norplant with only one pregnancy, compared to only 33% of 50 teens still using OCs, with 19 pregnancies having occurred. Cromer and coworkers (215) found that adolescents who selected Norplant or Depo-Provera were significantly more likely to have been pregnant than those choosing OCs. Weight gain has commonly been reported, although *actual* weights have not been obtained in all studies. In some adolescents, the weight gain is minimal; in others, major weight gain occurs. Kozlowski and colleagues (213) found weight gain to be greater in heavy girls and African Americans (5.4 kg) than in white girls (2.6 kg) at ≥8 months of followup. Removal requests may occur because of side effects but also because of uncertainty about whether another pregnancy is desired, a change in partners, adverse publicity about Norplant, or other less well-defined reasons (214).

In spite of the current controversy and adverse publicity about implant removal, long-acting subdermal implants can provide a good contraceptive option if patients are counseled about the irregular menses, other possible side effects, and the importance of ongoing contraceptive care. The teen needs to have access to removal so that the method is not coercive. Adolescents most likely to select this method are those who desire 3 to 5 years of contraception, have experienced failure with other methods of contraception (especially teen mothers), can tolerate a small surgical procedure, and have the financial resources (e.g., insurance, Medicaid, Norplant Foundation [Wyeth Ayerst]) to obtain the device. Some clinicians prescribe a POP (e.g., Ovrette) before insertion of the implants to see whether a patient is a suitable candidate. However, POPs in this situation are unlikely to mimic the extent of irregular menses that leads to dissatisfaction with Norplant and may leave the patient with less effective contraception while on the POP. However, this trial may be worthwhile in patients with a past history or concern about acne, headaches, weight gain, or depression while taking progestins.

Management of irregular menses is usually accomplished through counseling and observation, with exclusion of diagnoses such as pregnancy or a STD (e.g., chlamydia). With persistent problems, a trial of a nonsteroidal antiinflammatory agent (e.g., ibuprofen) or several months of a combined OC pill may improve the symptoms. Norplant has been used in a small number of women with mild to moderate SS disease without difficulty (223). Drug interactions are an important consideration with levonorgestrel implants, and lowered efficacy is noted with anticonvulsants (except valproate) and rifampin (1). Studies of increased or decreased condom use among Norplant users have yielded mixed results (28, 217,222).

Norplant II has two Silastic rods and is currently approved in Finland and China. Data support effectiveness for 3 years, but several studies have found low pregnancy rates at 5 years (0.65/100 users with a continuation rate of 65%) (224). Several biodegradable implants are also in research and development. One barrier to further development has been the concern that a rod should remain intact during the length of effectiveness of the device, so that it can be removed if desired by the woman. A caprolactone polymer with levonorgestrel (Capronor) (225) has been noted in several studies to have higher pregnancy rates than are desirable (226,227). Alzamer is a polymer that undergoes hydrolytic erosion in contact with tissue and releases levonorgestrel or norethindrone for 4 to 6 months.

INTRAUTERINE DEVICES

Currently available intrauterine devices (IUDs) are the progesterone-releasing device (Progestasert) and the copper T-380A (ParaGard) (227–231). The progesterone-releasing device must be replaced every 12 months, while the copper T-380A IUD is approved for 10 years of use. The pregnancy rate with Progestasert is 2.1 to 2.9/100 woman-years of use, and 0.2 to 0.5/100 woman-years for ParaGard (2.6/100 women over 10 years of use) (229–232). Although the use of IUDs is popular worldwide, it represents <2% of contraceptive use in the United States. Several new IUDs are in use or in clinical trials (229), including a levonorgestrel-releasing T-shaped device (LNg-20), which has a low pregnancy rate (1.1/100 woman-years of use at 7 years or an annual rate of 0.16/100 women) (232). The exact mechanism of action of the IUD is unknown. Although IUDs may work in part by causing a low-grade endometritis inhibiting implantation, IUDs have a direct contraceptive effect prior to fertilization. Increased leukocytes in the fallopian tubes, changes in tubal fluids, lowered number of viable sperm, and decreased fertilization of ova occur with IUD use (229,230). Progestasert releases small amounts of progesterone that have a local effect on the endometrium and cervical mucus in addition to the effect noted above. LNg-20 releases levonorgestrel directly into the uterine cavity and appears to reduce the incidence of PID and provide treatment for menorrhagia (31,229).

In our opinion, IUDs are primarily useful for women beyond the teenage years in stable monogamous relationships who have had at least one child or preferably have completed childbearing (30). Infection and its sequelae are the principal worry for IUD users. The increased risk of PID noted in earlier studies has been questioned because the results were based on the use of inappropriate controls (groups with lower risk, such as OC users), overdiagnosis of PID in IUD users, and lack of control for confounding factors such as number of sexual partners and exposure to STDs. In the Women's Health Study (233), the greatest risk of PID in IUD users was found in never-married women, while there was no significant increase among married and cohabiting women with only one recent sexual partner. Recent insertion within 20 days (or reinsertion) appears to be associated with an increased risk of infection, which quickly declines to baseline levels; the risk is inversely associated with age (231). Careful screening for STDs before insertion is important; prophylactic antibiotics at insertion do not appear to lessen complications (234). Women <25 years of age may be especially susceptible to complications, perhaps because they are more likely to have more than one sexual partner and have an increased risk of chlamydia and gonorrhea. IUDs are also generally not recommended for HIV-positive patients.

Side effects include increased vaginal discharge, heavy menses (with occasional anemia), dysmenorrhea, uterine perforation, and pregnancy (including ectopic pregnancy), as well as difficulty in removal because of loss of IUD strings. Progestin-containing devices usually reduce the amount of bleeding, but the duration of bleeding and incidence of spotting may increase (232). The risk of an extrauterine pregnancy occurring is higher in patients using the Progestasert IUD than copper-bearing IUDs. Although there is a reduction of ectopic pregnancies compared to women using no method (RR: 0.2; 95% CI: 0.1, 0.4), tubal pregnancy is more likely to occur in IUD users than OC users (RR: 3.8) and barrier-method users (RR: 3.6) (235).

FEMALE BARRIER METHODS

Options for female-controlled barrier methods have increased in the past few years and more methods are in development. Intravaginal nonhormonal methods include diaphragms, cervical caps, female condoms, sponges, and spermicides.

Because of the increased concerns about STDs, including HIV infection, young women who might previously have selected a diaphragm are now more likely to have their partner use condoms plus spermicide. Some mature adolescents in stable monogamous relationships who are comfortable with their bodies do select the diaphragm.

The diaphragm is fitted by the health care provider. There are four types of diaphragms available: arcing spring, coil spring, flat spring, and wide-seal rim (Fig. 2). Diaphragms come in sizes 50 to 95, with sizes 60 to 75 most often used by adolescents. Actual diaphragms rather than fitting rings should be used so that the patient can practice in the clinic.

The ring of the arcing spring diaphragm provides firm pressure on the lateral vaginal walls and is therefore especially good for patients with poor vaginal tone, mild uterine prolapse, or marked uterine anteflexion or retroversion. The All-Flex (Ortho) arcing spring diaphragm folds at any point along its rim and must be held in the center, whereas the Koro-Flex (Schmid Laboratories) arcing diaphragm folds at two points and can be more easily held at the end by the new user. The coil spring rim (Ortho Coil Spring Diaphragm, Koromex Coil Spring Diaphragm), which folds flat for insertion, can be used for most women with average vaginal tone and a normal pubic notch. The flat spring (Ortho-White Flat Spring Diaphragm) has a thin rim and is generally worn by nulliparous women with firm vaginal tone and a shallow arch behind the symphysis. The wide-seal rim (Milex) has a flexible flange on it to create a better seal and is available in arcing spring and coil spring. The arcing model folds in two places but has a light spring, which may make it useful for the adolescent who has experienced discomfort with other arcing spring diaphragms or who has had recurrent cystitis.

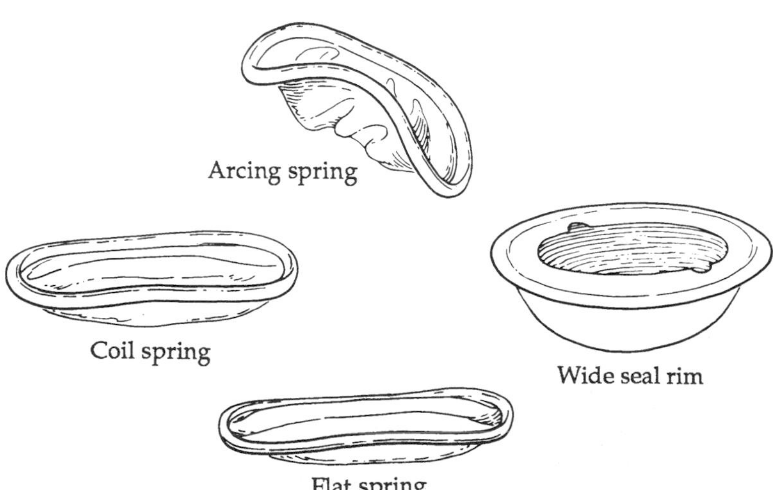

FIG. 2. Types of diaphragms. (From Hatcher RA, Trussell J, Stewart F, et al. *Contraceptive technology,* 16th ed. Atlanta, GA: Irvington, 1994; with permission.)

The size of the diaphragm is estimated by the examiner's placing a gloved index finger and middle finger in the vagina until they reach the posterior vaginal wall behind the cervix. The thumb is then placed on top of the index finger to mark the point at which the index finger touches the pubic bone. The fingers are removed in this position, and the diaphragm size is determined by placing the tip of the middle finger against the rim and the opposite rim against the spot on the index finger previously marked with the thumb (Fig. 3). The diaphragm should fit snugly, since vaginal size increases with sexual stimulation and coitus. Virginal patients who have a comfortably distensible hymen can be fitted but should have the size of the diaphragm checked after the first four to eight episodes of coitus. A too loose diaphragm will be displaced; a too large diaphragm can cause pressure, pain, and urinary tract infections.

The pregnancy rates reported with diaphragm use vary from 6 to 23/100 woman-years of use, with most studies reporting 10 to 18 pregnancies (31,

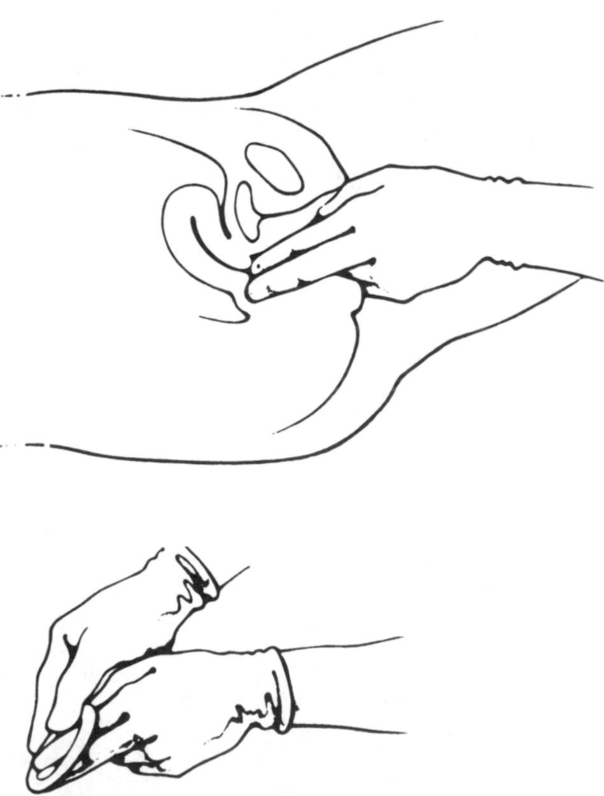

FIG. 3. Determining diaphragm size. (From *Ortho diaphragms.* Raritan, NJ: Ortho Pharmaceutical Corp, 1981; with permission.)

236). Trussell and associates (236) reported a pregnancy rate of 8% for perfect use in nulliparous women (15% for consistent use) versus 4% for perfect use in parous women (5% for consistent use). Causes of failure include nonuse, an incorrect fit, a flawed device, and failure to insert additional spermicide with a second episode of intercourse. Occasionally, adolescents cannot use a diaphragm because of poor vaginal tone, congenital anomalies, uterine prolapse, rectovaginal or vesicovaginal fistulas, or allergy to latex or spermicide. A 2- to 2.5-fold increased risk of urinary tract infections has been noted (237,238). Vaginal colonization with *Escherichia coli* was significantly greater in diaphragm users. A change in diaphragm type or size, postcoital antibiotics, or a change to a different method of contraception may be necessary in adolescents with recurrent urinary tract infections associated with diaphragm use.

Other problems with the diaphragm include foul-smelling vaginal discharge associated with prolonged wearing of the diaphragm, pelvic discomfort, and vaginal ulceration from excessive rim pressure. Because of the rare association of diaphragm use and toxic shock syndrome (see Chapter 11), patients should probably not leave a diaphragm in for >12 hours or use a diaphragm during menses (a condom should be used); they should also learn about warning signs of the disease.

Patients should be given careful instructions, preferably written, on the use and care of the diaphragm. Before a prescription is given, they should be shown how to feel for the cervix and should have an opportunity during the office visit to insert the diaphragm and remove it. Teaching aids such as the Ortho pelvic model are very helpful for adolescents to understand the location of the diaphragm. A return appointment 2 to 3 weeks later to check for proper fit of the prescribed size allows the clinician a chance to assess patients' understanding and acceptance of this form of contraception.

Patients are given the following instructions (31,239):

1. Before inserting, urinate and wash hands with soap and water.
2. Place 1 to 2 tsp of contraceptive jelly or cream inside the cup of the diaphragm and spread a small amount around the entire rim. The diaphragm can be inserted up to 6 hours prior to intercourse. If >6 hours have elapsed, an extra applicatorful of cream inserted into the upper vagina in front of the diaphragm provides added protection. (Many women routinely insert the diaphragm every night.) Never use Vaseline or petroleum products on the diaphragm.
3. For insertion, hold the diaphragm with the dome facing down, and press together the opposite sides of the rim. After inserting the diaphragm, check the cervix to make sure that it is covered by the diaphragm and that the diaphragm is locked in place behind the pubic bone.
4. Leave the diaphragm in place for at least 6 hours but not >12 hours after intercourse, and do not douche during the 6 hours after intercourse.

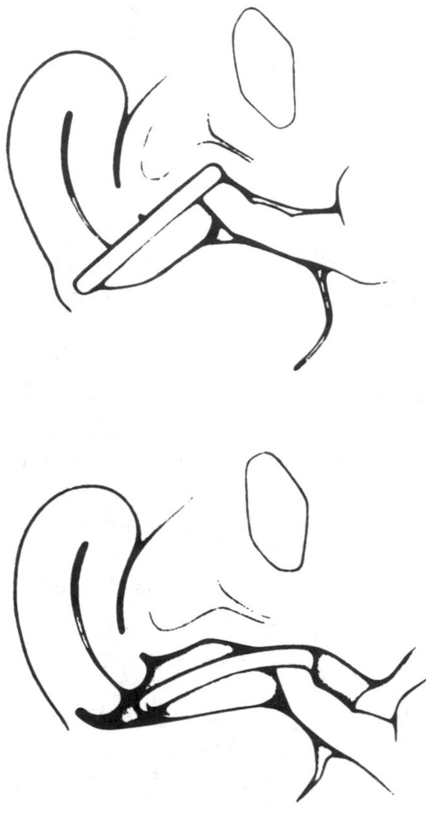

FIG. 4. A technique for removal of the diaphragm. (From *Ortho diaphragms.* Raritan, NJ: Ortho Pharmaceutical Corp, 1981; with permission.)

5. To remove the diaphragm, insert a forefinger up and over the top side of the diaphragm. Turn the palm of the hand downward and backward, hooking the finger firmly inside the top rim and breaking the suction. Pull the diaphragm down and out (Fig. 4).
6. After removal, wash the diaphragm with mild soap, dry it thoroughly, and store it in a cool, dry place.
7. Before each use, hold the diaphragm up to the light and check for holes.
8. The diaphragm should be replaced at least every 2 years and at any time a small tear or puckered appearance near the rim is noted. If a woman has a weight change of 10 lbs or has had a recent pregnancy, the clinician should be consulted to make sure that the diaphragm still fits.

Cervical Cap

A cervical cap is similar to a diaphragm except that it is made of rigid plastic and is designed to cover only the cervix (240,241). A small amount of spermicide is placed in the cap (about one-third full of a potent spermicide), and the cap is inserted onto the cervix; it is held in place by suction.

The Prentif Cavity-Rim Cervical Cap is available in four sizes. One-tenth to one-third of women cannot be fitted, although the introduction of custom molded caps may alleviate some of this problem. Patients need to feel comfortable with insertion of tampons or diaphragms into the vagina, before considering the cap. The device can be left in place for at least 8 hours (maximum of 48 hours) and should not be worn during menses. It is not necessary to reapply spermicide with repeated intercourse, but the cap should be checked before and after intercourse (especially in the first month of use) to make sure it has not been dislodged. Use of additional spermicide in the vagina and/or use of a condom seems prudent in the first 2 months after fitting and with a new position or new partner.

The pregnancy rates are similar to those with the diaphragm, with a range of 7.6 to 26/100 woman-years of use (237,242–245). In a study of >3400 women, Richwald and colleagues (242) estimated first year pregnancy rate to be 11.3% (8.3% and 3.8% for user and method failure, respectively). "Near-perfect" users had half the pregnancy rate of others (6.1% vs. 11.9%). Trussell and coworkers (237) have estimated a pregnancy rate of 16% for perfect use in nulliparous women (22% for consistent use) and 9% for perfect use in parous women (10% for consistent use). Because of questions in the initial trials related to Pap smear changes, the cap is contraindicated in patients with abnormal Pap smears. Other problems with the cap include odor, dislodgment, vaginal discharge, partner discomfort, and difficulty with insertion or removal. Contraindications to use of a cap include known or suspected uterine or cervical malignancy and current cervicovaginal infections. Practitioners usually wait 6 to 8 weeks postpartum and 3 to 4 weeks postabortion to fit a cap.

Two other devices similar to the cervical cap are Lea's shield and Femcap (246). Lea's shield is a one size fits all vaginal contraceptive that is made of silicone rubber and shaped like an elliptical bowl with a loop at the front end to aid removal; it has a valve to allow passage of cervical secretions and air to allow a better fit. More efficacy data is needed. The Femcap is another vaginal contraceptive made of silicone rubber that is shaped like a sailor's hat. The brim adheres and conforms to the vaginal walls. It can be used with a spermicide and in the future with microbiocides. Because it comes in two sizes, it requires fitting by a clinician. The device was in stage III clinical trials in late 1996.

Spermicides and Sponges

Spermicides include vaginal creams, jellies, foams, suppositories, and films. The most well known spermicide is nonoxynol-9. Spermicides have efficacy *in vitro* against the agents responsible for gonorrhea, chlamydia, genital herpes infections, trichomoniasis, syphilis, and HIV infection and *in vivo* effects against gonorrhea (247), chlamydia, and trichomoniasis (248). However, it remains unclear whether spermicides will change transmission of HIV *in vivo.* HIV transmission could be decreased because of the *in vitro* viricidal properties of the spermicide (249) or could be increased if the dose or frequent usage of spermicides results in irritation of the vaginal mucosa or the development of genital ulcers. Most studies suggest no additional protection above that provided by condoms.

Spermicidal methods are important for the adolescent because they are available over the counter without the necessity of a health care visit. The pregnancy rates for spermicides alone are in the range of 3 to 30/100 woman-years of use; the lower rate can be achieved by educated, motivated women in their 30s who are given specific in-office demonstration of appropriate use and application (high in the vagina) of spermicides (31,250). Whenever possible, adolescents choosing a spermicide should also have their partners use a condom.

The jellies, creams, and foams should be inserted no more than 30 minutes before intercourse and are effective within several minutes (foams are effectively immediately, but gels and creams need a few minutes to reach body temperature to melt). Suppositories require 10 to 15 minutes to melt or effervesce and appear more unpredictable in their dispersion. Patients using the effervescing Encare Ovals may notice vaginal warmth and burning. A vaginal contraceptive film (VCF) consists of a 2- × 2-inch flat package with wax paper-like tissues, each containing 72 mg of nonoxynol-9. The film is inserted on a dry fingertip up into the vagina at least 5 minutes before intercourse and remains effective for 2 hours.

Studies including FDA data have not found any link between spermicides and congenital anomalies (251,252). Patients may have difficulty with odor and allergic reactions to the spermicides; vaginal flora is altered with the use of spermicides and may increase the risk of urinary tract infections.

During counseling, specific names of foams (e.g., Emko, Delfen), suppositories (e.g., Semicid, Intercept), and film (e.g., VCF) should be mentioned. A demonstration of how to fill the applicator with foam is useful. Individual one-dose applicators (Conceptrol Jel) are convenient for adolescents but are also more expensive than the refillable applicators.

Our instructions to teenage girls are the following:

1. Be sure to read the instructions for the product you use before insertion. For example, films and suppositories must be inserted 5 to 15 minutes before intercourse to allow time to dissolve.
2. Insert the contraceptive foam, suppository, or film high into the vagina so that it will cover the cervix. Use the foam 30 minutes or less prior to intercourse—not after intercourse.
3. Do not douche for at least 6 hours after intercourse.
4. Wash the spermicide applicator with warm water and soap after each use.

5. Keep an extra condom with the contraceptive foam, since using the combination lessens the risk of failure.

The Today Vaginal Contraceptive Sponge (Whitehall Laboratories), a disposable polyurethane foam sponge impregnated with a high dose of nonoxynol-9, was voluntarily removed from the market in 1995. The Protectaid sponge is a new barrier method that acts as a physical barrier absorbing semen and as a chemical barrier with three spermicides (sodium cholate, nonoxynol-9, and benzalkonium chloride); it is currently available in Canada (246). The low concentrations of nonoxynol and the dispersing gel appear to markedly reduce vaginal irritation. It can be placed in the vagina up to 12 hours before intercourse.

Female Condom

The introduction of the female condom offers an additional alternative for patients, especially in the era of heightened awareness of STDs (Fig. 5). The Reality female condom is a loose-fitting, disposable polyurethane sheath with two diaphragm-like flexible rings at either end. The inner ring covers the cervix (similar to a diaphragm) and the outer ring fits against the vulva. In a 6-month trial involving 240 women, the pregnancy rate was estimated at 2.6% with perfect use and 12.4% with typical use (9.5% failure for women ≥25 years and 22.3% failure for women <25 years) (253,254). Trussell and colleagues (254) have estimated a 5.1% pregnancy/failure rate with perfect use; they also suggested that with perfect use the device would be 94% protective against HIV infection for women having intercourse twice a week with an infected partner. The female condom offers the advantage of female control over a barrier method that can aid in the prevention of STDs and does not change vaginal flora (255). The cost ($2.75 each) and the unusual appearance may be barriers to the widespread usage by teenagers. Some users complain that there is a "squeaking" sound with intercourse or that the female condom seems to be sticking to the penis; both problems can be addressed by the use of a vaginal lubricant (e.g., K-Y Jelly) on the inside of the device or on the penis.

Our instructions to patients are the following:

1. Find a comfortable position. You may want to stand with one foot on a chair, squat with knees apart, or lie down with legs bent and knees apart.
2. Hold the female condom with the open end hanging down. Squeeze the inner ring with your thumb and middle finger.
3. Holding the inner ring squeezed together, insert the ring into the vagina and push the inner ring and pouch into the vagina past the pubic bone.
4. When properly inserted, the outer ring will hang down slightly outside the vagina. During intercourse, when the penis enters the vagina, the slack will lessen.

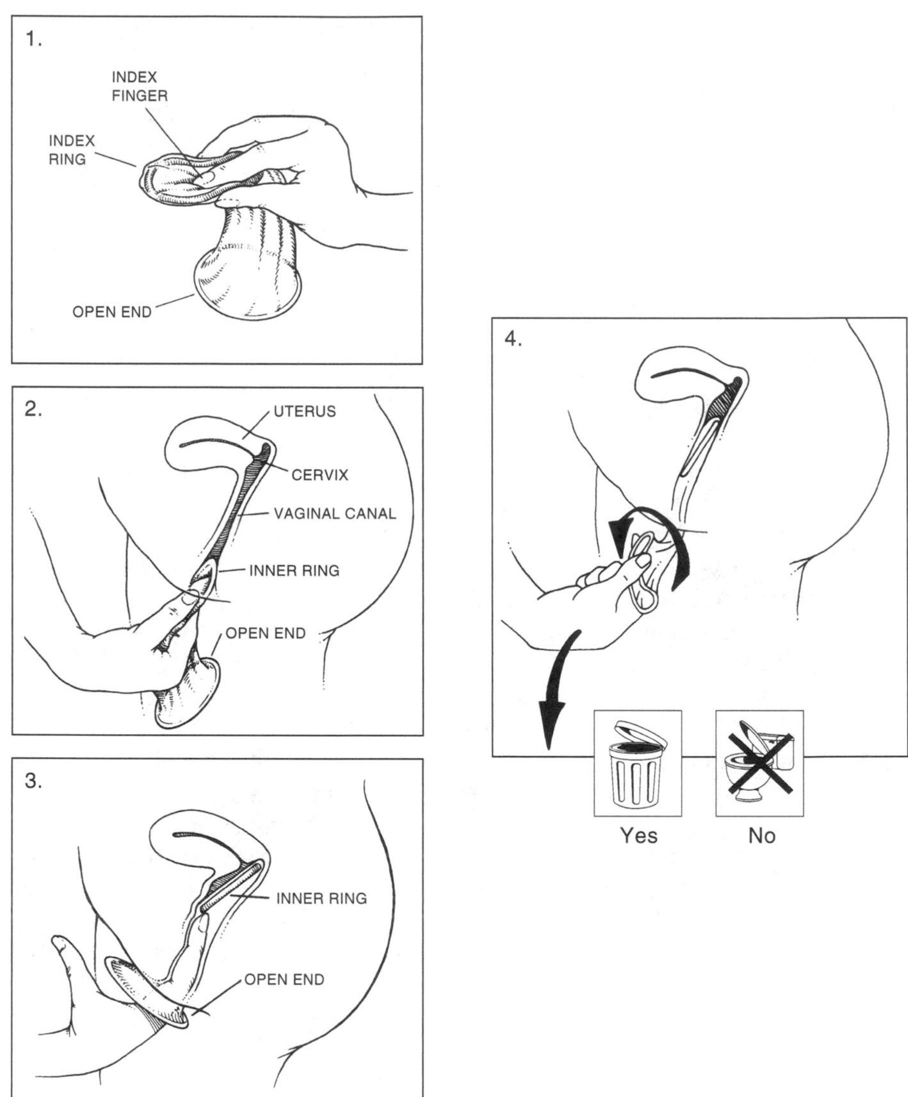

FIG. 5. The female condom. (From *Contracept Rep* 1994;5(6):8; with permission.)

5. To remove the device, squeeze and twist the outer ring to keep the sperm inside the pouch. Pull the condom out gently. Throw away in the garbage; do not flush down the toilet. Do not reuse.

Other female condom designs under development that both use latex include the Bikini condom (a panty with a covered perineal area) and Women's Choice (which requires an applicator for insertion).

CONDOMS

Recognition of the major threat posed by HIV infection and other STDs to the life and reproductive health of all sexually active people markedly increased condom usage between 1982 and 1988. From 1988 to 1991, Pleck and coworkers (256) reported that condom use among 17.5- to 19-year-old men remained about the same: 53% used a condom at last intercourse in 1988 and 56% in 1991. Among sexually experienced 9th to 12th grade students responding to the 1997 Youth Risk Behavior Survey, 50.8% of girls (58% of 9th graders, 43% of 12th graders) and 62.5% of boys (59.2% of 9th graders, 61.2% of 12th graders) reported condom use at last intercourse (3). The decline in consistent use with increasing age has been noted in other studies in the United States and abroad.

Major behavioral change requires skills-based learning, practice, empowerment of women, overcoming cultural barriers, and peer support (17,257–260). Orr and Langefeld (261) found that condom use was less likely among males with other health risk behaviors and more STD risk behaviors. Three reasons were noted to be highly predictive of condom use: STD prevention, birth control, and AIDS prevention. Creative approaches in clinics, advertising, and marketing based on an understanding of adolescent risk taking and motivational factors and barriers could improve condom rates among teens (262). Educational efforts to improve the image of condom users and increase the peer pressure to use condoms, as well as the availability of free condoms in drug stores, clinics, and schools, have increased usage in some settings.

Adolescent girls frequently are not assertive about the use of condoms when the male rejects the notion. It is helpful for the health care provider to give patients some ideas to bolster their self-esteem, as well as some catchy phrases such as "You don't know how? Allow me" or "My doctor says I must protect my cervix." Cultural barriers need to be understood and efforts framed within the context of realistic change that can occur for a given adolescent. Sexually active adolescent girls should be encouraged to purchase condoms and keep them with their spermicide or OC pills. Every girl must understand that hormonal agents do not protect against STDs. Some condoms are now marketed exclusively for women and are shelved in pharmacies with other feminine hygiene products. Many adolescents feel more comfortable purchasing contraceptive supplies from an unfamiliar pharmacy.

The pregnancy rate of condoms has varied in studies from 2 to 20/100 woman-years of use, with good usage resulting in pregnancy rates of 3 to 4/100 woman-years of use (31,33). A survey of 20- to 39-year-old men who had used a condom in the preceding 6 months showed that the average condom breakage rate was 2.9% and that 1.9% of all condoms used broke during that time (263). Men with low incomes and infrequent use of condoms were more likely to experience condom breakage and slippage (264,265). Similar findings were noted in a study of 177 couples, with a breakage rate of 5% and a slippage rate of 3.5% (265).

Condoms provide significant protection against STDs, including infection with *N. gonorrhoeae*, *C. trachomatis*, and HIV (31). Depending on the location of the lesions on the genitals, condoms can also provide some protection against herpes simplex and HPV infection. Because natural condoms have larger pores that can allow the smaller particles of hepatitis B virus or HIV to pass through, latex condoms should be used for the prevention of STDs. Whether the talc used on some condoms has any adverse effects is unknown but requires investigation; fewer condoms than several years ago have talc as part of the lubricant.

In August 1993, the FDA approved a new polyurethane condom (Avanti). Unlike latex condoms, this type of condom can be lubricated with oil-based lubricants. It is thinner and potentially provides greater sensitivity and comfort. The polyurethane condom is more expensive than latex condoms, and further testing is being undertaken to assess breakage, slippage, and pregnancy risks. A latex-free natural-rubber condom (Tactylon) is another option under study for latex-allergic patients (31).

Latex condoms that contain spermicides have the advantage of greater inactivation of sperm, as well as antiviral properties. *In vitro* studies of condoms containing nonoxynol-9 have demonstrated that condoms offer an excellent physical barrier against HIV and that the addition of a spermicide prevented the detection of HIV *in vitro* even after rupture of the condom (249) (see section on spermicides). Although epidemiologic studies have suggested that condoms are very effective in preventing HIV transmission in couples discordant for HIV infection (266,267), intercourse with an infected partner still poses a risk to the patient. Pregnant teenagers should also be encouraged to use condoms throughout pregnancy to prevent exposure to sexually transmitted infections.

Condoms may be lubricated or unlubricated, with the former being preferred by most adolescents. Condoms may also be lubricated with spermicide, which increases the cost but also the protection from pregnancy. Even higher pregnancy protection is achieved by the use of a vaginal spermicide (separate from the condoms) and a latex condom. It is unknown whether thick condoms offer any more protection than thin condoms with vaginal intercourse, although thin condoms may be more likely to tear. Instructions—with a demonstration if possible—are extremely important for adolescents to be able to use condoms correctly. Just the statement "Use condoms" may otherwise go unheeded. Condoms should not be exposed to excessive heat (i.e., in a wallet for >1 month or in a glove compartment).

Our recommendations to teenagers using condoms include the following (31,267):

1. Latex condoms are preferred because they offer greater protection against STDs.
2. Condoms should be stored in a cool, dry place.
3. Condoms in damaged packages (brittle, sticky, discolored) should not be used.
4. Condoms should be put on before any genital contact. The tip of the condom should be held and the condom unrolled onto the erect penis, leaving 1/4 to 1/2 inch of space at the tip to collect semen yet ensuring that no air is trapped in the tip.

5. Adequate lubrication should be used. Only water-based lubricants (e.g., K-Y Jelly, Surgilube) should be used, not petroleum-based lubricants such as Vaseline.
6. Use of condoms containing spermicide may offer greater pregnancy protection, although use of a vaginal spermicide is even better.
7. If the condom breaks, it should be replaced. If ejaculation occurs after breakage, immediate application of a spermicide has been suggested, although efficacy is unproved. Emergency contraception (postcoital contraception) should be strongly considered. (Some clinicians suggest that couples relying on condoms should have a supply of oral contraceptives for self-administration).
8. After ejaculation, the base of the condom should be held to prevent slippage. The penis should be withdrawn while still erect. Be careful not to let semen spill. Remove the condom, and dispose of it safely.

COITUS INTERRUPTUS

Withdrawal is a not an effective method of contraception, although it is practiced widely by adolescents who often believe that it offers significantly more protection than it does. Few adolescents have the ability to prevent ejaculation effectively, and thus even those who believe they can practice this method well often have difficulty. Couples are clearly not protected from STDs with the use of withdrawal, and pregnancy rates are high because the preejaculate may contain sperm from a previous ejaculation. The annual failure rate with typical use of this method has been estimated at 19% (31).

"NATURAL" FAMILY PLANNING OR FERTILITY AWARENESS

Calendars, basal body temperature charts, cervical mucus awareness, and hormonal testing have been used for both contraception and facilitation of conception in infertile couples (268,269). The advantages are the ease of the method and the fact that adolescents can be taught the method as a noncontroversial part of reproductive health. The major drawbacks of these methods are the high failure rate for pregnancies and the lack of protection against STDs. Although these methods do encourage communication between sexual partners, extensive records are required and sexual spontaneity is restricted. Calendar methods are less likely to help adolescents prevent pregnancy than adults because of the wider range of cycles in adolescents. The Billings method of cervical mucus awareness is based on determining ovulation by the change of mucus to abundant slippery mucus. Secretions can be affected by coitus, vaginitis, cervicitis, and vaginal medications and spermicides. Electronic hand-held computers can boost the reliability of the rhythm method. Most of the high-technology methods of hormonal assays are more appropriate for the treatment of infertile couples.

The pregnancy rates reported are variable, ranging from 6 to 38/100 woman-years of use (typical use 20) depending on the population studied and the method employed (31,268–271).

EMERGENCY CONTRACEPTION (POSTCOITAL CONTRACEPTION)

Emergency contraception (previously known as postcoital contraception or the "morning after pill") is an important yet underutilized method of contraception in the United States. Other countries such as Sweden, the Netherlands, and the United Kingdom have been more effective in popularizing and increasing availability of hormonal emergency contraception. Public knowledge with regard to availability and use of emergency contraception is limited, as is the practice of prescribing pills among obstetrician/gynecologists (272). All adolescents should be educated about the availability of this method in situations of unexpected coitus, broken condoms, rape, multiple missed OCs, dislodged diaphragm or cervical cap, exposure to a possible teratogen, etc. The most commonly used hormonal dosing is the Yuzpe regimen, which utilizes two tablets of Ovral (50 μg ethinyl estradiol/0.5 mg norgestrel per tablet) within 72 hours of unprotected intercourse, followed by two tablets 12 hours later (272,274). Five tablets of Alesse can be used similarly. Slightly higher doses of hormones can also be used including four tablets of Lo/Ovral, Levlen, or Nordette or the yellow tablets of Triphasil or Tri-Levlen followed by four tablets 12 hours later (31). A specially marketed formulation (Preven) comes with a pregnancy test. The pregnancy rate is 0.2% to 2.0% versus an expected rate of 4.7% to 6.8% (31,273–287), depending in part on how the studies were done and whether the day of cycle was controlled. Trussell and colleagues (286) have suggested that estimates of efficacy should consider the reduction in expected pregnancies; in reviewing ten studies of the Yuzpe regimen that contained data on the cycle day of unprotected intercourse, they estimated that effectiveness was 74% (95% CI: 68.2%, 79.3%). In a review of nine studies, Trussell and colleagues (287) found no difference in failure rates whether therapy was initiated on the first, second, or third day after unprotected intercourse.

Progestin-only therapies have had more variable efficacy but appear to be similar to the Yuzpe regimen (31,275–277). A regimen using 0.75 mg levonorgestrel within 48 hours and repeated 12 hours later has been reported to have a pregnancy rate of 2.9% (275); in the United States, a large number of progestin-only tablets of Ovrette would be needed to simulate this dose (20 tablets of Ovrette for each dose). However, the rates of both nausea and vomiting are considerably lower than with the Yuzpe regimen. Danazol has been reported to have efficacy in some but not other studies. Postcoital insertion of a copper T IUD has not been widely used, although it is effective.

A promising medication for emergency contraception is mifepristone (RU 486). Although not yet available in the United States, postcoital use of a single 600-mg dose of RU 486 has shown excellent results in preventing pregnancy with a low incidence of side effects. In a comparative study involving 800 women and adolescents treated within 72 hours of unprotected intercourse with the Yuzpe regimen or RU 486, Glasier and colleagues (277) found a pregnancy rate of 1% (4/398) with the Yuzpe regimen and 0/402 with RU 486. Vomiting occurred in 17% of those with the Yuzpe regimen and 3% of those with RU 486; delayed menses occurred in 13% of those following the Yuzpe method and in 42% of the RU 486 group. Current doses under study are 10 mg and 50 mg, with use up to 5 days after intercourse.

The clinician prescribing the Yuzpe regimen should consider whether the adolescent has any contraindications to the short-term use of high-dose estrogens, such as migraine headache with neurologic symptoms. Although the other contraindications to OCs, such as a history of thromboembolism, stroke, and breast cancer, may be considered contraindications to the Yuzpe regimen, there is insufficient evidence that short-term use has any significant risks with these conditions; however, progestin-only therapy is an alternative. Although there is no evidence that OCs are teratogenic, the possibility of pregnancy from the current or a prior episode of intercourse in the past 10 days should be discussed with the patient. At the time of the visit, the patient's history, her last menstrual period, number of hours since unprotected intercourse (and recent other unprotected intercourse), attitudes about pregnancy and contraceptive use, and risk factors should be reviewed. A sensitive urine pregnancy test and a blood pressure reading are indicated. A general physical examination and pelvic examination should be done at that visit or scheduled to provide ongoing preventive care. Since the Yuzpe regimen probably does not protect against tubal pregnancy, a prior tubal pregnancy is a cause for extra caution in followup. Although some clinicians advocate allowing patients to receive pills by phone prescription or having a package of pills at home available for self-administration, adolescents may be more likely to deny the possibility of preexisting pregnancy and, in most cases, benefit from direct counseling and medical assessment.

It is prudent to provide patients with extra pills so that if she vomits the initial dose within 2 hours, it can be repeated. It also makes sense to provide patients with an antiemetic, such as prochlorperazine (Compazine) 5 to 10 mg, trimethobenzamide (Tigan) 250 mg, dimenhydrinate (Dramamine) 50 mg, cyclizine (Marezine) 50 mg, or promethazine (Phenergan) 25 mg (warn patient about drowsiness), to use 1 to 2 hours prior to the second dose if needed. Others find it more effective to administer antiemetics prophylactically 1/2 hour before the first course and then every 4 to 8 hours as indicated to ensure better adherence to the regimen. Other possible side effects of high-dose OCs for postcoital therapy include fluid retention, headaches, dizziness, menstrual irregularities, and breast soreness. Patients are warned against having intercourse for the remainder of the cycle. A return visit 2 weeks later should be arranged for teens to repeat the pregnancy test and ensure that contraception is addressed for the future. The directory of sites providing emergency contraception in the United States is available through 1-800-584-9911 and 1-888-NOT-2-LATE or at the

World Wide Web site reachable through the universal resource locator (URL): http://opr.princeton.edu/ec.

FUTURE DEVELOPMENTS IN CONTRACEPTION

Contraceptive development has been slow in the United States in the past decade because of inadequate funding of research and fear of litigation. Additional methods that minimize side effects and provide women with protection against STDs are urgently needed. Methods that are female controlled and have viricidal and microbiocidal properties are under developement. Some of these products would be spermicides as well as microbiocides; others need to prevent infection and preserve fertility (278).

Hormonal methods include a two-rod levonorgestrel subdermal implant (Norplant II), currently approved in Finland and China, with efficacy for 3 to 5 years; one-rod implants using nomegestrol acetate (Uniplant), 3-keto-desogestrel (Implanon), or the progestin ST-1435 (registered as Nestorone by the Population Council); a biodegradable implant with levonorgestrel (Capronor); biodegradable norethindrone pellets; biodegradable injectable norethindrone microspheres; transdermal progestin contraceptives; vaginal rings impregnated with progestin alone or a combination of estrogen and progestin; injectable progestins and combination estrogens and progestins, and luteinizing hormone-releasing hormone analogs (31,227). Newer IUDs are also being developed, as well as new female barrier methods, new spermicides, disposable diaphragms, new cervical caps, vaccines, reversible sterilization, and a variety of potential methods for men (213).

REFERENCES

1. McCann MF, Potter LS. Progestin-only oral contraception: comprehensive review. *Contraception* 1994;50(suppl 1):1.
2. *Facts in brief: teenage reproductive health in the United States.* New York: The Alan Guttmacher Institute, 1994.
3. Centers for Disease Control and Prevention. Youth risk behavior surveillance—United States, 1997. *MMWR* 1998;47(SS-3):1.
4. Centers for Disease Control and Prevention. Trends in sexual risk behaviors among high school students—United States, 1991–1997. *MMWR* 1998;47(36):749.
5. Centers for Disease Control. Health risk behavior among adolescent who do not attend school—United States, 1992. *MMWR* 1994;43:129.
6. Abma JC, Chandra A, Mosher WD, et al. Fertility, family planning, and women's health: new data from the 1995 National Survey of Family Growth. National Center For Health Statistics. *Vital Health Stat* 1997;23.
7. Shrier A, Emans SJ, Woods ER, DuRant RH. The association of sexual risk behaviors and problem drug behaviors in high school students. *J Adolesc Health* 1997;20:377.
8. Rosenthal SL, Biro FM, Succop PA, et al. Age of first intercourse and risk of sexually transmitted disease. *Adolesc Pediatr Gynecol* 1994;7:210.
9. Forrest JD. Epidemiology of unintended pregnancy and contraceptive use. *Am J Obstet Gynecol* 1994:170:1485.
10. Mosher WD, Horn MC. First family planning visits by young women. *Fam Plann Perspect* 1988;20:33.

11. Chamie M, Eisman S, Forrest JD, et al. Factors affecting adolescents' use of family planning clinics. *Fam Plann Perspect* 1982;14:126.
12. Zabin LS, Clark SD. Institutional factors affecting teenagers' choice and reasons for delay in attending a family planning clinic. *Fam Plann Perspect* 1983;15:25.
13. Furstenberg FF, Shea J, Allison P, et al. Contraceptive continuation among adolescents attending family planning clinics. *Fam Plann Perspect* 1983;15:211.
14. Zelnik M, Koenig MA, Kim YJ. Sources of prescription contraceptives and subsequent pregnancy among young women. *Fam Plann Perspect* 1984;16:6.
15. Zabin LS, Clark DSD. Why they delay: a study of teenage family planning clinic patients. *Fam Plann Perspect* 1981;13:205.
16. Emans SJ, Grace E, Woods ER, et al. Adolescents' compliance with the use of oral contraceptives. *JAMA* 1987;257:3377.
17. Departments of Education and Public Health. *Massachusetts youth risk behavior survey, 1993.* Boston, MA, 1993.
18. Zabin LS, Stark HA, Emerson MR. Reasons for delay in contraceptive clinic utilization. *J Adolesc Health* 1991;12:225.
19. Durant RH, Jay MS, Linder CW, et al. Influence of psychosocial factors on adolescent compliance with oral contraceptives. *J Adolesc Health Care* 1984;5:1.
20. Scher PW, Emans SJ, Grace EM. Factors associated with compliance to oral contraceptive use in an adolescent population. *J Adolesc Health Care* 1982;3:120.
21. Litt IF. Know thyself: adolescents' self-assessment of compliance behavior. *Pediatrics* 1985;75:693.
22. Woods ER, Grace E, Havens KK, et al. Contraceptive compliance with a levonorgestrel triphasic and a norethindrone monophasic oral contraceptive pill in adolescent patients. *Am J Obstet Gynecol* 1992;166:901.
23. Adler NE, Kegeles SM, Irwin CE, Wibbelsman C. Adolescent contraceptive behavior: an assessment of decision process. *J Pediatr* 1990;116:463.
24. Kegeles SM, Adler NE, Irwin CE. Adolescents and condoms: associations of beliefs with intention to use. *Am J Dis Child* 1989;143:911.
25. DuRant RH, Sanders JM, Jay S, Levinson R. Analysis of contraceptive behavior of sexually active female adolescents in the United States. *J Pediatr* 1988;113:930.
26. DuRant RH, Sanders JM, Jay S. Adolescent contraceptive risk-taking behavior: a social psychological model of females' use of and compliance with birth control. *Adv Adolesc Mental Health* 1990;4:87.
27. Oakley D. Rethinking patient counselling techniques for changing contraceptive behavior. *Am J Obstet Gynecol* 1994:170:1585.
28. Rosenberg MJ, Waugh MS, Long S. Unintended pregnancies and use, misuse, and discontinuation of oral contraceptives. *J Reprod Med* 1995;40:355.
29. Potter L, Oakley D, Leon-Wong E, et al. Measuring compliance among oral contraceptive users. *Fam Plann Perspect* 1996;28:154.
30. Loeb L, Colacurio V, Atkinson E, Darney P. Concurrent condom use intentions and practice among adolescent users of hormonal contraceptives (abstract). Presented at the American Public Health Association (APHA), Nov 1994.
31. Hatcher RA, Trussell J, Stewart F, et al. *Contraceptive technology,* 16th ed. Atlanta, GA: Irvington, 1994.
32. Choice of contraceptives. *Med Lett* 1995;37:9.
33. Trussell J, Hatcher RA, Cates E, et al. A guide to interpreting contraceptive efficacy studies. *Obstet Gynecol* 1990;76:558.
34. Trussell J, Kost K. Contraceptive failure in the United States: a critical review of the literature. *Stud Fam Plann* 1987;18:237.
35. Davis A. The role of hormonal contraception in adolescents. *Am J Obstet Gynecol* 1994;170:1581.
36. Hillard PJA. Family planning in the teen population. *Curr Opin Obstet Gynecol* 1993;5:798.
37. Jones KP, Wild RA. Contraception for patients with psychiatric or medical disorders. *Am J Obstet Gynecol* 1994:170:1575.
38. Armstrong KA, Stover MA. Smart start: an option for adolescents to delay the pelvic examination and blood work in family planning clinics. *J Adolesc Health* 1994;15:389.
39. Goldzieher JW. Pharmacokinetics and metabolism of ethynyl estrogens. In: Goldzieher JW, Fotherby K, eds. *Pharmacology of the contraceptive steroids.* Philadelphia: Lippincott-Raven, 1994;127.
40. Brody SA, Turkes A, Goldzieher JW. Pharmacokinetics of three bioequivalent norethindrone/mestranol 50 μg pills and three norethindrone/ethinyl estradiol OC formulations: are "low-dose" pills really lower? *Contraception* 1989:40:269.

41. Fotherby K. Pharmacokinetics and metabolism of progestins in humans. In: Goldzieher JW, Fotherby K, eds. *Pharmacology of the contraceptive steroids.* Philadelphia: Lippincott-Raven, 1994;99.
42. Dorflinger LJ. Relative potency of progestins used in oral contraceptives. *Contraception* 1985; 31:557.
43. Gilmer MD. Progestogen potency in oral contraceptive pills. *Am J Obstet Gynecol* 1987;157:1040.
44. Runnebaum B, Rabe T. New progestogens in oral contraceptives. *Am J Obstet Gynecol* 1987; 157:1059.
45. Letterie GS, Chow GE. Effect of "missed" pills on oral contraceptive effectiveness. *Obstet Gynecol* 1992;79:979.
46. Grimes DA, Godwin AJ, Rubin A, et al. Ovulation and follicular development associated with three low-dose oral contraceptives: a randomized controlled trial. *Obstet Gynecol* 1994;83:29.
47. Archer DF, DelConte A. *The efficacy and safety of a new monophasic low-dose 21-day oral contraceptive containing levonorgestrel 100 µg and ethinyl estradiol 20 µg.* (abstract). American Society for Reproductive Medicine, Boston, November 1996.
48. Shoupe D. Multicenter randomized comparative trial of two low-dose triphasic combined oral contraceptives containing desogestrel and norethindrone. *Obstet Gynecol* 1994;83:679.
49. Speroff L, DeCherney A. Evaluation of a new generation of oral contraceptives. *Obstet Gynecol* 1993;81:1034.
50. Hanson MS, Stewart GK, Bechtel RC, et al. Planned Parenthood experience with Triphasil. *J Reprod Med* 1987;32:592.
51. Kafrissen ME. A norgestimate-containing oral contraceptive: review of clinical studies. *Am J Obstet Gynecol* 1992;167:1196.
52. Corson SL. Efficacy and clinical profile of a new oral contraceptive containing norgestimate. U.S. clinical trials. *Acta Obstet Gynecol Suppl* 1990:152:25.
53. Walling M. A multicenter efficacy and safety study of an oral contraceptive containing 150 µg desogestrel and 30 µg ethinyl estradiol. *Contraception* 1992;46:313.
54. Rekers H. Multicenter trial of a monophasic oral contraceptive containing ethinyl estradiol and desogestrel. *Acta Obstet Gynecol Scand* 1988;67:171.
55. Moore PJ, Adler NE, Kegeles SM. Adolescents and the contraceptive pill: the impact of beliefs on intentions and use. *Obstet Gynecol* 1996;88:48S.
56. Carpenter S, Neinstein LS. Weight gain in adolescent and young adult oral contraceptive users. *J Adolesc Health Care* 1986;7:342.
57. Grimes DA. The safety of oral contraceptive: insights from the first 30 years. *Am J Obstet Gynecol* 1992;166:1950.
58. Robinson TC, Plichta S. Weisman CS, et al. Dysmenorrhea and use of oral contraceptives in adolescent women attending a family planning clinic. *Am J Obstet Gynecol* 1992;166:578.
59. Potter L, Oakley D, de Leon-Wong E, et al. Measuring compliance among oral contraceptive users. *Fam Plann Perspect* 1996;28:154.
60. Krettek JE, Arkin SI, Chaisilwattana P, et al. *Chlamydia trachomatis* in patients who used oral contraceptives and had intermenstrual spotting. *Obstet Gynecol* 1993;81:728.
61. Casper RF, Powell AM. Evaluation and therapy of breakthrough bleeding in women using a triphasic oral contraceptive. *Fertil Steril* 1991;55:292.
62. Mattson RH, Rebar RW. Contraceptive methods for women with neurologic disorders. *Am J Obstet Gynecol* 1993;168:2027.
63. Meade TW. Update: cardiovascular effects of oral contraception and hormonal replacement therapy: risks and mechanisms of cardiovascular events in users. *Am J Obstet Gynecol* 1988;158:1646.
64. Porter JB, Hunter JR, Jick H, et al. Oral contraceptives and nonfatal vascular disease. *Obstet Gynecol* 1985;66:1.
65. Ramcharan S, Pellegrin FA, Ray RM, et al. The Walnut Creek contraceptive drug study: a prospective study of the side effects of oral contraceptives. *J Reprod Med* 1980;25(suppl 6):345.
66. Hirvonen E, Idanpaan-Heikkila JI. Cardiovascular death among women under 40 years of age using low-estrogen oral contraceptives and intrauterine devices in Finland from 1975. *Am J Obstet Gynecol* 1990;163:281.
67. Gerstman BB, Piper JM, Freiman JP, et al. Oral contraceptive oestrogen and progestin potencies and the incidence of deep venous thromboembolism. *Int J Epidemiol* 1990;19:931.
68. Gerstman BB, Piper JM, Tomita DK, et al. Oral contraceptive estrogen dose and the risk of deep venous thromboembolic disease. *Am J Epidemiol* 1991;133:32.
69. Sturtevant FM. Cardiovascular safety of oral contraceptives: a critical commentary. *Int J Fertil* 1991;36(suppl 3):32.

70. Beller FK. Cardiovascular system: coagulation, thrombosis, and contraceptive steroids—is there a link? In: Goldzieher JW, Fotherby K, eds. *Pharmacology of the contraceptive steroids.* Philadelphia: Lippincott-Raven, 1994;301.
71. Goldzieher JW. Hormonal contraception: benefits versus risks. *Am J Obstet Gynecol* 1987;157:1023.
72. Greene GR, Sartwell PE. Oral contraceptive use in patients with thromboembolism following surgery, trauma or infection. *Am J Public Health* 1972;62:680.
73. Alving BM, Comp PC. Recent advances in understanding clotting and evaluating patients with recurrent thrombosis. *Am J Obstet Gynecol* 1992;167:1184.
74. Notelovitz M, Zauner C, McKenzie L, et al. The effect of low-dose oral contraceptives on cardiorespiratory function, coagulation, and lipids in exercising young women: a preliminary report. *Am J Obstet Gynecol* 1987;156:591.
75. Bonnar J. Coagulation effects of oral contraception. *Am J Obstet Gynecol* 1987;157:1042.
76. World Health Organization Collaborative Study of Cardiovascular Disease and Steroid Hormone Contraception. Venous thromboembolic disease and combined oral contraceptives: results of an international multicentre case-control study. *Lancet* 1995;346;1575.
77. World Health Organization Collaborative Study of Cardiovascular Disease and Steroid Hormone Contraception. Effect of different progestagens in low-oestrogen oral contraceptives on venous thromboembolic disease. *Lancet* 1995;346;1582.
78. Jick H, Jick SS, Gurewich V, et al. Risk of idiopathic cardiovascular death and nonfatal venous thromboembolism in women using oral contraceptives with differing progestagen components. *Lancet* 1995;346;1589.
79. Bloemenkamp KW, Rosendaal FR, Helmerhorst FM, et al. Enhancement of factor V Leiden mutation of risk of deep-vein thrombosis associated with oral contraceptives containing a third-generation progestagen. *Lancet* 1995;346;1593.
80. Ridker PM, Miletich J, Hennekens CH, et al. Ethnic distribution of factor V Leiden in 4,047 men and women. *JAMA* 1997;277:1305.
81. Lewis MA, Heinemann LAJ, MacRae KD, et al. The increased risk of venous thromboembolism and the use of third-generation progestagens: role of bias in observational research. *Contraception* 1996;54:5.
82. Lewis MA, Spitzer WO, Heinemann LAJ, et al. Third-generation oral contraceptives and risk of myocardial infarction: an international case-control study. *BMJ* 1996;312:88.
83. Ginsberg JS. Management of venous thromboembolism. *N Engl J Med* 1996;335:1816.
84. Vessey MP, Doll R, Fairbairn AS, et al. Postoperative thromboembolism and the use of oral contraceptives. *BMJ* 1970;3:123.
85. Neinstein LS. *Issues in reproductive management.* New York: Thieme Medical Publishers, 1994.
86. Howard RJ, Tuck SM. Haematological disorders and reproductive health. *Br J Fam Plann* 1993; 19:147–150.
87. Howard RJ, Lillis C, Tuck SM. Contraceptives, counselling, and pregnancy in women with sickle cell disease. *BMJ* 1993;306:1735–1737.
88. Vessey M, Villard-Mackintosh L, McPherson K, et al. Mortality among oral contraceptive users: 20 year followup of women in a cohort study. *BMJ* 1989;299:1487.
89. Colditz GA. Oral contraceptive use and mortality during 12 years of follow-up: the Nurses Health Study. *Ann Intern Med* 1994;120:821.
90. WHO Collaborative Study of Cardiovascular Disease and Steroid Hormone Contraception. Ischaemic stroke and combined oral contraceptives: results of an international, multicentre, case-control study. *Lancet* 1996;348:498.
91. WHO Collaborative Study of Cardiovascular Disease and Steroid Hormone Contraception. Hemorrhagic stroke, overall stroke risk, and combined oral contraceptives: results of an international, multicentre, case-control study. *Lancet* 1996;348:505.
92. Petitti DB, Sidney S, Bernstein A, et al. Stroke in the users of low-dose oral contraceptives. *N Engl J Med* 1996;335:8.
93. Keefe D. Nervous system. In: Goldzieher JW, Fotherby K, eds. *Pharmacology of the contraceptive steroids.* Philadelphia: Lippincott-Raven, 1994;283.
94. Thorogood M, Vessey MP. An epidemiologic survey of cardiovascular disease in women taking oral contraceptives. *Am J Obstet Gynecol* 1990;163:274.
95. Stampfer MJ, Willett WC, Colditz GA. A prospective study of past use of oral contraceptive agents and risk of cardiovascular diseases. *N Engl J Med* 1988;319:1313.
96. Goldbaum GM, Kendrick JS, Hogelin GC, et al. The relative impact of smoking and oral contraceptive use on women in the United States. *JAMA* 1987;258:1339.

97. Hoyle M. Small bowel ischaemia and infarction in young women taking oral contraceptives and progestromal agents. *Br J Surg* 1977;64:533.
98. Perlman JA, Russell-Briefel R, Eczati T, et al. Oral glucose tolerance and the potency of contraceptive progestogens. *J Chronic Dis* 1985;38:857.
99. Spellacy WN, Birksa, Buggie J, et al. Prospective studies of carbohydrate metabolism in "normal" women using norgestrel for 18 months. *Fertil Steril* 1981;35:167.
100. Skouby SO, Molsted-Pedersen L, Kuhl C, et al. Oral contraceptives in diabetic women: metabolic effects of four compounds with different estrogen/progestogen profiles. *Fertil Steril* 1986; 46:858.
101. Skouby SO, Andersen O, Saurbrey N, et al. Oral contraception and insulin sensitivity: *in vivo* assessment in normal women and women with previous gestational diabetes. *J Clin Endocrinol Metab* 1987;64:519.
102. Krauss R, Burkman RT. The metabolic impact of oral contraceptives. *Am J Obstet Gynecol* 1992;167:1177.
103. Elkind-Hirsch K, Goldzieher JW. Metabolism: carbohydrate metabolism. In: Goldzieher JW, Fotherby K, eds. *Pharmacology of the contraceptive steroids.* Philadelphia: Lippincott-Raven, 1994;345.
104. Crook D, Godsland IF, Worthington M, et al. A comparative metabolic study of two low-estrogen-dose oral contraceptives containing desogestrel or gestodene progestins. *Am J Obstet Gynecol* 1993: 169:1183.
105. Radberg T, Gustafson A, Skryten A, et al. Oral contraception in diabetic women: a cross-over study on serum and high-density lipoprotein (HDL), lipids and diabetes control during progestogen and combined estrogen/progestogen contraception. *Horm Metab Res* 1982;14:61.
106. Klein BEK, Moss SE, Klein R. Oral contraceptives in women with diabetes. *Diabetes Care* 1990;13:895.
107. Garg SK, Chase HP, Marshall G. Oral contraceptives and renal and retinal complications in young women with insulin-dependent diabetes mellitus. *JAMA* 1994;271:1099.
108. Knopp RH, La Rosa JC, Burkman RT. Contraception and dyslipidemia. *Am J Obstet Gynecol* 1993;168:1994.
109. Crook D, Godsland IF, Wymann V. Oral contraceptives and coronary heart disease: modulation of glucose tolerance and plasma lipid risk factors by progestins. *Am J Obstet Gynecol* 1988;158:1612.
110. Burkman RT, Robinson JC, Kruszon-Moran D, et al. Lipid and lipoprotein changes associated with oral contraceptive use: a randomized clinical trial. *Obstet Gynecol* 1988;71:33.
111. Krauss RM, Roy S, Mishell DR, et al. Effects of two low-dose oral contraceptives on serum lipids and lipoproteins: differential changes in high-density lipoprotein subclasses. *Am J Obstet Gynecol* 1983;145:446.
112. Adams MR, Clarkson TB, Koritnik DR, et al. Contraceptive steroids and coronary artery disease in *Cynomolgus* macaques. *Fertil Steril* 1987;47:1010.
113. Davidoff F, Tishler S, Rosoff C. Hyperlipidemia and pancreatitis associated with oral contraceptive therapy. *N Engl J Med* 1973;289:552.
114. Miale JB, Kent JW. The effects of oral contraceptives on the results of laboratory tests. *Am J Obstet Gynecol* 1974;120:264.
115. Grace EA, Emans SJ, Drum D. Hematologic abnormalities in adolescents on birth control pills. *J Pediatr* 1982;101:771.
116. Amatayakul K. Metabolism: vitamins and trace elements. In: Goldzieher JW, Fotherby K, eds. *Pharmacology of the contraceptive steroids.* Philadelphia: Lippincott-Raven, 1994;363.
117. Chapdelaine A, Desmarais J-L, Derman RJ. Clinical evidence of the minimal androgenic activity of norgestimate. *Int J Fertil* 1989;34:347.
118. Becker H. Supportive European data on a new oral contraceptive containing norgestimate. U.S. clinical trials. *Acta Obstet Gynecol Scand Suppl* 1990;152:33.
119. Murphy AA, Cropp CS, Smith BS, et al. Effect of low-dose oral contraceptive on gonadotropins, androgens, and sex hormone binding globulin in nonhirsute women. *Fertil Steril* 1990;53:35.
120. Thijs C, Knipschild P. Oral contraceptives and the risk of gallbladder disease: a meta-analysis. *Am J Public Health* 1993;83:1113.
121. Vessey M, Painter R. Oral contraceptive use and benign gallbladder disease; revisited. *Contraception* 1994;50:167.
122. Grodstein F, Colditz GA, Hunter DJ, et al. A prospective study of symptomatic gallstones in women: relation with oral contraceptives and other risk factors. *Obstet Gynecol* 1994;84:207.
123. Logan RFA, Kay CR. Oral contraception, smoking and inflammatory bowel disease—findings in the Royal College of General Practitioners' oral contraception study. *Int J Epidemiol* 1989;18:105.

124. Vessey MP, Jewell D, Smith A, et al. Chronic inflammatory bowel disease, cigarette smoking and the use of oral contraceptives: findings in a large cohort study of women of childbearing age. *BMJ* 1986;292:1101.
125. Boyko EJ, Theis MK, Vaughan TL, et al. Increased risk of inflammatory bowel disease associated wtih oral contraceptive use. *Am J Epidemiol* 1994;140:269.
126. Fernandez E, LaVecchia C, D'Avanzo B, et al. Oral contraceptives, hormone replacement therapy and the risk of colorectal cancer. *Br J Cancer* 1996;73:1431.
127. Sillem MH, Teichmann AT. The liver. In: Goldzieher JW, Fotherby K, eds. *Pharmacology of the contraceptive steroids.* Philadelphia: Lippincott-Raven, 1994;247.
128. Chapel T, Burns R. Oral contraceptives and exacerbation of lupus erythematosus. *Am J Obstet Gynecol* 1971;110:366.
129. Julkunen HA, Kaaja R, Friman C. Contraceptive practice in women with systemic lupus erythematosus. *Br J Rheumatol* 1993;32:227.
130. Julkunen HA. Oral contraceptives in systemic lupus erythematosus: side-effects and influence on the activity of SLE. *Scand J Rheumatol* 1991;20:427.
131. Schuurs AH, Geurts TB, Goorissen EM, et al. Immunologic effects of estrogens, progestins, and estrogen-progestin combinations. In: Goldzieher JW, Fotherby K, eds. *Pharmacology of the contraceptive steroids.* Philadelphia: Lippincott-Raven, 1994;379.
132. Moskowitz MA, Jick SS, Burnside S, et al. The relationship of oral contraceptive use to rheumatoid arthritis. *Epidemiology* 1990;1:153.
133. Vandenbroucke JP, Witteman JCM, Valkenburg HA, et al. Noncontraceptive hormones and rheumatoid arthritis in perimenopausal and postmenopausal women. *JAMA* 1986;255:1299.
134. Del Junco DJ, Annegers JF, Luthra HS, et al. Do oral contraceptives prevent rheumatoid arthritis? *JAMA* 1985;254:1938.
135. Mattson RH, Cramer JA. Epilepsy, sex hormones and antiepileptic drugs. *Epilepsia* 1985;26(suppl 1):S40.
136. Dana-Haeri J, Richers A. Effects of norethindrone on seizures associated with menstruation. *Epilepsia* 1983;24:377.
137. Mattson RH, Cramer JA, Darney PD, et al. Use of oral contraceptives by women with epilepsy. *JAMA* 1986;256:238.
138. Crawford P, Chadwick D, Cleland P, et al. The lack of effect of sodium valproate on the pharmacokinetics of oral contraceptive steroids. *Contraception* 1986;33:23.
139. Crawford P, Chadwick DJ, Martin C, et al. The interaction of phenytoin and carbamazepine with combined oral contraceptive steroids. *Br J Clin Pharmacol* 1990;30:892.
140. Back DJ, Orme ML. Drug interactions. In: Goldzieher JW, Fotherby K, eds. *Pharmacology of the contraceptive steroids.* Philadelphia: Lippincott-Raven, 1994;407.
141. Geurts TBP, Goorissen EM, Sitsen JMA. *Summary of drug interactions with oral contraceptives.* New York: Parthenon Publishing Group, 1993.
142. Back DJ, Breckenridge AM, Crawford FE, et al. The effects of rifampicin on the pharmokinetics of ethinyl estradiol in women. *Contraception* 1980;21:135.
143. Szoka PR, Edgren RA. Drug interactions with oral contraceptives: compilation and analysis of an adverse experience report database. *Fertil Steril* 1988;49:318.
144. Murphy AA, Zacur HA, Chararche P, Burkman RT. The effect of tetracycline on levels of oral contraceptives. *Am J Obstet Gynecol* 1991;164:28.
145. Friedman CI, Huneke AL, Kim MH, et al. The effect of ampicillin on oral contraceptive effectiveness. *Obstet Gynecol* 1980;55:33.
146. Sparrow MJ. Pill method failures. *N Z Med J* 1987;100:102–105.
147. Sparrow MJ. Pregnancies in reliable pill takers. *N Z Med J* 1989;102:575.
148. Zamah NM, Humepl M, Kuhnz W, et al. Absence of an effect of high vitamin C dosage on the systemic availability of ethinyl estradiol in women using a combination oral contraceptive. *Contraception* 1993;48:377.
149. Hull MG. Normal fertility in women with post-pill amenorrhea. *Lancet* 1981;1:1329.
150. American College of Obstetricians and Gynecologists. Committee Opinion: Committee on Gynecologic Practice. Contraceptives and congenital anomalies. *Int J Gynaecol Obstet* 1993;42:316.
151. The Cancer and Steroid Hormone Study of the Centers for Disease Control and the National Institute of Child Health and Human Development. Oral-contraceptive use and the risk of breast cancer. *N Engl J Med* 1986;315:405.
152. Centers for Disease Control. Oral contraceptive use and the risk of breast cancer in young women. *MMWR* 1984;33:353.

153. Lipnick RJ, Buring JE, Hennekens CH, et al. Oral contraceptives and breast cancer: a prospective cohort study. *JAMA* 1986;255:58.
154. Stadel BV, Rubin GL, Webster LA, et al. Oral contraceptives and breast cancer in young women. *Lancet* 1985;2:970.
155. Beller FK, The female breast. In: Goldzieher JW, Fotherby K, eds. *Pharmacology of the contraceptive steroids.* Philadelphia: Lippincott-Raven, 1994;199.
156. Coker AL, Harlap S, Fortney JA. Oral contraceptives and reproductive cancers: weighing the risks and benefits. *Fam Plann Perspect* 1993;25:17.
157. Petitti DB, Porterfield D. Worldwide variations in the lifetime probability of reproductive cancer in women: implications of best-case, worst-case, and likely-case assumptions about the effect of oral contraceptive use. *Contraception* 1992;45:93.
158. Collaborative Group on Hormonal Factors in Breast Cancer. Breast cancer and hormonal contraceptives: collaborative reanalysis of individual data on 53,297 women with breast cancer and 100,239 women without breast cancer from 54 epidemiological studies. *Lancet* 1996;347:1713.
159. Collaborative Group on Hormonal Factors in Breast Cancer. Breast cancer and hormonal contraceptives: further results. *Contraception* 1996;54:1S.
160. Wingo PA, Lee NC, Ory HW, et al. Age-specific differences in the relationship between oral contraceptive use and breast cancer. *Obstet Gynecol* 1991;78:161.
161. Ebeling K, Nischan P, Schindler C. Use of oral contraceptives and risk of invasive cervical cancer in previously screened women. *Int J Cancer* 1987;39:427.
162. Valente PT, Hanjani P. Endocervical neoplasia in long-term users of oral contraceptives: clinical and pathologic observations. *Obstet Gynecol* 1986;67:695.
163. Irwin KL, Rosero-Bixby L, Oberle MW, et al. Oral contraceptives and cervical cancer risk in Costa Rica: detection bias or causal association? *JAMA* 1988;259:59.
164. Coker AL, McCann MF, Hulka BS, et al. Oral contraceptive use and cervical intraepithelial neoplasia. *J Clin Epidemiol* 1992;45:1111.
165. Ye Z, Thomas DB, Ray RM, et al. Combined oral contraceptives and risk of cervical carcinoma in situ. *Int J Epidemiol* 1995;24:19.
166. Kaufman DW, Shapiro S, Slone D, et al. Decreased risk of endometrial cancer among oral-contraceptive users. *N Engl J Med* 1980;303:1045.
167. Centers for Disease Control. Oral contraceptive use and the risk of endometrial cancer. *JAMA* 1983; 249:1600.
168. CASH, Cancer and Steroid Hormone Study of the Centers for Disease Control and the National Institute of Child Health and Human Development. Combination oral contraceptive use and the risk of endometrial cancer. *JAMA* 1987;257:796.
169. Johannisson E, Brosens I. The lower reproductive tract. In: Goldzieher JW, Fotherby K, eds. *Pharmacology of the contraceptive steroids.* Philadelphia: Lippincott-Raven, 1994;211.
170. Jick SS, Walker AM, Jick H. Oral contraceptives and endometrial cancer. *Obstet Gynecol* 1993;82:931.
171. Cramer DW, Hutchison GB, Welch WR, et al. Factors affecting the association of oral contraceptives and ovarian cancer. *N Engl J Med* 1982;307:1047.
172. The Cancer and Steroid Hormone Study of the Centers for Disease Control and the National Institute of Child Health and Human Development. The reduction in risk of ovarian cancer associated with oral contraceptive use. *N Engl J Med* 1987;316:650.
173. Centers for Disease Control. Oral contraceptive use and the risk of ovarian cancer. *JAMA* 1983; 249:1596.
174. Hankinson SE, Colditz, GA, Hunter DJ, et al. A quantitative assessment of oral contraceptive use and risk of ovarian cancer. *Obstet Gynecol* 1992;80:708.
175. Gross TP, Schlesselman JJ. The estimated effect of oral contraceptive use on the cumulative risk of epithelial ovarian cancer. *Obstet Gynecol* 1994;83:419.
176. Prentice RL. Epidemiologic data on exogenous hormones and hepatocellular carcinoma and selected other cancers. *Prev Med* 1991;20:38.
177. Harlap S, Kost K, Forrest JD. *Preventing pregnancy, protecting health: a new look at birth control choices in the United States.* New York: The Alan Guttmacher Institute, 1991.
178. World Health Organization Collaborative Study of Neoplasia and Steroid Contraceptives. Combined oral contraceptives and liver cancer. *Int J Cancer* 1989;43:254.
179. Rooks JB, Ory HW, Ishak KG. Epidemiology of hepatocellular adenomas. *JAMA* 1979;242:644.
180. Goodman ZD, Ishak KG. Hepatocellular carcinoma in women: probable lack of etiologic association with oral contraceptive steroids. *Hepatology* 1982;2:440.

181. Goldzieher JW. Effects on the skin. In: Goldzieher JW, Fotherby K, eds. *Pharmacology of the contraceptive steroids.* Philadelphia: Lippincott-Raven, 1994;271.
182. Shoupe D, Mishell Jr DR, Bopp BL, et al. The significance of bleeding patterns in Norplant implant users. *Obstet Gynecol* 1991;77:256.
183. Petursson GJ, Fraunfelder FT, Meyer SM. Oral contraceptives. *Ophthalmology* 1981;88:368.
184. Notelovitz M. Bone. In: Goldzieher JW, Fotherby K, eds. *Pharmacology of the contraceptive steroids.* Philadelphia: Lippincott-Raven, 1994;259.
185. Corson SL. Oral contraceptives for the prevention of osteoporosis. *J Reprod Med* 1993;38(12S);1015.
186. Recker RR, Davies M, Hinders SM, et al. Bone gain in young adult women. *JAMA* 1992;268:2403.
187. Klerrekoper M, Brienza RS, Schultz LR, Johnson CC. Oral contraceptive use may protect against low bone mass. *Arch Intern Med* 1991;151:1971.
188. Wolner-Hanssen P, Eschenbach DA, Paavonen J, et al. Decreased risk of symptomatic chlamydial pelvic inflammatory disease associated with oral contraceptive use. *JAMA* 1990;263:54.
189. Vessey MP, Lawless M, Yeates D, et al. Progestin-only oral contraception: findings in a large prospective study with special reference to effectiveness. *Br J Fam Plann* 1985;10:117.
190. Kaunitz AM. Injectable contraception. *Clin Obstet Gynecol* 1989;32:17.
191. Primiero FM, Benagiano G. Long-acting contraceptives. In: Goldzieher JW, Fotherby K, eds. *Pharmacology of the contraceptive steroids.* Philadelphia: Lippincott-Raven, 1994;153.
192. World Health Organization. A multicentered phase III comparative clinical trial of depot-medroxyprogesterone acetate given three-monthly at doses of 100 mg or 150 mg: contraceptive efficacy and side effects. *Contraception* 1986;34:223.
193. Jeppson S, Gerhagen S, Johansson EDB, Rannevik G. Plasma levels of medroxyprogesterone acetate (MPA), sex hormone binding globulin, gonadal steroids, gonadotropins and prolactin in women during long-term use of depo-MPA (Depo-Provera) as a contraceptive agent. *Acta Endocrinol* 1982;99:339.
194. Amatayakul K, Sirassomboom B, Singkamani R. Effects of MPA in serum lipids, protein, glucose tolerance and liver function in Thai women. *Contraception* 1980;21:283.
195. Skegg DCG, Noonan EA, Paul C, et al. Depot-medroxyprogesterone acetate and breast cancer. *JAMA* 1995;273:799.
196. Cundy T, Evans M, Roberts H, et al. Bone density in women receiving depot-medroxyprogesterone acetate for contraception. *BMJ* 1991;303:13.
197. Cromer BA, Blair JM, Mahan JD, et al. A prospective comparison of bone density in adolescent girls receiving depot medroxyprogesterone acetate (Depo-Provera), levonorgestrel (Norplant), or oral contraceptives. *J Pediatr* 1996;129:671.
198. Sangi-Haghpeykar H, Poindexter AN, Moseley DC, et al. Characteristics of injectable contraceptive users in a low-income population in Texas. *Fam Plann Perspect* 1995;27:208.
199. De Ceulaer K, Hayes R, Gruber C, Serjeant GR. Medroxyprogesterone acetate and homozygous sickle cell disease. *Lancet* 1982;2:229.
200. Smith RD, Cromer BA, Hayes JR, et al. Medroxyprogesterone (Depo-Provera) use in adolescents: uterine bleeding and blood pressure patterns, patient satisfaction, and continuation rates. *Adolesc Pediatr Gynecol* 1995;8:24.
201. World Health Organization. Multinational comparative trial of long-active injectable contraceptives: norethisterone enanthate given in two dosage regimens and depot-medroxyprogesterone acetate: final report. *Contraception* 1983;28:1.
202. Fraser IS. Vaginal bleeding patterns in women using once-a-month injectable contraceptives. *Contraception* 1994;49:399.
203. Segal S. A new delivery system for contraceptive steroids. *Obstet Gynecol* 1987;157:1090.
204. Darney PD, Atkinson E, Tanner S, et al. Acceptance and perceptions of Norplant among users in San Francisco, USA. *Stud Fam Plann* 1990;21:152.
205. Frank ML, Poindexter AN, Cornin LM, et al. One-year experience with subdermal contraceptive implants in the United States. *Contraception* 1993;48:229.
206. Shoupe D, Mishell DR. Norplant: subdermal implant system for long-term contraception. *Am J Obstet Gynecol* 1989;160:1286.
207. Grimes DA, ed. Insertion and removal of levonorgestrel subdermal implants. *Contracept Rep* 1994;5(5):4.
208. Sarma SP, Hatcher R. The Emory method: a modified approach to Norplant implants removal. *Contraception* 1994;49:551.

209. Darney PD, Klaisle CM, Walker DM. The pop-out method of Norplant removal. *Adv Contracept* 1992;8:188.
210. Praptohardjo U, Wibowo S. The "U" technique: a new method for Norplant implants removal. *Contraception* 1993;48:526.
211. Singh K, Viegas OAC, Loke DFM, et al. Effect of Norplant implants on liver, lipid, and carbohydrate metabolism. *Contraception* 1992;45:141.
212. Diaz S, Pavez M, Cardenas H, et al. Recovery of fertility and outcome of planned pregnancies after removal of Norplant subdermal implants or copper-T IUDs. *Contraception* 1987;35:569.
213. Kozlowski KJ, Rickert VI, Hendon AE, Davis P. Adolescents and Norplant: preliminary findings of side effects. *J Adolesc Health* 1995;16:373.
214. Glantz S, Schaff E, Campbell-Heider N, et al. Contraceptive implant use among inner city teens. *J Adolesc Health* 1995;16:389.
215. Cromer BA, Smith RD, Blair JA, et al. A prospective study of adolescents who choose among levonorgestrel implant (Norplant), medroxyprogesterone acetate (Depo-Provera), or the combined oral contraceptive pill as contraception. *Pediatrics* 1994;94:687.
216. Cullins VE, Remsburg R, Blumenthal PD, et al. Comparison of adolescent and adult experiences with Norplant levonorgestrel contraceptive implants. *Obstet Gynecol* 1994;83:1026.
217. Polaneczky M, Slap G, Forke C, et al. The use of levonorgestrel implants (Norplant) for contraception in adolescent mothers. *N Engl J Med* 1994:331:1201.
218. Berenson AB, Wiemann CM. Patient satisfaction and side effects with levonorgestrel implant (Norplant) use in adolescents 18 years of age or younger. *Pediatrics* 1993;92:257.
219. Rainey DY, Parsons LH, Kenney PG, Krowchuk DP. Compliance with return appointments for reproductive health care among adolescent Norplant users. *J Adolesc Health* 1995;16:385.
220. Rickert VI, Hendon AE, Davis P, Kozlowski KJ. Maternal influence on the decision to adopt Norplant. *J Adolesc Health* 1995;16:354.
221. O'Connell BJ, Bacon J, Klein-Havens K, et al. Norplant contraceptive use in the adolescent population (abstract). Presented at the North American Society for Pediatric and Adolescent Gynecology (NASPAG), Toronto, Ontario, Canada, April 1995.
222. Dinerman LM, Wilson MD, Duggan AK, Joffe A. Outcomes of adolescents using levonorgestrel implants vs. oral contraceptives or other contraceptive methods. *Arch Pediatr Adolesc Med* 1995; 149:967.
223. Ladipo OA, Faluci AG, Feldblum PJ, et al. Norplant use by women with sickle cell disease. *Int J Gynaecol Obstet* 1993;41:85.
224. Buckshee K, Chatterjee P, Dhall GI, et al. Phase III clinical trial with Norplant II (two covered rods): report on five years of use. *Contraception* 1993;48:120.
225. Ory S, Hammond C, Yancy S, et al. The effect of a biodegradable contraceptive capsule (Capronor) containing levonorgestrel on gonadotropin, estrogen, and progesterone levels. *Am J Obstet Gynecol* 1983;145:600.
226. Darney PD, Cook CE, Klaisle CM, et al. Evaluation of a 1-year levonorgestrel-releasing contraceptive implant: side effects, release rates and biodegradability. *Fertil Steril* 1992;58:137.
227. Mastroianni L. Future contraceptive methods. *Contracept Rep* 1994;5(4):4.
228. Hutchings JE, Benson PJ, Perkin GW, et al. The IUD after 20 years: a review. *Fam Plann Perspect* 1985;17:244.
229. Grimes D, ed. Highlights from an international symposium on IUDs. *Contracept Report* 1992;3(3):4.
230. Bronham DR. Intrauterine contraceptive devices—a reappraisal. *Br Med Bull* 1993;49:100.
231. Farley TM, Rosenberg MJ, Rowe PJ, et al. Intrauterine devices and pelvic inflammatory disease: an international perspective. *Lancet* 1992;339:785.
232. Sivin I, Stern J. Health during prolonged use of levonorgestrel 20 μg/d and the copper TCU 380 Ag intrauterine contraceptive devices: a multicenter study. International Committee for Contraception Research. *Fertil Steril* 1994;61:70.
233. Lee NC, Rubin GL, Borucki R. The intrauterine device and pelvic inflammatory disease revisited: new results from the Women's Health Study. *Obstet Gynecol* 1988;72:1.
234. Walsh, T, Grimes D, Frezieres R, et al. Randomised controlled trial of prophylactic antibiotics before insertion of intrauterine devices. *Lancet* 1998;351:1005.
235. Rossing MA, Daling JR, Voigt LF, et al. Current use of an intrauterine device and risk of tubal pregnancy. *Epidemiology* 1993;4:252.
236. Trussell J, Strickler J, Vaughan B. Contraceptive efficacy of the diaphragm, the sponge, and the cervical cap. *Fam Plann Perspect* 1993;25:100.

237. Fihn SD, Lathan RH, Roberts P, et al. Association between diaphragm use and the urinary tract infection. *JAMA* 1985;254:240.
238. Hooten TM, Hillier S, Johnson C, et al. *Escherichia coli* bacteremia and contraceptive method. *JAMA* 1991;265:64.
239. Patient update: how to use a diaphragm. *Contracept Rep* 1995;5.
240. Chalker R. *The complete cervical cap guide.* New York: Harper and Row, 1987.
241. Gallagher DM, Richwald GA. *Fitting the cervical cap: a handbook for clinicians.* Los Gatos, CA: Cervical Cap Ltd, 1989.
242. Richwald GA, Greenland S, Gerber M, et al. Effectiveness of the cavity rim cervical cap: results of a large clinical study. *Obstet Gynecol* 1979;74:143.
243. Koch JP. The Prentif cervical cap: acceptability aspects and their implications for future cap design. *Contraception* 1982;25:161.
244. Koch JP. The Prentif cervical cap: a contemporary study of its clinical safety and effectiveness. *Contraception* 1982;25:135.
245. Eliot J, Anderson L, Bernstein S. Progress report on a study of the cervical cap. *J Reprod Med* 1985;30:753.
246. Future barrier methods. *The Contraception Report* 1997;8(1):9.
247. Rosenberg MJ, Rojanapithayakorn W, Feldblum PJ, et al. Effect of the contraceptive sponge on chlamydial infection, gonorrhea and candidiasis: a comparative clinical trial. *JAMA* 1987;257:2308.
248. Weir S, Feldblum PJ, Zekeng L, et al. The use of nonoxynol-9 for protection against cervical gonorrhea. *Am J Public Health* 1994;84:910.
249. Rietmeijer CAM, Krebs JW, Foerino PM, et al. Condoms as physical and chemical barriers against human immunodeficiency virus. *JAMA* 1988;259:1851.
250. Squire JJ, Berger GS, Keith L. A retrospective clinical study of a vaginal contraceptive suppository. *J Reprod Med* 1977;22:319.
251. Warburton D, Neugut RH, Lustenberger A, et al. Lack of association between spermicide use and trisomy. *N Engl J Med* 1987;317:478.
252. Louik C, Mitchell AA, Werler MM, et al. Maternal exposure to spermicides in relation to certain birth defects. *N Engl J Med* 1987;317:474.
253. Farr G, Gabelnick H, Sturgen K, et al. Contraceptive efficacy and acceptability of the female condom. *Am J Public Health* 1994;84:1960.
254. Trussell J, Sturgen K, Strickler J, et al. Comparative contraceptive efficacy of the female condom and other barrier methods. *Fam Plann Perspect* 1994;26:66.
255. Soper DE, Brockwell NJ, Dalton HP. Evaluation of the effects of a female condom in the female lower genital tract. *Contraception* 1991;44:21.
256. Pleck JH, Sonenstein FL, Ku L. Changes in adolescent males' use of and attitudes toward condoms. *Fam Plann Perspect* 1993;25:106.
257. Hauser D, Pichaud PA. Does a condom-promoting strategy (the Swiss stop-AIDS campaign) modify sexual behavior among adolescents? *Pediatrics* 1994;93:580.
258. Joffe A. Adolescents and condom use. *Am J Dis Child* 1993;147:746.
259. Brown LK, Diclemente RJ, Park T. Predictors of condom use in sexually active adolescents. *J Adolesc Health* 1992;13:651.
260. Kegeles SM, Adler NE, Irwin CE. Sexually active adolescents and condoms: changes over one year in knowledge, attitudes and use. *Am J Public Health* 1988;78:460.
261. Orr DP, Langefeld CD. Factors associated with condom use by sexually active male adolescents at risk for sexually transmitted disease. *Pediatrics* 1993;91:873.
262. Langer LM, Zimmerman RS, Katz JA. Which is more important to high school students: preventing pregnancy or preventing AIDS? *Fam Plann Perspect* 1994;26:154.
263. Grady WR, Tanfer K. Condom breakage and slippage among men in the United States. *Fam Plann Perspect* 1994;26:107.
264. Sparrow MJ, Lavill K. Breakage and slippage of condoms in family planning patients. *Contraception* 1994;50:117.
265. Steiner M, Piedrahita C, Glover L, et al. Can condom users likely to experience condom failure be identified? *Fam Plann Perspect* 1993;25:220.
266. Cates W Jr, Stone KM. Family planning, sexually transmitted diseases and contraceptive choice: a literature update. *Fam Plann Perspect* 1992;24:75.
267. Centers for Disease Control. Condoms for prevention of sexually transmitted diseases. *MMWR* 1988;37:133.

268. Brown JB, Blackwell LF, Billings JJ, et al. Natural family planning. *Am J Obstet Gynecol* 1987; 157:1082.
269. Klaus H, Goebel J, Muraski B, et al. Use effectiveness and client satisfaction in six centers teaching the Billings ovulation method. *Contraception* 1979;19:497.
270. Wade ME, McCarthy P, Braunstein GD, et al. A randomized prospective study of the use-effectiveness of two methods of natural family planning. *Am J Obstet Gynecol* 1981;141:368.
271. Rice FJ, Lanctot CA, Garcia-Deversa C. Effectiveness of the symptothermal method of natural family planning: an international study. *Int J Fertil* 1981;26:222.
272. Delbanco SF, Mauldon J, Smith MD. Little knowledge and limited practice: emergency contraceptive pills, the public, and the obstetrician-gynecologist. *Obstet Gynecol* 1997;89:1006.
273. Yuzpe AA, Thurlow HJ, Ramzy I, et al. Postcoital contraception: a pilot study. *J Reprod Med* 1974; 13:53.
274. Yuzpe AA, Lancee WJ. Ethinyl estradiol and *dl*-norgestrel as a postcoital contraceptive. *Fertil Steril* 1977;28:932.
275. Ho PC, Kwan MSW. A prospective randomized comparison of levonorgestrel with the Yuzpe regimen in post-coital contraception. *Hum Reprod* 1993:8:389.
276. Webb AMC, Russell J, Elstein M. Comparison of Yuzpe regimen, danazol, and mifepristone (RU 486) in oral postcoital contraception. *BMJ* 1992;305:927.
277. Glasier A, Thong KJ, Dewar M, et al. Mifepristone (RU 486) compared with high-dose estrogen and progestogen for emergency postcoital contraception. *N Engl J Med* 1992;327:1041.
278. The search for microbiocides to prevent STDs. *The Contraception Report* 1997;8(1):4.
279. Schilling LH. An alternative to the use of high-dose estrogens for postcoital contraception. *J Am Coll Health Assoc* 1979;27:247.
280. Van Santen MR, Haspels AA. Interception II: postcoital low-dose estrogens and norgestrel combination in 633 women. *Contraception* 1985;31:275.
281. Trussell J, Stewart F, The effectiveness of postcoital hormonal contraception. *Fam Plann Perspect* 1992;24:262.
282. Hatcher RA, Trussell J, Stewart F, et al. *Emergency contraception: the nation's best-kept secret.* Atlanta GA: Bridging the GAP Communications, 1995.
283. Ellertson C. History and efficacy of emergency contraception: beyond Coca-Cola. *Fam Plann Perspect* 1996;28:44.
284. Glasier A, Ketting E, Ellertson C, Armstrong E. Emergency contraception in the United Kingdom and the Netherlands. *Fam Plann Perspect* 1996;28:48.
285. von Hertzen H, Nav Look PFA. Research on new methods of emergency contraception. *Fam Plann Perspect* 1996;28:52.
286. Trussell J, Ellertson C, Stewart F. The effectiveness of the Yuzpe regimen of emergency contraception. *Fam Plann Perspect* 1996;28:58.
287. Trussell J, Ellertson C, Rodriquez G. The Yuzpe regimen of emergency contraception: how long after the morning after? *Obstet Gynecol* 1996;88:151.

FURTHER READING

Adolescents' right to refuse long-term contraceptives. American College of Obstetricians and Gynecologists Committee Opinion, No. 139, June 1994.

Condom availability for adolescents. American College of Obstetricians and Gynecologists Committee Opinion, No 154, Apr 1995.

Emergency contraception. A resource manual for providers. Seattle, WA: Program for Appropriate Technology in Health (PATH), 1997.

Grimes D, Wallach M, et al. *Modern contraception.* Totowa, N.J.: Emron, 1997.

Improving the use of contraceptives. *Obstet Gynecol Suppl* 1996;88(3S).

Intrauterine contraception in the U.S. A current perspective. Conference Proceedings. January 20–21, 1996. University of Minnesota Office of Continuing Education.

Neinstein LS. *Issues in reproductive management.* New York: Thieme Medical Publishers, 1994.

Safety of oral contraceptives for teenagers. American College of Obstetricians and Gynecologists Committee Opinion, No 90, Feb 1991.

Speroff L, Darney P. *A clinical guide for contraception.* Baltimore, MD: Williams & Wilkins, 2nd ed, 1996.

18

Teenage Pregnancy

The diagnosis and management of unintended pregnancies among teenagers is a major issue for clinicians. Poverty and the change in sexual mores and behaviors (see Chapter 17), coupled with inconsistent contraceptive use, have resulted in a high adolescent pregnancy rate in the United States. The pregnancy rate is twice as high as in England and Wales, France, and Canada; three times as high as in Sweden; and seven times as high as in the Netherlands (1–3). The media, using both subtle and explicit advertisements, stories, and articles, has glorified sex at the same time that schools and other groups often have not adequately provided information on sexuality and birth control. Parents are frequently caught in the middle, uncomfortable with the change in sexual bchaviors and yet unable to initiate the necessary discussion about either abstinence or contraception. Health care providers are often called on to address these issues in the office setting. In addition, many clinicians are asked to be consultants to the community school system, even though they may not be experienced in discussing teenage sexuality or sexually transmitted diseases (STDs).

The task of clinicians has been made more challenging by new developments in the political, legal, social, and medical landscape of the United States. New approaches for schools and clinics are being advocated, and more rigorous evaluations are being initiated. At the same time, legislation and court decisions are limiting adolescent options as new requirements for parental involvement in pregnancy decision making are mandated and solutions such as cutting off aid to teenage mothers and their children are enacted. It becomes essential that clinicians move beyond the rhetoric and understand issues behind the high rate of school-age pregnancy in the United States. Factors associated with teenage pregnancy, including minority status, low socioeconomic status, low educational and career opportunities, residence in a single-parent home, and poor family relationships, are all inextricably intertwined (1–8). The presence of confounding factors needs to be kept in mind as the literature on causes and outcomes of teenage pregnancy is reviewed.

Many of the myths about adolescent pregnancy have been dispelled by recent research. For example, the high rates of adolescent sexual activity, pregnancy, and childbearing seen among minority youths in the United States probably have more to do with the low socioeconomic status than with minority status. Except in the case of very young adolescents, pregnant teenagers do not necessarily experience poor medical outcomes at delivery. Adolescent mothering, long thought to be a cause of educational failure, is now viewed as a possible outcome of academic difficulties. Adolescent pregnancy is not always unintended; an adolescent's desire to become pregnant may be fostered by her culture, her socioeconomic background, her peers, and her family expectations. Poor parenting by adolescents may be related not just to age but to socioeconomic background and other risk-taking and problem behaviors.

During the 1980s, more adolescents reported being sexually experienced; much of the increase occurred among white teenagers and those in higher-income families, narrowing the previous racial, ethnic, and income differences (1–3,9–13). In 1995, slightly fewer than 1 million teenage pregnancies

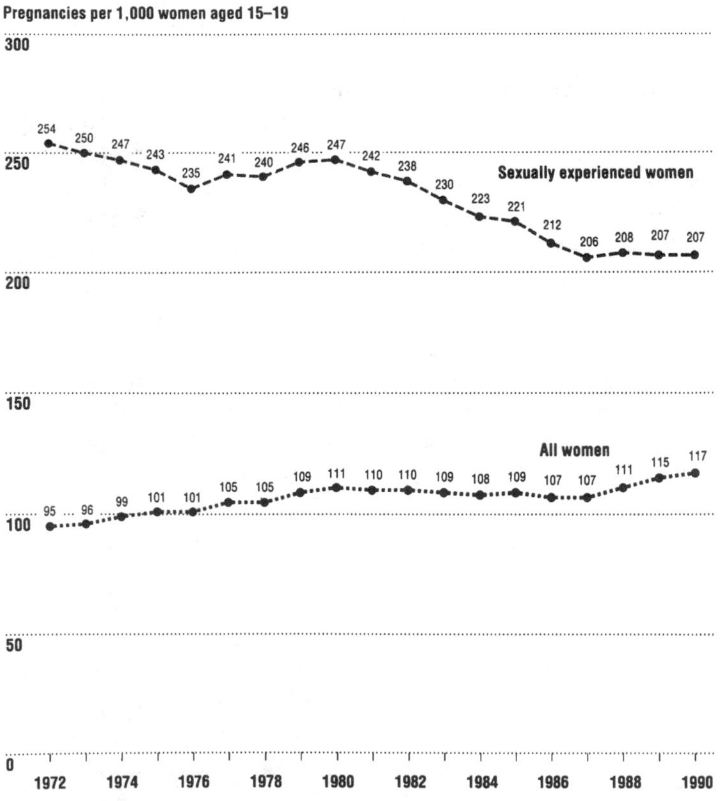

FIG. 1. Decline and rise of pregnancy rates among women age 15–19 years (1972–1990). (From *Sex and America's teenagers.* New York, Washington: The Allan Guttmacher Institute, 1994; with permission.) A subsequent decline occurred from 1990 to 1997.

occurred, including births, abortions, and fetal losses. These pregnancies resulted in 499,873 births to women <20 years of age. From 1980 to 1990, 21 states showed significant declines in their teenage pregnancy rates, while 12 states showed significant increases (10) (Fig. 1). Following a 24% increase in birth rates from 1986 through 1991 with a continuing decrease in abortions, the national birth rate for 15- to 19-year-olds decreased from 62.1/1,000 in 1991 to 56.8/1,000 in 1995 (11). The 1995 birth rate per 1,000 was 50.1 for whites, 96.1 for blacks, 78.7 for American Indians, 27.0 for Asian/Pacific Islanders, and 106.7 for all Hispanics. The birth rate for black teens declined 17% from 1991 to 1995 (11). From 1986 to 1991, birth rates for women aged 15 to 17 years increased 27%, declined 2% in 1992, and further declined in 1996 to 32.6 births per 1,000 (10,11–13). States show significant variations in pregnancy and abortion rates. For example, in 1992 pregnancy rates among 15- to 19-year-olds ranged from 53.7/1000 (Wyoming) to 106.9/1000 (Georgia). For those <15 years old, pregnancy rates ranged from 2.0/1000 (Idaho) to 10.9/1000 (Mississippi) (13). Overall, pregnancy rates for 15- to 19-year-olds declined from 1991 to 1992, with significant decline in 31 of 42 states for which age-specific data were available. In two states, rates increased significantly. The decrease in teenage pregnancy rates was reflected in both birth and abortion rates. Birth rates decreased significantly in 20 states; abortion rates decreased significantly in 31 of 42 states (15% to 27% in 15 states).

FACTORS IN TEENAGE PREGNANCY

The most obvious prelude to pregnancy in adolescents is early initiation of sexual activity. Low socioeconomic status, low future-achievement orientation, academic difficulties, few opportunities, and poor schools are major risk factors for the early initiation of sexual intercourse (7). Another important influence on adolescents' decision to engage in sex is influence from peers and sisters (14–17). An early adolescent surrounded by sexually active sisters and friends is more likely to be permissive with regard to premarital sex, sexual behavior, and, for virginal girls, their intentions to have sex (14). Adolescents who have a family history of early parenting are also at risk for adolescent pregnancy (18). Klerman (7) notes, "It takes an extraordinarily determined young woman to separate herself from her family, friends and neighbors and say, 'I am going to live differently.'" Adolescents surrounded by either pregnant or childbearing siblings and peers are likely to hold positive or ambivalent feelings about adolescent childbearing (14–17). While many adults may view adolescent pregnancy as a negative life event, this opinion is not necessarily held by all teens. The design of effective adolescent pregnancy prevention programs depends on a deeper understanding of why some adolescents welcome or at least do not actively work to prevent pregnancy (7).

Sexual behavior is also influenced by lack of family support and structure in adolescents' lives, as well as by glamorous portrayals in the media of sexual activity without consequences. Perceived emotional deprivation may cause adolescents to engage in sexual activity in search of emotional closeness. Early initiation of sexual activity has also been associated with other factors such as being a victim of sexual abuse or being involved in problem behaviors such as smoking, drinking, and drug use (19–24).

Sexual activity accompanied by improper or nonuse of contraceptives greatly contributes to the high rate of adolescent pregnancy in the United States. Recent evidence has suggested that despite myths to the contrary, adolescents use contraceptives as effectively as, and sometimes even better than, unmarried adults. At all ages, poor or low-income women have more difficulties in using contraceptives effectively (1). However, adolescents do face special challenges in using contraceptives. Cognitively immature adolescents may be unable to perceive the future consequences (pregnancy and/or STD) of current behavior (sexual intercourse) and thus choose not to use contraceptives. The maturation process during adolescence involves the formation of a stable self-image, a sexual identity, and a concept of self as separate from parents. This process does not occur in an orderly fashion, and thus an adolescent does not always see herself as a woman capable of fertility at the same time that she is in fact able to bear children and has become sexually mature. The consistency, responsibility, and planning necessary for effective contraceptive use are not always compatible with the stage of adolescent development at which the adolescent may have chosen to become sexually active. The limitation in cognitive development in young adolescents often makes it impossible for them to consider the feelings and values of their partner, or to recognize that a pregnancy can result and contraception is necessary. Although for older adolescents risk taking is less haphazard and behaviors and their consequences are more clearly connected, many continue to deny possible consequences of lack of contraceptive use.

Adolescents may deny their own risk of pregnancy and hold misconceptions, such as believing that only frequent sexual activity can lead to pregnancy. For some adolescents, their reluctance to acknowledge their sexuality impairs proper contraceptive usage. Denial of fertility is a common theme; statements such as "I didn't think it would happen to me," or "I had sex for 2 years and didn't get pregnant," or "I never thought I would get pregnant" are frequently expressed. Patients with medical conditions such as cystic fibrosis, diabetes mellitus, recurrent pelvic inflammatory disease, delayed development, or oligomenorrhea may take more risks because of their belief that they are unlikely to get pregnant.

Often, the longer that adolescents are sexually active without experiencing pregnancy, the more the risk-taking behavior is reinforced. Adolescents are usually unaware that with increasing gynecologic age, the chance of regular ovulatory cycles and thus fertility is greater. They are also often unable to identify the time of greatest risk in their menstrual cycle for fertility or to understand the impact of irregular cycles on ovulation. Including a simple factual explanation of the menstrual cycle in sexuality courses in schools and office-based interventions is important. Variable cycles and unreliable methods are thus important factors in unintended pregnancies.

Frequent office visits for pregnancy tests that all turn out negative have also been labeled a risk marker for teenage pregnancy (25,26). A study of adolescents visiting a clinic for pregnancy tests showed that those who receive negative pregnancy tests have much in common with those who receive positive pregnancy tests and choose to continue their pregnancies: academic difficulties, low socioeconomic status, and desire to conceive. Fifty-six percent of teens with a negative pregnancy test are pregnant within 18 months (27). Adolescents with a negative pregnancy test are good candidates for counseling and intervention to prevent future, unintended pregnancies.

Due to unequal gender relations and cultural and ethnic expectations of gender roles, female adolescents may find it difficult to discuss contraception with their male partners or to insist on use of a condom. Further, they may be unwilling or unable to say "No" to sexual intercourse, especially in the case of a much older partner (7). Seventy-four percent of women who had sex before age 14 and 60% of those who had sex before age 15 report having had sex involuntarily (1).

Adolescents often face the burden of their minor status in obtaining contraceptives. Fear of parental discovery and disapproval precludes some teenagers from seeking out contraceptives. Clinicians often do not initiate discussion about contraception and STDs, and adolescents may be too timid to raise the subject. Those who choose to obtain contraception may be hampered in their attempts by lack of transportation to and availability (free or low cost) of health care facilities that confidentially dispense contraceptives to adolescents. Between 1980 and 1992, Title X family planning program funding that provides support for clinics declined 72%, which has led to higher fees, shorter hours, and reduction in education and outreach efforts (1).

FACTORS IN ADOLESCENT CHILDBEARING

If an adolescent becomes pregnant, she has the options of continuing the pregnancy to term and parenting, terminating the pregnancy through abortion, or continuing the pregnancy and placing her child for adoption. Very few pregnant teenagers currently choose the last option; between 1982 and 1988, only 3% of never-married, non-Hispanic white women placed their children for adoption (1). As a result, most adolescents choose between abortion or childbearing with parenting. Approximately 51% of teenage pregnancies end in childbirth, 14% end in miscarriage, and 35% end in abortion.

The most important factor leading adolescents to choose childbearing is low socioeconomic status; 80% of all adolescents who give birth are poor or low income (1). Pregnant teenagers from advantaged families tend to have abortions. Klerman (7) asserts, "If poor adolescents are to act like nonpoor adolescents in regard to sexuality, pregnancy, and child rearing, society will need to offer them comparable life circumstances, for example, adequate family incomes, contact with positive role models, more adequate schools and better housing."

Many of the risks associated with adolescent pregnancy also put adolescents at high risk for adolescent childbearing. Adolescents with academic difficulties and lack of future orientation are more likely to become adolescent mothers. In a Rand Corporation study (28), single parenthood rates ranged from 1 in 1000 for white girls with high academic ability from upper income, intact families to 1 in 4 for black girls with low academic ability from poor, female-headed families. Risk factors for teenage parenthood varied with the ethnic group; for example, decreased risk was found in whites with good parent–child communication, in blacks with good parental supervision, and in Hispanics with increased religiosity. The presence of problem behaviors was a significant risk factor for Hispanics and whites to become pregnant. College plans reduced the likelihood of single parenthood in all groups but most significantly in blacks. Girls who have faced academic failure and hopelessness may find producing a healthy child a powerful, successful experience.

A family history of early parenting in mothers and sisters and positive or ambivalent feelings about childbearing are associated with adolescent childbearing. Using the experience from providing health care to >600 teenage mothers, Cox and colleagues (16) developed a model for examining the many factors that contribute to the high pregnancy rate among sisters (Fig. 2). Intrafamilial factors that promote early pregnancy include an early parenting age for mothers, permissive attitudes, lack of parental control, and the presence of a sibling parent. The influence of the sister may relate to the positive role of the teen mother

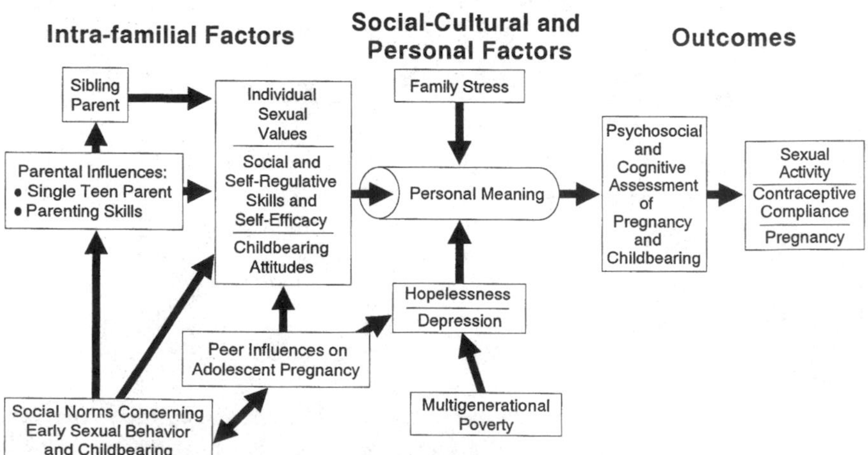

FIG. 2. Conceptual model of influences on siblings of teen parents. (From Cox JE, DuRant RH, Emans SJ, Woods ER. Early parenthood for the sisters of adolescent mothers: a proposed conceptual model of decision making. *Adolesc Pediatr Gynecol* 1995;8:188–194; with permission.)

within the household, more favorable attitudes toward early sexual activity, and shared activities. Sociocultural factors including community and social norms that favor early parenting interact with peer influences to affect social and self-regulative skills, feelings of self-efficacy, and individual sexual values. Personal factors such as depression and hopelessness are influenced by multigenerational poverty. Family stress such as high rates of family violence, sexual and physical abuse, and substance abuse may enhance the value of early pregnancy in the adolescent's life. The central integrative process of intrafamilial, sociocultural, and personal factors is personal meaning, "the inner subjective life of the adolescent." The meaning, combined with cognitive development, knowledge about risk, and skills to deal with risks, influences the adolescent's behavior in high-risk situations. She may then perceive various options, assign values to these options, and choose one that is preferable to others.

Several studies in the past decades indicate that many of the factors enumerated in the study of sibling pregnancy are associated with pregnancy in general. Emotional deprivation may cause adolescents to seek emotional closeness via early parenthood. In a study by Nadelson and coworkers (29), 37% of young women in a maternity home agreed with the statement, "Sometimes I feel so lonely that I would like to have a baby." Some teenagers also believe that a baby will help establish a lasting relationship with a boyfriend; repeat pregnancies are more common when the boyfriend desires the pregnancy.

The link between race and adolescent childbearing is a complicated one. In 1994, African-American teenagers between the ages of 15 and 19 years were two times more likely to give birth than white teenagers (11), but a majority of teen mothers are white. Differences among advantaged and disadvantaged Hispanic adolescents with regard to adolescent childbearing underscore the importance of economic issues (10,12,30,31). Mexican-American and Puerto Rican adolescents aged 15 to 19 years who tend to have low socioeconomic status have birth rates of 108.8/1000 and 110.4/1000, respectively. Cuban-American adolescents who generally are of a higher socioeconomic status have a birth rate of 26.3/1000. In 1993, Cuban-American 15- to 17-year-olds had a birth rate of 20.4/1000 compared to 73.4/1000 for Puerto Rican 15- to 17-year-olds (10,12). Poverty coupled with family and peer expectations plays a significant role in adolescent childbearing, and there is a dearth of research related to white pregnant and childbearing adolescents or African-American teenagers along the socioeconomic continuum.

DIAGNOSIS OF PREGNANCY

Since the most common cause of secondary amenorrhea is pregnancy, any adolescent who is late for a menstrual period should have a urine sample screened for human chorionic gonadotropin (hCG) (see Chapter 1). An adolescent who is 1 to 2 weeks late for a period and expresses concern about this should be seen by the clinician to consider the diagnosis of pregnancy. If the teenager is not pregnant, she may well be sexually active and in need of contraceptive counseling. Some adolescents will express the fear that they may be pregnant; others may request appointments with the hope that the physician may accidentally discover the pregnancy. Often, the patient's complaint is a minor stomach ache, constipation, or headache, and she later admits to having missed her period only after being directly questioned. Other adolescents may not have thought of the possibility and may have dizziness, syncope, nausea, or urinary frequency. Occasionally, a patient will experience a light period in the first trimester and therefore will be falsely reassured she is not pregnant.

Pregnancies are dated from first day of the last menstrual period, even though ovulation usually occurs at least 2 weeks later. Calculation of dates from the last menstrual period, along with a pelvic examination for uterine sizing, is necessary so that the clinician can discuss with the adolescent the possible options for the pregnancy. By rectal or vaginal examination, the 8-week uterus feels about the size of an orange; the 12-week uterus is approximately the size of a grapefruit. An abdominal examination with the patient supine helps in staging a later pregnancy; a 12-week uterus is just palpable at the symphysis pubis, a 20-week uterus at the level of the umbilicus, and a 16-week uterus midway between (Fig. 3). Because of the high prevalence of STDs in pregnant teenagers, endocervical tests for *Neisseria gonorrhoeae* and *Chlamydia trachomatis* should be obtained at the time of the examination. Other testing, including Papanicolaou (Pap) smears and serology for syphilis, rubella, Rh factor, hepatitis B surface antigen, and human immunodeficiency virus (HIV) (after counseling), should follow the guidelines of the American College of Obstetricians and Gynecologists.

Although adolescents can be quite uncertain about the date of their last menstrual period, other diagnoses need to be entertained if the uterus is small or large for dates given. If the uterus is smaller than expected, possible diagnoses include inaccurate dates (or oligomenorrhea and irregular ovulation), lab error, incomplete or missed abortion, ectopic pregnancy, or, rarely, other sources of hCG (tumors). A uterus felt to be larger than expected may be caused by inaccurate dates, twin pregnancy, leiomyomata, molar pregnancy, or a corpus luteum cyst of pregnancy, which may be mistaken initially as part of the enlarged uterus. Ultrasonography (including the use of a vaginal probe) and, if indicated, serial quantitative hCG measures are important in making the correct diagnosis. Vitamins with adequate content of folic acid should be provided to teenagers who are ambivalent or continuing their pregnancies to term to lessen the chance of neural tube defects, although folic acid is most effective if started prior to conception. Women should also be given advice about the use of prescribed and over-the-counter drugs. Drugs should be used with caution throughout pregnancy and given for a specific indication at the minimal effective dosage and for the shortest duration possible. Some drugs with known or suspected teratogenicity include anticonvulsants such as hydantoin and valproate sodium, anticoagulants, alcohol, folic acid antagonists (methotrexate and aminopterin), diethylstilbe-

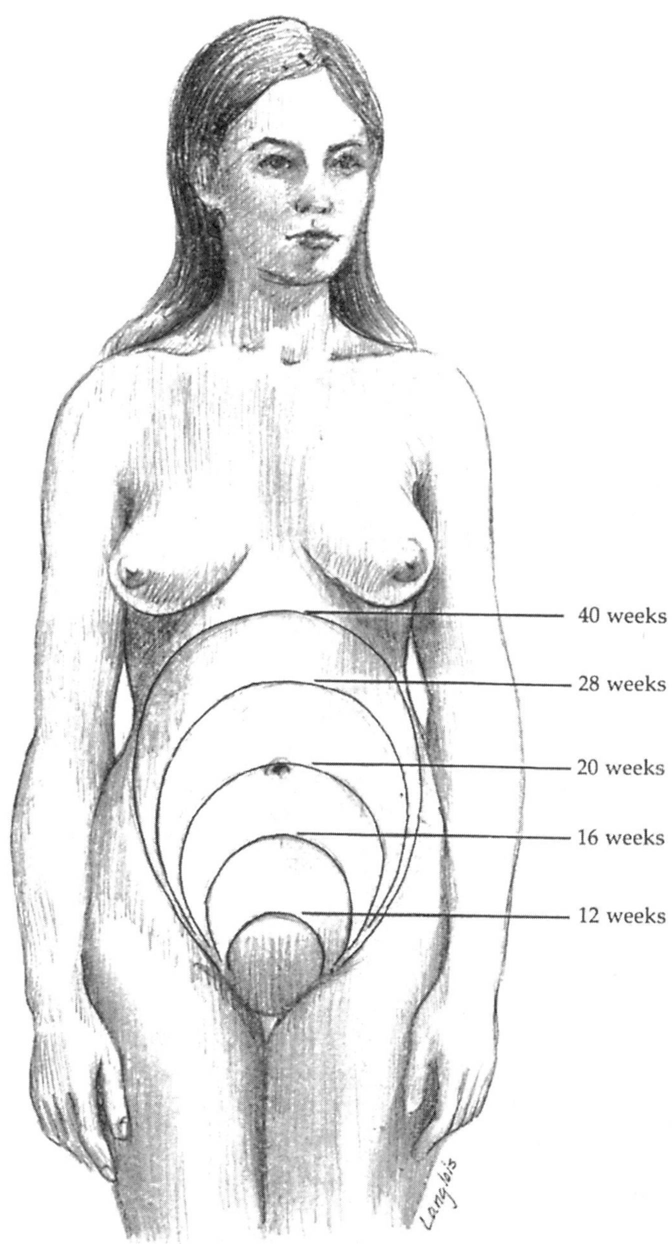

FIG. 3. Uterine size in pregnancy.

strol, isotretinoin, thalidomide, alkylating agents, and lithium carbonate (32). Teratogenic effects, including growth restriction, microcephaly, and mental retardation, can also occur in patients exposed to high-dose radiation (100 to 200 rad) (33). The greatest risk of central nervous system effects appears to be with exposure to >20 rad between 8 and 15 weeks of gestation, with no proven risk at <8 weeks or >25 weeks. Fetal risks do not appear to increase with radiation exposure <5 rad, a level above the range of *fetal* exposure in common diagnostic procedures (e.g., 0.02 to 0.07 mrad from a chest X-ray or 200 mrad from a hip X-ray); however, certain procedures do give higher doses (e.g., 2 to 4 rad from a barium enema or small bowel series or 3.5 rad from computed tomography of the abdomen and lumbar spine) (33).

COUNSELING THE PREGNANT ADOLESCENT

Counseling the pregnant teenager as an individual within a family context is essential to helping her with decision making and to determining her feelings toward the pregnancy—ambivalent, happy, depressed, anxious, quiet, worried, in denial. Adolescents benefit from being told by health care providers that they have spoken to other teens in the same situation and that they will provide support during the process of decision making and afterward, regardless of what decision is reached. We have found it helpful in providing care to pregnant adolescents to see them in clinic or communicate with them by telephone once a week, and sometimes more often, until they have made the decision and connected to the necessary services (prenatal clinic or abortion clinic). It is important for them to know that there is no "perfect" alternative to an unintended pregnancy. Options counseling in an unbiased and unhurried manner is essential and must include all three options open to women in the 1990s: continuing pregnancy to parent the child, continuing to term with adoption planning and placement, and abortion. With both adoption and abortion, pregnant teenagers must ultimately work through the feelings of loss. Those who elect to keep their babies may be emotionally unprepared to cope with the demands of child care.

When counseling pregnant teenagers, the clinician will sense striking differences between 11- to 14-year-olds and 17- or 18-year-old young women. The younger girls may not understand the symptoms of pregnancy, the meaning of gestational age, or the urgency for decision making, and may deny the pregnancy until quite late. Because of their lack of abstract thinking, these young adolescents may be unable to connect the pregnancy with the responsibility of motherhood. Sometimes their decisions about what to do with the pregnancy are related to angry feelings toward their parents that day, and thus several visits are often necessary before a referral for abortion or obstetric care is made. Pregnancy in the very young also may be the first clue to a rape or an abusive relationship within the family, and thus the counselor needs to be sensitive in approaching the source of the pregnancy. Problem behaviors including running away and substance abuse may also be signs of disturbed family relationships and/or sexual abuse (see Chapter 20). The 17- or 18-year-olds are usually better able to appreciate the consequences of their actions and to consider the choices available. Patients' needs, strengths, and defenses need to be assessed to formulate a plan.

In a study of 96 pregnant teens in a general adolescent clinic, Forman and colleagues (34) found that most patients followed the plan they had made at the initial visit. Among those who were unsure at the initial visit, 42% ultimately decided to terminate and 58% to continue to term. Those who planned to tell more people had a significantly higher rate of continuing to term.

Teenagers do have the final word on what decisions are to be made and must live with the decisions over a lifetime, but counseling needs to take into account their family, social, and economic context. Ambivalence about unintended pregnancies is universal. For those choosing abortion, the ambivalence is heightened by the conflict between the positive aspects of conception and pregnancy versus the frustration and sadness about making a choice to terminate a pregnancy. It is important that adolescents reach the point of acceptance and comfort with their decision in order to minimize emotional sequelae.

To be fair to teenagers, the clinician should be relatively unbiased about the ethics of abortion. If he or she is opposed to abortion and cannot present an unbiased view, then patients should be referred to an unbiased pregnancy counseling service. Likewise, it is often difficult to remain unbiased about the prospect of the very young adolescent continuing the pregnancy because problems with teenage marriages and single parenthood are so frequent.

The assessment of pregnant adolescents should focus on a number of important areas (Table 1). The interview that occurs when pregnancy is diagnosed lays the foundation for understanding patients and providing for their future needs. The personal history should include details of the current social situation, educational goals, self-esteem, previous psychiatric diagnoses and counseling, and financial status. Clarifying patients' educational plans before the unintended pregnancy occurred allows them to put the pregnancy in perspective and assess its potential impact on their life's goals. Asking questions about what they had planned to do (before the pregnancy was known) in 1 year and 5 years are important; this information should be recorded so that the clinician can help patients later to understand the reasons for their particular decision. Assessment of self-esteem allows the physician some estimate of postabortion and postpartum problems and contraceptive compliance. Since an unintended pregnancy can further the feeling that "Things just happen to me," it is important in the counseling process to foster in pregnant adolescents the concept of decision making and to stress their ability to intervene in their own lives. It may be the first time that they have been called on to make an important decision, especially one that will affect the rest of their life. Drawing a table of pros and cons using another common life example to explain the idea of weighing the benefits and the problems of a particular decision can be helpful for young adolescents. Young teens, who

TABLE 1. *Assessment and counseling of the pregnant teenager*

- Personal history
  - Social situation
    - Who currently lives with you?
    - Who is in your family?
    - In whom do you confide?
    - Who knows about the possible pregnancy?
  - Educational/life goals
    - Are you currently in school? How are you doing?
    - What do you want to do in 1 year? in 5 years?
  - Self-esteem/self-efficacy
    - What kinds of decisions have you made before?
  - Psychiatric history
    - Previous coping skills, counseling
    - Suicide attempts
  - Financial status/insurance
    - Do you have insurance? Can you access it without loss of confidentiality?
    - Are there resources for parenting or termination?
- Medical/gynecologic/sexual history
  - Current/prior medical problems and medications
  - Information level about conception and contraception
  - Previous contraceptive use
  - Previous pregnancies and outcomes
  - Previous sexually transmitted diseases
- Personal beliefs about parenting, abortion, adoption
  - Experiences with sisters, relatives, or friends who have been pregnant
  - What do you think is the best age to be pregnant?
  - What do you think is the best age to parent?
  - Religious/cultural beliefs
- Family/friend/partner influences and beliefs
  - Which adult can be supportive—i.e., parent, teacher, counselor, relative, partner
  - Whom do you plan to tell?
  - Attitudes/beliefs of others toward pregnancy, parenting, abortion, adoption
- Current pregnancy
  - Intended or unintended?
  - *Who* wants to continue to term?
  - *Who* wants an abortion?
  - Has adoption/placement been considered?
- Information about options
  - Concrete issues about termination and parenting
  - Health risks and costs
- Postpregnancy
  - Anticipatory guidance
  - Anticipation of feelings
  - Contraception
  - Health care options

tend to think concretely, need to understand the process of decision making before they begin to look at the options for their pregnancy.

Assessing patients' previous coping mechanisms for dealing with crisis and loss is important for those considering abortion or adoption. Those with anticipated difficulties may do better if the counselor's concerns are shared with them. It is often less frightening, and potentially a relief, for adolescents to understand the connection between their difficulty with acceptance of previous losses and the counselor's concern about what the loss of this pregnancy through abortion means to them. Availability for followup counseling after the abortion is crucial.

The health care provider should also be aware of patients' medical problems and whether they are currently taking medications, because preexisting medical problems may impact on the choice of abortion clinic, whether genetic counseling should be made available before a choice is made, and whether referral to a high-risk obstetrics clinic is necessary. In addition, patients who experience medical complications at the time of the abortion may have more difficulty in resolving the issue of abortion.

The level of information and the prior experience of patients should be assessed because myths and inaccurate information are still widespread, even among the college population. Pregnancy often results from the use of the less reliable methods of contraception, and misconceptions need to be corrected. A history of previous pregnancies and outcomes and STDs should be obtained.

It is important to explore patients' personal beliefs, as well as those of family, partners and friends, about parenting, adoption, and abortion. Some questions might include "What do you think is the best age to become pregnant?" "What do you think is the best age to become a parent?" "How will you manage child care? Your education?" The nature of the current relationship with the male partner should be discussed, and a patient should be encouraged to bring him in if she desires. Patients should be asked with whom they feel they can and will share the information about the pregnancy and who can provide them support. Family attitudes should be discussed, since if the family is strongly antiabortion or strongly against continuing to term, this may intensify a sense of guilt and secrecy in patients and delay access to services. Attitudes of friends influence decision making as well.

The actual details of how the unintended pregnancy occurred are important in making plans for preventing repeat pregnancies. It is essential to find out "Who wants this abortion?" and "Who wants to continue to term?" Adolescents sometimes have abortions to please their mothers or boyfriends and end up with another pregnancy very soon thereafter, because they did not fully work through the decision themselves. Likewise, other adolescents may feel pressured to continue to term by their partner and then find that he has disappeared soon after the initiation of prenatal care. Some adolescents may have intended to become pregnant and may already have made plans for school or child care that may or may not be realistic, especially if their mother has not been involved.

Concrete information about options should be presented. Fears concerning the actual abortion procedure need to be explored, since this remains a significant issue for a high percentage of adolescents. A clear understanding of and attention to the nature of their fears and fantasies will reduce anxiety. Patients are often afraid to ask questions about pain, anesthesia, subsequent fertility, and some of the details of the procedure. They often fantasize a more drastic procedure. It is important that the physician keep abreast of the available resources and the procedures done within the community, as well as safety at clinics and potential harassment by picketers. Adolescents also often have fantasies about childbirth and the realities of parenting that need to be addressed. They will feel most comfortable asking questions of a person whom they perceive as helpful, supportive, and understanding.

Feelings after the pregnancy and the need for contraceptives should be explored. For most, the overwhelming feeling after the abortion is relief. However, feelings of depression may be apparent, especially in adolescents with low self-esteem. Introducing the topic of birth control after the pregnancy is essential, for many teenagers and parents feel that "it won't happen again." Those with a prior abortion are not necessarily more successful contraceptive users than those who have never experienced a pregnancy (35). The likelihood of a repeat pregnancy should be emphasized to both those who have an abortion and those continuing to term. Discussions should be undertaken with adolescents at the time of referral to prenatal care as to whether they will be able to return to their primary care clinician who diagnosed the pregnancy or whether they will be referred to a postpartum adolescent clinic, teen-tot clinic, or other source of ongoing health care.

The issue of parental consent and responsibility for the notification of an abortion in teenagers is in considerable flux and is increasingly decided by the state legislatures. Teenagers may find it easier to have the health care provider help them tell parents of the diagnosis. The majority of young to midadolescents benefit from the support that parents, especially the mother, are able to provide. Effective counseling can then deal with the family issues that may have been important precipitants to the unplanned pregnancy. Parents may feel very guilty or very angry. It is important to state to the mother that if she expresses her demands for abortion or continuing the pregnancy too emphatically, she may push her daughter in the opposite direction. Teenagers often have unrealistic expectations that their mother will provide child care while they continue the tasks of adolescence. Since teenagers generally will continue to live with their parents, a solution acceptable to both parents and teenagers needs to be evolved through counseling. Mediation through state social agencies is occasionally needed if there is no agreement and placement of a teenager is needed.

Many teenagers are unable to talk to their parents about the issue of pregnancy, sometimes because of justified fear of physical or other abuse and sometimes out of fear that a pregnancy will announce to parents that they are sexually active. Teenagers unable to involve their parents should be informed by the clinician and counselors of legal alternatives to parental consent provisions within their state and neighboring states, including judicial bypass. It is essential to discourage adolescents from delaying obtaining adequate medical intervention or from seeking abortions in nonmedical facilities because they fear parental reprisals.

CONTINUING PREGNANCY TO TERM

Teenagers who desire to continue a pregnancy to term should receive special prenatal care. A first consideration for those providing prenatal care to adolescents is how barriers to access can be minimized, since inadequate prenatal care is a major determinant of poor pregnancy outcome among adolescent mothers. Kinsman and Slap (36) found that adolescents who received inadequate prenatal care identified confusion about available services, lack of health insurance, desire for adolescent-only clinics, negative attitudes toward physicians, perceived unimportance of first-trimester care, inexperience with pregnant friends, and late recognition of pregnancy as barriers to their early entry into prenatal care. Financial barriers and negotiating paperwork and secretaries are especially salient for adolescents. Timeliness of prenatal care has fortunately improved over the past few years but is still a problem for young teens. In 1992, prenatal care in the first trimester was received by 43% of teenagers <15 years old and 59.5% of those 15 to 19 years old, compared to 78% of all pregnant women. Seventeen percent of teenagers <15 years of age had no or only late prenatal care, compared to 10% of 15- to 19-year-old women and 5% of all women (10).

Adolescents have higher rates of delivering low-birth-weight babies than older women (4–6,20,21,37–43). Data have been conflicting as to whether the difference should be attributed more to poverty, closely spaced pregnancies, risk-taking behaviors, or inadequate prenatal care than to maternal age (41,42). The risk for low-birth-weight infants seems especially prominent in adolescents <15 years old and in multiparous adolescents. McAnarney (37) suggested that multiple maternal factors account for the finding of low birth weight (<2500 g) and neonatal mortality, including poor nutrition, substance use (cigarettes, alcohol, and illicit drugs), and genital infections. Adolescents in the first 2 years after menarche need more nutrients and are in competition for those needed by the developing fetus, and thus it seems more biologically plausible that there should be risk associated with age alone primarily or exclusively in young adolescents (42). In addition, low prepregnancy weight has been shown to be associated with poor outcomes in the first pregnancy, and young age is associated with maternal thinness (42,43). Shorter intervals between pregnancies also appear to be a major factor in low birth weight and preterm delivery and occur more commonly among black women than white women (44). A second child born to an adolescent mother is at high risk of low birth weight and prematurity (45). Inner city teenage mothers appear to initiate prenatal care later in their second pregnancy, even if they had received adequate prenatal care during the first pregnancy. This behavior leads to increases in adverse pregnancy outcomes, especially if there was a poor outcome during the first pregnancy.

The chance of a good outcome for pregnant adolescents and their babies can be improved with adequate weight gain and proper nutrition. There is some dispute as to what "adequate" weight gain is for pregnant adolescents (46–50). McAnarney and Stevens-Simon (46,47) took issue with the Institute of Medicine's recommendations that pregnant adolescents strive for weight gains at the upper end of the range. They argued that these new recommendations place teenagers at an increased risk for obesity and suggested that weight gain recommendations based on prepregnancy body mass index or weight-for-height percentile is reasonable for pregnant adolescents. The American Dietetic Association has proposed specific nutritional recommendations for pregnant adolescents, including full access to nutrition care by dietetic professionals in interdisciplinary prenatal programs specifically devoted to serving adolescents (49).

Providers of prenatal care to adolescents must be mindful of further issues endemic to adolescents. Pregnant adolescents are at high risk for urinary tract infections, STDs, and abnormal Pap smears. Condoms should be encouraged throughout pregnancy to prevent the acquisition of new infections including syphilis, gonorrhea, chlamydia, human papillomavirus, and HIV. Adolescents should be routinely screened for a history of current or past physical and/or sexual abuse (23,51–53). Berenson and colleagues (23) found that 25% of pregnant adolescents attending a teenage pregnancy clinic had experienced physical or sexual abuse during their pregnancies, especially from a partner. Parker and coworkers (51) also found abuse during pregnancy to be more common among teenagers (20.6%) than adults (14.2%). Abused teenagers had a significantly greater risk for poor weight gain, first- or second-trimester bleeding, smoking, alcohol and drug use, and suicide (51–53). Better screening for a history of violence coupled with effective interventions may prevent maternal and fetal injuries, as well as improving parenting outcomes. Substance use during pregnancy is also a problem for teenagers and is associated with difficulties in school, living apart from one's mother, prior cigarette smoking, and drug or cigarette use by friends or family (23). Interventions are urgently needed to help adolescents understand the adverse consequences for the fetus of smoking and substance abuse and to assist them in changing their behaviors.

Many special programs have been developed in this country to help prepare pregnant teenagers for delivery, motherhood, and future family planning. Adolescents are seen for frequent visits by a multidisciplinary team consisting of a physician and/or nurse practitioner, nurse, social worker, and nutritionist. Informal discussion groups, often led by a nurse, help educate adolescents in nutrition, basic physiology, types of anesthesia, fetal monitoring, breast- versus bottle-feeding, postpartum care, and use of contraceptives. Home visitations by social workers or nurses may be part of an adolescent prenatal care program. Data on the impact of adolescent-specific clinics for prenatal care are mixed but generally show a favorable effect (54–56). Felice and coworkers (56) reported that only 9.0% of infants born to teenage mothers in the special clinic weighed <2500 g as compared to 20.9% of infants in the regular clinic. Morris and associates (57) found that pregnant adolescents in a teen prenatal clinic began prenatal care earlier and had more visits than adolescents in a traditional prenatal setting, but the two groups had similar pregnancy outcomes. Although pregnancy outcomes were similar, Stevens-Simon and colleagues (58) found that adolescents in a comprehensive, adolescent-oriented prenatal care program were referred more frequently to community organizations and agencies providing emotional, legal, and financial assistance and were tested more frequently for STDs than were adolescent patients receiving adult care. Culturally sensitive and appropriate interventions are particularly important in providing prenatal care.

Obstetric complications are relatively uncommon for adolescent pregnant women given good prenatal care. In a study of nulliparas <15 years old compared to nulliparous controls aged 20 to 29 years, there were no differences in cervical dilatation at admission, frequency of labor induction, epidural anesthesia, mean birth weight, or preterm birth weight (59). The duration of the active phase of labor and the rate of cesarean delivery were actually lower in the young adolescents.

Postdelivery, poverty, depression, and social isolation are frequent problems of young parents (60). Substance use is associated with depression, stress, high support need, and peer group drug use (61). Young mothers may have no access to daycare or babysitting and may have lost the social contacts they had in school. Teenagers who give birth while in school or soon after quitting school are far less likely to graduate from high school than those who delay childbearing until their 20s. Merely having a teenage birth leads to a 50% reduction in the likelihood of high school completion, compared with not having a teenage birth. Family background characteristics, individual differences, and academic difficulties prior to the pregnancy arc also important variables in predicting high school completion (62). Even for young parents able to continue in school, extracurricular activities (especially sports) are often impossible.

Many programs have focused on the pregnancy and the immediate postpartum period when adolescents' needs are obviously long-term. In addition, adolescents may lose the nurturing, supportive relationships that they had with clinic personnel after they deliver, and this loss may tend to promote recidivism. A number of innovative approaches have been tried to deal with these problems (63–65). In Boston, a teen obstetrics service at the Brigham and Women's Hospital provides antenatal and postpartum care specifically for adolescents. At Children's Hospital in Boston, a young parents' program provides contraceptive services and other medical and social services to mothers whenever they bring in their infants for well-child care. A provider with expertise in both adolescent and pediatric health provides medical care to the family. Outreach workers and visiting nurses fill an important educational role, as well as helping adolescents overcome barriers to making clinic appointments.

Since children of adolescent mothers are at particular risk of behavioral and cognitive difficulties, efforts need to be made to help mothers interact with their children. McAnarney and colleagues (66) found that younger adolescent mothers tended to show less acceptance, sensitivity, and cooperation and more negative verbal communication with their 9- to 12-month-old infants than did older adolescent mothers. Pope and associates (67) noted that coresidence of adolescent mothers and their infants with the infants' grandmother was associated with improved cognitive and health outcomes for infants. This finding suggests that programs to help adolescent parents should also target and include the extended family, thereby acknowledging the impact of familial and environmental factors on adolescents and their children.

The involvement of fathers in intervention programs has increased in the past decade. Many young fathers suffer negative psychosocial consequences, including depression and social isolation (68). They may quit school to try to provide financial support, an effort that is often counterproductive in the long run because of limited skills. Since many teenage fathers tend to be involved with their children, inclusion in programs with job training would be ideal. In a study of adolescent mothers in a teen-tot clinic, Cox and Bithoney (69) reported that factors associated with at least monthly contact between a father and child during the first 24 months of life were attending at least one prenatal visit, seeing the newborn in the hospital, and a reported supportive relationship between the young mother's family and the father at the 2-week interview.

Interventions need to target adolescent mothers to prevent a subsequent adolescent birth, since approximately 25% of teenage mothers have a second child within 24 months of the first birth. Eighty percent of repeat pregnancies are unplanned (70). Kalmuss and Namerow (71) reported that teenagers whose first birth occurred before age 16 were at a higher risk of a closely spaced birth, and Hispanic, black, and poor white teenagers were at a higher risk of having a second birth within 24 months than a nonpoor white teenager. Teens who wanted the first birth and who had not completed high school by the first birth were more likely to have a closely spaced birth. In addition, involvement in school, whether continuing high school or pursuing postsecondary education, exerted an important impact on reducing the likelihood of a closely spaced birth (72,73).

Adolescents' best hope for the future is to avoid repeated pregnancies, since closely spaced children appear to sharply limit the options for the future in terms of school achievement, independence from welfare, and other goals, as well as posing a health threat to their babies. In a followup study of women who were teenage mothers in the 1960s, Furstenberg and associates (74) found that women who had more children in the 5 years after their first birth did less well in school, had lower aspirations, and came from more disadvantaged families. Women with better-educated parents who were more economically secure often were able to escape welfare, finish education, and find satisfying careers.

There has been little research devoted to examining the impact of adoption on adolescent mothers. The choice often allows adolescents to continue their education and career plans. However, little is known about how many adolescents experience depression and need help coping with the loss and how many cope effectively with the transition and look toward future options.

ELECTIVE PREGNANCY TERMINATION

In 1994, 1,267,415 legal abortions were reported to the Centers for Disease Control and Prevention (75). This total represented a 3.7% decrease from 1993. Females ≤19 years old accounted for 20% of these procedures. Of women who become pregnant as teenagers, 41% choose abortion (76). Women who obtained legal abortions in 1994 were predominately <25 years of age, white, and unmarried. However, the abortion rate for black women is approximately three times that for white women. The percentage of adolescents undergoing abortions has decreased since 1972, when adolescents accounted for 32.6% of all abortions in the United States. In a national survey of abortion patients in 1994 to 1995, more patients were using contraception during the month they became pregnant than in 1987 (58% vs. 51%), and the proportion of patients whose pregnancy was attributable to condom failure increased from 15% to 32% (77).

Curettage (suction and sharp) remained the primary abortion procedure, representing approximately 99% of all such procedures (78). As in previous years, approximately 54% of legal abortions were performed during the first 8 weeks of gestation: 16% of abortions were performed at ≤6 weeks, 16% at 7 weeks, and 22% at 8 weeks. Approximately 88% of abortions were performed during the first 12 weeks of pregnancy (75). Teenagers are more likely to have an abortion in the second 3 months of pregnancy than are older women (76,78). Reasons for delay in seeking abortion services include young age, irregular menses, failure to recognize pregnancy symptoms, ambivalence about pregnancy, low educational level, and lack of awareness and availability of a clinic (79). The reduction in the number of abortions may reflect changing attitudes toward abortion or childbirth outside of marriage, as well as the smaller number of clinicians and clinics providing services (79).

With legalization, abortion has become remarkably safe over the past two decades (79–81). The case fatality ratio of legal induced abortion decreased 90% from 1972 to 1987 with 0.4 deaths per 100,000 abortions in 1987 (80). Women ≥40 years of age had three times the risk of death of teenagers; black women and other minority races had 2.5 times the risk of white women. Abortions at ≥16-weeks of gestation had almost 15 times the risk of death of procedures at ≤12 weeks (80). Morbidity and mortality rise with increased gestational age, so that the risk approximately doubles with each 2-week delay beyond 8 weeks. The death-to-case rate for legal abortion in 1972 to 1987 was 0.4/100,000 for ≤8 weeks, 0.8/100,000 for 9 to 10 weeks, and 1.4/100,000 for 11 to 12 weeks.

The interview that occurs before an abortion is crucial in laying the foundation for understanding patients and providing for their future needs (Table 1). Among adolescents having abortions, three-quarters say they cannot afford to have a baby, and two-thirds think they are not mature enough (76). Case intervention for healthy patients may be brief and effective and can support strengths formed from earlier life situations. For those less healthy, ongoing support may be required that focuses on self-determination. Counseling is often helpful to enable adolescents to tolerate the delay between the time of the diagnosis and the actual abortion procedure. Adolescents tend to be considerably more verbal before an abortion than after the procedure, when they may express a reluctance to talk about what has happened to them. However, calling a day or two after the procedure to ask a few brief questions ("How did it go?" "How are you doing?" "How are you feeling?") can be extremely supportive. It is also a good time to make sure that patients know when to start their oral contraceptive pills (if that is the method chosen). Seeing patients again at 2 weeks is important for a checkup and to review contraceptive options.

Followup visits are usually scheduled at least every 3 months and allow patients a chance to verbalize their feelings. Ambivalence about the pregnancy and abortion may recur. Some teenagers may discontinue their pills for several days when ambivalent feelings emerge. The abortion date or due date itself may occasionally take on a magical quality for teenagers, and they may return 1 year after the abortion with psychosomatic complaints, depression, and, rarely, attempted suicide. Writing down some of the details of the decision-making process at the time of the initial interviews allows the clinician subsequently, even a year or two later, to be able to clarify with adolescents that they made the best decision at that particular time, taking into account their educational plans, goals for the future, and plans for a job or financial independence. This discussion often helps patients resolve feelings of ambivalence.

The physician may be confronted with counseling boyfriends as well. They may feel prematurely trapped by a relationship in which important decisions about a pregnancy may affect their life. Boyfriends are frequently called on to be strong and supportive at a time when they are working through their own feelings and guilt about the situation.

First-Trimester Pregnancy Termination

The evaluation of adolescents planning to have an elective pregnancy termination should include a history and physical examination. An accurate assessment and correlation of gestational age and uterine size are necessary, as many adolescents will have irregular cycles, making dating difficult. If an adequate uterine sizing cannot be obtained, an ultrasound is necessary so that patients can be offered safe options prior to initiating a surgical procedure. Laboratory testing should include a documented positive pregnancy test, a Pap smear (within 1 year), endocervical tests for *N. gonorrhoeae* and *C. trachomatis,* hematocrit, urinalysis, Rh determination, and, in most adolescents, a serology for syphilis. HIV testing may be a consideration but in general is nonurgent and should be preceded by access to high-quality counseling. If cultures are done with sufficient time to obtain results before the procedure, treatment with antibiotics can be instituted for positive results. Many clinics prefer to give prophylactic tetracycline or doxycycline for 4 to 7 days in high-risk patients, including adolescents and those with a history of previous pelvic inflammatory disease (PID). In a study in Sweden (82), a single dose of doxycycline 10 to 12 hours before a first-trimester abortion resulted in a lower rate of postabortion endometritis/PID (2.1% vs. 6.2% for placebo; $p < 0.01$) but more nausea and vomiting. All Rh-negative women should receive immune globulin at the time of the abortion to prevent possible sensitization and resulting erythroblastosis fetalis with future pregnancies (see section on Prevention of D Isoimmunization).

In the first 12 weeks of gestation, the most commonly used method for abortion in the United States is suction curettage. Suction curettage, or dilatation and evacuation (D&E), involves mechanical cervical dilatation. Clinicians currently follow their individual preferences as to the use or nonuse of laminaria, since controlled studies of complications and morbidity are conflicting. Laminaria are seaweed or synthetic sticks that are hydrophilic, absorb water, and thus result in a mechanical dilatation of the uterine cervix. They must be put in place in the endocervical canal 3 to 24 hours before the procedure, and thus cause delay and an added procedure for patients. Use of laminaria may lessen the risk of cervical lacerations and uterine perforation, as these complications are most likely during the dilatation portion of the procedure.

Patients are instructed that a D&E feels like a very intense and severe menstrual cramp. The suction procedure itself lasts only a few minutes, but the uterine cramping, although brief, can be severe. The procedure can be performed with a local paracervical block and/or intravenous sedation in a freestanding clinic or hospital-based ambulatory setting. It is essential that patients be calm so that movement is limited during the procedure in order to decrease the risk of uterine perforation. Very young adolescents or victims of rape may prefer general anesthesia, as the pelvic examination alone may be difficult. General anesthesia is associated with a two- to fourfold increase in the risk of death compared to local anesthesia, and a higher rate of uterine perforation and hemorrhage, intraabdominal hemorrhage, and cervical trauma (83). Inhalational anesthetics relax the uterus, which may cause a larger blood loss.

After the procedure, patients should be informed that they may have bleeding like a "heavy period" that may continue for several days and up to 2 weeks after the procedure. They are encouraged to start their birth control pills within 3 days or on the Sunday after the procedure. The products of conception should always be carefully examined (and optimally sent to pathology) to make sure that a pregnancy has been completely terminated and to rule out a molar gestation (gestational trophoblastic disease). Failure to detect fetal parts or villi and an implantation site should prompt the clinician to consider diagnoses such as ectopic pregnancy, a false-positive pregnancy test (rare with the new kits), unrecognized early spontaneous abortion, uninterrupted intrauterine pregnancy, uterine anomaly with a continued pregnancy, or incomplete evacuation of the uterus. Repeat pregnancy test, curettage, ultrasonography, and laparoscopy are tools for making the correct diagnosis. When an early pregnancy (5 to 6 weeks) is terminated by menstrual extraction, it is especially important to consider the possibility of a failed abortion. No matter what type of abortion is performed, the patient must be seen in 2 weeks for followup to avoid missing a failed abortion with ongoing pregnancy, ectopic pregnancy, pathologic identification of trophoblastic disease, or other complications.

Complications of first-trimester abortion include excess blood loss resulting in transfusion, perforation of the uterus, postabortion hematometra, cervical trauma, infection, retained products of conception, and failed abortion (83). Immediately after the procedure, oxytocic agents may decrease blood loss and are used primarily in second-trimester abortions and with general anesthesia. Women with retained products of conception usually complain of heavy bleeding and cramps, with or without fever, in the first week after the abortion and require repeat curettage. Pelvic infection following an abortion is a potentially serious problem because of the risks of subsequent tubal disease, Asherman's syndrome (intrauterine adhesions), and infertility. Risk factors for postabortion endometritis or PID include late gestational age, endocervical gonorrhea or chlamydial infection, and intraamniotic instillations for induction of the abortion. Patients with infections typically complain of fever and bleeding 3 to 7 days after the abortion and have uterine tenderness and sometimes adnexal tenderness on examination. Antibiotics for the treatment of PID (see Chapter 12) should be instituted, and if retained products of conception are present, repeat curettage should be performed.

The data on the long-term medical and psychological effects of first-trimester abortion are reassuring (84,86). There is no conclusive evidence of an increase in miscarriages, ectopic pregnancy, or adverse late pregnancy outcomes in patients with one previous induced abortion (85). The use of gentle cervical dilatation techniques in the past decade should lessen the previously noted increased risk of midtrimester spontaneous abortions (84). Two or more induced abortions may slightly increase subsequent pregnancy loss (86). Any change in ectopic pregnancy rate is likely to be confined to women who have had a postabortal infection or multiple abortions. In a Danish study (87), postabortal pelvic infection was associated with a higher rate of spontaneous abortion, secondary infertility, dyspareunia, and chronic pelvic pain than uncomplicated abortion. Prophylactic antibiotics at the time of the abortion decreased the rates of later spontaneous abortion and dyspareunia.

A new approach to first-trimester abortion is the use of the synthetic progesterone antagonist mifepristone (RU 486) (88–91). A single dose administered to women at <50 days from the last menstrual period was effective and safe in causing abortion in most patients; efficacy was 100% with an initial β-hCG level <5000 mIU/ml compared to 81% at >20,000 mIU/ml (88). Overall 45 of 50 patients aborted, with only one of these requiring a suction curettage. The five patients who did not abort underwent a suction curettage without complications. The most serious side effect was bleeding, with a mean decrease in hemoglobin of 0.4 g/dl and bleeding lasting up to 16 days in some patients. Only two patients had a decrease >3 g/dl. Similar findings were reported by Couzinet and associates (89) in France with the recommendation that this drug be used only under close medical supervision because of the risk of bleeding. Recent trials have shown high success in the induction of abortion with the use of RU 486 and oral or vaginal misoprostol (90) and with methotrexate and misoprostol (92–93). Misoprostol alone is successful in only 60% of cases, all within 24 hours (94). Advances in the safe medical induction of abortion will hopefully decrease the emotional, physical, and political risk to women making the choice of terminating a pregnancy.

Second-Trimester Abortion

Second-trimester abortions (≥13 weeks) account for only about 10% of abortions in the United States. These later abortions carry higher risks to the patient and have more ethical issues and emotional consequences. Due to normally irregular menstrual periods, an adolescent may not be concerned about a late period and thus lengthen the time to confirmation of the pregnancy. Unfortunately, the political climate, the restriction of funding for indigent patients, the lack of convenient access to first-trimester abortion in some communities, and the legislation related to parental consent in some states may delay adolescents' decisions and result in more late abortions. Age is a major factor in delay; in 1991, 23% of abortions performed on girls <15 years of age were midtrimester, compared to 15.7% for 15- to 19-year-old adolescents and 8% for 30- to 34-year-old women (78). Another reason for delay is serious psychological problems resulting in denial of the pregnancy.

Techniques of performing second-trimester abortions have significantly evolved over the past 15 years, as studies in the 1970s revealed that D&E was significantly safer than intraamniotic instillation. From 1974 to 1991, the percentage of second-trimester abortions performed by D&E increased from 31% to 92%, and the percentage performed by intrauterine instillation decreased from 57% to 5% (78). For terminations between weeks 16 and 20 in 1991, 86.6% were performed using curettage, 5.4% with intrauterine saline instillation, and 4.1% with intrauterine prostaglandin instillation. The risks of cervical injury are lessened if laminaria are used before dilatation, and new materials continue to be investigated. Placement of laminaria overnight followed by D&E can be used up to 21 weeks (depending on state laws) by an appropriately skilled surgeon. A combination of urea and prostaglandin appears to be particularly useful when D&E is not available. Most clinicians feel that intravenous sedation with local anesthesia is the safest for patients to lessen the chance of uterine perforation. Ultrasound determination of gestational age is extremely useful in pregnancies at ≥13 weeks and should be done in all gestations of >20 weeks to prevent ethical, legal, and medical complications. Intraoperative ultrasound, particularly in terminations at ≥18 weeks, has proved invaluable to ensure that the uterine cavity is empty.

Although second-trimester abortions constituted only 10% of abortions between 1972 and 1981, they accounted for half of the mortality from abortions. Causes of death included infection (30%), amniotic fluid embolism, hemorrhage, disseminated intravascular coagulation, pulmonary embolism, and anesthetic complications. Potential problems encountered with second-trimester abortion methods included difficulties in the instillation, excessive bleeding, retained placenta, failed abortion, uterine rupture, and disseminated intravascular coagulation (95). Cervical incompetence and later spontaneous losses may be associated with forceful dilatation of the cervix.

Health care providers need to know in detail the medical procedures done in their community (including the availability and type of abortion done between 16 and 20 weeks of gestation) in order to do adequate counseling and to refer patients to appropriate centers. The telephone numbers and the fees (and types of insurance accepted) should be updated once a year.

DISORDERS OF EARLY PREGNANCY

Adolescents can experience the same difficulties during early pregnancy as adults, including ectopic pregnancy, molar pregnancy, and threatened, missed, or incomplete abortion. The difference is that adolescents may not have previously thought that they were pregnant before presenting to the emergency department with heavy bleeding, irregular menses, or pelvic pain. In addition, they may have a preexisting cervical infection with *N. gonorrhoeae* or *C. trachomatis* and may therefore be at increased risk for endometritis and salpingitis, although PID in pregnancy is uncommon.

With the advent of sensitive pregnancy testing, it is clear that early pregnancy loss is more common than previously thought. Wilcox and colleagues (96) found that the rate of pregnancy loss after implantation, including clinically recognized spontaneous abortions, was 31%. Twenty-two percent of the pregnancies ended before a pregnancy was detected clinically. Although this observation is important, the possibility of an ectopic pregnancy always needs to be kept in mind.

The sharp rise in the incidence of ectopic pregnancy noted in the 1970s and 1980s has been attributed to a number of factors including the increased incidence of salpingitis, the use of intrauterine devices, the delay in childbearing until the 30s (an age with a higher rate of ectopic pregnancy), tubal surgery including tubal sterilization, the earlier detection of pregnancy with the use of sensitive urine and blood tests of hCG, and the use of progestin-only birth control pills (see Chapter 17) (97–99). The rate should, however, be stated in relation to *all* pregnancies, not just live births, to take into account induced abortions. With the rising number of cases of STDs and PID in adolescents, the clinician needs to consider an ectopic pregnancy, when evaluating adolescents with irregular bleeding and/or abdominal pain. In addition, girls may have more than one diagnosis (e.g., ectopic pregnancy and PID) at the time of presentation to the clinic. The health care provider's detailed history should include questions relating to ectopic risk factors: previous ectopic pregnancy, history of PID, STDs, previous intraabdominal or pelvic surgery, reproductive tract congenital anomalies, and a history of intrauterine device use.

Mortality rates from ectopic pregnancy have declined in the past decade but are higher for black women than white women, especially among teenagers and older women (100). Blacks are less likely to seek prenatal care in the first trimester of pregnancy, and black teenagers may have less adequate access to gynecologic services. Non-English-speaking patients, patients with cognitive delay and psychiatric illness, and substance abusers are at increased risk of late ectopic pregnancy diagnosis.

The classic history of ectopic pregnancy includes pelvic pain, amenorrhea, and irregular vaginal bleeding. However, many patients do not have all or, in fact, any of these symptoms, in part because of earlier diagnosis with the use of sensitive pregnancy tests and ultrasonography. A missed menstrual period or irregular spotting or bleeding are the most frequent presenting complaints. Adolescents may give vague histories of the timing of the last menstrual period and may accept menstrual irregularity as a normal event. Some patients do not skip menses. In the past, acute pelvic pain was reported in 96% to 99% of patients, but that presentation is much less frequent today. Nausea, vomiting, and fainting can also occur. Acute tubal rupture with hemorrhage can cause shock and death.

The physical examination may show helpful signs for the clinician but also may be nonspecific for other diagnoses. In acute, ruptured ectopic pregnancy, signs of intraperitoneal hemorrhage and shock are found. In unruptured ectopic pregnancy, findings are much more subtle. Abdominal tenderness and rebound tenderness may be found. Adnexal tenderness may prevent adequate assessment for the presence of a pelvic mass, which in fact may not be palpable for early diagnosis. Bimanual examination should be performed gently in these patients. The uterus may be enlarged, simulating an early intrauterine pregnancy.

The hCG level is the mainstay of diagnosis in combination with ultrasonography and laparoscopy (101–104). The clinician needs to decide whether the pregnancy is intrauterine or ectopic and, if intrauterine, whether or not it is developing normally. The differential diagnosis must include a nonviable intrauterine pregnancy, as well as a spontaneous abortion. A patient's desire for the pregnancy should be a factor in the approach to intervention, even though clinicians frequently assume that all adolescent pregnancies are unwanted. A sensitive urine pregnancy test can detect levels of hCG as low as 10 to 25 mIU/ml. Only an extremely rare lesion without trophoblastic tissue or with apparent defects in hCG production would be expected to have no detectable hCG. A very early ectopic or intrauterine pregnancy can have a level of hCG <50 mIU/ml, but the likelihood of symptomatology is low. Quantitative serum tests should help the clinician to elucidate the diagnosis (104). To rely on the results of the urine pregnancy testing, the physician must feel comfortable that the urine belongs to the patient and has not been altered because of her fear of testing for illicit drugs.

Some centers have found that serum progesterone levels are helpful in making the diagnosis of ectopic pregnancy (105,106,125). In one study, women with normal intrauterine pregnancies had serum progesterone levels >20 ng/ml and those with ectopic pregnancies had levels <15 ng/ml (106). Another study found that the probability of an abnormal pregnancy outcome (spontaneous abortion, ectopic pregnancy) with a serum progesterone ≤6 ng/ml at 8 weeks of gestation was 81% (106). In addition, molar pregnancies, gestational trophoblastic neoplasia, and some ovarian tumors and central nervous system dysgerminonas also produce hCG.

The management of unstable or "shocky" patients with a positive pregnancy test and ectopic pregnancy is clearly different from the evaluation of stable or asymptomatic adolescents with a positive pregnancy test and vaginal bleeding. Unstable patients require surgical intervention with immediate laparoscopy; young women in shock must be treated for the shock and taken to the operating room for laparotomy.

Most patients do not require immediate surgical intervention, and the treatment is guided by clinical assessment and measurement of quantitative hCG levels. During the evaluation, patients need to understand the nature of the differential diagnosis; they should receive careful instructions on warning signs of ectopic pregnancy and spontaneous abortion (107). Thus, if adolescents present with vaginal spotting or pain and have a positive pregnancy test, the possibility of an ectopic or threatened abortion needs to be determined. Serial serum quantitative hCG levels must be done in the same laboratory with the same reference preparation so that changes can be used to guide the clinician (see Table 4, Chapter 1). Above an hCG of 100 mIU/ml, doubling time of hCG is approximately 2.3 days in early gestation. Mean doubling time is 1.6 days for 23 to 35 days of gestation, 2.0 days for 35 to 42 days of gestation, and 3.4 days for 41 to 50 days (108). As gestational age is unlikely to be known precisely, the clinician typically uses the lower limits of a 48-hour interval. Between 5 and 8 weeks, the hCG should increase by 29% in 24 hours, 66% at 48 hours, 114% in 72 hours, 175% in 96 hours, and 255% in 120 hours (109); an increase less than this increment should alert the clinician to the possibility of a failed intrauterine or ectopic pregnancy (109–111). Clinical assessment is important because 6% to 15% of normal pregnancies do have a lag in doubling, and 13% of ectopic pregnancies will initially show a normal increase.

Ultrasonography has proved to be a valuable tool in the diagnosis of normal and abnormal pregnancies (112). The so-called discriminatory zone is a key concept and depends on the medical center, the ultrasound equipment, the type of ultrasound (abdominal vs. vaginal), and the radiologist. A gestational sac can optimally be visualized by abdominal ultrasound using the latest scanning equipment at approximately 4000 to 6000 mIU/ml hCG (International Reference Preparation [IRP]) (5 to 6 weeks from last menstrual period [LMP]) and at approximately 1000 to 1500 mIU/ml hCG by transvaginal ultrasonography. Sometimes an ectopic pregnancy will be associated with a pseudodecidual reaction of the endometrium within the uterus that may mimic an intrauterine gestational sac. Fossum and associates (113) reported finding a gestational sac at 34.8 ± 2.2 days from LMP, at which time hCG was 1398 ± 155 mIU/ml (IRP); a fetal pole at 40.3 ± 3.4 days from LMP with hCG at 5113 ± 298 mIU/ml; and fetal heartbeat at 46.9 ± 6.0 days from LMP with hCG at 17,208 ± 3772 mIU/ml. The location of a fetal heart (5.5 to 7 weeks from LMP) is conclusive evidence of an intrauterine pregnancy by ultrasound; it is extremely rare for intrauterine and ectopic (heterotopic) pregnancies to coexist (1/30,000). An ectopic pregnancy may occasionally be visualized by sonography as a heart beat in the adnexa. A noncystic adnexal mass is suggestive of an ectopic pregnancy but not conclusive. Free fluid in the cul-de-sac may be associated with a ruptured simple ovarian cyst, a ruptured hemorrhagic corpus luteum, a leaking ectopic pregnancy, or a ruptured ectopic pregnancy. Culdocentesis may be done to determine whether the free fluid is nonclotting blood or clear cyst fluid. Communication with the ultrasonographer and correlation with the quantitative hCG are critical in the care of patients suspected of having an ectopic pregnancy.

Clinical management thus depends on the status of the patient, the levels of hCG, the desire to continue an intrauterine pregnancy, and the ultrasound results. In *asymptomatic* adolescents who have *falling* hCG levels, the clinician should follow the hCG levels to zero to make sure that whatever process there was (tubal pregnancy, missed abortion, abortion) has totally resolved. If the hCG results show a *constant* plateaued level or *subnormal increase,* the intervention depends in part on whether the pregnancy is desired. Another hCG reading may be required along with a repeat ultrasound done at the discriminatory zone if a normal pregnancy with initial slightly subnormal increases in hCG is suspected. If the hCG is above the discriminatory zone and no intrauterine gestational sac is seen on ultrasound, the diagnosis is most likely an ectopic pregnancy, unless the hCG is elevated due to multiple or a molar gestation. If the pregnancy is desired but the clinician suspects an ectopic pregnancy (noncystic adnexal mass or subnormal increases in hCG), laparoscopy is done first. If the pregnancy is *not* desired, a D&E is done first. If no villi from an intrauterine pregnancy are identified grossly or by pathology at the time of D&E, then treatment for the ectopic pregnancy must be undertaken.

Treatment of ectopic pregnancy should aim at timely intervention and preservation of future fertility (114). Laparoscopic salpingostomy with preservation of the fallopian tube is classically used for the treatment of ectopic pregnancy. After salpingostomy, reapproximation of the fallopian tube is not necessary, as spontaneous closure and healing will result in less likelihood of tubal scarring or adhesions. Laparoscopic salpingectomy is reserved for the fallopian tube that is felt to be irreversibly destroyed by the ectopic pregnancy or for cases in which hemostasis cannot be achieved with salpingostomy. Free fluid or blood in the pelvis is not a contraindication to a laparoscopic approach, unless the patient is hypotensive. Many young women will be orthostatic but not hypotensive, and thus a laparoscopic approach is not contraindicated.

Medical management of ectopic pregnancies is rapidly gaining approval within the United States (114–116). With increased experience with the use of methotrexate, many clinical guidelines have been developed for the medical management of ectopic pregnancies including the use of intravenous, intramuscular, and oral methotrexate with and without the use of citrovorum factor rescue (117–120). Most protocols have found that the highest treatment success rates occur in cases in which the ectopic pregnancy is <3 to 5 cm on ultrasound, no evidence of tubal rupture exists, and no fetal cardiac activity is found within the fallopian tube. Outpatient single-dose methotrexate therapy of 1 mg/kg body weight or 50 mg/m^2 body surface area without citrovorum factor rescue appears to be safe and is rapidly gaining in popularity (114, 120–122). Compliance with followup is a must, as some medically treated ectopic pregnancies will rupture even in the situation of a declining hCG level. Levels of hCG are expected to fall by 1 log value within 18 days. If the hCG level plateaus or has an initial fall followed by an increase, a second treatment with methotrexate may be required. Of note, it has been shown that *some* ectopic pregnancies <2 cm with no pain and with β-hCG <1000 mIU/ml resolve spontaneously without surgery; however, some patients entered into the trial required surgical treatment (122). Due to issues of compliance with adolescents and the need to adhere to a rigid protocol, more studies are needed before clinicians routinely convert current surgical intervention in the care of adolescents with ectopic pregnancies to medical therapy (123).

In all cases, after surgical therapy for ectopic pregnancy, hCG levels should be checked 2 weeks later to be sure that the levels have fallen to zero, and, if not, they should be followed to zero. Most patients have a negative titer by 12 days (104). There is a small chance of regrowth of trophoblastic tissue with a procedure of less than a total salpingectomy. Methotrexate can also be used for the management of the postsurgical persistent ectopic pregnancy.

Timely intervention has clearly improved the prognosis of patients. Many young women are able to conceive, but there is an increased risk (10% to 16%) of repeat ectopic pregnancy. Adolescents with tubal disease sufficient to cause an ectopic pregnancy are at high risk of future tubal disease, and therefore total salpingectomy should be avoided, if possible, to leave open the options for future fertility repair. In cases in which the fallopian tubes are diseased or have been removed, patients should be made aware of advances in and the availability of assisted reproductive technologies (*in vitro* fertilization).

Spontaneous Abortion, or Blighted Ovum (Nonviable Pregnancy)

The treatment of the nonviable intrauterine pregnancy depends on several factors. As with the management of ectopic pregnancies, declining or plateaued hCG levels must be from the same laboratory in order to establish that the pregnancy is nonviable. Patients without significant trophoblastic tissue and low levels of hCG can be followed without operative intervention, provided heavy bleeding does not occur and the hCG declines to zero. Rh status should be assessed at initial presentation and Rh^0 (D) immune globulin administered as indicated. In spontaneous abortion, the hCG is usually near zero by 19 days. In contrast, following elective first-trimester abortion, patients will have a slower decline of hCG to zero because of high initial levels; hCG is detectable for 16 to 60 days after D&E, with a mean of 30 days.

Two treatment options may be considered for adolescents with a nonviable pregnancy, intrauterine products of conception, a closed cervix, and declining hCG levels: observation or D&E. If observation is chosen, patients must be followed closely and be able to return promptly for curettage if there is excessive bleeding with the spontaneous passage of tissue. The open os makes the procedure less risky, but adolescents may have difficulty arranging transportation to the hospital. Electively scheduled D&E avoids adolescents' having to carry a nonviable pregnancy and having to go to the emergency department for sudden profuse bleeding. Many hospital emergency departments are now set up to offer immediate suction curettage. Cultures for *N. gonorrhoeae* and *C. trachomatis* should be done at the time of the examination, and consideration given to prescribing prophylactic antibiotics (doxycycline 100 mg twice daily for 5 to 7 days) following D&E.

Adolescents seen for irregular bleeding at followup after a spontaneous abortion, term pregnancy, or elective termination of pregnancy should always have a pregnancy test done at the appropriate interval when it would be expected to be negative. Irregular bleeding should not be assumed to be due to breakthrough bleeding from oral contraceptives. A positive pregnancy test should raise the possibility of a new pregnancy (normal or abnormal), retained products of conception, or gestational neoplasia.

Gestational Trophoblastic Disease Including Molar Pregnancy

Gestational trophoblastic disease (GTD) is a spectrum of disease processes involving abnormal placental tissue. The term incorporates the following histologically distinct entities: complete hydatidiform mole, partial hydatidiform mole, invasive mole, placental site trophoblastic tumor, and choriocarcinoma (124). In the United States, hydatidiform moles are identified in 1 in 600 therapeutic abortions and in 1 in 1000 to 1200 pregnancies (126). A complete mole is characterized by hydropic (swollen) chorionic villi, diffuse trophoblastic hyperplasia, and no identifiable embryonic or fetal tissue. Complete moles have a diploid karyotype, and all chromosomes are of paternal origin. Most often, a haploid (23,X) sperm fertilizes an anuclear ovum and then replicates its own chromosomes. A partial mole is characterized by focal swelling of the chorionic villi, focal trophoblastic hyperplasia, and presence of embryonic or fetal tissues. Partial moles usually have a triploid karyotype derived from the fertilization of a normal ovum by two spermatozoa. Approximately 20% of patients with primary hydatidiform mole will develop malignancies. Choriocarcinoma occurs in 1 in 20,000 to 40,000 pregnancies. Approximately 50% develop after a term pregnancy. It has been noted that there is an increased prevalence of molar disease in both older and adolescent women.

Hydatidiform mole is usually diagnosed in the first trimester of pregnancy. A woman may present with irregular bleeding or uterine size greater than that expected by the dates given, or may be found to have an abnormally high hCG level. In addition, the diagnosis may be made on a pathologic specimen from a therapeutic or spontaneous abortion. Ultrasound will show the classic snowstorm appearance of the cystic tissue. When a diagnosis of hydatidiform mole is made, the treatment is uterine evacuation with a suction D&E. As Rh^0D factor is expressed on trophoblasts, patients who are Rh negative should receive Rh^0 (D) immune globulin. Prior to evacuation, the following evaluation should be completed: complete blood cell count, platelet count, clotting function tests, renal and liver function tests, blood type and antibody screen, and a sensitive quantitative hCG. A chest X-ray should also be obtained. A physician familiar with this disease process should manage the patient. A quantitative hCG level should be obtained 48 hours after the evacuation, every 1 to 2 weeks until the levels are normal, and then at 1- to 2- month intervals for an additional 6 months. Contraception is recommended for 1 year after remission. An excellent review of the management of complete and partial molar pregnancy has recently been published (127). If the hCG level rises, additional evaluation and therapy will be initiated by the gynecologic oncologist. The malignant GTDs include invasive mole, gestational choriocarcinoma, and placental site trophoblastic tumor. With medical advances for diagnosis (sensitive hCG testing) and therapies, most women with all forms of GTD can be successfully treated while maintaining subsequent reproductive function.

Prevention of D Isoimmunization

The administration of Rh^0 (D) immune globulin can be very successful in preventing isoimmunization to the D antigen. To reduce future risk of Rh hemolytic disease, health care providers must identify women at risk, those who are Rh negative, and provide treatment with D immunoglobulin. The treatment should be given in the following clinical scenarios: bleeding in early pregnancy; spontaneous abortion; therapeutic abortion; ectopic pregnancy; molar pregnancy; at the time of amniocentesis, chorionic villus sampling, percutaneous umbilical cord blood sampling, or fetal surgery or manipulation; at 28 to 29 weeks of gestation; and at delivery (128). Therapy is indicated when a patient's blood type is Rh negative and the father's blood type is Rh positive or unknown. A 50-μg dose of Rh^0 (D) immune globulin (MICRhoGAM) is usually given for bleeding in early pregnancy, ectopic pregnancy, or spontaneous or therapeutic abortion (<13 weeks of gestation). For spontaneous or therapeutic abortion after 13 weeks of gestation or at later times of pregnancy for other indications, a 300-μg dose is used.

ADOLESCENT PREGNANCY PREVENTION

Various programs have been implemented throughout the United States to reduce the number of adolescent pregnancies, but there is no consensus as to how to best prevent teenagers from becoming pregnant (1,7,129–133). Some feel that abstinence should be the only message imparted to teenagers. Others feel that abstinence is the ideal, but the reality of large numbers of teenagers engaged in sexual intercourse requires instruction in responsible sexual behavior and access to contraception. Financing of pregnancy prevention programs is a major issue, and a program must also garner the support of the community to be successful. Ethnically, racially, and socioeconomically different groups of teenagers may require different types of programs. Analysis of the success or failure of a program is difficult and expensive.

The Postponing Sexual Involvement (PSI) program, a project run by the Emory University School of Medicine/Grady Memorial Hospital Teen Services Program in Atlanta, Georgia, is an example of a successful adolescent pregnancy-prevention program (131). During the early 1970s, Grady Memorial Hospital created the Teen Services Program and developed an outreach program in the Atlanta public schools, with 8th-grade students' having classroom periods covering basic human sexuality, decision-making information, how to postpone sexual intercourse, and family planning information. The PSI program is an experiential effort led by 11th- and 12th-grade girls and boys trained by the hospital staff. The older teenagers work with the 8th graders to identify instances of peer pressure, role-play responses to pressures, develop assertiveness skills, and discuss problem situations. Through skits, younger teenagers practice skills for resisting peer pressure and saying "No" to sex. The use of older teenagers shows the younger teens that those who abstain from sex can be admired and liked by others.

The PSI program has been shown to be effective in postponing sexual involvement among those who had not already had intercourse. Among the initially nonsexually active, 17% of girls and 39% of boys involved in PSI became sexually active by the end of ninth grade, compared to a control group in which 27% of girls and 61% of boys became sexually active (131). Fewer pregnancies occurred among the girls in the program, since there were fewer who were sexually involved. The program was not effective for young people who had begun sexual activity prior to the program (132).

Reducing the Risk is another curriculum that has been used in 9th- and 10th-grade classes in California and involves 15 classes; components of the program include abstinence, life skills, and contraception and access to services on site or nearby (132,134). Among those with no sexual experience, 29% of girls became sexually active at followup, compared to 38% in a control group.

The Teen Primary Pregnancy Prevention Program of the Children's Aid Society (CAS) in Harlem is another example of a successful intervention (135). Designed and implemented by Michael A. Carrera, PhD, this program started in

1985 with 22 teenagers and 12 parents. As of 1994, about 200 youths and parents had been served at three locations in New York City. The philosophy behind the program is that a climate must be created in which positive change can occur and direction can be given to young people: "The most powerful contraceptive is knowing that you're a valuable person and can make something of yourself" (135). The CAS program, a holistic, multidimensional approach to preventing adolescent pregnancy, consists of seven components: (a) a family life and sex education unit, (b) academic assessment, homework help, and guaranteed admission to Hunter College, (c) on-site primary health care services, (d) self-esteem enhancement, (e) a job club and career awareness program, (f) individual counseling, and (g) skills training in individual sports that emphasize self-discipline and self-control.

Although no controlled group studies have been conducted to evaluate the CAS program, the results are promising. During the first 5 years of the program, eight teenagers became pregnant, and two males caused pregnancies. The teenagers in the program were attending junior and senior high school. In the fall of 1994, 75 students attended Hunter College. By April 1994, ten New York City agencies and ten cities outside of New York were replicating the CAS model. Despite the program's positive impact, concerns have been raised that the program is highly labor- and cost-intensive for a relatively small group of teens ($1500 per student annually).

The Teen Choice program of Inwood House, a voluntary social service agency, also seeks to reduce teenage pregnancy in New York City through a school-based program (135) by providing accurate information on human sexuality and STDs and enhancing self-esteem, self-reflection, values clarification, and decision-making skills. A 1984 to 1987 longitudinal study of the Teen Choice program found that it was effective in reaching and recruiting adolescents at high risk of unintended pregnancy and that students were more knowledgeable about contraception and had responsible attitudes about the use of birth control, with reduced frequency of unprotected sexual intercourse.

Another approach aimed at reducing adolescent pregnancy has been to place health clinics at or very near school sites (136–141). Zabin and colleagues (136–138) reported on a school-based program that was carried out in a junior and senior high school in inner-city Baltimore. Over three school years, students were provided with education about sexuality and contraception, individual and group counseling at school, and medical and contraceptive services in a clinic across the street. Significant changes in contraceptive and sexual knowledge occurred, and young men made significantly more visits to the clinic than had occurred before the intervention. For 8th-grade boys, the number attending the birth control clinic increased from 24% to 62% and for 12th-grade boys from 14% to 64%. Eighth-grade girls increased attendance from 33% to 64%, and 12th-grade girls from 69% to 75%. Students at the two control schools that did not receive the intervention did not see any changes in the number of students using services. The mean age of coitus was delayed slightly, not advanced, as some opponents of the school-based clinics have feared. Students were more likely to seek contraceptives before intercourse or during the early months of sexual activity than before the intervention.

School-based health clinics do not necessarily lead to declines in adolescent pregnancy rates, as hoped (141,142). School-based clinics in St. Paul, Minnesota, that have existed in the city for almost two decades have not significantly lowered school-wide birth rates. However, studies have not looked specifically at the birth rates of the adolescent females known to have visited the clinic to evaluate the impact of them. It is also unknown whether provision of prenatal care and help for teens in obtaining social services encourage them to view pregnancy as more acceptable or feasible (142,143). To increase the effectiveness of school-based clinics, Kirby and associates (141) have recommended: (a) giving a high priority to pregnancy prevention and AIDS prevention, (b) conducting more outreach in schools, (c) developing programs to delay and reduce sexual activity, (d) identifying and targeting students engaged in sexual activity, (e) making contraceptives available through the clinics, (f) conducting effective followup procedures, and (g) emphasizing condoms and male responsibility. Program directors have found that enlisting the support of the community is crucial to the success of these programs. Providing comprehensive health services and improving overall health, not just reducing pregnancy rates, makes the clinic more attractive to students. Although some clinicians have rightly worried about clinics that are not open at night, weekends, or summers, practical solutions can be found, especially by using linkages with existing neighborhood services. In addition, creative solutions are needed to reach teenagers who do not attend school, a particularly high-risk group.

A successful intervention program in a South Carolina county provides insight into the difficulties of accurately assessing all the factors responsible for the outcome. In the original report, Vincent and associates (144) designed an innovative pregnancy prevention program to target parents, teachers, ministers, community leaders, and children enrolled in public schools. An integrated curriculum of sex education was implemented in all grades from kindergarten to grade 12, with objectives of improved decision making and communication skills, enhanced self-esteem, alignment of personal values with those of the family, church, and community, and increased knowledge of human reproduction and contraception. Further education occurred through churches and community groups, and the message was promoted in newspapers and radio. The estimated pregnancy rate for girls 14 to 17 years old declined significantly during the intervention period (25/1000) in comparison to preintervention statistics (62/1000) and was markedly lower than in similar counties in the area (49 to 59/1000). A reevaluation of this intervention demonstrated that the estimated pregnancy rates for females declined during the intervention period (37/1000) in comparison to preintervention statistics (77/1000) and was markedly lower than in similar counties in the area (67 to 87/1000) (138); however, the program components were not solely responsible for the decline. Instead, the intervention was assisted by the activities of a school nurse who provided contraceptive counseling and supplies to students. When the clinic was no longer able to provide supplies without parental consent for those <16 years old, the school nurse left the school system, the momentum of the intervention ceased, and the pregnancy rate returned to 66/1000.

In contrast to these successful programs, Stevens-Simon and colleagues (146), using a prospective randomized design, could not demonstrate that the popular Dollar-A-Day Program (a peer-based incentive program) in Colorado was effective in reducing pregnancy although the incentives were effective in increasing attendance at peer groups (146). In addition, replication in a new site of a successful program, such as PSI, mentioned earlier, may not yield similar outcomes. In a large-scale study of the PSI curriculum in California, given in five sessions with 90% adult leaders (rather than peers), a positive effect could not be found at the 17-month followup, and the project was terminated (147). The authors of the evaluation have suggested that a longer intervention was likely needed including booster sessions and that all curricula require continuing revision and evaluation.

In 1996, President Clinton launched a national strategy to prevent out-of-wedlock teen pregnancy and to ensure that more communities had teen pregnancy prevention programs in place. Many programs have now been evaluated in a Program Archive on Sexuality, Health, and Adolescence collection (148).

Prevention of unintended pregnancy among adolescents thus represents a major challenge for health care providers, educators, policymakers, and society in general. Programs are needed to enhance educational and life opportunities for these young people, to help them postpone becoming sexually active, and to assist them to use effective contraception when they initiate sexual activity. Concerned clinicians play a vital role in counseling young women who do become pregnant during their school-age years.

REFERENCES

1. *Sex and America's teenagers.* New York, Washington: The Alan Guttmacher Institute, 1994.
2. *Facts in brief: teenage sexual and reproductive behavior in the United States.* New York: The Alan Guttmacher Institute, 1994.
3. *Teenage pregnancy: the problem that hasn't gone away.* New York: The Alan Guttmacher Institute, 1980.
4. Zuckerman BS, Walker DK, Frank DA, et al. Adolescent pregnancy: biobehavioral determinants of outcome. *J Pediatr* 1985;105:857.
5. McAnarney ER. Adolescent pregnancy and childbearing: new data, new challenges (commentaries). *Pediatrics* 1985;75:973.
6. Spivak H, Weitzman M. Social barriers faced by adolescent parents and their children. *JAMA* 1987;258:1500.
7. Klerman LV. Adolescent pregnancy and parenting: controversies of the past and lessons for the future. *J Adolesc Health* 1993;14:553.
8. Spitz AM, Velebil P, Koonin LM. Pregnancy, abortion, and birth rates among U.S. adolescents: 1980, 1985, and 1990. *JAMA* 1996;275:989.
9. Centers for Disease Control and Prevention. Teenage pregnancy and birth rates—United States, 1990. *MMWR* 1993;42:734.

10. Wegman ME. Annual summary of vital statistics—1993. *Pediatrics* 1994;94:792.
11. Guyer B, Strobino DM, Ventura S, et al. Annual summary of vital statistics—1995. *Pediatrics* 1996;98:1007.
12. Guyer B, MacDorman MF, Martin JA, et al. Annual summary of vital statistics—1997. *Pediatrics* 1998;102:1333.
13. Centers for Disease Control and Prevention. State-specific pregnancy and birth rates among teenagers—United States, 1991–1992. *MMWR* 1995;44:677.
14. East PL. Do adolescent pregnancy and childbearing affect younger siblings? *Fam Plann Perspect* 1996;28:148.
15. Cox J, Emans SJ, Bithoney W. Sisters of teen mothers: increased risk for adolescent parenthood. *Adolesc Pediatr Gynecol* 1993;6:138.
16. Cox JE, DuRant RH, Emans SJ, Woods ER. Early parenthood for the sisters of adolescent mothers: a proposed conceptual model of decision-making. *Adolesc Pediatr Gynecol* 1995;8:188.
17. Friede A, Hogue C, Doyle L, et al. Do sisters of childbearing teenagers have increased rates of childbearing? *Am J Public Health* 1986;76:1121.
18. Furstenberg FF, Levine JA, Brooks-Gunn J. The children of teenage mothers: patterns of early childbearing in two generations. *Fam Plann Perspect* 1990;22:54.
19. Hechinger FM. *Fateful choices healthy youth for the 21st century.* New York: Carnegie Corporation of New York, 1992.
20. Hayes CD, ed. *Risking the future: adolescent sexuality, pregnancy, and childbearing.* Washington, DC: National Academy Press, 1987.
21. Lancaster JB, Hamburg BA, eds. *School-age pregnancy and parenthood.* Hawthorne, NY: Aldine de Gruyter, 1986.
22. Stevens-Simon C, Reichert S. Sexual abuse, adolescent pregnancy, and child abuse: a developmental approach to an intergenerational cycle. *Arch Pediatr Adolesc Med* 1994;148:26.
23. Berenson AB, San Miguel VV, Wilkinson GS. Prevalence of physical and sexual assault in pregnant adolescents. *J Adolesc Health* 1992;13:468.
24. Kokotailo PK, Adger H, Duggan AK, et al. Cigarette, alcohol, and other drug use by school-age pregnant adolescents: prevalence, detection, and associated risk factors. *Pediatrics* 1992;90:332.
25. Zabin LS, Emerson MR, Ringers PA, et al. Adolescents with negative pregnancy test results. *JAMA* 1996;275:113.
26. Zabin LS, Hirsch MB, Boscia JAB. Differential characteristics of adolescent pregnancy test patients: abortion, childbearing and negative test groups. *J Adolesc Health* 1990;11:112.
27. Zabin LS, Sedivy V, Emerson MR. Subsequent risk of childbearing among adolescents with a negative pregnancy test. *Fam Plann Perspect* 1994;26:212–217.
28. Abrahamse AF, Morrison PA, Waite LJ, et al. *Beyond stereotypes:* who *becomes a single teenage mother?* Santa Monica, CA: Rand Corporation, 1988. Publication R-3489-HHS-NICHD.
29. Nadelson CC, Notman MT, Gillon JW. Sexual knowledge and attitudes of adolescents: relationship to contraceptive usage. *Obstet Gynecol* 1980;55:340.
30. Wegman ME. Annual summary of vital statistics—1992. *Pediatrics* 1993;92:744.
31. Centers for Disease Control and Prevention. Childbearing patterns among selected racial/ethnic minority groups—United States, 1990. *MMWR* 1993;42:400.
32. Iams JD, Rayburn WF, Zuspan FP. Drug effects on the fetus. In: Rayburn WF, Zuspan ZP, ed. *Drug therapy in obstetrics and gynecology,* 2nd ed. Norwalk, CT, Appleton-Century-Croft, 1986:13–23.
33. *Guidelines for diagnostic imaging during pregnancy.* American College of Obstetricians and Gynecologists Committee Opinion, No. 158:1–3, Sept 1995.
34. Forman SF, Aruda MM, Emans SJ, et al. Followup of pregnant teens at a hospital-based clinic. *J Adolesc Health* 1995;17:193.
35. Scher P, Emans SJ, Grace E. Factors associated with compliance to oral contraceptive use in an adolescent population. *J Adolesc Health Care* 1982;3:120.
36. Kinsman SB, Slap GB. Barriers to adolescent prenatal care. *J Adolesc Health* 1992;13:153.
37. McAnarney ER. Young maternal age and adverse neonatal outcome. *Am J Dis Child* 1987;141:1053.
38. Leppert PC, Namerow PB, Barker D. Pregnancy outcomes among adolescent and older women receiving comprehensive prenatal care. *J Adolesc Health Care* 1986;7:112.
39. Slap GB, Schwartz JS. Risk factors for low birth weight to adolescent mothers. *J Adolesc Health Care* 1989;10:267.
40. Scholl TO, Hediger ML, Huang J, et al. Young maternal age and parity: influences on pregnancy outcome. *Ann Epidemiol* 1992;2:572.

41. Fraser AM, Brockert JE, Ward RH. Association of young maternal age with adverse reproductive outcomes. *N Engl J Med* 1995;332:1113.
42. Goldenberg R, Klerman LV. Adolescent pregnancy—another look (editorial). *N Engl J Med* 1995;332:1161.
43. Stevens-Simon C, Kaplan DW, McAnarney ER. Factors associated with preterm delivery among pregnant adolescents. *J Adolesc Health* 1993;14:341.
44. Rawlings JS, Rawlings VB, Read JA. Prevalence of low birth weight and preterm delivery in relation to the interval between pregnancies among white and black women. *N Engl J Med* 1995; 332:69.
45. Blankson ML, Cliver SP, Goldenberg RL, et al. Health behavior and outcomes in sequential pregnancies of black and white adolescents. *JAMA* 1993;269:1401.
46. McAnarney ER, Stevens-Simon C. First, do no harm: low birth weight and adolescent obesity. *Am J Dis Child* 1993;147:984.
47. Stevens-Simon C, McAnarney ER. Adolescent pregnancy: gestational weight gain and maternal and infant outcomes. *Am J Dis Child* 1992;146:1363.
48. Segel JS, McAnarney ER. Adolescent pregnancy and subsequent obesity in African-American girls. *J Adolesc Health* 1994;15:491.
49. The American Dietetic Association. Position of the American Dietetic Association: nutrition care for pregnant adolescents. *J Am Diet Assoc* 1994;94:450.
50. Gutierrez Y, King JC. Nutrition during teenage pregnancy. *Pediatr Ann* 1993;22:99.
51. Parker B, McFarlane J, Soeken K. Abuse during pregnancy: effects on maternal complications and birth weight in adult and teenage women. *Obstet Gynecol* 1994;84:323.
52. Berenson AB, San Migul VV, Wilkinson GS. Violence and its relationship to substance abuse in adolescent pregnancy. *J Adolesc Health* 1992;134:470.
53. Bayatpour M, Wells RD, Holford S. Physical and sexual abuse as predictors of substance abuse and suicide among pregnant teenagers. *J Adolesc Health* 1992;13:131.
54. Scholl TO, Hediger ML, Belsky DH. Prenatal care and maternal health during adolescent pregnancy: a review and metaanalysis. *J Adolesc Health* 1994;15:444.
55. McAnarney ER, Roghmann KJ, Adam BN et al. Obstetric, neonatal and psychosocial outcome of pregnant adolescents. *Pediatrics* 1978;61:199.
56. Felice ME, Granados JL, Ances IG, et al. The young pregnant teenager: impact of comprehensive prenatal care. *J Adolesc Health Care* 1981;1:193.
57. Morris DL, Berenson AB, Lawson J, et al. Comparison of adolescent pregnancy outcomes by prenatal source. *J Reprod Med* 1993;38:375.
58. Stevens-Simon C, Fullar S, McAnarney ER. Tangible differences between adolescent-oriented and adult-oriented prenatal care. *J Adolesc Health* 1992;13:300.
59. Lubarsky SL, Schiff E, Friedman SA, et al. Obstetric characteristics among nulliparas under age 15. *Obstet Gynecol* 1994;84:365.
60. Panzarine S, Slater E, Sharps P. Coping, social support and depressive symptoms in adolescent mothers. *J Adolesc Health* 1995;17:113.
61. Barnet B, Duggan AK, Wilson MD, Joffe A. Association between postpartum substance use and depressive symptoms, stress, and social support in adolescent mothers. *Pediatrics* 1995;96:659.
62. Ahn N. Teenage childbearing and high school completion: accounting for individual heterogeneity. *Fam Plann Perspect* 1994;26:17.
63. Centers for Disease Control. Pregnant adolescent group for education and support—Illinois. *MMWR* 1987;36:549.
64. Warrick L, Christianson JB, Walruff J, Cook PC. Educational outcomes in teenage pregnancy and parenting programs: results from a demonstration. *Fam Plann Perspect* 1993;25:148.
65. Stevens-Simon C, O'Connor P, Bassford K. Incentives enhance postpartum compliance among adolescent prenatal patients. *J Adolesc Health* 1994;15:396.
66. McAnarney ER, Lawrence RA, Ricciuti HN, et al. Interactions of adolescent mothers and their 1-year-old children. *Pediatrics* 1986;78:585.
67. Pope SK, Whiteside L, Brooks-Gunn J, et al. Low birth weight infants born to adolescent mothers: effects of coresidency with grandmother on child development. *JAMA* 1993;269:1399.
68. Rivara FP, Sweeney PJ, Henderson BF. Black teenage fathers: what happens when the child is born? *Pediatrics* 1986;78:151.
69. Cox JE, Bithoney WG. Fathers of children born to adolescent mothers: predictors of contact with their children at 2 years. *Arch Pediatr Adolesc Med* 1995;149:962.

70. Ford K. Second pregnancies among teenage mothers. *Fam Plann Perspect* 1983;15:268.
71. Kalmuss DS, Namerow PB. Subsequent childbearing among teenage mothers: the determinants of a closely spaced second birth. *Fam Plann Perspect* 1994;26:153.
72. Linares LO, Leadbeater BJ, Jaffe L, et al. Predictors of repeat pregnancy outcomes among black and Puerto Rican adolescent mothers. *Dev Behav Pediatr* 1992;13:93.
73. Maynard R, Rangarajan A. Contraceptive use and repeat pregnancies among welfare-dependent teenage mothers. *Fam Plann Perspect* 1994;26:198.
74. Furstenberg FF, Brooks-Gunn J, Morgan SP. Adolescent mothers and their children in later life. *Fam Plann Perspect* 1987;19.142.
75. Centers for Disease Control and Prevention. Abortion surveillance: preliminary data—United States, 1994. *MMWR* 1997;45:1123.
76. *Facts in brief: abortion in the United States.* New York, Washington: The Alan Guttmacher Institute 1994.
77. Henshaw SK, Kost K. Abortion patients in 1994–1995: characteristics and contraceptive use. *Fam Plann Perspect* 1996;28:140.
78. Centers for Disease Control and Prevention. Abortion surveillance—United States, 1991. *MMWR* 1995;44(SS-2):23.
79. Henshaw SK, Van Vort J. Abortion services in the United States, 1991 and 1992. *Fam Plann Perspect* 1994;26:140.
80. Lawson HW, Frye A, Atrash HK, et al. Abortion mortality, United States, 1972 through 1987. *Am J Obstet Gynecol* 1994;171:1365.
81. Frye AA, Atrash HK, Lawson HW, McKay T. Induced abortion in the United States: a 1994 update. *J Am Med Wom Assoc* 1994;49:131–136.
82. Darj E, Stralin EB. The prophylactic effect of doxycycline on postoperative infection rate after first-trimester abortion. *Obstet Gynecol* 1987;70:755.
83. Kaunitz AM, Grimes DA. First-trimester abortion technology. In: Corson SL, Derman RJ, Tyrer LB, eds. *Fertility control.* Boston: Little, Brown, 1985;63.
84. Harlap S, Shiono P, Ramcharan S, et al. A prospective study of spontaneous fetal losses after induced abortions. *N Engl J Med* 1979;301:677.
85. Atrash HK, Strauss LT, Kendrick JS, et al. The relation between induced abortion and ectopic pregnancy. *Obstet Gynecol* 1997;89:512.
86. Levin AA, Schoenbaum SC, Monson RR, et al. Association of induced abortion with subsequent pregnancy loss. *JAMA* 1980;243:2495.
87. Heisterberg L, Hebjorn S, Andersen LF, Petersen H. Sequelae of induced first-trimester abortion: a prospective study assessing the role of postabortal pelvic inflammatory disease and prophylactic antibiotics. *Am J Obstet Gynecol* 1986;155:76.
88. Grimes DA, Mishell DR, Shoupe D, Lacarra M. Early abortion with a single dose of the antiprogestin RU-486. *Obstet Gynecol* 1988;158:1307.
89. Couzinet B, LeStrat N, Ulmann A, et al. Termination of early pregnancy by the progesterone antagonist RU 486 (mifepristone). *N Engl J Med* 1986;315:1565.
90. El-Refaey H, Dhamnasekar R, Abdalla M, et al. Induction of abortion with mifepristone (RU 486) and oral or vaginal misoprostol. *N Engl J* Med 1995;332:983.
91. Grimes DA. Medical abortion in early pregnancy: a review of the evidence. *Obstet Gynecol* 1997; 89:790.
92. Hausknecht RU. Methotrexate and misoprostol to terminate early pregnancy. *N Engl J Med* 1995;333:537.
93. Methotrexate and misoprostol for abortion. *Med Lett* 1996;38:39.
94. Koopersmith TB, Mishell DR. The use of misoprostol for termination of early pregnancy. *Contraception* 1996;53:237.
95. Stubblefield PG. Induced abortion in the mid-trimester. In: Corson SL, Derman RJ, Tyrer LB, eds. *Fertility control.* Boston: Little, Brown, 1985;77.
96. Wilcox AJ, Weinberg CR, O'Connor JF, et al. Incidence of early loss of pregnancy. *N Engl J Med* 1988;319:189.
97. Marchbanks RA, Annegers JF, Coulam CB, et al. Risk factors for ectopic pregnancy: a population-based study. *JAMA* 1988;259:1823.
98. Sauer MV. New methods for diagnosis and management of ectopic pregnancy. *Resid Staff Phys* 1987;33:39.
99. Goldner TE, Lawson HW, Xia Z, et al. Surveillance for ectopic pregnancy—United States, 1970–1979. *MMWR CEC Surveill Summ* 1993;42:73.

100. Atrash HK, Friede A, Hogue CJ. Ectopic pregnancy mortality in the United States, 1980–1983. *Obstet Gynecol* 1987;80:817.
101. Kim DS, Chung SR, Park MI, et al. Comparative review of diagnostic accuracy in tubal pregnancy: a 14-year survey of 1040 cases. *Obstet Gynecol* 1987;70:547.
102. DeCrespigny LC. Early diagnosis of pregnancy failure with transvaginal ultrasound. *Am J Obstet Gynecol* 1988;159:408.
103. Leach RE, Ory SJ. Modern management of ectopic pregnancy. *J Reprod Med* 1989;34:324.
104. David AJ, O'Boyle EA, Reindollar RH. Human chorionic gonadotropin in pediatric and adolescent gynecology. *Adolesc Pediatr Gynecol* 1989;1:207.
105. Matthews CP, Coulson PB, Wild RA. Serum progesterone levels as an aid in the diagnosis of ectopic pregnancy. *Obstet Gynecol* 1986;68:390–392.
106. Daily CA, Laurent SL, Nunley WC. The prognostic value of serum progesterone and quantitative human chorionic gonadotropin in early human pregnancy. *Am J Obstet Gynecol* 1994;171:380–384.
107. Ammerman S, Shafer M, Snyder D. Ectopic pregnancy in adolescents: a clinical review for pediatricians. *J Pediatr* 1990;117:677.
108. Hatcher RA, Trussett J, Stewart F, et al. *Contraceptive technology,* 16th ed. New York: Irvington Publishers, 1994.
109. Kadar N, Burton VC, Romero R. A method of screening for ectopic pregnancy and its indications. *Obstet Gynecol* 1981;58:162.
110. Cartwright PS, DiPietro DL. Ectopic pregnancy: changes in serum human chorionic gonadotropin concentration. *Obstet Gynecol* 1984;63:76.
111. Shepherd RW, Patton PE, Novy MJ, Burry KA. Serial β-hCG measurements in the early detection of ectopic pregnancy. *Obstet Gynecol* 1990;75:417.
112. Bateman BG, Nunley WC, Kolp LA, et al. Vaginal sonography findings and hCG dynamics of early intrauterine and tubal pregnancies. *Obstet Gynecol* 1990;75:421.
113. Fossum GT, Davajan V, Kletzky OA. Early detection of pregnancy with transvaginal ultrasound. *Fertil Steril* 1988;49:788
114. Yao M, Twandi T. Current status of surgical and nonsurgical management of ectopic pregnancy. *Fertil Steril* 1997;67:421.
115. Ory SJ. New options for diagnosis and treatment of ectopic pregnancy. *JAMA* 1992;267:534.
116. Carson SA, Buster JE. Ectopic pregnancy. *N Engl J Med* 1993;329:1174.
117. Sauer MV. Nonsurgical management of unruptured ectopic pregnancy: an extended clinical trial. *Fertil Steril* 1987;48:752.
118. Stovall TG, Ling FW, Gray LA, et al. Methotrexate treatment of unruptured ectopic pregnancy: a report of 100 cases. *Obstet Gynecol* 1991;77:749.
119. Pansky M, Golan A, Bukovsky I, Caspi E. Nonsurgical management of tubal pregnancy: necessity in view of the changing clinical appearance. *Am J Obstet Gynecol* 1991;164:888.
120. Stovall TG, Ling FW. Single-dose methotrexate: an expanded clinical trial. *Am J Obstet Gynecol* 1993;168:1759.
121. Fernandez H, Bourget P, Ville Y, et al. Treatment of unruptured tubal pregnancy with methotrexate: pharmokinetic analysis of local versus intramuscular administration. *Fertil Steril* 1994;62:943.
122. Fernandez H, Rainhorm JD, Papiernik E, et al. Spontaneous resolution of ectopic pregnancy. *Obstet Gynecol* 1988;71:717.
123. McCord ML, Muram D, et al. Methotrexate therapy for ectopic pregnancy in adolescents. *J Pediatr Adolesc Gynecol* 1996;9:71.
124. Berkowitz RS, Goldstein DP. Chorionic tumors. *N Engl J Med* 1996;335:1740.
125. Yeko TR, Gorrill MJ, Hughes LH, et al. Timely diagnosis of early ectopic pregnancy using a single blood progesterone measurement. *Fertil Steril* 1987;48:1048.
126. *Management of gestational trophoblastic disease.* ACOG Technical Bulletin 178. Washington, DC: American College of Obstetricians and Gynecologists, 1993.
127. Goldstein DP, Berkowitz RS. Current management of complete and partial molar pregnancy. *J Reprod Med* 1994;39:139.
128. *Prevention of D isoimmunization.* ACOG Technical Bulletin 147. Washington, DC: American College of Obstetricians and Gynecologists, 1990.
129. Jones EF, Forrest JD, Goldman N, et al. *Teenage pregnancy in industrialized countries.* New Haven, CT: Yale University Press, 1986.
130. McAnarney ER, Hendee WR. The prevention of adolescent pregnancy. *JAMA* 1989;262:78.

131. Howard M, McCabe JB. Helping teenagers postpone sexual involvement. *Fam Plann Perspect* 1990;22:21.
132. Frost H, Howard, Howard M, McCabe JB. An information and skills approach for younger teens: postponing sexual involvement program. In: Miller BC, et al, eds. *Preventing adolescent pregnancy*. Newbury Park, CA: Sage Publications, 1992:83–109.
133. Grimes DA. Unplanned pregnancies in the United States. *Obstet Gynecol* 1986;67:438.
134. Barth RP. *Reducing the risk: building skills to prevent pregnancy, STD, and HIV,* 2nd ed. Santa Cruz, CA: ETR Associates, 1993.
135. Adolescent pregnancy prevention programs. *The Contraception Report* 1994;5:10.
136. Zabin LS, Hirsch MB, Smith EA, et al. Evaluation of a pregnancy prevention program for urban teenagers. *Fam Plann Perspect* 1986;18:119.
137. Zabin LS, Hirsch MB, Streett R, et al. The Baltimore pregnancy prevention program for urban teenagers I: how did it work? *Fam Plann Perspect* 1988;20:182.
138. Zabin LS, Hirsch MB, Smith EA. The Baltimore pregnancy prevention program for urban teenagers II: what did it cost? *Fam Plann Perspect* 1988;20:188.
139. Dryfoos JG. School-based health clinics: three years of experience. *Fam Plann Perspect* 1988;20:193.
140. Kirby D, Resnich MD, Downes B, et al. The effects of school-based health clinics in St. Paul on school-wide birthrates. *Fam Plann Perspect* 1993;25:16.
141. Kirby D, Waszak C, Ziegler J. Six school-based clinics: their reproductive health services and impact on sexual behavior. *Fam Plann Perspect* 1991;23:16.
142. Sauer MV, Vermesh M, Anderson RE, et al. Rapid measurement of urinary pregnanediol glucuronide to diagnose ectopic pregnancy. *Am J Obstet Gynecol* 1988;159:1531.
143. Stevens-Simon C, Boyle C. Gravid students: characteristics of nongravid classmates who react with positive and negative feelings about conception. *Arch Pediatr Adolesc Med* 1995;149:272–275.
144. Vincent ML, Clearie AF, Schluchter MD. Reducing adolescent pregnancy through school and community-based education. *JAMA* 1987;257:3382.
145. Koo HP, Dunteman GH, George C, et al. Reducing adolescent pregnancy through a school- and community-based intervention: Denmark, South Carolina, revisited. *Fam Plann Perspect* 1994;26:206–217.
146. Stevens-Simons C, Dolgan IJ, Kelly L, et al. The effect of monetary incentives and peer support on repeat adolescent pregnancies. *JAMA* 1997;277:977.
147. Kirby D, Korpi M, Barth RP, et al. The impact of the postponing sexual involvement curriculum among youths in California. *Fam Plann Perspect* 1997;29:100.
148. Card BJ, Niego S, Mallari A, Farrell WS. The Program Archive on Sexuality, Health, and Adolescence: promising "prevention programs in a box." *Fam Plann Perspect* 1996;28:210.

FURTHER READING

American Academy of Pediatrics Committee on Adolescence. The adolescent's right to confidential care when considering abortion. *Pediatrics* 1996;97:746.

Brown SS, Eisenberg L. *The best intentions: unintended pregnancy and the well-being of children and families*. Washington, DC: National Academy Press, 1995.

Kaufman RB, Spitz AM, Strauss LT, et al. The decline of U.S. teen pregnancy rates, 1990–1995. *Pediatrics* 1998;102:1141.

Moore KA, Driscoll AK, Lindberg LD. A statistical portrait of adolescent sex, contraception, and childbearing. Washington DC: National Campaign to Prevent Teen Pregnancy, 1998. (www.teenpregnancy.org).

U.S. Department of Health and Human Services, Public Health Service, National Center for Health Statistics. *Report to Congress on out-of wedlock childbearing.* Hyattsville, MD: Department of Health and Human Services, 1995. DHHS publication PHS 95-1257.

19

Gynecologic Issues in Young Women with Chronic Diseases

Tremendous medical advances have improved the quality of life of patients with chronic disease as well as their life expectancies. This chapter focuses on gynecologic health issues for these young women, including pubertal development, menstrual function, fertility, and pregnancy. Contraception is discussed in Chapter 17.

CANCER

Advances in diagnosis and therapies have greatly enhanced the life expectancy of children and adolescents with malignancies. While the cancers themselves may have an impact on reproductive function, the treatment-specific therapies (chemotherapy and radiation) have produced the major long-term sequelae (1).

Pubertal Development and Menstrual Function

Radiation therapy can result in permanent ovarian damage and ovarian failure. In a study of long-term survivors of childhood malignancies, Stillman and colleagues (2) reported that ovarian failure occurred in 68% of patients with both ovaries within the radiation field, in 14% whose ovaries were at the edge of the treatment beam, and in none with one or both ovaries outside the field. Ovarian function is directly related to the dose of radiation and the age of the patient at the time of treatment (3–5). The median lethal dose (LD_{50}) for the human oocyte has been estimated to be approximately 400 rad. A single dose of 250 to 500 rad results in menstrual irregularities in all women; up to 60% to 70% of women 15 to 40 years of age and 100% of women >40 years will be permanently sterilized (Fig. 1). Women aged 20 to 30 years can tolerate 2000 rad fractionated over 5 to 6 weeks with less risk of sterility than women >40 years, in whom 600 rad will

Ovarian dose (rads)	Results
60	No deleterious effect
150	No deleterious effect in young women; some risk for sterilization women older than 40
250–500	In women aged 15 to 40, 60% permanently sterilized; remainder may suffer temporary amenorrhea. In women older than 40, 100% permanently sterilized
500–800	In women aged 15 to 40, 60% to 70% permanently sterilized; remainder may experience temporary amenorrhea. No data available for women over 40
>800	100% permanently sterilized

FIG. 1. Effects of ionizing radiation on ovarian function. (From Damewood MD. What factors underlie premature ovarian failure? *Contemp Obstet Gynecol* 1990:31; with permission.)

induce menopause (6–8). Thus, children and adolescents have a better prognosis for preservation of reproductive function than women >40 years of age (3,6).

Radiation to areas outside the pelvis can also affect reproductive function. Dysfunction of the hypothalamic–pituitary axis resulting in hypogonadotropic amenorrhea is a common sequela of cranial tumors treated with surgery and/or radiation. Hall and colleagues (9) administered a physiologic replacement regimen of exogenous gonadotropin-releasing hormone (GnRH) to survivors of brain tumors, based on the hypothesis that the defect would be hypothalamic rather than pituitary in origin. Ovulation occurred in 78% of the nine patients. Hyperprolactinemia may also occur secondary to whole-brain irradiation for brain tumors. Early and precocious puberty may occur in girls who received hypothalamic–pituitary radiation for acute lymphoblastic leukemia (10). Radiation to the neck can result in hypothyroidism in as many as one-third to one-half of patients who received doses >3500 cGy, resulting in delayed maturation and poor linear growth if undiagnosed (11) (see Chapter 6).

Chemotherapeutic agents affect ovarian function and fertility in a dose-dependent fashion. The marked cytotoxicity of most anticancer drugs, in particular the alkylating agents, can have adverse affects on reproductive potential. Cytotoxic agents produce azoospermia and compromised Leydig cell function in males and perifollicular agenesis progressing to premature ovarian failure in females. Chemotherapeutic agents that have been associated with premature ovarian failure in adults include cyclophosphamide, chlorambucil, busulfan, and melphalan (L-PAM), and the combination regimens MOPP (mechlorethamine, vincristine, procarbazine, and prednisone), MVPP (nitrogen mustard, vinblastine, procarbazine, and prednisolone), and ChlVPP/EVA (chlorambucil, vinblastine, prednisolone, procarbazine, doxorubicin, and etoposide) (2–4,12–14).

The severity of gonadal dysfunction is a function of the chemotherapeutic regime and total dose in both sexes, as well as the age of the patient at the time of therapy (15,16) (Fig. 2). Children and adolescents appear more resistant to the deleterious effects of these agents, although long-term effects have not been fully assessed. In a review of 30 studies that evaluated patients who had received chemotherapy for renal disease (cyclophosphamide), Hodgkin's disease, or acute lymphocytic leukemia, Rivkees and Crawford (13) concluded that chemotherapy-induced damage was more likely to occur in sexually mature females and with higher doses of alkylating agents. They found gonadal dysfunction at followup in none of the girls given cyclophosphamide during prepuberty and mid-

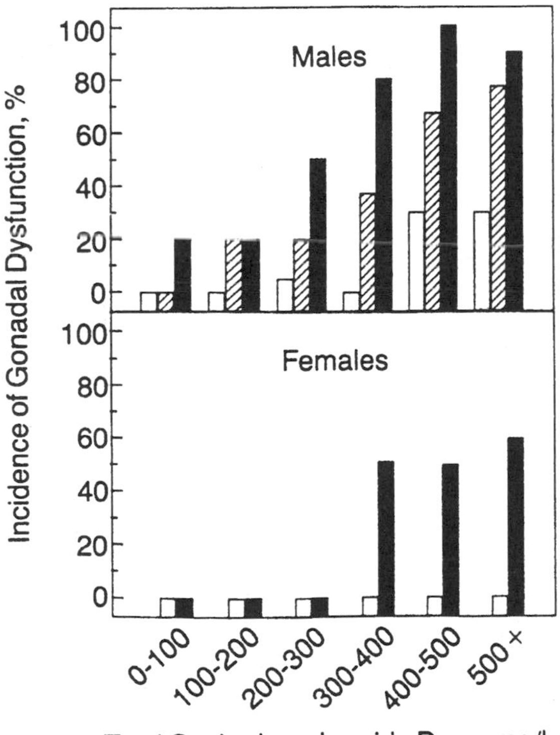

FIG. 2. Incidence of chemotherapy-induced gonadal dysfunction as related to pubertal stage during therapy and total dose of cyclophosphamide administered for treatment of renal disease. *Open bars* indicate prepubertal; *slashed bars,* midpubertal; and *solid bars,* sexually mature. Midpubertal females are not included due to insufficient data. (From Rivkees SA, Crawford JD. The relationship of gonadal activity and chemotherapy-induced gonadal damage. *JAMA* 1988;259: 2123; with permission.)

puberty compared with 58% of those who were sexually mature. For Hodgkin's disease, 7% of those treated in midpuberty and 71% of the sexually mature had gonadal dysfunction. For leukemia, the percentages were 10% for those treated before puberty, 36% for midpuberty, and 22% for those sexually mature. For cyclophosphamide, a dose of 5.2 g is associated with amenorrhea in women >40 years, whereas a dose of 20.4 g is associated with the same effect in women 20 to 29 years of age (17). Even in girls who appear to go through a normal or early puberty, prior chemotherapy for acute lymphocytic leukemia can result in elevated follicle-stimulating hormone levels and decreased plasma inhibin levels, despite normal plasma estradiol levels (18,19).

The combination of chemotherapy and radiation therapy, especially in Hodgkin's disease, often significantly impairs ovarian function. Patients <30 years of age have the best chance for recovery of ovarian function (20). In a long-term followup study of 92 girls treated for Hodgkin's disease at age ≥15 years, 87% had normal menstrual function: 83% following pelvic irradiation, 94% following chemotherapy, and 67% following combined modality treatment (21). None of the girls who had subtotal lymphoid irradiation alone (mantle or spade field) or those who received three cycles or less of MOPP developed ovarian failure. Among 1067 5-year cancer survivors with disease diagnosed at 13 to 19 years of age and still menstruating at age 21, Byrne and associates (22) noted the

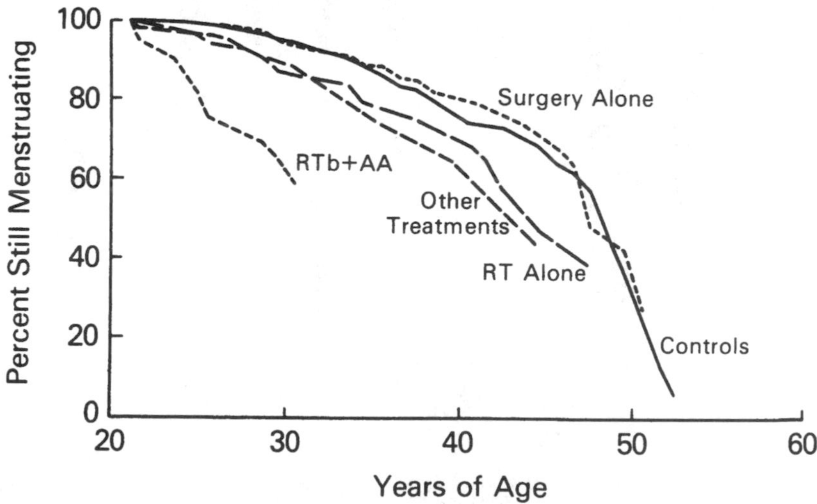

FIG. 3. Proportion still menstruating among cancer survivors diagnosed between ages 13 and 19 years grouped by type of treatment received compared with proportion of controls still menstruating (Kaplan-Meier curves). Survivor and control cohorts only (RTb + AA, radiotherapy below diaphragm plus alkylating agents; RT, radiotherapy). (From Byrne J, Fears TR, Gail MH. Early menopause in long-term survivors of cancer during adolescence. *Am J Obstet Gynecol* 1992;166:788; with permission.)

risk of early menopause was four times greater than that of control women 21 to 25 years of age (Fig. 3). The relative risk (RR) for early menopause was increased with radiation treatment alone (RR: 3.7; 95% confidence interval [CI]: 1.3,10.0), with alkylators alone (RR: 9.2; 95% CI: 2.7, 31.5), and combined modality of radiation below the diaphragm and alkylating agents (RR: 27.4; 95% CI: 12.4, 60.4), when compared to controls. It is thus important to counsel long-term cancer survivors that, even if they have regular menses and ovulatory function, they may undergo a premature menopause and they should consider not delaying pregnancies.

Although bone marrow transplantation (BMT) has been life saving in girls with advanced cancer, as well as for those with metabolic and hematologic diseases, significant gonadal damage may result from preconditioning therapies (23–29). Spinelli and colleagues (25) calculated that among 79 females undergoing allogeneic BMT with total body irradiation, the actuarial chance of having a menstrual period at 10 years after BMT was 43%. Four of five girls who received BMT in the premenarcheal age started menses. Immediately after BMT, all adult women had clinical evidence of ovarian insufficiency. Ten (13.5%) of 74 postmenarcheal women showed ovarian recovery ranging from 21 to 87 months. Patients <18 years of age had a much better prognosis than those >18 years. In a study of 44 postpubertal women after allogeneic BMT, Schubert and coworkers (27) reported that 80% (35/44) had reduced vaginal elasticity and rugal folds, small vaginal, uterine, and cervical size, atrophic vulvovaginitis, introital stenosis, and/or loss of pubic hair. Even prepubertal girls treated with BMT for sickle cell disease or thalassemia and given standard preconditioning therapies may have significant gonadal damage (24,28,29).

Cancer survivors are also at risk for the development of a second malignancy, often 10 years or more after completion of therapy for the primary neoplasm (30–33). The Late Effects Study Group (34) followed a cohort of 1380 children with Hodgkin's disease and found 88 second neoplasms compared with 4.4 expected in the general population: 56 had solid cancers, 26 had leukemia, and 6 had non-Hodgkin's lymphoma. The estimated actuarial incidence of a second neoplasm 15 years after the diagnosis of Hodgkin's disease was 7.0% (95% CI: 5.2, 8.8%); the incidence of solid tumors was 3.9% (95% CI: 2.3, 5.5%). Breast cancer was the most common solid tumor, with an estimated actuarial incidence in women that approached 35% (95% CI: 17.4, 52.6%) by age 40 years. Older age (10 to 16 years vs. <10 years) at the time of radiation treatment (RR: 1.9) and a higher dose (2000 to 4000 vs. <2000 cGy) of radiation (RR: 5.9) were associated with a significantly increased risk of breast cancer. High cure rates should continue to be the essential priority in the management of childhood Hodgkin's disease; however, better strategies need to be developed to maintain lifelong followup of treated patients in order to minimize their risks from any of these treatment modalities (35).

Adolescents with impaired or absent ovarian function may experience no secondary sexual development or may have some development and subsequently present with primary or secondary amenorrhea. Replacement therapy with estrogen and progestin can provide normal secondary sexual development (see Chapter 6).

Young women newly diagnosed with a malignancy may experience a spectrum of menstrual disorders. Adolescents with leukemia and thrombocytopenia may present with heavy or prolonged menses. Menarcheal females undergoing treatments for active disease may experience significant bone marrow suppression that may also lead to severe dysfunctional uterine bleeding. Once pathology is excluded, an oral contraceptive (OC) can be prescribed in a continuous fashion using packages containing 21 days of active pills (and no placebos). OCs are continued until the platelet count is >50,000/mm^3 (36) and it is deemed safe for the patient to have menses. At this point, these girls can be changed to cyclic therapy with a low-dose progestin-dominant OC. Medroxyprogesterone acetate (e.g., Provera, Cycrin) 10 mg (tapered to 5 mg) daily has been used in some centers to induce amenorrhea for months and even years, but breakthrough bleeding is common (36,37). Patients who have weight loss with resultant hypothalamic amenorrhea from radiation or chemotherapy may not require hormonal therapy during the time interval of thrombocytopenia.

Because of the problems associated with cancer treatments, investigators have looked toward preventive measures. Several procedures have been proposed to lessen the exposure of the ovaries to radiation, including ovarian suspension (also termed "transposition of the ovaries" or "oophoropexy"). The ovaries are shielded or moved out of the radiation field. In a study of Hodgkin's disease, none of the girls treated with pelvic radiation without oophoropexy maintained ovarian function (21). For those with optimal oophoropexy, the

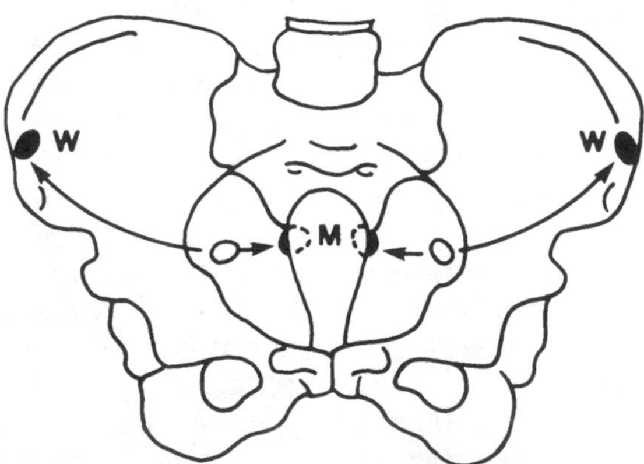

FIG. 4. Oophoropexy sites (M, medial displacement; W, wide lateral displacement). (From Damewood MD. What factors underlie premature ovarian failure? *Contemp Obstet Gynecol* 1990:31; with permission.)

ovarian doses ranged between 6% and 14% (38). Thibaud and colleagues (6) studied 18 girls (12 prepubertal and 6 postmenarcheal) who had ovarian transposition (15 bilateral, 3 unilateral) before external-beam irradiation (11 patients) or vaginal implants (7 patients). At a mean followup of 8.6 ± 0.9 years after ovarian transposition, 16 had menstruated and two remained amenorrheic. Ovulation was documented in seven, and two pregnancies had occurred. Complications of the ovarian transposition in four patients included intestinal occlusion, dyspareunia, and pelvic adhesions with tubal obstruction. The ovary may be pexed to different locations depending on the planned radiation field. Historically, oophoropexy for Hodgkin's disease utilized medial transposition, in which the ovary is mobilized on a vascular pedicle and placed medially by

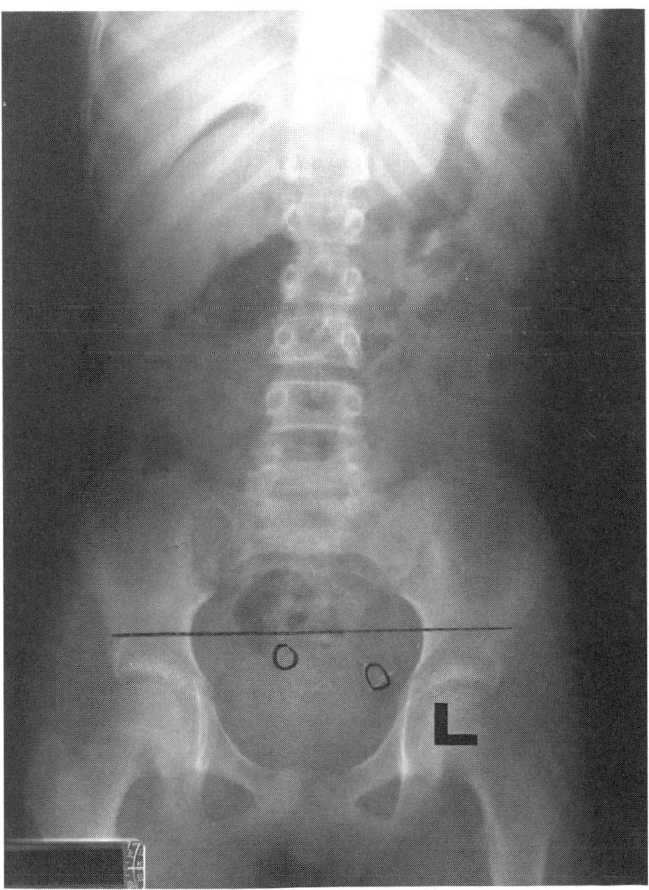

FIG. 5. Postoperative KUB film showing the location of the right ovary and the pexed left (*L*) ovary, with demonstration of the radiation beam edge. (From Laufer MR, Billett AL, Diller L, et al. A new technique for laparoscopic prophylactic oophoropexy before craniospinal irradiation in children with medulloblastoma. *Adolesc Pediatr Gynecol* 1995;8:81; with permission.)

suturing it to the serosal surface of the uterus (8,39) (Fig. 4). Recently, Hadar and Loven (40) reported using the lateral transposition approach for Hodgkin's patients, in which the ovary and its vascular pedicle are placed retroperitoneally by suturing the ovary to the peritoneum lateral to the colon and superior to the iliac crest (Fig. 4). Laufer and associates (41) described an outpatient laparoscopic technique for oophoropexy with marking of both ovaries with titanium clips in order to calculate the radiation dose to each ovary (Fig. 5). The right ovary was marked and the left ovary was attached to the anterior peritoneum, both with 4.8-mm titanium staples (Fig. 6). All patients underwent craniospinal irradiation for medulloblastoma after recovery from the oophoropexy. The authors calculated that if the pexed ovary is moved 2 cm outside of a megavoltage radiation beam, the dosage is reduced to <5% of the total exposed dose. To date, two girls in their series of three (ages 5, 7, and 9 years at the time of the procedure) have reported the onset of normal puberty.

To prevent the detrimental effects of chemotherapy on ovarian function, several hormonal therapies have been investigated. The potential for preserving reproductive function through the suppression of ovarian activity using OCs is not well studied. Chapman and Sutcliffe (42) reported in 1981 ovarian function to be normal in five women treated for Hodgkin's disease who were concomitantly treated with OCs. Use of a long-acting GnRH agonist to induce amenorrhea prior to the

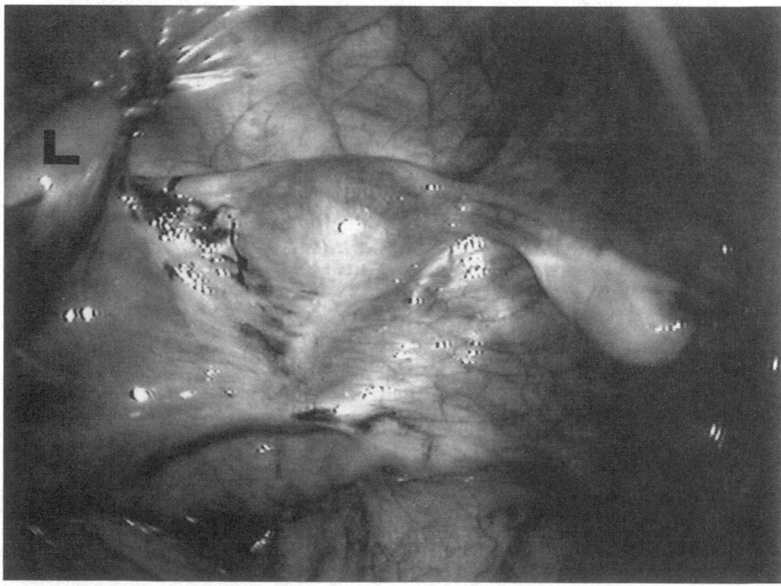

FIG. 6. Postoophoropexy showing the location of the right ovary and the pexed left (L) ovary. (From Laufer MR, Billett AL, Diller L, et al. A new technique for laparoscopic prophylactic oophoropexy before craniospinal irradiation in children with medulloblastoma. *Adolesc Pediatr Gynecol* 1995;8:81; with permission.)

chemotherapy is an option for controlling menstrual bleeding and possibly preserving ovarian function (43). GnRH agonists produce an initial increase in gonadotropins and gonadotropic steroids that is followed in approximately 3 weeks by suppression of the gonadotropins and their associated steroids and a resulting menstrual period; GnRH agonists are thus initiated at least 3 to 4 weeks before conditioning therapy for BMT (44). If a GnRH "antagonist" was commercially available, immediate suppression of the gonadotropins and their steroids would result, avoiding this initial surge that can produce significant vaginal bleeding (36). To maintain suppression after BMT, U.S. Food and Drug Administration–approved methods of administration (subcutaneous, intranasal, and intramuscular) may not be advisable in a neutropenic and thrombocytopenic patient. The use of intravenous leuprolide acetate for patients in these restricted states is under investigation. In small studies (44,45), intravenous therapy appears to be a safe alternative in which a 1-mg per day dose is given as a rapid intravenous bolus.

Fertility and Pregnancy

In a large National Cancer Institute study of 2283 adult survivors of childhood and adolescent cancer (diagnosed in the period 1945 to 1975) that included both sexes and a variety of treatment agents (46), the overall crude relative fertility of survivors of cancer as compared with their sibling controls was 0.88. The male survivors had a greater fertility deficit than the female survivors (relative fertility: 0.83 vs. 0.94, respectively) (Fig. 7). Treatment effects were pronounced, with increased infertility in those treated with a combination of radiation and alkylating agents (1). Other studies have also found increased infertility (47).

Lacher and Toner (48) found better fertility rates and better pregnancy outcomes in patients with Hodgkin's disease treated with a limited field of radiation and chemotherapy with thiotepa, vinblastine, vincristine, procarbazine, and prednisone, when compared with the results published in the Horning et al (20) review of 103 women treated with multiple modalities of chemotherapy with or without total body irradiation after oophoropexy.

For adolescents who are already pubertal and in whom the potential for permanent gonadal failure from therapy exists, the cryopreservation of nonfertilized oocytes is now a possibility (49,50,51). In addition to the utilization of current assisted reproductive techniques, donor- or partner-inseminated oocytes can be cryopreserved as embryos for later implantation and gestation.

For those cancer survivors who retain their fertility after treatment excluding those who have received direct pelvic high-dose radiation, complications of pregnancy, spontaneous abortions, or congenital abnormalities are not increased compared to pregnancies in the general population (3,47,52,53). The health of offspring of childhood survivors of cancer is usually normal (1,39,47,54,55). However, in a study of 202 pregnancies in 100 survivors, 2 of 20 offspring born to eight women treated with dactinomycin had structural cardiac defects: a ventricular septal defect and a tetralogy of Fallot (55). Although these data are not

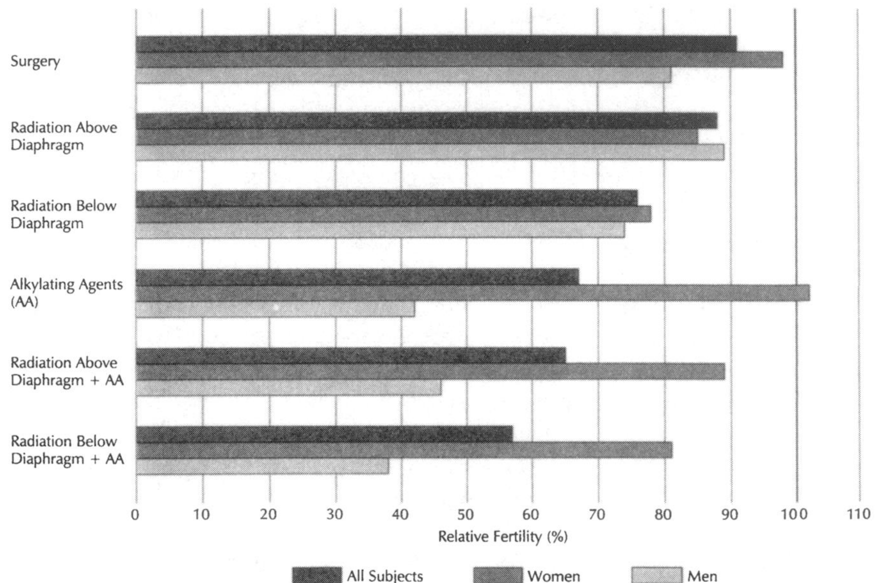

FIG. 7. Association between treatment of childhood cancer and subsequent loss of fertility was explored in 2283 cancer survivors who had undergone various therapies. Each treatment impaired fertility: surgery least of all, and radiation less than alkylating agents. Most deleterious were combinations of radiation and alkylating agents. The effect of the drugs was most pronounced in men. In contrast, radiotherapy affected both sexes more or less equally. Relative fertility was the frequency of a first pregnancy achieved by married couples in which one partner was a survivor of childhood cancer, compared with the frequency achieved in marriages by sibling controls (with adjustment for years of marriage and age at marriage). The study was done by Julianne Byrne of the National Cancer Institute and colleagues at five U.S. cancer centers. In order to quantify the unsuspected consequences of cancer therapy, subjects were excluded if they did not want children or knew they were sterile. (From Meadows AT. Follow-up and care of childhood cancer survivors. *Hosp Pract* 1991;26:99; with permission.)

conclusive, given the small numbers, fetal echocardiogram may be useful in screening those mothers who have been treated with dactinomycin.

Iodohippurate sodium ^{131}I in standard doses of 250 mCi to treat thyroid cancer 1 year or more before conception is not associated with any long-term risks (56). Two children born to mothers treated in pregnancy or 6 months before conception showed fetal brain deformities. Most health care providers now recommend waiting 1 year after therapy before women become pregnant.

Survivors of Wilms' tumor who had received abdominal radiation therapy have been noted to have an eightfold RR for perinatal mortality and a fourfold RR of low birth weight in their offspring (57). Among the survivors of Wilms' tumor who were included in the Five Center Study (58), women had four times more adverse pregnancy outcomes (defined as miscarriage, preterm delivery, or infants with birth defects) than did controls. Radiation-induced damage of the uterus may impair adequate expansion, possibly leading to premature delivery (59). The rate for malformations was not increased (1).

Data are limited on pregnancies after BMT. In a series reported by Hinterberger-Fischer and associates (60), three patients who received transplants for severe aplastic anemia (two female, one male) parented four healthy children, but offspring complications included persistence of fetal circulation, erythroblastosis fetalis, and prolonged newborn icterus. Others have reported pregnancies with successful outcomes in women following allogeneic BMT for acute leukemia (61,62). At our adult Center for Reproductive Medicine at Brigham and Women's Hospital, there are a number of BMT cancer survivors who have conceived either spontaneously or with assisted fertility methods (utilizing either their own or donor oocytes or sperm) and have had successful pregnancies.

Additional investigation with such assisted reproductive techniques as ovulation induction, ovum donation, and *in vitro* fertilization needs to be undertaken in this group of patients.

CYSTIC FIBROSIS

In the last 35 years, the life expectancy of persons with cystic fibrosis (CF) has greatly increased. National median survival was 10.6 years in 1966, 20 years in 1981, and 29.4 years in 1992. At the end of 1992, 33% of individuals with CF in the United States were 18 years of age or older (63). As a result, reproductive health needs have increased for this population.

Pubertal Development and Menstrual Function

In young women with CF, Neinstein and coworkers (64) noted a mean age of menarche of 14.4 years versus 12.9 years for controls. Adolescent girls with CF often have low weight for height and chronic pulmonary infections that may significantly delay pubertal development and menarche (64,65,66). A recent study of Swedish girls with CF found that pubertal and menarcheal delay was still present even with improved nutritional and clinical status; the mean age of peak height velocity was 12.9 ± 0.8 years and the mean age of menarche was 14.9 ± 1.4 years. Patients who were homozygous for δ F508 and those with abnormal oral glucose tolerance tests were most likely to have pubertal delay (65).

Fertility and Pregnancy

Young women with CF generally initiate sexual activity at the same age as other healthy young women but may be less likely to use contraception than control subjects (67). Pregnancies in women with CF are frequently unplanned, and some women may assume they are infertile. Most adolescents can use hormonal contraceptives successfully.

Although chronic illness and poor nutritional state may lower the fertility of an individual woman with CF (68–70), some have postulated that the thick cervical mucus (lower water content) may also be a barrier to sperm (71). A woman with CF has approximately a 1:40 chance of having an affected offspring if the carrier status of the father is unknown, and a 50% chance if the father is a heterozygote (72). There are now reports of combining *in vitro* fertilization and preimplantation diagnostic testing for CF that have resulted in normal offspring (73).

Successful pregnancies have been reported in women with CF (74–79). In a 1980 review of 119 CF centers, 129 pregnancies were reported in 100 patients (74); 97 pregnancies were completed with 86 viable infants. The mean age at delivery was 20.7 years, and 27% delivered at a gestation <37 weeks. The average maternal weight gain was <4.5 kg. Individuals with more advanced disease had a worse pregnancy course. In a review of 20 reports of 217 pregnancies in 162 women, Kent and Farquharson (75) reported that 24% were preterm and the perinatal death rate was 7.9%. Between 1986 and 1990, the annual number of pregnancies reported to the CF patient registry in the United States doubled (77). Recent studies confirm that pregnancy is well tolerated by women with mild disease but that both maternal and fetal outcomes are more guarded for those with moderate to severe disease (78). In a retrospective study of the case notes of 22 pregnancies in 20 patients with CF, the prepregnancy parameter that showed the best correlation with maternal weight gain, gestation, birth weight, and maternal survival was the forced expiratory volume in 1 second (79). Whether pregnancy adversely affects the course of disease in the mother is still unclear. Careful medical assessment of the cardiac, pulmonary, and nutritional status is important before patients undertake a planned pregnancy (77).

Other Issues

A pseudopolypoid cervical ectropion has been noted in CF patients, in both users and nonusers of OCs (80,81).

GASTROINTESTINAL DISEASE

Pubertal Development and Menstrual Function in Inflammatory Bowel Disease

Adolescents with inflammatory bowel disease (IBD) may experience growth failure and delay of puberty and menarche. Delayed growth may be the first sign of IBD, especially in Crohn's disease (Fig. 8), and may overshadow symptoms of

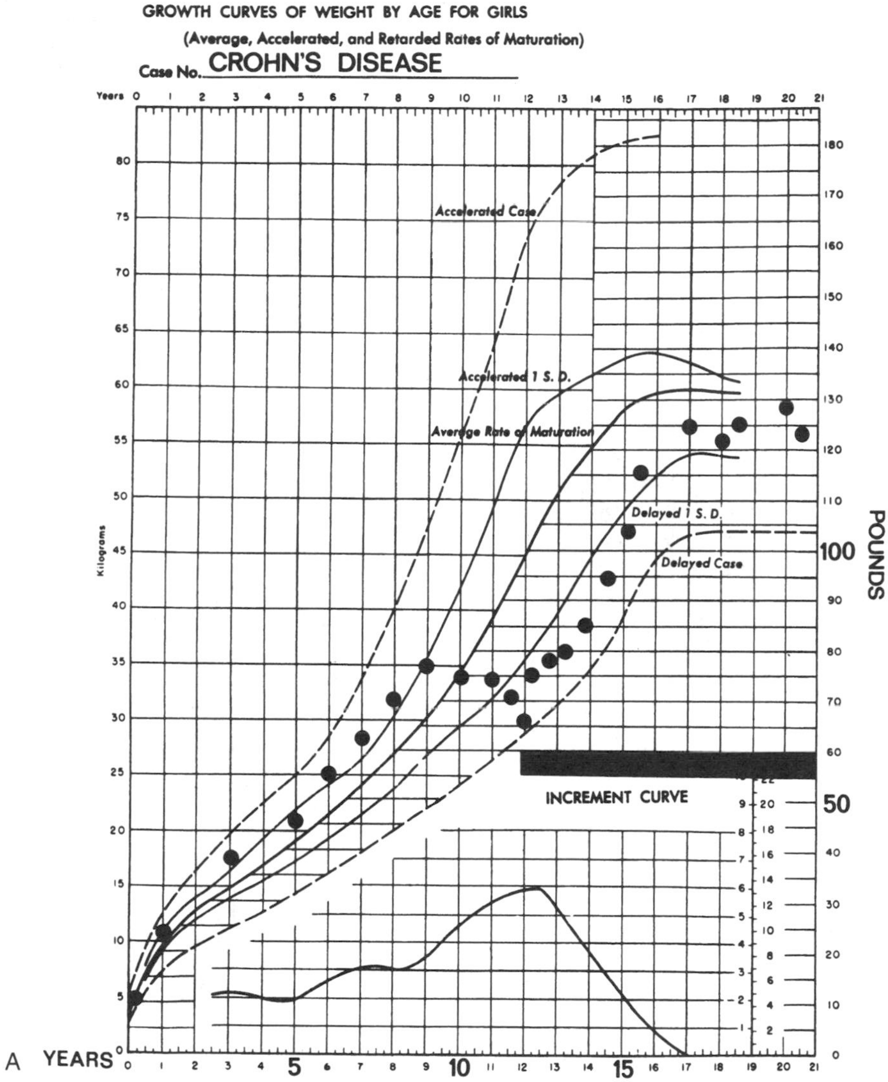

GROWTH CURVES OF WEIGHT BY AGE FOR GIRLS
(Average, Accelerated, and Retarded Rates of Maturation)
Case No. CROHN'S DISEASE

Accelerated Case
Accelerated 1 S. D.
Average Rate of Maturation
Delayed 1 S. D.
Delayed Case
INCREMENT CURVE
Kilograms
POUNDS
A YEARS

FIG. 8. Growth chart of a patient with Crohn's disease; *bar* represents treatment with prednisone. **(A)** Weight.

the gastrointestinal dysfunction. In girls with IBD, gonadotropin and estrogen levels are low, implying a depressed hypothalamic–pituitary axis. Nutritional and medical therapy, and sometimes surgery to treat active bowel disease, are important to ensure normal pubertal growth and development and regular menses. Although excess corticosteroids may impair growth, when the illness is adequately treated, the patient often has a growth spurt (70).

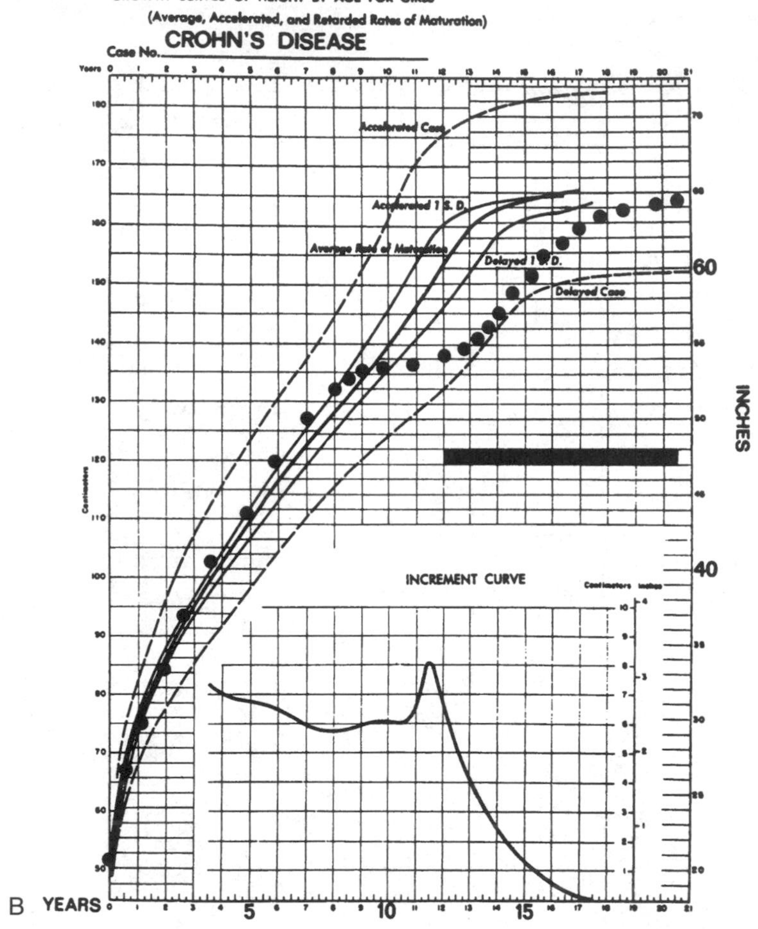

FIG. 8. *Continued.* **(B)** Height.

Fertility and Pregnancy in IBD

Several studies have suggested subfertility in women with IBD (82,83); however, many of these reports failed to adjust for factors such as smoking, age, or whether the patient was attempting to conceive. A woman's fertility does not appear to be affected by the presence of ulcerative colitis; 90% of patients with this disorder will be able to conceive if pregnancy is desired (83,84). There are conflicting data regarding fertility in women with Crohn's disease, with factors such as lack of a desire for intercourse, occlusion of fallopian tubes, and perineal fistula affecting conception rates (85,86). Diagnosis during pregnancy or activation of disease during pregnancy may increase the risk of spontaneous abortion (87).

The common medications used to treat IBD, sulfasalazine and corticosteroids, are usually well tolerated in pregnancy. The majority of women with either ulcerative colitis or Crohn's disease complete normal full-term pregnancies with healthy offspring. Ninety percent of women with inactive ulcerative colitis complete a full-term pregnancy; those with active colitis do not do as well (88). Successful pregnancy outcome in women with Crohn's disease also reflects the predominance of women with inactive disease in these studies (83,84,89). Active Crohn's disease probably results in a higher incidence of spontaneous abortion and prematurity (90). It has been estimated that 15% to 40% of patients with Crohn's disease will have an exacerbation during their pregnancy and about an equal number will remain unchanged or improved (87). The absence of gastrointestinal problems in a pregnancy does not predict the course of IBD in future pregnancies. Postpartum, the patients usually return to their prepregnancy gastrointestinal state.

Other Issues

In Crohn's disease, ulcers of the perineum may mimic herpetic lesions but in fact are granulomatous lesions. They may last for weeks to months and can progress to fistula tracts that may require long-term antibiotic therapy (e.g., metronidazole) or even surgery (91). The possible association of IBD and OCs is discussed in Chapter 17.

Peutz-Jeghers syndrome has been found to be associated with an increased risk of malignant neoplasia. The associated gynecologic malignancies that have been reported are ovarian and cervical. The ovarian tumors include Sertoli cell tumors (92), mucinous adenocarcinoma, mucinous cystadenoma (93), and sex cord tumors (94). The associated cervical neoplasia is a specific type of adenocarcinoma termed *adenoma malignum* (94). Breast carcinoma has also been reported (95). Regular yearly gynecologic examinations are essential in this at-risk population.

LIVER DISEASE

Pubertal Development and Menstrual Dysfunction

Women with chronic liver disease may have irregular menses, particularly amenorrhea that resolves if the liver disease improves. Amenorrhea has also been noted to resolve when spironolactone, an androgen inhibitor, was discontinued (96). Women with severe liver disease may also present with severe menorrhagia due to thrombocytopemia and the decreased production of clotting factors. Treatment of menorrhagia should be directed at treating the underlying disease and replacing clotting factors. Patients with this condition may not do well with oral estrogen therapy, as their liver dysfunction precludes adequate metabolism (97). Other possibilities of hormonal control of the bleeding with liver failure include medroxyprogesterone acetate (Provera), GnRH analogs, and the estrogen patch with an added oral progestin (97–99). The estrogen patch has an advantage over oral conjugated estrogens, as it avoids the liver "first-pass" effect. In the rare occasion hormonal manipulation fails, a dilatation and curettage with adequate preoperative coagulation factor replacement may be necessary.

Fertility and Pregnancy

Chronic liver disease is associated with anovulation and decreased fertility. Amenorrhea is commonly seen. Pregnancy can only be expected if the liver dysfunction can be reversed.

Wilson's disease, a disorder of copper metabolism, is treated with chelation therapy, which should be maintained during the pregnancy. No teratogenicity has been associated with penicillamine, the primary chelator (100,101).

SICKLE CELL DISEASE

Pubertal Development and Menstrual Function

In a study of >2000 patients with homozygous SS disease (SS), sickle C disease (SC), sickle β^+-thalassemia (Sβ^+), and sickle β^0-thalassemia (Sβ^0), patients with SS and Sβ^0 were shorter on cross-sectional growth data than those with SC and Sβ^+. The weight curves followed a similar but more pronounced pattern than the heights: SS and Sβ^0 patients weighed less than SC and Sβ^+ patients. Analysis of Tanner staging showed that patients with SS and Sβ^0 were less sexually developed than those with Sβ^+ and SC disease. When age and weight were included in the statistical model, menarcheal status did not differ among the various hemoglobinopathies (102).

This notable delay in growth in sickle cell disease is associated with a delay in menarche (103–105). Mann (103) reported a mean age of menarche to be 11.6 years versus 15 years for SS disease and 11 years in girls with SC thalassemia. In a sample of Jamaican women with SC disease >15 years of age (range, 15 to 65 years), Alleyne and coworkers (104) reported a mean age of menarche of 15.4 ± 1.7 years compared to 13.1 ± 1.7 years in a control population.

An analysis of the growth of young children with homozygous β-thalassemia treated for 36 months with deferoxamine (106) concluded that abnormalities occurred in metaphyseal growth plates in 11 of 37 patients in whom a significant decline in mean height percentile was also noted (107).

Fertility and Pregnancy

Although an earlier study reported fetal wastage rates to be 19.7% versus 9.5% in the general population (104), maternal and perinatal morbidity and mortality among pregnant patients with sickle cell disease have been decreasing in the past two decades with the coordinated efforts of the obstetric and hematologic teams (108). Despite this effort, women with sickle cell anemia are 2.5 times more likely to bear newborns who are small for gestational age than are women with other types of sickle cell disease, sickle trait, or C trait (109). In a retrospective analysis of records of patients with the sickle hemoglobinopathies (SS and SC diseases), there was a high occurrence of preterm labor, preeclampsia, pain crisis, pulmonary complications, and cesarean sections (110). An average of 2 units of blood was required by 43.1% of the patients. Two patients with SS disease had unpreventable deaths, and there were two intrauterine fetal deaths and two neonatal deaths (perinatal mortality was 10.5% for SS disease and 2.9% for SC disease). The role of partial prophylactic red cell exchange transfusion in the management of pregnant patients with major sickle hemoglobinopathies is unclear (111,112). In a series of 131 patients with major sickle hemoglobinopathies studied over a 10-year period, transfusion provided a benefit in terms of lowering the number of preterm deliveries, the prevalence of low-birth-weight infants, and the perinatal death rate (111). However, a smaller series by Howard and colleagues (112) could not demonstrate a direct relationship between uteroplacental circulation (measured by Doppler ultrasound) and the use of prophylactic blood transfusion in these pregnancies. Contraceptive choices for sickle cell disease are discussed in Chapter 17.

Major problems for women with β-thalassemia major seeking fertility treatment are hypogonadism, diabetes, and cardiomyopathy. In a study of 16 pregnancies in 11 women with β-thalassemia major, Jensen and colleagues (113) found no increased obstetric complications except a high cesarean section rate (10/13) felt to be primarily due to cephalopelvic disproportion. In a review of the literature, however, Savona-Ventura and Bonello (114) felt that pregnant mothers with thalassemia faced deleterious consequences resulting from chronic anemia, including a poor fetal outcome with greater fetal loss, preterm labor, and intrauterine growth retardation. Nonsplenectomized patients had an increased risk of a hypersplenic crisis.

RENAL DISEASE

Pubertal Development and Menstrual Function

Patients with renal disease, as with other chronic diseases, often have a delay in pubertal growth and development and menarche. The constellation consisting of uremic syndrome, metabolic acidosis, chronic malnutrition, chronic infection, and interference with bone growth and mineralization contributes to the growth failure.

Patients on chronic dialysis do not usually have regular menses. In a survey of 17 premenopausal patients, only 1 had regular menses, 6 had irregular menses with occasional spotting to dysfunctional uterine bleeding, and 10 were amenorrheic. Follicle-stimulating hormone (FSH) levels were comparable to those of normal women; luteinizing hormone (LH) levels were normal or increased and showed an absence of cyclicity (115–118). Prolactin levels are often elevated in uremic patients on hemodialysis because of impaired renal clearance, and the hyperprolactinemia may contribute to persistent amenorrhea. Lim and colleagues (117) reported prolactin levels of 41.4 ± 5.8 ng/ml in uremic women versus 11.7 ± 1.1 ng/ml in controls; 7 of 17 women had galactorrhea (117,119). Administration of bromocriptine to three patients led to resumption of menstruation in only one.

Since the studies indicate that most women on dialysis are anovulatory despite the type of menstrual pattern, a progestin should be administered cyclically. Patients on dialysis with significant menorrhagia often require treatment with an OC.

Fertility and Pregnancy

Most patients with chronic renal failure are anovulatory and therefore subfertile, but dialysis and transplantation may correct this problem (118). Sexual dysfunction and decreased libido have been described in female patients undergoing dialysis, and thus the quality of sexual function should be addressed with the patient who presents for contraceptive counseling (118,120).

Pregnant women with mild renal insufficiency (serum creatinine <1.4 mg/dl) appear to have only mildly reduced fetal survival and experience no effect on the underlying disease. In contrast, Jones and Hayslett (121) recently reported that among 67 women with moderate or severe renal insufficiency, serum creatinine increased from a mean of 1.9 ± 0.8 mg/dl in early pregnancy to 2.5 ± 1.3 mg/dl in the third trimester, hypertension increased from 28% to 48%, and high-grade proteinuria from 23% to 41%. Pregnancy-related loss of renal function occurred in 43% of women, often irreversibly. For those with initial serum creatinine >2 mg/dl, 65% had worsening of renal function, and 35% had end-stage renal failure necessitating dialysis. Preterm delivery occurred in 59% and growth retardation in 37%, but infant survival was 93%. Thus, young women with moderate to severe renal disease need sensitive counseling about the risks of undertaking pregnancy (122).

Patients on dialysis rarely conceive, but if they do, special considerations must be undertaken (123–124), including longer and more frequent periods of dialysis and strict adherence to diet. Aggressive blood pressure control and prompt diagnosis and treatment of bleeding episodes are essential, although severe complications may occur (125). Of dialysis patients who conceive, 20% to 50% will have a successful pregnancy. In a survey of U.S. centers providing women with continuous peritoneal dialysis, 44 pregnancies were identified. Two-thirds of the pregnancies were complicated by hypertension; 48% of pregnancies resulted in surviving infants with all but one premature (125.) Whether erythropoietin will improve further the currently poor outcome is unclear (126). Up to 46% of reported pregnancies are delivered by cesarean section, usually for worsening fetal or maternal condition (118,127). Reasons for early delivery include premature labor (often complicated with polyhydramnios), placental abruption, ruptured membranes, fetal distress, growth retardation, worsening maternal hypertension, and preeclampsia (118,127,128).

Many patients after transplantation have the return of ovulation and fertility within 6 months of a successful procedure. Pregnancies should be carefully planned. Patients should have good renal status for a minimum of 1 year after a transplant before attempting pregnancy (129–131).

By 1981, 440 pregnancies had been reported in transplantation patients, with a 70% successful outcome of those carrying to term. Since that time, experience has continued to accumulate on pregnancy in transplantation patients and the potential complications (129,130). In a survey of 2309 pregnancies in 1594 women with renal transplants, 60% of the pregnancies were completed, and of those 92% ended successfully (132). In most, renal function increased in pregnancy, with transient deterioration occurring in late pregnancy. Permanent renal impairment occurred in 15% of pregnancies, and there was a 30% chance of developing hypertension, preeclampsia, or both. Preterm delivery occurred in 50%, and intrauterine growth retardation in 25%. The transplanted kidney rarely produced obstetrical fetal/pelvic dystocia and was not injured during vaginal delivery.

Among women with autosomal-dominant polycystic kidney disease (ADPKD), normotensive women usually have successful, uncomplicated pregnancies, but hypertensive women are at an increased risk for fetal and maternal complications (133,134). Measures should be taken to prevent the development of preeclampsia in these women. Any patient with ADPKD should be counseled that the disease can be transmitted genetically in an autosomal-dominant pattern leading to a 50% risk of having an affected offspring.

DIABETES MELLITUS

Pubertal Development and Menstrual Function

Girls with insulin-dependent diabetes mellitus (IDDM) may have a later onset of puberty and menarche, although most do not vary from the norm (70). Insulin resistance develops at the time of puberty, associated with increased production of growth hormone, and thus increases in daily insulin may be required for glucose control (135–137). Impaired growth, hepatomegaly, and delayed puberty have been described in children with poorly controlled diabetes (Mauriac's syndrome). Other disorders such as hypothyroidism and Addison's disease can cause the same constellation of symptoms and occur with an increased frequency in patients with IDDM. The effect of diabetes on both longitudinal growth and specific growth phases has been studied, with conflicting results. In a longitudinal study, DuCaju and colleagues (138) concluded that diabetic children have a normal height at the onset of the disease, that final height in girls is reduced from target height, and that girls have a tendency to become obese during puberty.

While this study did not find a correlation between growth velocity or attainment of final height and metabolic control, other reports have shown improvement of growth with tight control of diabetes (107,139).

Menstrual function in IDDM is usually normal, but irregular cycles can occur, especially in girls with elevated glycosylated hemoglobin and poor diabetic control (141,142). In a study of 24 type I diabetics, irregular cycles were associated with higher hemoglobin A1c (HbA1c) and body mass index, a lower sex hormone–binding globulin, a higher LH/FSH ratio, and polycystic ovaries on ultrasound (140).

The literature is conflicting on the effect of the menstrual cycle on glucose homeostasis. In the majority of women, there appears to be no change in insulin requirements during the menstrual cycle. However, a subgroup of patients shows worsening premenstrual hyperglycemia and significantly decreased insulin sensitivity during the luteal phase (142,143). Many women also report an increased appetite accompanied by greater food consumption during this phase. Brown and colleagues (144) reported a small series of seven diabetic girls who presented with cyclical disturbance of diabetic control before the menarche, usually hyperglycemia occurring at 21- to 34-day intervals and lasting 2 to 5 days. The precise mechanism for this disturbance is unknown. Contraceptive options for diabetics are discussed in Chapter 17.

Fertility and Pregnancy

In a survey of infertility and pregnancy outcomes in an unselected group of women with IDDM, Kjaer and associates (145) found that the ability to conceive was normal but fewer pregnancies and fewer births per pregnancy occurred than in normal controls. Offspring of women with IDDM have a significantly lower risk of IDDM than the offspring of men with IDDM (146). In a study of 304 offspring of women with IDDM, the risk of IDDM for the offspring by age 20 was 6.0% ± 2.4% for those born at maternal ages <25 years, whereas the risk was significantly lower (0.7% ± 0.7%) for those born at older maternal ages ($p = 0.03$) (146).

The importance of planning pregnancies in diabetic women cannot be too strongly emphasized. Diabetic women need effective diabetic control, reflected in a normal glycosylated hemoglobin level, so that when they become pregnant, good metabolic control will help lessen the risk of fetal congenital malformations and prematurity (147,148). Rosenn and colleagues (149) reported that women with IDDM with initial HbA1c concentrations >12% or median first-trimester preprandial glucose concentrations >120 mg/dl have an increased risk of abortion and malformations.

Other Issues

In diabetic adolescents, persistent candidal vulvovaginitis is often associated with poor control. The use of topical antifungal therapy is preferred, and weekly therapy may be indicated. Oral fluconazole should be used only as needed to prevent chronic use (see Chapter 11).

THYROID DISEASE

Pubertal Development and Menstrual Function

Thyroid disease may be associated with delayed development, precocious puberty, amenorrhea, and irregular menses (see Chapters 5 and 6) (150,151). Patients with acquired hypothyroidism associated with growth deceleration and retarded skeletal maturation during late childhood or early adolescence may experience rapid growth acceleration and pubertal advance when euthyroidism is restored with appropriate doses of levothyroxine (152).

Menstrual irregularities are common in hypothyroid women. Amenorrhea can be a consequence of hypothyroidism; prolactin levels may be elevated because of thyrotropin-releasing hormone–induced increases (37). Menstrual changes associated with hyperthyroidism are unpredictable, ranging from amenorrhea to normal cycles to dysfunctional uterine bleeding. These menstrual changes usually resolve when the euthyroid state is restored.

Fertility and Pregnancy

In response to the metabolic demands of pregnancy, there are increases in the basal metabolic rate, iodine uptake, and the size of the thyroid gland (caused by hyperplasia and increased vascularity). However, a pregnant woman is euthyroid with normal levels of thyroid-stimulating hormone (TSH), free T_4, and free triiodothyronine (T_3); thyroid nodules or goiter require further evaluation. In normal pregnancies, placental transfer of TSH, T_4, and T_3 is severely limited in both directions (37).

Untreated thyrotoxicosis in pregnancy is associated with a higher risk of preeclampsia, heart failure, intrauterine growth retardation, and stillbirth (153). Heart failure is a consequence of the demands of pregnancy superimposed on the hyperdynamic cardiovascular state induced by the increased thyroid hormone (154). Although the most common cause of thyrotoxicosis in pregnancy is Graves' disease, trophoblastic disease can cause hyperthyroidism due to the cross-reactivity between TSH and human chorionic gonadotropin. The aim of treatment of Graves' disease should be to maintain mild hyperthyroidism in the mother to avoid thyroid dysfunction in the fetus (37). Treatment of maternal hyperthyroidism with propylthiouracil is preferred, as methimazole crosses the placenta more readily (155). Followup assessment of children whose mothers received propylthiouracil during pregnancy has indicated normal intellectual development (156). Although small amounts of antithyroid drugs are transmitted in breast milk, the amount has no impact on neonatal thyroid function and breast-feeding can be encouraged (37). Once the pregnancy and breast-feeding are completed, definitive treatment with radioactive iodine can be undertaken, if indicated.

Preeclampsia and intrauterine growth retardation are more frequent in women with significant hypothyroidism (157). Women being treated for hypothyroidism may require a small increase in levothyroxine during pregnancy, and TSH should be monitored through the pregnancy to keep the level in the normal range (158).

Autoimmune thyroid disease is suppressed to some degree by the immunologic changes of pregnancy (159). Thus, postpartum thyroiditis is not uncommon 3 to 6 months after delivery, manifested by either hyperthyroidism or hypothyroidism (160). Women at risk for postpartum thyroiditis are those with a personal or family history of autoimmune disease or with a previous postpartum episode. The symptoms usually last 1 to 3 months, and most women return to normal thyroid function (37,161).

CONNECTIVE TISSUE DISEASES

Pubertal Development and Menstrual Function

As with other chronic diseases, delayed growth and sexual development may occur in adolescents with systemic lupus erythematosus (SLE), juvenile rheumatoid arthritis, and other connective tissue disorders. Rarely is there an autoimmune disorder of the ovary associated with these conditions (see Chapter 6).

Fertility and Pregnancy

Autoimmune rheumatic diseases (ARDs) are known to occur predominantly in women. Fertility in patients with an ARD does not seem to be impaired. On the other hand, long-term uses of some of the medical treatments, specifically cyclophosphamide, are associated with gonadal dysfunction and infertility.

Spontaneous abortion, premature deliveries, and intrauterine growth retardation are frequently encountered in pregnant women with SLE. The increased incidence of fetal loss in patients with SLE has been attributed to the presence of placental vasculitis and infarctions. Other factors that have been associated are maternal autoantibody responses, including immune complex deposition, and the cross-reaction of lymphocytotoxic antibodies with trophoblasts (162–164). Neonatal lupus syndrome and cardiac conduction defects may occur.

With systemic sclerosis (scleroderma), the reports of pregnancies are few. An increased incidence of maternal complications of hypertension and preeclampsia and perinatal mortality in scleroderma has been reported (165,166).

Neither rheumatoid arthritis nor scleroderma seem to be exacerbated by pregnancy (166,167). Symptoms from ankylosing spondylitis either stay the same or are slightly aggravated during the course of pregnancy (168). Patients with psoriatic arthritis have been reported to improve or even have remission of symptoms during pregnancy (169).

CARDIOVASCULAR DISEASE

Pubertal Development and Menstrual Function

Significant congenital cardiac anomalies commonly lead to decreased height and weight, with weight more often retarded than height. The retardation of growth seems to be more profound in early childhood than in adolescence. Skeletal growth and maturation are also delayed. The more severe and prolonged the cardiac failure, the greater is the effect on growth (63) and puberty.

Fertility and Pregnancy

Pregnancy is associated with major hemodynamic changes in the cardiovascular system that can contribute to greater morbidity and mortality in women with underlying heart disease (170). Knowledge of the specific congenital cardiac lesion is essential (171–174).

Pregnancy in Marfan's syndrome is associated with several problems, including the potential for catastrophic aortic dissection and the 50% risk for having a child with the syndrome. Gestation seems to be safer in women without preexisting cardiovascular disease; a preconceptual transesophageal echocardiogram is helpful in delineating aortic disease. However, the absence of any vascular pathology does not preclude complications. The prophylactic use of β-blockers may help in preventing aortic dilatation (175).

Pregnancies complicated by hypertension require a well-formulated management plan. At the onset of pregnancy, women should be classified as having low-risk or high-risk hypertension, with the latter requiring medication. Those classified as low-risk should have a favorable perinatal outcome. Both classes of hypertensive disorders are at risk for preeclampsia (176).

COAGULATION DISORDERS

Pubertal Development and Menstrual Function

Rigorous double-blind trials have not been conducted in adolescents with known or potential coagulation disorders to define the best medical management to control menstrual bleeding. For adolescents with von Willebrand's disease and other factor deficiencies, consultation with a hematologist is critical in making a plan for menarche and subsequent cycles (177). In addition to the use of desmopressin and coagulation factors, most girls benefit from the prophylactic management of menses using low-dose cyclic combined OCs. We typically prescribe OCs with moderate progestin potency and low-dose estrogen to lessen the chance of breakthrough bleeding (e.g., Lo/Ovral, Triphasil, and Tri-Levlen).

The use of a GnRH agonist may avoid recurrent heavy bleeding in patients with an underlying hematologic disorder (36). This therapy requires advanced planning, as suppression with a GnRH agonist takes approximately 3 weeks (43). In the case of acute bleeding, stability can be gained with conventional hormone (OC) therapy, and long-term prevention can be initiated with a GnRH agonist (36). Conventional OC therapy can subsequently be discontinued with a limited, if any, withdrawal bleed (36). The use of long-term GnRH agonist therapy (i.e., >6 months) with estrogen add-back treatment may be a long-term solution for patients with an underlying coagulopathy and recurrent life-threatening dysfunctional uterine bleeding (DUB). Rau and Muram (178) reported the successful use of medroxyprogesterone and intranasal GnRH agonist in controlling severe DUB in a young woman with thrombotic thrombocytopenic purpura and abnormal liver function tests.

Oral anticoagulation is not a contraindication to OCs. OCs reduce the chance of serious hemorrhage during ovulation and lessen the risk of unplanned pregnancy (179).

Fertility and Pregnancy

In a retrospective review over 30 years (177), the pregnancies of 18 obligate carriers of hemophilia A, five carriers of Christmas disease, and eight patients with von Willebrand's disease were reported. In 14 pregnancies in seven patients with von Willebrand's disease, there were four primary and four secondary postpartum hemorrhages and one perineal hematoma. These problems occurred despite the endogenous rise in coagulation factor VIIIc seen with pregnancy. In 43 pregnancies in the carriers of hemophilia A and Christmas disease, there were five postpartum hemorrhages and one perineal hematoma (177).

SEIZURE DISORDERS

Pubertal Development and Menstrual Function

Studies of gynecologic issues in young women with seizure disorders are few. Although there are some reports of menstrual dysfunction, it is difficult to establish whether the etiology is the neurologic disorder, its treatment, or both. Higher incidences of polycystic ovary disease and hypogonadotropic hypogonadism have been suggested (180–182). Phenytoin has been reported to cause hirsutism, and valproate has been reported to be associated with polycystic ovary disease (see Chapter 7). Seizure frequency may increase in the luteal or menstrual phase of the cycle (183).

Fertility and Pregnancy

Women with epilepsy account for approximately 0.5% of all pregnancies (184). Clinicians and their female patients with epilepsy face difficult decisions. Antiepileptic drugs, including valproate and carbamazepine, increase the risk of major malformations, minor anomalies, neonatal hemorrhage, and delayed fetal growth and development. Maternal seizures also appear to be disadvantageous to the fetus, increasing the risk of miscarriage, premature labor, intracranial hemorrhage, and, perhaps, developmental or learning difficulties. Clinicians caring for pregnant women with epilepsy are therefore faced with a dilemma and must carefully chart a middle ground, providing effective seizure control while minimizing fetal exposure to antiepileptic drugs (185,186).

NEUROLOGIC DEFICITS AND MENTAL RETARDATION

Upper and lower urogenital tract dysfunction often occurs in adolescents with neurologic deficits, including those with central nervous system lesions (developmental delay and/or cerebral palsy), spinal cord lesions from congenital anomalies (spina bifida or sacral agenesis), or lesions acquired from trauma or neoplasm.

Pubertal Development and Menstrual Function

Major concerns in adolescents with these disorders include management of bladder and bowel control, control and management of menses, and sexual function. In a study of 25 patients with spina bifida, Furman and Mortimer (187) reported an earlier mean age of menarche (10.3 years) for these patients compared to mothers (11.9 years) and unaffected sisters (12.3 years). There was no difference with respect to dysmenorrhea, premenstrual syndrome (PMS), and irregular menses.

If perineal hygiene becomes a problem, induction of amenorrhea with continuous OC therapy or depot-medroxyprogesterone injection (Depo-Provera) may be indicated. Although some have suggested endometrial ablation as an alternative to hysterectomy for severe problems with menstrual bleeding or hygiene (188), we recommend medical management with Depo-Provera before surgical intervention is undertaken.

The gynecologic examination is often frightening to adolescents but more so to the developmentally disabled who cannot fully understand the importance of such an examination. Presenting the examination in a relaxed setting, as recommended with the prepubertal population, is useful with this group as well. The use of smaller swabs and instruments is also recommended. Rectoabdominal examination, pelvic ultrasound, and occasionally examination under anesthesia may be utilized (see Chapter 1 and Appendix 1 for resources).

Calendars to document menstrual problems, including irregularity and behavioral symptoms (tantrums, crying spells, self-abusive behavior, and seizures) suggestive of PMS or dysmenorrhea, are essential to provide optimal care to developmentally disabled young women. Nonsteroidal antiinflammatory drugs are first-line treatment, followed by the use of OCs or long-acting progestins such as depot-medroxyprogesterone injection (see Chapter 17).

Fertility and Pregnancy

It is important to address issues of sexual function and sexuality, when appropriate, with adolescents and their parents. For adolescents with mental retardation, special social and sexuality programs have been developed. For example, the Edwards assessment of social-sexual skills has photo cards that allow the student to learn the concepts of private and public places for behaviors (189,190).

In a study of female adolescents with spina bifida in Louisiana, the sexuality dimension of the self-image profile was significantly below normal compared to the other 10 dimensions that were normal (191). In a retrospective interview, 24 of 35 female patients aged ≥16 years with myelomeningocele were sexually active, and 12 had become pregnant (192). In Furman and Mortimer's study (187), only 4 of 20 young women with spina bifida were offered family planning counseling, although 13 desired it.

With more aggressive surgical management, patients with spina bifida may now reach adulthood and achieve pregnancy (192,193). Preconceptual genetic counseling and folic acid supplementation should be strongly recommended. Special care is needed during pregnancy in the management of urologic, obstetric, neurologic, and anesthetic problems. Compromise of urologic function may occur, including obstruction of the urinary tract (194). The incidence of preterm labor is increased. Although there is a risk of a contracted pelvis, vaginal delivery should be allowed if the head engages normally and the labor pattern proceeds appropriately.

Cerebrospinal fluid shunts may malfunction and cause focal neurologic problems, and cerebral peritoneal shunt malfunction may appear as uterine size increases. In those patients with a shunt, vaginal delivery is preferable, and pushing during the second stage is not contraindicated (195). Peripartum prophylactic antibiotics may be indicated, and special care is exercised if epidural analgesia and cesarean section are necessary (195).

MENTAL HEALTH DISORDERS

Approximately 22% of Americans will experience a psychiatric disorder within the span of their lifetime. Anxiety disorders will afflict some 14% of the general population, and depression 8% to 10%. These numbers increase when concomitant illicit drug abuse is included.

Pubertal Development and Menstrual Function

Women taking psychotropic drugs such as phenothiazines or tricyclic antidepressants may have elevated prolactin levels, leading to galactorrhea, anovulation, and amenorrhea. OCs may be beneficial in reversing the amenorrhea and hypoestrogenization.

Contraception

Barriers to effective use of contraception by mentally ill patients are sometimes magnified by their inability to establish reliable, long-term approaches to pregnancy prevention. A contraceptive program tailored to the individual needs of patients is essential. Whereas laws vary from state to state, the criteria for informed consent always should include an explanation of risks, benefits, and alternatives, as well as a determination of whether the patient is competent to understand the informed consent. Mental and reproductive health professionals must collaborate with legal professionals in making this determination.

Several factors need to be addressed in choosing a specific hormonal preparation. Hepatic enzyme induction by antiepileptic agents can result in increased contraceptive failures with OCs, and women taking such agents may do better with an alternative contraceptive method (196). In the institutionalized patient, who is accustomed to long-term drug regimens, an OC would be an appropriate choice in the absence of risk factors. Compliance is more difficult to ensure in the outpatient psychiatric patient. In these situations, the progestin-only injectables or implants may be considered. However, the side effect of irregular bleeding may be perceived as a sign of "ill health" and less tolerated in these women (197). Some women who use progestin-only preparations may experience depressed mood. To alleviate confusion between an underlying depressive condition and the possible medication effect, we often initiate a trial of a progestin-only pill—e.g., Ovrette or Micronor—for a month or longer before using an injectable or implant. The need to take oral medication at the same time every day and the use of condoms must be emphasized.

Fertility and Pregnancy

Areas that should be included in discussions with patients considering pregnancy and, if possible, their partners are heritability of the underlying mental health disorder, risks during pregnancy, and risks during the postpartum period (198). Although women with serious mental illness have normal fertility rates, multiple risk factors and a paucity of emotional and economic support during the initial phases of parenthood may be present (199). These risks are significantly multiplied when one factors in the issues of pregnancy in adolescence (200) (see Chapter 18).

Although pregnancy is often believed to be a time of emotional well-being, many women develop or have a recurrence of psychiatric illness during this time. The risks associated with not treating a woman during pregnancy are potentially substantial and must be weighed against the risks of exposing the fetus to potentially teratogenic medications. Studies have suggested a relative safety of use of tricyclic antidepressants during pregnancy (201). Data on neuroleptics, lithium, and benzodiazepines are mixed but suggest an increased risk of congenital malformations if these drugs are used in the first trimester of pregnancy (201).

STERILIZATION

Sterilization of young nulliparous women arises on rare occasions as an adjunct to the management of certain chronic conditions such as cardiac, pulmonary, and renal impairment, genetic diseases, and neuromuscular and severe seizure disorders, as well as in women with substantial developmental delays. Use of reversible contraception may become a problem because the choice is limited by numerous contraindications and patient compliance. Consequently, these patients may resort to less than optimal methods of birth control, even though their needs may be as real as those of healthy teenagers. Frequently, these young women develop tremendous anxiety regarding pregnancy because it could result in deterioration of their medical condition or in the birth of a baby affected by a genetically transmitted disease or teratogenic medications.

In a review of patients undergoing tubal ligation from 1977 to 1984 at Children's Hospital, Boston, there were 27 patients ranging in age from 15 to 28 years (mean, 21.8 years) (202). Tubal ligations were carried out by laparoscopy: 19 with Falope rings, 6 with Hulka clips, and 2 by electrocoagulation and division. General anesthesia was used in 25 patients and local anesthesia in 2 patients. There were two major postoperative complications, both of which involved excessive bleeding in patients who were anticoagulated. The first patient had bleeding from the necrosis of the Falope ring. Due to that complication, Hulka clips were substituted for Falope rings in the second patient with a bleeding complication. However, this patient also developed postoperative bleeding that was found to be from the infraumbilical trocar site. Since the report of that study, we predominantly use Falope rings for laparoscopic tubal ligation due to the improved success with pregnancy after tubal reversal if the patient should desire fertility at a future time.

The issue of sterilization of young women may represent an uncomfortable subject for the gynecologist, as well as for patients and their families. With modern medical advances in the treatment of these diseases, as well as in the refinement of the progestin-only injectables, the requests may be decreasing. However, in those few situations when a mature young woman unwilling to take the risks or comply with the physical restrictions of a high-risk pregnancy requests sterilization, that request needs to be respected. Consultation with the primary provider who is well acquainted with her medical and emotional status is essential. Even if the physician feels that sterilization is the optimal contraceptive modality, the patient should never be rushed into making this decision. In most instances, it is wise to have the patient seen by a mental health professional who can assist with the evaluation and provide subsequent emotional support (203) (see Chapter 21 for discussion of legal issues).

The procedure should be performed when the primary disease is under optimal control. The choice of the technique utilized depends on the gynecologist, who should opt for a method requiring the shortest anesthesia time with which he or she feels comfortable.

SUMMARY

Given recent advances in the health care field, persons with chronic diseases are experiencing improved life expectancies. More young women with chronic diseases are now dealing with gynecologic, sexuality, and fertility issues (199). These concerns present new challenges to health care providers. Further experience and study are needed to improve long-term reproductive health for this unique group of patients.

REFERENCES

1. Nicholson HS, Byrne J. Fertility and pregnancy after treatment for cancer during childhood or adolescence. *Cancer* 1993;71:3392.
2. Stillman RJ, Schinfeld JS, Schiff I, et al. Ovarian failure in long-term survivors of childhood malignancy. *Am J Obstet Gynecol* 1981;139:62.
3. Damewood MD, Grochow LB. Prospects for fertility after chemotherapy or radiation for neoplastic disease. *Fertil Steril* 1986;45:443.
4. Bookman MA, Longo DL, Young RC. Late complications of curative treatment in Hodgkin's disease. *JAMA* 1988;260:680.
5. Hammond CB, Maxson WS. *Current concepts. Physiology of the menopause: premature menopause*. Kalamazoo, MI: Upjohn Co, 1983.
6. Thibaud E, Ramirez M, Brauner R, et al. Preservation of ovarian function by ovarian transposition performed before pelvic irradiation during childhood *J Pediatr* 1992;121:880.
7. Gradishar WJ, Schilsky RL. Ovarian function following radiation and chemotherapy for cancer. *Semin Oncol* 1989;16:425.
8. Damewood MD. What factors underlie premature ovarian failure? *Contemp Obstet Gynecol* 1990:31.
9. Hall JE, Martin KA, Whitney HA, et al. Potential for gonadotropin-releasing hormone in long-term female survivors of cranial tumors. *J Clin Endocrinol Metab* 1994;79:1166.
10. Oberfield SE, Soranno D, Nirenberg A, et al. Age at onset of puberty following high-dose central nervous system radiation therapy. *Arch Pediatr Adolesc Med* 1996;150:589.
11. Meadows AT. Follow-up and care of childhood cancer survivors. *Hosp Pract* 1991;26:99.
12. Watson AR, Taylor J, Rance CP, et al. Gonadal function in women treated with cyclophosphamide for childhood nephrotic syndromea: a long-term follow-up study. *Fertil Steril* 1986;46:331.
13. Rivkees SA, Crawford JD. The relationship of gonadal activity and chemotherapy-induced gonadal damage. *JAMA* 1988;259:2123.
14. Clark ST, Radford JA, Crowther D, et al. Gonadal function following chemotherapy for Hodgkin's disease: a comparative study of MVPP and a seven-drug hybrid regimen. *J Clin Oncol* 1995;13:134.
15. Schilsky RL, Schering RJ, Hubbard SM. Long-term follow-up of ovarian function in women treated with MOPP chemotherapy for Hodgkin's disease. *Am J Med* 1981;71:552.

16. Whitehead G, Shalet SM, Blackledge G, et al. The effect of combination chemotherapy on ovarian function in women treated for Hodgkin's disease. *Cancer* 1983;52:988.
17. Shalet SM. Effects of cancer chemotherapy on gonadal function of patients. *Cancer Treat* 1980;7: 141.
18. Quigley C, Cowell C, Jimenez M, et al. Normal or early development of puberty despite gonadal damage in children treated for acute lymphoblastic leukemia. *N Engl J Med* 1989;321:143.
19. Dacou-Voutetakis C, Kitra V, Grafakos S, et al. Auxologic data and hormonal profile in long-term survivors of childhood acute lymphoid leukemia. *Am J Pediatr Hematol Oncol* 1993;15:227.
20. Horning SJ, Hoppe RT, Kaplan HS, et al. Female reproductive potential after treatment for Hodgkin's disease. *N Engl J Med* 1981;304:1377.
21. Ortin TTS, Shostak CA, Donaldson SS. Gonadal status and reproductive function following treatment for Hodgkin's disease in childhood: the Stanford experience. *Int J Radiat Oncol Biol Phys* 1990;19:873.
22. Byrne J, Fears TR, Gail MH. Early menopause in long-term survivors of cancer during adolescence. *Am J Obstet Gynecol* 1992;166:788.
23. Sanders JE, Buckner CD, Leonard JM, et al. Late effects on gonadal function of cyclophosphamide, total body irradiation and marrow transplantation. *Transplantation* 1983;36:252.
24. Cohen MT, Van-Lint A, Lavagetto S, et al. Pubertal development and fertility in children after bone marrow transplantation. *Bone Marrow Transplant* 1991;8(suppl):16.
25. Spinelli S, Chiodi S, Bacigalupo A, et al. Ovarian recovery after total body irradiation and allogeneic bone marrow transplantation: long-term follow-up of 79 females. *Bone Marrow Transplant* 1994;14: 373.
26. Ogilby-Stuart AL, Clark DJ, Wallace WHB, et al. Endocrine deficit after fractionated total body irradiation. *Arch Dis Child* 1992;67:1107.
27. Schubert MA, Sullivan KM, Schubert MM, et al. Gynecological abnormalities following allogenic bone marrow transplantation. *Bone Marrow Transplant* 1990;5:425.
28. Vergauwen P, Ferster A, Valsamis J, et al. Primary ovarian failure after prepubertal marrow transplant in a girl. *Lancet* 1994;343:125.
29. DeSanctis V, Galimberti M, Lucarelli G, et al. Gonadal function after allogenic bone marrow transplantation for thalassemia. *Arch Dis Child* 1991;66:517.
30. Mike V, Meadows AT, D'Angio GJ. Incidence of second malignant neoplasms in children: results of an international study. *Lancet* 1982;2:1326.
31. Coleman CN, Kaplan HS, Cox R, et al. Leukaemias, non-Hodgkin's lymphoma and solid tumours in patients treated for Hodgkin's disease. *Cancer Surv* 1982;1:733.
32. Boivin JF, Hutchison GB, Lyden M, et al. Second primary cancers following treatment of Hodgkin's disease. *J Natl Cancer Inst* 1984;72:233.
33. Tucker MA, Meadows AT, Boice JD Jr, et al. Leukemia after therapy with alkylating agents for childhood cancer. *J Natl Cancer Inst* 1987;78:459.
34. Bhatia S, Robison LL, Oberlin O, et al. Breast cancer and other second neoplasms after childhood Hodgkin's disease. *N Engl J Med* 1996;334:745.
35. Donaldson SS, Hancock SL. Second cancers after Hodgkin's disease in childhood (editorial). *N Engl J Med* 1996;334:792.
36. Laufer MR, Rein MS. Treatment of abnormal uterine bleeding with gonadotropin-releasing hormone analogues. *Clin Obstet Gynecol* 1993;36:678.
37. Speroff L, Glass RH, Kase NG. *Clinical gynecologic endocrinology and infertility*, 5th ed. Baltimore, MD: Williams & Wilkins, 1994.
38. Lefloch O, Conaldson SS, Kaplan HS. Pregnancy following oophoropexy and total nodal irradiation in women with Hodgkin's disease. *Cancer* 1976;38:2263.
39. Byrne J, Mulvihill JJ. Long-term survivors of childhood and adolescent cancer: their fertility and the health of their offspring. In: Plowman PN, McElwain IT, Meadows AT, eds. *Complications of cancer management*. Gunford, UK: Butterworth Scientific Ltd, 1991.
40. Hadar H, Loven D. An evaluation of lateral and medial transposition of the ovaries out of radiation fields. *Cancer* 1994;74:779.
41. Laufer MR, Billett AL, Diller L, et al. A new technique for laparoscopic prophylactic oophoropexy before craniospinal irradiation in children with medulloblastoma. *Adolesc Pediatr Gynecol* 1995;8: 81.
42. Chapman RM, Sutcliffe SB. Protection of ovarian function by oral contraceptive use in women receiving chemotherapy for Hodgkin's disease. *Blood* 1981;58:851.

43. Blumenfeld Z, Avivi I, Linn S, et al. Prevention of irreversible chemotherapy-induced ovarian damage in young women with lymphoma by gonadotropin-releasing hormone agonist in parallel to chemotherapy. *Hum Reprod* 1996;19:1620.
44. Laufer MR, Townsend NL, Parons KE, et al. Inducing amenorrhea during bone marrow transplantation. *J Reprod Med* 1997;42:537.
45. Ghalie R, Porter C, Radwanska E, et al. Prevention of hypermenorrhea with leuprolide in premenopausal women undergoing bone marrow transplantation. *Am J Hematol* 1993;42:350.
46. Byrne J, Mulvihill JJ, Myers MH, et al. Effects of treatment of fertility in long-term survivors of childhood or adolescent cancer. *N Engl J Med* 1987;317:1315.
47. Aisner J, Wiernik PH, Pearl P. Pregnancy outcome in patients treated for Hodgkin's disease. *J Clin Oncol* 1993;1:507.
48. Lacher MJ, Toner K. Pregnancies and menstrual function before and after combined radiation (RT) and chemotherapy (TVPP) for Hodgkin's disease. *Cancer Invest* 1986;4:93.
49. Gook DA, Osborn SM, Bourne H, Johnston WIH. Fertilization of human oocytes following crypopreservation; normal karyotypes and absence of stray chromosomes. *Hum Reprod* 1994;9:684.
50. Gook DA, Scheiwe MC, Osborn SM, et al. Intracytoplasmic sperm injection and embryo development of human oocytes cryopreserved using 1,2-propanedioc. *Hum Reprod* 1995;10:2637.
51. Toth TL, Lanzendorf SE, Sandow BA, et al. Cryopreservation of human prophase I oocytes collected from unstimulated follicles. Fertilization and in vitro development of cryopreserved human prophase I oocytes. *Fertil Steril* 1994;61:896.
52. Dein RA, Mennuti M, Kovach P, Gabbe SG. The reproductive potential of young men and women with Hodgkin's disease. *Obstet Gynecol Surv* 1984;39:474.
53 Dodds L, Marrett LD, Tomkins DJ, et al. Case-control study of congenital anomalies in children of cancer patients. *BMJ* 1993;307:164.
54. Green DM, Fiorello A, Zevon MA, et al. Birth defects and childhood cancer. *Arch Pediatr Adolesc Med* 1997;151:379.
55. Green DM, Aevon MA, Lowrie G, et al. Congenital anomalies in children of patients who received chemotherapy for cancer in childhood and adolescence. *N Engl J Med* 1991;325:141.
56. Smith MB, Xue H, Takahashi H, et al. Iodine 131 thyroid ablation in female children and adolescents: long-term risks of infertility and birth defects. *Ann Surg Oncol* 1994;1:128.
57. Li FP, Gimbrere K, Gelber RD, et al. Outcome of pregnancy in survivors of Wilms' tumor. *JAMA* 1987;257:216.
58. Byrne J, Mulvihill JJ, Connelly RR, et al. Reproductive problems and birth defects in survivors of Wilms' tumor and their relatives. *Med Pediatr Oncol* 1988;16:233.
59. Hawkins MM, Smith FA. Pregnancy outcomes in childhood cancer survivors: probable effects of abdominal irradiation. *Int J Cancer* 1989;43:399.
60. Hinterberger-Fisher M, Kier P, Kahls P. Fertility, pregnancies and offspring complications after bone marrow transplantation. *Bone Marrow Transplant* 1991;7:5.
61. Russell JA, Hanley DA. Full-term pregnancy after allogeneic transplantation for leukemia in a patient with oligomenorrhea. *Bone Marrow Transplant* 1989;4:579.
62. Miliken S, Powles R, Parikh M, et al. Successful pregnancy following bone marrow transplantation for leukemia. *Bone Marrow Transplant* 1990;5:135.
63. Rudolph A. *Rudolph's pediatrics*, 20th ed. Norwalk, CT: Appleton & Lange, 1996.
64. Neinstein LS, Stewart D, Wang C, et al. Menstrual dysfunction in cystic fibrosis. *J Adolesc Health Care* 1983;4:153.
65. Johannesson M, Gottlieb C, Hjelte L. Delayed puberty in girls with cystic fibrosis despite good clinical status. *J Pediatr* 1997;99:29.
66. Reiter ED, Stern RL, Root AW. The reproductive endocrine system in cystic fibrosis I: basal gonadotropins and sex steroid levels. *Am J Dis Child* 1981;135:422.
67. Sawyer SM, Phelan PD, Bowles G. Reproductive health in young women with cystic fibrosis: knowledge, attitudes and behavior. *J Adolesc Health* 1995;17:46.
68. Sawyer SM. Reproductive health in young people with cystic fibrosis. *Curr Opin Pediatr* 1995;7:376.
69. Stern RC. Cystic fibrosis and the reproductive systems. In: Davis PB, ed. *Cystic fibrosis*. New York: Marcel Dekker, 1993.
70. Emans SJ. Gynecologic problems in adolescents with chronic diseases. In: Goldstein DP, ed. *Gynecologic disorders of children and adolescents*. New York: Elsevier 1989;1:171.
71. Kopito LE, Losasky HJ, Shwachman H. Water and electrolytes in cervical mucus from patients with cystic fibrosis. *Fertil Steril* 1973;24:512.

72. diSant'Agnese PA, Davis DB. Cystic fibrosis in adults. *Am J Med* 1979;66:121.
73. Handyside AH, Lesko JG, Tarin JJ, et al. Birth of a normal girl after *in vitro* fertilization and preimplantation diagnostic testing for cystic fibrosis. *N Engl J Med* 1992;327:905.
74. Cohen LF, diSant'Agnese PA, Friedlander J. Cystic fibrosis and pregnancy: a national survey. *Lancet* 1980;2:842.
75. Kent NE, Farquharson DF. Cystic fibrosis in pregnancy. *Can Med Assoc J* 1993;149:809.
76. Palmer J, Dillon-Baker C, Tecklin JS, et al. Pregnancy in patients with cystic fibrosis. *Ann Intern Med* 1983;99:596.
77. Kotloff RM, FitzSimmons SC, Fiel SB. Fertility and pregnancy in patients with cystic fibrosis. *Clin Chest Med* 1992;13:623.
78. Canny GL, Corey M, Livingstone RA, et al. Pregnancy and cystic fibrosis. *Obstet Gynecol* 1991;77:850.
79. Edenborough FP, Stableforth DE, Webb AK, et al. Outcome of pregnancy in women with cystic Fibrosis. *Thorax* 1995;50:170.
80. Dooley RR, Braunstein H, Osher AB. Polypoid cervicitis in cystic fibrosis patients receiving oral contraceptives. *Am J Obstet Gynecol* 1974;118:971.
81. Fitzpatirick SB, Stokes DC, Rosenstein BJ, et al. Use of oral contraceptives in women with cystic fibrosis. *Chest* 1984;86:863.
82. Banks BM, Korelitz BI, Zetzel L. The course of nonspecific ulcerative colitis: review of twenty years' experience and late results. *Gastroenterology* 1980;32:983.
83. Hanan IM. Inflammatory bowel disease in the pregnant woman. *Compr Ther* 1983;19:91.
84. Korelitz BI. Inflammatory bowel disease in pregnancy. *Gastroenterol Clin North Am* 1992;21:827.
85. Khosia R, Willoughby CP, Jewell DP. Crohn's disease and pregnancy. *Gut* 1984;25:52.
86. Mayberry JF, Weterman IT. European survey of fertility and pregnancy in women with Crohn's disease: a case-control study by European collaborative group. *Gut* 1986;27:821.
87. Vender FJ, Spiro HM. Inflammatory bowel disease and pregnancy. *J Clin Gastroenterol* 1982;4:231.
88. Nielsen OH, Andreasson B, Bondesen S, et al. Pregnancy in ulcerative colitis. *Scand J Gastroenterol* 1983;18:735.
89. Baiocco PJ, Korelitz BI. The influence of inflammatory bowel disease and its treatment on pregnancy and fetal outcome. *J Clin Gastroenterol* 1984;6:211.
90. Federkow DM, Persaud D, Nimrod MB. Inflammatory bowel disease: a controlled study of late pregnancy outcome. *Am J Obstet Gynecol* 1989;160:998.
91. Kremer M, Nussenson E, Steinfeld M, et al. Crohn's disease of the vulva. *Am J Gastroenterol* 1984;79:376.
92. Ferry JA, Young RH, Engel G, Scully RE. Oxyphilic Sertoli cell tumor of the ovary: a report of three cases, two patients with the Peutz-Jeghers syndrome. *Int J Gynecol Pathol* 1994;13:259.
93. Young RH, Scully RE. Mucinous ovarian tumors associated with mucinous adenocarcinomas of the cervix: a clinicopathological analysis of 16 cases. *Int J Gynecol Pathol* 1988;7:99.
94. Srivatsa PJ, Keeney GL, Podratz KC. Disseminated cervical adenoma malignum and bilateral ovarian sex cord tumors with annular tubules associated with Peutz-Jeghers syndrome. *Gynecol Oncol* 1994;53:256.
95. Martin-Odegard B, Svane S. Peutz-Jeghers syndrome associated with bilateral synchronous breast carcinoma in a 30-year-old woman. *Eur J Surg* 1994;160:511.
96. Potter C, Willis D, Sharp HL, Scharzengerg SJ. Primary and secondary amenorrhea associated with spironolactone therapy in chronic liver disease. *J Pediatr* 1992;121:141.
97. Nicholas SL, Rulin MC. Acute vaginal bleeding in women undergoing liver transplantation. *Am J Obstet Gynecol* 1994;170:733.
98. Chetkowski RJ, Meldrum DR, Steingold KA, et al. Biologic effects of transdermal estradiol. *N Engl J Med* 1986;314:1615.
99. Blumfeld Z, Enat R, Brandes JM, Baruch Y. Gonadotropin-releasing hormone analogues for dysfunctional bleeding in women after liver transplantation: a new application. *Fertil Steril* 1992;57:1121.
100. Scheinler IH, Sternlieb I. *Wilson's disease*. Philadelphia: WB Saunders, 1984.
101. Riely CA. Hepatic disease in pregnancy. *Am J Med* 1994;96:18.
102. Platt OS, Rosenstock W, Espeland MA. Influence of sickle hemoglobinopathies on growth and development. *N Engl J Med* 1984;311:7.
103. Mann J. Sickle cell haemoglobinopathies in England. *Arch Dis Child* 1981;56:676.
104. Alleyne R, Rauseo R, Serjeant G. Sexual development and fertility of Jamaican female patients with homozygous sickle cell disease. *Arch Intern Med* 1981;141:1295.

105. Balgir RS. Age at menarche and first conception in sickle cell hemoglobinopathy. *Ind Pediatr* 1994; 31:827.
106. Olivieri NF, Koren G, Harris J, et al. Growth failure and bony changes induced by deferoxamine. *Am J Pediatr Hematol Oncol* 1992;14:48.
107. Jackson RL. Growth and maturation of children with insulin-dependent diabetes mellitus. *Pediatr Clin North Am* 1984;31:545.
108. Koshy M, Burd L. Management of pregnancy in sickle cell syndromes. *Hematol Oncol Clin North Am* 1991;5:585.
109. Brown AK, Sleeper LA, Peglow CH, et al. The influence of infant and maternal sickle disease on birth outcome and neonatal course. *Arch Pediatr Adolesc Med* 1994;148:1156.
110. Seoud MA, Cantwell D, Nobles G, Levy DL. Outcome of pregnancies complicated by sickle cell and sickle-C hemoglobinopathies. *Am J Perinatol* 1994;11:187.
111. Morrison JC, Morrison FS, Floyd RC, et al. Use of continuous flow erythrocytapheresis in pregnant patients with sickle cell disease. *J Clin Apheresis* 1991;6:224.
112. Howard RJ, Tuck SM, Pearson TC. Blood transfusion in pregnancies complicated by maternal sickle cell disease: effects on blood rheology and uteroplacental Doppler velocimetry. *Clin Lab Hematol* 1994;16:253.
113. Jensen CE, Tuck SM, Wonke B. Fertility in beta-thalassemia major: a report of 16 pregnancies, preconceptual evaluation and a review of the literature. *Br J Obstet Gynaecol* 1995;102:625.
114. Savona-Ventura C, Bonello F. Beta-thalassemia syndromes and pregnancy. *Obstet Gynecol Surv* 1994;49:129.
115. Morley JE, Distiller LA, Epstein S, et al. Menstrual disturbance in chronic renal failure. *Horm Metab Res* 1979;11:68.
116. Perez, RJ, Lipner H, Abdfulla J, et al. Menstrual dysfunction of patients undergoing chronic hemodialysis. *Obstet Gynecol* 1978;51:552.
117. Lim VS, Henriquez C, Stevertson G, et al. Ovarian function in chronic renal failure: evidence suggesting hypothalamic anovulation. *Ann Intern Med* 1980;93:21.
118. Ginsburg ES, Owen WF. Reproductive endocrinology and pregnancy in women on hemodialysis. *Semin Dial* 1993;6:105.
119. Gomez F, de la Cueva R, Wauters JP, et al. Endocrine abnormalities in patients undergoing long-term hemodialysis: the role of prolactin. *Am J Med* 1980;93:21.
120. Levy NB. Sexual adjustment to maintenance hemodialysis and renal transplantation. National survey by questionnaire: preliminary report. *Trans Am Soc Artif Intern Organs* 1973;19:138.
121. Jones DC, Hayslett JP. Outcome of pregnancy in women with moderate or severe renal insufficiency. *N Engl J Med* 1996;335:226.
122. Brown MA, Whitworth JA. The kidney in hypertensive pregnancies—victim and villain. *Am J Kidney Dis* 1992;20:427.
123. Registration Committee of EDTA. Successful pregnancies in women treated by dialysis and kidney transplantation. *Br J Obstet Gynaecol* 1980;87:839.
124. Souquiyyeh MZ, Huraib SO, Saleh AGM, Aswas S. Pregnancy in chronic hemodialysis patients in the Kingdom of Saudi Arabia. *Am J Kidney Dis* 1992;19:235.
125. Okundaye I, Hou S. Management of pregnancy in women undergoing continuous ambulatory peritoneal dialysis. *Adv Perit Dial* 1996;12:151.
126. Scott LL, Ramin SM, Richey M, et al. Erythropoietin use in pregnancy: two cases and a review of the literature. *Am J Perinatol* 1995;12:22.
127. Hou S. Pregnancy in women requiring dialysis for renal failure. *Am J Kidney Dis* 1987;9:368.
128. Kincaid-Smith P, Fairley KF, Bullen M. Kidney disease and pregnancy. *Med J Aust* 1967;2:1155.
129. Fine RN. Pregnancy in renal allograft recipients. *Am J Nephrol* 1982;2:117.
130. Whetham JC, Cardella C, Harding M. Effect of pregnancy on graft function and graft survival in renal cadaver transplant patients. *Am J Obstet Gynecol* 1983;145:193.
131. Dafnis E, Sabatini S. The effect of pregnancy on renal function: physiology and pathology. *Am J Med Sci* 1992;303:184.
132. Davison JM. Dialysis, transplantation, and pregnancy. *Am J Kidney Dis* 1991;17:127.
133. Chapman AB, Johnson AM, Gabow PA. Pregnancy outcome and its relationship to progression of renal failure in autosomal-dominant polycystic kidney disease. *J Am Soc Nephrol* 1994;5: 1178.
134. Alcalay M, Blau A, Barkai G, et al. Successful pregnancy in a patient with polycystic kidney disease and advanced renal failure: the use of prophylactic dialysis. *Am J Kidney Dis* 1992;19:382.

135. Caprio S, Cline G, Boulware SD, et al. Effects of puberty and diabetes on insulin-sensitive fuels. *Am J Physiol* 1994;266:885.
136. Rother KI, Levitsky LL. Diabetes mellitus during adolescence. *Endocrinol Metab Clin North Am* 1993;22:553.
137. Amiel SA, Sherwin RS, Cimonson DC, et al. Impaired insulin action in puberty: a contributing factor to poor glycemic control in adolescents. *N Engl J Med* 1986;31:215.
138. DuCaju MVL, Rooman RP, DeBeeck LO. Longitudinal data on growth and final height in diabetic children. *Pediatr Res* 1995;38:607.
139. Wise J, Kolb E, Sauder S. Effect of glycemic control on growth velocity in children with IDDM. *Diabetes Care* 1992;15:826.
140. Adcock CJ, Perry LA, Lindsell DR, et al. Menstrual irregularities are more common in adolescents with type 1 diabetes: association with poor glycemic control and weight gain. *Diabet Med* 1994;11:465.
141. Kjaer K, Hagen C, Sando SH, et al. Epidemiology of menarche and menstrual disturbances in an unselected group of women with insulin-dependent diabetes mellitus compared to controls. *J Clin Endocrinol Metab* 1992;75:524.
142. Widom B, Diamond MP, Simonson DC. Alterations in glucose metabolism during menstrual cycle in women with IDDM. *Diabetes Care* 1992;15:213.
143. Cawood EH, Bancroft J, Steel JM. Perimenstrual symptoms in women with diabetes mellitus and the relationship to diabetic control. *Diabet Med* 1993;10:444.
144. Brown KC, Darby CW, Ng SH. Cyclical disturbance of diabetic central injuries before the menarche. *Arch Dis Child* 1991;66:1279.
145. Kjaer K, Hagen C, Sando SH, et al. Infertility and pregnancy outcome in an unselected group of women with insulin dependent diabetes mellitus. *Am J Obstet Gynecol* 1992;166:1412.
146. Warram JH, Martin BC, Krolewski AS. Risk of IDDM in children of diabetic mothers decreases with increasing maternal age at pregnancy. *Diabetes* 1991;40:1679.
147. Reece EA, Homko CJ. Assessment and management of pregnancies complicated by pregestational and gestational diabetes mellitus. *J Assoc Acad Minor Phys* 1994;5:87.
148. Kappy MS. Diabetes in pregnancy: rationale and guidelines for care. *Compr Ther* 1991;17:50.
149. Rosenn B, Miodovnik M, Combs CA, et al. Glycemic thresholds for spontaneous abortion and congenital malformations in insulin-dependent diabetes mellitus. *Obstet Gynecol* 1994;84:515.
150. Longcope C. The male and female reproductive systems in thyrotoxicosis. In: Braverman LE, Tigier RD, eds. *Werner and Ingbar's the thyroid*, 6th ed. Philadelphia: JB Lippincott, 1991.
151. Foley TP. Effects of thyroid on gonadal and reproductive function. In: Sanfilippo JS, ed. *Pediatric and adolescent gynecology*. Philadelphia: WB Saunders, 1994.
152. Rivkees SA, Bode HH, Crawford JD. Long-term growth in juvenile acquired hypothyroidism: the failure to achieve normal adult stature. *N Engl J Med* 1988;318:599.
153. Davis LE, Lucas MJ, Hankins GV, et al. Thyrotoxicosis complicating pregnancy. *Am J Obstet Gynecol* 1989;160:63.
154. Easterling TR, Chmucker BC, Carlson KL, et al. Maternal hemodynamics in pregnancies complicated by hyperthyroidism. *Obstet Gynecol* 1991;78:348.
155. Cheron RG, Kaplan MM, Larsen PR, et al. Neonatal thyroid function after propylthiouracil therapy for maternal Graves' disease. *N Engl J* Med 1981;304:525.
156. Mitsuda N, Tamaki H, Amino N, et al. Risk factors for developmental disorders in infants born to women with Graves' disease. *Obstet Gynecol* 1992;80:359.
157. Leung AS, Millar LK, Koonings PP, et al. Perinatal outcome in hypothyroid pregnancies. *Obstet Gynecol* 1993;8:349.
158. Mandel SJ, Larsen PR, Seely EW, Brent GA. Increased need for thyroxine during pregnancy in women with primary hypothyroidism. *N Engl J* Med 1990;323:91.
159. Roti E, Emerson CH. Clinical review 29: postpartum thyroiditis. *J Clin Endocrinol Metab* 1992;74:3.
160. Vargas MT, Bariones-Urbina R, Bladman D, et al. Antithyroid microsomal autoantibodies and HLA-DR5 are associated with postpartum thyroid dysfunction: evidence supporting an autoimmune pathogenesis. *J Clin Endocrinol Metab* 1988;67:327.
161. Walfish PG, Chan YYC. Postpartum hyperthyroidism. *Clin Endocrinol Metab* 1985;14:417.
162. Siamopoulou-Mavridou A, Manoussakis MN, Mavridis AK, Moutsopoulos HM. Outcome of pregnancy in patients with autoimmune rheumatic disease before the disease onset. *Ann Rheum Dis* 1988;47:982–7.

163. Petri M, Golbus M, Anderson R, et al. Antinuclear antibody, lupus anticoagulant, and anticardiolipin antibody in women with idiopathic habitual abortion. *Arthritis Rheum* 1987;30:602.
164. Lockshin MD, Harpel PC, Druzin ML, et al. Lupus pregnancy. *Arthritis Rheum* 1985;28:58.
165. Ballou SP, Morley JJ, Kushner I. Pregnancy and systemic sclerosis. *Arthritis Rheum* 1984;37:295.
166. Gimovsky ML, Montoro M. Systemic lupus erythematosus and other connective tissue disease in pregnancy. *Clin Obstet Gynecol* 1991;34:35.
167. Ostensen M. Pregnancy in patients with a history of juvenile rheumatoid arthritis. *Arthritis Rheum* 1991;34:881.
168. Ostensen M, Husby G. A prospective clinical study of the effect of pregnancy on rheumatoid arthritis and ankylosing spondylitis. *Arthritis Rheum* 1983;26:9.
169. Ostenson M. The effect of pregnancy on ankylosing spondylitis, psoriatic arthritis and juvenile rheumatoid arthritis. *Am J Reprod Immunol* 1992;28:235.
170. Bhagwat AR, Engel PJ. Heart disease and pregnancy. *Cardiol Clin* 1995;13:163.
171. Mendelson MA. Pregnancy in the woman with congenital heart disease. *Am J Card Imaging* 1995; 9:44.
172. Perloff JK. Congenital heart disease and pregnancy. *Clin Cardiol* 1994;17:579.
173. Hess DB, Hess LW. Management of cardiovascular disease in pregnancy. *Obstet Gynecol Clin North Am* 1991;18:237.
174. Clark SL. Cardiac disease in pregnancy. *Crit Care Clin* 1991;7:777.
175. Elkayam U, Ostrzega E, Shotan A, Mehra A. Cardiovascular problems in pregnant women with the Marfan syndrome. *Ann Intern Med* 1995;123:117.
176. Sibai BM. Hypertension in pregnancy. *Obstet Gynecol Clin North Am* 1992;19:615.
177. Greer IA, Lowe GD, Walker JJ, Forbes CD. Haemorrhagic problems in obstetrics and gynaecology in patients with congenital coagulopathies. *Br J Obstet Gynaecol* 1991;98:909.
178. Rau FJ, Muram D. Control of uterine bleeding in a patient with gonadotropin-releasing hormone agonists. *Adolesc Pediatr Gynecol* 1992;5:256.
179. Comp PC, Zacur HA. Contraceptive choices in women with coagulation disorders. *Am J Obstet Gynecol* 1993;168:1990.
180. Herzog AG, Seibel MM, Schomer DL, et al. Reproductive endocrine disorders in women with partial seizures of temporal lobe origin. *Arch Neurol* 1986;43:341.
181. Bilo L, Meo R, Nappi C, et al. Reproductive endocrine disorders in women with primary generalized epilepsy. *Epilepsia* 1988;29:612.
182. Isojarvi JI, Laatikainen TJ, Pakarinen AJ, et al. Menstrual disorders in women with epilepsy receiving carbamazepine. *Epilepsia* 1995;36:676.
183. Herzog AG. Reproductive endocrine considerations and hormonal therapy for women with epilepsy. *Epilepsia* 1991;32(suppl):S27.
184. Yerby MS. Pregnancy and epilepsy. *Epilepsia* 1991;32(suppl):S51.
185. Yerby MS. Epilepsy and pregnancy. New issues for an old disorder. *Neurol Clin* 1993;11:777.
186. Hiilesmaa VK. Pregnancy and birth in women with epilepsy. *Neurology* 1992;42(suppl):8.
187. Furman L, Mortimer JC. Menarche and menstrual function in patients with myelomeningocele. *Dev Med Child Neurol* 1994;36:910.
188. Wingfield M, McClure N, Mamers P, et al. Endometrial ablation: an option for the management of menstrual problems in the intellectually disabled. *Med J Aust* 1994;160:533.
189. Edwards J, Wapnick S. *Being me: a social/sexual training program for the developmentally disabled.* Austin, TX: Pro-ed, 1988.
190. Edwards JP, Elkins TE. *Just between us: a social sexual training guide for parents and professionals with concerns for persons with developmental disabilities.* Austin, TX: Pro-ed, 1988.
191. Cartright DB, Joseph AS, Grenier CE. A self-image profile analysis of spina bifida adolescents in Louisiana. *J La State Med Soc* 1993;145:394.
192. Cass AS, Bloom BA, Luxenberg M. Sexual function in adults with myelomeningocele. *J Urol* 1986; 136:425.
193. Rietberg CC, Lindhout D. Adult patients with spina bifida cystica: genetic counselling, pregnancy and delivery. *Eur J Obstet Gynecol Reprod Biol* 1993;52:63.
194. Farine D, Jackson U, Portale A, et al. Pregnancy complicated by maternal spina bifida: a report of two case. *J Reprod Med* 1988;33:323.
195. Cusimano MD, Meffe FM, Gentili F, Sermer M. Management of pregnant women with cerebrospinal shunts. *Pediatr Neurosurg* 1991;17:10.
196. Speroff L, Darney P. *A clinical guide for contraception.* Baltimore, MD: Williams & Wilkins, 1992.

197. Hankoff LD, Darney PD. Contraceptive choices for behaviorally disordered women. *Am J Obstet Gynecol* 1993;168:1986.
198. Packer S. Family planning for women with bipolar disorder. *Hosp Community Psychiatry* 1992;43: 479.
199. Mowbray CT, Oyserman D, Zemencuk JK, Ross SR. Motherhood for women with serious mental illness: pregnancy, childbirth, and the postpartum period. *Am J Orthopsychiatry* 1995;65:21.
200. Trad PV. Mental health of adolescent mothers. *J Am Acad Child Adolesc Psychiatry* 1995;34:130.
201. Altshuler LL, Szuba MP. Course of psychiatric disorders in pregnancy: dilemmas in pharmacologic management. *Neurol Clin* 1994;12:613.
202. Goldstein DP, Pinsonneault O. Sterilization of the unusual adolescent female. In: Goldstein DP, ed. *Gynecologic disorders of children and adolescents*. 1989;1:167.
203. Peterson K. The family v. the family court: sterilisation. *Aust J Public Health* 1992;16:196.

20

Sexual Abuse

The past two decades have witnessed an increasing awareness of the broad spectrum of problems that are seen under the term *sexual abuse* (1–113). The health care provider may be involved in the detection and diagnosis of sexual abuse cases, the evaluation of adolescents who are victims of sexual assault, and the followup of children and adolescents with psychological sequelae. In 1993, there were 330,000 reports of child sexual abuse, of which 150,000 were substantiated (11). In 1990, the U.S. Department of Justice reported the annual incidence of sexual assault to be 80 per 100,000 women. The peak of reported rapes occurs among young women 16 to 19 years of age; the frequency of date rape also peaks in late adolescence.

The percentage of adult women disclosing histories of sexual abuse ranges from 2% to 62%, with most estimates at 20% or more; for adult men, 3% to 16% have a history of abuse, with most estimates at 5% to 10% (12). The definition of abuse, methodologic approach, and quality of surveys vary. Surveys of children and adolescents suggest a high prevalence of nonconsensual sexual contact. In surveys of middle and high school students, 18% of females have reported a history of unwanted sexual activity, the majority of episodes occurring between ages 13 and 16 years (14). Finkelhor (15) found that 15% of college women reported some type of sexual experience (usually fondling or touching with siblings) during childhood. One-quarter of these incidences could be classified as exploitive because they involved force or age discrepancy. In the 1995 National Survey of Family Growth, among women whose first sexual intercourse occurred under age 16 years, the first intercourse was not voluntary in 16% of women (20). Children are particularly likely to be abused between age 8 and 12 years (8).

Problem behaviors and suicide have been associated with sexual abuse in cross-sectional studies (16–19). In a study of 8th to 10th graders in Alabama, Nagy and colleagues (16) reported that 13% of girls and 7% of boys said that they had been sexually abused; both boys and girls who were abused were significantly more likely to report risky behaviors such as drug and alcohol use. Sexually abused girls were more likely to have been pregnant, to have initiated sexual intercourse at a younger age, and to express more frequent suicidal ideation (17).

Sexual abuse is generally defined as the involvement of developmentally immature children or adolescents in sexual activities that they do not fully comprehend, to which they are unable to give informed consent, or that violate taboos of family relationships. Sexual abuse may include exhibitionism, fondling and manipulation, genital viewing, oral–genital contact, insertion of objects, or vaginal or rectal penetration. The contact may be a single event between the child and a stranger occurring with or without the use of force, or it may be a long-standing sexualized relationship between a father, stepfather, or other known individual and a child and may involve repeated encounters over months to years. The sexual interaction may start with touching or fondling and progress over the course of months to vulvar coitus and penetration. The assailant is known to the child in 70% to 90% of cases, and in half of cases a relative is involved (12,21,22). Most (90%) of sexual abuse is committed by men (1,12,19).

Sexual assault is defined as any sexual act performed by one person on another without that person's consent. The use or threat of force may be involved, or the person may not be able to give consent because of age, mental or physical capacity, or impairment with drugs or alcohol. A child who is unconscious or intoxicated cannot give consent. Different states have varying legal definitions of sexual assault and sexual abuse. For example, in the California penal code, sexual abuse is defined as any penetration of the vagina or anal opening of a child by the penis of another person; any sexual contact between the genitals or anal opening of one person and the mouth or tongue of another person; any intrusion by one person into the genitals or anal opening of another person, including the use of any object for this purpose (except as performed for a valid medical purpose); the intentional touching of the genitals or intimate parts (including the breasts, genital area, groin, inner thighs, and buttocks), or the clothing covering them, of a child or of the perpetrator by a child for purposes of sexual arousal or gratification (the statute specifies that this does not include normal caretaker responsibilities or interactions with or demonstrations of affection for the child or acts performed for a valid medical purpose); and the intentional masturbation of the perpetrator's genitals in the presence of a child. Sexual exploitation of children is also covered and includes activities such as pornography and prostitution. Crimes of indecent exposure also apply when an adult exposes his or her private parts to a child (11).

Reported cases of sexual abuse represent a small percentage of actual events. Clinicians should ask questions that would reveal the possibility of sexual abuse at the routine physical examination, especially in children and adolescents with somatic complaints, nightmares, running away, "acting out," or pregnancy. Patients should be reassured that the questions posed to them are the same as asked of all patients. For adolescents, these questions can be included in the menstrual and sexual history: "Have you ever been touched in your private parts or sexually when you did not want to be touched?", "Have you ever been forced to have sex?", or "Have you ever felt that someone older than you made inappropriate sexual advances?" Acknowledging that some youngsters may have felt embarrassed or unable to tell another person in the past can relieve anxiety. Younger children with unexplained somatic symptoms or any evidence of genital infection, pain, or bleeding can be asked: "Has an adult or someone you know ever touched the vaginal area or your private parts?", "If you were ever touched, whom would you tell?" If a child can mention her mother, father, or other trusted adult without hesitation, clinicians can feel at least some reassurance that lines of communication are available.

The recognition of sexual abuse is frequently prompted by a child's disclosure to a parent, friend, teacher, or health professional. The disclosure may be purposeful or accidental. For example, a child may have told a peer about abuse, and the peer may subsequently tell her own mother, who reports the case. In most cases, the child does not anticipate the sequelae of the allegation. Sexual abuse may become evident during an evaluation for somatic symptoms or behavioral difficulties. Girls with vaginal bleeding, foreign bodies in the vagina (24), condyloma acuminata, genital herpes, *Trichomonas vaginalis* or *Chlamydia trachomatis* infection, or gonococcal vulvovaginitis need an especially careful history for sexual abuse, and the history is often best obtained without the parents present (see Assessment of the Prepubertal Child). Occasionally, a pregnancy in a young adolescent is the first sign of long-standing incest.

Because clinicians frequently feel uncomfortable about the diagnosis of incest or sexual abuse, even obvious problems are sometimes overlooked. Most children who disclose sexual abuse are telling the truth, and it is highly unlikely for a child to make up the concrete details of sexual involvement unless a sexually stimulating experience has occurred. Even if one encounters the rare circumstance in which a child has not had the sexual experience alleged, most likely something sexually stimulating occurred that is unhealthy for the child's development. In cases of incest, there is a great deal of pressure from families to have the child retract the story to prevent disruption of the family unit and possible incarceration of the father. Thus, clinicians must be prepared to file the necessary report with child protective services, support the youngster in her original story, and proceed with an appropriate referral to a mental health facility capable of dealing with the issues of sexual abuse or to a sexual abuse treatment team in a hospital setting. Interdisciplinary teams that include a social worker, psychologist, psychiatrist, nurse, and physician are extremely helpful in sorting out the complex issues involved in child sexual abuse cases, including decreasing the number of interviews for the child, identifying the perpetrator, and pressing charges (22,23,25). Custody battles may be particularly problematic (26).

In all cases of sexual abuse, it is extremely important that patients be given sympathetic medical care. All patients with an episode of sexual abuse should be seen promptly by their primary care clinician. If a sexual assault has occurred within hours or days, the clinician will probably want to make use of an emergency department setting or specially equipped clinic to collect the necessary forensic evidence in the event that prosecution is undertaken.

PATTERNS OF SEXUAL ABUSE

It is important for physicians to understand some of the patterns of sexual abuse of children and to realize that all cases cannot be considered in the same way. Evaluation and treatment are quite different in the various forms of abuse. Becker (27) used the term *child molester* to refer to perpetrators who choose child victims and the term *sex offender* more broadly to refer to those who offend against adult victims, child victims, or both. *Pedophilia* is the preference of an adult for sexual contact with a child. It may involve genital fondling, genital contact, or genital viewing. Finkelhor (28) theorized that four factors are necessary before pedophilic fantasies turn to action: (a) the adult finds that it is emotionally satisfying to relate to children; (b) the adult experiences a physiologic response to a child, for example, erection; (c) the adult is blocked in his or her ability to get needs met by an adult; and (d) the individual may have poor impulse control or may utilize substances such as drugs or alcohol to lower inhibitions (27,28). There is clearly no one causative factor but rather multiple pathways of development. Several models have been developed that take into account individual characteristics, family variables, and socioeconomic factors, but none has been validated empirically (27). Traditionally, it was thought that incest offenders were exclusively incestuous, but more recent studies have found that many sex offenders are engaged in both intrafamilial and extrafamilial abuse (12,27). The onset of deviant sexual interest often begins in adolescence, predating any family disruption or dysfunction in adult life. In addition, many apprehended sex offenders are adolescents, and they may offend against peers, younger children, and adults. Few studies have been done of these individuals, although many have histories of depression and of having been sexually abused themselves. Many lack social skills and impulse control.

Knight and associates (29) proposed that nonincestuous child molesters can be classified on the basis of their degree of fixation on children and their behavior during the molestation. At one extreme are interpersonal offenders who develop a relationship with a child, and the sexual contact is typically nongenital and nonorgasmic. At the other end of the spectrum are offenders who rarely have nonsexual contact with children, choose strangers as victims, and often have a history of violent acts that are sexually arousing.

In many cases, offenders attempt to entice or entrap a youngster through the use of money, candy, or other bribes without resorting to physical force. Very often, victims and offenders know each other as neighbors or relatives. The involvement can continue over a long period of time or can involve a single episode. Although some offenders may not intend actual injury, victims may end up harmed or with a hymenal laceration because they resist or their anatomy does not permit penetration. Additionally, many child molesters do resort to force (27). Child molesters may target children of both sexes, although it is more typical for only females to be targeted (30).

In its broadest definition, *incest* means a sexual relationship between people who are related and cannot legally marry. It generally refers to relationships between members of the immediate nuclear family, such as between father and daughter, mother and son, father and son, mother and daughter, or between siblings. Although sexual involvement between a stepparent and child is not traditional incest, it has many of the same psychodynamics and problems for management and treatment as do other forms of incest. Most referred cases of incest involve sexual offenses committed by the father against a child, usually the daughter. Mother–son incest is reported very infrequently; generally, either the mother or the son has major psychopathology or psychosis. Brother–sister incest is not frequently reported because of the assumption by many that it represents normal sexual play; however, it often occurs as an exploitive situation when the brother is considerably older than the sister (15). Incestuous relations may also include grandparents, uncles, and cousins. A sexual relationship between a stepfather and child or between a mother's boyfriend and child is sometimes called "functional parent incest." In parental incest, there is some form of major family dysfunction. Isolation and depression are frequently present. The child learns to adapt to the sexual expectations of the relationship. The mother may be involved in conscious or unconscious complicity, and by frequent absences from the home, she may allow a relationship to develop between the father and the daughter, keeping the family together.

Incestuous relationships may start in the early childhood years and continue through adolescence. Often, the daughter feels the threat of family disruption if she were to tell the secret. A crisis may occur if there is sudden disclosure of the situation when the child is in late puberty or adolescence; the youngster may begin to feel that her involvement is no longer age appropriate and may wish to have more meaningful relationships with her peer group.

An extraordinary number of families who are involved in incestuous situations will recount similar situations in their own childhood. Although incest is reported more frequently in chaotic families of lower socioeconomic status, it may be that such families are more likely to come to the attention of child-abuse workers because of their prior involvement with welfare and other social agencies. Clearly, incest occurs in all socioeconomic groups; however, the secret may remain within the family for years, and it may only be disclosed when a young woman is in psychotherapy during her young adult years. Any disclosure of incestuous relationships should be taken seriously, and appropriate evaluation and treatment undertaken. Often, the adults involved in the incest will show little remorse or shame and will typically deny or minimize the behavior.

Little research has been done on recidivism, but rates appear to be 30% to 40% for perpetrators overall and 10% for perpetrators involved in incest (27). Those who target both males and females and pre- and postpubertal victims appear to have the highest recidivism rate (75%). A prior criminal record is a strong predictor of repeat offenses.

PATIENT ASSESSMENT

Due to the legal implications, medical data should be carefully collected and recorded in all cases of alleged rape or sexual abuse (9,23,31). The aim of the evaluation is to document what has happened, obtain adequate medicolegal evidence, and provide patients with medical and psychological followup. Clinicians should avoid trying to decide whether rape actually occurred or whether there is sufficient evidence for a verdict.

The timing and the extent of the physical examination depend on the history. Any child who has pain, vaginitis, bleeding, dysuria, or a history of trauma or has been abused within the past 72 hours should be seen immediately for an assessment. Physical findings that may corroborate a sexual assault must be documented. Since children often have difficulty disclosing a full history of the nature of the abuse, a complete physical examination is always indicated. A standard protocol is available in most emergency departments and should be followed so that forensic evidence can be passed directly to a police officer to maintain a legal "chain of evidence." Protocols that include drawings of male and female genitalia are excellent for documenting abnormalities (see Appendix 5).

Patients who were abused weeks to months before seeking help should be interviewed as soon as is practical. The physical examination is done at the completion of the initial assessment, but samples for sperm are not obtained.

Sexually Transmitted Diseases and Sexual Assault

Parents and health care providers often ask about the risk of acquiring a sexually transmitted disease (STD) in the context of sexual abuse, especially with the increasing prevalence of herpes, human papillomavirus, and human immunodeficiency virus (HIV). The estimate of the risk also determines which, if any, infections should be treated with prophylactic medications at the time of the initial evaluation (32–56) (see Chapters 3, 11, and 12). The implications of commonly encountered STDs from the 1991 American Academy of Pediatrics statement are shown in Table 1.

Jenny and associates (38,39,42,45) have reviewed the risk of STDs in children and adults with histories of sexual abuse. Importantly, Jenny has distinguished between infections noted at the initial evaluation and those found at followup visits. This distinction is particularly relevant in the care of adolescents, since adolescent assault victims who come to medical attention in hospital settings may have a preexisting STD (36–39,50). However, it should be noted that not all infections noted at baseline are necessarily preexisting infections since it is possible that a culture could be positive as a result of exposure to the male ejaculate (48). At least one STD is present at the time of evaluation in 29% to 43% of patients (45,47).

Studies of sexual assault victims have found *Neisseria gonorrhoeae* to be present in 2.4% to 12.0% of patients at initial evaluation; studies of patients who

TABLE 1. *Implications of commonly encountered sexually transmitted diseases (STDs) for the diagnosis and reporting of sexual abuse of prepubertal infants and children*

STD confirmed	Sexual abuse	Suggested action
Gonorrhea[a]	Certain	Report[b]
Syphilis[a]	Certain	Report
Chlamydia trachomatis[a]	Probable[c]	Report
Condyloma acuminata[a]	Probable	Report
Trichomonas vaginalis	Probable	Report
Herpes simplex virus type 1 (genital)	Possible	Report[d]
Herpes simplex virus type 2	Probable	Report
Bacterial vaginosis	Uncertain	Medical followup
Candida albicans	Unlikely	Medical followup

[a]If not perinatally acquired.
[b]To agency mandated in community to receive reports of suspected sexual abuse.
[c]Culture only reliable diagnostic method.
[d]Unless there is a clear history of autoinoculation.
(From American Academy of Pediatrics Committee on Child Abuse and Neglect. Guidelines for the evaluation of sexual abuse of children. *Pediatrics* 1991;87:254; with permission.)

are negative at the initial visit have noted positive gonorrhea cultures in 2.6% to 4% of patients at followup (37,38,45). The Centers for Disease Control and Prevention (CDC) have estimated the risk of acquiring gonorrhea to be 6% to 12% (51). In sexually abused children, a positive culture for gonorrhea has been reported in 0% to 26.7%, with a usual rate of 2% to 5% (Table 2). Although a positive gonorrhea culture in prepubertal girls is almost always associated with vaginal discharge at presentation or by history (52–54), the infection may occasionally be asymptomatic (56). In Muram et al's series (55), 1.4% (12/865) of prepubertal girls seen within 72 hours of assault were positive, and all had signs of acute vulvovaginitis. In a series of 2731 girls (age 1 to 12 years) referred to the Child Sexual Abuse Team and who had vaginal cultures performed, Ingram and colleagues (58) identified 84 girls with vaginal gonococcal infections; 80 had vaginitis, 2 had a history of vaginal intercourse with a perpetrator with gonorrhea, 1 had *N. gonorrhoeae* isolated from a urine culture, and 1 had a sister with gonorrhea.

Jenny and colleagues (45) reported that 10% of women were positive for *C. trachomatis* at the initial visit for evaluation of a sexual assault; at followup, 2% of women with initially negative cultures who had not been given antibiotics were positive. In a study of 76 postpubertal women seen within 60 hours of sexual assault, Glaser and coworkers (48) found that 20 (26%) had chlamydial infection by culture (11), a fourfold rise in serologic titer (6), or both (3). The finding of serologic evidence of infection suggested that the identification of *C. trachomatis* immediately after assault may in fact signify that some positive cultures at baseline are the result of acquisition during the assault (48). The risk of acquiring chlamydial infection has been estimated to be 4% to 17% (51). In the Glaser et al (48) study, 11% of assault victims developed pelvic inflammatory disease (four of whom had gonorrhea or *Chlamydia*).

C. trachomatis has been reported in 2% to 17% of prepubertal girls, depending on the population studied (see Table 2). Embree and colleagues (59) used a vaginal wash technique in 138 prepubertal girls and detected 4 girls (2.8%) with positive polymerase chain reaction (PCR) tests for *C. trachomatis*; only 2 had positive *Chlamydia* cultures and thus more data on the very sensitive molecular amplification tests are needed. As noted in Chapter 3, *C. trachomatis* may persist after birth for a number of months. Because the majority of girls will have been treated with antibiotics to which the organism is sensitive by 1 to 3 years of age, the issue of persistence often becomes less likely and the potential for sexual transmission as the source of infection becomes much greater.

The risk of syphilis appears to be low and is estimated by the CDC at 0.5% to 3% (51), although in patients with other STDs the risk is increased (40). White and coworkers (35) reported that 6 (5.5%) of 108 children had positive serologies for syphilis but this group of children had a positive gonorrhea rate of 26.7%. Lande and colleagues (60) identified syphilis in 1 (0.7%) of 139 children (ages 10 months to 13 years) in the period 1984 to 1987, and Ingram and associates (57) reported that 0.1% of abused children had syphilis (see Table 2).

Bacterial vaginosis and *T. vaginalis* infection have been found in 5% to 42% and 6% to 20%, respectively, of postpubertal assault victims (48). Jenny and colleagues (45) found that 15% of women had vaginal trichomoniasis at baseline evaluation for sexual assault and 12% had new infections at followup. Bacterial vaginosis was noted in 34% at baseline and 19% at followup. Glaser and coworkers (48) found bacterial vaginosis in 38 women (50%) in their study, of whom 21% (8/38) appeared to have been infected during the assault. Trichomoniasis was found in 17 women (22%), with 29% (5/17) having acquired it during the assault. Data on prepubertal girls are sparse. *Trichomonas* can be transmitted at the time of birth and cause vaginitis and nasal discharge, but the organism usually disappears spontaneously with waning estrogen effects on the vaginal mucosa or with treatment. Trichomoniasis can rarely occur in the vagina of prepubertal girls and is usually associated with sexual abuse (61). Bacterial vaginosis has also been noted at followup in children with a history of acute vaginal assault. Conflicting studies have provided data on the prevalence of *Gardnerella vaginalis* in prepubertal girls (see Chapter 3).

TABLE 2. *Sexually transmitted diseases in 1538 children (ages 1–12 years) evaluated for sexual abuse 1981–1991*

Neisseria gonorrhoeae	2.8%
Chlamydia trachomatis	1.2%
Human papillomavirus	1.8%
Treponema pallidum	0.1%
Herpes simplex virus	0.1%

(From Ingram DL, Everett VD, Lyna PR. Epidemiology of adult sexually transmitted disease agents in children being evaluated for sexual abuse. *Pediatr Infect Dis J* 1992;11:945; with permission.)

Other organisms have also been studied in relation to child sexual abuse. A single case report has associated a urinary tract infection with *Staphylococcus saprophyticus* in a sexually abused 26-month-old child (62). In general, however, although urinary tract symptoms are common following sexual abuse, actual urinary tract infection is uncommon (63).

Jenny and coworkers (45) reported positive herpes simplex virus (HSV) cultures from 2% of adolescents at the initial visit and none at followup. Studies in children have noted that genital herpes can be acquired through self-inoculation from oral–genital contact (HSV type 1 gingivostomatitis occurring simultaneously with genital lesions), but sexual abuse may result in infections with either HSV type 1 or type 2 (see Chapter 3).

The risk of acquiring HPV from sexual abuse is unknown, but we and others have seen adolescents with a single rape episode develop cervical dysplasia associated with HPV infection (61). Studies of prepubertal children beyond the first 2 years of life have indicated that a substantial number of infections are associated with sexual abuse and thus a careful history is mandatory (see Chapter 13).

The potential transmission of HIV to victims of sexual abuse and sexual assault has received increasing attention in the last few years. In the survey by Gellert and colleagues (43), 28 HIV-infected children with sexual abuse as their exclusive risk factor were detected from 5622 HIV-antibody tests during 113,198 sexual abuse assessments (a total of 41 HIV-infected children were identified). Another STD was present in 33%. The reasons for HIV testing were physical findings suggestive of HIV infection in 32%, HIV-seropositive or high-risk perpetrator in 21%, and another STD in 14%. Penile–vaginal and/or –rectal penetration was reported in only 50%. Fifty-eight percent of perpetrators had behavioral risk factors or signs and symptoms of HIV infection, and the serostatus was known in 67% of cases. Although the authors estimated the prevalence risk at 3.55 per 1000 HIV-antibody tests and 0.25 per 1000 sexual abuse assessments conducted (65), the children who were tested in the survey were not randomly selected.

Guidelines for counseling and testing children who have a history of sexual abuse continue to be debated (43,65–68). Recommendations have varied from testing no one, because the risk is small, to universal testing. Experts generally agree that victims who have been involved in behaviors that place them at risk, have symptoms of HIV infection, have been abused by a perpetrator who is HIV positive, or have an STD should have HIV counseling and testing (43,67,68). Children who have had exposure, particularly of long duration, to semen through oral, genital, or anal sex acts are at increased risk of acquiring HIV. Rarely, children have become infected after being injected with intravenous drugs using contaminated needles preceding the sexual abuse. Although recognizing constraints within the legal system, Gutman, Rimsza, and others (44,67,69) have advocated the importance of testing the perpetrator to avoid venipuncture in the child. Not only are prospective studies of HIV risk in sexually abused children needed, but clinicians must remain vigilant in exploring the possibility of sexual abuse in any child who tests positive for HIV and in maintaining surveillance of other children in the households of index cases of HIV infection. Because of the potential for transmission of HIV during sexual assault, protocols are being developed for postexposure prophylaxis of victims. Although much more data are needed, recent reviews have suggested that the estimated probability of HIV transmission associated with unprotected receptive anal intercourse with an HIV-infected person is 0.008 to 0.032 and with vaginal intercourse is 0.0005 to 0.0015 (70). Postexposure prophylaxis has to take into account the type and timing of exposure and the likelihood of HIV infection in the perpetrator. Protocols similar to those used for occupational needlestick exposure prophylaxis (zidovudine and lamivudine) are increasingly being used, and clinicians need to keep up to date with CDC recommendations.

Given the incubation times of STDs (see Chapters 11–13), it is clear that initial cultures may miss many infections depending on the number of hours, days, or months the examination is done after sexual contact. Prepubertal children frequently come for examination weeks to months after the abusive episode(s), and thus a single set of cultures is adequate. In contrast, adolescents often come to medical attention shortly after the assault, and thus followup cultures and wet preparations for *Trichomonas* infection and bacterial vaginosis are necessary to detect infections acquired at the time of the assault, unless they are treated at the time of the examination. Whether all prepubertal children need to be tested for STDs continues to be debated. Some infections are asymptomatic, but the cost of testing all victims in multiple sites, the low risk of infection, and the potential discomfort remain barriers to universal culturing (53–56,71,72). On the other hand, a positive culture finding can be very helpful in confirming the diagnosis of sexual abuse.

The CDC recommendations for considering testing are outlined in Table 3. Siegel and colleagues (53) have argued that prevalence rates of STDs among prepubertal girls are low (3.2% overall, 3.1% with *N. gonorrhoeae*, 0.8% with *C. trachomatis*, and 0% with syphilis, trichomoniasis, or HIV infection), even using the guidelines of testing only prepubertal girls with a history of genital discharge or contact with the perpetrator's genitalia or when an examination finds genital discharge or trauma. Hymel and Jenny (54) have proposed that STD screening be done at the time of the assault in prepubertal girls who have a history or physical examination indicative of penetrating trauma, have been molested by a perpetrator at high risk of STD, or have a vaginal discharge or history of vaginal discharge. In low-risk prepubertal patients, they have suggested deferring the cultures to two weeks after an acute assault. In contrast to selective testing of prepubertal girls, there is broad consensus on the need to culture *all* postpubertal girls because of the high prevalence of STDs.

If tests for STDs are to be obtained, the recommended laboratory tests are given in Table 3. Vaginal secretions are examined for *Trichomonas* and clue cells (including a "whiff" test; see Chapter 11). Culture of *G. vaginalis* is not indicated. Some centers also culture the rectum for *C. trachomatis;* more studies are needed on normal populations to use a positive rectal culture of *Chlamydia* as confirmatory evidence of sexual abuse. Nonculture immunoassays and DNA

TABLE 3. *Recommendations for testing prepubertal children for sexually transmitted diseases (STDs)*

The decision should be individualized

Situations involving a high risk for STDs and a strong indication for testing include the following:
- A suspected offender is known to have an STD or to be at high risk for STDs (e.g., multiple partners or past history of STDs)
- The child has symptoms or signs of an STD
- There is a high STD prevalence in the community
- Evidence of oral or genital penetration or ejaculation

Recommended laboratory tests, if testing is done, include the following:
- Cultures for *Neisseria gonorrhoeae* from pharynx, anus, and vagina
- Cultures for *Chlamydia trachomatis* from the vagina and anus
- Wet mount and culture for *Trichomonas vaginalis*
- Collection of frozen serum sample
- Inspection of genital, perianal, and oral area for human papillomavirus
- Herpes simplex virus culture for ulcerative lesions
- Serologic testing for syphilis, human immunodeficiency virus, and/or hepatitis B if risk factors or epidemiologic evidence

[From Centers for Disease Control. 1998 STD treatment guidelines. *MMWR* 1998;47(RR-1):111.]

probes for *C. trachomatis* should not be used for abuse evaluations. Lesions suggestive of HSV infection should be cultured for this virus.

A serologic test for syphilis can be done initially and then 8–12 weeks later if prophylactic antibiotics are not administered. Because of the low risk of acquiring this infection, many centers do selective testing. The low risk of HIV infection should be discussed with parents and child (if old enough), and the benefits and risks of testing made clear. Patients and families may wish to make use of confidential or anonymous counseling and testing centers.

Tests for Semen

Several tests are available for identifying the presence of semen in assault victims. Acid phosphatase tests can be helpful but may be negative during the first 3 hours; the test is positive in about 50% of vaginal swabs at 12 hours and can be positive for up to 48 hours (73–76). Acid phosphatase from vaginal sources or plant materials may give false-positive results, and thus the qualitative test is presumptive, not diagnostic, evidence of semen. Quantitative assays for acid phosphatase can be more definitive, but specific tests are still recommended. The semen protein antigen p30 of prostatic origin is found in the semen of both normal and vasectomized men, but not in body fluids of women, and is thus more sensitive and specific than acid phosphatase (76). p30 is undetectable in the vagina by 48 hours after intercourse. The p30 enzyme-linked immunosorbent assay (ELISA) has been estimated to be 100-fold more sensitive than counterimmunoelectrophoresis (77). The MHS-5 test is an ELISA based on a monoclonal antibody to a seminal vesicle–specific antigen (78–80). MHS-5 does not cross-react with other biologic fluids and appears to be stable on clothes for months.

Swabs obtained during an evaluation should be immediately air-dried and then frozen or maintained in a desiccated chamber at ambient temperature. The use of both p30 and MHS-5 should provide a high level of confidence. Blood group antigens can also be evaluated by many forensic laboratories. DNA mapping of semen, blood, and other bodily fluids has been increasingly used in forensic medicine and provides courts with more precise estimation of odds for a particular perpetrator (75,81). DNA typing using PCR methodology has also been used to determine paternity in prenatal cases and could be applied to sexual assault cases that result in pregnancy (82).

Wood's lamp fluorescence (white, yellow-green, or blue-green) can aid in the detection of areas of the body that should be tested for semen. However, urine and other substances that can occur in the genital area of children and adolescents may also fluoresce, and thus the test should only be used to aid in collecting adequate forensic specimens. In addition, the intensity of the fluorescence of semen can diminish markedly and disappear on skin by 24 hours, even though the actual semen is still present and detectable by other, much more sensitive and specific tests using p30 and MHS-5 (77). Thus, for forensic evaluation, swabs of the perineal area, inner thighs, and buttocks should be obtained even when the Wood's lamp examination is negative.

Data vary on the length of time that motile and nonmotile sperm may be found in the vagina or cervical mucus. Soules and coworkers (73) found that in adults with voluntary intercourse only 50% of the specimens examined had motile sperm 3 hours after intercourse, whereas at 72 hours nonmotile sperm could be detected on a fixed preparation in nearly 50%. All specimens contained whole sperm up to 18 hours after intercourse and sperm heads up to 24 hours. Since the staining technique in this study was very sensitive, physicians need to know data from the police laboratory performing the test. Duenhoelter and associates (74) found motile sperm in 31.7% of the victims within 6 hours of the alleged sexual assault and in 18% of those examined 7 to 24 hours after the incident. However, the latter group contained three patients in whom the sperm were detected in cervical mucus; sperm may remain motile longer in cervical mucus (up to 2 to 5 days). Nonmotile sperm may be present in the vagina for 3 to 5 days and in the endocervical canal for up to 17 days (83,84). It should be remembered that the absence of sperm should not be taken as evidence against a sexual assault; up to 50% of specimens obtained from victims of acute rape may have no motile sperm either because the offender has sexual dysfunction or oligospermia or because detection techniques are insensitive (85).

Normal and Abnormal Anogenital Findings in Children and Adolescents

Some examples of the normal and abnormal hymenal and vulvar findings are shown in Color Plates 1 to 22 and in Chapters 1, 3, and 8. The percentage of sexually abused children with a "normal" examination has varied from 16% to 90%, depending on the case mix, age of patients, definition of normal versus abnormal, and examiners (86–94).

Several other volumes with extensive photographs are available to clinicians (1–3). The American Professional Society on the Abuse of Children* has been working in consensus groups to further the definitions that can be useful to practicing clinicians. Accurate descriptions of genital findings are essential. (For terminology, figures, and photographs, see Figs. 1 and 2, Chapter 1, Color Plates, and Appendix 4.)

The use of the colposcope has greatly increased physicians' knowledge of normal anatomy and fine-tuned visual skills. The advantages of the colposcope are that the hymen and vulva can be greatly magnified to detect small changes not easily visible with the naked eye and photographs are easily taken at the time of the examination to provide future documentation. The latter prevents the need for repeated examinations when the presence of physical findings is disputed. Cross-sectional data and observations on genital anatomy have improved substantially in the past 10 years (89,96–105). Several longitudinal studies of girls with changes in hymenal anatomy have also been reported (107–113).

An early study by Jenny and associates (114) confirmed that all 1131 newborn female infants in the study were born with hymens. Berenson and coworkers (101) extended this observation by observing the hymenal configuration and number and location of clefts, bumps, tags, and ridges in 468 neonates (photographs were taken in 449 neonates) (Figs. 1 and 2). Most infants had an annular hymen with a central or ventral orifice. Clefts were observed only on the ventral half of the hymen and were noted in 34%; 56% had a longitudinal intravaginal ridge, 87% an external hymenal ridge, and 13% a tag extending from a rim or a ridge. In a longitudinal study of girls examined at birth and 1 year of age, Berenson (111) reported that 8% of the girls developed labial adhesions, 58% had a decrease in the amount of hymenal tissue, more infants at 1 year had crescentic configurations, and significantly fewer had an external ridge (82% vs. 14%). Inferior notches between 4 and 8 o'clock were not observed at either age. In a second longitudinal study of girls examined at ≤2 months and again at 3 years, Berenson (110) observed that the hymenal configuration changed in 65% of subjects, usually from annular or fimbriated to crescentic. External ridges observed at birth usually disappeared by age 3 years. Intravaginal ridges were observed more often at age 3, perhaps in part because observation was easier in the 3-year-old with an unestrogenized hymen. Nine tags formed during the followup interval. No notches were noted between 5 and 7 o'clock at initial or followup study in any of the girls. The mean transhymenal diameters increased during the interval.

Studies have also looked at the older prepubertal child. In an early study (87), we compared children presenting with a history of sexual abuse with children seen for routine examinations and for genital complaints. Among 127 girls (mean age 3.8 years) seen for routine physical examination, erythema was noted in 13%, labial adhesions in 7%, "attenuated" hymen in 4%, bumps in 24%, clefts in 13%, and scars in 1%; in contrast, among 119 girls with history of sexual abuse (mean

*American Professional Society on the Abuse of Children, 407 South Dearborn, Suite 1300, Chicago IL 60605; phone: 312-554-0166.

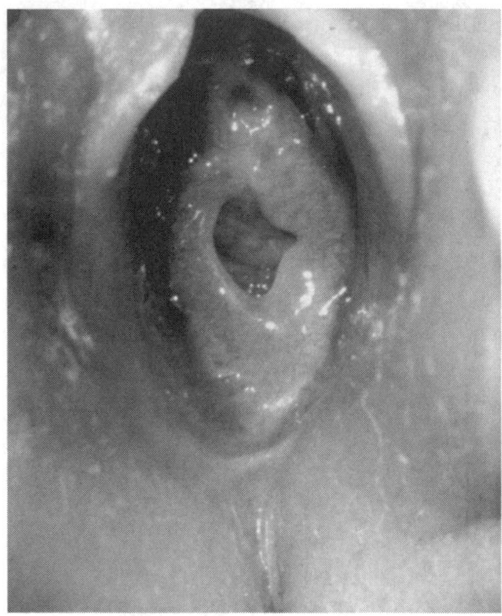

FIG. 1. Hymenal cleft at 3 o'clock in a 3-year-old girl.

age 5.8 years), erythema was noted in 34%, "attenuated" hymen in 18%, scars in 9%, a transection at 6 o'clock in 3%, and a transection at 4 and 8 o'clock in 1%. Hymenal transections, condyloma, and/or abrasions occurred only among the sexually abused girls (9/119). Although we originally used the term "attenuated" to describe hymens with narrow rims, this terminology has been replaced with more descriptive terminology to denote whether the rim appears sharply defined or thickened and rounded, a determination often made best using the knee-chest position. A narrow rim hymen that is rounded, thickened, absent, and/or blends into the vagina has been associated with sexual abuse. In contrast, narrow, sharply defined posterior rim hymens can occur in both nonabused populations and in sexually abused girls although it appears more commonly in the latter. More data on the prevalence of this variant in nonabused populations followed prospectively are needed. We have also observed that girls presenting with vaginitis to our clinic may be more likely to have a sharply defined but narrow posterior rim hymen; it is possible either that some of these girls have undisclosed abuse or that this particular variant predisposes girls to vaginal contamination and symptoms.

In 1990, McCann et al (100) published an important study examining the genital findings in 93 girls (mean age 5 years, 6 months; range 10 months to 10 years, 4 months) who gave no history of sexual abuse (Table 4). In 1992, Berenson (102), in collaboration with several investigators including Heger and Emans, published a study of 211 girls (mean age 21 months; range, 1 month to 7 years) with no history of sexual abuse and noted bumps in 7%, notches in 8% (none were observed between 4 and 8 o'clock), extensive labial agglutination in 5%, partial labial agglutination in 17%, hymenal tags in 3%, vaginal ridges in 25%, external ridge in 15%, attenuated hymen in 2%, and transection in 0.5%.

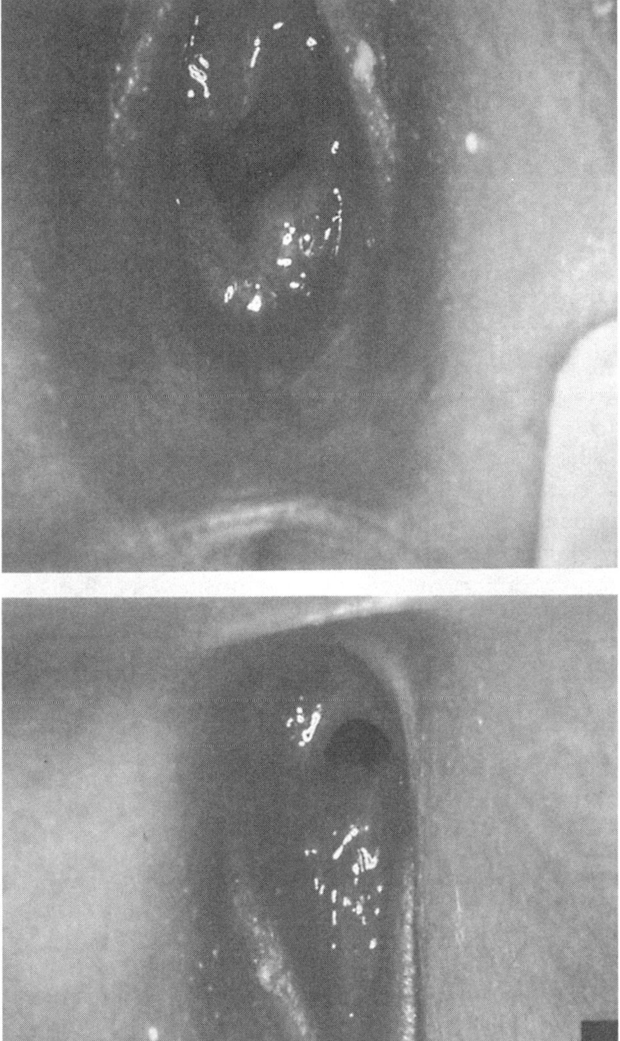

FIG. 2. In the supine position **(top)**, a bump is observed between the 3 and 9 o'clock positiion; however, in knee-chest position **(bottom)** the bump disappears and a normal hymenal border is observed. (From Heger AH, Emans SJ, et al, eds. *Evaluation of the sexually abused child: medical textbook and photographic atlas.* New York; Oxford University Press, 1992; with permission.)

A hymen with a narrow rim and transection was not felt to be normal, but the child could not be located for further history and evaluation for sexual abuse. A fimbriated hymen was the most common in girls ≤12 months, and a crescentic hymen was most common in girls >24 months of age.

Kellogg and Parar (103) described in newborns and children a normal structure termed *linea vestibularis*, also called midline sparing, white median raphe, or midline avascular area (see Color Plate 5). In a study of 123 newborns, 10% were noted to have the white linear structure; a white spot, termed a *partial linea vestibularis*, was noted in 14%. The prominence increased in some and decreased in others over time (113).

Hymenal findings in adolescents have recently been examined by our center (115). In a study of 300 girls (100 who denied sexual activity and had never used tampons, 100 who denied sexual activity and had used tampons, and 100 consensually active adolescent girls), we found that sexually active girls were significantly more likely to have complete clefts between the 2 and 10 o'clock positions than nonsexually active girls (Table 5). Among the nonsexually active girls, only 3% had a complete cleft between 4 and 8 o'clock and only one had a complete cleft at 6 o'clock (0.5%; 95% confidence interval: 0.01, 2.75). We hypothesized that the few girls with complete clefts between 4 and 8 o'clock likely had unreported consensual or nonconsensual sexual intercourse. Tampon use, sports participation (including gymnastics), and prior pelvic examination did not increase the number of complete clefts observed. Among the sexually active group, 74% had complete clefts on the lower half of the hymen between 3 and 9 o'clock. Median hymenal diameter was greater in the sexually active group, but there was overlap between the groups, and exact measurement of an elastic hymenal orifice is problematic. Only sexually active girls had evidence of "attenuation" or "myrtiform caruncles" (rounded hymenal remnants separated on both sides by complete clefts). Girls who had been sexually active for >3 years or were over age 20 years were more likely to have these findings (Table 6).

Dermatoses, other genital conditions, and accidental genital trauma offer a challenge to the clinician who is called upon to assess whether the genital find-

TABLE 4. *Frequency of hymenal findings by examination method*[a]

Findings	Separation	Traction	Knee-chest
Hymenal edge			
Sharp	38/75 (50.7)	43/79 (54.4)	68/79 (86.1)
Thickened	39/76 (51.3)	43/80 (53.8)	21/80 (26.3)
Rolled[b]	14/76 (18.4)	19/80 (23.8)	5/80 (6.3)
Mounds	18/76 (23.7)	27/80 (33.8)	14/78 (17.9)
Projections	16/76 (21.1)	26/78 (33.3)	25/75 (33.3)
Tags	20/82 (24.4)	20/82 (24.4)	16/81 (19.8)
Perihymenal bands	8/83 (9.6)	13/81 (16.0)	9/79 (11.4)
"Septal remnants"	0/83 (0.0)	7/81 (8.6)	15/81 (18.5)
Septa	1/82 (1.1)	2/80 (2.5)	1/81 (1.2)
Notches	3/74 (4.1)	5/76 (6.6)	2/90 (2.2)
Synechiae	2/84 (2.4)	2/83 (2.4)	3/78 (3.8)
Anterior clefts	0/81 (0.0)	1/82 (1.2)	0/79 (0.0)
Vascularity (irregular)	21/67 (31.3)	21/68 (30.9)	22/76 (28.9)
Isolated vascularity	12/86 (13.9)	13/81 (16.0)	18/79 (22.8)

[a]Results are given as number (%) of subjects.
[b]Localized areas of rolled edges.
(From McCann J, Wells R, Simon M, Voris J. Genital findings in prepubertal girls selected for nonabuse: a descriptive study. *Pediatrics* 1990;86:438; with permission.)

TABLE 5. *Genital findings observed in 300 female patients in two adolescent medicine practices: 200 subjects not sexually active, by choice of menstrual hygiene product, and 100 sexually active subjects*

	Not sexually active			
	Pad users (n = 100)	Tampon users (n = 100)	Sexually active (n = 100)	p^*
Subjects with complete clefts (no.)	6	14	84[a]	<0.001[b]
Subjects with complete clefts (2–10 o'clock) (no.)	5	11	81[a]	0.001[b]
Complete hymenal clefts per patient (no.)	0 (0–2)	0 (0–2)	2 (0–4)[a]	<0.0001[c]
Median hymenal diameter (cm) (range)	1.2 (0.2–2.0)[a]	1.5 (0.3–0.25)[a]	2.5 (1.5–3.5)[a]	<0.0001[c]

*p < 0.01
Ranges are shown in parentheses.
[a]Different from others at $p < 0.05$ (Duncan, chi-square test).
[b]Chi-square test.
[c]Kruskal-Wallis test.
(From Emans SJ, Woods ER, Allred EN, Grace E. Hymenal findings in adolescent women: impact of tampon use and consensual sexual activity. *J Pediatr* 1994;125:153; with permission.)

ings noted are the result of child sexual abuse. Conditions such as lichen sclerosus (see Color Plates 3 and 4), urethral prolapse (see Chapter 3), failure of midline fusion from the anus to the posterior fourchette (see Color Plate 6), localized vulvar pemphigoid (116), phytophotodermatitis, linear IgA dermatosis, Crohn's disease, herpes zoster, allergic contact dermatitis, psoriasis, Ehlers-Danlos syndrome, and ulcerating hemangioma have been confused with trauma from physical and sexual abuse (117).

Genital trauma may be accidental or secondary to sexual abuse (117, 118–122). Straddle injuries usually cause trauma to the soft tissues over the symphysis pubis, the ischiopubic ramus, or adductor longus tendon. These injuries are usually unilateral and anterior and cause damage to the external rather than internal genital structures. The history is usually striking for a fall or trauma. Vaginal lacerations and rectovaginal injuries can occur in girls who fall astride sharp objects (117). In a large study on unintentional perineal injury in 56 prepubertal girls (ages 1 to 12 years), the labia minora were most commonly involved, and the majority of the injuries were anterior or lateral to the hymen (119). In 34%, the injuries involved areas posterior to the hymen. In only one patient was the hymen involved; the patient was 2 years old and fell at a park, abducting her legs in a splits-type mechanism. Among 72 females seen for straddle injuries, 79% had minor lacerations or abrasions of the labia majora or minora; 16% had injuries to the posterior fourchette, and 9% had vulvar hematomas (119). Vaginal injury occurred in seven patients, and two had hymenal injuries (three had penetrating injuries and two others fell on a crossbar or curb). Thus penetrating trauma sexual abuse needs to be strongly considered in the presence of a posterior hymenal transection and absence of a convincing history of accidental trauma.

TABLE 6. *Genital findings observed in 300 female patients in two adolescent medicine practices*[a]

	Not sexually active (n = 200)	Sexually active (n = 100)	p*
Attenuation	0	37%	<0.001
SA ≤3 yr		19/63 (30%)	
SA >3 yr		18/37 (49%)	0.09
Myrtiform caruncles	0	21%	<0.001
SA ≤3 yr		8/63 (13%)	
SA >3 yr		13/37 (35%)	0.009
Age ≤20 yr old		9/61 (15%)	
Age >20 yr old		12/39 (31%)	0.049

[a]Data are number/total, with percent in parentheses.
*Chi-square test; SA, sexually active.
(From Emans SJ, Woods ER, Allred EN, Grace E. Hymenal findings in adolescent women: impact of tampon use and consensual sexual activity. *J Pediatr* 1994;125:153; with permission.)

Several classification systems have been proposed for child sexual abuse (Table 7) (89,91,92,123), and variable percentages of girls with a history of sexual abuse have been noted to have abnormal examinations (86,87,92,107,124). It is important to remember that a normal examination (Category 1) does not confirm or disprove a history of sexual abuse (92). Definitive and specific findings are more common in those who reported genitogenital assault (86%) than in those who reported digital assault (16%) (92). In a study of physical findings in 31 sexual assault victims (1 to 17 years old) based on offenders' confessions, Muram (123) noted that specific findings suggesting sexual abuse occurred in only 45% of the patients; findings occurred in 11 (61%) of 18 girls when the perpetrator confessed to penetration, compared to 3 (23%) of 13 when penetration was denied. Thus, 7 (39%) of 18 girls in whom the perpetrator confessed to penetration had a normal examination or nonspecific findings. However, both perpetrators and victims may report "vaginal penetration" when vulvar coitus has occurred.

A subsequent study by Adams and associates (91) examined the genital and anal findings in children (mean age 9.0 years; range, 8 months to 17 11/12 years) who were victims of child sexual abuse and whose abusers were convicted. The type of molestation described by children was fondling in 36%, oral–genital contact in 31%, digital–vaginal penetration in 44%, and penile–vaginal penetration in 63%. Using the definition they originally published in 1992 (126) and modified for the current study (91), Adams et al. reported that the hymen was normal in 50%, erythema was present in 32%, increased vascularity in 25%, and labial adhesions in 17% (nonspecific findings). In addition, they found that a hymenal rim <1 mm was present in 6% and acute abrasions were present in 2% (suspicious findings); there were two or more genital findings in 4% (suggestive), and the hymen was absent in 4% and transected in 5% (clear evidence). Using their classification schema for genital examination, they considered the findings normal in 28%, nonspecific in 49%, suspicious in 9%, and abnormal in 14%. Abnormal anal findings were present in only 1% of patients. An abnormal examination was more common for girls who were examined within 72 hours than for those exam-

TABLE 7. *Two systems for classification of anogenital findings in children with suspected sexual abuse*

Muram's classification	
Category 1	Normal-appearing genitalia
Category 2	Nonspecific findings: abnormalities of the genitalia that could have been caused by sexual abuse, but also often seen in girls who are not victims of sexual abuse (e.g., inflammation and scratching). These findings may be the sequelae of poor perineal hygiene or nonspecific infection. Included in this category are redness of the external genitalia, increased vascular pattern of the vestibular and labial mucosa, presence of purulent discharge from the vagina, small skin fissures or lacerations in the area of the posterior fourchette, and agglutination of the labia minora
Category 3	Specific findings: the presence of one or more abnormalities strongly suggesting sexual abuse. Such findings include recent or healed lacerations of the hymen and vaginal mucosa, enlarged hymenal opening of ≥1 cm[a], procto-episiotomy (a laceration of the vaginal mucosa extending to the rectal mucosa), and indentations in the skin indicating teeth marks (bite marks). The category also includes patients with laboratory confirmation of a venereal disease
Category 4	Definitive findings: any presence of sperm
Adams' classification	
Class I	Normal—periurethral (or vestibular) bands; longitudinal intravaginal ridges or columns; hymenal tags; hymenal bump or mound; linea vestibularis; hymenal cleft/notch in the anterior (superior) half of the hymenal rim, on or above the 3 o'clock and 9 o'clock line, patient supine, estrogen changes
Class 2	Nonspecific or normal variants: findings that may be the result of sexual abuse, depending on the timing of the examination with respect to the abuse, but which may also be due to other causes or may be variants of normal—septate hymen; failure of midline fusion; diastasis ani; perianal skin tag; increased perianal skin pigmentation; erythema (redness) of the vestibule or perianal tissues; increased vascularity ("dilatation of existing blood vessels") of vestibule; labial adhesion; vaginal discharge; lesions of condyloma acuminata in a child <2 years of age; anal fissures; flattened anal folds; anal dilatation with stool present; venous congestion, or venous pooling, in perianal tissues
Class 3	Concerning for abuse: findings that have been noted in children with documented abuse, and may be suspicious for abuse, but for which insufficient data exist to indicate that abuse is the only cause; enlarged hymenal opening—a measurement of the transverse, horizontal opening of the hymen, which is greater than two standard deviations above the mean for age; immediate anal dilatation of at least 20 mm, with stool not visible *or* palpable in rectal vault; hymenal notch/cleft in the posterior (inferior) portion of the hymenal rim; apparent condyloma acuminata in a child >2 years of age; acute abrasions, lacerations, or bruising of labia or perihymenal tissues—history is crucial in determining overall significance
Class 4	Suggestive of abuse/penetration: findings that can only reasonably be explained by postulating that abuse or penetrating injury has occurred—scar or fresh laceration of the posterior fourchette, not involving the hymen; perianal scar

(*Continued on next page*)

TABLE 7. *Continued*

Class 5	Clear evidence of blunt force or penetrating trauma: findings that can have no explanation other than trauma to the hymen or perianal tissue—laceration of the hymen, acute; ecchymosis (bruising) on the hymen; perianal lacerations extending deep to the external anal sphincter; hymenal transection (healed). An area where the hymen has been torn through, to the base, so there is no hymenal tissue remaining between the vaginal wall and the fossa or vestibular wall.This finding has also been referred to as a "complete cleft" in adolescent and young adult women; absence of hymenal tissue. Wide areas in the posterior (inferior) half of the hymenal rim with an absence of hymenal tissue, extending to the base of the hymen, which is confirmed in the knee–chest position

[a]The enlarged opening is not a criteria for the 1997 revision.

(**Muram:** from Muram D. Classification of genital findings in prepubertal girls who are victims of sexual abuse. *Adolesc Pediatr Gynecol* 1988;1:151. **Adams:** from Adams JA. Sexual abuse and adolescents. *Pediatr Ann* 1997;26:299; and Adams JA, Harper K, Knudson S. A proposed system for classification of anogenital findings in children with suspected sexual abuse. *Adolesc Pediatr Gynecol* 1992;5:73; with permission.)

ined later (42% vs. 8%) and more common in those who reported blood being observed at the time of the molestation than those who did not (46% vs. 8%).

Another study by Adams and Knudson (106) of 204 girls aged 9 to 17 years with a reported history of penile–vaginal penetration found abnormal genital findings in only 32%; findings were more common in those with bleeding and an examination within 72 hours of abuse. Transections were noted in only 8%. Kerns and colleagues (107) noted that concave hymenal variations were present in 12.6% of suspected female child and adolescent sexual abuse victims and concluded that concavity with a posterolateral location, angular contour, and rim irregularity were associated with prior hymenal trauma. A normal genital examination was found in 60% of cases in which a perpetrator confessed (62% of digital–vaginal penetrations and 18% of penile–vaginal penetrations) (124).

Healing of genital injuries from sexual abuse occurs promptly in most situations, and thus residua may not be present (108,109). In a complete followup with photographs of three girls, McCann and associates (108) observed that the signs of acute injuries disappeared rapidly but that some changes, including hymenal transection, persisted throughout the pubertal years. The most persistent findings were irregular hymenal edges and narrow rims at the point of injury. The jagged angular margins smoothed off. Injuries to the posterior fourchette healed with minimal scar tissue and left only the slightest evidence of trauma. Finkel (109) observed that wound healing by the process of regeneration might be complete in 48 to 72 hours. Complete restoration of epithelial tissues can take 6 weeks (112). Children with epithelial healing had no residua apparent to the naked eye or at ten-fold magnification at followup. When injuries are more serious, healing involves repair with formation of granulation tissue and a subsequent scar. Since the linear scar may be only a fraction of the width of the original injury, this too may be difficult for clinicians to detect at followup (109).

A discussion of various methods of measurement of the diameter of the hymenal orifice, as well as the pitfalls of using exact cutoff numbers without more normative data, is in several recent reviews (1,122,125,127). The position of measurement (knee-chest vs. supine) and the amount and duration of traction are important in the amount of dilatation. The opening is larger in the knee-chest position than in the supine position using gentle separation only (not retraction). The type of hymen is also important; a posterior rim hymen has a larger orifice than a redundant hymen. The older the child and the more relaxed, the larger the opening. Techniques such as the colposcope have allowed more precise measurements, but it is important to note that since the hymen is elastic, digital penetration is possible even if the *measured* diameter is only 5 mm. The passage of time, healing, variations in measurement technique, and error can lead to changing, especially decreasing, hymenal orifice diameters in serial examinations. The measurements taken by McCann (100), Berensen (102), and colleagues are shown in Tables 8 and 9. A 1-cm hymenal opening in a 4-year-old and a 1.5-cm opening in an 8-year-old are abnormal, but a diagnosis of sexual abuse requires more than the diameter of a hymenal opening and must be consistent with the rest of the total assessment of the child (125). A much more important clinical finding is the presence of the enlarged orifice in association with the presence of defects or transections on the lower half of the hymen (8). Importantly, physicians should be comfortable with their own measurements in normal and sexually abused girls.

Over the past few years, data on perianal findings in nonabused and abused children have been published (98,104,105,128). McCann and coworkers (104) collected data on 267 prepubertal children felt to be nonabused and ranging in age from 2 months to 11 years (Tables 10 and 11). Berenson and colleagues (105) examined 89 female infants ≤18 months of age and reported a smooth area adjacent to the perianal folds in 26%, changes in pigmentation in 10%, erythema in 7%, a skin tag at the 6 or 12 o'clock position in 3%, and a fissure in 1%.

Perianal injuries that result from sexual abuse heal rapidly. In a followup of four children with perianal injuries from sexual abuse documented with photographs, McCann and Voris (112) described initial findings including erythema, edema of the skin folds, localized venous engorgement, dilatation of the external anal sphincter, and lacerations. The superficial lacerations healed in 1 to 11 days; the second-degree wounds in two children healed by the 1- to 5-week return visits, leaving narrow bands of scar tissue. By 12 to 14 months after the assaults, the signs from these two injuries and one surgically repaired injury had virtually disappeared. A skin tag that resulted from the initial injury was persistent, although less evident over time.

Importantly, many children with a history of anal assault have no abnormal findings. Specific findings include scars, sphincter tears, and distortion of the anus, although the latter can also occur with inflammatory bowel disease. Fissures can result from sexual abuse and from constipation.

It is essential for clinicians involved in the evaluation of children for alleged sexual abuse to remember that despite the increasing information on associated

TABLE 8. *Colposcopic transhymenal diameter means and ranges by age group and examination method (n = 72)*[a]

Age group (yr)	Method	Plane	No.	Mean ± SD (mm)	Range (mm)
Preschool (2–4 11/12)	Separation	Vertical	21	5.5 ± 2.2	2.5–10.0
		Horizontal	21	3.9 ± 1.4	1.0–5.5
	Traction	Vertical	24	5.5 ± 1.7	3.0–8.5
		Horizontal	24	5.2 ± 1.4	2.0–8.0
	Knee-chest	Vertical	29	6.3 ± 1.7	3.0–10.0
		Horizontal	29	4.6 ± 1.3	2.5–7.5
Early school age (5–7 11/12)	Separation	Vertical	39	5.6 ± 2.3	1.0–11.0
		Horizontal	39	4.2 ± 1.7	1.0–8.0
	Traction	Vertical	43	6.1 ± 2.1	1.0–10.0
		Horizontal	43	5.6 ± 1.8	1.0–9.0
	Knee-chest	Vertical	41	7.0 ± 2.0	3.0–11.5
		Horizontal	41	5.6 ± 1.5	2.5–8.5
Preadolescent (8 to Tanner II)	Separation	Vertical	19	8.4 ± 2.2	5.0–13.5
		Horizontal	19	5.7 ± 1.6	3.0–8.5
	Traction	Vertical	20	8.3 ± 2.8	2.0–15.0
		Horizontal	20	6.9 ± 2.0	2.5–10.5
	Knee-chest	Vertical	21	8.7 ± 2.6	5.0–15.0
		Horizontal	21	7.3 ± 1.7	4.0–11.0

[a]Infant age group not included because of small number.

(From McCann J, Wells R, Simon M, Voris J. Genital findings in prepubertal girls selected for nonabuse: a descriptive study. *Pediatrics* 1990;86:428; with permission.)

TABLE 9. *Measurements of inferior rim and transhymenal diameters of annular and crescentic hymens in prepubertal girls by age*

	Age (mo)				
	1–12	13–24	25–48	49–81	p[a]
Horizontal diameter (mm)					
No.	35	26	27	25	
Mean ± SD	2.5 ± 0.8	2.9 ± 1.2	2.9 ± 1.0	3.6 ± 1.2	.003
Range	1.0–3.5	1.5–6.5	1.0–6.5	2–4.8	
Vertical diameter (mm)[b]					
No.	11	8	14	6	
Mean ± SD	3.4 ± 1.4	2.8 ± 1.0	3.6 ± 1.2	3.9 ± 2.7	NS
Range	1.8–6.0	1.0–4.3	1.0–6.0	1.0–8.8	
Inferior rim (mm)					
No.	28	26	29	24	
Mean ± SD	2.8 ± 0.8	2.7 ± 1.1	2.7 ± 0.9	2.7 ± 0.7	NS
Range	1.5–4.5	0.9–5.0	0.9–5.0	1.0–3.8	

[a]NS, not significant.

[b]Includes annular hymens only.

(From Berenson AB, Heger AH, Hayes JM, Bailey RK, Emans SJ. Appearance of the hymen in prepubertal girls. *Pediatrics* 1992;89:387; with permission.)

physical findings, the history is the most important element (129). Tables 12 and 13 provide information for probability of sexual abuse and the American Academy of Pediatrics guidelines for reporting child sexual abuse combining physical examination, history, and behavioral indicators.

TABLE 10. *Frequency of perianal findings for total sample[a]*

Findings	Subjects observed (no.)[b]	Subjects with positive findings	
		No.	%
Erythema	168	68	41
Pigmentation	251	74	30
Venous congestion			
Beginning	113	8	7
Midpoint	113	59	52
End	113	83	73
Anal dilatation	267	130	49
Intermittent anal dilatation	130[c]	81	62
Configuration during dilatation			
Oval	94	84	89
Round	94	8	9
Irregular	94	2	2
Smooth area	81	21	26
Dimple/depression	81	15	18
Skin tags	164	18	11
Scars	240	4[d]	2

[a]No abrasions, hematomas, fissures, or hemorrhoids were discovered in the 267 subjects.
[b]The number of observed subjects varied due to missing data as a result of changes over time in the number of variables assessed.
[c]Includes only those subjects whose anus dilated.
[d]May include "smooth area" on anal verge; no photographs available to recheck findings.
(From McCann J, Voris J, Simon M, et al. Perianal findings in prepubertal children selected for nonabuse: a descriptive study. *Child Abuse Negl* 1989;13:179; with permission.)

TABLE 11. *Comparison of diameter of anal orifice with presence of stool in rectal ampulla*

Vertical diameter (mm)	Stool in rectal ampulla			Total subjects[a]
	Yes	No	UTD	
<5.0	2	4	1	7 (9%)
5.0–9.9	2	4	13	19 (23%)
10.0–14.9	18	8	8	34 (42%)
15.0–19.9	7	6	1	14 (17%)
20.0–24.9	6	1[b]	0	7 (9%)
>25.0	0	0	0	0 (0%)
Total	35 (44%)	23 (28%)	23 (28%)	81 (100%)

UTD, unable to detect.
[a]49 of the 130 children with anal dilatation who were examined in the early part of the study were not included due to the lack of notations regarding the presence/absence of stool in the rectal ampulla.
[b]Abnormal behavioral and emotional response profile just below criteria used for exclusion.
(From McCann J, Voris J, Simon M, et al. Perianal findings in prepubertal children selected for nonabuse: a descriptive study. *Child Abuse Negl* 1989;12:179; with permission.)

ASSESSMENT OF THE PREPUBERTAL CHILD

The clinician should take the history from the parents and the child separately, if possible. If there was a forceful assault, the child may feel more comfortable being interviewed with the mother or other caretaker present. The interview should remain unhurried and calm, and a patient–provider relationship should be

TABLE 12. *A proposed system for assessing the probability of child sexual abuse, using the classification scheme for genital findings in Table 7*

Class 1—no evidence of abuse
Normal examination, no history of abuse, no behavioral changes, no witnessed abuse
Nonspecific findings with another known or likely explanation and no history of abuse or behavior changes
Child considered at risk for sexual abuse but gives no history and has only nonspecific behavior changes
Physical findings of injury consistent with history of accidental injury, which is clear and believable
Class 2—possible abuse
Class 1 or 2 findings in combination with significant behavior changes, especially sexualized behaviors, but child unable to give a history of abuse
Condyloma acuminata or herpes type 1 anogenital lesions in a prepubertal child, in the absence of a history of abuse, and with an otherwise normal examination
Child has made a statement, but the statement is either not sufficiently detailed given the child's developmental level, or is not consistent
Class 3 findings with no disclosure of abuse or behavior changes
Class 3—probable abuse
Child gives clear, consistent, detailed description of being molested, with or without physical findings
Class 4 findings in a child, with or without a history of abuse and with no history of accidental penetrating injury
Positive culture (not rapid antigen test) for *Chlamydia trachomatis* from genital area in a prepubertal children >2 years of age
Positive culture for HSV type 2 from genital lesions
Trichomonas infection diagnosed by wet mount or culture
Class 4—definite evidence of abuse or sexual contact
Class 5 physical findings with no history of accident
Finding sperm or seminal fluid in or on a child's body
Pregnancy (from nonconsensual intercourse)
Positive, confirmed cultures for *Neisseria gonorrhoeae* from genital, anal, or pharyngeal source
Syphilis acquired after delivery (i.e., not prenatally acquired)
Witnessed abuse or cases in which photographs or videotapes show child being abused
Confession by the alleged perpetrator to the acts described by the child
Human immunodeficiency virus infection with no documented means of transmission other than sexual contact

(From Adams JA. Sexual abuse and adolescents. *Pediatr Ann* 1997;26:299; with permission.)

established before questions are broached on the issue of the abuse. The review should include the child's past medical history and an assessment of her development and family and social history (10). The clinician should establish credibility with the child by showing interest and telling her that other children with similar problems have been helped. The clinician should remain nonjudgmental and not presuppose that the experience was bad or painful for the child. It may have been neutral or even pleasurable, and the child may not have experienced guilt or anger. In speaking, the clinician should use words that are familiar to the child; it is often helpful to repeat some of the questions during the actual physical examination to make sure the youngster understands what parts of the anatomy are being questioned. The history, written in the child's words, should include such details as time, place, circumstances, others present, and resistance.

TABLE 13. *Guidelines for making the decision to report child sexual abuse*

Data available			Response	
History	Physical	Laboratory	Level of concern about sexual abuse	Action
None	Normal examination	None	None	None
Behavioral changes	Normal examination	None	Low (worry)	± Report,[a] follow closely (possible mental health referral)
None	Nonspecific findings	None	Low (worry)	± Report,[a] follow closely
Nonspecific history by child or history by parent only	Nonspecific findings	None	Possible (suspect)	± Report,[a] follow closely
None	Specific findings	None	Probable	Report
Clear statement	Normal examination	None	Probable	Report
Clear statement	Specific findings	None	Probable	Report
None	Normal examination, nonspecific or specific findings	Positive culture for gonorrhea; positive serologic test for syphilis; presence of semen, sperm, acid phosphatase	Definite	Report
Behavioral changes	Nonspecific changes	Other sexually transmitted diseases	Probable	Report

[a]A report may or may not be indicated. The decision to report should be based on discussion with local or regional experts and/or child protective services agencies.

(From American Academy of Pediatrics Committee on Child Abuse and Neglect. Guidelines for the evaluation of sexual abuse of children. *Pediatrics* 1991;87:25; with permission.)

Dating the time of the abuse may be easier by referring to a grade in school or a birthday. The child is asked to tell as much about the episode as she remembers. Leading questions should be avoided. Appropriate questions include the following: "Do you know why you are here today?", "Can you tell me what happened?", "How did it begin? What happened?", "Did anything change? Where?", "Where was everyone else?", "Why tell now? Has anybody told you to keep it a secret?", "Have you been hurt lately?" It is important to remember that the first report is almost never the first incident. The interviewer should then ask questions such as: "And then what happened?", "What were you wearing?", "What did the room look like?" Older children may be aware of whether ejaculation occurred. The clinician should try to document whether vulvar, vaginal, or rectal penetration has occurred or whether there has been any evidence of oral contact. The child should be asked about any pain or injuries occurring at the time of the episode. Any symptoms that have occurred following the assault such as sore throat, dysuria, enuresis, vaginal discharge or bleeding, rectal bleeding or pain, abdominal pain, nightmares, or changes in school performance should be recorded.

It is important to establish whether the relationship was prolonged and whether the child has been involved with more than one adult. The child should be asked if she received any gifts or remuneration from the adult and whether she knew the adult. It is important to know whether she told the parent of the event immediately after its occurrence. Often children have been threatened and sworn to secrecy. The clinician should make it clear to the child that the incident is not her fault. It is important to concentrate on what happened rather than why (e.g., "Why did you get in the car?"). A young child may feel more comfortable using a doll, puppet, or picture and explaining how the doll feels about the incident. However, dolls are best used by those with training in this area (130). The presence of genitalia in a child's drawing may be associated with a history of sexual abuse (131). The child should be told what information needs to be shared, with whom, and why, and she needs a chance to ask her own questions both before and after the examination.

The child's history is an extraordinarily important part of the evaluation (132). If the initial disclosure can be videotaped, the child may not have to relate the story over and over again. The validation of the story involves looking for behavioral clues, the occurrence of multiple episodes over time, a progression from fondling to penetration, an element of secrecy fostered by coercion, and explicit details of the abuse. Mental health workers with expertise in child sexual abuse can be extremely helpful in the evaluation of the child and her parents. Children's memories about genital touch have been found to be remarkably accurate, especially with direct questioning. In a study of 5- and 7-year-old children, half of whom had an anogenital examination and half a scoliosis examination, the majority of errors to direct questions were omission errors. One child (2.8%) affirmed vaginal touch when it was not part of the examination, and two children (5.6%) gave false reports of anal touch, but two of the three were unable to provide any details (133). Older children (7 years old) answered misleading questions more correctly than did 5-year-olds. To lessen stress in the child and the risk of suggestibility, the number of interviews and interviewers should be minimal, and only interviewers who have skill in eliciting information, are not attached to a particular hypothesis, and are nonjudgmental should be involved (12,134,135). The most problematic cases are those involving child-custody disputes, especially visitation rights. In Paradise and coworkers' study (26), a custody dispute occurred in 39% of 31 sexual abuse complaints against parents. Sexual abuse allegations were substantiated less frequently in cases involving parental conflict than other cases of sexual abuse (67% vs. 95%). These disputes often involve very young children, so the issues are difficult to resolve.

Parents should be allowed to tell their own story separately from the child and to air their feelings without traumatizing the child. In sexual abuse cases involving nonforceful abuse of a child by a stranger, parents may need more counseling and reassurance than the child. The parental response may greatly influence the reaction of the child to the event (136). The child needs to know that parental anger is directed toward the assailant and not toward her.

The physical examination of the young child should be done in a relaxed setting with the mother, father, or other supportive caretaker in the room. An assistant can help in the collection of samples and can reassure the child. It is extremely important to elicit the cooperation of the child. The steps for an acute assault are outlined here, although most cases seen by clinicians in the office setting will probably involve long-standing abuse by a known individual, and the need to obtain specimens for STD testing is discussed under Sexually Transmitted Diseases and Sexual Assault. Hymel and Jenny (54) have suggested that in addition to the guidelines for selective testing for STDs outlined in Table 3 initial STD screening should occur at the time of the event in girls with a history or physical examination indicative of penetrating trauma or with a history or examination consistent with vaginitis but that for low-risk prepubertal girls the cultures can be delayed to 2 weeks after acute sexual assault. Muram et al (55) have suggested that culturing for gonorrhea only those seen at the 2-week visit with symptoms may be a reasonable alternative to initial cultures in low-risk prepubertal girls. Specimens should be collected so that the legal evidence is preserved if the family decides to press charges (1–3,136,137). Photographs are optional (138) but can be helpful for reexamination by others.

The physical examination should include the following steps:

1. Description of the patient's general appearance, emotional state, and condition of thc clothing (neat, disheveled, torn, blood-stained). She should be asked if she has changed clothes or bathed since the assault. If the clothing was worn at the time of the incident, the clothing should be placed in a paper bag. All debris observed during the gross examination of the patient, such as grass, sand, or hair fibers, should be enclosed in a paper container.
2. General physical examination with notation of hematomas, bruises, edema, abrasions, lacerations, bite marks, and other evidence of struggle, such as hair or skin beneath the fingernails or scratches. The size and color of any hematomas should be recorded on a sketch of the child. Photographs should be taken of any contusions. The areas related to the history of assault should receive close attention (e,g., bruise marks around the neck from strangulation, hand marks on the inner thighs from forced abduction, bruises or petechiae on the gums from a hand over the mouth). Bruises may not appear for 24 hours. After marking the locations where the specimens were obtained, any area of dried secretions such as saliva from bite marks, blood, or semen should be swabbed with a slightly moistened gauze pad or swabs and retained as evidence. A Wood's lamp can detect areas of semen by fluorescence.
3. Genital examination with careful inspection of the perineum, noting bleeding, hematomas, lacerations, hymenal transections, vulvar erythema, condyloma acuminata, and any evidence of dried secretions. The hymen and posterior fourchette should be carefully examined using magnification with a

hand-held lens, otoscope, or colposcope. Acute assaults may be accompanied by extensive hymenal and perineal lacerations or ecchymoses. Dried secretions are collected with a slightly moistened gauze pad. The size of the hymenal opening should be recorded, as well as the position used. The vagina can be visualized in the knee-chest position, and any abnormal hymenal configuration, discharge, bleeding, or foreign bodies should be noted. One study found that application of toluidine blue to the vulva of girls seen within 48 hours of abuse may aid in the detection of posterior fourchette lacerations (139); many centers use magnified visualization in the green spectrum of the colposcope.

Specimens to check for the presence of sperm and cultures if indicated can be obtained with a saline-moistened Calgiswab, soft plastic Clinitest eye dropper, a small French catheter gently inserted through the hymenal opening, or a piece of intravenous tubing inside a catheter. We find the moistened Calgiswab easiest in most situations. A wet preparation should be done to look for motile sperm, trichomonads, and clue cells, and a "whiff" test should be done. Specimens should be streaked onto glass slides and allowed to air-dry. A swab should be collected for sending to the police laboratory for semen testing (see Tests for Semen). Any genital or anal discharge should be Gram-stained. Woodling and Kossoris (83) suggested another method to obtain specimens from a prepubertal child; while the child is in a semireclining position on a bedpan, a rubber catheter is used to obtain vaginal washing. Muram has also described a vaginal wash technique (see Chapter 1). Such washings must be refrigerated or frozen immediately. Urine can be examined for white cells, trichomonads, and sperm.

If a bleeding laceration cannot be properly assessed or the child has been too traumatized to cooperate with an examination, a brief examination under anesthesia is preferable to further trauma.

4. Inspection of the perianal area. If anal assault is suspected, specimens for detection of semen should be collected from the rectum. Rectal sphincter tone should be assessed.
5. Oral swabs are obtained for forensic studies if oral–genital contact within 24 hours is suspected.
6. Blood drawn for a serologic test for syphilis (rapid plasma reagin [RPR] test).
7. Serum frozen to do future testing for HIV and hepatitis B, if needed.
8. Cultures can be individualized in prepubertal children. As noted above, in Table 3 and in section on STDs earlier in this chapter, positive cultures are uncommon and therefore selective screening is acceptable. If cultures are obtained, samples for *N. gonorrhoeae* culture are obtained from the vagina, rectum, and throat, and samples for *Chlamydia trachomatis* culture from the vagina (and rectum, if possible). Genital vesicles and ulcers should be cultured for HSV.

9. Prophylaxis. In the asymptomatic prepubertal child involved in chronic or prior abuse, treatment is usually prescribed only if a positive culture is found. In the acute situation of sexual assault by a stranger, prophylaxis for gonorrhea and chlamydial infection can be instituted (although the risk is low) by giving ceftriaxone 125 mg followed by erythromycin 50 mg/kg/day for 7 days, azithromycin 20 mg/kg (max 1 g) single dose, or doxycycline if the patient is >9 years old. A short course of stool softeners may be prescribed for sodomy cases, and phenazopyridine for girls with vulvar trauma and dysuria. Tetanus toxoid is given according to standard pediatric guidelines following acute injuries. HIV prophylaxis should be individualized.

The child should be seen for medical followup after the evaluation for the acute assault to assess healing of injuries, document physical findings (if still present) noted in the emergency department, and check the results of the initial cultures. If no prophylactic antibiotics were given at the time of an acute assault, cultures for *N. gonorrhoeae* and *C. trachomatis* can be repeated at the followup visit. If, however, 1 to 2 weeks have elapsed between the incident of abuse and the initial evaluation, cultures need not be repeated. Vaginal secretions should be examined for trichomoniasis and bacterial vaginosis. Repeat serology for syphilis and possibly HIV testing can be obtained at a followup 12 weeks later. HIV testing can be repeated 6 to 12 months later.

Most cases of sexual abuse in young children involve episodes that occurred weeks to months before the actual examination. In such cases, the examination should still include a general physical examination to look for signs of neglect or abuse and a genital examination that includes inspection of the perineum, magnification of the hymen and posterior fourchette, visualization of the vagina in the knee-chest position (if possible), measurement of the hymenal opening, and anal assessment, and, if indicated, tests for STDs. Signs of previous abuse may include scars, hymenal remnants or transections, which may heal in a V or U shape. In cases of long-standing abuse, genital fondling, oral–genital contact, or penile contact with either the vulva or the abdomen may have occurred without penile–vaginal penetrations; therefore, many sexually abused prepubertal girls have a normal genital examination or minimal signs of irritation. Thus, the finding of a normal examination should in no way preclude the diagnosis of sexual abuse.

At the conclusion of the examination, it is extremely important to discuss with the child and parent(s) the clinical findings, since many assume the child is "damaged goods." Parents are greatly relieved to be told that their child is normal and healthy. Before the examination, parents often express extreme anxiety over the possible loss of virginity and reproductive potential and are greatly reassured by a careful discussion. When there has been an injury, the treatment and followup plan of care should be outlined. Most minor trauma heals without visible sequelae.

All cases of sexual abuse in children must be reported to the child protective services. Optimally, children should have a psychological evaluation at the time of the history and physical examination. In intrafamilial situations, it is important to establish whether the child can be safely returned to the family environment; the alleged perpetrator should not be confronted in an intrafamilial situation until the clinician is sure that the child is protected.

The need for long-term psychological support for the child depends on the individual case and the presence of preexisting psychological problems and psychosocial circumstances (6,140–145). Briere and Elliott (143) have identified some broad categories of problems, including posttraumatic stress, cognitive distortions, emotional pain (depression, anxiety, anger), impaired sense of self, avoidance, and interpersonal difficulties. Both a child's stage of development and the nature of the encounter determine the impact on the child. In situations of one-time nonforceful exposure (fondling, touching), a careful history, genital examination, and reassurance for the family are important. Most of the followup counseling is directed to the parents, since if they can remain unambiguously supportive, the impact on the child is usually minimal. In cases involving a caregiver and/or repetitive abuse, the child and family should receive counseling directed to their needs. Young children may have a high level of anxiety and be manifesting somatic and behavioral symptoms. The child may have difficulty separating from her mother and be exceptionally clinging. Sorting out good and bad feelings toward the perpetrator, mother, and others involved is important. Children may need to relearn the ability to trust and to display affection; self-esteem needs to be fostered and increased. Allowing the child to make choices can empower her to realize that she can believe in herself and make wise choices in the future.

Cases involving long-standing intrafamilial abuse are particularly problematic. Clinicians need legal and psychological services within the community prepared to deal long-term with these difficult situations. The aim of incest treatment must be to stop the incest and to treat all the family members. The mother must be willing and able to protect her children, and both parents have to admit to the problem and have a desire to remedy it either by improving their marriage or divorcing. The best interests of the child must be foremost, not the reuniting of the family. Long-term outcomes are variable, and clearly the inability of parents to provide the necessary protection for the child may cause long-term problems. The continuation of incest during adolescence appears to be particularly damaging and may result in conversion hysteria, promiscuity, phobias, suicide attempts, and psychosis.

Increased court involvement and prosecution have been useful in the resolution of some cases. Children can be helped through the court process by sensitive victim–witness advocates, district attorneys, and mental health professionals. Unfortunately, the long, drawn-out process and the need for the child to confront the defendant directly rather than by videotape have made the judicial process difficult for many (146,147). A not-guilty verdict can be devastating to the victim, who feels she has not been believed. On the other hand, a guilty verdict can be helpful in the child's recovery. Runyan and coworkers (148) reported that testimony in court that helped the resolution of anxiety but protracted criminal proceedings had the potential for an adverse effect. Psychotherapy should not await a court verdict but should be ongoing from the time of the disclosure. More attention also needs to be focused on offenders, many of whom were previously sexually abused themselves. Physicians and nurse practitioners often find the task of testifying in court problematic because of lack of experience and interruptions to their usual patient schedule. Proper preparation is essential (1,149).

ASSESSMENT OF THE ADOLESCENT

In contrast to the pattern of sexual abuse in prepubertal children, sexual abuse during adolescence is more likely to be a one-time assault by a stranger and involve vaginal intercourse. Thus, a rape kit for collection of forensic specimens is more likely to be necessary for this evaluation. Even among adolescents, the rape may involve an acquaintance or someone whom the teenager had seen in her neighborhood or school and who was assumed to be a safe individual. In these cases, the adolescent may accept a ride with that individual and then later be forced into a sexual relationship, often involving intercourse. Risk-taking behaviors such as alcohol and drug use and hitchhiking may make certain adolescents more vulnerable (150–152). In one college study, 73% of assailants and 55% of victims had used drugs, alcohol, or both immediately before a sexual assault (151). In other cases, the developmental changes that take place during adolescence may make a long-standing incestuous relationship intolerable; the adolescent may then respond with a sudden disclosure, may seek medical care for somatic symptoms such as abdominal pain or headache, or may become involved in impulsive behavior such as running away. A pregnancy may be the first sign of a previous rape or chronic sexual abuse. It is therefore important to ask the adolescent not only whether she has ever had sexual relations but also whether she has ever been forced into a sexual relationship.

In recording the history of the adolescent with alleged sexual assault, clinicians should follow a similar outline to that described in the above section Assessment of the Prepubertal Child. It is important to record the date of the visit and sources of the history, as well as who brought the patient in and who knows of the current situation. The date, time, and place of the sexual assault(s) should be recorded. In acute situations, the patient should be asked if she has bathed, douched, or urinated since the assault. A menstrual and contraceptive history should be obtained. Clinicians should not try to decide whether rape has occurred on the basis of the patient's emotional response to the trauma, for clearly some patients will be tearful, tense, and hysterical, and others will appear controlled or subdued. Questions should focus on what happened and whether vaginal, rectal, or oral penetration occurred (terms understood by the patient should be used). These questions may need to be repeated during the examination when the adolescent is more familiar with the anatomic terms. She should be asked if she is aware of any other injuries or symptoms following the attack. A rape protocol should be used to collect evidence. It is extremely helpful if a nurse, preferably an experienced rape-victim counselor, can be assigned to the adolescent throughout the 2- to 4-hour stay in the emergency department and can be present during the history taking, physical examination, and police interviews. The rape-victim counselor can provide the patient with information on the details of the physical examination and be an ally to the patient. A number of general hospitals now have a rotating system of nurses who have had special training in rape counseling and who are on-call to provide such support for sexual abuse victims. Other cities have established separate rape crises centers (e.g., Memphis, Tennessee). A police officer should not be present during the medical evaluation.

After the history is obtained, the patient should be told of the need for a thorough physical examination to assess injuries and collect laboratory specimens, including tests for STDs. Each part of the examination should be discussed in advance, and the patient should be given a sense of control over the tempo of the examination. She should be told that the examination is important but that the examiner can stop if the patient wishes and finish at another time. Anatomic pictures or a plastic model (Ortho) can be used to familiarize the adolescent with the type of examination. The following assessment applies to the acute sexual assault. When there is a history of an ongoing incestuous relationship in which intercourse has occurred >5 days before the physical examination, the search for motile sperm is omitted (see previous section for discussion of semen tests).

The physical examination should include the following seven steps:

1. A description should be recorded of the patient's general appearance, emotional state, and especially the condition of the clothing. Any clothing that might provide evidence in a legal case should be included in the rape-evidence clothing bag.
2. A general physical examination should note any evidence of bruises, scratches, or lacerations. As noted in the examination of the prepubertal child (see above), debris and dried secretions should be properly collected. The Tanner stages of sexual development should be noted. If the history indicates any attempt by the patient to scratch or fight her assailant, fingernail scrapings should be obtained with a wooden applicator stick and saved in an envelope. Head-hair combings and a head-hair standard (clipped close to the scalp) are included in many rape kits. Hair samples can be deferred until clearly needed as long as the patient does not cut, color, or chemically process her hair.
3. The pelvic examination should include a careful inspection of the perineum, noting any evidence of bleeding or lacerations. A gauze pad or cotton swab lightly moistened with nonbacteriostatic sterile saline should be used to wipe the vulva. The location of any dried secretions should be marked on a sketch. A collection paper should be placed under the buttocks of the patient and the pubic hair combed toward the paper to collect any debris. The debris should be placed in the collection envelope. If any foreign hairs are noted, 8 to 25 pubic hairs of the patient should be cut near the surface of the skin and included in a separate envelope. Soules and associates (73) found no hair transfer in 15 patients studied after intercourse.

The hymenal border can be examined for tears by running a saline-moistened cotton-tipped applicator around the edges or by using a Foley bladder catheter (see Chapter 1). A hand-held lens or colposcope can aid in the evaluation. Small abrasions or telangiectasia in the posterior fourchette may be identified with magnification or toluidine blue (49). The size of the hymenal opening should be noted in millimeters. Vaginal swabs for semen can be obtained by gently inserting a cotton-tipped applicator through the hymenal ring. In most protocols, the swabs are then smeared on two dry slides (frosted at one end so that the patient's name and date can be recorded) and allowed to air-dry. The swabs are protected in a test tube and saved for transport to a police laboratory, where they and the slides can be examined using specific semen tests. A moistened cotton-tipped applicator can be used to obtain further vaginal samples to look for the presence of motile sperm, trichomonads, and clue cells. A "whiff" test is also done on this specimen. Any genital discharge should be Gram-stained. Genital ulcers suggestive of genital herpes should be cultured.

In most pubertal adolescent girls, a gentle vaginal examination can be done with a water-moistened (Huffman) small speculum. If the hymen is too tight, cultures for *C. trachomatis* and *N. gonorrhoeae* can be obtained from the vagina. It is extremely important to examine the teenager gently so that the examination does not represent a further trauma. With the speculum in place, the vagina is inspected for injury and the presence of semen or vaginal discharge, and endocervical specimens for cultures are obtained. A purulent endocervical discharge should be Gram-stained to look for white cells and gram-negative intracellular diplococci. If cervical smears are also taken to check for motile sperm, the wet and dry smears should be appropriately marked. Approximately 1% of victims have moderate or severe genital injuries that require surgical intervention. Upper vaginal lacerations usually require laparotomy.

4. The anus should be inspected, and any discharge swabbed and Gram-stained. Specimens for sperm should be obtained if there is a history of rectal assault within 24 hours. Perianal swabs are collected using cotton swabs lightly moistened with saline; anorectal swabs are not moistened prior to collection. A culture for *N. gonorrhoeae* (and *C. trachomatis*) is obtained. Anoscopy should be done if rectal bleeding is present or the rectal examination reveals fecal occult blood. A bimanual rectoabdominal or rectovaginal–abdominal examination should be done gently to make sure that there is no tenderness or enlargement of the uterus to suggest infection or pregnancy. Rectal sphincter tone should be assessed since patients subjected to chronic rectal sexual abuse may have reflex relaxation.
5. If oral–genital contact has occurred, specimens from the girl's mouth should be obtained. A throat swab should be plated for *N. gonorrhoeae*. Oral swabs are obtained for detection of semen and other foreign matter if oral–genital contact occurred within 24 hours. Dry swabs are wiped on the areas between

the lips and gums and along the tooth and gum lines. A saliva sample is also obtained for secretor status (even if no oral contact occurred).

6. Blood should be drawn for a serologic test for syphilis (RPR or VDRL) and serum frozen to do future testing for HIV and hepatitis B, if indicated. A blood sample is also frequently included in rape kits for the police laboratory to do ABO blood typing of the victim.
7. A sensitive urine or serum pregnancy test should be done to detect a preexisting pregnancy.

If the patient was unconscious during the assault, samples should be obtained from vagina, rectum, and mouth.

All specimens for the pathology laboratory or the police should be delivered personally by the doctor or nurse involved in the case, and properly signed receipts should be obtained. Use of a rape-evidence kit or rape protocol does not imply that the family or patient must proceed with prosecution; however, reporting the rape and using a protocol to collect the evidence ensures that the evidence has been appropriately handled and will be admissible in court if prosecution is to occur. Under the stress of the crisis, many families may have difficulty deciding whether prosecution will be sought; it therefore behooves clinicians to obtain evidence that is medically and legally appropriate.

In cases of acute rape, the decision to prescribe antibiotics should be individualized and based on the risks of acquiring an STD. The benefits of prophylactic treatment for syphilis, gonorrhea, *Chlamydia,* and trichomoniasis should be discussed with the patient. In asymptomatic adolescents with long-standing incestuous relationships, clinicians may wait for the results of cultures and blood tests before initiating treatment (unless the perpetrator is known to be infected). For the adolescent victim of acute assault, we believe that antibiotics should be given to prevent sequelae, such as pelvic inflammatory disease, and to lessen the need for repeat cultures 2 weeks later, because patients are often lost to followup. The patient should be informed that not all organisms are covered by antibiotics and followup is essential. For therapy, a single intramuscular dose of ceftriaxone 125 mg, followed by metronidazole 2 g orally in a single dose *plus* 7 days of doxycycline 100 mg twice a day for 7 days or azithromycin 1 g single dose (55) is recommended. It is likely that cefixime 400 mg and azithromycin 1 g orally, both in single doses, followed in 1 day with the metronidazole would be another option. Alternatively, the metronidazole could be given as 500 mg twice a day for 7 days (48).

If the initial RPR test is negative, a followup serologic test at 12 weeks for syphilis is necessary if spectinomycin is chosen as an alternative for gonococcal prophylaxis or no prophylaxis is given. Tetanus toxoid should be given following standard pediatric guidelines for injuries. Prophylaxis against hepatitis B has not been studied in the context of assault. Prophylaxis would require administration of hepatitis B immune globulin in a single intramuscular dose; a series of vaccinations would be added for future immunity. The adolescent population should be soon immunized if universal immunization for hepatitis B is accomplished.

The efficacy of HIV prophylaxis is unknown. Gostin and colleagues (153) suggested that introduction of information about "unsubstantiated prevention of an already small risk may create both added anxiety and unsubstantiated hope." However, the potential for transmission of HIV during sexual assault does need to be considered and protocols are being developed for postexposure prophylaxis of victims, taking into account the type and timing of exposure and the likelihood of HIV infection in the perpetrator. Clinicians need to keep up to date with CDC recommendations and studies of efficacy and cost.

Emergency postcoital contraception with "morning-after" hormonal therapy should be offered to the postpubertal adolescent who was raped within the last 72 hours (see Chapter 17). A sensitive (urine or blood) pregnancy test should be done before hormonal medication is given.

A current telephone number of the patient should be verified, and a followup appointment should be arranged for 2 weeks later. A repeat pelvic examination is done to assess healing of injuries and to look for vaginal trichomoniasis and bacterial vaginosis if not treated. It should be remembered that absence of injuries does not preclude the possibility of rape. In Cartwright's (154) study of sexual assault victims >10 years of age, 40% sustained nongenital and 16% genital injuries. Repeat cultures for *N. gonorrhoeae* and *C. trachomatis* should be done if initial cultures were positive (and treated) or if prophylaxis was not given. A sensitive pregnancy test should be done 2 to 3 weeks after the rape, regardless of whether postcoital hormonal therapy was given. Testing for HIV and hepatitis B can be performed at 12 weeks post assault and, if positive, compared with the serum frozen from the initial visit. If HIV testing is negative, it can be repeated 12 months post assault. At long-term followup, the patient should be examined for HIV infection, and Pap smear screening should be initiated.

The patient should be reassured about the findings on genital examination. Patients greatly benefit from drawings to show them the range of hymenal sizes and configurations. The virginal adolescent who has had a forced episode of sexual intercourse may feel considerably relieved to understand that her external genitalia is not very different from some adolescents who have not had intercourse. She needs to be reassured that the assault in no way changes her ability to have normal sexual intercourse in the future or to have normal, healthy children. Teenagers may have unprotected intercourse because of concern that a rape that occurred when they were 12 or 13 years old markedly diminished their reproductive potential. It is not unusual for a patient to have somatic reactions in the first several weeks following a rape—muscle soreness, headaches, fatigue, stomach pain, dysuria, sleep disturbances, and nightmares. Most rape victims express an extreme fear of physical violence and death. Many older women move and change their telephone numbers (155).

The extent of counseling in the aftermath of a sexual assault depends on the initial encounter. For example, in the situation of an isolated episode of exhibitionism or nonforceful genital fondling by a stranger or neighbor, counseling should help integrate the event with a strongly positive view of the future. A case of a long-standing incestuous relationship requires a long-term treatment program. If the young adolescent has been trained to be a sexual object and to give and receive sexual pleasure in order to get approval, the outcome is often poor and sexual exploitation may continue in other settings.

For the victim of acute sexual assault, clinicians should provide information about the legal system and discuss the benefits of counseling. Even if the girl seems nonverbal or appears to be coping well, the counselor can often play an educational and supportive role in the initial interviews, reassuring the girl about her intactness and her femininity. The teen may need the opportunity to tell and retell her story to a caring, sympathetic person. Ideally, the same counselor is available at the time the rape is reported and is able to followup with visits and telephone calls. Despite the need to work through issues both at the time of crisis and in later years, a teenager may express reluctance to continue followup care because repeated encounters with the hospital setting may remind her of the original incident. Thus, the initial counseling interviews are critical in assessing the patient's strengths in coping with stress and emphasizing the availability of followup or referral. Involving a friend or relative whom the patient views as supportive is often helpful.

During counseling, the patient needs to hear that she may feel vulnerable and helpless or have fears of violence or death and that the rape incident may interfere in the short term with her ability to form trusting relationships, especially with men. It is not unusual for women to experience extreme shame, guilt, and loss of self-esteem after a rape and to insist that they might have somehow avoided the incident. Self-blame may, however, have an adaptive value for the victim as she identifies factors of the assault that she could control, thus permitting her to feel in greater control of situations in the future. The response of parents, doctors, and friends often fosters this guilt in the victim and forces her to regard the rape as a sexual act rather than the violent crime she perceived.

Physicians should work with the parents to help them support their daughter. Even when the daughter has been a victim of forced rape, parents may feel that the style of dress, the acceptance of a ride, or other behavior meant the teen was "asking for it." The clinician should make it clear to the parents that the teenager will deal with the crisis considerably better if she has their support.

Also, parents and boyfriends may respond by being overprotective at a time when the teenager is striving for independence; her sense of adequacy is thus further questioned. The young adolescent is often reluctant to return to school because of the fear that peer groups "will whisper behind her back." Stating this as a problem and suggesting that some of this behavior may be related to their feelings may relieve the patient of some of her anxiety. Preventive measures, such as avoiding walking alone or hitchhiking, can be emphasized in such a way that the patient does not feel that she shares the blame for the incident.

It is difficult to predict the long-term sequelae of a rape because victims cope with stress in many different ways. However, it is clear that later sexual disturbances are common when the first sexual experience occurs in the context of violence and degradation. The other issues that tend to emerge later include (a) mistrust of men, (b) phobic reactions, and (c) neurotic symptoms of anxiety and depression precipitated by events that remind the victim of the original episode (156). A "rape trauma syndrome" has been described by a number of authors, and the long-term reactions have characteristics of post-traumatic stress disorder (155–159). The syndrome consists of reexperiencing the traumatic event by intrusive thoughts, dreams, or flashbacks; an avoidance of previously pleasurable activities; an avoidance of the place or circumstances in which the rape occurred; and an increased state of psychomotor arousal leading to difficulty with sleep and memory. Patients may have difficulty with pelvic examinations done months to years after the rape episode.

In general, responsibility for reporting the incident to law enforcement officials belongs to the patient and her parents (if the patient is <18 years old). Although improvements are in sight, prosecution may intensify the guilt and shame of the victim. Questions such as "What were you doing out late?", "What did you expect?", or "Why didn't you struggle?" may force the patient to feel that she was somehow responsible for the rape. On the other hand, unless rapes are reported and prosecuted, the prevention of further violence is jeopardized. A counselor for the victim should ideally accompany the teenager through the legal process and explain the involvement of prosecutors, judges, and courts.

SEXUAL ABUSE PREVENTION

With the recognition by health care professionals and educators of the widespread problem of sexual abuse, efforts have been made in the area of prevention. Jenny and associates (160) outlined a protocol for pediatric visits (Table 14). The American Academy of Pediatrics has published a brochure—*Child Sexual Abuse: What It Is and How to Prevent It*—in consultation with the National Committee for Prevention of Child Abuse. The pamphlet outlines steps for suspecting abuse, dealing with a disclosure, and planning prevention. The AAP encourages parents to make sure their schools have prevention programs for students and teachers, to discuss the subject with their children, to teach their children about body parts, to be good listeners, and to know with whom their children are spending time. Young children should have sufficient knowledge of their bodies to know what types of behavior from adults to avoid or report. Children need to know that they can refuse demands for physical closeness, even from friends or relatives. They should be told early to avoid accepting rides from strangers or candy or money in exchange for close relationships. Most programs include the following topics: the distinction between good, bad, and questionable touching; the rights of children to control who touches their bodies; the importance of children's telling a responsible adult if someone inappropriately touches them; assertive skills; and support systems (161).

Reality dictates that children understand what are threats from others, but placing undue burdens on children's comprehension or ability to protect themselves is not helpful. Measuring effectiveness of prevention programs is a difficult task. Young preschool children lack the developmental level to understand many of the concepts that are included in curricula, and thus programs are better targeted to older children. A review of 17 programs found that some children had modest increases in knowledge and were more likely to disclose prior sexual abuse following a prevention program, but a small number of children were more worried following the intervention (161). These studies have not demonstrated the effectiveness of curricula in actually helping children resist or prevent sexual abuse. Daro (161) suggested that prevention programs for 7- to 12-year-olds have the potential for the greatest magnitude of effect and that the promising programs have the following characteristics: role playing of prevention strategies; curricula tailored to the age group and learning abilities; material presented in a varied and stimulating manner; generic concepts such as assertive behavior, decision-making skills, and communication skills that can be used in other daily activities; emphasis on telling when touch makes them uncomfortable; and longer programs that are integrated into the school curricula. Prevention efforts should be broadened to include programs to improve parenting; life-skills training for adolescents to help potential offenders develop empathy for peers; support services for families and children, especially for those in transition and vulnerable children and adults; and enhanced supervision for children (161).

Programs have been initiated in many communities to help young women deal with rape prevention. Since rape commonly occurs among college students and other young women who have recently moved to a new location where environmental cues may not be so apparent, prevention programs stress the need for young women to learn about safe versus unsafe areas, to walk in a purposeful way, and to be constantly aware of dark corners and people who may be walking near them. Particular risk factors for adolescents who have been victims of sexual assault are voluntarily agreeing to go to the house or apartment or in the car of a young man that they have known for <24 hours, impairment with drugs or alcohol, and hitchhiking (150). If a threatening situation arises, women are instructed to run toward traffic areas or lighted areas where other people are present. If self-defense measures are used initially, women should then run as soon as possible. Women living alone may wish to change their mailboxes to read "Mr. and Mrs.", instead of listing their first name or an initial. The American College of Obstetricians and Gynecologists has developed a number of recommendations to prevent rape (152).

Although this chapter has dealt only with girls because the focus of this volume is gynecology, boys, too, may be subject to intrafamilial and stranger homosexual and heterosexual abuse; they need the same type of education and meaningful medical care during childhood as their female counterparts.

TABLE 14. *Protocol for sex education and abuse prevention in well-child care*

Age	Developmental issues	Prevention plan
Newborns	Complete dependency	Discuss choosing daycare and babysitter
6 mo	Discovery of pleasant feelings associated with genitals	Talk about normalcy of infant genital exploration and self-stimulation
18 mo	Beginning of language development	Encourage parents to teach children normal anatomic terms for body parts
2½–4 yr	Establishment of gender identity	Identify children with sex role confusion
3–5 yr	Increasing independence of child, beginning of oedipal stage, recognition of sexual differences	Encourage parents to give child permission to say "No" to advances, teach children about "private places," reassure parents about normalcy of sexual curiosity and play, encourage parents to give their children straightforward answers about sex
5–8 yr	Developing increasing independence and accomplishments, beginning school	Discuss safety away from home, encourage parents to teach children safe behaviors, reinforce self-protective behaviors and difference between good touch and bad touch, encourage children to talk about frightening experiences
8–12 yr	Developing sexuality, the time of highest incidence of child sexual abuse	Parental planning for sex education for their children, reinforce personal safety education
13–18 yr	Development of adult identity, increasing independence from family, beginning of normal sexual experimentation	Discuss personal safety and risk-taking behavior including alcohol and drug abuse; discuss sexuality, birth control, and sexually transmitted diseases

(From Jenny C, Sutherland SE, Sandahl BB. Developmental approach to preventing the sexual abuse of children. *Pediatrics* 1987;78:1034; with permission.)

REFERENCES

1. Heger AH, Emans SJ, et al., eds. *Evaluation of the sexually abused child: a medical textbook and photographic atlas.* New York: Oxford University Press, 1992.
2. Chadwick D, Berkowitz C, Kerns D. *Color atlas of child sexual abuse.* Chicago: Year Book Medical Publishers, 1989.
3. Finkel, M. Medical findings in child sexual abuse. In: Reece RM, ed. *Child abuse*. Baltimore, MD: Williams & Wilkins, 1994.
4. Burgess AW, Groth AN, Holmstrom LL, et al. *Sexual assault of children and adolescents.* Lexington, MA: Lexington Books, 1978.
5. Finkelhor D. *Sexually victimized children.* New York: The Free Press, 1979.
6. Sgroi S. *Handbook of clinical interventions in child sexual abuse.* Lexington, MA: Lexington Books, 1984.
7. Kempe CH. Sexual abuse, another hidden pediatric problem. *Pediatrics* 1978;62:382.
8. Hymel KP, Jenny C. Child sexual abuse. *Pediatr Rev* 1996;17:236.

9. American Academy of Pediatrics Committee on Child Abuse and Neglect. Guidelines for the evaluation of sexual abuse of children. *Pediatrics* 1991;87:254.
10. Berkowitz CD. Child sexual abuse. *Pediatr Rev* 1992;13:443.
11. Larson CS, Terman DL, Gomby DS, et al. Sexual abuse of children: recommendations and analysis. *Future of Children* 1994;4:4
12. Finkelhor D. Current information on the scope and nature of child sexual abuse. *Future of Children* 1994;4:31.
13. Finkelhor D, Dzxiuba-Leatherman J. Children as victims of violence: a national survey. *Pediatrics* 1994;94:413.
14. Erickson PI, Rapkin AJ. Unwanted sexual experiences among middle and high school youth. *J Adolesc Health* 1991;12:319.
15. Finkelhor D. Sex among sibships: a survey on prevalence, rarity, and effects. *Arch Sex Behav* 1980; 3:171.
16. Nagy S, Adcock AG, Nagy MC. A comparison of risky health behaviors of sexually active sexually abused, and abstaining adolescents. *Pediatrics* 1994;93:570.
17. Nagy S, DiClemente R, Adcock AG. Adverse factors associated with forced sex among southern adolescent girls. *Pediatrics* 1995;96:944.
18. Hibbard RA, Brack CJ, Rauch S, et al. Abuse, feelings, and health behaviors in a student population. *Am J Dis Child* 1988;142:326.
19. Hibbard RA, Ingersoll GM, Orr DP. Behavioral risk, emotional risk, and child abuse among adolescents in a nonclinical setting. *Pediatrics* 1990;86:896.
20. Abma JC, Chandra C, Mosher WD, et al. Fertility, family planning, and women's health: new data from the 1995 National Survey of Family Growth. National Center for Health Statistics. *Vital Health Stat* 23(19), 1997.
21. Orr DP, Prietto SV. Emergency management of sexually abused children. *Am J Dis Child* 1979;33: 628.
22. Dubowitz H, Black M, Harrington D. The diagnosis of child sexual abuse. *Am J Dis Child* 1992;146: 688.
23. Committee on Adolescence. Sexual assault and the adolescent. *Pediatrics* 1994;94:761.
24. Herman-Giddens ME. Vaginal foreign bodies and child sexual abuse. *Arch Pediatr Adolesc Med* 1994;148:195.
25. Kienberger Jaudes P, Martone M. Interdisciplinary evaluations of alleged sexual abuse cases. *Pediatrics* 1992;89:1164.
26. Paradise JE, Rostain AL, Nathanson M. Substantiation of sexual abuse charges when parents dispute custody or visitation. *Pediatrics* 1988;81:835.
27. Becker JV. Offenders: characteristics and treatment. *Future of Children* 1994;4:176.
28. Finkelhor D. *Child sexual abuse: new theory and research*. New York: Free Press, 1984.
29. Knight R, Cater D, Prentky R. A system of classification of child molesters. *J Interpersonal Violence* 1989;4:3.
30. Abel G, Becker J, Cunningham-Rathner J, et al. Multiple paraphilic diagnoses among sex offenders. *Bull Am Acad Psychiatry Law* 1988;16:153-168.
31. Schetsky DH, Green AH. *Child sexual abuse: a handbook for health care and legal professionals*. New York: Brunner/Mazel, 1988.
32. Fuster CD, Neinstein LS. Vaginal *Chlamydia trachomatis* prevalence in sexually abused prepubertal girls. *Pediatrics* 1987;79:235.
33. Glaser JB, Hammerschlag MR, McCormack WM. Sexually transmitted diseasea in victims of sexual abuse. *N Engl J Med* 1986;313:625.
34. Hammerschlag MR, Cummings M, Doraiswamy B, et al. Nonspecific vaginitis following sexual abuse. *Pediatrics* 1985;75:1028.
35. White ST, Loda FA, Ingram DL. Sexually transmitted diseases in sexually abused children. *Pediatrics* 1983;72:16.
36. Jones JG, Jamauchi T, Lambert B. *Trichomonas vaginalis* infestation in sexually abused girls. *Am J Dis Child* 1985;139:846.
37. Dattel BJ, Landers DV, Coulter K, et al. Isolation of *Chlamydia trachomatis* from sexually abused female adolescents. *Obstet Gynecol* 1988;72:240.
38. Jenny C. Sexual assault and STD. In: Holmes KK, Mårdh P-A, Sparling PF, et al, eds. *Sexually transmitted diseases*, 2nd ed. New York: McGraw-Hill, 1990.
39. Jenny C. Child sexual abuse and STD. In: Holmes KK, Mårdh P-A, Sparling PF, et al, eds. *Sexually transmitted diseases*, 2nd ed. New York: McGraw-Hill, 1990.

40. Rawstron SA, Bromberg K, Hammerschlag MR. STD in children: syphilis and gonorrhoea. *Genitourin Med* 1993;69:66.
41. Shapiro RA, Schubert CJ, Myers PA. Vaginal discharge as an indicator of gonorrhea and chlamydia infection in girls under 12 years old. *Pediatr Emerg Med* 1993;9:341.
42. Jenny C. Sexually transmitted diseases and child abuse. *Pediatr Ann* 1992;21:497.
43. Gellert GA, Durfee MJ, Berkowitz CD, et al. Situational and sociodemographic characteristics of children infected with human immunodeficiency virus from pediatric sexual abuse. *Pediatrics* 1993; 91:39.
44. Gutman LT, St Claire KK, Weedy C, et al. Human immunodeficiency virus transmission by child sexual abuse. *Am J Dis Child* 1991;145:137.
45. Jenny C, Hooton TM, Bowers BA, et al. Sexually transmitted diseases in victims of rape. *N Engl J Med* 1990;322:713.
46. Kellogg ND, Huston RL, Foulds DM. *Chlamydia trachomatis* infections in children evaluated for sexual abuse. *Fam Med* 1991;23:59.
47. Estreich S, Forster GE, Robinson A. Sexually transmitted diseases in rape victims. *Genitourin Med* 1990;66:433.
48. Glaser JB, Schachter J, Benes S, et al. Sexually transmitted diseases in postpubertal female rape victims. *J Infect Dis* 1991;164:726.
49. Hampton HL. Care of the woman who has been raped. *N Engl J Med* 1995;332:234.
50. Sturm JT, Carr ME, Luxenberg MG, et al. The prevalence of *Neisseria gonorrhoeae* and *Chlamydia trachomatis* in victims of sexual assault. *Ann Emerg Med* 1990;19:597.
51. Schwarcz SK, Whittington WL. Sexual assault and sexually transmitted diseases: detection and management in adults and children. *Rev Infect Dis* 1990;12(suppl 6):S682.
52. Sicoli RA, Losek JD, Hudlett JM, Smith D. Indications for *Neisseria gonorrhoeae* cultures in children with suspected sexual abuse. *Arch Pediatr Adolesc Med* 1995;149:86.
53. Siegel RM, Schubert CJ, Myers PA, et al. The prevalence of sexually transmitted diseases in children and adolescents evaluated for sexual abuse in Cincinnati: rationale for limited STD testing in prepubertal girls. *Pediatrics* 1995;96:1090.
54. Hymel KP, Jenny C. Child sexual abuse. *Pediatr Rev* 1996;17:236.
55. Muram D, Speck PM, Dockter M. Child sexual abuse examination: is there a need for routine screening for *N. gonorrhoeae? J Pediatr Adolesc Gynecol* 1996;9:79.
56. Centers for Disease Control and Prevention. 1998 STD treatment guidelines. *MMWR* 1998;47 (RR-1):1.
57. Ingram DL, Everett VD, Lyna PR. Epidemiology of adult sexually transmitted disease agents in children being evaluated for sexual abuse. *Pediatr Infect Dis J* 1992;11:945.
58. Ingram DL, Everett D, Flick AR, et al. Vaginal gonococcal cultures for sexual abuse evaluations: evaluation of selective criteria in pre-teenaged girls. *Pediatrics* 1997;99:(6). URL: http://www.pediatrics.org/cgi/content/full/99/6/e8
59. Embree JE, Lindsay D, Williams T, et al. Acceptability and usefulness of vaginal washes in premenarcheal girls as a diagnostic procedure for sexually transmitted diseases. *Pediatr Infect Dis J* 1996;15:662.
60. Lande MB, Richardson AC, White KC. The role of syphilis serology in the evaluation of suspected sexual abuse. *Pediatr Infect Dis J* 1992;11:125.
61. Ross JDC, Scott GR, Busuttil A. *Trichomonas vaginalis* infection in pre-pubertal girls. *Med Sci Law* 1993;22:82.
62. Goldenring JM. *Staphylococcus saprophyticus* urinary tract infection in a sexually abused child. *Pediatr Infect Dis J* 1988;7:73.
63. Klevan JL, DeJong AR. Urinary tract symptoms and urinary tract infection following sexual abuse. *Am J Dis Child* 1990;144:242.
64. Kellogg ND, Parro JM. The progression of human papillomavirus lesions in sexual assault victims. *Pediatrics* 1995;96:1163.
65. Gellert G. Pediatric acquired immunodeficiency syndrome: testing as a barrier to recognizing the role of child sexual abuse (editorial). *Arch Pediatr Adolesc Med* 1994;148:766.
66. Gutman LT, Herman-Giddens ME, McKinney RE. Pediatric acquired immunodeficiency syndrome: barriers to recognizing the role of child sexual abuse. *Am J Dis Child* 1993;147:775.
67. Rimsza ME. Words too terrible to hear: sexual transmission of human immunodeficiency virus to children (editorial). *Am J Dis Child* 1993;147:711.
68. Gellert GA, Durfee MJ, Berkowitz CD. Developing guidelines for HIV antibody testing among victims of pediatric sexual abuse. *Child Abuse Negl* 1990;14:9.
69. Gutman LT, St Claire KK, Weedy C, et al. Sexual abuse of human immunodeficiency virus-positive

children: outcomes for perpetrators and evaluation of other household children. *Am J Dis Child* 1992;146:1185.
70. Katz MH, Gerberding JL. Postexposure treatment of people exposed to the human immunodeficiency virus through sexual contact or injection-drug use. *N Engl J Med* 1997;336:1097.
71. Dattel BJ, Landers DV, Coulter K, et al. Isolations of *Chlamydia trachomatis* and *Neisseria gonorrhoeae* from the genital tract of sexually abused prepubertal females. *Adolesc Pediatr Gynecol* 1989; 2:217.
72. Sirotnak AP. Testing sexually abused children for sexually transmitted diseases: who to test, when to test, and why. *Pediatr Ann* 1994;23:370.
73. Soules MR, Pollard AA, Brown KM, et al. The forensic laboratory evaluation of evidence in alleged rape. *Am J Obstet Gynecol* 1978;130:142.
74. Duenhoelter JH, Stone IC, Santos-Ramos R, et al. Detection of seminal fluid constituents after alleged sexual assault. *J Forensic Sci* 1978;4:824.
75. Jenny C. Forensic examination: the role of the physician as "medical detective." In: Heger AH, Emans SJ, et al, eds. *Evaluation of the sexually abused child: a medical textbook and photographic atlas*. New York: Oxford University Press, 1992:51.
76. Graves HC, Sensabaugh GF, Blake ET. Postcoital detection of a male-specific semen protein. *N Engl J Med* 1985;312:330.
77. Gabby T, Winkleby MA, Boyce WT, et al. Sexual abuse of children: the detection of semen on skin. *Am J Dis Child* 1992;146:700.
78. Evans RJ, Herr JC. Immunohistochemical localization of the MHS-5 antigen in principal cells of human seminal vesicle epithelium. *Anat Rec* 1986;214:372.
79. Herr JC, Woodward MP. An enzyme-linked immunosorbent assay (ELISA) for human semen identification based on a biotinylated monoclonal antibody to a seminal vesicle-specific antigen. *J Forensic Sci* 1987;32:346.
80. Herr JC, Summers TA, McGee RS. Characterization of a monoclonal antibody to a conserved epitope on human seminal vesicle-specific peptides: a novel probe/marker system for semen identification. *Biol Reprod* 1986;35:773.
81. Annas GJ. Setting standards for the use of DNA-typing results in the courtroom—the state of the art. *N Engl J Med* 1992;326:1641.
82. Hammond HA, Redman JB, Caskey CT. *In utero* paternity testing following alleged sexual assault: a comparison of DNA-based methods. *JAMA* 1995;273:1774.
83. Woodling B, Kossoris P. Sexual abuse: rape, molestation, and incest. *Pediatr Clin North Am* 1981; 28:481.
84. Dahlke MC, Cooke C, Cunnanne M, et al. Identification of semen in 500 patients seen because of rape. *Am J Clin Pathol* 1977;68:740.
85. Groth AN, Burgess AW. Sexual dysfunction during rape. *N Engl J Med* 1977;297:764.
86. Rimsza MR, Niggemann EH. Medical evaluation of sexually abused children: a review of 311 cases. *Pediatrics* 1982;69:8.
87. Emans SJ, Woods ER, Flagg NT, et al. Genital findings in sexually abused, symptomatic and asymptomatic girls. *Pediatrics* 1987;79:778.
88. Woodling BA, Heger A. The use of the colposcope in the diagnosis of sexual abuse in the pediatric age group. *Child Abuse Negl* 1986;10:111.
89. Muram D. Classification of genital findings in prepubertal girls who are victims of sexual abuse. *Adolesc Pediatr Gynecol* 1988;1:151.
90. Muram D. Child sexual abuse: relationship between genital findings and sexual acts. *Child Abuse Negl* 1989;13:211.
91. Adams JA, Harper K, Knudson S, et al. Examination findings in legally confirmed child sexual abuse: it's normal to be normal. *Pediatrics* 1994;94:310.
92. Muram D, Speck PM, Gold SS. Genital abnormalities in female siblings and friends of child victims of sexual abuse. *Child Abuse Negl* 1991;15:105.
93. Muram D. Child sexual abuse—genital tract findings in prepubertal girls. I. The unaided medical examination. *Am J Obstet Gynecol* 1989;160:328.
94. Muram D, Elias S. Child sexual abuse—genital tract findings in prepubertal girls. II. Comparison of colposcopic and unaided examinations. *Am J Obstet Gynecol* 1989;160:333.
95. Brayden RM, Altemeier WA III, Yeager T, Muram D. Interpretations of colposcopic photographs: evidence for competence in assessing sexual abuse? *Child Abuse Negl* 1991;15:69.
96. Herman-Giddens ME, Frothingham TC. Prepubertal female genitalia: examination for evidence of sexual abuse. *Pediatrics* 1987;80:203.

97. Enos FW, Conrath TB, Byer JC. Forensic evaluation of the sexually abused child. *Pediatrics* 1986; 78:385.
98. Teixeira W. Hymenal colposcopic examination in sexual abuse. *Am J Forensic Med Pathol* 1980;2:209.
99. Pokorny SF, Kozinetz CA. Configuration and other anatomic detail of the prepubertal hymen. *Adolesc Pediatr Gynecol* 1988;1:97.
100. McCann J, Wells R, Simon M, Voris J. Genital findings in prepubertal girls selected for nonabuse: a descriptive study. *Pediatrics* 1990;86:428.
101. Berenson AB, Heger AH, Andrews S. Appearance of the hymen in newborn. *Pediatrics* 1991;87:458.
102. Berenson AB, Heger AH, Hayes JM, Bailey RK, Emans SJ. Appearance of the hymen in prepubertal girls. *Pediatrics* 1992;89:387.
103. Kellogg, Parra JM. Linea vestibularis: a previously undescribed normal genital structure in female neonates. *Pediatrics* 1991;87:926.
104. McCann J, Voris J, Simon M et al. Perianal findings in prepubertal children selected for nonabuse: a descriptive study. *Child Abuse Negl* 1989;13:179.
105. Berenson AB, Somma-Garcia A, Barnett S. Perianal findings in infants 18 months of age or younger. *Pediatrics* 1993:91;838.
106. Adams JA, Knudson S. Genital findings in adolescent girls referred for suspected abuse. *Arch Pediatr Adolesc Med* 1996;150:850.
107. Kerns DL, Ritter ML, Thomas RG. Concave hymenal variations in suspected child sexual abuse victims. *Pediatrics* 1992;90:265.
108. McCann J, Voris J, Simon M. Genital injuries resulting from sexual abuse: a longitudinal study. *Pediatrics* 1992;89:307.
109. Finkel MA. Anogenital trauma in sexually abused children. *Pediatrics* 1989;84:317.
110. Berenson AB. A longitudinal study of hymenal morphology in the first 3 years of life. *Pediatrics* 1995;95:490.
111. Berenson AB. Appearance of the hymen at birth and one year of age: a longitudinal study. *Pediatrics* 1993;91:820.
112. McCann J, Voris J. Perianal injuries resulting from sexual abuse: a longitudinal study. *Pediatrics* 1993;91:390.
113. Kellogg ND, Parra JM. Linea vestibularis: followup of a normal genital structure. *Pediatrics* 1993; 92:453.
114. Jenny C, Kuhns ML, Abrahams F. Hymens in newborn female infants. *Pediatrics* 1987;80:399.
115. Emans SJ, Woods ER, Allred EN, Grace E. Hymenal findings in adolescent women: impact of tampon use and consensual sexual activity. *J Pediatr* 1994;125:153.
116. Levine V, Sanchez M, Nestor M. Localized vulvar pemphigoid in a child misdiagnosed as sexual abuse. *Arch Dermatol* 1992;128:804.
117. Bays J, Jenny C. Genital and anal conditions confused with child sexual abuse trauma. *Am J Dis Child* 1990;144:1319.
118. Bond GR, Dowd MD, Landsman I, Rimsza M. Unintentional perineal injury in prepubescent girls: a multicenter, prospective report of 56 girls. *Pediatrics* 1995;95:628.
119. Dowd MD, Fitzmaurice L, Knapp J, et al. The interpretation of urogenital findings in children with straddle injuries. *J Pediatr Surg* 1994;29:7.
120. Pokorny S, Pokorny W, Kramer W. Acute genital injury in the prepubertal girl. *Am J Obstet Gynecol* 1992;166:1461.
121. Hostetler BR, Muram D, Jones CE. Sharp penetrating injury to the hymen. *J Adolesc Pediatr Gynecol* 1994;7:94.
122. Heger AH, Emans SJ. Introital diameter as the criterion for sexual abuse. *Pediatrics* 1990;85:222.
123. Muram D. Child sexual abuse: relationship between genital findings and sexual acts. *Child Abuse Negl* 1989;13:211.
124. Kerns DL, Ritter ML. Medical findings in child sexual abuse with perpetrator confessions (abstract). *Am J Dis Child* 1992;146:494.
125. Paradise JE. Predictive accuracy and the diagnosis of sexual abuse: a big issue about a little tissue. *Child Abuse Negl* 1989;13:169.
126. Adams JA, Harper K, Knudson S. A proposed system for classification of anogenital findings in children with suspected sexual abuse. *Adolesc Pediatr Gynecol* 1992;5:73.
127. McCann J, Voris J, Simon M, et al. Comparison of genital examination techniques in prepubertal girls. *Pediatrics* 1990;85:182.
128. Muram D. Anal and perianal abnormalities in prepubertal victims of sexual abuse. *Am J Obstet Gynecol* 1989;161:278.

129. DeJong AR, Rose M. Legal proof of child sexual abuse in the absence of physical evidence. *Pediatrics* 1991;88:506.
130. Goldberg CC, Yates A. The use of anatomically correct dolls in the evaluation of sexually abused children. *Am J Dis Child* 1990;144:1334.
131. Hibbard RA, Roghmann K, Hoekelman RA. Genitalia in children's drawings: an association with sexual abuse. *Pediatrics* 1987;79:129.
132. Myers JEB. Role of physician in preserving verbal evidence of child abuse. *J Pediatr* 1986;109:409.
133. Saywitz KJ, Goodman GS, Nicholas E, Moan SF. Children's memories of a physical examination involving genital touch: implications for reports of child sexual abuse. *J Consult Clin Psychol* 1991; 59:682.
134. Myers JEB. Adjudication of child sexual abuse cases. *Future of Children* 1994;4:84.
135. Melton GB. Doing justice and doing good: conflicts for mental health professionals. *Future of Children* 1994;4:102.
136. DeJong AR. Maternal responses to the sexual abuse of their children. *Pediatrics* 1988;81:14.
137. Bays J, Chadwick D. Medical diagnosis of the sexually abused child. *Child Abuse Negl* 1993;17:91.
138. Muram D. Child sexual abuse. *Adolesc Pediatr Gynecol* 1992;19:193.
139. American Professional Society on the Abuse of Children (APSAC) Practice Guidelines. Photographic documentation of child abuse: statement of purpose. APSAC:1.
140. McCauley J, Gorman RL, Guzinski G. Toluidine blue in the detection of perineal lacerations in pediatric and adolescent sexual abuse victims. *Pediatrics* 1986;78:1039.
141. Paradise J, Rose L, Sleeper L, Nathanson M. Behavior, family function, school performance, and predictors of persistent disturbance in sexually abused children. *Pediatrics* 1994;93:452.
142. Beutler LAE, Williams RA, Zetzer HA. Efficacy of treatment for victims of child sexual abuse. *Future of Children* 1994;4:156.
143. Briere JN, Elliott DM. Immediate and long-term impacts of child sexual abuse. *Future of Children* 1994;4:54.
144. Koverola C. Psychological effects of child sexual abuse. In: Heger A, Emans SJ et al, eds. *Evaluation of the sexually abused child: a medical textbook and photographic atlas.* New York: Oxford University Press, 1992:15.
145. Wells RD, McCann J, Adams J, et al. Emotional, behavioral, and physical symptoms reported by parents of sexually abused, nonabused, and allegedly abused prepubescent females. *Child Abuse Negl* 1995;19:155.
146. Landwirth J. Children as witnesses in child sexual abuse trials. *Pediatrics* 1987;60:585.
147. Berliner L, Barbieri MK. The testimony of the child victim of sexual assault. *J Soc Issues* 1984;40:125.
148. Runyan DK, Everson MD, Edelsohn GA, et al. Impact of legal intervention on sexually abused children. *Pediatrics* 1988;113:647.
149. Kerns DL, Terman DL, Larson CS. The role of physicians in reporting and evaluating child sexual abuse cases. *Future of Children* 1994;4:119.
150. Jenny C. Adolescent risk-taking behavior and the occurrence of sexual assault. *Am J Dis Child* 1988; 142:770.
151. Abbey A. Acquaintance rape and alcohol consumption on college campuses: how are they linked? *J Am College Health* 1991;39:165.
152. Committee on Adolescent Health Care No. 122, American College of Obstetricians and Gynecologists. Adolescent acquaintance rape. *Int J Gynaecol Obstet* 1993;42:209.
153. Gostin LO, Lazzarini Z, Alexander D, et al. HIV testing, counseling, and prophylaxis after sexual assault. *JAMA* 1994;271:1436.
154. Cartwright PS. Factors that correlate with injury sustained by survivors of sexual assault. *Obstet Gynecol* 1987;70:44.
155. Burgess A, Holmstrom L. Rape trauma syndrome. *Am J Psychiatry* 1974;131:981.
156. Notman M, Nadelson C. The rape victim: psychodynamic considerations. *Am J Psychiatry* 1976; 133:408.
157. Moscarello R. Posttraumatic stress disorder after sexual assault: its psychodynamics and treatment. *J Am Acad Psychoanal* 1991;19:235.
158. Bownes IT, O'Gorman EC, Sayers A. Assault characteristics and posttraumatic stress disorder in rape victims. *Acta Psychiatr Scand* 1991;83:27.
159. Dahl S. Acute response to rape—a PTSD variant. *Acta Psychiatr Scand Suppl* 1989;80:56.
160. Jenny C, Sutherland SE, Sandahl BB. Developmental approach to preventing the sexual abuse of children. *Pediatrics* 1987;78:1034.
161. Daro DA. Prevention of child sexual abuse. *Future of Children* 1994;4:198.

21

Legal Issues in Pediatric and Adolescent Gynecology

This chapter focuses on legal issues in pediatric and adolescent gynecology. The legal complexity of these issues is compounded by social, psychological, and moral questions (teenage sex); the perceived need for parents to be aware of the behavior of children; the authority to consent to medical intervention; the point at which life begins; the desirability of preventing birth through contraception, abortion, or sterilization; and issues of quality of life.

NATURE AND SOURCES OF LAW

Law emanates from both the state and federal levels of government. In the medical area, state law is generally the more important source of legal guidelines and constraints. It is important to remember that, unlike federal law, state law varies by jurisdiction. Therefore, it is necessary to know the laws of the state in which you practice before making treatment decisions. It is equally important to understand that when state and federal law conflict, federal law under the doctrine of preemption usually takes precedence. Thus, for example, if the federal government permits abortions and state law does not, the federal law controls.

Both state and federal laws have similar sources. The United States Constitution, of course, is interpreted by the federal courts, including the U.S. Supreme Court, while state courts interpret the state constitutions. Constitutional rights may differ between the state and federal levels, with state rights being either broader or narrower when compared with the federal Constitution.

Law that is made or interpreted by judges is called *case law*. Judges, in deciding a particular case, are guided by legal precedents. The process of using decisions of prior courts to decide a case is called *stare decisis*. Much legal debate exists as to whether the proper function of judges is to interpret narrowly existing case law and statutes or actually to create law in response to a matter before them. Those who oppose "judicial legislation" argue that courts have as their sole responsibility the interpretation of legislative action, that is, the action of elected representatives.

Laws promulgated by the legislature are called *statutes* and usually appear in bound volumes under various chapters and sections. Generally, when one wishes to clarify the law in a certain area, the first step is to find out whether there is a statute dealing with the issues.

In addition to constitutional law, case law, and statutes are laws promulgated by the executive branch of government called *executive orders*. There are also laws created by state or federal agencies called *regulations*. State agencies such as a department of public health or a department of mental health and federal agencies such as the Federal Trade Commission enact regulations that serve to clarify and interpret statutes. These regulations of executive agencies have the force and effect of law.

A final distinction of importance is that between civil and criminal law. *Civil law* involves such actions as medical malpractice, where a plaintiff, the alleged victim, brings suit against a defendant, the alleged wrongdoer, seeking monetary damages for harmful acts. In civil actions, the burden of proof is on the plaintiff who must prove his or her case by a preponderance of the evidence, that is, more evidence showing that the plaintiff has been wronged than evidence legally exculpating the defendant. In a *criminal* case, the state acts as the prosecutor and must prove criminal wrongdoing beyond a reasonable doubt. While the primary purpose of a civil suit is to recover damages for an injured plaintiff, the primary purpose of criminal action is to punish a guilty defendant. Such punishment, of course, can range from a fine to death.

CONSENT TO MEDICAL CARE

The general rule regarding consent to medical care is that anyone who has reached the age of majority, usually 18 or 21 years, may consent to treatment. If a patient is under the age of majority, a parent or legal guardian must usually consent to medical intervention. Every legal rule, however, has exceptions. In the case of an emergency, for example, consent is implied, and neither a parent, legal guardian, nor patient need explicitly authorize the medical care. It is important, however, to document that an emergency existed and what efforts were made to notify the parents of a minor patient. It is also necessary to determine how state law defines an emergency. For example, in Massachusetts, an emergency is defined as the following: "When delay in treatment will endanger the life, limb or mental well-being of the patient" (1). The definition of an emergency may vary from state to state but generally involves the same concept.

In addition to the emergency exception, minors are legally capable of consenting to their own health care if they are emancipated. Emancipation generally has two statutory definitions. The first is a minor fulfilling an adult status. If a patient, for example, is a member of the armed forces, is a parent of a child, is married, widowed, or divorced, or is living separately from and is financially independent of parents, he or she may consent to intervention without informing the parent or guardian.

The second basis of emancipation is where the minor's health may be endangered and the state wishes to encourage the minor to seek help despite possible parental resistance. Such areas where a minor may consent to treatment under state law include pregnancy, diseases dangerous to the public health, and alcohol or drug dependency. Reasoning that getting treatment is more important than obtaining parental consent, the state in these areas encourages the minor to seek intervention on his or her own authority by allowing treatment without parental consent. Unlike minors fulfilling an adult status, who generally may consent to any kind of medical care, minors in the second category generally may only consent to treatment for the specific condition creating emancipation.

The separate concept of mature minor, moreover, has received increasing judicial approval. Courts have recognized that there may be situations not otherwise controlled by statute in which it is in the best interest of the minor not to notify parents of the intended medical treatment. If the minor is able to give informed consent to the intended treatment, the mature minor rule may apply.

The initial determination of whether a minor is mature or not usually rests with the treating health care provider, who assesses the nature of the procedure, its likely benefit, and the capacity of the particular minor to understand fully what the medical procedure involves. Thus, in a situation where a minor is not emancipated, it may still be possible to enter into a provider–patient relationship with the minor and without parental consent on the basis of the provider's assessment that the minor is mature.

Generally, a health care provider will not be held liable for providing medical treatment without parental consent if he or she relies in good faith on the minor's reasonable representation that he or she is emancipated. Consents obtained from emancipated and mature minors, and any interventions resulting from such consents, moreover, are confidential. Parents should not be informed unless the minor agrees. Such agreements should be documented in the patient's medical record.

Some states require health care providers treating minors to inform the parent if the minor's condition is endangering of life or limb. Under such circumstances, the situation should be discussed with the minor before informing the parent, and this discussion should be documented in the patient's record. Under circumstances not endangering to life or limb, no information should be shared with the parent without the consent of the minor patient, and billings should not be mailed to parents if they undermine or are likely to undermine the confidentiality of the relationship.

In medical management, disagreements may arise among care providers, minor patients, and their parents. For example, an adolescent diagnosed with an ovarian tumor may resist chemotherapy that her parent requests; or both parents and patient may refuse surgery that physicians feel is medically necessary. Hopefully, these conflicts will resolve with ongoing dialogue and the obtaining of second opinions. If consensus does not emerge, however, the legal options vary, depending on such factors as the age of the patient, the seriousness of the underlying condition, the nature and variety of possible interventions, their contraindications, and the probability of their success.

Courts, for example, would likely order treatment in a minor's "best interest" if her parents are unwilling to consent to treatment, the underlying condition is potentially fatal, the recommended treatment is the only one available or is clearly preferred, and the risks of treatment are minimal (2).

Health care providers should obviously resist the coercive imposition of treatment on a minor. If, however, the patient is not "mature," the underlying condition is serious, and the parents are consenting to its use, the parents' desires can legally "trump" the minor's right to refuse.

Obtaining informed consent is a process that involves four distinct steps. The first step, which has already been discussed, is determining who has the authority to consent. The second step is determining whether the person with the authority to consent is competent to consent. Legally, a person is presumed competent until demonstrated otherwise. Thus, for example, parents of a mentally retarded patient who has reached the age of majority do not automatically become their child's legal guardian. They must be appointed by a court, and without such judicial appointment, they do not have the legal authority to consent to their child's treatment. The provider should be cautious about providing treatment if there is any question regarding a person's capacity to understand the nature and consequences of a proposed procedure. Such reasons may include mental retardation, inebriation, or drug usage.

The third step in obtaining informed consent involves providing the person who has the authority to consent with all the material information necessary for a reasonable person to make an informed decision. Generally speaking, the patient or parent/guardian must be informed of the nature of the patient's condition, the nature and probability of the risks, the benefits to be reasonably expected, the inability of the treater to predict results, the reversibility of the procedure, the likely result of no treatment, and the alternatives to the proposed treatment, including the risks and benefits of such alternatives. The provider should keep in mind that the more elective a proposed treatment, the more necessary it is to disclose all risks.

The final step in the informed consent process is obtaining the agreement of the person with the authority to consent. The person with legal authority to consent should sign the consent form agreeing to any interventions after such interventions have been fully communicated and understood. It is important to note that merely obtaining the signature of the person with authority to consent, without going through the other steps in the process, does not constitute informed consent. It is advisable therefore to make a note in the medical record documenting the informed consent process.

Finally, it is necessary for the practitioner to be aware of special situations where the general rules of consent may not apply. Such situations include a child's being in the custody of the state or a divorce situation where one parent may have physical care of a child but both parents may have legal custody or decision-making responsibility. Other special situations may include abortion, sterilization, management of child abuse cases, and consent to human immunodeficiency virus (HIV) testing (to be discussed subsequently).

To illustrate a special situation, if the Massachusetts Department of Social Services (DSS) has legal custody of a child, it is authorized to consent to the youngster's routine medical care (e.g., immunizations, preventive health services, and treatment of illnesses). If, however, the required medical interventions are "extraordinary"—for example, "do not resuscitate" orders, the giving or withholding of life-prolonging medical treatment, or the use of antipsychotic medications—the DSS cannot consent but will seek judicial approval before proceeding.

CONFIDENTIALITY OF PATIENT INFORMATION

As a general rule, medical records and communications between providers and patients and their families are confidential and should not be released without the written authorization of the patient/guardian or a proper judicial order. Even though parents, including noncustodial parents, usually have access to medical information of their minor children, certain situations may mandate a denial of access. As indicated previously, mature minors and emancipated minors who consent to treatment need not reveal either the consent or the treatment to their parents. Later sections will discuss other exceptions to parental notification, including the prescription of contraceptives to unemancipated minors.

Physicians and other care providers should learn whether statutory or common law privileges protect the confidentiality of a patient relationship. In some jurisdictions, for example, statutory privileges exist between psychotherapists and patients, physicians and patients, and social workers and clients. These privileges prevent professionals from revealing any information about their patients without specific authorization. Case law may further prohibit a professional's ability to disclose information without written consent.

Regardless of maturity, emancipation, or privilege, teenagers may hesitate to reveal sensitive information to care providers if it is automatically shared with their parents. At the beginning of the professional relationship, therefore, the physician should consider negotiating ground rules with families: that before any sharing, the older minor will be notified as to what will be communicated and why and that to maintain a teenager's trust, parents will only receive information that is legally or clinically necessary to share—for example, indications of serious illness or potentially life-threatening behavior.

Though all clinical information in a patient's chart is confidential, recorded data concerning such matters as psychiatric history and HIV status are especially sensitive. To facilitate increased protection of these notes, care providers might stamp the word "confidential" on the relevant pages.

SEXUAL ABUSE

Reporting statutes exist in every state that require various professionals to report sexual abuse to state agencies, usually a department of social services or its equivalent. Physicians, nurses, and other medical professionals are *mandated* reporters. The standard employed for determining whether the state agency should be notified is reasonable belief or suspicion that a child has suffered sexual abuse. Knowledge of incest or sexual abuse is not required because very rarely is a professional certain that sexual abuse has occurred. Symptoms such as fear of men, nightmares and sleep disturbances, stomachaches, and headaches are symptomatic but not diagnostic of sexual exploitation and may require reporting.

Generally, reports of abuse have no statute of limitations requirement. State child protection agencies, however, are understandably reluctant to accept filings that are difficult to investigate because the alleged events occurred in the past. They may also refuse to accept reports in which the suspected perpetrator is a stranger to the child rather than a care provider (e.g., a parent or family member, babysitter, or school bus driver) with legitimate authority over him/her. Under these circumstances, the professional may defer to the agency's decision, documenting in the patient's chart the agency's refusal to become involved, or file the report regardless, requesting protective services to forward it to law enforcement.

From a legal point of view, if a mandated reporter has concerns about sexual abuse of a patient, it is generally safer to file a report than to withhold filing. Most states, for example, have an immunity provision protecting from suit or liability those professionals who file a report that is later proved erroneous. On the other hand, there are sanctions for mandated reporters who fail to fulfill their statutory responsibility to report.

After child abuse reports are received by state agencies, the agency must investigate the allegedly abusive family to determine whether a child is at risk. Assuming that a report is corroborated, the state agency has an obligation to monitor the child's safety, to provide services that may protect a child from future harm, and, in certain circumstances, to refer the case for possible criminal prosecution, or to remove the child from biologic parents for placement in foster care. Most states waive any privileges that otherwise may exist between the professional and patient in order to encourage reporting; in other words, the confidentiality that usually exists within a relationship is waived by law in the case of child abuse.

In addition to mandatory reporting statutes, states may have other legislation relevant to the management of sexual abuse. For example, statutes often exist that allow a health care provider serving in a hospital or health center to prevent a child from being removed by his or her caretaker if the child is in imminent and serious danger because of abuse and neglect. Legislation may also exist that allows professionals to petition juvenile or family courts if they feel that parental unfitness is causing harm to a child. Under such circumstances, the courts may remove legal custody from biologic parents, place it with the state, and order that such children be placed in foster care or another more secure environment.

Because sexual abuse is more often criminally prosecuted than physical abuse, physicians and medical personnel may need to testify in prosecutions of alleged abusers. Sometimes they serve as expert witnesses who, though uninvolved in the direct care of the child, have reviewed records and will offer opinions to the court. At other times, though having expertise, they essentially serve as fact witnesses who communicate what they did or observed in their professional role (e.g., the diagnostic tests performed and treatment given). Clearly, these two categories of testimony overlap.

It is imperative for health care providers to keep complete and accurate records of any examinations conducted on children who have been victimized. Before testifying, health care providers should "refresh their recollection" of the case by reviewing their notes and should seek legal consultation and advice, if it is available. The professional should also make certain that no privileges exist that impede communication without the consent of patient or parent.

On the witness stand the physician should not use jargon or overly complex language; if professional terms are necessary, they require clarification. A witness should answer only the specific question asked, should not respond to a question beyond his/her knowledge or expertise, and should refrain from argumentative or clearly partisan communications.

It should be understood that cases of child sexual abuse can be very difficult to prosecute successfully because of the child's age and frequent lack of physical evidence. In criminal matters, the state must prove a defendant guilty beyond a reasonable doubt, and this standard can be difficult to reach in sexual abuse cases.

CONTRACEPTION

The provision of contraception to minors raises two legal issues: consent and the need for parental notification. In regard to consent, in 1977 the U.S. Supreme Court in *Carey* v *Population Serv Int'l* (3) invalidated a New York statute that prohibited the distribution or sale of contraceptives to minors under the age of 16. The court ruled that the New York law violated the privacy rights of minors, which included the right to make procreative decisions. Such decisions, of course, should be based on informed consent, and a medical practitioner should review state law to ascertain whether additional requirements need to be met before contraceptives are prescribed. With the subdermal implant contraceptive

(Norplant System), for example, consent of the parent/guardian of a minor patient is generally recommended, because insertion requires a surgical procedure and, practically, because the device is unlikely to go unnoticed.

Even if unemancipated minors can obtain contraceptives without parental consent, state law may require a provider to notify parents of the provision of contraceptives. In 1980, a U.S. Appeals Court in the case of *Doe* v *Irwin* (4) found that parents did not have a right to notification when minors voluntarily sought contraceptive devices from publicly operated family planning centers. This decision finds support in more recent cases that find it is not in the best interest of the minor to breach a confidential relationship between the minor and the family planning service.

Since some contraceptives can have harmful side effects, it is important to assess possible risks, to communicate them to the patient, to properly implement the contraceptive, and to monitor the patient for adverse reactions.

STERILIZATION

The sterilization of minors is almost exclusively a matter of state law. Because sterilization, if successful, ends the minor's reproductive capability, it is strictly regulated or prohibited outright. In some states, a mentally retarded child or adult may be sterilized, but only after a formal proceeding to ensure protection of the incompetent's best interest. In other states, there is no legal basis for performing sterilization procedures on incompetents. The general rule is that neither courts nor a guardian can authorize voluntary sterilization of minors without specific statutory authority.

A private hospital may prohibit its medical staff from performing voluntary sterilization. Some states, moreover, have so-called conscience clauses that allow individual physicians or nurses to refuse participation in sterilization or abortion procedures if such procedures are performed in the facility in which they work.

ABORTION

In 1973, the U.S. Supreme Court in *Roe* v *Wade* (5) held that the "fundamental right" of privacy included the right of abortion. It then developed a trimester system that made the woman's health and viability of the fetus key decision points. In the first trimester of pregnancy, the abortion decision is primarily between a woman and her health care provider. In the second trimester, the state has an increasing interest in the woman's health and can regulate the conditions under which an abortion is performed. In the third trimester, because the fetus is viable and can generally survive separate and apart from its mother, the state develops a "compelling interest" in the life of the fetus and can prohibit abortions except if the mother's life or health is endangered.

In the case of *Webster* v *Reproductive Health Services* (6), the Court upheld a Missouri statute requiring doctors to test for fetal viability in any fetus thought to be at least 20 weeks old and forbidding public facilities and employees (doctors, nurses, and other health care providers) from performing abortions other than those to save the life of the mother. Though not specifically overruling the *Roe* v *Wade* decision, Chief Justice Rehnquist, writing for a plurality of the Court, attacked its trimester structure as "unsound" and "unworkable." He said there is "no reason why the state's compelling interest in protecting potential human life should not extend throughout pregnancy rather than coming into existence only at the point of viability." While the Roe case functioned to keep states from restricting most abortions, the Webster decision allows states much greater license to regulate and curtail abortions.

Prior to Webster, the Supreme Court had consistently struck down regulations and procedures that inhibit a woman's access to abortion. Impermissible restrictions include requirements that all second trimester abortions be performed in a hospital, that minors obtain either parental or judicial consent for abortions, and that women wait a minimum of 24 hours after signing a consent form before an abortion can occur. The Seventh Circuit U.S. Court of Appeals, for example, struck down an Illinois statute imposing a 24-hour waiting period on minors seeking abortion (7).

In the 1992 case of *Planned Parenthood of Southeastern Pennsylvania* v *Casey* (8), however, the U.S. Supreme Court declared that a 24-hour waiting period between information disclosed for a woman's "informed consent" and the performance of an abortion is constitutional as long as the delay may be voided in a medical emergency and does not create any appreciable health risk to the patient. Generally, statutes requiring parental consent as a precondition to abortion have been struck down. In the case of *Planned Parenthood of Central Missouri* v *Danforth* (9), the Supreme Court held unconstitutional a statute requiring parental consent to abortions for unmarried women under age 18. Some states, however, have enacted legislation allowing minors seeking abortions to apply for judicial consent as an alternative to parental consent. In the Massachusetts case of *Bellotti* v *Baird* (10), the court ruled that the state must provide a pregnant minor with a timely and confidential opportunity to show she is mature and informed enough to make her own abortion decision in consultation with her health care provider. If the court finds the minor not sufficiently mature to give consent, it must authorize an abortion if this is found to be in her best interest. If state legislation contains these two provisions, then according to the Baird case, requiring parental consent would not constitute the absolute and arbitrary veto that was found unconstitutional in *Danforth*.

In addition to the issue of parental consent for a minor's abortion is the question of parental notification. In *H.L.* v *Matheson* (11), the Supreme Court upheld a Utah statute that required physicians to "notify if possible" the parents or guardian of an unmarried minor who sought an abortion. The Court stated that the statute served an important state interest in protecting family integrity, safeguarding adolescents, and providing parents the opportunity to supply essential psychological and medical information to their child's physician. Although most parental notification statutes have been found constitutional, those that require more than simple notification have been struck down. For example, in *Hodgson* v *Minnesota* (12), the U.S. Court of Appeals for the Eighth Circuit ruled that a judicial consent alternative must be an option in abortion statutes that require parental notification. The court wished to ensure that the notice requirement was not unduly burdensome to the pregnant minor attempting to obtain an abortion. To ensure that the parental notification requirement is not unduly burdensome, the minor must be given the option of an alternative court procedure in which she can show her maturity or demonstrate that performance of an abortion is in her best interest.

Given the current Congressional balance and the political strength of some antiabortion groups, abortions may be increasingly restricted or curbed. Controversial issues include a ban on abortions in overseas military hospitals, the prohibition of abortion coverage in federal employees' health insurance except in cases of life endangerment, state authorization to eliminate Medicaid funding for abortions for low-income women who are pregnant from rape or incest, the ending of federal funding for human embryo research, and the outlawing of late-term abortions. The ultimate fate of these measures depends on the responses of the U.S. House of Representatives and Senate, the willingness of the President to exercise his veto, and, assuming constitutional challenge, the ultimate holdings of the Supreme Court.

SEXUALLY TRANSMITTED DISEASES

States commonly require that health care professionals report cases of venereal disease or diseases dangerous to the public health to a state or local board of health. For example, in Massachusetts, a physician treating a patient with acquired immunodeficiency syndrome (AIDS) must report the fact of AIDS to the local board of health. Gonorrhea and syphilis, on the other hand, are reported directly to the state Department of Public Health. As indicated earlier, a minor who believes that he or she is suffering from a sexually transmitted disease usually can consent to treatment without the authorization of a parent or guardian.

HIV AND AIDS

The statutes on HIV infection and AIDS are of recent origin and, like other laws, vary by state. Four important issues that arise are testing, confidentiality, universal precautions, and documentation. To test for the presence of HIV antibody, voluntary and informed consent of the patient and/or parent/guardian usually is required. As a matter of public policy, many states prohibit mandatory, coerced, or secret testing of individual patients for AIDS.

Many states, moreover, require that HIV testing and test results be maintained in confidence. In these states, the fact and the results of such testing cannot be disclosed without the subject's written informed consent. This confidentiality requirement may conflict with the professional's perceived duty to warn a party who may be exposed to HIV or AIDS. For example, a teenager who has used drugs and tests positive on an HIV test may request that her boyfriend not be informed of the test results. The health care provider may feel strongly that the boyfriend is entitled to the test information so that he also may be tested, receive medical and psychiatric intervention, and take prophylactic action regarding other sexual partners. The health care provider should learn whether a state confidentiality statute exists for HIV infection or AIDS.

The Occupational Safety and Health Administration of the U.S. Department of Labor requires the implementation of universal precautions in health care settings. Use of universal precautions makes mandatory testing less necessary to protect hospital staff. If professionals assume that blood and body fluids of all patients need to be avoided, the rationale for universal mandatory testing becomes less salient.

Though health care providers need to maintain the confidentiality of HIV testing and results, it is necessary to document the fact and the results of testing in hospital and private patient records. Documentation is necessary so that professionals can provide the best and most appropriate care for a patient. The confidentiality concern is not met by failing to record medical information. It is fulfilled by giving access only to those who have a clinical or administrative need to know.

SUMMARY

Minors are generally not capable of consenting to their own health care. In an emergency situation, however, consent of a parent or a guardian is not required. Furthermore, if a minor is mature (close to the age of majority and capable of reasonable decision making), he or she may consent to care without parental involvement if the mature minor doctrine is recognized by the state courts. If the minor is emancipated under state statute (has an adult status or a condition that is health endangering, such as pregnancy, venereal disease, or drug dependency), the teen is empowered to consent to treatment.

Parents generally have access to the medical and other information of their children. However, if a statutory privilege exists such as between social worker and client or psychotherapist and patient or if common law requires that a physician not disclose patient data, the confidential relationship between the professional and minor must be maintained. Confidentiality also must be respected if the minor is defined as mature or emancipated.

All 50 states have child-abuse reporting statutes that require professionals to report cases of incest and sexual abuse to government agencies. State law may also allow or require professionals to obtain restraining orders to protect victims of sexual exploitation who are in imminent and serious danger. Legislation may also exist that allows minors to be placed in the temporary custody of the state for their protection.

The Supreme Court has upheld the right of minors to make procreative decisions and has forbidden states from prohibiting the distribution of contraceptives to them. In terms of notification, a U.S. Court of Appeals has ruled that parents have no constitutional right to be advised when a public facility distributes contraceptives to their children.

In the case of *Peck* v *Califano* (13), it was held that sterilization of persons under 21 years of age may not lawfully be funded with federal money. This decision supports social policy restricting a minor's access to sterilization.

The Supreme Court decisions in *Roe* v *Wade* (5) and *Doe* v *Bolton* (14) essentially permit abortions to occur during the first two trimesters of pregnancy. States may not promulgate regulations or procedures that restrict the constitutionally protected right of privacy unless a compelling state interest overrides that right. Generally, statutes requiring parental consent as a precondition to an abortion have been struck down by courts. Some states, however, have passed laws allowing minors seeking abortions to apply for the consent of a judge as an alternative to parental consent.

Certain sexually transmitted diseases must be reported to local or state public health agencies. HIV testing generally requires the voluntary informed and written consent of the patient and/or parent/guardian. The testing itself and the test results usually are confidential, but a duty to warn may exist if someone is in danger of contagion. Universal precautions as specified by the federal Centers for Disease Control and Prevention should be followed, and HIV or AIDS testing and treatment should be properly documented in a medical record.

REFERENCES

1. Massachusetts General Law, C112, sec 12F.
2. Bourne R. Coerced treatment of adolescents. In: Ventrell MR, ed. *Children's law, policy and practice*. Denver: National Association of Counsel for Children, 1995.
3. *Carey* v *Population Serv Int'l,* 431 US 678, 97 SCt 2010 (1977).
4. *Doe* v *Irwin*, 615 F2d 1162 (6th Cir 1980).
5. *Roe* v *Wade*, 410 US 113, 93 SCt 705 (1973).
6. *Webster* v *Reproductive Health Services*, 109 SCt 3040 (1989).
7. *Zbarez* v *Hartigan*, 763 F2d 1532 (7th Cir 1985).
8. *Planned Parenthood of Southeastern Pennsylvania* v *Casey*, 120 LEd 2d 674 (1992).
9. *Planned Parenthood of Central Missouri* v *Danforth*, 428 US 52, 96 SCt 2831 (1976).
10. *Bellotti* v *Baird*, 443 US 622, 99 SCt 3035 (1979).
11. *H.L.* v *Matheson*, 450 US 398, 1101 SCt 1164 (1981).
12. *Hodgson* v *Minnesota*, 827 F2d 1191 (8th Cir 1987).
13. *Peck* v *Califano*, 454 F Supp 484 (1977).
14. *Doe* v *Bolton*, 410 US 179, 93 SCt 739 (1973).

22

Sexuality Education

Sexuality, as explained by the Sex Information and Education Council of the United States (SIECUS), refers to the totality of being a person. Sexuality reflects human character, the way in which people interact. Sexuality education is the lifelong process of acquiring information and developing values about one's identity, relationships, and intimacy. It includes learning about sexual development, reproductive health, interpersonal relationships, affection, body image, and gender roles. Sexuality is a multidimensional concept with ethical, psychological, biological, and cultural dimensions (1). As young children and adolescents grow and develop physically and cognitively, they are exposed to and receive sexuality education from multiple sources: classrooms, home and family, the streets, the media, medical settings, and work and play among peers and friends. As health care providers, it is critical to recognize the messages our youth are receiving about sexuality and help them with their process of self-discovery and self-determination.

By giving children, teens, and young adults correct information, the opportunity to develop their own values, attitudes, and insights, and the skills with which to effectively communicate and make decisions, parents and professionals involved with young people can contribute significantly to their well-being.

SEXUALITY EDUCATION AT HOME

True sexuality education begins much earlier than school programs, and the primary instructors are parents. As children grow, become curious about their bodies and sexual issues, and develop relationships within and outside of the family, they glean information with which to develop their belief systems and patterns of behavior from their most valued role models. When parents are uncomfortable discussing sex and sexuality, either the physical or more emotional dimensions, this discomfort may be transmitted and incorporated by the child. Children who are uncomfortable with sexuality topics may be less tolerant of sexuality differences among others and may be less likely to discuss and seek help for concerns about sexuality. Family values and communication about sex and sexuality can have a significant impact on the initiation of sex and use of contraception among youths (2).

The parental responses to children's early questions can establish the tone of future interactions and discussions about sexuality. Educational programs for parents have been shown to facilitate parent–child communication about sex (3). Young parents should be encouraged to know the facts about sex, develop comfort with issues of sexuality, be honest and open with children on an age-appropriate level (i.e., use appropriate names for body parts in lieu of made-up names that may relay a message of discomfort with the facts), and avoid judgmental or argumentative discussions about sex. It is helpful for parents to anticipate the role that the media will play in their children's attitudes about sex; parents may want to watch some of those messages with children and use the media as a means to discuss sex within a context in which parents can introduce their own values and attitudes. As children develop physically, it is important to provide them with communication skills. Children are not cognitively able to anticipate situations, including sexual situations, in which they might be placed; one skills-building strategy is to role-play various age-appropriate scenarios. Five-year-olds might benefit from role-playing a scenario of what to say to someone who wanted to touch them where they did not want to be touched, and adolescents might learn from a scenario where a partner refuses to wear a condom. By thinking about possible responses to such situations, youths can be prepared to react nonimpulsively and in ways consistent with their own developing belief systems to any unanticipated predicaments.

SEXUALITY EDUCATION IN SCHOOL

Organized sexuality education in the schools and/or community groups represents an important part of a child's education. Despite some controversy about specific course content, 87% to 90% of parents, both urban and rural, approve of school-based sexuality education, and a significant proportion endorse starting such education in the elementary grades (4,5).

The content of traditional sex education is controversial, and the goals and means of evaluating this education are murky and sometimes confused as well. Teaching healthy attitudes, feelings, and behaviors about sex and sexuality is not everyone's goal, and achievement of healthy feelings about sexuality is an ambiguous measure to evaluate. Articles evaluating sex education programs frequently focus on statistics about the high rates of teen sexually transmitted disease and sexual activity, early age of sexual debut, and high rates of pregnancies and abortions. This creates a difficult standard by which to evaluate sex education programs in the schools. Sexual behavior and the consequences of such behavior have multifactorial causes in this country, including the biological urges, cognitive developmental stage, and natural desire for experimentation among teens, as well as more pervasive political, socioeconomic, moral, and financial concerns. These latter concerns are inextricably intertwined with the type of formal education provided to youth, and they affect the way parents teach children at home. Although it is difficult to evaluate the efficacy of sexuality education without examining behavioral outcomes, it is critical when discussing traditional educational programs to understand the shortcomings of this means of evaluation.

Approaches to sex education have evolved through several "generations" (6). First-generation programs imparted knowledge about sexuality, pregnancy, and birth control. Second-generation programs continued to focus on knowledge but also included values clarification, decision making, and communication-skills building. Evaluations of both first- and second-generation programs demonstrated that they had no effect, positive or negative, on adolescent sexual behavior (6). Third-generation programs were a departure from the path of program development, arising in opposition to sex education and emphasizing a moral message of abstinence, often eliminating "conflictual" information from the curriculum about contraception and "safe sex." The limited evaluation of these programs that has been done reveals that they do not reduce the age of sexual debut or the frequency of intercourse among youth (6). A study of an abstinence-based program, Sex Respect, found that the program had significant limitations in content (7). It is important to note that evaluative studies of all three of these early generations of sex education programs were not always methodologically sound (6), and this limitation may have contributed to some of the null findings. The methodology within this field of research has been found to be weak in several areas, most notable being the lack of control groups and failure to present pre- and postintervention data (6,8). Oakley and colleagues (8) reported that only 18% of the educational outcome evaluation studies published since 1982 were methodologically sound.

The most recent, fourth-generation educational programs were based initially on the health-belief model, which emphasizes the importance of the perceived risk/benefit ratio to young persons in health decision making, and more recently on social learning theory, which includes the concept that societal pressures and interaction play a role in the young person's health decisions. The newer educational programs acknowledge and address the adolescent developmental and motivational framework (6). They emphasize delaying intercourse as a safe and wise decision yet also provide information about contraception and safe sex. There is a strong component of experiential skills building within the curriculum for teens to learn how to avoid unwanted or unprotected intercourse. This format allows adolescents to practice and develop confidence with these skills. Learning and practicing these skills via various media (i.e., role playing, computer simulation games) not only teach decision-making skills but stimulate discussion of these issues with peers and parents, an important advantage of such exercises (9). Several of these programs have been rigorously evaluated and have been found to be effective in decreasing pregnancy rates, reducing the proportion of adolescents initiating sexual activity, and/or increasing the rates of contraception use (10,11). The most successful fourth-generation programs incorporate many of the educational strategies found to be most effective in the evaluation literature (see Chapter 18) (10,11):

1. They provide a narrow focus on reducing sexual risk-taking behaviors, including behaviors increasing the likelihood of pregnancy or sexually transmitted diseases including human immunodeficiency virus (HIV) infection.
2. They provide social learning theory as the foundation of the program.
3. They include accurate information as well as experiential activities to personalize and reinforce information.
4. They address the social and media influences on sexual behavior.
5. They reinforce clear values and group attitudes about unsafe sexual practices.
6. They provide modeling of and practice in communication and negotiation skills (i.e., role-play activities).

Although few studies have been done, it appears that linking these educational programs to a school-based clinic that may or may not distribute contraception does not increase the frequency of risky sexual behaviors. In fact, the presence of school-based clinics may increase the use of condoms and other forms of contraception (12).

WHAT TO TEACH AND WHEN TO TEACH IT

Sexuality education is most effective if it takes place prior to a young person's sexual debut (6,12). Ideally, sexuality education is a lifelong endeavor, not a 10-week intervention at school. If sexuality education is taught at home or in health professionals' offices and is incorporated throughout the school years, progress toward healthier sexual behaviors is more likely.

Sexuality education must be approached like any other educational program: the information must be developmentally appropriate, culturally sensitive, inclusive of people who are traditionally disenfranchised (i.e., mentally and physically challenged populations, chronically ill people), and free of biases, including heterosexual bias (i.e., discussing only heterosexual couples as the basis for family development). It is important throughout sexuality education to teach, as well as model, tolerance for differences among various types of people and lifestyles.

The content of any sexuality education program is best determined by the community for which it is being developed. Sexuality education is optimal if taught in kindergarten through the 12th grade. No one can determine at what ages every topic should optimally be addressed among youth; however, there are some general guidelines. Young children (ages 3 to 5 years) learn primarily through life itself (13). Exploration of their bodies is normal at this age. Information imparted in response to behaviors or questions should be factually correct, short, and simple. Sexuality needs to be an acceptable and comfortable topic of conversation. Scolding children for questioning or exploring aspects of themselves may be detrimental. Children, even at this age, are also entitled to a measure of privacy (13). Some of the most common issues at this age include body-part naming, recognizing the roles of family members, developing self-esteem, and understanding that living things grow, reproduce, and die.

In early elementary school (ages 5 to 8 years), children become more interested in how the body functions, the differences between males and females, child abuse, and family responsibilities and relationships, including divorce. Many of the questions asked at this time revolve around babies (how are babies born, how many babies can a woman have, do babies come from eggs?), adoption, twins, and marriage (13); thus, the curriculum for this age group should reflect these concerns.

Between the ages 9 and 12 years, many physical and emotional changes begin to take place, thus initiating new questions and concerns about sexuality. Children are noticing that others are developing at different rates. Youngsters display more interest in reproduction (how does the sperm get to the egg, do boys menstruate?), and self-consciousness about the other sex begins. Important issues for this age group include how families can be happy together, including nontraditional families (i.e., same-sex parents, single-parent families, communal families), teenage pregnancy, interest in boy–girl relationships, and preventing divorce. Important topics to cover in the education of this period include the following (13):

1. Biologic information including the endocrine system, menstruation, birth and pregnancy, nocturnal emissions, masturbation, body differences, responses to sexual stimulation, birth control, and abortion.
2. Interpersonal relationship information including heterosexual feelings, homosexual feelings, emotions' effects on the way the body functions, and changing roles and relationships within the family.
3. Self-concept development, the interpretation of people's reactions, reacting to others, self-image, and the changing feelings toward others.

During the early teen years (ages 12 to 14 years), physical changes and curiosity about sex abound. It is critical that young teens know the facts about sex, pregnancy, and birth control, not just the information that their friends have given them. They need the tools and skills to decide how intimate they want to become with others and when they want to become intimate (why do some people choose to date and others don't?). It is also the time to discuss variations in sexual behaviors in a nonjudgmental yet informative way. Teens need the skills to be able to postpone sexual intercourse and to make healthy choices. Again, understanding the differences among people in an atmosphere of tolerance is critical in the healthy development of sexuality.

Curricula for adolescents can include issues of dating behaviors, refusal skills and ways of dealing with coercive situations, premarital sex, contemporary marriage patterns, living together, sexual myths, moral decisions, control of sex drives, parenthood, and cultural aspects of sexuality (13). By the mid to late teenage years, more details about sexual information are necessary, and the more community and global aspects of sexual behavior can be addressed. Research on birth control, population dynamics, sexual response, sexual dysfunction, pornography, and sexuality education itself are appropriate topics. As teens evolve toward adulthood and achieve emotional maturity and abstract thought processes, these discussions regarding the societal concerns and consequences of sexual behaviors become more relevant.

SEXUALITY EDUCATION FOR ALL

This same educational process must be available for youth with both mental and physical disabilities. People with emotional and mental disabilities are also sexual beings and often have unmet needs for sexuality education; programs that address this special population's needs are needed to protect the rights of this group in our society and help them function to achieve their highest potential for social interaction (14). Materials need to be taught more slowly and graphically, but in general the same topics are appropriate for this special group of students (13).

Young people with physical disabilities and chronic illnesses have sometimes been seen as asexual; their disability may be the focus during health care interactions and their need for sexuality education ignored (15–17). Young people with sensory impairments may require specialized teaching techniques.

It is also critical to be sensitive to cultural diversity among sexuality education students and encourage community participation. It is important for programs to (18,19):

1. Use appropriate and understandable language.
2. Choose appropriate staff who are familiar with the culture of the student.
3. Choose the goals of prevention based on the culture.
4. Try to reflect the given culture in the activities and materials chosen for the program.
5. Promote positive self-images and relationships with others.
6. Examine the expectations for the intervention (program directors should expect equal learning from all groups, and programs may need adjustment to attain such a goal in various situations.)

Bias can plague a sexuality education curriculum, especially heterosexual bias that alienates and excludes an estimated 10% of adolescents who are questioning their sexual orientation (20). Issues of sexual orientation (the physical/emotional attraction to members of the same or other sex) and gender identity (one's feelings of maleness or femaleness) surface during adolescence and should be addressed in a sexuality education curriculum. As children enter adolescence, they begin to experiment with their sexual roles in society. This experimentation does not necessarily predict their sexual preferences in the future, and experimentation is thought by most experts to represent normative adolescent behavior and sexual-identity formation. Gender identity disorders range from transvestitism (cross-dressing that is linked to sexual excitement) to transgenderism (a profound discomfort with one's anatomic body to the point of seeking surgical/hormonal gender reassignment), and these behaviors and feelings evolve during the adolescent years. This group of teens needs support during this time of change in their lives. It has been estimated that 30% of teen suicides result from worry and depression about sexual identity (21), and despair can also lead to acting out or involvement in high-risk behaviors.

One final, critical element to include in a sexuality education curriculum is the element of eroticism. Given the dangers of unsafe sex, talk about sex and sexuality has necessarily become very medicalized. Relationship "instructions" include quizzing partners about their sexual histories and maintaining safe behaviors (22). The element of desire and intimacy can easily get lost, given the current goals of sex education. Examining the topics of intimacy, desire, and effective yet open and gratifying interpersonal communication may help students foster the elements of healthy decision making and desire in their sexual relationships.

ROLE OF THE HEALTH CARE PROVIDER

The health care provider plays an important role in the sexuality education of youth. Health care providers are seen as the logical choice of professionals to discuss these health issues with children and teens. Parents, however, may perceive that some health care providers have varying degrees of comfort with sexuality issues (23). Many professionals use "medicalese" and terms that are unfamiliar to patients and parents when discussing sexual issues, and many adolescent patients do not fully understand the information being imparted to them (24).

Discussing sex should be a routine part of a medical assessment. It is critical that health care professionals explore and understand their own feelings about sexuality topics so that they can feel more comfortable counseling parents of young children and their adolescent patients about sexuality and health. Although it is important for providers to understand how their own biases may affect counseling, appropriate counseling should focus on the personal values of the patient.

As children begin to enter adolescence, the patient–provider relationship changes. Patients need to have private and confidential time with a provider. Asking less personally intrusive questions about a patient's life and circumstances helps establish a relationship with the patient prior to asking questions about sexuality. Adolescents may need help broaching these topics; providers need to ask appropriate questions about sexual behaviors, sexual orientation, and history of sexual abuse or coercion. Adolescents may initially feel awkward or be unresponsive, but if clinicians routinely ask questions in a comfortable and nonjudgmental manner, patients sense their interest and concern and receive the message that they are available and willing to discuss those issues. In some cases, it may be helpful to role-play scenarios of sexual decision making (i.e., what would you say if your partner refused to wear a condom?) with teens to help them develop communication and refusal skills. The Guidelines for Adolescent Preventive Services and Bright Future Health Supervision Guidelines (see Chapter 1) delineate specific recommendations regarding sexuality screening and anticipatory guidance about responsible sexual behaviors, avoidance of alcohol and other drugs prior to or during sex, sexual orientation, abstinence, the correct use of condoms, contraceptive information, the prevention of sexually transmitted diseases including HIV infection, sexual exploitation, and sexual abuse.

When providers preface a screening and counseling conversation with statements such as "I ask everyone all of these questions" it prevents patients from feeling that they have been prejudged in some way. Heterosexually biased phrasing of questions such as "Do you have a boyfriend/girlfriend?" should be avoided. It is less biased to ask, "Is there someone with whom you are in a sexual relationship? Tell me about your partner." Or if the patient is sexually involved, one can ask, "With males, females, or both?" If some patients laugh or scoff at these questions, this provides clinicians with an opportunity to model tolerance and an appreciation for personal differences. Asking these questions allows teens to seek the support they need. The goal of counseling should be to guide them to appropriate resources.

HEALTH CARE PROVIDER AS SEXUALITY EDUCATION ADVOCATE

Health care providers can serve as strong community advocates for sexuality education. Clinicians see the effects of inadequate health education daily; they are well qualified to speak out for the education of our youth.

Talking to parents and teens either in a clinical setting or through community groups about the sexuality education needs of the community allows the provider to work in concert with the community for change. This method also empowers parents and teens to organize their own thoughts and campaigns for what they would like to see happen in the schools and community. Providers can initiate improvements in sexuality education on multiple levels. Talking to small groups of youths in focus groups or developing peer leadership groups are effective in directly educating young people about how to teach themselves and each other accurate sexuality information, behaviors, and skills. Community organizations such as the neighborhood boys or girls clubs could benefit from a health care provider knowledgeable in sexuality serving as advisor or perhaps sitting on the board. Materials are available for providers to use for their own and their patients' education through several organizations (see Appendix 1).

Providers are also needed at parent–teacher organizations, both as information resources and as advocates for appropriate sexuality education curricula in the schools. Clinicians can offer their services in the media, writing letters and speaking out when misinformation or biased views on sexuality education are expressed. Several sources that have compiled specific responses to arguments against sexuality education are available to health care providers (13,25).

Clinicians can have a strong voice in government policy that is rarely heard. Without health care professionals' expert advice, community and state representatives have no guidance on sexuality education issues. Advocacy is a role for which most providers feel untrained, yet health care providers are perhaps the most appropriate experts to speak out about the importance of effective sexuality education. Clinicians need to become more adept at advocacy to help shape the sexuality education that is required to protect the youth of this generation.

REFERENCES

1. *Sexuality education and the schools: fact sheet.* New York: Sex Information and Education Council of the U.S.
2. Hofferth SL. Factors affecting the initiation of sexual intercourse. In: *Risking the future: adolescent sexuality, pregnancy, and childbearing*, vol. 2. Washington, DC: National Academy Press, 1987.
3. Huston RL, Martin LJ, Foulds DM. Effect of a program to facilitate parent-child communication about sex. *Clin Pediatr* 1990;29:626.
4. Sex in America. *Gallup Poll Monthly* 1991;56:1.
5. Welshimer KJ, Harris SE. A survey of rural parents' attitudes toward sexuality education. *J Sch Health* 1994;64:347.
6. Stout JW, Kirby D. The effects of sexuality education on adolescent sexual activity. *Pediatr Ann* 1993; 22:120.
7. Goodson P, Edmundson E. The problematic promotion of abstinence: an overview of Sex Respect. *J Sch Health* 1994;64:205
8. Oakley A, Fullerton D, Holland J, et al. Sexual health education interventions for young people: a methodological review. *BMJ* 1995;310:158.
9. Alemi F, Cherry F, Meffert G. Rehearsing decisions may help teenagers: an evaluation of a simulation game. *Comput Biol Med* 1989;19:283.
10. Frost JJ, Forrest JD. Understanding the impact of effective teenage pregnancy prevention programs. *Fam Plann Perspect* 1995;27:188.
11. Kirby D, Short L, Collins J, et al. School-based programs to reduce sexual risk behaviors: a review of effectiveness. *Public Health Rep* 1994;109:339.
12. Kirby D, Waszak C, Ziegler J. Six school-based clinics: their reproductive health services and impact on sexual behavior. *Fam Plann Perspect* 1991;23:6.
13. Bruess CE, Greenberg JS. *Sexuality education: theory and practice.* New York: MacMillan, 1988.
14. McCabe MP. Sex education programs for people with mental retardation. *Ment Retard* 1993;31:377.
15. Anderson MM. Principles of care for the ill adolescent. *Adolesc Med* 1991;2:441.
16. Cromer BA, Enrile B, McCoy K, et al. Knowledge, attitudes and behavior related to sexuality in adolescents with chronic disability. *Dev Med Child Neurol* 1990;32:603.
17. Coupey SM, Alderman EM. Sexual behavior and related health care for adolescents with chronic medical illness. *Adolesc Med State of the Art Reviews* 1992;3:317.
18. Pittman KJ, Wilson PM, Adams-Taylor S, Randolph S. Making sexuality education and prevention programs relevant for African-American youth. *J Sch Health* 1992;62:339.
19. Walters JL, Canady R, Stein T. Evaluating multicultural approaches in HIV/AIDS educational material. *AIDS Educ Prev* 1994;6:446.
20. Remafedi G, Resnick M, Blum R, Harris L. Demography of sexual orientation in adolescents. *Pediatrics* 1992;89:714.
21. Committee on Adolescence. Homosexuality and adolescence. *Pediatrics* 1993;92:631.

22. Adelman MB. Sustaining the passion: eroticism and safe-sex talk. *Arch Sex Behav* 1992;21:481.
23. Croft CA, Assmussen L. A developmental approach to sexuality education: implications for medical practice. *J Adolesc Health* 1993;14:109.
24. Ammerman SD, Perelli E, Adler N, Irwin CE. Do adolescents understand what physicians say about sexuality and health? *Clin Pediatr* 1992;31:590.
25. *HIV Prevention: looking back, looking ahead: does sex education work?* San Francisco: University of California Center for AIDS Prevention Studies, 1994.

Appendix 1

Sexuality: Additional Resources

Clinicians interested in providing educational materials for their patients should consult their public library and peruse the materials available for parents, children, and adolescents to become familiar with the content. It is useful to order many different pamphlets and read them before selecting several to have available in the office. Pamphlets and videos are for different age groups and different levels of sophistication and often have different messages on the important issues of sexuality, contraception, and abortion. The following is a partial list, and more extensive lists can be obtained from local Planned Parenthood clinics, the Sexuality Information and Education Council of the United States (SIECUS), the American Academy of Pediatrics (AAP), and the American College of Obstetricians and Gynecologists (ACOG). Physicians working with developmentally disabled patients will find the SIECUS bibliographies especially helpful. The addresses for obtaining these materials, as well as other sources, are found at the end of this section. Many of the pharmaceutical firms that make contraceptives and medications for vaginitis also have free pamphlets available.

FOR CHILDREN UNDER 10

Books

Aho JJ, Petras JW. *Learning about sex: a guide for children and their parents.* New York: Holt, Rinehart, and Winston, 1978.
Andry A, Schepp S. *How babies are made.* Boston: Little, Brown, 1984.
Blank J. *A kid's first book about sex.* San Francisco: Yes Press, 1983.
Cole J. *How you were born.* New York: William Morrow, 1984.
Gordon S. *Girls are girls and boys are boys, so what's the difference?: a nonsexist sexuality education book for children.* Buffalo, NY: Prometheus Books, 1991.
Gordon S, Gordon J. *Did the sun shine before you were born?* Buffalo, NY: Prometheus Books, 1992.
Gruenberg S. *The wonderful story of how you were born.* New York: Doubleday, 1970.
Jennings DA. *Baby Brendon's busy day: a sexuality primer.* Tallahassee, FL: Goose Pond Publishing, 1993.
May J. *How we are born.* Chicago: Follett, 1969.
Meredith S. *Where do babies come from?* Tulsa, OK: EDC Publishing, 1991.
Portal C. *The beauty of birth.* New York: Knopf, 1971.

Ratner M, Chamlins S. *Straight talk: sexuality education for parents and kids 4-7.* Planned Parenthood of Westchester, New York, 1985.
Sanchez G J. *Let's talk about sex and loving.* Milpitas: Empty Nest Press, 1994.
Showers D, Showers K. *Before you were a baby.* New York: Crowell, 1968.
Stein S. *Making babies.* New York: Walker, 1974.

FOR PRETEENS AND YOUNG TEENAGERS

Books

Bourgeois P. *Changes in you and me: a book about puberty, mostly for girls.* Kansas City: Andrews & McMeel, 1994.
Cole J. *Asking about sex and growing up.* New York: Morrow Junior Books, 1988.
Gardner-Loulan J, Lopez B, Quackenbush M. *Period.* San Francisco: Volcano Press, 1981.
Harris RH. *It's perfectly normal growing up: changing bodies, sex and sexual health.* Cambridge, MA: Candlewick Press, 1994.
Johnson EW. *Love and sex in plain language.* New York: Bantam, 1988.
Johnson EW. *People, love, sex, and families: answers to questions preteens ask.* New York: Walker, 1985.
Madaras L. *My body, myself: the "What's happening to my body" workbook for girls.* New York: Newmarket Press, 1993.
Madaras L. *My feelings, my self: Lynda Madaras' growing-up guide for girls.* New York: Newmarket Press, 1993.
Madaras L. *"What's happening to my body" for girls: a growing up guide for parents and daughters,* 2nd ed. New York: Newmarket Press, 1988.
Mayle P. *What's happening to me?: the answers to some of the world's most embarrassing questions.* New York: Carol Publishing Group, 1995.
McCoy K. *Changes and choices: a junior high survival guide.* New York: Perigee Books, 1989.
McCoy K, Wibblesman C. *Growing and changing: a handbook for preteens.* New York: Perigee Books, 1986.
Westheimer RK. *Dr. Ruth talks to kids: where you came from, how your body changes, and what sex is all about.* New York: Macmillan, 1993.

Pamphlets

American College of Obstetricians and Gynecologists (ACOG):
Growing up
Menstruation and the menstrual cycle
Planned Parenthood Federation of America (PPFA):
About menstruation
Feeling good about growing up
Having your period
ETR Associates *(see page 819)*
Menstruation: Talking with your daughter

FOR MIDDLE TO OLDER TEENAGERS AND SEXUALLY ACTIVE TEENAGERS

Books

Basso MJ. *The underground guide to teenage sexuality.* Minneapolis: Fairview Press, 1997.
Bell R. Boston Women's Health Book Collective. *Changing bodies, changing lives.* New York: Random House, 1988.

Boston Children's Hospital with Robert Masland. *What teenagers want to know about sex.* Boston: Little, Brown, 1992.
Boston Women's Health Book Collective. *The new our bodies, ourselves.* New York: Simon and Schuster, 1996.
Breitman P, Knutson K, Reed P. *How to persuade your lover to use a condom... and why you should.* Rocklin, CA: Prima Publishing, 1994.
Gordon S. *Facts about sex for today's youth.* Buffalo, NY: Prometheus Books, 1992.
Harris RH. *It's perfectly normal: a book about changing bodies, growing-up, sex, and sexual health.* Cambridge, MA: Candlewick Press, 1994.
Heron A, ed. *Two teenagers in 20: writings by gay and lesbian youth.* Boston: Alyson Publications, 1994.
Landers A. *Ann Landers talks to teenagers about sex.* New York: Ballantine Books, 1983.
McCoy K, Wibbelsman C. *The new teenage body book.* New York: The Body Press/Perigee Books, 1992.
McCoy K, Wibbelsman C. *Life happens.* New York: Perigee Books, 1996.
Pipher MB. *Reviving Ophelia: saving the selves of adolescent girls.* New York: Putnam, 1994.

Pamphlets

AAP:
Deciding to wait: what you need to know
Making the right choice—facts young people need to know about avoiding pregnancy
ACOG:
Being a teenager: you and your sexuality
Birth control
Birth control pills
Chlamydial infections
Contraception: which method for you
Detecting and treating breast problems
Dysmenorrhea
Genital herpes
Genital warts
How to prevent sexually transmitted diseases
Human papillomavirus (HPV) infections
The Pap test
Sexually transmitted diseases
Advocates for Youth:
Advice from teens on buying condoms
American Social Health Association (ASHA):
Chlamydia: what you should know
Condoms: contraceptives and STD's
For teens
HPV and genital warts questions/answers
P.I.D. questions and answers
STD (VD) questions/answers
Telling your partner about herpes
Vaginitis: what every woman should know
When your partner has herpes
Association of Reproductive Health Professionals:
Choosing a birth control method
Channing L. Bete Co, Inc:
Making decisions about sex
Saying "no" to sex
ETR Associates:
Birth control/pregnancy
Am I parent material?
Are you ready to be pregnant?
Babies and relationships

Birth control facts
Birth control: talking with your daughter
Birth control: talking with your parents
Birth control: talking with your partner
Birth control: talking with your son
The condom
Condoms: talking with your partner
Condoms: think about it
If you are a man... understanding birth control
Pregnancy: get real!
Pregnancy options: pamphlet set
Pregnant?
Sex and birth control
Sex and you
Talking about birth control: pamphlet set
The truth about babies
What about adoption?
What is an abortion?

Rape
Acquaintance rape
Date rape!: Terri and J.R. talk to teens

Sexual abstinence
101 ways to make love without doin' it
101 ways to say no to sex
Abstinence ABC's
Abstinence and HIV
Abstinence: Think about it
The choice to abstain
It's about sex!
Not everyone's doin' it
Sex and abstinence
Sex? Let's wait!
Worth waiting!

STD/vaginitis
Chlamydia
Genital warts
Gonorrhea
Herpes
NGU (nongonococcal urethritis)
PID (pelvic inflammatory disease)
Sex and STD
STD, you and others
Syphilis
Vaginitis

PPFA:
Chlamydia: questions and answers
The condom: what it is, what it is for, how to use it
Your contraceptive choices
Herpes: questions and answers
HPV and genital warts: questions and answers
Is Depo-Provera for you?
Your key to good health: the gynecologic exam
Sex—safer and satisfying
Sexually transmitted infections: the facts
Smoking on the pill

Teen sex? It's okay to say: no way!
What if I am pregnant?
You and the pill
Journeyworks Publishing:
Am I ready for sex?
The condom quiz
The good reasons not to be a teenage parent
How to say no and keep your boyfriend
March of Dimes Birth Defects Foundation:
Teens talk sex
U.S. Department of Health and Human Services:
Many teens are saying "no"

AIDS AND HIV

Books

Blake J. *Risky times.* New York: Workman, 1990.
Hein K, DiGeronimo TM, editors of Consumer Books. *AIDS: trading fears for facts,* 3rd ed. New York: Consumer Reports Books, 1993.
Kittredge M. *Teens with AIDS speak out.* Thorndike, ME: Thorndike Press, 1993.
Madaras L. *Lynda Madaras talks to teens about AIDS: an essential guide for parents, teachers and young people.* New York: Newmarket Press, 1994.

Pamphlets

ASHA:
HIV/AIDS: questions and answers
HIV negative: when are you free from HIV?
Positive living
ETR Associates:
Abstinence and HIV
After the test
Answers for women
The antibody test
Condoms: think about it
Drugs and HIV: think about it
Get the answers
HIV ABC's
HIV/AIDS: am I at risk?
HIV and the immune system
HIV: think about it
Safer sex can be fun!
Safer sex: talking with your partner
Sex and HIV
Teens and HIV!
What if I'm positive?
What is safer sex?
PPFA:
AIDS and HIV: questions and answers

Pamphlets from the AAP on other common health issues for teens:

Acne treatment and control
Alcohol: your child and drugs
Cocaine: your child and drugs
Deciding to wait: what you need to know
Marijuana: your child and drugs
The risks of tobacco use: a message to parents and teens
Smoking: straight talk for teens
Teens who drink and drive: reducing the death toll

FOR PARENTS

Books

Bernstein A. *The flight of the stork: what children think (and when) about sex and family building.* New York: Perspective Press, 1994.

Calderone M. *Talking with your child about sex:* New York: Ballantine, 1994.

Calderone M, Johnson EW. *The family book about sexuality.* New York: Harper Collins, 1990 (out-of-print; may be available at your library).

Cassell C. *Straight from the heart: how to talk to your teenager about love and sex.* New York: Simon and Schuster, 1987.

Edwards JP, Elkins TE. *Just between us: a social sexual training guide for parents and professionals with concerns for persons with developmental disabilities.* Austin, TX: Pro-ed, 1988.

Fairchild B, Hayward N. *Now that you know: what every parent should know about homosexuality.* New York: Harcourt Brace Jovanovich, 1990.

Flowers JV, Horsman J, Schwartz B. *Raising your child to be a sexually healthy adult.* Englewood Cliffs, NJ: Prentice-Hall, 1982.

Gale J. *A parent's guide to teenage sexuality.* New York: Henry Holt, 1989.

Gitchel S, Foster L. *Let's talk about… S-E-X, a read-and-discuss guide for people nine to twelve and their parents.* Planned Parenthood Center of California, 1995.

Gochros J. *What to say after you clear your throat.* Kailua, HA: Press Pacifica, 1980.

Gordon S, Gordon J. *Raising a child conservatively in a sexually permissive world.* New York: Simon and Schuster, 1986.

Hacker SS. *What every teenager really wants to know about sex: with the startling new information every parent should read.* NewYork: Carroll & Graf, 1993.

Kohner N. *What shall we tell the children? Talking with your children about sex.* Great Britain, BBC Books, 1993.

Lewis H. *Sex education begins at home: how to raise sexually healthy children.* Norwalk, CT: Appleton-Century-Crofts, 1983.

Lewis HR, Lewis ME. *The parent's guide to teenage sex and pregnancy.* New York: St. Martin's Press, 1980.

McKee L, Blacklidge V. *An easy guide for caring parents: sexuality and socialization. A book for parents of people with mental handicaps.* Walnut Creek, CA: Planned Parenthood, 1986.

Miller PM. *Sex is not a four-letter word: talking sex with your children made easier.* New York: Crossroad, 1994.

Parents, Families and Friends of Lesbian and Gays (PFLAG). Our *daughters and sons: questions and answers for parents of gay, lesbian and bisexual people.* Washington, DC: PFLAG Publications

Planned Parenthood, Wattleton F, Keiffer E. *How to talk with your child about sexuality.* New York: Planned Parenthood Federation of America and Doubleday, 1986.

Somers L. *Talking to your children about love and sex.* New York: New American Library, 1989.

Stark P. *Sex is more than a plumbing lesson: a parent's guide to sexuality education for infants through the teen years.* Dallas, TX: Preston Hollow Enterprises, 1990.

Strasburger V. *Getting your kids to say "no" in the 90's when you said "yes" in the 60's.* New York: Fireside Books, 1993.

Pamphlets

ACOG:
Teaching your child about sexuality
ASHA:
Askable parent
ETR Associates:
HIV: talking with your child
HIV: talking with your teen
The National Parent–Teachers Association:
How to talk to your preteen and teen about sex: a guide for parents
PPFA:
How to be a good parent
How to talk to your teen about the facts of life
How to talk with your child about sexuality: a parent's guide
Human sexuality: what children should know and when they should know it
Kids and AIDS: a guide for parents
Channing L. Bete Co, Inc:
About helping your child grow up drug-free
Talking to adolescents about sex
Talking with your child about AIDS
SIECUS:
Now what do I do? How to give your pre-teens your message
Gordon S, Dickman I:
Sex education: the parents' role. Public Affairs Pamphlet No. 549.

FOR PROVIDERS

AAP and ACOG. *Adolescent sexuality: guides for professional involvement.* AAP and ACOG, 1992. (Modules for presentations, including slides, are available from either organization.)
Alan Guttmacher Institute. *Sex and America's teenagers.* New York: Alan Guttmacher Institute, 1995.
Haffner D. *Facing facts: sexual health for America's adolescent.* New York: SIECUS, 1995.
AAP. *Practicing adolescent medicine: a collection of resources.* AAP, 1994.

BIBLIOGRAPHIES

AAP:
Sex education: a bibliography of educational materials for children, adolescents, and their families. (Single copies are available for $1.95.)
ACOG:
Adolescent special needs packet: references and resources on care for adolescents with physical or mentally handicapping conditions or chronic disease
SIECUS:
Bibliographies are available for $2.50 each plus 15% postage and handling.
AIDS and safer sex education (1988)
Bibliography of religious publications on sex education and sexuality (1987)
Child sexual abuse and prevention (1986)
Human sexuality: a bibliography for everyone (1987)
Publications for professionals (1989)

Sexuality and the developmentally disabled (1988)
Sexuality and family life education: an annotated bibliography of curricula for sale (1985)
Sexuality education pamphlets (1986)

VIDEOTAPES

Women's Healthcare Video Library, Inc:
Adolescence: a woman's first transition. Children's Hospital, Boston, Divisions of Gynecology and Adolescent Medicine, and Women's Healthcare Video Library, Inc. ($29.95 plus shipping and handling.)
Ortho Pharmaceutical Corp:
Videotapes for examination:
The pelvic examination: a practical guide
From childhood through adolescence: issues in gynecologic care
Terrorism in the home: responding to the victim of domestic violence
Patients with mental retardation: issues in gynecologic care
Patients with physical disabilities: issues in gynecologic care
Straight talk
Others:
Health care issues for gay, lesbian, bisexual and transgender youth. Distributed by Wolfe Video (CA) (408-268-6782).
Teen AIDS—in focus. Produced by the Kenwood Group for San Francisco Department of Public Health and San Francisco Unified School District.

ADDRESSES

Advocates for Youth
1025 Vermont Avenue NW
Washington, DC 20005
202-347-5700

The Alan Guttmacher Institute
120 Wall Street, 21st Floor
New York, NY 10005
212-248-1111

American Academy of Pediatrics (AAP)
Division of Publications
141 Northwest Point Blvd.
PO Box 927
Elk Grove Village, IL 60009-0927
708-228-5005

American College of Obstetricians and Gynecologists (ACOG)
Distribution Center
409 12th Street SW
Washington, DC 20024-2188
202-638-5577

American Medical Association (AMA)
515 N State Street
Chicago, IL 60610
312-464-5570

American Social Health Association (ASHA)
PO Box 13827
Research Triangle Park, NC 27709
800-783-9877

Channing L. Bete Co, Inc
200 State Road
South Deerfield, MA 01373
800-628-7733

Education Programs Associates (EPA)
One West Campbell, Suite 40
Campbell, CA 95008
408-374-3720

ETR Associates
PO Box 1830
Santa Cruz, CA 95061-1830
800-321-4407

Harvard Community Health Plan Foundation
185 Dartmouth Street
Boston, MA 02116-3502
617-859-5036

Journeyworks Publishing
PO Box 8466
Santa Cruz, CA 95061-8466
800-775-1998

March of Dimes Birth Defects Foundation
1275 Mamaroneck Avenue
White Plains, NY 10605
800-367-6630

The National Parent-Teachers Association (PTA)
330 N Wabash Avenue, Suite 2100
Chicago, IL 60611-6783
312-670-6782

Ortho-McNeil Pharmaceutical Corporation
US Route 202
PO Box 303
Raritan, NJ 08869
908-218-6000

Parents, Families and Friends of
Lesbians and Gays (PFLAG)
1101 14th Street NW, Suite 1030
Washington, DC 20005
202-638-4200

Planned Parenthood Federation of
America, Inc (PPFA)
810 Seventh Avenue
New York, NY 10019
800-669-0156

Sexuality Information and Education
Council of the United States (SIECUS)
Publication Department
130 West 42nd Street, Suite 350
New York, NY 10003
212-819-9770

Tambrands, Inc
1 Marcus Avenue
Lake Success, NY 11042

U.S. Department of Health and Human Services
Public Health Service
Health Services Administration
Bureau of Community Health Services
5600 Fishers Lane
Rockville, MD 20857

Women's Healthcare Video Library, Inc
55 Pond Avenue
Brookline, MA 02146
800-300-TAPE

Appendix 2

Informed Consent for Oral Contraceptives

Check the space after reading the statements.

I have discussed the methods of birth control and have chosen to take the birth control pill. _____

I understand the Pill is very effective birth control, but occasionally women might get pregnant while taking it. I know there is less chance of this happening if I take the Pill correctly and do not skip or miss taking any pills. I understand I should not begin to take the Pill if I am pregnant. _____

I understand that Pill users may have a slightly greater chance than nonusers of developing certain serious problems, including blood clots, that may become fatal in very rare cases. I will read the complete package insert. _____

I understand that the chance of developing serious health problems increases with age and when certain other health risk factors are present such as:

- smoking more than 15 cigarettes a day
- age 35 or older
- high blood pressure
- high levels of blood cholesterol
- diabetes _____

I understand that I should not use the Pill if I have had, now have, or develop in the future:

- blood clots
- inflammation in the veins (phlebitis) _____

I understand that some minor side effects of the Pill may include:
nausea, vomiting
breast tenderness
weight gain or loss
spotting between periods
headaches ______

I know when taking the Pill I should watch for these danger signals:
A — abdominal pain
C — chest pain or shortness of breath
H — headaches that are severe
E — eye problems such as blurring or double vision
S — severe depression
S — severe leg pain/swelling
and report them immediately to my doctor, nurse, or other health care provider. ______

I understand I need regular check-ups while taking the Pill including a physical exam, pelvic exam, and lab tests. ______

I understand that I should do a monthly breast self-examination. ______

I understand that there may be less protection from pregnancy when the Pill is taken with some drugs, including drugs to control seizures and certain antibiotics. I understand that I should talk to my doctor about taking any other medicines with the Pill. ______

I understand that in addition to its benefit as a method of birth control, some women experience the following benefits from using the Pill:
decreased menstrual cramps and blood loss
predictable, regular menstrual cycles
less iron deficiency anemia
less acne
some protection from noncancerous breast tumors and ovarian cysts
some protection from ovarian and uterine lining cancer
decreased risk of infection of the pelvis, uterus or tubes (pelvic inflammatory disease)
fewer ectopic pregnancies ______

I understand that if I see a doctor for any reason, I should tell him/her that I am on the Pill. ______

I understand that the Pill does not protect me from getting sexually transmitted diseases (STDs) and it is recommended that condoms be used with each occurrence of vaginal intercourse. ______

I know that if I have any questions or problems, a health care provider is available to me by phone, or by page, or in the Emergency Room. ______

Signature of Patient	Date	Signature of Witness

Telephone Number

UPDATES

Signature of Patient	Date	Signature of Witness
Signature of Patient	Date	Signature of Witness
Signature of Patient	Date	Signature of Witness
Signature of Patient	Date	Signature of Witness

Appendix 3

Instruction Sheet for Taking 28-Day Oral Contraceptive Pills

1. The name of your birth control pill is ______________________

2. A. Sunday start:

   If you are taking pills for the first time, take the first pill of your first package on the *Sunday* following the first day of your next period, even if you have stopped bleeding before that day. If your period begins on Sunday, start taking the pill that same day.

If menstrual flow starts on	*Pill-taking begins on*
Monday	
Tuesday	
Wednesday	Following
Thursday	Sunday
Friday	
Saturday	
Sunday	*That* Sunday

   B. First-day start:

   Start your pills on the *first day* of your next period, then take one pill a day. Because you start the pill on the first day of your period, you will have two periods your first package (1st week and 4th week). After that, you will have only one period each package (4th week).

3. Take one pill every day without fail. When you finish your last pill in the package, start the first pill in a new package the next day. This means that you will be taking the pills even during the days you are having a period. *Never skip a day.*

4. Always take the pill at approximately the same time each day. The best time is 1/2 hour after a good meal or snack or at bedtime, but whatever schedule you set up, you should stick to it. Try to think of something you do every day, so you can take your pill at the same time (such as brushing your teeth). You may have mild nausea the first month. This usually disappears with time. You are less likely to have this problem if you take your pill in the evening.

5. **If you forget pills:**

   If you *forget 1 pill*—take the pill you forgot *as soon as you remember*; then take your regular pill for that day at the same time you usually take your pill.

   If you *forget 2 pills in a row in the first 2 weeks*—take 2 pills on the day you remember and 2 pills the next day. Take 1 pill per day until the pack is finished. Use condoms for at least 7 days.

   If you *forget 2 pills in a row in the third week OR you miss 3 pills or more in a row* at any time:

   Sunday starter: Keep taking a pill every day until Sunday. On Sunday, throw away the unused portion of the pack and start a new pack. Use condoms for at least 7 days.

   Non-Sunday starter: Throw out the rest of the current pack. Start a new pack the same day. Use condoms for at least 7 days.

6. If you have vomiting or diarrhea or are taking a course of antibiotics, the pill may be less effective. Use a back-up method such as condoms.

7. **Remember the pill does *not* protect you from AIDS or sexually transmitted diseases, and we advise that you ALWAYS use condoms.**

8. If you miss a period and have taken every pill on time, begin your next pack as usual, but call or come into the clinic for a pregnancy test. If you miss a period and may have forgotten or been late with one or more pills, call your health care professional immediately to make arrangements to come in.

9. **Extra bleeding while taking the 21 hormone tablets**

   Breakthrough bleeding is *very common* in the first 3 months of taking birth control pills, especially if pills are missed or taken late. The bleeding usually occurs during the second week of taking the hormone tablets and may be light (spotting for a few days) or heavy (like a normal menstrual period). The bleeding *can usually be ignored* and will become less of a problem by the third cycle.

   If light bleeding persists for more than 5 days or heavy bleeding lasts for more than 2 days, you can take two hormone tablets each day (one in the morning and one in the evening). The extra tablet needed each day should be drawn from an *extra* package of pills. You should continue taking two tablets per day until you have stopped bleeding for 1 day. Normally, you will need to take the extra medicine for 2 or 3 days. Please call your health care provider with any questions.

10. **DANGER SIGNALS**

    1. *SEVERE* ABDOMINAL PAIN
    2. *SEVERE* CHEST PAIN
    3. *SEVERE* HEADACHES
    4. BLURRED VISION, LOSS OF SIGHT, FLASHING LIGHTS, OR YELLOWING OF THE EYEBALLS
    5. *SEVERE* LEG PAIN (IN CALF OR THIGH)

    Please call and ask to speak to a health care provider. At night, ask the answering service to page the physician on call.

11. Benefits of the Pill—Birth control pills lower your chance of acquiring cancer of the uterus or ovary and make you less likely to have anemia, ovarian cysts, or menstrual cramps. They also improve acne and may protect your bones.

12. While you arc on the Pill, you should be seen for a visit every 6 months, unless told otherwise by the doctor or nurse. Call to make an appointment. If you have a scheduled appointment, please keep it. If you are unable to keep the appointment, please call and cancel at least 24 hours in advance.

13. If you purchase your pills in 3-month supplies, you must keep the pharmacy label from the first package and bring it with you when you go to the pharmacy to get refills. This label has your prescription number on it.

Appendix 4

American Professional Society on the Abuse of Children: Definitions of Anatomical Terms

The forensic medical evaluation of suspected child sexual abuse victims has developed into a specialized field of practice in the last 10 years. Pediatricians, gynecologists, nurse practitioners, and physician assistants may all be called on to examine children for suspected sexual abuse and describe their findings. The records of such examinations then become medicolegal documents.

Precision in documentation is critical for all who must communicate and understand medical findings. These terminology guidelines were developed to assist professionals actively involved in the medical diagnosis and treatment of child sexual abuse to establish a shared vocabulary that is clear, precise, and easily communicated. This shared vocabulary will enable those in child protection, law enforcement, and the courts to understand previously confusing and at times inconsistent terminology. Consistency in terminology will also assist in the development of a research language.

The terminology presented in these guidelines emanates primarily from medical dictionary definitions, anatomy texts, and clinicians actively involved in the care of sexually abused children. Unless otherwise noted, definitions are from *Stedman's Medical Dictionary* (1). As experience and scientific knowledge expand, further revision of these guidelines is expected.

ANATOMICAL STRUCTURES

Anal skin tag A protrusion of anal verge tissue that interrupts the symmetry of the perianal skin folds.

Anal verge The tissue overlying the subcutaneous external anal sphincter at the most distal portion of the anal canal (anoderm) and extending exteriorly to the margin of the anal skin.

Anterior commissure The union of the two labia minora anteriorly (toward the clitoris).

Anus The anal orifice, which is the lower opening of the digestive tract, lying in the fold between the buttocks, through which feces are extruded (9).

Clitoris A small cylindrical erectile body situated at the anterior (superior) portion of the vulva, covered by a sheath of skin called the clitoral hood; homologous with the penis in the male (9).

Fossa navicularis/posterior fossa Concavity on the lower part of the vestibule, situated posteriorly (inferiorly) to the vaginal orifice and extending to the posterior fourchette (posterior commissure).

Glans penis The cap-shaped expansion of the corpus spongiosum at the end of the penis; also called balanus (9). It is covered by a mucous membrane and sheathed by the prepuce (foreskin) in uncircumcised males.

Genitalia (external) The external sexual organs; in males, includes the penis and scrotum; in females, includes the contents of the vulva.

Hymen This membrane (external vaginal plate or urogenital septum) partially or rarely completely covers the vaginal orifice. This membrane is located at the junction of the vestibular floor and the vaginal canal.

Labia majora ("outer lips") Rounded folds of skin forming the lateral boundaries of the vulva.

Labia minora ("inner lips") Longitudinal thin folds of tissue enclosed within the labia majora. In the pubertal child, these folds extend from the clitoral hood to approximately the midpoint on the lateral wall of the vestibule. In the adult, they enclose the structures of the vestibule.

Median raphe A ridge or furrow that marks the line of union of the two halves of the perineum (9).

Mons pubis The rounded, fleshy prominence created by the underlying fat pad that lies over the symphysis pubis (pubic bone) in females.

Pectinate/dentate line The saw-toothed line of demarcation between the distal (lower) portion of the anal valves and the pectin, the smooth zone of stratified epithelium that extends to the anal verge (9). This line is apparent when the external and internal anal sphincters relax and the anus dilates.

Penis Male sex organ composed of erectile tissue through which the urethra passes (homologous with the clitoris in the female) (9).

Perianal folds Wrinkles or folds of the anal verge skin radiating from the anus, created by contraction of the external anal sphincter. (Definition not found in *Stedman's*.)

Perineal body The central tendon of the perineum located between the vulva and the anus in females and between the scrotum and anus in males.

Perineum The external surface or base of the perineal body, lying between the vulva and the anus in females and between the scrotum and the anus in males (1). Underlying the external surface of the perineum is the pelvic floor and its associated structures occupying the pelvic outlet, which is bounded anteriorly by the pubic symphysis (pubic bone), laterally by the ischial tuberosity (pelvic bone), and posteriorly by the coccyx (tail bone).

Posterior commissure The union of the two labia majora posteriorly (toward the anus).

Posterior fourchette The junction of two labia minora posteriorly (inferiorly). This area is referred to as a posterior commissure in the prepubertal child, as the labia minora are not completely developed to connect inferiorly until puberty, when it is referred to as the fourchette.

Scrotum The pouch containing the testicles and their accessory organs (9).

Urethral orifice External opening of the canal (urethra) from the bladder.

Vagina The uterovaginal canal in females, an internal structure extending from the uterine cervix to the inner aspect of the hymen.

Vaginal vestibule An anatomic cavity containing the opening of the vagina, the urethra, and the ducts of Bartholin's glands, bordered by the clitoris anteriorly, the labia laterally, and the posterior commissure (fourchette) posteriorly (inferiorly). The vestibule encompasses the fossa navicularis immediately posterior (inferior) to the vaginal introitus.

Vulva The external genitalia or pudendum of females; includes the clitoris, labia majora, labia minora, vaginal vestibule, urethral orifice, vaginal orifice, hymen, and posterior fourchette (or commissure) (9).

HYMENAL MORPHOLOGY (2)

Annular Circumferential; hymenal membrane tissue extends completely around the circumference of the entire vaginal orifice.

Crescentic Hymen with attachments at approximately the 11 and 1 o'clock positions without tissue being present between the two attachments.

Cribriform Hymen with multiple small openings.

Imperforate Hymenal membrane with no opening.

Septate The appearance of the hymenal orifice when it is bisected by a band of hymenal tissue creating two or more orifices.

DESCRIPTIVE TERMS RELATING TO THE HYMEN

Estrogenized Effect of influence by the female sex hormone estrogen resulting in changes to the genitalia: the hymen takes on a thickened, redundant, pale appearance. These changes are observed in neonates, with the onset of puberty, and as the result of exogenous estrogen.

Fimbriated/denticular Hymen with multiple projections and indentations along the edge, creating a ruffled appearance.

Membrane thickness The relative amount of tissue between the internal and external surfaces of the hymenal membrane.

Narrow/wide hymenal rim The width of the hymenal membrane as viewed in the coronal plane, i.e., from the edge of the hymen to the muscular portion of the vaginal introitus.

Redundant Abundant hymenal tissue that tends to fold back on itself or protrude.

OTHER STRUCTURES OR FINDINGS

Acute laceration A tear through the full thickness of the skin or other tissue.

Attenuated Used to describe areas where the hymen is narrow. However, the term should be restricted to indicate a documented change in the width of the posterior portion of the hymen following an injury.

Diastasis ani A congenital midline smooth depression that may be V or wedge shaped, located either anterior or posterior to the anus; due to a failure of fusion of the underlying corrugator external anal sphincter muscle (5).

Erythema Redness of tissues.

External hymenal ridge A midline longitudinal ridge of tissue on the external surface of the hymen. May be either anterior or posterior. Usually extends to the edge of the membrane (2).

Friability of the posterior fourchette/commissure A superficial breakdown of the skin in the posterior fourchette (commissure) when gentle traction is applied, causing slight bleeding (11).

Hymenal cleft An angular or V-shaped indentation on the edge of the hymenal membrane (9). When curved, it creates a hollowed or U-shaped depression on the edge of the membrane that has been referred to as a "concavity" (10,11).

Hymenal cyst A fluid-filled elevation of tissue, confined within the hymenal tissue (2).

Labial agglutination (labial adhesion) The result of adherence (fusion) of the adjacent edges of the mucosal surfaces of the labia minora. This may occur at any point along the length of the vestibule, although it most commonly occurs posteriorly (inferiorly) (6).

Linea vestibularis A vertical pale/avascular line across the posterior fourchette and/or fossa, which may be accentuated by putting lateral traction on the labia major (4,11,12).

O'clock designation A method by which the location of structures or findings may be designated by using the positions of the numerals on the face of a clock. The 12 o'clock position is always superior (up). The 6 o'clock position is always inferior (down). The position of a patient must be indicated when using this designation.

Perineal groove Developmental anomaly, also called "failure of midline fusion" (7). This skin and mucosal defect may be located anywhere from the fossa to the anus (11).

Projections

1. **Hymenal tag** An elongated projection of tissue rising from any location on the hymenal rim. Commonly found in the midline and may be an extension of a posterior vaginal column (6,11).
2. **Mound/bump** A solid elevation of hymenal tissue wider than or as wide as it is long, located on the edge of the hymenal membrane. This structure may be seen at the site where an intravaginal column attaches to the hymen (2,3,11).

Scar Fibrous tissue which replaces normal tissue after the healing of a wound (6).

Synechia Any adhesion that binds two anatomic structures through the formation of a band of tissue (1). A synechia can result in the healing process following an abrasion of tissues.

Transection of hymen (complete) A tear or laceration through the entire width of the hymenal membrane extending to (or through its attachment) to the vaginal wall.

Transection of hymen (partial) A tear or laceration through a portion of the hymenal membrane not extending to its attachment to the vaginal wall.

Vaginal columns (columnae rugarum vaginae) Raised (sagittally oriented) columns, most prominent on the anterior wall with less prominence on the posterior wall. May also be observed laterally (2,3).

Vaginal rugae (rugae vaginales) Folds of epithelium (rugae) running circumferentially from vaginal columns. These rugae account in part for the ability of the vagina to distend (11).

Vascularity (increased) Dilatation of existing superficial blood vessels.

Vestibular bands

1. **Perihymenal bands (pubovaginal)** Bands lateral to the hymen connecting to the vestibular wall.
2. **Periurethral bands** Small bands lateral to the urethra that connect the periurethral tissues to the anterior lateral wall of the vestibule. These bands are usually symmetrical and frequently create a semilunar-shaped space between the bands on either side of the urethral meatus. Also called urethral supporting ligaments (11).

DESCRIPTIVE TERMS FOR VARIATIONS IN PERIANAL ANATOMY

Anal dilatation Opening of the external and internal anal sphincters with minimal traction on the buttocks (5,6).

Anal fissure A superficial break (split) in the perianal skin that radiates out from the anal orifice (6,11).

Flattened anal folds A reduction or absence of the perianal folds or wrinkles, noted when the external anal sphincter is partially or completely relaxed.

Venous congestion Pooling of venous blood in the perianal tissues resulting in a purple discoloration, which may be localized or diffuse (6).

REFERENCES

1. *Stedman's medical dictionary,* 22nd ed. Baltimore, MD: Williams & Wilkins, 1972.
2. Berenson A, Heger A, Andrews S. Appearance of the hymen in newborns. *Pediatrics* 1991;87:458.
3. Berenson AB, Heger AH, Hayes JM, Bailey RK, Emans SJ. Appearance of the hymen in prepubertal girls. *Pediatrics* 1992:89:387.
4. McCann J, Wells R, Simon M, Voris J. Genital findings in prepubertal children selected for non-abuse: a descriptive study. *Pediatrics* 1990;86:428.
5. McCann J, Voris J, Simon M, Wells R. Perianal findings in prepubertal children selected for non-abuse: a descriptive study. *Child Abuse Negl* 1989;12:179.
6. Chadwick D, Berkowitz CD, Kerns D, et al. *Color atlas of child sexual abuse*. Chicago: Year Book Medical Publishers, 1989.
7. McCann J. Use of the colposcope in childhood sexual abuse examination. *Pediatr Clin North Am* 1990;37:863–880.
8. Adams JA, Phillips P, Ahmad M. The usefulness of colposcopic photographs in the evaluation of suspected child abuse. *Adolesc Pediatr Gynecol* 1990;3:75.
9. *Dorland's illustrated medical dictionary,* 27th ed. Philadelphia: WB Saunders, 1988.
10. Kerns DL, Ritter ML, Thomas RG. Concave hymenal variations in suspected child sexual abuse. *Pediatrics* 1992;90:265.
11. Heger A, Emans SJ, et al. *Evaluation of the sexually abused child: a medical textbook and photographic atlas*. New York: Oxford University Press, 1992.
12. Kellogg ND, Parra JM. Linea vestibularis: a previously undescribed normal genital structure in female neonates. *Pediatrics* 1991;87:926.
13. Giardino AP, Finkel M, Giardino ER et al. *A practical guide to the evaluation of sexual abuse in the prepubertal child.* Newbury Park, CA: Sage Publications, 1992.
14. Finkel M, DeJong AR. Medical findings in child sexual abuse. In: Reece RM. *Child abuse: medical diagnosis and management.* Philadelphia: Lea & Febiger, 1994.

ACKNOWLEDGMENTS

These guidelines were produced by the Terminology Subcommittee of the APSAC Task Force on Medical Evaluation of Suspected Child Abuse. The Terminology Subcommittee is chaired by Joyce Adams, M.D. The Terminology Subcommittee held open meetings at the San Diego, CA, Conference on Responding to Child Maltreatment in January of 1991, 1992, 1993, and 1995 to review and reach consensus on the terms listed. Active members of the subcommittee include Martin Finkel, D.O.; Mary Gibbons, M.D.; Marcia Herman-Giddens, P.A., Dr.P.H.; Susan Horowitz, M.D.; John McCann, M.D.; Margaret Moody, M.D.; David Muram, M.D.; Sue Perdew, R.N., Ph.D.; Sue Ross, R.N., P.N.P.; Sara Schuh, M.D.; Rizwan Shah, M.D.; and Elizabeth Young, M.D.. Valuable contributions were also made by Carol Berkowitz, M.D.; S. Jean Emans, M.D.; Dirk Huyer, M.D.; Carole Jenny, M.D., M.B.A.; and Susan Pokorny, M.D..

From the American Professional Society on the Abuse of Children; with permission.

Appendix 5

Sexual Abuse Protocol of the State of California

D. OBTAIN PATIENT HISTORY. RECORDER SHOULD ALLOW PATIENT OR OTHER PERSON PROVIDING HISTORY TO DESCRIBE INCIDENT(S) TO THE EXTENT POSSIBLE AND RECORD THE ACTS AND SYMPTOMS DESCRIBED BELOW. DETERMINE AND USE TERMS FAMILIAR TO THE PATIENT. FOLLOW-UP QUESTIONS MAY BE NECESSARY TO ENSURE THAT ALL ITEMS ARE COVERED.

1. Name of person providing history	Relationship to child	Address	City	County	State	Phone (W) (H)

2. Chief complaint(s) of person providing history

3. Chief complaint(s) in child's own words

4. ☐ Less than 72 hours since incident(s) took place
Date/time/location

☐ Over 72 hours since incident(s) took place
Date(s) or time frame/location

5. Identity of alleged perpetrator(s), if known	Age	Sex	Race	Relationship to child

6. Acts described by patient and/or other historian

	Described by patient Yes	No	Unk	Described by historian Yes	No	Unk
Vaginal contact						
Penis						
Finger						
Foreign object						
Describe the object						
Anal contact						
Penis						
Finger						
Foreign object						
Describe the object						
Oral copulation of genitals						
of victim by assailant						
of assailant by victim						
Oral copulation of anus						
of victim by assailant						
of assailant by victim						
Masturbation						
of victim by assailant						
of assailant by victim						
other						
Did ejaculation occur outside a body orifice?						
If yes, describe the location on the body:						
Foam, jelly, or condom used (circle)						
Lubricant used						
Fondling, licking or kissing (circle)						
If yes, describe the location on the body:						
Other acts:						
Was force used upon patient? If yes, describe:						

7. Post-assault hygiene/activity
( ) Not applicable if over 72 hours

	Described by patient Yes	No	Unk	Described by historian Yes	No	Unk
Urinated						
Defecated						
Genital wipe/wash						
Bath/shower						
Douche						
Removed/inserted tampon						
Brushed teeth						
Oral gargle/swish						
Changed clothing						

8. Symptoms described by patient and/or other historian

	Described by patient Yes	No	Unk	Described by historian Yes	No	Unk
Physical symptoms						
Abdominal/pelvic pain						
Vulvar discomfort or pain						
Dysuria						
Urinary tract infections						
Enuresis (daytime or nighttime)						
Vaginal itching						
Vaginal discharge						
Describe color, odor and amount below.						
Vaginal bleeding						
Rectal pain						
Rectal bleeding						
Rectal discharge						
Constipation						
Incontinent of stool (daytime or nighttime)						
Lapse of consciousness						
Vomiting						
Physical injuries, pain, or tenderness. Describe below.						
Behavioral/emotional symptoms						
Sleep disturbances						
Eating disorders						
School						
Sexual acting out						
Fear						
Anger						
Depression						
Other symptoms						

Additional information:

HOSPITAL IDENTIFICATION INFORMATION

OCJP 925

86 96690

E. OBTAIN PERTINENT PAST MEDICAL HISTORY

1. Menarche age ( ) N/A	Date of last menstrual period ( ) N/A	Use of tampons ( ) Yes ( ) No ( ) N/A	History of Vaginitis ( ) Yes ( ) No ( ) N/A

2. Note pre-existing physical injuries ( ) N/A

3. Pertinent medical history of anal-genital injuries, surgeries, diagnostic procedures, or medical treatment? ( ) Yes ( ) No If yes, describe

4. Previous history of child abuse? ( ) Yes ( ) No ( ) Unknown. If known, describe

F. CONDUCT A GENERAL PHYSICAL EXAM AND RECORD FINDINGS. COLLECT AND PRESERVE EVIDENCE FOR EVIDENTIAL EXAM.

1. Blood pressure	Pulse	Temperature	Respiration	Include percentiles for children under six Height Weight

2. Record general physical condition noting any abnormality ( ) Within normal limits

- Record injuries and findings on diagrams: erythema, abrasions, bruises (detail shape), contusions, induration, lacerations, fractures, bites, and burns.
- Record size and appearance of injuries. Note swelling and areas of tenderness.
- Examine for evidence of physical neglect.
- Take a GC culture from the oropharynx as a base line. Take other STD cultures as indicated. Provide prophylaxis.

IF EXAMINED WITHIN 72 HOURS OF ALLEGED INCIDENT(S):

- Note condition of clothing upon arrival (rips, tears, or foreign materials) if applicable. Use space below to record observations.
- Collect outer and underclothing if worn during or immediately after the incident.
- If applicable, collect fingernail scrapings.
- Collect dried and moist secretions, stains, and foreign materials from the body including the head, hair, and scalp. Identify location on diagrams.
- Scan the entire body with a Wood's Lamp. Swab each suspicious substance or fluorescent area with a separate swab. Label Wood's Lamp findings "W.L."
- Examine the oral cavity for injury and the area around the mouth for seminal fluid. Note frenulum trauma. If indicated by history: Swab the area around the mouth. Collect 2 swabs from the oral cavity up to 6 hours post-assault for seminal fluid. Prepare two dry mount slides.
- Collect saliva and head hair reference samples at the time of the exam if required by crime lab and if there is a need to compare them to a suspect.
- Record specimens collected on Section 7.

HOSPITAL IDENTIFICATION INFORMATION

Optional: Take photographs of genitals before and after exam.

Record injuries and findings on anal-genital diagrams: abrasions, erythema, bruises, tears/transections, scars, distortions or adhesions, etc. Use anal-genital chart on next page to record additional descriptive information.

3. External genitalia
- Examine the external genitalia and perianal area including inner thighs for injury.
- For boys, take a GC culture from the urethra. Take other STD cultures as indicated. Provide prophylaxis.

IF EXAMINED WITHIN 72 HOURS OF INCIDENT:
- Collect dried and moist secretions and foreign materials. Identify location on diagrams.
- Pubertal children: Cut matted pubic hair. Comb pubic hair to collect foreign materials. Collect pubic hair reference samples at time of exam if required by crime lab and if there is a need to compare them to a suspect.
- Scan area with Wood's Lamp. Swab each suspicious substance or fluorescent area. Label Wood's Lamp findings "W.L."
- For boys, collect 2 penile swabs if indicated. Collect one swab from the urethral meatus and one swab from the glans and shaft. Take a GC culture from the urethra. Take other STD cultures as indicated. Provide prophylaxis.
- Record specimens collected on Section 7.

4. Vagina
- Examine for injury and foreign materials.
- Pre-pubertal girls with intact hymen/normal vaginal orifice: No speculum exam necessary.
- Pre-pubertal girls with non-intact hymen and/or enlarged vaginal orifice: Only conduct a speculum exam if major trauma is suspected and use pediatric speculum.
- Take a GC culture from the vaginal introitus in pre-pubertal girls with intact hyman/normal vaginal orifice; from the vagina in pre-pubertal girls with non-intact hymen and/or enlarged vaginal orifice; and, the endocervix in adolescents. Take other STD cultures as indicated. Provide prophylaxis.
- Obtain pregnancy test (blood or urine) from pubertal girls.

IF EXAMINED WITHIN 72 HOURS OF INCIDENT:
- Pre-pubertal girls with intact hymen/normal vaginal orifice: Collect 2 swabs from the vulva.
- Adolescents or pre-pubertal girls with non-intact hymen and/or enlarged vaginal orifice: Collect 3 swabs from vaginal pool. Prepare 1 wet mount and 2 dry mount slides. Examine wet mount for sperm and trichomonas.
- Record specimens collected on Section 7.

5. Anus and rectum
- Examine the buttocks, perianal skin, and anal folds for injury.
- Conduct an anoscopic or proctoscopic exam if rectal injury is suspected.
- Take a GC culture from the rectum. Take other STD cultures as indicated. Provide prophylaxis.
- Take blood for syphilis serology. Provide prophylaxis.

IF EXAMINED WITHIN 72 HOURS OF ALLEGED INCIDENT:
- Collect dried and moist secretions and foreign materials. Foreign materials may include lubricants and fecal matter.
- If indicated by history and/or findings: Collect 2 rectal swabs and prepare 2 dry mount slides. Avoid contaminating rectal swabs by cleaning the perianal area and relaxing the anus using the lateral or knee-chest position prior to insertion of swabs.
- Record specimens collected on Section 7.

DRAW SHAPE OF ANUS AND ANY LESIONS ON GENITALIA, PERINEUM, AND BUTTOCKS

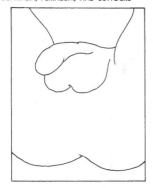

DRAW SHAPE OF HYMEN AND ANUS AND ANY LESIONS ON GENITALIA, PERINEUM, OR BUTTOCKS

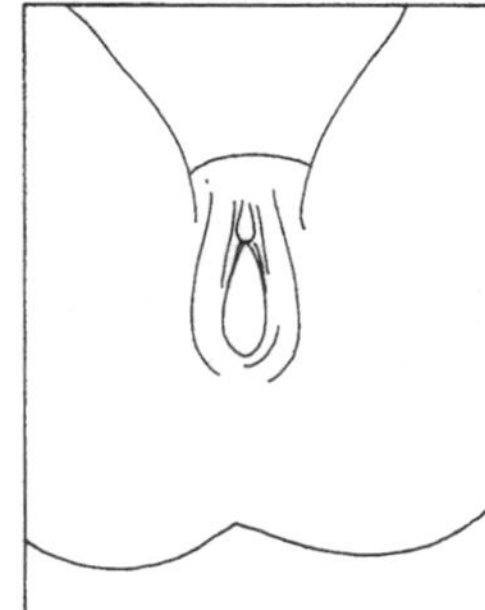

HOSPITAL IDENTIFICATION INFORMATION

OCJP 925

86 96698

6. Anal-genital chart

Female/Male General	WNL	ABN	Describe
Tanner stage			
Breast 1 2 3 4 5	☐	☐	
Genitals 1 2 3 4 5	☐	☐	
Inguinal adenopathy	☐	☐	
Medial aspect of thighs	☐	☐	
Perineum	☐	☐	

	Yes	No	
Vulvovaginal/urethral discharge	☐	☐	
Condyloma acuminata	☐	☐	

Female	WNL	ABN	Describe
Labia majora	☐	☐	
Clitoris	☐	☐	
Labia minora	☐	☐	
Periurethral tissue/ urethral meatus	☐	☐	
Perihymenal tissue (vestibule)	☐	☐	
Hymen Record diameter of hymen and check measurement used: ☐ Horizontal ☐ Vertical	☐	☐	
Posteriour fourchette	☐	☐	
Fossa Navicularis	☐	☐	
Vagina	☐	☐	
Other			

Exam position used:
☐ Supine
☐ Knee chest

Male	WNL	ABN	Describe
Penis Circumcised ☐ Yes ☐ No	☐	☐	
Urethral Meatus	☐	☐	
Scrotum	☐	☐	
Testes	☐	☐	

Female/Male Anus	WNL	ABN	Describe
Buttocks	☐	☐	
Perianal skin	☐	☐	
Anal verge/ folds/rugae	☐	☐	
Tone	☐	☐	

Anal spasm
☐ Yes ☐ No
Anal laxity
☐ Yes ☐ No
Note presence of stool in rectal ampulla
☐ Yes ☐ No
Method of exam for anal tone (discretion of examiner)
☐ Observation
☐ Digital exam
Exam position used:
☐ Supine
☐ Prone
☐ Lateral recumbent
Anoscopic exam
☐ Yes ☐ No ☐ N/A
Proctoscopic exam
☐ Yes ☐ No ☐ N/A

Genital exam done with:
Direct visualization ☐
Colposcope ☐
Hand held magnifier ☐

HOSPITAL IDENTIFICATION INFORMATION

7. Record evidential and specimens collected.

FOR EVIDENTIAL EXAMS CONDUCTED WITHIN 72 HOURS OF ALLEGED INCIDENT

ALL SWABS AND SLIDES MUST BE AIR DRIED PRIOR TO PACKAGING (PENAL CODE § 13823.11). AIR DRY UNDER A STREAM OF COOL AIR FOR 60 MINUTES. Swabs and slides must be individually labeled, coded to show which slides were prepared from which swabs, and time taken. All containers (tubes, bindles, envelopes) for individual items must be labeled with the name of the patient, contents, location of body where taken, and name of hospital. Package small containers in a larger envelope and record chain of custody. See the State of California Medical Protocol for Examination of Sexual Assault and Child Sexual Abuse Victims published by the state Office of Criminal Justice Planning, 1130 K Street, Sacramento, California 95814 (916) 324-9100 for additional information.

SPECIMENS FOR PRESENCE OF SEMEN, SPERM MOTILITY, AND TYPING TO CRIME LAB

	Swabs	Dry Mount Slides	Yes	No	N/A	Taken by	Time
Oral							
Vaginal							
Rectal							
Vulvar							
Penile							

	Yes	No	N/A	Taken by	Time
Vaginal wet mount slide examined for spermatozoa and trichomonas, dried, and submitted to crime lab					
Motile sperm observed					
Non-motile sperm observed					

OTHER EVIDENCE TO CRIME LAB

	Yes	No	N/A	Taken by
Clothing				
Fingernail scrapings				
Foreign materials on body				
Blood				
Dried secretions				
Fiber/loose hair				
Vegetation				
Dirt/gravel/glass				
Matted pubic hair cuttings				
Pubic hair combings				
Comb				
Swabs of bite marks				
Control swabs				
Photographs				

Area of body __________

Type of camera __________

Other __________

REFERENCE SAMPLES AND TOXICOLOGY SCREENS TO CRIME LAB

Reference samples can be collected at the time of the exam or at a later date according to crime lab policies if there is a need to compare them to a suspect. Toxicology screens should be collected at the time of the exam upon the recommendation of the physical examiner, law enforcement officer, or child protective services.

Reference samples	Yes	No	N/A	Taken by
Blood typing (yellow top tube)				
Saliva				
Head hair				
Pubic hair				
Toxicology screens				
Blood/alcohol toxicology (grey top tube)				
Urine toxicology				

OCJP 925

CLINICAL EVIDENCE TO HOSPITAL LAB

	Yes	No	N/A	Taken by
Syphilis serology (red top tube)				
STD culture				
Oral				
Vaginal				
Rectal				
Penile				
Pregnancy test Blood (red top tube) or urine				

PERSONNEL INVOLVED (print)		PHONE
History taken by:		
Physical examination performed by:		
Specimens labeled and sealed by:		
Assisting nurse:		
Family assessment taken by: ( ) N/A ( ) Report attached		
Additional narrative prepared by physician: ( ) N/A ( ) Report attached		

FINDINGS AND FOLLOW-UP

Report of child sexual abuse, exam reveals:

☐ PHYSICAL FINDINGS
- ☐ Exam consistent with history
- ☐ Exam inconsistent with history

☐ NO PHYSICAL FINDINGS
- ☐ Exam consistent with history
- ☐ Exam inconsistent with history

SUMMARY OF PHYSICAL FINDINGS:

☐ Oral trauma ☐ Genital trauma
☐ Perineal trauma ☐ Anal trauma
☐ Hymenal trauma
☐ Other findings consistent/inconsistent (circle one) with history as follows:

____

Follow-up arranged: ( ) Yes ( ) No

Child released to: __________

PHYSICAL EXAMINER

Print name of examiner

Signature of examiner

License number of examiner

LAW ENFORCEMENT/CHILD PROTECTIVE SERVICES

I have received the indicated items of evidence and the original of this report.

Law enforcement officer or child protective services

Agency ID number Date

HOSPITAL IDENTIFICATION INFORMATION

86 96698

Appendix 6

Methods for Estimating Percentage Body Fat from Skinfold Measurements in Girls

1. Percentage of body fat can be estimated based on measurements of triceps and subscapular skinfolds. For females (1):

$$\% \text{ body fat} = 1.33 \text{ (triceps + subscapular)} - 0.013 \text{ (triceps + subscapular)}^2 - 2.5$$

For women in whom the sum of triceps and subscapular skinfold measurements is >35 mm, the following equation is recommended:

$$\% \text{ body fat} = 0.546 \text{ (triceps + subscapular)} + 9.7$$

2. Lohman's table (Table 1) for estimating body fat using the sum of triceps and subscapular skin folds (2).

TABLE 1. *The use of the sum of triceps plus subscapular skinfolds in girls to estimate body fat percentage (2)*

Skinfolds (mm)	5	10	15	20	25	30	35	40	45	50	55	60
	Very low 6%		Low	Optimal range		Moderately high		High			Very high	
% Fat	4	10	15	20	24	28	30	33	33.5	38	40	

(From Lohman TG. The use of skinfold to estimate body fatness in children and youth. *JOPERD* 1987:98; with permission.)

3. Duerenberg and associates (3) calculated body fat percentages using additional skinfold measurements from girls at different levels of maturation (Table 2).

TABLE 2. *Percentage body fat estimated from the sum of biceps, triceps, suprailiac, and subscapular skinfolds in girls of different maturation levels*[a]

Sum of skinfolds	Prepubertal 10.5 yr (SE 1.6)		Pubertal 13.1 yr (SE 1.3)		Postpubertal 16.8 yr (SE 2.1)	
	Mean	95% CI	Mean	95% CI	Mean	95% CI
15	9.2	8.3–10.1	9.3	8.6–10.0	—	—
20	13.0	12.1–13.9	12.3	9.6–13.0	—	—
25	15.9	15.0–16.8	14.6	13.9–15.3	11.1	9.9–12.3
30	18.2	17.3–19.1	16.5	15.8–17.2	14.1	12.9–15.3
35	20.2	19.5–21.1	18.1	17.4–18.8	16.8	15.6–18.0
40	22.0	21.1–22.9	19.5	18.8–20.2	19.0	17.8–20.2
45	23.5	22.6–24.4	20.7	20.0–21.4	21.0	19.8–22.2
50	24.8	23.9–25.7	21.8	21.1–22.5	22.8	21.6–24.0
55	26.1	25.2–27.0	22.8	22.1–23.5	24.4	23.2–25.6
60	27.2	26.3–28.1	23.7	23.0–24.4	25.9	24.7–27.1
65	28.2	27.3–29.1	24.5	23.8–25.2	27.2	26.0–28.4
70	29.2	28.3–30.1	25.3	24.6–26.0	28.5	27.3–29.7
75	30.1	29.2–31.0	26.0	25.3–26.7	29.7	28.5–30.9
80	30.9	30.0–31.8	26.7	26.0–27.4	30.8	29.6–32.0
85	31.7	30.8–32.6	27.3	26.6–28.0	31.8	30.6–33.0
90	32.5	31.6–33.4	27.9	27.2–28.6	32.8	31.6–34.0
95	33.2	32.3–34.1	28.5	27.8–29.2	33.7	32.5–34.9

[a]95% CI, 95% confidence interval; SE, standard error.

(From Duerenberg P, Pieters JJL, Hautvast JG. The assessment of the body fat percentage by skinfold thickness measurements in childhood and young adolescence. *Br J Nutr* 1990;63: 293; with permission.)

REFERENCES

1. Slaughter MH, Lohman TG, Boilezu RA, et al. Skinfold equations for estimation of body fitness in children and youth. *Hum Biol* 1988;60:709.
2. Lohman TG. The use of skinfold to estimate body fatness in children and youth. *JOPERD* 1987;98.
3. Duerenberg P, Pieters JJL, Hautvast JG. The assessment of the body fat percentage by skinfold thickness measurements in childhood and young adolescence. *Br J Nutr* 1990;63:293.

Appendix 7

Bone Age Predictions for Final Height

TABLE 1. *Average girls—percentages and estimated mature heights for girls with skeletal ages within 1 year of their chronological ages: skeletal ages 6–11 years*

	Skeletal age (yr-mo)																							
	6-0	6-3	6-6	6-10	7-0	7-3	7-6	7-10	8-0	8-3	8-6	8-10	9-0	9-3	9-6	9-9	10-0	10-3	10-6	10-9	11-0	11-3	11-6	11-9
% of mature height	72.0	72.9	73.8	75.1	75.7	76.5	77.2	78.2	79.0	80.1	81.0	82.1	82.7	83.6	84.4	85.3	86.2	87.4	88.4	89.6	90.6	91.0	91.4	91.8
Height (inches)																								
37	51.4																							
38	52.8	52.1	51.5																					
39	54.2	53.5	52.8	52.0	51.5	51.0																		
40	55.6	54.9	54.2	53.3	52.8	52.3	51.8	51.2																
41	56.9	56.2	55.6	54.6	54.2	53.6	53.1	52.4	51.9	51.2														
42	58.3	57.6	56.9	55.9	55.5	54.9	54.4	53.7	53.2	52.4	51.9	51.2												
43	59.7	59.0	58.3	57.3	56.8	56.2	55.7	55.0	54.4	53.7	53.1	52.4	52.0	51.4										
44	61.1	60.4	59.6	58.6	58.1	57.5	57.0	56.3	55.7	54.9	54.3	53.6	53.2	52.6	52.1	51.6	51.0							
45	62.5	61.7	61.0	59.9	59.4	58.8	58.3	57.5	57.0	56.2	55.6	54.8	54.4	53.8	53.3	52.8	52.2	51.5						
46	63.9	63.1	62.3	61.3	60.8	60.1	59.6	58.8	58.2	57.4	56.8	56.0	55.6	55.0	54.5	53.9	53.4	52.6	52.0	51.3				
47	65.3	64.5	63.7	62.6	62.1	61.4	60.9	60.1	59.5	58.7	58.0	57.2	56.8	56.2	55.7	55.1	54.5	53.8	53.2	52.5	51.9	51.6	51.4	51.2
48	66.7	65.8	65.0	63.9	63.4	62.7	62.2	61.4	60.8	59.9	59.3	58.5	58.0	57.4	56.9	56.3	55.7	54.9	54.3	53.6	53.0	52.7	52.5	52.3
49	68.1	67.2	66.4	65.2	64.7	64.1	63.5	62.7	62.0	61.2	60.5	59.7	59.3	58.6	58.1	57.4	56.8	56.1	55.4	54.7	54.1	53.8	53.6	53.4
50	69.4	68.6	67.8	66.6	66.1	65.4	64.8	63.9	63.3	62.4	61.7	60.9	60.5	59.8	59.2	58.6	58.0	57.2	56.6	55.8	55.2	54.9	54.7	54.5
51	70.8	70.0	69.1	67.9	67.4	66.7	66.1	65.2	64.6	63.7	63.0	62.1	61.7	61.0	60.4	59.8	59.2	58.4	57.7	56.9	56.3	56.0	55.8	55.6
52	72.2	71.3	70.5	69.2	68.7	68.0	67.4	66.5	65.8	64.9	64.2	63.3	62.9	62.2	61.6	61.0	60.3	59.5	58.8	58.0	57.4	57.1	56.9	56.6
53	73.6	72.7	71.8	70.6	70.0	69.3	68.7	67.8	67.1	66.2	65.4	64.6	64.1	63.4	62.8	62.1	61.5	60.6	60.0	59.2	58.5	58.2	58.0	57.7
54		74.1	73.2	71.9	71.3	70.6	69.9	69.1	68.4	67.4	66.7	65.8	65.3	64.6	64.0	63.3	62.6	61.8	61.1	60.3	59.6	59.3	59.1	58.8
55			74.5	73.2	72.7	71.9	71.2	70.3	69.6	68.7	67.9	67.0	66.5	65.8	65.2	64.5	63.8	62.9	62.2	61.4	60.7	60.4	60.2	59.9
56				74.6	74.0	72.2	72.5	71.6	70.9	69.9	69.1	68.2	67.7	67.0	66.4	65.7	65.0	64.1	63.3	62.5	61.8	61.5	61.3	61.0
57						74.5	73.8	72.9	72.2	71.2	70.4	69.4	68.9	68.2	67.5	66.8	66.1	65.2	64.5	63.6	62.9	62.6	62.4	62.1
58								74.2	73.4	72.4	71.6	70.6	70.1	69.4	68.7	68.0	67.3	66.4	65.6	64.7	64.0	63.7	63.5	63.2
59									74.7	73.7	72.8	71.9	71.3	70.6	69.9	69.2	68.4	67.5	66.7	65.8	65.1	64.8	64.6	64.3
60										74.9	74.1	73.1	72.6	71.8	71.1	70.3	69.6	68.7	67.9	67.0	66.2	65.9	65.6	65.1
61												74.3	73.8	73.0	72.3	71.5	70.8	69.8	69.0	68.1	67.3	67.0	66.7	66.4
62														74.2	73.5	72.7	71.9	70.9	70.1	69.2	68.4	68.1	67.8	67.5
63															74.6	73.9	73.1	72.1	71.3	70.3	69.5	69.2	68.9	68.6
64																	74.2	73.2	72.4	71.4	70.6	70.3	70.0	69.7
65																		74.4	73.5	72.5	71.7	71.4	71.1	70.8
66																			74.7	73.7	72.9	72.5	72.2	71.9
67																				74.8	74.0	73.6	73.3	73.0
68																						74.7	74.4	74.1

(From Bayley N, Pinneau SR. Tables for predicting adult height from skeletal age: revised for use with the Greulich-Pyle hand standards. *J Pediatr* 1952;40:423; with permission.)

TABLE 2. *Average girls—percentages and estimated mature heights for girls with skeletal ages within 1 year of their chronological ages: skeletal ages 12–18 years*

	Skeletal age (yr-mo)																						
	12-0	12-3	12-6	12-9	13-0	13-3	13-6	13-9	14-0	14-3	14-6	14-9	15-0	15-3	15-6	15-9	16-0	16-3	16-6	16-9	17-0	17-6	18-0
% of mature height	92.2	93.2	94.1	95.0	95.8	96.7	97.4	97.8	98.0	98.3	98.6	98.8	99.0	99.1	99.3	99.4	99.6	99.6	99.7	99.8	99.9	99.95	100.0
Height (inches)																							
47	51.0																						
48	52.1	51.5	51.0																				
49	53.1	52.6	52.1	51.6	51.1																		
50	54.2	53.6	53.1	52.6	52.2	51.7	51.3	51.1	51.0														
51	55.3	54.7	54.2	53.7	53.2	52.7	52.4	52.1	52.0	51.9	51.7	51.6	51.5	51.5	51.4	51.3	51.2	51.2	51.2	51.1	51.1	51.0	51.0
52	56.4	55.8	55.3	54.7	54.3	53.8	53.4	53.2	53.1	52.9	52.7	52.6	52.5	52.5	52.4	52.3	52.2	52.2	52.2	52.1	52.1	52.0	52.0
53	57.5	56.9	56.3	55.8	55.3	54.8	54.4	54.2	54.1	53.9	53.8	53.6	53.5	53.5	53.4	53.3	53.2	53.2	53.2	53.1	53.1	53.0	53.0
54	58.6	57.9	57.4	56.8	56.4	55.8	55.4	55.2	55.1	54.9	54.8	54.7	54.5	54.5	54.4	54.3	54.2	54.2	54.2	54.1	54.1	54.0	54.0
55	59.7	59.0	58.4	57.9	57.4	56.9	56.5	56.2	56.1	56.0	55.8	55.7	55.6	55.5	55.4	55.3	55.2	55.2	55.2	55.1	55.1	55.0	55.0
56	60.7	60.1	59.5	58.9	58.5	57.9	57.5	57.3	57.1	57.0	56.8	56.7	56.6	56.5	56.4	56.3	56.2	56.2	50.2	56.1	56.1	56.0	56.0
57	61.8	61.2	60.6	60.0	59.5	58.9	58.5	58.3	58.2	58.0	57.8	57.7	57.6	57.5	57.4	57.3	57.2	57.2	57.2	57.1	57.1	57.0	57.0
58	62.9	62.2	61.6	61.1	60.5	60.0	59.5	59.3	59.2	59.0	58.8	58.7	58.6	58.5	58.4	58.3	58.2	58.2	58.2	58.1	58.1	58.0	58.0
59	64.0	63.3	62.7	62.1	61.6	61.0	60.6	60.3	60.2	60.0	59.8	59.7	59.6	59.5	59.4	59.4	59.2	59.2	59.2	59.1	59.1	59.0	59.0
60	65.1	64.4	63.8	63.2	62.6	62.0	61.6	61.3	61.2	61.0	60.9	60.7	60.6	60.5	60.4	60.4	60.2	60.2	60.2	60.1	60.1	60.0	60.0
61	66.2	65.5	64.8	64.2	63.7	63.1	62.6	62.4	62.2	62.1	61.9	61.7	61.6	61.6	61.4	61.4	61.2	61.2	61.2	61.1	61.1	61.0	61.0
62	67.2	66.5	65.9	65.3	64.7	64.1	63.7	63.4	63.3	63.1	62.9	62.8	62.6	62.6	62.4	62.4	62.2	62.2	62.2	62.1	62.1	62.0	62.0
63	68.3	67.6	67.0	66.3	65.8	65.1	64.7	64.4	64.3	64.1	63.9	63.8	63.6	63.6	63.4	63.4	63.3	63.3	63.2	63.1	63.1	63.0	63.0
64	69.4	68.7	68.0	67.4	66.8	66.2	65.7	65.4	65.3	65.1	64.9	64.8	64.6	64.6	64.4	64.4	64.3	64.3	64.2	64.1	64.1	64.0	64.0
65	70.5	69.7	69.1	68.4	67.8	67.2	66.7	66.5	66.3	66.1	65.9	65.8	65.7	65.6	65.5	65.4	65.3	65.3	65.2	65.1	65.1	65.0	65.0
66	71.6	70.8	70.1	69.5	68.9	68.3	67.8	67.5	67.3	67.1	66.9	66.8	66.7	66.6	66.5	66.4	66.3	66.3	66.2	66.1	66.1	66.0	66.0
67	72.7	71.9	71.2	70.5	69.9	69.3	68.8	68.5	68.4	68.2	68.0	67.8	67.7	67.6	67.5	67.4	67.3	67.3	67.2	67.1	67.1	67.0	67.0
68	73.8	73.0	72.3	71.6	71.0	70.3	69.8	69.5	69.4	69.2	69.0	68.8	68.7	68.6	68.5	68.4	68.3	68.3	68.2	68.1	68.1	68.0	68.0
69	74.8	74.0	73.3	72.6	72.0	71.4	70.8	70.6	70.4	70.2	70.0	69.8	69.7	69.6	69.5	69.4	69.3	69.3	69.2	69.1	69.1	69.0	69.0
70			74.4	73.7	73.1	72.4	71.9	71.6	71.4	71.2	71.0	70.8	70.7	70.6	70.5	70.4	70.3	70.3	70.2	70.1	70.1	70.0	70.0
71				74.7	74.1	73.4	72.9	72.6	72.4	72.2	72.0	71.9	71.7	71.6	71.5	71.4	71.3	71.3	71.2	71.1	71.1	71.0	71.0
72						74.5	73.9	73.6	73.5	73.2	73.0	72.9	72.7	72.7	72.5	72.4	72.3	72.3	72.2	72.1	72.1	72.0	72.0
73							74.9	71.6	74.5	74.3	74.0	73.9	73.7	73.7	73.5	73.4	73.3	73.3	73.2	73.1	73.1	73.0	73.0
74												74.9	74.7	74.7	74.5	74.4	74.3	74.3	74.2	74.1	74.1	74.0	74.0

(From Bayley N, Pinneau SR. Tables for predicting adult height from skeletal age: revised for use with the Greulich-Pyle hand standards. *J Pediatr* 1952;40:423; with permission.)

TABLE 3. *Accelerated girls—percentages and estimated mature heights for girls with skeletal ages 1 year or more advanced over their chronological ages: skeletal ages 7–11 years*

	Skeletal age (yr-mo)																			
	7-0	7-3	7-6	7-10	8-0	8-3	8-6	8-10	9-0	9-3	9-6	9-9	10-0	10-3	10-6	10-9	11-0	11-3	11-6	11-9
% of mature height	71.2	72.2	73.2	74.2	75.0	76.0	77.1	78.4	79.0	80.0	80.9	81.9	82.8	84.1	85.6	87.0	88.3	88.7	89.1	89.7
Height (inches)																				
37	52.0	51.2																		
38	53.4	52.6	51.9	51.2																
39	54.8	54.0	53.3	52.6	52.0	51.3														
40	56.2	55.4	54.6	53.9	53.3	52.6	51.9	51.0												
41	57.6	56.8	56.0	55.3	54.7	53.9	53.2	52.3	51.9	51.3										
42	59.0	58.2	57.4	56.6	56.0	55.3	54.5	53.6	53.2	52.5	51.9	51.3								
43	60.4	59.6	58.7	58.0	57.3	56.6	55.8	54.8	54.4	53.8	53.2	52.5	51.9	51.1						
44	61.8	60.9	60.1	59.3	58.7	57.9	57.1	56.1	55.7	55.0	54.4	53.7	53.1	52.3	51.4					
45	63.2	62.3	61.5	60.6	60.0	59.2	58.4	57.4	57.0	56.3	55.6	54.9	54.3	53.5	52.6	51.7	51.0			
46	64.6	63.7	62.8	62.0	61.3	60.5	59.7	58.7	58.2	57.5	56.9	56.2	55.6	54.7	53.7	52.9	52.1	51.9	51.6	51.3
47	66.0	65.1	64.2	63.3	62.7	61.8	61.0	59.9	59.5	58.8	58.1	57.4	56.8	55.9	54.9	54.0	53.2	53.0	52.7	52.4
48	67.4	66.5	65.6	64.7	64.0	63.2	62.3	61.2	60.8	60.0	59.3	58.6	58.0	57.1	56.1	55.2	54.4	54.1	53.9	53.3
49	68.8	67.9	66.9	66.0	65.3	64.5	63.6	62.5	62.0	61.3	60.6	59.8	59.2	58.3	57.2	56.3	55.5	55.2	55.0	54.6
50	70.2	69.3	68.3	67.4	66.7	65.8	64.9	63.8	63.3	62.5	61.8	61.1	60.4	59.5	58.4	57.5	56.6	56.4	56.1	55.7
51	71.6	70.6	69.7	68.7	68.0	67.1	66.1	65.1	64.6	63.8	63.0	62.3	61.6	60.6	59.6	58.6	57.8	57.5	57.2	56.9
52	73.0	72.0	71.0	70.1	69.3	68.4	67.4	66.3	65.8	65.0	64.3	63.5	62.8	61.8	60.7	59.8	58.9	58.6	58.4	58.0
53	74.4	73.4	72.4	71.4	70.7	69.7	68.7	67.6	67.1	66.3	65.5	64.7	64.0	63.0	61.9	60.9	60.0	59.8	59.5	59.1
54		74.8	73.8	72.8	72.0	71.1	70.0	68.9	68.4	67.5	66.7	65.9	65.2	64.2	63.1	62.1	61.2	60.9	60.6	60.2
55				74.1	73.3	72.4	71.3	70.2	69.6	68.8	68.0	67.2	66.4	65.4	64.3	63.2	62.3	62.0	61.7	61.3
56					74.7	73.7	72.6	71.4	70.9	70.0	69.2	68.4	67.6	66.6	65.4	64.4	63.4	63.1	62.8	62.4
57							73.9	72.7	72.2	71.3	70.5	69.6	68.8	67.8	66.6	65.5	64.6	64.3	64.0	63.5
58								74.0	73.4	72.5	71.1	70.8	70.0	69.0	67.8	66.7	65.7	65.4	65.1	64.7
59									74.7	73.8	72.9	72.0	71.3	70.2	68.9	67.8	66.8	66.5	66.2	65.8
60											74.2	73.3	72.5	71.3	70.1	69.0	68.0	67.6	67.3	66.9
61												74.5	73.7	72.5	71.3	70.1	69.1	68.8	68.5	68.0
62													74.9	73.7	72.4	71.3	70.2	69.9	69.6	69.1
63														74.9	73.6	72.4	71.3	71.0	70.7	70.2
64															74.8	73.6	72.5	72.2	71.8	71.3
65																74.7	73.6	73.3	72.9	72.5
66																	74.7	74.4	74.1	73.6
67																				74.7

(From Bayley N, Pinneau SR. Tables for predicting adult height from skeletal age: revised for use with the Greulich-Pyle hand standards. *J Pediatr* 1952;40:423; with permission.)

TABLE 4. *Accelerated girls—percentages and estimated mature heights for girls with skeletal ages 1 year or more advanced over their chronological ages: skeletal ages 12–17 years*

	Skeletal age (yr-mo)																					
	12-0	12-3	12-6	12-9	13-0	13-3	13-6	13-9	14-0	14-3	14-6	14-9	15-0	15-3	15-6	15-9	16-0	16-3	16-6	16-9	17-0	17-6
% of mature height	90.1	91.3	92.4	93.5	94.5	95.5	96.3	96.8	97.2	97.7	98.0	98.3	98.6	98.8	99.0	99.2	99.3	99.4	99.5	99.7	99.8	99.95
Height (inches)																						
46	51.1																					
47	52.2	51.5																				
48	53.3	52.6	51.9	51.3																		
49	54.4	53.7	53.0	52.4	51.9	51.3	50.9															
50	55.5	54.8	54.1	53.5	52.9	52.4	51.9	51.7	51.4	51.2	51.0											
51	56.6	55.9	55.2	54.5	54.0	53.4	53.0	52.7	52.5	52.2	52.0	51.9	51.7	51.6	51.5	51.4	51.4	51.3	51.3	51.2	51.1	51.0
52	57.7	57.0	56.3	55.6	55.0	54.5	54.0	53.7	53.5	53.2	53.1	52.9	52.7	52.6	52.5	52.4	52.4	52.3	52.3	52.2	52.1	52.0
53	58.8	58.1	57.4	56.7	56.1	55.5	55.0	54.8	54.5	54.2	54.1	53.9	53.8	53.6	53.5	53.4	53.4	53.3	53.3	53.2	53.1	53.0
54	59.9	59.1	58.4	57.8	57.1	56.5	56.1	55.8	55.6	55.3	55.1	54.9	54.8	54.7	54.5	54.4	54.4	54.3	54.3	54.2	54.1	54.0
55	61.0	60.2	59.5	58.8	58.2	57.6	57.1	56.8	56.6	56.3	56.1	56.0	55.8	55.7	55.5	55.4	55.4	55.3	55.3	55.2	55.1	55.0
56	62.2	61.3	60.6	59.9	59.3	58.6	58.2	57.9	57.6	57.3	57.1	57.0	56.8	56.7	56.5	56.5	56.4	56.3	56.3	56.2	56.1	56.0
57	63.3	62.4	61.7	61.0	60.3	59.7	59.2	58.9	58.6	58.3	58.2	58.0	57.8	57.7	57.6	57.5	57.4	57.3	57.3	57.2	57.1	57.0
58	64.4	63.5	62.8	62.0	61.4	60.7	60.2	59.9	59.7	59.4	59.2	59.0	58.8	58.7	58.6	58.5	58.4	58.3	58.3	58.2	58.1	58.0
59	65.5	64.6	63.9	63.1	62.4	61.8	61.3	61.0	60.7	60.4	60.2	60.0	59.8	59.7	59.6	59.5	59.4	59.4	59.3	59.2	59.1	59.0
60	66.6	65.7	64.9	64.2	63.5	62.8	62.3	62.0	61.7	61.4	61.2	61.0	60.9	60.7	60.6	60.5	60.4	60.4	60.3	60.2	60.1	60.0
61	67.7	66.8	66.0	65.2	64.6	63.9	63.3	63.0	62.8	62.4	62.2	62.1	61.9	61.7	61.6	61.5	61.4	61.4	61.3	61.2	61.1	61.0
62	68.8	67.9	67.1	66.3	65.6	64.9	64.4	64.0	63.8	63.5	63.3	63.1	62.9	62.8	62.6	62.5	62.4	62.4	62.3	62.2	62.1	62.0
63	69.9	69.0	68.2	67.4	66.7	66.0	65.4	65.1	64.8	64.5	64.3	64.1	63.9	63.8	63.6	63.5	63.4	63.4	63.3	63.2	63.1	63.0
64	71.0	70.1	69.3	68.4	67.7	67.0	66.5	66.1	65.8	65.5	65.3	65.1	64.9	64.8	64.6	64.5	64.4	64.4	64.3	64.2	64.1	64.0
65	72.1	71.2	70.3	69.5	68.8	68.1	67.5	67.1	66.9	66.5	66.3	66.1	65.9	65.8	65.7	65.5	65.5	65.4	65.3	65.2	65.1	65.0
66	73.3	72.3	71.4	70.6	69.8	69.1	68.5	68.2	67.9	67.6	67.3	67.1	66.9	66.8	66.7	66.5	66.5	66.4	66.3	66.2	66.1	66.0
67	74.4	73.4	72.5	71.7	70.9	70.2	69.6	69.2	68.9	68.6	68.4	68.2	68.0	67.8	67.7	67.5	67.5	67.4	67.3	67.2	67.1	67.0
68		74.5	73.6	72.7	72.0	71.2	70.6	70.2	70.0	69.6	69.4	69.2	69.0	68.8	68.7	68.6	68.5	68.4	68.3	68.2	68.1	68.0
69			74.7	73.8	73.0	72.3	71.7	71.3	71.0	70.6	70.4	70.2	70.0	69.8	69.7	69.6	69.5	69.4	69.3	69.2	69.1	69.0
70				74.9	74.1	73.3	72.7	72.3	72.0	71.6	71.4	71.2	71.0	70.8	70.7	70.6	70.5	70.4	70.3	70.2	70.1	70.0
71						74.3	73.7	73.3	73.0	72.7	72.4	72.2	72.0	71.9	71.7	71.6	71.5	71.4	71.4	71.2	71.1	71.0
72							74.8	74.4	74.1	73.7	73.5	73.2	73.0	72.9	72.7	72.6	72.5	72.4	72.4	72.2	72.1	72.0
73										74.7	74.5	74.3	74.0	73.9	73.7	73.6	73.5	73.4	73.4	73.2	73.1	73.0
74														74.9	74.4	74.6	74.5	74.4	74.4	74.2	74.1	74.0

(From Bayley N, Pinneau SR. Tables for predicting adult height from skeletal age: revised for use with the Greulich-Pyle hand standards. *J Pediatr* 1952;40:423; with permission.)

TABLE 5. *Retarded girls—percentages and estimated mature heights for girls with skeletal ages 1 year or more retarded for their chronological ages: skeletal ages 6–11 years*

	Skeletal age (yr-mo)																							
	6-0	6-3	6-6	6-10	7-0	7-3	7-6	7-10	8-0	8-3	8-6	8-10	9-0	9-3	9-6	9-9	10-0	10-3	10-6	10-9	11-0	11-3	11-6	11-9
% of mature height	73.3	74.2	75.1	76.3	77.0	77.9	78.8	79.7	80.4	81.3	82.3	83.6	84.1	85.1	85.8	86.6	87.4	88.4	89.6	90.7	91.8	92.2	92.6	92.9
Height (inches)																								
38	51.8	51.2																						
39	53.2	52.6	51.9	51.1																				
40	54.6	53.9	53.3	52.4	51.9	51.3																		
41	55.9	55.3	54.6	53.7	53.2	52.6	52.0	51.4																
42	57.3	56.6	55.9	55.0	54.5	53.9	53.3	52.7	52.2	51.7	51.0													
43	58.7	58.0	57.3	56.4	55.8	55.2	54.6	54.0	53.5	52.9	52.2	51.4	51.1											
44	60.0	59.3	58.6	57.7	57.1	56.5	55.8	55.2	54.7	54.1	53.5	52.6	52.3	51.7	51.3									
45	61.4	60.6	59.9	59.0	58.4	57.8	57.1	56.5	56.0	55.4	54.7	53.8	53.5	52.9	52.4	52.0	51.5							
46	62.8	62.0	61.3	60.3	59.7	59.1	58.4	57.7	57.2	56.6	55.9	55.0	54.7	54.1	53.6	53.1	52.6	52.0	51.3					
47	64.1	63.3	62.6	61.6	61.0	60.3	59.6	59.0	58.5	57.8	57.1	56.2	55.9	55.2	54.8	54.3	53.8	53.2	52.5	51.8	51.2	51.0		
48	65.5	64.7	63.9	62.9	62.3	61.6	60.9	60.2	59.7	59.0	58.3	57.4	57.1	56.4	55.9	55.4	54.9	54.3	63.6	52.9	52.3	52.1	51.8	51.7
49	66.9	66.0	65.2	64.2	63.6	62.9	62.2	61.5	60.9	60.3	59.5	58.6	58.3	57.6	57.1	56.6	56.1	55.4	54.7	54.0	53.4	53.1	52.9	52.7
50	68.2	67.4	66.6	65.5	64.9	64.2	63.5	62.7	62.2	61.5	60.8	59.8	59.5	58.8	58.3	57.7	57.2	56.6	55.8	55.1	54.5	54.2	54.0	53.8
51	69.6	68.7	67.9	66.8	66.2	65.5	64.7	64.0	63.4	62.7	62.0	61.0	60.6	59.9	59.4	58.9	58.4	57.7	56.9	56.2	55.6	55.3	55.1	54.9
52	70.9	70.1	69.2	68.2	67.5	66.8	66.0	65.2	64.7	64.0	63.2	62.2	61.8	61.1	60.6	60.0	59.5	58.8	58.0	57.3	56.6	56.4	56.2	56.0
53	72.3	71.4	70.6	69.5	68.8	68.0	67.3	66.5	65.9	65.2	64.4	63.4	63.0	62.3	61.8	61.2	60.6	60.0	59.2	58.4	57.7	57.5	57.2	57.1
54	73.7	72.8	71.9	70.8	70.1	69.3	68.5	67.8	67.2	66.4	65.6	64.6	64.2	63.5	62.9	62.4	61.8	61.1	60.3	59.5	58.8	58.6	58.3	58.1
55		74.1	73.2	72.1	71.4	70.6	69.8	69.0	68.4	67.7	66.8	65.8	65.4	64.6	64.1	63.5	62.9	62.2	61.4	60.6	59.9	59.7	59.4	59.2
56			74.6	73.4	72.7	71.9	71.1	70.3	69.7	68.9	68.0	67.0	66.6	65.8	65.3	64.7	64.1	63.3	62.5	61.7	61.0	60.7	60.5	60.3
57				74.7	74.0	73.2	72.3	71.5	70.9	70.1	69.3	68.2	67.8	67.0	66.4	65.8	65.2	64.5	63.6	62.8	62.1	61.8	61.6	61.4
58						74.5	73.6	72.8	72.1	71.3	70.5	69.4	69.0	68.2	67.6	67.0	66.4	65.6	64.7	63.9	63.2	62.9	62.6	62.4
59							74.9	74.0	73.4	72.6	71.7	70.6	70.2	69.3	68.8	68.1	67.5	66.7	65.8	65.0	64.3	64.0	63.7	63.5
60									74.6	73.8	72.9	71.8	71.3	70.5	69.9	69.3	68.7	67.9	67.0	66.2	65.4	65.1	64.8	64.6
61											74.1	73.0	72.5	71.7	71.1	70.4	69.8	69.0	68.1	67.3	66.4	66.2	65.9	65.7
62												74.2	73.7	72.9	72.3	71.6	70.9	70.1	69.2	68.4	67.5	67.2	67.0	66.7
63													74.7	74.0	73.4	72.7	72.1	71.3	70.3	69.5	68.6	68.3	68.0	67.8
64															74.6	73.9	73.2	72.4	71.4	70.6	69.7	69.4	69.1	68.9
65																	74.4	73.5	72.5	71.7	70.8	70.5	70.2	70.0
66																		74.7	73.7	72.8	71.9	71.6	71.3	71.0
67																			74.8	73.9	73.0	72.7	72.4	72.1
68																					74.1	73.8	73.4	73.2
69																						74.8	74.5	74.3

(From Bayley N, Pinneau SR. Tables for predicting adult height from skeletal age: revised for use with the Greulich-Pyle hand standards. *J Pediatr* 1952;40:423; with permission.)

TABLE 6. *Retarded girls—percentages and estimated mature heights for girls with skeletal ages 1 year or more retarded for their chronological ages: skeletal ages 12–17 years*

	Skeletal age (yr-mo)																				
	12-0	12-3	12-6	12-9	13-0	13-3	13-6	13-9	14-0	14-3	14-6	14-9	15-0	15-3	15-6	15-9	16-0	16-3	16-6	16-9	17-0
% of mature height	93.2	94.2	94.9	95.7	96.4	97.1	97.7	98.1	98.3	98.6	98.9	99.2	99.4	99.5	99.6	99.7	99.8	99.9	99.9	99.95	100.0
Height (inches)																					
48	51.5	51.0																			
49	52.6	52.0	51.6	51.2																	
50	53.6	53.1	52.7	52.2	51.9	51.5	51.2	51.0													
51	54.7	54.1	53.7	53.3	52.9	52.5	52.2	52.0	51.9	51.7	51.6	51.4	51.3	51.3	51.2	51.2	51.1	51.1	51.1	51.0	51.0
52	55.8	55.2	54.8	54.3	53.9	53.6	53.2	53.0	52.9	52.7	52.6	52.4	52.3	52.3	52.2	52.2	52.1	52.1	52.1	52.0	52.0
53	56.9	56.3	55.8	55.4	55.0	54.6	54.2	54.0	53.9	53.8	53.6	53.4	53.3	53.3	53.2	53.2	53.1	53.1	53.1	53.0	53.0
54	57.9	57.3	56.9	56.4	56.0	55.6	55.3	55.0	54.9	54.8	54.6	54.4	54.3	54.3	54.2	54.2	54.1	54.1	54.1	54.0	54.0
55	59.0	58.4	58.0	57.5	57.1	56.6	56.3	56.1	56.0	55.8	55.6	55.4	55.3	55.3	55.2	55.2	55.1	55.1	55.1	55.0	55.0
56	60.1	59.4	59.0	58.5	58.1	57.7	57.3	57.1	57.0	56.8	56.6	56.5	56.3	56.3	56.2	56.2	56.1	56.1	56.1	56.0	56.0
57	61.2	60.5	60.1	59.6	59.1	58.7	58.3	58.1	58.0	57.8	57.6	57.5	57.3	57.3	57.2	57.2	57.1	57.1	57.1	57.0	57.0
58	62.2	61.6	61.1	60.6	60.2	59.7	59.4	59.1	59.0	58.8	58.6	58.5	58.3	58.3	58.2	58.2	58.1	58.1	58.1	58.0	58.0
59	63.3	62.6	62.2	61.7	61.2	60.8	60.4	60.1	60.0	59.8	59.7	59.5	59.4	59.3	59.2	59.2	59.1	59.1	59.1	59.0	59.0
60	64.4	63.7	63.2	62.7	62.2	61.8	61.4	61.2	61.0	60.9	60.7	60.5	60.4	60.3	60.2	60.2	60.1	60.1	60.1	60.0	60.0
61	65.5	64.8	64.3	63.7	63.3	62.8	62.4	62.2	62.1	61.9	61.7	61.5	61.4	61.3	61.2	61.2	61.1	61.1	61.1	61.0	61.0
62	66.5	65.8	65.3	64.8	64.3	63.9	63.5	63.2	63.1	62.9	62.7	62.5	62.4	62.3	62.2	62.2	62.1	62.1	62.1	62.0	62.0
63	67.6	66.9	66.4	65.8	65.3	64.9	64.5	64.2	64.1	63.9	63.7	63.5	63.4	63.3	63.3	63.2	63.1	63.1	63.1	63.0	63.0
64	68.7	67.9	67.4	66.9	66.4	65.9	65.5	65.2	65.1	64.9	64.7	64.5	64.4	64.3	64.3	64.2	64.1	64.1	64.1	64.0	64.0
65	69.7	69.0	68.5	67.9	67.4	66.9	66.5	66.3	66.1	65.9	65.7	65.5	65.4	65.3	65.3	65.2	65.1	65.1	65.1	65.0	65.0
66	70.8	70.1	69.5	69.0	68.5	68.0	67.6	67.3	67.1	66.9	66.7	66.5	66.4	66.3	66.3	66.2	66.1	66.1	66.1	66.0	66.0
67	71.9	71.1	70.6	70.0	69.5	69.0	68.6	68.3	68.2	68.0	67.7	67.5	67.4	67.3	67.3	67.2	67.1	67.1	67.1	67.0	67.0
68	73.0	72.2	71.7	71.1	70.5	70.0	69.6	69.3	69.2	69.0	68.8	68.6	68.4	68.3	68.3	68.2	68.1	68.1	68.1	68.0	68.0
69	74.0	73.2	72.7	72.1	71.6	71.1	70.6	70.3	70.2	70.0	69.8	69.6	69.4	69.3	69.3	69.2	69.1	69.1	69.1	69.0	69.0
70		74.3	73.8	73.1	72.6	72.1	71.6	71.4	71.2	71.0	70.8	70.6	70.4	70.4	70.3	70.2	70.1	70.1	70.1	70.0	70.0
71			74.8	74.2	73.6	73.1	72.7	72.4	72.2	72.0	71.8	71.6	71.4	71.4	71.3	71.2	71.1	71.1	71.1	71.0	71.0
72					74.7	74.2	73.7	73.4	73.3	73.0	72.8	72.6	72.4	72.4	72.3	72.2	72.1	72.1	72.1	72.0	72.0
73							74.7	74.4	74.3	74.0	73.8	73.6	73.4	73.4	73.3	73.2	73.1	73.1	73.1	73.0	73.0
74											74.8	74.6	74.4	74.4	71.3	74.2	74.1	74.1	74.1	74.0	74.0

(From Bayley N, Pinneau SR. Tables for predicting adult height from skeletal age: revised for use with the Greulich-Pyle hand standards. *J Pediatr* 1952;40:423; with permission.)

Appendix 8

Calcium Handout

MILK GROUP

Most of the calcium in the American food supply comes from foods in the milk group. It's very difficult to get all the calcium you need without eating milk group foods.

While the milk group supplies 75% of the calcium in our food supply, it only supplies 12% of the fat. If you're watching your fat intake, look for foods with an asterisk (*).

Foods in this group are also a major source of riboflavin, protein, and vitamin D.

Milk group

Your calcium options	Calcium (mg)
Yogurt, plain, nonfat (1 cup)*	452
Yogurt, plain, low-fat (1 cup)*	415
Cheese, Swiss (1 1/2 oz)	408
Milkshake, chocolate (10 fl oz)	319
Yogurt, fruit-flavored, low-fat (1 cup)*	314
Cheese, cheddar (1 1/2 oz)	306
Milk, skim (1 cup)*	302
Milk, 1% low-fat (1 cup)*	300
Milk, 2% low-fat (1 cup)*	297
Milk, whole (1 cup)*	291
Buttermilk (1 cup)*	285
Milk, chocolate, 2% low-fat (1 cup)*	284
Milk, chocolate, whole (1 cup)	280
Cheese, mozzarella, part skim (1 1/2 oz)	275
Cheese, American (1 1/2 oz)	261
Pudding, cooked (1/2 cup)	152
Ice cream, soft serve (1/2 cup)	113
Yogurt, frozen, vanilla (1/2 cup)*	103
Ice cream, hardened, 16% fat (1/2 cup)	87
Ice cream, hardened, 10% fat (1/2 cup)	85
Cheese, cottage 2% low-fat (1/2 cup)*	77

*Lower in fat (≤5 g of fat per serving).

MEAT, VEGETABLE, AND GRAIN GROUPS

The meat group supplies about 9% of the calcium in the American food supply. Foods in this group are also a major source of protein, niacin, iron, and thiamine.

The vegetable and grain groups supply even less calcium than the meat group. However, vegetables are a major source of vitamin A, vitamin C, and fiber, and grains are a major source of carbohydrate, thiamine, iron, niacin, and fiber.

A few foods in each of these groups contain calcium. For example, canned salmon and sardines supply calcium when you eat the bones. Some leafy green vegetables contain calcium, too. So do some grain products.

Meat group

Your calcium options	Calcium (mg)
Tofu, with calcium sulfate (1/2 cup)	434
Sardines, canned, with bones (3 oz)	321
Salmon, canned, with bones (3 oz)	203
Tofu, without calcium sulfate (1/2 cup)	130
Perch, baked (3 oz.)*	117
Almonds (1/3 cup)	114
Vegetable group	
Spinach, fresh, cooked (1/2 cup)**	122
Turnip greens, fresh, cooked (1/2 cup)*	99
Okra, frozen, cooked (1/2 cup)*	88
Beet greens, fresh, cooked (1/2 cup)*	82

**The calcium in spinach is very poorly absorbed.

Grain group

Your calcium options	Calcium (mg)
Waffle, homemade (7-in waffle)	191
Biscuit, from mix (1 biscuit)	105

*Lower in fat (≤5 g of fat per serving).

COMBINATION FOODS AND FAST FOODS

Combination foods are made with foods from more than one food group. It's the foods from the milk group that make these combination foods good sources of calcium. Combination foods are also good sources of many other nutrients.

Combination foods/fast foods

Your calcium options	Calcium (mg)
Lasagna (2 1/2 × 2 1/4 in)	460
Macaroni and cheese, homemade (1 cup)	362
Enchilada, cheese (1 enchilada)	324
Taco Bell's® Chili Cheese Burrito	300
Chef's salad, without dressing (1 1/2 cups)	235
Quiche (1/8 pie)	211
Pizza, meat and veg., thin crust (1/4 of 12-in pie)	201
McDonald's Big Mac® (1 sandwich)	200
Cheeseburger, regular (1 sandwich)	182
Tomato soup, with milk (1 cup)	159
McDonald's Egg McMuffin® (1 sandwich)	150
Burger King's Croissan'wich® (1 sandwich)	150
Spaghetti with meat balls (1 cup)	124
Wendy's broccoli and cheese potato (1)	100
McDonald's Filet-o-Fish (1 sandwich)	100
Submarine sandwich (3–4-in sub)	95

CALCIUM-FORTIFIED FOODS

Calcium is sometimes added to orange juice, bread, soft drinks, cereal, milk, yogurt, and other foods. The amount of calcium in these foods is listed on the label. Keep in mind that calcium-fortified foods can increase your calcium intake. However, they do not provide the body with other nutrients supplied by dairy foods.

CALCIUM SUPPLEMENTS

There is a wide variety of calcium supplements on the market. The amount of calcium in these supplements is listed on the label. There are no benefits for taking more than your recommended daily allowance (RDA) for calcium. In fact, high doses of calcium may interfere with the absorption of other nutrients, like iron. Pills are not a substitute for a nutritionally adequate diet. Talk to your health care provider or dietitian before taking a calcium supplement.

Adapted from *The All-American Guide to Calcium-Rich Foods, 2nd ed.,* National Dairy Council, 1995; with permission.

Appendix 9

Topical Steroid Preparations

Classification of topical steroid preparations by potency

Low potency
- Alclometasone dipropionate 0.05%
- Dexamethasone phosphate 0.1%
- Fluocinolone acetonide 0.01%
- Hydrocortisone base or acetate 0.5%
- Hydrocortisone base or acetate 1%
- Hydrocortisone base or acetate 2.5%
- Triamcinolone acetonide 0.025%

Intermediate potency
- Desonide 0.05%
- Desoximetasone 0.05%
- Fluocinolone acetonide 0.025%
- Flurandrenolide 0.025%
- Flurandrenolide 0.05%
- Flurandrenolide 0.25%
- Fluticasone propionate 0.005%
- Fluticasone propionate 0.05%
- Hydrocortisone valerate 0.2%
- Mometasone furoate 0.1%
- Prednicarbate 0.1%
- Triamcinolone acetonide 0.1%
- Triamcinolone acetonide 0.2%

High potency
- Amcinonide 0.1%
- Betamethasone dipropionate, augmented 0.05%
- Desoximetasone 0.25%
- Diflorasone diacetate 0.05%
- Fluocinonide 0.05%
- Fluocinolone acetonide 0.2%
- Halcinonide 0.1%
- Triamcinolone acetonide 0.5%

Superhigh potency
- Betamethasone dipropionate, augmented 0.05%
- Clobetasol propionate 0.05%
- Diflorasone diacetate 0.05%
- Halobetasol propionate 0.05%

Subject Index

Subject Index